# ENCYCLOPEDIA OF

# BIOETHICS

**3**RD EDITION

# EDITORIAL BOARD

# ENCYCLOPEDIA OF
# BIOETHICS

## 3RD EDITION

EDITED BY

STEPHEN G. POST

VOLUME

I

A – C

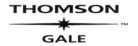

MACMILLAN
REFERENCE
USA™

THOMSON
GALE

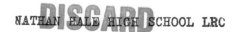

New York • Detroit • San Diego • San Francisco • Cleveland • New Haven, Conn. • Waterville, Maine • London • Munich

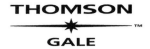

**Encyclopedia of Bioethics, 3rd edition**

Stephen G. Post

Editor in Chief

**Library of Congress Cataloging-in-Publication Data**

Encyclopedia of bioethics / Stephen G. Post, editor in chief.— 3rd ed.
    p. cm.
Includes bibliographical references and index.
    ISBN 0-02-865774-8 (set : hardcover : alk. paper) — ISBN
0-02-865775-6 (vol. 1) — ISBN 0-02-865776-4 (vol. 2) — ISBN
0-02-865777-2 (vol. 3) — ISBN 0-02-865778-0 (vol. 4) — ISBN
0-02-865779-9 (vol. 5)
    1. Bioethics—Encyclopedias. 2. Medical ethics—Encyclopedias. I.
Post, Stephen Garrard, 1951-
QH332.E52 2003
174′.957′03—dc22

2003015694

This title is also available as an e-book.
ISBN 0-02-865916-3 (set)
Contact your Gale sales representative for ordering information.

Printed in the United States of America
10 9 8 7 6 5 4 3 2 1

Front cover photos (from left to right): Custom Medical Stock;
Photo Researchers; Photodisc; Photodisc; AP/Worldwide Photos.

# CONTENTS

# EDITORIAL AND PRODUCTION STAFF

Monica M. Hubbard
*Project Editor*

Nicole Watkins
*Project Associate Editor*

Mark Drouillard, Melissa Hill,
Diane Sawinski
*Editorial Support*

Elizabeth B. Inserra, Peter J.
Jaskowiak, Christine Kelley,
Eric Lowenkron, David E.
Salamie
*Copyeditors*

John Krol, Dorothy Bauhoff
*Proofreaders*

Laurie Andriot
*Indexer*

Kate Scheible
*Art Director*

Autobookcomp and GGS, Inc.
*Typesetters*

Mary Beth Trimper
*Manager, Composition*

Evi Seoud
*Assistant Manager, Composition*

Rita Wimberly
*Buyer*

### MACMILLAN REFERENCE USA

Frank Menchaca
*Vice President*

Hélène Potter
*Director, New Product
Development*

# PREFACE

At the time of the first publication of the *Encyclopedia of Bioethics* in 1978, the then fledgling field of bioethics was neither well defined nor widely recognized. Warren Thomas Reich, then Senior Research Scholar in the Kennedy Institute of Ethics at Georgetown University, envisioned a major reference work that would contribute significantly to the establishment of bioethics as a field by integrating historical background, current issues, future implications, ethical theory, and comparative cultural and religious perspectives. Professor Reich became the editor in chief for the first edition, a four-volume set that, as he foresaw, was immediately acknowledged as a landmark reference work defining the field.

The 1978 edition received the American Library Association's 1979 Dartmouth Medal for outstanding reference work of the year, as well as widespread critical acclaim. The eminent bioethicist Daniel Callahan, writing for *Psychology Today* in March of 1979, entitled his stellar review of the *Encyclopedia* "From Abortion to Rejuvenation: A Summa of Medical Ethics." *Choice* declared the work "an outstanding achievement." *Social Science* described the work as "magnificent," and the *Hastings Center Report* acknowledged it as both "an astonishing achievement" and "a major event." Throughout the 1980s, as programs in bioethics and medical humanities proliferated in professional schools, undergraduate and graduate school curricula, "think tanks," and academic societies, the first edition of the *Encyclopedia* was considered the essential reference work in the field, and contributed significantly to intellectual vitality.

While the 1978 first edition will always be essential and fascinating reading for anyone interested in the history of bioethics, it was, by the late 1980s, in need of a revision. A reference work at the interface of biology, technology, healthcare and ethics becomes dated due to the fast pace of biotechnological development, changes in the healthcare delivery system, and the emergence of important new voices in a rapidly expanding field. Although in certain respects the modern bioethics movement began in the United States, it took root in many countries around the world during the 1980s, requiring the inclusion of scholarship from other nations and cultures in order to properly reflect worldwide growth. Professor Reich impressed all those working on the second edition with his remarkable grasp of the history of medical ethics, of the modern bioethics movement, of European thinkers, of religious ethics and moral philosophy, and of salient clinical issues.

The revised edition included various topic areas including: professional–patient relationship; public health; ethical theory; religious ethics; bioethics and the social sciences; healthcare; fertility and human reproduction; biomedical and behavioral research; history of medical ethics; mental health and behavioral issues; sexuality and gender; death and dying; genetics; population; organ and tissue transplantation and artificial organs; welfare and treatment of animals; environment; and codes, oaths, and other directives. All of these topics are retained and enhanced in the third edition.

The five-volume revised edition, which was carefully planned at editorial meetings in the spring and fall of 1990, was supported by both the National Endowment for the Humanities and the National Science Foundation, in addition to several private foundations and individual donors. The Joseph P. Kennedy, Jr. Foundation was a major funder of both the first and the revised editions. Published in 1995 by Macmillan Reference Division, it received the same high level of acclaim as the first edition.

## Development of a Third Edition

Yet with the passing of the 1990s, the *Encyclopedia* again required a thorough revision and update. Warren Reich, professor *emeritus* at Georgetown and deeply engaged with a new project on the history of "care," decided not to prepare the third edition. He recommended Stephen Garrard Post—who had served as his associate editor in the preparation of the second edition—for the position of editor in chief of the third edition. Subsequently, Macmillan Reference, after consulting with Georgetown University (which had sponsored the first edition), offered the position of editor in chief to Post.

This invitation was accepted with the understanding that a third edition could only emerge from the already remarkable scope and framework of the revised edition, and would be much indebted to all those responsible for that extraordinary work, including the following area editors: Dan E. Beauchamp, Arthur L. Caplan, Christine K. Cassel, James F. Childress, Allen R. Dyer, John C. Fletcher, Stanley M. Hauerwas, Albert R. Jonsen, Patricia A. King, Loretta M. Kopelman, Ruth B. Purtillo, Holmes Rolston III, Robert M. Veatch, and Donald P. Warwick.

There are more than 110 new article titles in the third edition, and approximately the same number of new articles appearing under old titles. Thus, half of the third edition is entirely new, while half consists of deeply revised and updated articles from the earlier edition. There isn't a single article that was not thoroughly updated, even if only at the level of bibliographies. The least revision was needed in the topic areas of environmental ethics, population ethics, and the history of medical ethics. For all necessary revisions, we went back to the articles' original authors, whenever possible, and many accepted to undertake the revision work. In those cases where the original authors were not available, new authors were asked to complete the work. Both original and new authors are acknowledged and their contributions clearly identified in the bylines. A small but exceptional set of articles from the revised edition were designated by the editorial board as *classics,* and are retained in the third edition unchanged. These articles were selected because they were written by a distinguished contributor to the field and were still deemed definitive. For example, Daniel Callahan's article on "Bioethics" was retained as a classic, as was Reich's "Care: I: History of the Notion." Also included without revision are those articles under the title "Medical Ethics, History of," which do not pertain to the contemporary period. But all articles dealing with the contemporary period were significantly revised in order to be current with the many developments in bioethics over the past decade in countries and regions across the world.

EDITORIAL BOARD. The development of this third edition of the *Encyclopedia* was facilitated by a new editorial board consisting of area editors David Barnard, Dena S. Davis,

Eric T. Juengst, Loretta M. Kopelman, Maxwell J. Mehlman, Kenneth F. Schaffner, Bonnie Steinbock, Leonard J. Weber, and Stuart J. Youngner. These editors were selected because their particular expertise—as philosophers, ethicists, healthcare professionals, and teachers—was needed to revise and expand those topic areas from the revised edition where new developments had been particularly rapid over the 1990s. The Editor in Chief and the Editorial Board were responsible for the intellectual planning of the third edition, including all decisions about contents and authorship, as well as for reviewing and approving all manuscripts. Mark Aulisio served as associate editor for ethical theory and clinical ethics.

CONSULTANTS. William Deal, Patricia Marshall, Carol C. Donley, Sana Loue, Robert H. Binstock, and Barbara J. Daly made significant contributions to the quality of the overall work as editorial consultants. Carrie Zoubol assisted with bibliographical updating.

The Appendix, found in volume five of the *Encyclopedia,* consists largely of an exhaustive collection of historical and contemporary codes and oaths across all the healthcare professions, as well as research ethics guidelines and regulations. The remarkable collection of primary documents in the revised edition was thoroughly updated by Kayhan Parsi of the Neiswanger Institute for Bioethics and Health Policy at the Stritch School of Medicine of Loyola University. This was a major task because there have been so many revisions of contemporary documents since the early 1990s, as well as the introduction of many new policy and ethical statements from a wide array of professional organizations. Carol C. Donley contributed an annotated bibliography on literature and medicine from the Center for Literature, Medicine, and the Healthcare Professions at Hiram College. Emily Peterson added an annotated bibliography on law and medicine. Doris M. Goldstein, Director of Library and Information Services at the Kennedy Institute of Ethics, Georgetown University, thoroughly updated the section on "Additional Resources in Bioethics," which she had prepared for the revised edition. Volume five is the fruit of much labor and will be a definitive resource for the field over the next decade.

## Acknowledgments

The day-to-day work of preparing the third edition entailed close collaboration with the publisher's team in New York and Michigan. None of this work would have been possible without a publisher able to efficiently implement the intellectual plan. The Macmillan team commissioned all the articles, maintained contact with all authors, coordinated reviews, copy edited all manuscripts, checked revised manuscripts and bibliographies, and prepared all materials for production. In particular, Hélène G. Potter, Editor in Chief of Macmillan Reference USA, provided vision and managerial insight for the development of the third edition—as well as many thoughtful perspectives. Similarly, Monica M. Hubbard, Senior Editor with Macmillan Reference USA, provided excellent leadership in implementing all the operational aspects of the project. Before the revision project began in earnest, Elly Dickason, prior to her retirement from Macmillan Reference USA, provided her usual thoughtful guidance.

The Department of Bioethics, School of Medicine, Case Western Reserve University, provided a collegial environment for a number of those involved as editors, consultants, authors and reviewers. The School of Medicine has a long tradition of humanism in medicine that creates a welcome atmosphere for the *Encyclopedia.*

We wish to acknowledge support for both the revised and third editions from The Alton F. and Carrie S. Davis Fund of the Cleveland Foundation. In addition, the John Templeton Foundation provided Stephen Post with a generous grant in 2002 in support of a research institute on altruism and compassion, "The Institute for Research on Unlimited Love—Altruism, Compassion, Service," which allowed him to devote additional editorial time to related themes in the third edition, especially as these pertain to the ongoing dialogue between science and religion.

STEPHEN G. POST
EDITOR IN CHIEF
SEPTEMBER 2, 2003

# INTRODUCTION

In the Introduction to the 1995 revised edition of the *Encyclopedia of Bioethics*, Warren Thomas Reich, Editor in Chief, defined bioethics as "*the systematic study of the moral dimensions—including moral vision, decisions, conduct, and policies—of the life sciences and health care, employing a variety of ethical methodologies in an interdisciplinary setting.*" This definition shapes the third edition, which continues the broad topical range of earlier editions.

The word *bioethics* was coined in the early 1970s by biologists in order to encourage public and professional reflection on two topics of urgency: (1) the responsibility to maintain the generative ecology of the planet, upon which life and human life depends; and (2) the future implications of rapid advances in the life sciences with regard to potential modifications of a malleable human nature. In his book entitled *Bioethics: Bridge to the Future,* published in 1971, Van Rensselaer Potter focused on evolutionary biology, a growing human ability to alter nature and human nature, and the implications of this power for our global future. Other life scientists at that time, such as Bentley Glass, Paul Berg, and Paul Ehrlich were among many similarly interested in spurring thought on the biological revolution with regard to eugenics, the engineering of new life forms, and population ethics. Bioethics, then, emerged from biologists who felt obliged to address the moral meaning of the biosphere, and to reflect on the remarkable implications of their discoveries and technological innovations.

Alongside of bioethics as an intellectual movement among life scientists there emerged the field of medical ethics, which was both old and new. It was old in the sense that physicians had reflected perennially on their professional duties from within the narrow confines of the guild. It was new in that now this reflection was occurring in open dialogue with theologians and philosophers, and attentive to

widening public concerns in a time of civil rights and "the twilight of authority." The emerging discussion quickly included all the significant healthcare professions. Physicians focusing on medical ethics were in conversation with the accumulated wisdom of Catholic, Jewish, and Protestant reflection on medical ethics, as well as with moral philosophy. Many philosophers in this early period engaged in fruitful and mutually enriching dialogue with religious thinkers. Such dialogue not only contributed to the vitality of the field, but also reflected the dynamics of a liberal democracy in which citizens of all backgrounds and persuasions were, by the early 1970s, becoming awakened to the important moral questions surrounding developments in healthcare, medicine, research, and the professional–patient relationship.

Bioethics, as the tradition of the *Encyclopedia* defines it, developed then from these two central lineages, and includes both. The *Encyclopedia* integrates all aspects of healthcare and medical ethics, without losing sight of the wider context provided by the life scientists of the early 1970s, including their environmental and public health concerns.

The earlier editions of the *Encyclopedia* remain the key historical documents defining the field in its initial stages. Many elegantly written and authoritative articles included in these editions represent the thought of a generation of remarkable thinkers whose intellectual creativity, scholarly breadth, and openness to dialogue across traditions may never be surpassed. These thinkers were relatively free of any conventional literature of the field of "bioethics" as we would now be able to describe it; they were generally free from the internal status hierarchies and concerns with legitimization in academic medical centers that can sometimes limit creativity; they were almost entirely free from conflicts of interest, a serious concern in current bioethics, in response to which this third edition has required full disclosure from all authors.

## Bioethics, Pluralism and Public Discourse

The tradition of the *Encyclopedia* makes an instructive contribution to the future of bioethics in the academy because it includes the full spectrum of voices addressing the questions of bioethics, consistent with diversity in the public square of liberal democracies. The academic field of bioethics, in order to remain both relevant and creative, is wise to include thoughtful representatives from this full spectrum.

As Alasdair MacIntyre has pointed out, every system of philosophical or religious ethics has its own foundational assumptions about human nature and the human good, its unique historical context and questions, and its inherent conceptual limits. Bioethics is therefore enhanced by dialogue between different traditions of thought, both secular and religious, reflecting the diversity of the public square. Such dialogue requires a set of core virtues—mutual respect, tolerance, civility, and an openness to modification of one's perspectives based on the clarification of empirical fact and the persuasiveness of others. These virtues pertain not only to discourse within the Western context, but to global discourse. Whether African, Asian, Middle Eastern, or Native American, religious perspectives and the philosophical systems that have emerged from them need to be respected and engaged. Secular or religious monism—the view that only one voice is valid—eliminates meaningful dialogue, inhibits full participation, and thwarts conceptual growth.

Even within the particularistic scope of contemporary Western moral philosophy, whether utilitarian, Kantian, or contractarian, there is a need for dialogue with equally useful schools of thought, such as Aristotelian reflection on the virtues and final causality, natural law thought on essential human goods and correlative moral obligations, existential concern with the emotional underpinnings of human action such as hope or "the will to power," phenomenological description of the transition from solipsism to the "discovery of the other as other," feminist reflection grounded in the experience of women, and many other Western philosophical traditions that raise significant and yet very distinctive questions. Depth discussion requires an appreciation for different systems of moral thought, each of which raises a unique set of questions that those inculcated in other systems may miss.

Secular monists hold that religious ethics should be privatized and excluded from bioethical and public discourse; that religion should be a purely internal affair, no more relevant to public discourse than one's culinary tastes;

that religious voices result in a discordant mixture that means nothing. Public debate requires, it is said, common secular language; religious language constitutes bad taste. While it is true that religious voices can be "conversation-stoppers"—to use the philosopher Richard Rorty's pejorative term—secular voices can be just as easily so. A great many religious voices are respectful, diplomatic, and contributory to deeper levels of discourse on public issues; they are often conversation-starters rather than conversation-stoppers by virtue of raising unique questions of human nature and destiny. In a liberal and robust bioethics, an opinion is no more disqualified for being *religious* than for being atheistic, psychoanalytic, feminist, Marxist, or secular existentialist.

The *Encyclopedia of Bioethics* is unique because it has always included many voices and traditions in an effort to foster dialogue, prevent the narrowing of the field, and engage a wide international readership. This edition, like previous ones, embraces cross-cultural approaches, the full history of bioethics, comparative religious and philosophical ethics, and global perspectives. The articles on the history of medical ethics are exemplary efforts to highlight the degree to which our contemporary theories of ethics and bioethics evolve from particular social, cultural–religious, and historical contexts. Moreover, the historical articles on "the contemporary period" provide important information on developments such as population ethics in China, assisted suicide in the Netherlands, and brain death legislation in Japan.

Yet the array of materials presented is not intended to imply moral relativism, even as it conveys the substantial reality of ideational difference. Many articles, while balanced and expository, do highlight areas where those in search of a common morality can find respite. In the classical dialectic between the One and the Many, or between moral objectivism and moral relativism, there are some areas in which no agreement is either likely or necessary. There are other areas, however, such as the wrongness of genocide or the sexual abuse of children, where agreement is both expected and imperative. Most of us are partial relativists, which is also to say that we are partial objectivists. When an incompetent physician lies by claiming competence and as a result inflicts avoidable harm on a patient, or when a researcher refuses to halt a study despite the intolerable suffering of subjects as they perceive it, ethics is objective and we can speak with authority of a common morality. Yet in other areas, such as brain definitions of death or certain reproductive technologies, few would assume moral objectivism. There are also difficult disagreements as to whether we should attempt to significantly modify human nature itself through advanced biotechnology.

The third edition of the *Encyclopedia* was animated by the recognition that no other work presents bioethics in its fullness, both with regard to definition, methods, and contents. It is this fullness that makes the *Encyclopedia* of continuing international value in maintaining the open and expansive nature of the field.

## New Points of Emphasis

The third edition includes a wide array of new titles ranging from "Bioterrorism," "Holocaust," and "Immigration, Ethical and Health Issues of," to "Artificial Nutrition and Hydration," "Cancer, Ethical Issues Related to Diagnosis and Treatment," "Dementia," "Dialysis, Kidney," "DNR—Do Not Resuscitate," and sets of articles under "Cloning" and "Pediatrics." Topic areas such as Reproduction and Fertility, Organ and Tissue Transplantation, Death and Dying, Ethical Theory, Law and Bioethics, Mental Health, Genetics, Religion and Ethics, and alike have been thoroughly redesigned, and are essentially new. As mentioned in the Preface, half of the third edition is entirely new, while half consists of deeply revised and updated articles from the earlier edition. There isn't a single article that was not thoroughly updated, even if only at the level of bibliographies, unless it is designated as *classic*.

Some new points of thematic emphasis in the third edition can be highlighted and commented on, although the revised edition was comprehensive with regard to general topic areas within the field of bioethics.

## Posthumanism and Anti-Posthumanism

The reader will find new articles entitled "Transhumanism and Posthumanism," "Cybernetics," "Cloning," "Human Dignity," "Embryo and Fetus: III. Embryonic Stem Cell Research," "Enhancement Uses of Medical Technology," "Nanotechnology," and "Aging and the Aged: VI. Anti-Aging Interventions: Ethical and Social Issues." Collectively, these articles and others accentuate the question of what it means to be human.

Posthumanism (or sometimes "transhumanism") is a pure scientism that endorses fundamental alterations in human nature (see, e.g., <www.betterhumans.com>, <www.transhumanism.org>, <www.forsight.org>). Off with biological constraints! Transcend humanness by technology! The posthumanist embraces the eventual goal of decelerated and even arrested aging, but only as a small part of a larger vision to re-engineer human nature, and thereby to create biologically and technologically superior human beings that we humans today will design for tomorrow. As such, posthumans would no longer be humans. Genetics,

nanotechnology, cloning, cybernetics, and computer technologies are all part of the posthuman vision, which even includes the idea of downloading of synaptic connections in the brain to form a computerized human mind freed of mortal flesh, and thereby immortalized. Posthumanists do not believe that biology is destiny, but rather something to be overcome, for there is, they argue, no "natural law," but only human malleability and morphological freedom. Their appeal lies in the fact that, within the boundaries of technology, humans have been reinventing themselves anyway through applied technologies for millennia. Science is moving so rapidly that serious conversation is required to distinguish salutary from destructive transformations.

Human nature as we know it is, for the posthumanist mind, a mere constraint to be overcome. To use Walt Whitman's language, theirs is a "Song of the Open Road." After all, it is argued, there was a time when the very idea of human beings trying to fly was deemed heretical hubris in the light of eternity—*sub specie aeternitatis*. Now are the posthumanists to be deemed the new heretics in the light of evolution—*sub specie evolutionis*? Or shall we set aside trepidation and with confidence rethink ourselves in the light of human creativity and so-called "superbiology?" Indeed, Francis Bacon, a founder of the scientific method, in his millennialist and utopian essay *The New Atlantis* (1627), set in motion a biological mandate for boldness that included both the making of new species or "chimeras," organ replacement, and the "Water of Paradise" that would allow the possibility to "indeed live very long."

One of the wiser minds of the last century, Hans Jonas (d. 1993), an intellectual inspiration for today's anti-posthumanists, articulated the ethical questions around human malleability with thoroughness. He asked how desirable would the potential power to slow or arrest aging be for the individual and for the species? Do we want to tamper with the delicate biological balance of death and procreation, and preempt the place of youth? Would the species gain or lose? Jonas, by merely raising these questions, meant to cast significant doubt on the anti-aging enterprise. In current discussion, debate grows over cybernetics, nanotechnology, genetic enhancement, reproductive cloning, therapeutic stem cell cloning, life span extension, and new forms of behavior control. For some, the ambitions of posthumanists to create a new posthuman who is no longer human are, it is argued, arrogant, pretentious, and lacking in fundamental appreciation for natural human dignity. And yet others see potential for progress in these developing technological powers.

Ours is an age that is seriously beginning to consider "transhuman" possibilities through biotechnological enhancements in human biological capacities such as lifespan, personality type, and intelligence. What will be the status of the altruistic generativity that Erik Erikson associated with old age as adventurous human beings begin to experiment with efforts to alter their lifespan? Will compassion be left behind in favor of the biotechnological pursuit of bigger muscles, prolongevity, happy dispositions, and unfading beauty? Or are the care and compassion that lie within us the "ultimate human enhancement"? Readers of the *Encyclopedia* are encouraged to reflect on such questions and draw their own conclusions.

## Business Ethics in Healthcare

The reader of the third edition will find new articles with titles such as "Corporate Compliance," "Health Insurance," "Health Policy in the United States," "Health Services Management Ethics," "Healthcare Institutions," "Just Wages and Salaries," "Labor Unions in Healthcare," "Managed Care," "Medicaid," "Mergers and Acquisitions," "Organizational Ethics in Healthcare," "Private Ownership of Inventions," and "Profit and Commercialism."

This new feature of the *Encyclopedia* grew from the concern throughout the 1990s and beyond with the ways in which healthcare has become a business ruled by corporate executives and the bottom line of economic profit. While the nonprofit context of healthcare delivery is still significant, even there the freedom of the physician to focus on the best interests of the patient has been to varying degrees compromised by sometimes necessary cost cutting. Many professionals have struggled to retain the moral core of commitment to beneficence and the well-being of patients as even the time allowed for each patient visit has been dramatically contracted, compromising the time to establish an empathic and compassionate relationship. With the restructuring of healthcare along corporate lines, and with the emergence of for-profit healthcare systems answerable to stock holders and Wall Street forces, business ethics in healthcare becomes a significant addition to the *Encyclopedia*.

The article entitled "Conflict of Interest" raises a question of significance for the field of bioethics itself. Increasingly, especially in academic medical centers at major universities, bioethicists have themselves accepted lucrative financial benefits from pharmaceutical companies and biotech firms. While this does not mean that some bioethicists are no longer free to think for themselves about ethical issues, it does mean that they are subject to various pressures and should fully disclose any financial interests whatsoever that might influence their opinions. Of all fields, bioethics should remain untainted by financial conflict of interest, for its public credibility is always at risk.

## Basic Approaches to Ethics

The *Encyclopedia* has, in its earlier editions, always been strong in providing the reader with background articles in ethical theory. The third edition enhances this aspect of the work with articles including "Conscience, Rights of," "Contractarianism and Bioethics," "Ethics Committees and Ethics Consultation," "Human Dignity," "Human Rights," "Moral Status," "Principlism," "Utilitarianism and Bioethics," and "Value and Healthcare," among others. In addition, new articles dealing with religious ethical approaches have been added, such as "Authority in Religious Traditions," "Christianity, Bioethics in," "Circumcision, Religious Aspects of," "Compassionate Love," "Jehovah's Witness Refusal of Blood Products," "Mormonism, Bioethics in," and related topics. Additional articles on anthropology and bioethics have also been developed.

## Organization of the *Encyclopedia*

Entries are arranged alphabetically. Some *entries* are comprised of several *subentries*. For example,

Aging and the Aged

I. Theories of Aging and Life Extension

II. Life Expectancy and Life Span

III. Societal Aging

IV. Old Age

V. Anti-Aging Interventions: Ethical and Social Issues

The reader wishing to study ethical aspects of aging and anti-aging research would do well to read all five of these interlocking articles.

Cross-references are provided for each article. However, for a complete perspective on the thematic relationships between articles, please see the "Topical Outline" in the front of the first volume following the "List of Contributors."

The bibliographies following each article are an important resource. These were prepared by the authors, or otherwise updated with approval by the Editor in Chief. The bibliographies are necessarily selective rather than completely exhaustive due to the volume of significant new books and articles relevant to each article.

The lengthy collection of codes, oaths, and policies in the fifth volume is of great value. Readers will benefit from reviewing these contents as they pertain to a specific topic of interest. Various annotated bibliographies in law and medicine, literature and medicine, and in bioethics should also be consulted. The section on "Additional Resources in Bioethics" is especially important for its thoroughness and its international aspects, including current websites worldwide that are easily available to students.

A special effort has been made to keep these volumes free from technical jargon. The articles should be accessible to students at the high school, college, and graduate levels, as well as to interested lay readers. They are written in such a manner as to be authoritative for professionals wishing to gain a clear perspective on how ideas have evolved.

## Bioethics, Civil Discourse, and a Common Humanity

Because the issues with which bioethics grapples are profoundly relevant to the future of nature, human nature, and healthcare, they are often contentious. Moreover, in the dialectic between moral objectivism and moral relativism, while many of these issues allow for plausible resolutions, there are others for which no resolutions emerge. Tolerance, civility, respect, and the willingness to seriously engage with the views of others who work out of different traditions, both secular and religious, are necessary virtues and habits of mind. Bioethics is inevitably subject to criticism by those who believe that answers to the many new questions brought on by the accelerating biological and healthcare revolutions are immediately and simply apparent. But what, after all, is a good ethicist, whether secular or religious, if not the person who asks an unsettling new question that no one else envisioned, and thereby prompts renewed debate as an alternative to superficiality.

While this *Encyclopedia* does not include biographies of bioethicists who were also moral leaders attempting to influence the world of science, healthcare, and public opinion, the list would be extensive and pluralistic. Many of the finest contributors to the field of bioethics are actively engaged in the service of needful constituencies, involved with voluntary associations, and otherwise engaged in practice. As appropriate, they move beyond the mere exposition of the essential inventory of existing thoughts on a topic, and argue persuasively for a normative viewpoint. Indeed, those who read these volumes will hopefully be motivated by a sense of responsibility and service, as well as by intellectual curiosity. For the purpose of liberal education and learning is not only the enhancement of knowledge, but also progress in benevolence, creative altruism, and commitment to a common humanity.

As Editor in Chief, I hope that readers of these volumes become better informed participants in a respectful public dialogue over a set of issues that increasingly must be understood and appreciated by all citizens of a liberal democracy. The gravity and significance of these bioethical issues for the future of our generative planet, of life itself, and of humankind might impress the reader so as to inspire purposeful educational and life pursuits.

STEPHEN G. POST
EDITOR IN CHIEF, THIRD EDITION
SEPTEMBER 2, 2003

# LIST OF ARTICLES

# LIST OF CONTRIBUTORS

Donald C. Ainslie
*University of Toronto*
PRINCIPLISM

Anita L. Allen
*University of Pennsylvania, School of Law*
ABORTION: II. CONTEMPORARY ETHICAL AND
    LEGAL ASPECTS: B. LEGAL AND REGULATORY
    ISSUES
PRIVACY IN HEALTHCARE

Darrel W. Amundsen
*Western Washington University*
MEDICAL ETHICS, HISTORY OF THE NEAR AND
    MIDDLE EAST: I. ANCIENT NEAR EAST (1995)
MEDICAL ETHICS, HISTORY OF EUROPE: I. ANCIENT
    AND MEDIEVAL A. GREECE AND ROME (1995)
MEDICAL ETHICS, HISTORY OF EUROPE: I. ANCIENT
    AND MEDIEVAL B. EARLY CHRISTIANITY (1995)
MEDICAL ETHICS, HISTORY OF EUROPE: I. ANCIENT
    AND MEDIEVAL C. MEDIEVAL CHRISTIAN EUROPE
    (1995)

Gerard F. Anderson
*Johns Hopkins Bloomberg School of Public Health*
HEALTHCARE SYSTEMS
HEALTH POLICY IN INTERNATIONAL PERSPECTIVE

Martha Anderson
*Musculoskeletal Transplant Foundation*
TISSUE BANKING AND TRANSPLANTATION, ETHICAL
    ISSUES IN

Georgia J. Anetzberger
*Case Western Reserve University*
ABUSE, INTERPERSONAL: III. ELDER ABUSE

George J. Annas
*Boston University Medical Center*
PATIENTS' RIGHTS: I. ORIGIN AND NATURE OF
    PATIENTS' RIGHTS (1995)

Kiley Ariail
*Oregon Health and Science University*
GENETIC TESTING AND SCREENING:
    I. REPRODUCTIVE GENETIC SCREENING

Robert Arking
*Wayne State University*
AGING AND THE AGED: I. THEORIES OF AGING AND
    LIFE EXTENSION

Robert M. Arnold
*University of Pittsburgh*
ADVANCE DIRECTIVES AND ADVANCE CARE
    PLANNING
BIOETHICS EDUCATION: I. MEDICINE
INFORMED CONSENT: IV. CLINICAL ASPECTS OF
    CONSENT IN HEALTHCARE

Mila A. Aroskar
*University of Minnesota*
BIOETHICS EDUCATION: II. NURSING (1995)

Mark P. Aulisio
*MetroHealth Medical Center, Case Western Reserve
    University*
CLINICAL ETHICS: I. DEVELOPMENT, ROLE AND
    METHODOLOGIES
DOUBLE EFFECT, PRINCIPLE OR DOCTRINE OF
ETHICS COMMITTEES AND ETHICS CONSULTATION

Osman Bakar
*Center for Muslim-Christian Understanding*
ABORTION: III. RELIGIOUS TRADITIONS: D. ISLAMIC
    PERSPECTIVES (1995)

John D. Banja
*Emory University*
REHABILITATION MEDICINE

Joanne Trautmann Banks
*Pennsylvania State University, College of Medicine*
LITERATURE AND HEALTHCARE

Annette Baran
*Psychotherapist, Los Angeles*
ADOPTION

David Barnard
*University of Pittsburgh*
PALLIATIVE CARE AND HOSPICE

William W. Bassett
*University of San Francisco*
EUGENICS AND RELIGIOUS LAW: II. CHRISTIANITY
(1995)

Margaret Pabst Battin
*University of Utah*
POPULATION POLICIES, STRATEGIES FOR FERTILITY
CONTROL IN
SUICIDE

Ronald Bayer
*Columbia University*
AIDS: I. PUBLIC HEALTH ISSUES

Corrine Bayley
*St. Joseph Health System, Orange, California*
HOSPITAL, CONTEMPORARY ETHICAL PROBLEMS OF
THE (1995)

Françoise Baylis
*Dalhousie University*
MEDICAL ETHICS, HISTORY OF THE AMERICAS:
III. CANADA

Dan E. Beauchamp
*State University of New York, Albany*
LIFESTYLES AND PUBLIC HEALTH (1995)
PUBLIC HEALTH: III. PHILOSOPHY (1995)
PUBLIC HEALTH LAW: II: LEGAL MORALISM AND
PUBLIC HEALTH (1995)

Tom L. Beauchamp
*Georgetown University*
INFORMED CONSENT: I. HISTORY OF INFORMED
CONSENT (1995)
INFORMED CONSENT: II. MEANING AND ELEMENTS
(1995)
PATERNALISM (1995)

Solomon R. Benatar
*Groote Schuur Hospital, Observatory*
MEDICAL ETHICS, HISTORY OF AFRICA: II. SOUTH
AFRICA (1995)

Martin Benjamin
*Michigan State University*
CONSCIENCE (1995)

Janet Bickel
*Faculty Career and Diversity Consultant*
WOMEN AS HEALTH PROFESSIONALS,
CONTEMPORARY ISSUES OF

Barbara Bowles Biesecker
*National Human Genome Research Institute, NIH*
GENETIC COUNSELING, PRACTICE OF

Robert H. Binstock
*Case Western Reserve University School of Medicine*
HEALTH POLICY IN THE UNITED STATES

Anne H. Bishop
*Lynchburg College*
NURSING, PROFESSION OF (1995)
NURSING, THEORIES AND PHILOSOPHY OF

Laura Jane Bishop
*Georgetown University*
MEDICAL ETHICS, HISTORY OF EUROPE:
CONTEMPORARY PERIOD: VI. GERMAN-SPEAKING
COUNTRIES AND SWITZERLAND (1995)

Bela Blasszauer
*University of Pécs, Faculty of Medicine*
MEDICAL ETHICS, HISTORY OF EUROPE:
CONTEMPORARY PERIOD VIII. CENTRAL AND
EASTERN EUROPE

Sidney Bloch
*Centre for the Study of Health and Society, University of
Melbourne, Australia*
PSYCHIATRY, ABUSES OF

Samuel W. Bloom
*Mount Sinai Medical Center*
PROFESSIONAL–PATIENT RELATIONSHIP:
II. SOCIOLOGICAL PERSPECTIVES (1995)

Alberto Bondolfi
*University of Zurich, Switzerland*
MEDICAL ETHICS, HISTORY OF EUROPE:
CONTEMPORARY PERIOD: VI. GERMAN-SPEAKING
COUNTRIES AND SWITZERLAND (1995)

John Bongaarts
*Policy Research Division Population Council*
POPULATION POLICIES, DEMOGRAPHIC ASPECTS OF

Andrea L. Bonnicksen
*Northern Illinois University*
REPRODUCTIVE TECHNOLOGIES: IX. IN VITRO
FERTILIZATION AND EMBRYO TRANSFER (1995)

Charles L. Bosk
*University of Pennsylvania*
HEALTH AND DISEASE: II. SOCIOLOGICAL
PERSPECTIVES
MISTAKES, MEDICAL

Jeffrey R. Botkin
*Primary Children's Medical Center*
CIRCUMCISION, MALE

Scott Bottenfield
TISSUE BANKING AND TRANSPLANTATION, ETHICAL
ISSUES IN

Cindy Bouillon-Jensen
*Washington State Department of Social and Health Services*
INFANTICIDE (1995)

Marilyn J. Boxer
*San Francisco State University*
WOMEN, HISTORICAL AND CROSS-CULTURAL
PERSPECTIVES (1995)

Roy Branson
*Georgetown University*
PRISONERS AS RESEARCH SUBJECTS (1995)

Troyen A. Brennan
*Harvard University*
INFORMED CONSENT: VI. ISSUES OF CONSENT IN
MENTAL HEALTHCARE (1995)
MALPRACTICE, MEDICAL (1995)

Lester Breslow
*University of California, Los Angeles*
PUBLIC HEALTH: I. DETERMINANTS (1995)

Gert H. Brieger
*The Johns Hopkins University*
MEDICINE, PROFESSION OF

Dan W. Brock
*National Institutes of Health*
LIFE SUSTAINING TREATMENT AND EUTHANASIA:
I. ETHICAL ASPECTS OF
PUBLIC POLICY AND BIOETHICS
SURROGATE DECISION-MAKING

Baruch A. Brody
*Baylor College of Medicine*
LAW AND MORALITY (1995)

Howard Brody
*Michigan State University*
CLINICAL ETHICS: I. DEVELOPMENT, ROLE AND
METHODOLOGIES (1995)
COMMERCIALISM IN SCIENTIFIC RESEARCH
PATIENTS' RESPONSIBILITIES: I. DUTIES OF
PATIENTS (1995)
PLACEBO

J. Pat Browder
*Doctor's Health Plan, Inc.*
HEALING (1995)

Alan P. Brown
*University of Massachusetts*
INFORMED CONSENT VI. ISSUES OF CONSENT IN
MENTAL HEALTHCARE (1995)

Roger J. Bulger
*Association of Academic Health Centers*
HEALTHCARE INSTITUTIONS

Chester R. Burns
*University of Texas Medical Branch*
MEDICAL ETHICS, HISTORY OF THE AMERICAS:
I. COLONIAL NORTH AMERICA AND
NINETEENTH-CENTURY UNITED STATES (1995)

Jeffrey P. Burns
*Children's Hospital, Boston Harvard Medical School*
DNR (DO NOT RESUSCITATE)

Lisa Sowle Cahill
*Boston College*
ABORTION: III. RELIGIOUS TRADITIONS: B. ROMAN
CATHOLIC PERSPECTIVES

Daniel Callahan
*Hastings Center*
BIOETHICS (1995)

J. Baird Callicott
*University of North Texas*
ENVIRONMENTAL ETHICS: I. OVERVIEW
ENVIRONMENTAL ETHICS: III. LAND ETHICS

Nigel M. de S. Cameron
*Council for Biotechnology Policy, Centre for Bioethics and
Public Policy*
CHRISTIANITY, BIOETHICS IN

Courtney S. Campbell
*Oregon State University*
MORMONISM (CHURCH OF JESUS CHRIST OF
LATTER-DAY SAINTS), BIOETHICS IN

Norman L. Cantor
*Rutgers University, School of Law*
LIFE, QUALITY OF: III. QUALITY OF LIFE IN LEGAL
PERSPECTIVE

Arthur L. Caplan
*University of Pennsylvania*
ARTIFICIAL HEARTS AND CARDIAC ASSIST DEVICES

Alexander Morgan Capron
*University of Southern California*
DEATH, DEFINITION AND DETERMINATION OF:
II. LEGAL ISSUES IN PRONOUNCING DEATH
LAW AND BIOETHICS (1995)

George J. Caranasos
*University of Florida, Gainesville*
PHARMACEUTICS, ISSUES IN PRESCRIBING (1995)

Michele A. Carter
*Institute for the Medical Humanities. University of Texas
    Medical Branch*
MENTAL HEALTH SERVICES: II. ETHICAL ISSUES

Christine K. Cassel
*University of Chicago*
HEALTHCARE INSTITUTIONS

Eric J. Cassell
*Cornell University Medical Center*
MEDICINE, ART OF (1995)

PAIN AND SUFFERING (1995)

Peter Caws
*George Washington University*
PSYCHOANALYSIS AND DYNAMIC THERAPIES

Louisa E. Chapmann
*Centers for Disease Control and Prevention, Atlanta,
    Georgia*
XENOTRANSPLANTATION

Christopher Key Chapple
*Loyola Marymount University*
JAINISM, BIOETHICS IN (1995)

R. Alta Charo
*University of Wisconsin, Law School*
REPRODUCTIVE TECHNOLOGIES: IV. LEGAL AND
    REGULATORY ISSUES (1995)

James F. Childress
*University of Virginia*
METAPHOR AND ANALOGY (1995)

Nicholas A. Christakis
*University of Pennsylvania*
RESEARCH, MULTINATIONAL (1995)

Tom Christoffel
*University of Illinois, Chicago*
HOMOSEXUALITY: I. CLINICAL AND BEHAVIORAL
    ASPECTS (1995)

Larry R. Churchill
*University of North Carolina*
BENEFICENCE (1995)

J. Richard Ciccone
*University of Rochester Medical Center*
EXPERT TESTIMONY (1995)

Ellen Wright Clayton
*Vanderbilt University*
GENETIC TESTING AND SCREENING: II. NEWBORN
    GENETIC SCREENING

Cynthia B. Cohen
*Kennedy Institute of Ethics, Georgetown University,
    Washington, D.C.*
REPRODUCTIVE TECHNOLOGIES: V. GAMETE
DONATION
REPRODUCTIVE TECHNOLOGIES: VII. SPERM, OVA,
AND EMBRYOS (1995)
REPRODUCTIVE TECHNOLOGIES: VIII. ETHICAL
ISSUES (1995)

Rachel Cohon
*University at Albany/SUNY*
DISABILITY: I. ETHICAL AND SOCIETAL
    PERSPECTIVES

Thomas R. Cole
*University of Texas Medical Branch Institute for the
    Medical Humanities*
AGING AND THE AGED: V. OLD AGE

Ronald Cole-Turner
*Pittsburgh Theological Seminary, Pennsylvania*
EMBRYO AND FETUS: IV. RELIGIOUS PERSPECTIVES

Harold J. Cook
*University College London*
MEDICAL ETHICS, HISTORY OF EUROPE:
    II. RENAISSANCE AND ENLIGHTENMENT (1995)

Ronald E. Cranford
*University of Minnesota, Twin Cities*
DEATH, DEFINITION AND DETERMINATION OF:
    I. CRITERIA FOR DEATH

Thomas J. Csordas
*Case Western Reserve University*
BODY: II. CULTURAL AND RELIGIOUS PERSPECTIVES
    (1995)

Charles M. Culver
*Barry University*
ELECTROCONVULSIVE THERAPY

MENTAL INSTITUTIONS, COMMITMENT TO

Abdallah S. Daar
*University of Toronto Joint Centre for Bioethics*
XENOTRANSPLANTATION

Teodoro Forcht Dagi
*Uniformed Services University of the Health Sciences*
AUTOEXPERIMENTATION (1995)

Clare Dalton
*American University*
SEXUALITY, LEGAL APPROACHES TO (1995)

Barbara J. Daly
*Case Western Reserve University*
NURSING, PROFESSION OF

Kurt Darr
*The George Washington University Medical Center*
HEALTH SERVICES MANAGEMENT ETHICS

Anne J. Davis
*University of California, San Francisco*
BIOETHICS EDUCATION II. NURSING

Dena S. Davis
*Clevland State University*
CIRCUMCISION, RELIGIOUS ASPECTS OF

John K. Davis
*Brody School of Medicine*
AUTOEXPERIMENTATION

William E. Deal
*Case Western Reserve University*
BUDDHISM, BIOETHICS IN

Ralph Dell
*Institute of Laboratory Animal Resources, Washington, D.C.*
ANIMAL RESEARCH: III. LAW AND POLICY (1995)

Anne M. Dellinger
*Hogan and Hartson, Washington, D.C.*
INFANTS, PUBLIC POLICY AND LEGAL ISSUES (1995)

Prakash N. Desai
*VA Medical Center, Psychiatry*
MEDICAL ETHICS, HISTORY OF SOUTH AND EAST ASIA: II. INDIA (1995)

Kenneth Allen de Ville
*East Carolina University*
COMMERICALISM IN SCIENTIFIC RESEARCH (1995)

Douglas S. Diekema
*University of Washington, School of Medicine*
PEDIATRICS, PUBLIC HEALTH ISSUES IN

Kenneth J. Doka
*The Hospice Foundation of America, Washington, D.C.*
*The College of New Rochelle*
GRIEF AND BEREAVEMENT

Dolores Dooley
*National University of Ireland, Cork*
MEDICAL ETHICS, HISTORY OF EUROPE: CONTEMPORARY PERIOD V. REPUBLIC OF IRELAND

Charles J. Dougherty
*Duquesne University*
CLINICAL ETHICS: III. INSTITUTIONAL ETHICS COMMITTEES (1995)
WHISTLEBLOWING IN HEALTHCARE (1995)

Derek Doyle
*Oxford Textbook in Palliative Medicine, Edingurgh, UK*
PALLIATIVE CARE AND HOSPICE

James F. Drane
*Edinboro University of Pennsylvania*
ALTERNATIVE THERAPIES: II. ETHICAL AND LEGAL ISSUES (1995)

Theresa Drought
*Kaiser Permanente*
BIOETHICS EDUCATION: II. NURSING

Nancy Neveloff Dubler
*Montefiore Medical Center*
FERTILITY CONTROL: III. LEGAL AND REGULATORY ISSUES (1995)
PRISONERS, HEALTHCARE ISSUES OF

John Duffy
*University of Maryland*
PUBLIC HEALTH: II. HISTORY (1995)

Annette Dula
*Independent Scholar*
BIOETHICS: AFRICAN-AMERICAN PERSPECTIVES

Julie Dunlap
*Freelance writer, Columbia, Maryland*
ANIMAL WELFARE AND RIGHTS: V. ZOOS AND ZOOLOGICAL PARKS (1995)

Troy Duster
*New York University*
EUGENICS: II. ETHICAL ISSUES

Allen R. Dyer
*East Tennessee State University*
ADVERTISING
DIVIDED LOYALTIES IN MENTAL HEALTHCARE

Rem B. Edwards
*The University of Tennessee*
BEHAVIORISM: II. PHILOSOPHICAL ISSUES
FREEDOM AND FREE WILL

Rebecca S. Eisenberg
*University of Michigan*
PATENTING ORGANISMS AND BASIC RESEARCH (1995)

Carl Elliott
*University of Minnesota, Center for Bioethics*
MENTALLY DISABLED AND MENTALLY ILL PERSONS: II. RESEARCH ISSUES

Jean Bethke Elshtain
*Vanderbilt University*
ETHICS: IV. SOCIAL AND POLITICAL THEORIES (1995)

H. Tristram Engelhardt, Jr.
*Rice University*
HEALTH AND DISEASE: IV. PHILOSOPHICAL
PERSPECTIVES

MEDICINE, PHILOSOPHY OF (1995)

Pedro Laín Entralgo
PROFESSIONAL–PATIENT RELATIONSHIP:
I. HISTORICAL PERSPECTIVES (1995)

Phyllis Griffin Epps
*University of Houston*
GENETIC DISCRIMINATION

John L. Esposito
*Georgetown University*
POPULATION ETHICS: III. RELIGIOUS TRADITIONS:
B. ISLAMIC PERSPECTIVES (1995)

Richard J. Evans
*University of London, England*
EPIDEMICS

Ruth R. Faden
*Johns Hopkins University*
INFORMED CONSENT: I. HISTORY OF INFORMED
CONSENT (1995)

INFORMED CONSENT: II. MEANING AND ELEMENTS
(1995)

Charles J. Fahey
*Milbank Memorial Fund*
CHRONIC ILLNESS AND CHRONIC CARE

Margaret A. Farley
*Yale Divinity School*
SEXUAL ETHICS (1995)

David M. Feldman
*Jewish Center of Teaneck*
EUGENICS AND RELIGIOUS LAW: I. JUDAISM (1995)

POPULATION ETHICS: III. RELIGIOUS TRADITIONS:
C. JEWISH PERSPECTIVES (1995)

Gary B. Ferngren
*Oregon State University*
MEDICAL ETHICS, HISTORY OF THE NEAR AND
MIDDLE EAST (1995)

Joseph J. Fins
*Cornell University Medical College*
*The Hastings Center*
DEEP BRAIN STIMULATION

Gary S. Fischer
*University of Pittsburgh*
ADVANCED DIRECTIVES AND ADVANCED CARE
PLANNING

Annette Flanagin
*American Medical Association, Chicago*
SCIENTIFIC PUBLISHING (1995)

Leonard M. Fleck
*Michigan State University*
GENETICS AND HUMAN BEHAVIOR:
II. PHILOSOPHICAL AND ETHICAL ISSUES

John C. Fletcher
*University of Virginia*
CLINICAL ETHICS: I. DEVELOPMENT, ROLE AND
METHODOLOGIES (1995)

David P. Folsom
*University of California, San Diego*
PSYCHOPHARMACOLOGY

Mary Ford
EMBRYO AND FETUS: III. STEM CELL RESEARCH AND
THERAPY

Lachlan Forrow
*Harvard University*
BIOETHICS EDUCATION: I. MEDICINE

Daniel M. Fox
*Milbank Memorial Fund*
CHRONIC ILLNESS AND CHRONIC CARE

Renée C. Fox
*University of Pennsylvania*
ORGAN TRANSPLANTS, SOCIOCULTURAL
ASPECTS OF

Joel E. Frader
*Feinberg School of Medicine, Northwestern University*
MISTAKES, MEDICAL

Sarah Franklin
*Fairfield University, Fairfield, CT*
HEALTHCARE PROFESSIONALS, LEGAL
REGULATION OF

LIFE (1995)

Cyril M. Franks
*Rutgers University*
BEHAVIOR MODIFICATION THERAPIES

Benjamin Freedman
*The Sir Mortimer B. Davis Jewish General Hospital*
RESEARCH, UNETHICAL (1995)

R. G. Frey
*Bowling Green State University*
UTILITARIANISM AND BIOETHICS

Emily Friedman
*Independent Health Policy and Ethics Analyst*
*Boston University, School of Public Health*
ACCESS TO HEALTHCARE

Sara T. Fry
*Boston College of Nursing*
NURSING ETHICS

K.W.M. Fulford
*University of Warwick*
*University of Oxford*
MENTAL ILLNESS: I. DEFINITION, USE AND
MEANING

Robert C. Fuller
*Bradley University*
ALTERNATIVE THERAPIES: I. SOCIAL HISTORY (1995)

Atwood D. Gaines
*Case Western Reserve University*
MENTAL ILLNESS: II. CULTURAL PERSPECTIVES
RACE AND RACISM (1995)

James Garbarino
*Cornell University*
CHILDREN: IV. MENTAL HEALTH ISSUES (1995)

Michael J. Garland
*Oregon Health & Science University, Department of Public
Health and Preventive Medicine*
HEALTH INSURANCE

Bernard Gert
*Dartmouth College*
VALUE AND HEALTHCARE

Karen G. Gervais
*Minnesota Center for Health Care Ethics*
*St. Olaf College*
DEATH, DEFINITION AND DETERMINATION OF:
III. PHILOSOPHICAL AND THEOLOGICAL
PERSPECTIVES
MANAGED CARE

Raanan Gillon
*Imperial College of Science, Technology & Medicine*
MEDICAL ETHICS, HISTORY OF EUROPE:
CONTEMPORARY PERIOD IV. UNITED KINGDOM

Richard M. Glass
*Journal of the American Medical Association*
SCIENTIFIC PUBLISHING (1995)

Shimon M. Glick
*Ben Gurion University of the Negev*
MEDICAL ETHICS, HISTORY OF THE NEAR AND
MIDDLE EAST: V. ISRAEL (1995)

Jacqueline J. Glover
*George Washington University*
HEALTHCARE SYSTEMS (1995)

Mark S. Gold
*University of Florida, McKnight Brain Institute*
ADDICTION AND DEPENDENCE

Elisa J. Gordon
*Neiswanger Institute for Bioethics and Health Policy,
Stritch School of Medicine, Loyola University*
HEALTH AND DISEASE: III. ANTHROPOLOGICAL
PERSPECTIVES
HOSPITAL, CONTEMPORARY ETHICAL PROBLEMS
OF THE

Lawrence O. Gostin
*Georgetown University, Center for Law and the Public's
Health*
DISABILITY: II. LEGAL ISSUES

Diego Gracia
*Instituto de Bioética*
MEDICAL ETHICS, HISTORY OF EUROPE:
CONTEMPORARY PERIOD II. SOUTHERN EUROPE

Teresa Gracia
*Complutense University of Madrid, Spain*
MEDICAL ETHICS, HISTORY OF EUROPE:
CONTEMPORARY PERIOD II. SOUTHERN EUROPE

Frank P. Grad
*Columbia University*
PUBLIC HEALTH LAW: I. THE LAW OF PUBLIC
HEALTH

Ronald M. Green
*Dartmouth College*
POPULATION ETHICS: I. ELEMENTS OF POPULATION
ETHICS: A. DEFINITION OF POPULATION ETHICS
POPULATION ETHICS: III. RELIGIOUS TRADITIONS:
A. INTRODUCTION

Jennifer K. Greene
*JKG St. Edward's University, Austin TX*
SEXUAL IDENTITY

Merwyn R. Greenlick
*Oregon Health Sciences University*
HEALTH INSURANCE

John A. Grim
*Bucknell University*
NATIVE AMERICAN RELIGIONS, BIOETHICS IN (1995)

Rita M. Gross
*University of Wisconsin*
AUTHORITY IN RELIGIOUS TRADITIONS

R. Kent Guy
*University of Washington*
MEDICAL ETHICS, HISTORY OF SOUTH AND EAST
ASIA: I. GENERAL SURVEY

Robert T. Hall
*West Virginia State College*
ORGANIZATIONAL ETHICS IN HEALTHCARE

Stanley S. Harakas
*Holy Cross School of Theology*
EASTERN ORTHODOX CHRISTIANITY, BIOETHICS IN
POPULATION ETHICS: III. RELIGIOUS TRADITIONS:
E. EASTERN ORTHODOX PERSPECTIVES (1995)

John M. Harris
*University of Manchester*
EMBRYO AND FETUS: III. EMBRYONIC STEM CELL
RESEARCH

Beverly Wildung Harrison
*Union Theological Seminary*
ABORTION: III. RELIGIOUS TRADITIONS: C.
PROTESTANT PERSPECTIVES

Jacqueline Hart
*University of Pennsylvania*
HEALTH AND DISEASE: II. SOCIOLOGICAL
PERSPECTIVES

Hassan Hathout
*Islamic Center of Southern California*
MEDICAL ETHICS, HISTORY OF THE NEAR AND
MIDDLE EAST: IV. CONTEMPORARY ARAB WORLD
(1995)

Stanley M. Hauerwas
*Duke University*
VIRTUE AND CHARACTER (1995)

Joseph M. Hawes
*University of Memphis*
CHILDREN: I. HISTORY OF CHILDHOOD (1995)

J. Bryan Hehir
*Harvard University*
POPULATION ETHICS: III. RELIGIOUS TRADITIONS:
D. ROMAN CATHOLIC PERSPECTIVES (1995)

Michael J. Herkov
*University of Florida, College of Medicine*
ADDICTION AND DEPENDENCE

David Heyd
*Hebrew University*
OBLIGATION AND SUPEREROGATION (1995)

N. Ray Hiner
*University of Kansas, Lawrence*
CHILDREN: I. HISTORY OF CHILDHOOD (1995)

Russell Hittinger
*University of Tulsa, College of Law*
NATURAL LAW (1995)

James G. Hodge, Jr.
*Center for Law and the Public's Health at Georgetown &*
*Johns Hopkins Universities*
GENETIC TESTING AND SCREENING: IV. PUBLIC
HEALTH CONTEXT

Catherine Hoffman
*Institute for Health and Aging, San Francisco*
MEDICAID (1995)

Angela Roddey Holder
*Duke University Medical Center*
INFORMED CONSENT: V. LEGAL AND ETHICAL
ISSUES OF CONSENT IN HEALTHCARE
(POSTSCRIPT)
PEDIATRICS, ADOLESCENTS

Suzanne Holland
*University of Puget Sound*
HOMOSEXUALITY: III. RELIGIOUS PERSPECTIVES

Dennis Hollinger
*Messiah College*
LIFE, SANCTITY OF

Martha Holstein
*University of Texas, Galveston*
AGING AND THE AGED: V. OLD AGE (1995)

C. Christopher Hook
*Mayo Clinic, Rochester, MN*
CYBERNETICS
NANOTECHNOLOGY
TRANSHUMANISM AND POSTHUMANISM

Jonathan P. Horenstein
*Oakwood Healthcare Inc.*
CORPORATE COMPLIANCE

Allan V. Horwitz
*Rutgers University, Institute for Health, Healthcare Policy,*
*and Aging Research*
MENTAL HEALTH SERVICES: I. SETTINGS AND
PROGRAMS

Paul W. Humphreys
*University of Virginia, Concoran Department of Philosophy*
SCIENCE, PHILOSOPHY OF

Kathryn Montgomery Hunter
*Northwestern University Medical School*
NARRATIVE (1995)

Rodney J. Hunter
*Emory University, Candler School of Theology*
PASTORAL CARE AND HEALTHCARE CHAPLAINCY

Sara Iden
*Columbia University*
ABORTION: I. MEDICAL PERSPECTIVES (1995)

Alison M. Jaggar
*University of Colorado, Boulder*
HUMAN NATURE (1995)

Andrew Jameton
*University of Nebraska Medical Center*
INFORMATION DISCLOSURE, ETHICAL ISSUES OF (1995)
MEDICAL ETHICS, HISTORY OF THE AMERICAS: II. THE UNITED STATES IN THE TWENTY-FIRST CENTURY

Dale Jamieson
*National Center for Atmospheric Research*
CLIMATE CHANGE

Nancy S. Jecker
*University of Washington, School of Medicine*
AGING AND THE AGED: III. SOCIETAL AGING
CARE: III. CONTEMPORARY ETHICS OF CARE

Bruce Jennings
*The Hastings Center*
MEDICAID

Dilip V. Jeste
*University of California, San Diego*
PSYCHOPHARMACOLOGY

Dawn E. Johnsen
*U.S. Department of Justice*
MATERNAL–FETAL RELATIONSHIP: III. LEGAL AND REGULATORY ISSUES (1995)

L. Syd M. Johnson
*University of Albany*
*State University of New York*
ABORTION: II. CONTEMPORARY ETHICAL AND LEGAL ASPECTS: A. ETHICAL PERSPECTIVES

Albert R. Jonsen
*University of Washington, School of Medicine*
CASUISTRY (1995)
MEDICAL ETHICS, HISTORY OF THE AMERICAS: II. THE UNITED STATES IN THE TWENTY-FIRST CENTURY
MEDICAL ETHICS, HISTORY OF SOUTH AND EAST ASIA: III. CHINA. B. CONTEMPORARY CHINA (1995)

Eric T. Juengst
*Case Western Reserve University*
AGING AND THE AGED: VI. ANTI-AGING INTERVENTIONS: ETHICAL AND SOCIAL ISSUES
DNA IDENTIFICATION
ENHANCEMENT USES OF MEDICAL TECHNOLOGY
GENETIC TESTING AND SCREENING: III. POPULATION SCREENING

Jeffrey Kahn
*University of Minnesota*
ANIMAL RESEARCH: III. LAW AND POLICY
ORGAN AND TISSUE PROCUREMENT: II. ETHICAL AND LEGAL ISSUES REGARDING LIVING DONORS

Rosalie A. Kane
*University of Minnesota, Center for Biomedical Ethics and School of Public Health*
LONG-TERM CARE: I. CONCEPTS AND POLICIES

George A. Kanoti
*Cleveland Clinic Foundation*
CLINICAL ETHICS: II. CLINICAL ETHICS CONSULTATION (1995)

Marshall B. Kapp
*Wright State University, School of Medicine*
IMPAIRED PROFESSIONALS

Jay Katz
*Duke University*
INFORMED CONSENT: V. LEGAL AND ETHICAL ISSUES OF CONSENT IN HEALTHCARE (1995)

James W. Kazura
*Case Western Reserve University, School of Medicine*
INTERNATIONAL HEALTH

Stephen R. Kellert
*Yale University*
ANIMAL WELFARE AND RIGHTS: V. ZOOS AND ZOOLOGICAL PARKS

Maureen Kelley
*University of Alabama at Birmingham*
CONTRACTARIANISM AND BIOETHICS

Kevin V. Kelly
*Cornell University*
*Columbia University*
PSYCHOANALYSIS AND DYNAMIC THERAPIES (1995)

M. Lynne Kesel
*Colorado State University, Fort Collins*
VETERINARY ETHICS (1995)

Daniel J. Kevles
*California Institute of Technology*
EUGENICS: I. HISTORICAL ASPECTS (1995)

John F. Kilner
*Center for Bioethics and Human Dignity (www.cbhd.org)*
HEALTHCARE RESOURCES, ALLOCATION OF: I. MACROALLOCATION
HEALTHCARE RESOURCES, ALLOCATION OF: II. MICROALLOCATION
HUMAN DIGNITY

Rihito Kimura
*School of Human Science, Waseda University*
MEDICAL ETHICS, HISTORY OF SOUTH AND EAST ASIA: IV. JAPAN. B. CONTEMPORARY JAPAN

Nancy M. P. King
*University of North Carolina, Chapel Hill*
PRIVACY AND CONFIDENTIALITY IN RESEARCH

Russell Kirkland
*University of Georgia*
DAOISM, BIOETHICS IN (1995)

Joseph Mitsuo Kitagawa
*University of Chicago*
MEDICAL ETHICS, HISTORY OF SOUTH AND EAST
ASIA: IV. JAPAN. A. JAPAN THROUGH THE
NINETEENTH CENTURY (1995)

Arthur Kleinman
*Case Western Reserve University*
MEDICINE, ANTHROPOLOGY OF (1995)

Lonnie D. Kliever
*Southern Methodist University*
DEATH: IV. WESTERN RELIGIOUS THOUGHT (1995)

James Allen Knight
*Texas A&M University*
DIVIDED LOYALTIES IN MENTAL HEALTHCARE
(1995)

Eric D. Kodish
*Rainbow Babies and Children's Hospital, Cleveland, Ohio*
CANCER, ETHICAL ISSUES RELATED TO DIAGNOSIS
AND TREATMENT
GENETIC TESTING AND SCREENING: VI. PEDIATRIC
GENETIC TESTING
PEDIATRICS, OVERVIEW OF ETHICAL ISSUES IN

Barbara A. Koenig
*Stanford University*
ANTROPOLOGY AND BIOETHICS
DEATH: I. CULTURAL PERSPECTIVES

Loretta M. Kopelman
*Eastern Carolina University*
CHILDREN: III. HEALTHCARE AND RESEARCH ISSUES
CIRCUMCISION, FEMALE (UPDATE)
RESEARCH METHODOLOGY: II. CLINICAL TRIALS
RESEARCH POLICY: II. RISK AND VULNERABLE
GROUPS

Louis E. Kopolow
*George Washington University*
PATIENTS' RIGHTS: II. MENTAL PATIENTS' RIGHTS
(1995)

Greg Koski
*Institute for Health Policy*
*Massachusetts General Hospital*
*Harvard Medical School*
RESEARCH POLICY: I. GENERAL BACKGROUND
STUDENTS AS RESEARCH SUBJECTS

Olayinka A. Koso-Thomas
*University of Nairobi, Kenya*
CIRCUMCISION, FEMALE (1995)

Mark G. Kuczewski
*Loyola University Chicago Stritch School of Medicine*
COMMUNITARIANISM AND BIOETHICS

Patricia C. Kuszler
*University of Washington, School of Law*
INFANTS, PUBLIC POLICY AND LEGAL ISSUES

Pedro Laín Entralgo
*University of Complutense*
PROFESSIONAL–PATIENT RELATIONSHIP:
I. HISTORICAL PERSPECTIVES (1995)

H. Richard Lamb
*University of Southern California, Keck School of Medicine*
INSTITUTIONALIZATION AND
DEINSTITUTIONALIZATION

John D. Lantos
*University of Chicago*
ABUSE, INTERPERSONAL: I. CHILD ABUSE
INFANTS, MEDICAL ASPECTS AND ISSUES IN THE
CARE OF

David R. Larson
*Loma Linda University*
INFANTICIDE

Paul Lauritzen
*John Carroll University*
CLONING: III. RELIGIOUS PERSPECTIVES

Michael Lavin
*University of Arizona*
SMOKING (1995)

Karen Lebacqz
*Pacific School of Religion*
PATIENTS' RESPONSIBILITIES: II. VIRTUES OF
PATIENTS (1995)
SEXUAL ETHICS AND PROFESSIONAL
STANDARDS (1995)

Drew Leder
*Loyola College, Baltimore*
BIOETHICS EDUCATION: III. SECONDARY AND
POSTSECONDARY EDUCATION
HEALTH AND DISEASE: V. THE EXPERIENCE OF
HEALTH AND ILLNESS

Susan E. Lederer
*Yale University, School of Medicine*
MILITARY PERSONNEL AS RESEARCH SUBJECTS

Sandra Soo-Jin Lee
*Stanford University*
GENETICS AND RACIAL MINORITIES

Charles Levenstein
*University of Massachusetts Lowell*
OCCUPATIONAL SAFETY AND HEALTH: I. ETHICAL ISSUES (1995)

Carol Levine
*United Hospital Fund*
RESEARCH METHODOLOGY: III. SUBJECTS (1995)
RESEARCH POLICY: III. SUBJECTS

Robert J. Levine
*Yale University*
INFORMED CONSENT: III. CONSENT ISSUES IN HUMAN RESEARCH
RESEARCH ETHICS COMMITTEES
RESEARCH, MULTINATIONAL (1995)

Judith Lichtenberg
*University of Maryland, College Park*
POPULATION POLICIES, MIGRATION AND REFUGEES IN (1995)

Charles W. Lidz
*University of Massachusetts Medical School*
COERCION
INFORMED CONSENT: IV. CLINICAL ASPECTS OF CONSENT IN HEALTHCARE

Victor Lidz
*Medical College of Pennsylvania Hahnemann University*
DEATH: V. DEATH IN THE WESTERN WORLD (POSTSCRIPT)

Betty Jean Lifton
*Psychologist, New York*
ADOPTION

B. I. B. Lindahl
*Stockholm University*
MEDICAL ETHICS, HISTORY OF EUROPE: CONTEMPORARY PERIOD VII. NORDIC COUNTRIES

Andrew Linzey
*University of Oxford*
ANIMAL WELFARE AND RIGHTS: II. VEGETARIANISM (1995)
ANIMAL WELFARE AND RIGHTS: IV. PET AND COMPANION ANIMALS (1995)

Bernard Lo
*University of California, San Francisco*
AIDS: II. HEALTHCARE AND RESEARCH ISSUES

Sana Loue
*Case Western Reserve University*
HOMICIDE
HOMOSEXUALITY: I. CLINICAL AND BEHAVIORAL ASPECTS
IMMIGRATION, ETHICAL AND HEALTH ISSUES OF

Robin W. Lovin
*Southern Methodist University*
ETHICS: V. RELIGION AND MORALITY (1995)

David T. Lowenthal
*University of Florida*
PHARMACEUTICS, ISSUES IN PRESCRIBING (1995)

Anne Drapkin Lyerly
*Duke University Medical Center, Durham NC*
ABORTION: I. MEDICAL PERSPECTIVES
FETAL RESEARCH

Anne Lyren
*Rainbow Babies and Children's Hospital, Cleveland, Ohio*
PEDIATRICS, OVERVIEW OF ETHICAL ISSUES IN

M. Therese Lysaught
*University of Dayton*
HUMAN GENE TRANSFER RESEARCH

Barbara MacKinnon
*University of San Francisco*
CLONING: II. REPRODUCTIVE

Ruth Macklin
*Albert Einstein College of Medicine*
RESEARCH, MULTINATIONAL

Andreas-Holger Maehle
*University of Durham*
MEDICAL ETHICS, HISTORY OF EUROPE: III. NINETEENTH CENTURY A. EUROPE (1995)

David Magnus
*Stanford University Center for Bioethics*
BIOLOGY, PHILOSOPHY OF

José Alberto Mainetti
*Instituo de Bioetica y Humanidades Medicas, Fundacion Mainetti, Centro Oncologico de Excelencia*
MEDICAL ETHICS, HISTORY OF THE AMERICAS: IV. LATIN AMERICA

Stephen P. Marks
*Harvard University*
HUMAN RIGHTS

Theodore Marmor
*Yale University, School of Management*
MEDICARE

Patricia A. Marshall
*Case Western Reserve University*
ANTHROPOLOGY AND BIOETHICS

DEATH: I. CULTURAL PERSPECTIVES

Rebecca Marsick
*Case Western Reserve University*
GENETIC TESTING AND SCREENING: VI. PEDIATRIC
GENETIC TESTING

Luigi Mastroianni, Jr.
*University of Pennsylvania Medical Center*
REPRODUCTIVE TECHNOLOGIES: I. INTRODUCTION

Alexandre Mauron
*University of Geneva, Switzerland*
EMBRYO AND FETUS: I. DEVELOPMENT FROM
FERTILIZATION TO BIRTH

Stephanie L. Maxwell
*Johns Hopkins University*
HEALTH POLICY IN INTERNATIONAL PERSPECTIVE

Thomas May
*Center for the Study of Bioethics, Medical College of
Wisconsin*
CONSCIENCE, RIGHTS OF

John S. Mbiti
*Princeton Theological Seminary*
AFRICAN RELIGIONS (1995)

Lawrence B. McCullough
LONG-TERM CARE: II. NURSING HOMES

W. H. McLeod
*University of Otago*
SIKHISM, BIOETHICS IN (1995)

John McMillan
*University of Cambridge, United Kingdom*
REPRODUCTIVE TECHNOLOGIES: II. SEX SELECTION

William Meadow
*University of Chicago*
INFANTS, MEDICAL ASPECTS AND ISSUES IN THE
CARE OF

David Mechanic
*Rutgers University*
MEDICINE, SOCIOLOGY OF (1995)

Maxwell Mehlman
*Case Western Reserve University*
MALPRACTICE, MEDICAL

Alan Meisel
*University of Pittsburgh, School of Law and Center for
Bioethics and Health Law*
RIGHT TO DIE: POLICY AND LAW

Paul T. Menzel
*Pacific Lutheran University*
ECONOMIC CONCEPTS IN HEALTHCARE

Harold Merskey
*University of Western Ontario, London, Canada*
PSYCHOSURGERY, ETHICAL ASPECTS OF

Barbara D. Miller
*George Washington University*
POPULATION ETHICS: III. RELIGIOUS TRADITIONS:
G. HINDU PERSPECTIVES (1995)

Bruce L. Miller
*Michigan State University*
AUTONOMY (1995)

STUDENTS AS RESEARCH SUBJECTS (1995)

Timothy S. Miller
*Salisbury State University*
HOSPITAL, MEDIEVAL AND RENAISSANCE HISTORY
OF THE (1995)

Nancy Milliken
*UCSF Women's Health—Daly City Resource Ctr*
MATERNAL–FETAL RELATIONSHIP: I. MEDICAL
ASPECTS (1995)

Carl Mitcham
*Pennsylvania State University*
TECHNOLOGY: II. PHILOSOPHY OF MEDICAL
TECHNOLOGY (1995)

Richard W. Momeyer
*Miami University*
DEATH: III. WESTERN PHILOSOPHICAL THOUGHT

Allison W. Moore
*Church of the Good Shepherd*
ABUSE, INTERPERSONAL: II. ABUSE BETWEEN
DOMESTIC PARTNERS

Jonathan D. Moreno
*University of Virginia*
BIOTERRORISM

CONSENSUS, ROLE AND AUTHORITY OF

Derek Morgan
*Cardiff Law School, United Kingdom*
EMBRYO AND FETUS: III. STEM CELL RESEARCH AND
THERAPY

E. Haavi Morreim
*University of Tennessee, College of Medicine*
CONFLICT OF INTEREST

LIFE, QUALITY OF: II. QUALITY OF LIFE IN
HEALTHCARE ALLOCATION

Kathryn L. Moseley
*Henry Ford Hospital, Detroit*
INFANTS, MEDICAL ASPECTS AND ISSUES IN CARE
OF (1995)

Alvin H. Moss
*West Virginia University*
DIALYSIS, KIDNEY

Arno G. Motulsky
*University of Washington*
GENETICS AND ENVIRONMENT IN HUMAN HEALTH
(1995)

Timothy F. Murphy
*University of Illinois, College of Medicine*
GENDER IDENTITY
HOMOSEXUALITY: II. ETHICAL ISSUES

Robert F. Murray, Jr.
*Howard University*
GENETIC COUNSELING, ETHICAL ISSUES IN (1995)

Thomas H. Murray
*Case Western Reserve University*
SPORTS, BIOETHICS OF (1995)

David F. Musto
*Yale School of Medicine*
HARMFUL SUBSTANCES, LEGAL CONTROL OF

Carol C. Nadelson
*Brigham and Women's Hospital*
WOMEN AS HEALTH PROFESSIONALS, HISTORICAL
ISSUES OF

Arne Naess
*University of Oslo*
ENVIRONMENTAL ETHICS: II. DEEP ECOLOGY (1995)

Jeckoniah O. Ndinya-Achola
*University of Nairobi, Kenya*
MEDICAL ETHICS, HISTORY OF AFRICA: I. SUB-
SAHARAN COUNTRIES (1995)

Hilde Lindemann Nelson
*Michigan State University*
FAMILY AND FAMILY MEDICINE
FEMINISM
REPRODUCTIVE TECHNOLOGIES: VI. CONTRACT
PREGNANCY

James Lindemann Nelson
*Hastings Center, Briarcliff Manor, New York*
REPRODUCTIVE TECHNOLOGIES: VI. CONTRACT
PREGNANCY

Lisa H. Newton
*Fairfield University*
HEALTHCARE PROFESSIONALS, LEGAL
REGULATION OF

Linda J. Nicholson
*State University of New York, Albany*
SEXUAL IDENTITY

Malkah T. Notman
*Harvard University*
WOMEN AS HEALTH PROFESSIONALS, HISTORICAL
ISSUES OF (1995)

David Novak
*University of Toronto*
JUDAISM, BIOETHICS IN (1995)

Vivian-Lee Nyitray
*University of California, Riverside*
CONFUCIANISM, BIOETHICS IN

John C. Oakley
*Northern Rockies Pain & Palliative Treatment Center*
PSYCHOSURGERY, MEDICAL AND HISTORICAL
ASPECTS OF

Justin Oakley
*Monash University*
MEDICAL ETHICS, HISTORY OF AUSTRALIA AND
NEW ZEALAND

Michelle Oberman
*DePaul University, College of Law*
MATERNAL–FETAL RELATIONSHIP: III. LEGAL AND
REGULATORY ISSUES

Thomas W. Ogletree
*Yale Divinity School*
RESEARCH METHODOLOGY: III. SUBJECTS (1995)
RESPONSIBILITY (1995)
VALUE AND VALUATION (1995)

S. Jay Olshansky
*University of Chicago, NORC Population Research Center*
AGING AND THE AGED: II. LIFE EXPECTANCY AND
LIFE SPAN (1995)

Gilbert S. Omenn
*University of Washington*
GENETICS AND ENVIRONMENT IN HUMAN HEALTH
(1995)

Richard W. Osborne
*Saratoga Therapy and Training, New York*
ALCOHOLISM (1995)

David T. Ozar
*Loyola University Chicago*
DENTISTRY
PROFESSION AND PROFESSIONAL ETHICS

Lisa S. Parker
*University of Pittsburgh, Center for Bioethics and Health Law*
INFORMED CONSENT: VI. ISSUES OF CONSENT IN MENTAL HEALTHCARE

Susan Parry
*University of Minnesota, Twin Cities*
ANIMAL RESEARCH: III. LAW AND POLICY

MENTALLY DISABLED AND MENTALLY ILL PERSONS: II. RESEARCH ISSUES

ORGAN AND TISSUE PROCUREMENT: II. ETHICAL AND LEGAL ISSUES REGARDING LIVING DONORS

Talcott Parsons
*Harvard University*
DEATH: V. DEATH IN THE WESTERN WORLD (1995)

Frances Partridge
PROFESSIONAL–PATIENT RELATIONSHIP: I. HISTORICAL PERSPECTIVES (TRANSLATION)

L. Gregory Pawlson
*George Washington University*
HEALTHCARE SYSTEMS (1995)

Edmund D. Pellegrino
*Georgetown University, Center for Clinical Bioethics*
MEDICAL EDUCATION (1995)

Philip J. Peters, Jr.
*University of Missouri-Columbia*
FUTURE GENERATIONS, REPRODUCTIVE TECHNOLOGIES AND OBLIGATIONS TO

William Petersen
*Ohio State University*
POPULATION ETHICS: I. ELEMENTS OF POPULATION ETHICS: C. HISTORY OF POPULATION THEORIES

Varduhi Petrosyan
*Johns Hopkins Bloomberg School of Public Health*
HEALTHCARE SYSTEMS

HEALTH POLICY IN INTERNATIONAL PERSPECTIVE

Jessica Pierce
*University of Colorado, Boulder*
ENVIRONMENTAL HEALTH

Michael S. Policar
*Solano Partnership Healthplan, Suisun, California*
FERTILITY CONTROL: I. MEDICAL ASPECTS (1995)

Roy Porter
*Wellcome Institute for the History of Medicine, London, England*
MEDICAL ETHICS, HISTORY OF EUROPE: III. NINETEENTH CENTURY B. GREAT BRITAIN (1995)

Stephen G. Post
*Case Western Reserve University*
DEMENTIA

Gail J. Povar
*George Washington University*
WOMEN AS HEALTH PROFESSIONALS, CONTEMPORARY ISSUES OF (1995)

Kathleen E. Powderly
*State University of New York, Downstate Medical Center*
FERTILITY CONTROL: II. SOCIAL AND ETHICAL ISSUES

Nancy Press
*Oregon Health & Science University*
GENETIC TESTING AND SCREENING: I. REPRODUCTIVE GENETIC TESTING

Ivor Anton Pritchard
*Institute of Education Sciences, U.S. Department of Education*
STUDENTS AS RESEARCH SUBJECTS

Jeffrey M. Prottas
*Brandeis University*
ORGAN AND TISSUE PROCUREMENT: I. MEDICAL AND ORGANIZATIONAL ASPECTS

Laura Purdy
*Wells College*
SEXISM

Ruth B. Purtilo
*Creighton University, Center for Health Policy and Ethics*
BIOETHICS EDUCATION: IV. OTHER HEALTH PROFESSIONS

PROFESSIONAL–PATIENT RELATIONSHIP: III. ETHICAL ISSUES

TEAMS, HEALTHCARE (1995)

Ren-Zong Qiu
*Chinese Academy of Social Sciences*
MEDICAL ETHICS, HISTORY OF SOUTH AND EAST ASIA: III. CHINA. B. CONTEMPORARY CHINA (1995)

Kimberly A. Quaid
*Indiana University, School of Medicine and Center for Bioethics*
GENETIC TESTING AND SCREENING: V. PREDICTIVE GENETIC TESTING

William Quigley
*Loyola University*
JUST WAGES AND SALARIES

Michael J. Quirk
*New School for Social Research*
ETHICS: II. MORAL EPISTEMOLOGY (1995)

Arti K. Rai
*Duke Law School*
PATENTING ORGANISMS AND BASIC RESEARCH
PRIVATE OWNERSHIP OF INVENTIONS

Pinit Ratanakul
*Mahidol University*
MEDICAL ETHICS, HISTORY OF SOUTH AND EAST
ASIA: V. SOUTHEAST ASIAN COUNTRIES (1995)
POPULATION ETHICS: III. RELIGIOUS TRADITIONS:
H. BUDDHIST PERSPECTIVES (1995)

Frederic G. Reamer
*Rhode Island College*
SOCIAL WORK IN HEALTHCARE (1995)

Geoffrey P. Redmond
*Foundation for Developmental Endocrinology, Cleveland,
Ohio*
EUGENICS AND RELIGIOUS LAW: IV. HINDUISM AND
BUDDHISM (1995)

Thomas Regan
*North Carolina State University*
ANIMAL WELFARE AND RIGHTS: I. ETHICAL
PERSPECTIVES ON THE TREATMENT AND STATUS
OF ANIMALS

Warren Thomas Reich
*Georgetown University*
CARE: I. HISTORY OF THE NOTION OF CARE (1995)
CARE: II. HISTORICAL DIMENSIONS OF AN ETHIC OF
CARE IN HEALTHCARE (1995)
CARE: III. CONTEMPORARY ETHICS OF CARE (1995)

Stanley Joel Reiser
*University of Texas, Houston*
TECHNOLOGY: I. HISTORY OF MEDICAL
TECHNOLOGY (1995)

Arnold S. Relman
*Harvard Medical School, Boston, MA*
PROFIT AND COMMERCIALISM

David B. Resnik
*The Brody School of Medicine, East Carolina University,
Greenville*
GENETIC ENGINEERING, HUMAN

Jill A. Rhymes
*Baylor College of Medicine*
LONG-TERM CARE: II. NURSING HOMES

Günter B. Risse
*University of California, San Francisco*
HOSPITAL, MODERN HISTORY OF THE (1995)

Laura Weiss Roberts
*University of New Mexico*
DIVIDED LOYALTIES IN MENTAL HEALTHCARE

John A. Robertson
*University of Texas*
REPRODUCTIVE TECHNOLOGIES: VII. SPERM, OVA,
AND EMBRYOS (1995)

Daniel N. Robinson
*Georgetown University*
*Oxford University*
BEHAVIORISM: I. HISTORY OF BEHAVIORAL
PSYCHOLOGY

William J. Rold
*New York, NY*
PRISONERS, HEALTHCARE ISSUES OF

Bernard E. Rollin
*Colorado State University*
ANIMAL WELFARE AND RIGHTS: VI. ANIMALS IN
AGRICULTURE AND FACTORY FARMING (1995)

Holmes Rolston III
*Colorado State University, Fort Collins*
ANIMAL WELFARE AND RIGHTS: III. WILDLIFE
CONSERVATION AND MANAGEMENT (1995)
ENDANGERED SPECIES AND BIODIVERSITY

Robin Room
*Stockholm University, Center for Social Research on Alcohol
and Drugs*
ALCOHOL AND OTHER DRUGS IN A PUBLIC HEALTH
CONTEXT

Allan Rosenfield
*Columbia University*
ABORTION: I. MEDICAL PERSPECTIVES (1995)

Sue V. Rosser
*Georgia Institute of Technology*
BIAS, RESEARCH

Frederick Rotgers
*Philadelphia College of Osteopathic Medicine*
BEHAVIOR MODIFICATION THERAPIES

David J. Rothman
*Columbia University*
RESEARCH, HUMAN: HISTORICAL ASPECTS (1995)

Diane Rowland
*Johns Hopkins University*
MEDICAID (1995)

David J. Roy
*Clinical Research Institute of Montreal, Canada*
MEDICAL ETHICS, HISTORY OF THE AMERICAS:
III. CANADA (1995)

Michael Ruse
*Florida State University*
HUMAN EVOLUTION AND ETHICS

Laura A. Russell
*Sanctuary for Families, New York*
ABUSE, INTERPERSONAL: II. ABUSE BETWEEN
DOMESTIC PARTNERS

Jeremy Sable
*University of California, San Diego*
PSYCHOPHARMACOLOGY

Abdulaziz Sachedina
*University of Virginia*
EUGENICS AND RELIGIOUS LAW: III. ISLAM (1995)
ISLAM, BIOETHICS IN (1995)
MEDICAL ETHICS, HISTORY OF THE NEAR AND
MIDDLE EAST: II. IRAN (1995)

Greg A. Sachs
*University of Chicago*
AGING AND THE AGED: IV. HEALTHCARE AND
RESEARCH ISSUES

John Z. Sadler
*University of Texas Southwestern, Medical Center at Dallas*
MENTAL ILLNESS: III. ISSUES IN DIAGNOSIS

Mark Sagoff
*Institute for Philosophy & Public Policy, University of Maryland*
AGRICULTURE AND BIOTECHNOLOGY
ENVIRONMENTAL POLICY AND LAW

Kamran Samakar
*University of Minnesota, Twin Cities*
INFORMED CONSENT: VI. ISSUES OF CONSENT IN
MENTAL HEALTHCARE

Nil Sari
*Cerrahpasa Medical Faculty, Istanbul, Turkey*
MEDICAL ETHICS, HISTORY OF THE NEAR AND
MIDDLE EAST: III. TURKEY (1995)

Hans-Martin Sass
*Ruhr University, Bochum, Germany*
MEDICAL ETHICS, HISTORY OF EUROPE:
CONTEMPORARY PERIOD VI. GERMAN-SPEAKING
COUNTRIES AND SWITZERLAND (1995)

Todd L. Savitt
*East Carolina University*
MINORITIES AS RESEARCH SUBJECTS

Kenneth F. Schaffner
*George Washington University*
GENETICS AND HUMAN BEHAVIOR: I. SCIENTIFIC
AND RESEARCH ISSUES
RESEARCH METHODOLOGY: I. CONCEPTUAL ISSUES

Thomas F. Schindler
*University of Detroit Mercy*
LABOR UNIONS IN HEALTHCARE

Angela J. Schneider
*The University of Western Ontario*
SPORTS, BIOETHICS OF

Richard Schneider
MEDICAL ETHICS, HISTORY OF EUROPE:
CONTEMPORARY PERIOD IX. RUSSIA (1995
TRANSLATION)

Bettina Schoene-Seifert
*University of Muenster*
HARM
MEDICAL ETHICS, HISTORY OF EUROPE:
CONTEMPORARY PERIOD VI. GERMAN-SPEAKING
COUNTRIES AND SWITZERLAND

Francis Schrag
*Columbia University*
CHILDREN: II. RIGHTS OF CHILDREN (1995)

Giles R. Scofield
*Pace University, White Plains, New York*
IMPAIRED PROFESSIONALS (1995)

Larry D. Scott
*University of Texas*
ARTIFICIAL NUTRITION AND HYDRATION

John R. Scudder, Jr.
*Lynchburg College*
NURSING, THEORIES AND PHILOSOPHY OF

George E. Seidel, Jr.
*Colorado State University*
CLONING: I. SCIENTIFIC BACKGROUND

Renie Shapiro
TISSUE BANKING AND TRANSPLANTATION, ETHICAL
ISSUES IN

Richard R. Sharp
*Baylor College of Medicine, Center for Medical Ethics and Health Policy*
GENETICS AND ENVIRONMENT IN HUMAN HEALTH

Nancy Sherman
*Georgetown University*
EMOTIONS

Kristin Shrader-Frechette
*University of Notre Dame*
HAZARDOUS WASTES AND TOXIC SUBSTANCES

Miriam Shuchman
*State University of New York at Buffalo, Center for Clinical Ethics and Humanities in Health Care*
MENTALLY DISABLED AND MENTALLY ILL PERSONS:
I. HEALTHCARE ISSUES

Richard A. Shweder
*University of Chicago*
GENETICS AND HUMAN BEHAVIOR:
II. PHILOSOPHICAL AND ETHICAL ISSUES (1995)

Victor W. Sidel
*Einstein College of Medicine*
SOCIAL MEDICINE
WARFARE: II. MEDICINE AND WAR
WARFARE: IV. CHEMICAL AND BIOLOGICAL
WEAPONS

George A. Silver
*Yale University*
SOCIAL MEDICINE (1995)

Laura A. Siminoff
*Case Western Reserve University*
EMPIRICAL METHODS IN BIOETHICS

Christian M. Simon
*Case Western Reserve University*
CANCER, ETHICAL ISSUES RELATED TO DIAGNOSIS
AND TREATMENT

Peter Singer
*Princeton University*
ANIMAL RESEARCH: II. PHILOSOPHICAL ISSUES

Jacquelyn Slomka
*University of Texas, Health Science Center, Houston*
SMOKING

Michael A. Slote
*University of Maryland*
ETHICS: I. TASK OF ETHICS (1995)

Martin L. Smith
*University of Texas, M. D. Anderson Cancer Center*
JEHOVAH'S WITNESS REFUSAL OF BLOOD
PRODUCTS

Mary M. Solberg
MEDICAL ETHICS, HISTORY OF THE AMERICAS:
IV. LATIN AMERICA (TRANSLATION)

Robert C. Solomon
*University of Texas, Austin*
SEXUAL IDENTITY

W. David Solomon
*University of Notre Dame*
ETHICS: III. NORMATIVE ETHICAL THEORIES (1995)

Tom Sorell
*University of Essex*
DEATH PENALTY (1995)

Colin L. Soskolne
*University of Alberta, Edmonton, Canada*
PUBLIC HEALTH: IV. METHODS (1995)

Sandro Spinsanti
*Institute for the Social Study of the State, Rome*
MEDICAL ETHICS, HISTORY OF EUROPE:
CONTEMPORARY PERIOD I. INTRODUCTION

Bonnie Steinbock
*SUNY at Albany*
MATERNAL–FETAL RELATIONSHIP: II. ETHICAL
ISSUES (1995)

James P. Sterba
*University of Notre Dame*
JUSTICE

Nathaniel Stewart
*Case Western Reserve University*
CLONING: III. RELIGIOUS PERSPECTIVES
FERTILITY CONTROL: III. LEGAL AND REGULATORY
ISSUES
SEXUALITY, LEGAL APPROACHES TO

Calvin R. Stiller
*University of Western Ontario*
ORGAN TRANSPLANTS, MEDICAL OVERVIEW OF

Karsten J. Struhl
*Adelphi University*
HUMAN NATURE (1995)

Mark D. Sullivan
*University of Washington*
MENTAL HEALTH THERAPIES

Judith P. Swazey
*Acadia Institute, Bar Harbor, Maine*
ORGAN TRANSPLANTS, SOCIOCULTURAL
ASPECTS OF

Carol A. Tauer
*University of Minnesota, Center for Bioethics*
EMBRYO AND FETUS: II. EMBRYO RESEARCH

Michael D. Teret
*Johns Hopkins University*
INJURY AND INJURY CONTROL (1995)

Stephen P. Teret
*Johns Hopkins University*
INJURY AND INJURY CONTROL

Michael J. Toole
*Macfarlane Burnet Institute for Medical Research*
WARFARE: III. PUBLIC HEALTH AND WAR

Robert Truog
*Harvard Medical School & Childrens Hospital Boston*
PEDIATRICS, INTENSIVE CARE IN

James B. Tubbs, Jr.
*University of Detroit Mercy*
MERGERS AND ACQUISITIONS

James A. Tulsky
*VA Medical Center*
*Duke University*
ADVANCED DIRECTIVES AND ADVANCED CARE
    PLANNING

Lynn G. Underwood
*Fetzer Institute*
COMPASSIONATE LOVE

Paul U. Unschuld
*Institut für Geschichte der Medizin*
MEDICAL ETHICS, HISTORY OF SOUTH AND EAST
    ASIA: III. CHINA. A. PRE-REPUBLICAN CHINA (1995)

Richard Vance
*Bowman Gray School of Medicine*
HEALING (1995)

Gerard Vanderhaar
*Christian Brothers University, Memphis TN*
WARFARE: I. INTRODUCTION

Harold Y. Vanderpool
*University of Texas Medical Branch, Galveston*
LIFE SUSTAINING TREATMENT AND EUTHANASIA:
    IL. HISTORICAL ASPECTS

Robert M. Veatch
*Georgetown University*
MEDICAL CODES AND OATHS: I. HISTORY (1995)
MEDICAL CODES AND OATHS: II. ETHICAL ANALYSIS
    (1995)

Benedetto Vitiello
*National Institute of Mental Health*
CHILDREN: IV. MENTAL HEALTH ISSUES

Dietrich von Engelhardt
*Medical University of Luebeck*
HEALTH AND DISEASE: I. HISTORY OF THE
    CONCEPTS
MEDICAL ETHICS, HISTORY OF EUROPE:
    CONTEMPORARY PERIOD I. INTRODUCTION

Maurice A. M. de Wachter
*Bioethics Consultant, Brussels, Belgium*
MEDICAL ETHICS, HISTORY OF EUROPE:
    CONTEMPORARY PERIOD II. THE BENELUX
    COUNTRIES

Bailus Walker, Jr.
*Howard University*
OCCUPATIONAL SAFETY AND HEALTH:
    II. OCCUPATIONAL HEALTHCARE PROVIDERS
    (1995)

William J. Wall
*University of Western Ontario*
ORGAN TRANSPLANTS, MEDICAL OVERVIEW OF

Edwin R. Wallace IV
*Medical College of Georgia*
MENTAL HEALTH, MEANING OF MENTAL HEALTH
MENTAL HEALTH, MEANING OF MENTAL HEALTH
    (POSTSCRIPT)

Ernest Wallwork
*Syracuse University*
SEXUAL BEHAVIOR, SOCIAL CONTROL OF

James J. Walter
*Loyola University of Chicago*
LIFE, QUALITY OF: I. QUALITY OF LIFE IN CLINICAL
    DECISIONS (1995)

James W. Walters
*Loma Linda University*
MORAL STATUS

LeRoy Walters
*Georgetown University*
FETAL RESEARCH (1995)

Karen J. Warren
*Macalester College*
ENVIRONMENTAL ETHICS: IV. ECOFEMINISM (1995)

Donald P. Warwick
*Harvard University*
POPULATION ETHICS: I. ELEMENTS OF POPULATION
    ETHICS: A. DEFINITION OF POPULATION ETHICS
    (1995)
POPULATION ETHICS: I. ELEMENTS OF POPULATION
    ETHICS: B. IS THERE A POPULATION PROBLEM?
    (1995)
POPULATION ETHICS: II. NORMATIVE APPROACHES
    (1995)

Leonard J. Weber
*University of Detroit Mercy*
PHARMACEUTICAL INDUSTRY
PHARMACEUTICS, ISSUES IN PRESCRIBING
SUSTAINABLE DEVELOPMENT (1995)
WHISTLEBLOWING IN HEALTHCARE

Robert F. Weir
*University of Iowa*
INFANTS, ETHICAL ISSUES WITH (1995)

Mitchell G. Weiss
*Swiss Tropical Institute*
HINDUISM, BIOETHICS IN (1995)

David E. Weissman
*Froedtert Hospital- East*
DEATH: VI. PROFESSIONAL EDUCATION

Peter S. Wenz
*Sangamon State University*
ENVIRONMENTAL HEALTH (1995)

Terrie Wetle
*University of Connecticut*
LONG-TERM CARE: III. HOME CARE (1995)

Robert M. Wettstein
*University of Pittsburgh*
COMPETENCE (1995)
INSANITY AND THE INSANITY DEFENSE

Caroline Whitbeck
*Case Western Reserve University*
*Online Ethics Center for Engineering & Science*
BIOMEDICAL ENGINEERING
TRUST (1995)

Amanda White
*Montefiore Medical Center, Bronx, New York*
FERTILITY CONTROL: III. LEGAL AND REGULATORY
ISSUES (1995)

Gladys B. White
*National Center for Ethics in Health Care (10AE)*
REPRODUCTIVE TECHNOLOGIES: III. FERTILITY
DRUGS

Glayde Whitney
*Florida State University*
GENETICS AND HUMAN BEHAVIOR: I. SCIENTIFIC
AND RESEARCH ISSUES (1995)

James C. Whorton
*University of Washington*
ANIMAL RESEARCH: I. HISTORICAL ASPECTS

Daniel Wikler
*University of Wisconsin, Madison*
LIFESTYLES AND PUBLIC HEALTH (1995)

Kevin Wm. Wildes
*Georgetown University*
HEALTH AND DISEASE: IV. PHILOSOPHICAL
PERSPECTIVES
MEDICINE, PHILOSOPHY OF (1995)

John R. Williams
*Canadian Medical Association, Ontario*
MEDICAL ETHICS, HISTORY OF THE AMERICAS:
III. CANADA

William J. Winslade
*University of Texas Medical Branch*
CONFIDENTIALITY (1995)

Gerald R. Winslow
*Loma Linda University*
TRIAGE

J. Philip Wogaman
*Wesley Theological Seminary*
POPULATION ETHICS: III. RELIGIOUS TRADITIONS:
F. PROTESTANT PERSPECTIVES (1995)

Leslie E. Wolf
*University of California, San Francisco*
AIDS: II. HEALTHCARE AND RESEARCH ISSUES

Rosalie S. Wolf
*Medical Center of Central Massachusetts, Worcester*
ABUSE, INTERPERSONAL: III. ELDER ABUSE (1995)

Paul Root Wolpe
*University of Pennsylvania, Center for Bioethics*
HOLOCAUST
NEUROETHICS

Allan Young
*McGill University, Montreal, Canada*
HEALTH AND DISEASE: III. ANTROPOLOGICAL
PERSPECTIVES (1995)

Katherine K. Young
*McGill University, Montreal, Canada*
DEATH: II. EASTERN THOUGHT (1995)

Stuart J. Youngner
*Case Western Reserve University*
CLINICAL ETHICS: II. CLINICAL ETHICS
CONSULTATION (1995)
MEDICAL FUTILITY
TISSUE BANKING AND TRANSPLANTATION, ETHICAL
ISSUES IN

Boris Yudin
*Russian Academy of Sciences, Moscow*
MEDICAL ETHICS, HISTORY OF EUROPE:
CONTEMPORARY PERIOD IX. RUSSIA (1995)

Richard M. Zaner
*Vanderbilt University*
BODY: I. EMBODIMENT IN THE
PHENOMENOLOGICAL TRADITION (1995)

Sheldon Zink
*Vanderbilt University*
ARTIFICIAL HEARTS AND CARDIAC ASSIST DEVICES

Laurie Zoloth
*Northwestern University*
ABORTION: III. RELIGIOUS TRADITIONS: A. JEWISH
PERSPECTIVES
GENETICS AND HUMAN SELF-UNDERSTANDING

# TOPICAL OUTLINE

*The classification of articles that follows provides a thematic view of the Encyclopedia's contents, depicting overall coverage in various divisions of the field of bioethics. It is also intended to assist the user, whether researcher or browser, in locating articles broadly related to a given topic. Because the topic headings are not mutually exclusive, certain entries are listed more than once.*

ABORTION

Abortion
Adoption
Autonomy
Buddhism, Bioethics in
Christianity, Bioethics in
Conscience, Rights of
Double Effect, Principle or Doctrine of
Embryo and Fetus
Feminism
Fertility Control
Freedom and Free Will
Genetic Testing and Screening: Reproductive Genetic Testing
Harm
Healing
Hinduism, Bioethics in
Homicide
Human Dignity
Human Rights
Infanticide
Islam, Bioethics in
Jainism, Bioethics in
Judaism, Bioethics in
Law and Morality
Life
Life, Sanctity of
Literature and Healthcare
Maternal–Fetal Relationship
Medical Codes and Oaths
Medical Ethics, History of
Medicine, Profession of
Mental Illness
Moral Status

Nursing, Profession of
Patients' Rights
Population Policies, Strategies for Fertility Control in
Professional–Patient Relationship
Reproductive Technologies: Fertility Drugs
Responsibility
Sexual Behavior, Social Control of
Sexual Ethics
Virtue and Character
Women, Historical and Cross-Cultural Perspectives

ABUSE AND HARM

Abuse, Interpersonal
Autoexperimentation
Bioterrorism
Circumcision
Cloning: Reproductive
Coercion
Double Effect, Principle or Doctrine of
Electroconvulsive Therapy
Embryo and Fetus
Eugenics: Historical Aspects
Genetic Discrimination
Harm
Harmful Substances, Legal Control of
Holocaust
Infanticide
Injury and Injury Control
Malpractice, Medical
Military Personnel as Research Subjects
Minorities as Research Subjects
Mistakes, Medical
Pain and Suffering

Psychiatry, Abuses of
Psychosurgery, Ethical Aspects of
Psychosurgery, Medical and Historical Aspects of
Race and Racism
Research, Unethical
Sexism
Smoking
Students as Research Subjects
Suicide
Transhumanism and Posthumanism
Warfare

### AFRICAN AMERICANS

African Religions
Anthropology and Bioethics
Bioethics: African-American Perspectives
Christianity, Bioethics in
Dialysis, Kidney
Genetic Discrimination
Genetic Testing and Screening: Population Screening
Health and Disease: Anthropological Perspectives
Healthcare Resources, Allocation of
Holocaust
Human Dignity
Human Rights
Islam, Bioethics in
Justice
Medical Ethics, History of Africa
Mental Illness: Cultural Perspectives
Metaphor and Analogy
Organ and Tissue Procurement
Organ Transplants
Pastoral Care and Healthcare Chaplaincy
Patients' Rights: Origins and Nature of Patients' Rights
Public Health
Race and Racism
Research Policy: Risk and Vulnerable Groups
Research, Unethical
Smoking
Trust

### AGING

Advance Directives and Advance Care Planning
Aging and the Aged
Artificial Nutrition and Hydration
Body
Care
Chronic Illness and Chronic Care
Confucianism, Bioethics in
Death
Dementia
Disability
Informed Consent
Justice
Life, Quality of

Long-Term Care
Medicaid
Medicare
Moral Status
Paternalism
Patients' Rights
Surrogate Decision-Making
Technology
Virtue and Character

### ANIMAL RESEARCH AND ANIMAL RIGHTS

Animal Research: Historical Aspects
Animal Research: Philosophical Issues
Animal Research: Law and Policy
Animal Welfare and Rights: Ethical Perspectives on the
    Treatment and Status of Animals
Animal Welfare and Rights: Vegetarianism
Animal Welfare and Rights: Wildlife Conservation and
    Management
Animal Welfare and Rights: Pet and Companion
    Animals
Animal Welfare and Rights: Zoos and Zoological Parks
Animal Welfare and Rights: Animals in Agriculture and
    Factory Farming

### BUSINESS ETHICS IN HEALTHCARE

Advertising
Commercialism in Scientific Research
Conflict of Interest
Corporate Compliance
Economic Concepts in Healthcare
Healthcare Institutions
Healthcare Systems
Health Insurance
Health Policy in the United States
Hospital
Just Wages and Salaries
Labor Unions in Healthcare
Pharmaceutical Industry
Pharmaceutics, Issues in Prescribing
Privacy in Healthcare
Profit and Commercialism
Research Policy

### CHILDREN AND INFANTS

Abortion
AIDS
Care
Children
Compassionate Love
Disability
Eugenics
Family and Family Medicine
Future Generations, Reproductive Technologies and
    Obligations to

INFORMED CONSENT

INTERNATIONAL PERSPECTIVES ON HEALTH

LAW AND BIOETHICS

Abortion
Autonomy
Coercion
Fertility Control
Human Rights
Immigration, Ethical and Health Issues of
Infanticide
International Health
Population Ethics
Population Policies, Demographic Aspects of
Population Policies, Migration and Refugees in
Population Policies, Strategies for Fertility Control in
Race and Racism
Reproductive Technologies
Sexism
Sustainable Development
Warfare

## PROFESSIONS AND PROFESSIONAL–PATIENT RELATIONSHIP

Alternative Therapies
Autonomy
Beneficence
Care
Compassionate Love
Confidentiality
Conscience, Rights of
Divided Loyalties in Mental Healthcare
Emotions
Epidemics
Healing
Healthcare Professionals, Legal Regulation of
Healthcare Resources, Allocation of
Health Insurance
Impaired Professionals
Information Disclosure, Ethical Aspects of
Informed Consent
Labor Unions in Healthcare
Malpractice, Medical
Managed Care
Medical Codes and Oaths
Medical Education
Medical Ethics, History of
Medicine, Art of
Medicine, Profession of
Mistakes, Medical
Nursing Ethics
Nursing , Profession of
Nursing, Theories and Philosophy of
Obligation and Supererogation
Pastoral Care and Healthcare Chaplaincy
Paternalism
Patients' Responsibilities
Patients' Rights
Pharmaceutical Industry
Pharmaceutics, Issues in Prescribing

Principlism
Privacy in Healthcare
Profession and Professional Ethics
Responsibility
Social Medicine
Teams, Healthcare
Trust
Veterinary Ethics

## PUBLIC HEALTH

Access to Healthcare
AIDS
Autonomy
Beneficence
Coercion
Confidentiality
Communitariansim and Bioethics
Conflict of Interest
Conscience, Rights of
Corporate Compliance
Environmental Ethics
Environmental Policy and Law
Epidemics
Eugenics
Hazardous Wastes and Toxic Substances
Healthcare Resources, Allocation of
Healthcare Systems
Homicide
International Health
Lifestyles and Public Health
Medical Codes and Oaths
Medical Ethics, History of
Medicine, Philosophy of
Population Ethics
Public Health
Public Health Law
Public Policy and Bioethics
Sexual Behavior, Social Control of
Suicide
Warfare: Public Health and War
Xenotransplantation

## RELIGIOUS ISSUES

Abortion: Jewish Perspectives
Abortion: Roman Catholic Perspectives
Abortion: Protestant Perspectives
Abortion: Islamic Perspectives
Body: Cultural and Religious Perspectives
Circumcision
Cloning: Religious Perspectives
Conscience, Rights of
Death: Western Religious Thought
Death, Definition and Determination of: Philosophical and Theological Perspectives
Embryo and Fetus: Religious Perspectives

# A

# ABORTION

• • •

## I. MEDICAL PERSPECTIVES

Medical information and perspectives on abortion are not just data untinged by values. Throughout history medical facts and moral values regarding abortion have been inextricably intertwined, and the current era is no exception.

People interested in the ethics of abortion turn to medicine and medical practitioners for the following sort of information and perspectives, which will be considered in this entry :

1. whether medical knowledge clarifies the moral status of the fetus as a human being;

2. whether medical information on abortion confirms it to be safe for the woman;

3. what the medical perspectives are on performing early versus late abortions, particularly in light of controversies regarding *partial birth abortion*;

4. what the public health and international perspectives are on abortion.

## Medical Knowledge Regarding Status of the Fetus

However much information biomedical investigation may provide regarding pregnancy, fetal development, and abortion, it cannot provide a determination as to when human life begins. The answer to that question—which deals with the moral status of the fetus—is arrived at by a process that entwines medical facts with experiences, values, religious and philosophical beliefs and attitudes, perceptions of meaning, and moral argument. Such a process extends beyond the special competency of medicine. For example, medicine has never had the ability to establish when ensoulment—an ancient criterion involving the *infusion* of the soul into the body of the fetus, thus conferring moral status on the fetus—occurs. Similarly there is disagreement among some physicians over the moral status of the fetus and the permissibility of abortion.

There is some confusion about the definition of abortion. Spontaneous abortion, or what is commonly termed a miscarriage, refers to a spontaneous loss of a pregnancy before viability (at about twenty-four weeks of gestation). Losses after that point in a pregnancy are termed *preterm deliveries,* or, in the case of the delivery of a fetus who has already died, *stillbirths.* The terminology commonly used in relation to induced abortion is different. Here, viability is not the key point. Rather, any termination of a pregnancy by medical or surgical means is termed an abortion, regardless of the stage of the pregnancy.

## Safety and Harm for the Woman

**POSSIBLE PHYSICAL HARM.** There is a close tie between medical information on the safety of abortion practices and ethical positions on abortion. For example, at a time when abortions were frequently harmful to women—such as when legal restrictions increased recourse to untrained practitioners—opponents of abortion appealed to information on the likelihood of medical harm to the woman and risks of future pregnancies as arguments against abortion (Kunins and Rosenfield).

As of 2003, induced abortions performed within the first twelve weeks of pregnancy are among the safest and simplest forms of surgery and, based on maternal mortality ratios (number of deaths per 100,000 live births), both first- and second-trimester abortions, when performed by properly trained personnel, in general are safer than carrying a pregnancy to term (Cates and Grimes). As a result, ethical arguments against abortion tend to be restricted to areas other than maternal safety. Nonetheless, some aspects of medical safety and harm—including possible complications and psychological sequelae—continue to be important for ethical discourse, especially since a basic tenet of medical ethics is to avoid harm.

The major immediate complications of induced abortion, listed in order of frequency, are infection, hemorrhage, uterine perforation, and anesthesia-related complications. Overall complication rates for legal first-trimester abortions are less than 0.5 deaths per 100,000 abortions performed (as compared to more than four per 100,000 in the early 1970s, before the U.S. Supreme Court decision *Roe v. Wade* [1973] permitted medically supervised abortions). Medical complications associated with induced abortion are directly related to gestational age and the type of procedure used to terminate the pregnancy. Most abortions (over 90%) done in the United States are performed within the first twelve weeks of pregnancy, when abortion is safest. More serious complications may occur in procedures done later in pregnancy.

ABORTION PROCEDURES. Information on abortion procedures often sheds light on questions of safety as well as on other aspects of abortion that are relevant to ethics. The most common early-trimester abortion procedure (done between seven and twelve weeks' gestation) is suction curettage, in which a thin plastic tube (canula) is inserted through the cervix and, by negative pressure vacuum, the contents of the uterus are aspirated. Usually, following the aspiration procedure, a curettage (using a sharp, spoon-shaped surgical instrument, a curette) is performed to ensure that all fetal tissue has been removed.

Complications of suction curettage procedures are rare, and even when they occur, are usually not serious. General anesthesia is considered by many to be an unnecessary additional risk, since local anesthesia, injected into the cervix, often is quite effective (Grimes et al.). A short course of prophylactic antibiotics is sometimes prescribed, although

postabortion infection is uncommon with suction curettage. Because of its safety, suction curettage is performed most often in free-standing clinics or outpatient centers in hospitals.

At twelve to twenty weeks' gestation, the most common method used for abortion is dilation and evacuation (D&E), which uses specially designed forceps in conjunction with vacuum aspiration to facilitate the removal of the uterine contents. Prior to initiating the procedure, the cervix is dilated gradually over a number of hours using sponge-like materials that expand as they absorb local cervical fluids. Though still considered a minor surgical procedure, D&E is clearly more involved and invasive than suction curettage, and a trained and skilled clinician is essential. Although it is possible to use only local anesthesia for D&E, the procedure is considerably more uncomfortable than suction curettage, and general anesthesia is often used, making the procedure more risky. The D&E procedure can be performed in free-standing clinics, but often ambulatory surgical services in a hospital setting are chosen for the procedures performed later in pregnancy (after the fourteenth week) because emergency care can be quickly provided in case of a complication. Informed-consent procedures require that the various methods of abortion be discussed as well as the possible anesthesia alternatives.

The other abortion procedure used fairly commonly in the second trimester is instillation abortion, in which a solution instilled into the amniotic cavity through the abdomen via amniocentesis results in the death of the fetus and termination of the pregnancy. Uterine contractions signaling labor begin twelve to twenty-four hours later and culminate with the expulsion of the fetus. Anesthesia is not commonly used for instillation procedures. Discomfort varies widely among patients, usually in relation to the length of labor and the time before complete expulsion of the fetus and placenta. More serious complications can occur during instillation procedures, including inadvertent introduction of the solution into the mother's bloodstream, excessive bleeding at the time of expulsion of the fetus, or retention of placenta, and for this reason hospital admission is usually advised. Instillation procedures are used mainly for procedures beyond the twentieth week of gestation. All late-pregnancy abortion procedures carry significant risk if carried out by physicians not specially trained in the technique.

A promising alternative to surgical abortion for early first-trimester terminations of pregnancy is chemical abortion. For example, the antiprogestin drug RU-486 works by blocking progesterone production by the ovaries, an essential hormone in the early stages of pregnancy and in the implantation of the embryo. The drug is given within the first forty-nine days of a confirmed pregnancy and is used in conjunction with a prostaglandin, which produces uterine contractions and subsequent expulsion of the uterine contents. A follow-up visit is necessary eight to twelve days later to ensure that complete termination of the pregnancy has occurred.

On September 28, 2000, the U.S. Food and Drug Administration (FDA) approved RU–486 for use in the United States, and it has been distributed since the following November by Danco Laboratories, LLC under the brand name Mifeprex. According to the guidelines set forth by the FDA, it has been distributed only to physicians and is not available through pharmacies; furthermore, the FDA has approved a specific regimen for the use of RU–486. Three visits are necessary for this medical means of pregnancy termination: the first to make the diagnosis and to give the RU–486, the second, two days later, for the prostaglandin, and the third within two weeks for the final follow-up. In France, a fourth visit is required by law since a one-week delay between the diagnosis of pregnancy and the initiation of an abortion procedure is mandated.

As a result of the requirement for three visits (or four in France), because there may be a few days before the abortion occurs and as many as ten or more days of vaginal bleeding thereafter, and because it may be more expensive than surgical abortion, many women in France and the United States still prefer suction curettage as their method of choice (Kolata). However, there is anticipation that as awareness grows, many women will still prefer a medical means of abortion, not wishing to undergo surgery (albeit a minor procedure) or to be subjected to the harassment that may occur outside some clinic facilities.

Successful termination has been shown to occur in 97 percent of patients using the RU-486 regimen, with the remaining patients requiring suction curettage for complete removal of the products of conception. In comparison, for surgical procedures, less than 1 percent of patients require a second curettage because the procedure was incomplete. Most women develop strong cramping after taking the prostaglandin (because the drug induces uterine contractions) and usually have the abortion within a few hours after receiving prostaglandin. In France, RU-486 is therefore provided only through clinic facilities and in this setting, the abortion often occurs during the same four hours women remain in the clinic after taking the prostaglandin. However, some French physicians believe that a clinic setting is not essential. In the United States, specific requirements for facilities providing abortion vary from state to state. Federal guidelines, however, require only that RU-486 be prescribed by or under the supervision of a physician who can diagnose the duration of pregnancy accurately, diagnose an ectopic pregnancy, and either can provide surgical intervention in cases of incomplete abortion or who has made arrangements to provide such care through others.

While studies have demonstrated the safety and effectiveness of RU-486 as a *morning after* pill for use after unexpected midcycle intercourse (Ashok), preparations containing the same hormones as are found in oral contraceptive pills (estrogen and progestin or progestin alone) have been approved for this purpose. Furthermore, the copper-T intrauterine device (IUD) can be inserted up to five days after unprotected intercourse to prevent pregnancy. Both emergency contraceptive pills (ECPs) and the IUD are more readily available and remain the standard of care for postcoital contraception in the United States (American College of Obstetricians and Gynecologists [ACOG], 2001).

**AVAILABILITY OF ABORTION PROVIDERS.** The majority of abortion procedures in the United States are provided by obstetrician-gynecologists, with a small percentage performed by other providers such as family practice physicians, midwives, or nurse practitioners. There are serious concerns about the provision of abortion procedures in the future for several reasons. Although most obstetrician-gynecologists believe that women should have the right to choose to terminate a pregnancy, at the same time, most do not wish to perform abortions. As a result, approximately 84 percent of counties in the United States do not have an abortion facility, and the number rises to 94 percent outside metropolitan areas.

Many ob-gyn residency training programs do not offer abortion training routinely and as a result, many graduating residents have little or no training in this area. However, over the last decade there has been an increase in the number of residency programs providing training in abortion procedures. In 1996, the Accreditation Council for Graduate Medical Education required ob-gyn residency programs to include family planning and abortion training for its students, though abortion is generally still presented as an elective part of training. The impact of these requirements was demonstrated in a survey conducted by the National Abortion Federation (NAF). The investigators of the NAF report found that from 1992 to 1998, ob-gyn residency programs reporting routine first trimester abortion training increased almost fourfold, from 12 percent to 46 percent, and routine second trimester abortion training from 7 percent to 44 percent (Almeling et al.).

Finally, even where training has taken place, the increasing incidence of harassment and even violence (including the 1993 and 1994 murders of abortion providers in Florida) has resulted in more reluctance on the part of physicians to be involved in the provision of this service. In response to the escalating violence, Congress enacted the

*Freedom of Access to Clinic Entrances Act,* or *FACE,* in 1994. This statute established federal criminal penalties and civil remedies for violent, obstructionist, or damaging conduct affecting reproductive healthcare providers and recipients, and supplemented the penalties available under then-existing federal criminal statutes such as the Hobbs Act, the Travel Act, and federal arson and firearms statutes. Rising violence as well as the federal response highlight serious ethical questions as to the social responsibility of professionals in this field to make certain that this procedure is available to all patients.

POSSIBLY HARMFUL EFFECTS ON SUBSEQUENT PREG-
NANCIES. Questions have been raised about possible long-term harmful effects of induced abortion, especially for women who have had multiple abortions. Much of the concern centers on subsequent pregnancies, following one or more induced abortions. Medical evidence has consistently shown that a woman who has one properly performed induced abortion in the first trimester of pregnancy has the same chance of a normal outcome of a subsequent pregnancy as a woman who has never had an abortion. The evidence is less definitive for women who have had more than one induced abortion or an abortion with complications, although there is no reason to believe that additional abortion procedures, carried out by well-trained professionals, will have a long-term adverse effect. Overall, in terms of medical risk, abortion procedures, particularly those carried out in the first trimester of pregnancy, are among the safest of all surgical procedures.

PSYCHOLOGICAL EFFECTS. A much grayer area is that of the psychological consequences of induced abortion. It is difficult to generalize about the emotional responses of patients to pregnancy termination but, like physical complications, psychological complications may be related to the type of procedure and the gestational age at the time of termination, with earlier suction curettage theoretically leading to fewer psychological complications than later procedures. However, most studies in this area suffer from methodological problems, including a lack of consensus about symptoms, inadequate study design, and lack of adequate follow-up. Furthermore, the so-called postabortion syndrome does not meet the American Psychiatric Association's definition of trauma (Gold).

Despite the many problems with most investigations, "the studies are consistent in their findings of relatively rare instance of negative responses after abortion and of decreases in psychological distress after abortion compared to before abortion" (Adler et al., p. 42). Former U.S. Surgeon General C. Everett Koop, at the request of the White House,

undertook a major assessment of the literature on this topic and concluded in a 1989 congressional hearing that "the data were insufficient ... to support the premise that abortion does or does not produce a postabortion syndrome and that emotional problems resulting from abortion are minuscule from a public health perspective" (Human Resources and Intergovernmental Relations Subcommittee of the Committee on Governmental Operations, p. 14). Given Koop's personal opposition to abortion, the conclusions of his assessment are of particular importance.

Approximately 10 percent of induced abortions in the United States take place between twelve and twenty weeks of gestation, and less than 1 percent take place between twenty and twenty-four weeks. This means that more than 150,000 second-trimester procedures occur each year, a much larger number than in other developed nations where abortion is legal. Most would agree that decreases in the total numbers of abortions would be highly desirable, particularly decreases in second-trimester procedures.

The most common reasons for these later procedures, particularly among younger teens, are indecision about termination and failure to recognize (or denial of) pregnancy. A smaller percentage of these later abortions occur because of medical or genetic reasons, which theoretically may correlate with greater psychological distress. Although techniques such as nuchal translucency measurement with serum screening, chorionic villus sampling, and early amniocentesis have allowed earlier diagnosis, the results of more commonly used techniques of antenatal fetal diagnosis with midtrimester amniocentesis are generally not available until well into the second trimester.

Choosing to terminate a pregnancy is a serious decision that is rarely made lightly. In addition to complete information about abortion procedure options, counseling should be made available to women faced with a decision about an unplanned pregnancy.

## Early Versus Late Abortions: Controversies in Medicine

Medical attitudes toward abortion have constantly been shaped by the medical profession's knowledge of and attitude toward the stage of development of the fetus, interacting with local cultural, religious, and legal ideas and beliefs. Together, these factors have had a significant impact on medical practice. Medical practitioners often have more difficulty with late abortions as compared to earlier ones, because the procedures are more difficult to perform in late abortions, because of the more advanced state of fetal development, and because of the political climate surrounding so-called *partial-birth abortion.*

Prior to the latter half of the nineteenth century, abortion was available in the United States under the doctrines of British common law that permitted termination of a pregnancy until the time of *quickening* (detection of fetal movement). However, medical knowledge available at that time made it difficult to confirm a pregnancy with certainty prior to quickening, for it was only this detection of fetal movement that confirmed the existence of a living human fetus. There is little in the historical literature that describes how physicians in that era actually felt about abortions, although based on the information discussed below, one can assume that there were concerns about abortion.

By the second half of the nineteenth century, as scientific knowledge grew, so did the realization that fetal development occurs on a continuum, suggesting that the fetus is a living entity before fetal movement is felt. Prompted by this new medical knowledge, physicians, particularly those who were members of the newly formed American Medical Association (AMA), began openly to oppose abortion and urged its criminalization as an immoral practice. As a basis for this change, the Hippocratic Oath was used to oppose abortion at any time during pregnancy.

The concept of the fetus as a human entity separate from the mother has long been the subject of ethical concern within the medical profession. The AMA's Principles of Medical Ethics permit physicians to perform abortions, provided they are done in accordance both with the law and with *good medical practice* (Council on Ethical and Judicial Affairs, Opinion 2.01). In general, for the last 100 years or more, and especially since the U.S. Supreme Court decision in *Roe v. Wade* greatly liberalized the legal permissibility of abortion, medical practitioners have tended to place the value of the life of the mother above that of the fetus and there has been general agreement that late abortion is permissible in those cases where medical judgment deems that the health of the mother is seriously compromised by a pregnancy.

However, just as *Roe v. Wade* allowed for some restrictions on abortions after fetal viability, so the medical profession has shown a reluctance to perform abortions later in pregnancy, even early in the second trimester. In addition to new ethical dilemmas over fetal and maternal rights, many medical professionals remain ambivalent about the morality of abortion, a conflict that is heightened both by increased technological sophistication in the field of perinatology and genetics and the current political climate.

Depending on the technology available to a physician and the condition of the individual fetus (gestational age and any developmental deformity), it is often possible, depending on the availability of neonatal intensive support, to save the lives of premature babies born at twenty-seven weeks gestation. Babies born at twenty-four to twenty-six weeks and earlier have survived with intensive neonatal intervention and support, though often with some degree of functional impairment. With abortions occasionally performed up to twenty-four weeks gestation, one can see the conflict within medicine: Fetuses that might be aborted by one group of physicians are aggressively supported as patients by another group.

Physicians who provide abortion services prefer to do early abortions, that is, up to twelve weeks, for several reasons. First, it is generally agreed that, though a fetus may exhibit primitive reflexes before twenty weeks gestation, there is no evidence that the brain and neurological system are developed enough even at twenty-four weeks for the fetus to experience pain. Second, as discussed earlier, second-trimester techniques that might appear to be more humane or to show more respect for the fetus generally entail more danger for the woman. Third, the physicians who are committed to offering abortion procedures are intent on offering the safest procedures for the woman and regard the benefit to the woman as superseding the goal of minimalization of harm to the fetus.

Most recently, the debate over partial birth abortion has presented significant challenges to physicians, other providers of abortion services, and proponents of a woman's right to choose to terminate a pregnancy. While legislation to ban this procedure has been proposed and debated in Congress, in several state legislatures, and finally in the Supreme Court, the vagueness of the definition of partial-birth abortion (which is not a term used by medical professionals), the failure to allow physicians to protect a woman's health after a fetus becomes viable, and the application of the ban before fetal viability has resulted in the failure of these bans to be constitutionally upheld (Annas, 1998).

In March 1995, the first Partial-Birth Abortion Ban Act was introduced in the U.S. Congress to make it a federal crime to perform "an abortion in which the person performing the abortion partially vaginally delivers a living fetus before killing the fetus and completing the delivery." In April 1996 President Clinton vetoed the bill because of its failure to include an exception allowing the procedure to prevent *serious, adverse health consequences to the mother* (Remarks on Returning without Approval to the House of Representatives Partial Birth Abortion Legislation, pp. 643–647); he vetoed a revised bill in October 1997 for the same reason (Message to the House of Representatives Returning without Approval Partial Birth Abortion Legislation, p. 1545).

Over the interim between the two bills, medical organizations took conflicting positions. In contrast with the AMA, which endorsed the federal bill, the ACOG executive board urged the president to veto the bill. The executive board understood the term partial birth abortion to describe a method members of the ACOG would understand as *intact dilation and extraction,* one method of terminating a pregnancy after sixteen weeks' gestation and specifically involving "1. deliberate dilation of the cervix, usually over a sequence of days; 2. instrumental conversion of the fetus to a footling breech; 3; breech extraction of the body excepting the head; and 4. partial evacuation of the intracranial contents of the living fetus to effect vaginal delivery of dead but otherwise intact fetus" (ACOG p. 2). While the committee could identify no specific circumstance where this method would be the only option to preserve the health of the woman, they stated that "only the doctor, in consultation with the patient, based upon the woman's particular circumstances can make this decision" (ACOG, 1997, p. 3).

Similar laws have since been passed in more than two dozen states and found unconstitutional; the most significant decision was issued by the Supreme Court in a challenge to Nebraska's Partial-Birth Abortion law in the case of *Stenberg v. Carhart* in 2000 (Annas, 2001). The case involved Dr. Leroy Carhart, a Nebraska physician who sued in federal court to have Nebraska's law declared unconstitutional because it endangered women's lives and was void because of its vagueness in that physicians could not know exactly what procedure was proscribed. Ultimately, the Supreme Court ruled on June 28, 2000, that the Nebraska law and all other laws banning partial birth abortion are unconstitutional. The majority opinion held that the law was unconstitutional for two reasons. First, it did not provide an exception to protect the health of the woman as required by *Roe v. Wade.* Second, the law imposed an undue burden (as proscribed in *Planned Parenthood v. Casey*) because it was written so broadly as to ban not only the rarely used dilation and extraction (D&X) procedures but also dilation and evacuation (D&E) so commonly used to terminate pregnancies even early in the second trimester. Ultimately, the *Stenberg* decision reinforced the important position that decisions regarding how abortions can most safely and satisfactorily be performed should be made by women and their physicians.

## Public Health and International Perspectives

Abortion is widely available with varying restrictions throughout the industrialized world. In recent years, there also has been a trend toward liberalization of abortion laws in many developing countries, such as in India, where abortion has been legalized; and in Bangladesh, where an early first-trimester procedure called menstrual regulation (which is really an early suction curettage) has been officially sanctioned by the government even though abortion per se has not been legalized. Abortion laws are most restrictive in Latin America, sub-Saharan Africa, and Central Asia.

Many of the countries in these regions have high rates of maternal mortality, and complications of illegal abortions are one of its leading causes. According to the World Health Organization (WHO), as many as 100,000 or more maternal deaths occur each year as a result of complications of an unsafe, usually illegal abortion. Even in the United States, some illegal abortions continue to be performed in cases where women are without the resources to obtain a legal abortion. Although reliable incidence data are lacking as to the number of illegal abortions performed worldwide, there clearly is a strong demand for abortion, a demand that will probably always exist. As evidenced by the estimated number of women who undergo illegal abortion, most women who are determined to terminate a pregnancy will attempt to do so either by themselves or with assistance.

Consequently, the public-health concerns about the complications of unsafe abortion, coupled with the complex issues relating to the reproductive and autonomy rights of women versus the rights of the fetus, suggest the continuing importance that must be given by the field of bioethics to abortion, particularly to the question of whether and by what means abortion should be made available equally to all persons requesting it, regardless of national citizenship, ethnic or racial identity, or economic status.

ALLAN ROSENFIELD
SARA IDEN (1995)
REVISED BY ANNE DRAPKIN LYERLY

**SEE ALSO:** *Embryo and Fetus; Fertility Control; Reproductive Technologies;* and other *Abortion* subentries

### BIBLIOGRAPHY

Adler, Nancy E.; David, Henry P.; and Major, Brenda N.; et al. 1990. "Psychological Responses After Abortion." *Science* 248: 41–44.

Almeling, Rene; Tews, Laureen; and Dudley, Susan. 2000. "Abortion Training in U.S. Obstetrics and Gynecology Residency Programs, 1998." *Family Planning Perspectives* 32 (6): 268–271.

American College of Obstetricians and Gynecologists. 1997. *Statement on Intact D&X.* Washington, D.C.: The American College of Obstetricians and Gynecologists.

American College of Obstetricians and Gynecologists. 2001. *Emergency Oral Contraception,* ACOG Practice Bulletin, Number 25. Washington, D.C.: The American College of Obstetrics and Gynecologists.

Annas, George J. 1998. "Partial Birth Abortion, Congress, and the Constitution." *New England Journal of Medicine* 339(4): 279–283.

Annas, George J. 2001. "*Partial Birth Abortion* and the Supreme Court." *New England Journal of Medicine* 344(2): 152–156.

Ashok, Premila W.; Wagaarachchi, Prabath T.; Flett, Gillian M.; et al. 2001. "Mifepristone as a Late Post-Coital Contraceptive." *Human Reproduction* 16: 72–75.

Berger, Gary S.; Brennar, William E.; and Keith, Louis G., eds. 1981. *Second Trimester Abortion.* Littleton, MA: Wright-PSG.

Cates, Willard, Jr., and Grimes, David A. 1981. "Morbidity and Mortality of Abortion in the United States." In *Abortion and Sterilization: Medical and Social Aspects,* ed. Jane E. Hodgson. London: Academic Press.

Corson, Stephen L.; Sedlacek, Thomas V.; and Hoffman, Jerome J. 1986. "Suction Dilation and Evacuation." In *Greenhill's Surgical Gynecology,* 5th edition, ed. Richard H. Lampert. Chicago: Year Book Medical.

Council on Ethical and Judicial Affairs, American Medical Association. 1994. *Code of Medical Ethics: Current Opinions with Annotations: Including the Principles of the Medical Ethics, Fundamental Elements of the Patient-Physician Relationship, and Rules of the Council on Ethical and Judicial Affairs.* Chicago: Author.

Gold, Rachel Benson. 1990. *Abortion and Women's Health: A Turning Point for America?* New York: Alan Guttmacher Institute.

Grimes, David A. 1992. "Surgical Management of Abortion." In *Te Linde's Operative Gynecology,* 8th edition, ed. John D. Thompson and John A. Rock. Philadelphia: J. B. Lippincott.

Grimes, David A. 1998. "The Continuing Need for Late Abortions." *Journal of the American Medical Association* 280(8): 747–750.

Grimes, David A.; Schultz, Kenneth F.; Cates, Willard, Jr.; et al. 1979. "Local Versus General Anesthesia: Which Is Safer for Performing Suction Curettage Abortions?" *American Journal of Obstetrics and Gynecology* 135(8): 1030–1035.

Henshaw, Stanley K. 1990. "Induced Abortion: A World Review, 1990." *Family Planning Perspectives* 22(2): 76–89.

House Human Resources and Intergovernmental Relations Subcommittee of the Committee on Governmental Operations: Hearings on the Federal Role in Determining the Medical and Psychological Impact of Abortions on Women. 101st Congress, 1st session, 1989, p. 14.

Kolata, Gina. "Abortion Pill Slow to Win Users among Women and their Doctors." *New York Times,* September 25, 2002.

Koop, C. Everett. 1989. *Medical and Psychological Effects of Abortion on Women.* Washington, D.C.: U.S. Department of Health and Human Services.

Kunins, Hillary, and Rosenfield, Allan. 1991. "Abortion: A Legal and Public Health Perspective." *Annual Review of Public Health* 12: 361–382.

Message to the House of Representatives Returning without Approval Partial Birth Abortion Legislation. Weekly Compilation of Presidential Documents. October 10, 1997, p. 1545.

*Planned Parenthood of Southeastern Pennsylvania v. Casey,* 502 U.S. 1056 (1992).

Remarks on Returning without Approval to the House of Representatives Partial Birth Abortion Legislation. Weekly Compilation of Presidential Documents. April 10, 1996, pp. 643–647.

*Roe v. Wade.* 410 U.S. 113 (1973).

*Stenberg v. Carhart.* 530 U.S. 914 (2000).

INTERNET RESOURCE

U.S. Federal Drug Administration. *Approval Letter for Mifepristone,* September 28, 2000. Available from <http://www.fda.gov/cder/drug/infopage/mifepristone/default.htm>.

## II. CONTEMPORARY ETHICAL AND LEGAL ASPECTS: A. ETHICAL PERSPECTIVES

Abortion is widely regarded as one of the most intractable problems in bioethics. It is certainly true that few issues in bioethics have inspired as much discussion, debate, and open conflict as abortion, in part because the abortion controversy, unlike many others in ethics, has not been limited to scholars and practitioners, but has been engaged on numerous fronts in the United States. Churches and religious organizations, political office holders and candidates, the courts, and the general public have all taken a stand on abortion. In the decades since the U.S. Supreme Court, in its historic 1973 *Roe v. Wade* decision, effectively legalized abortion through the second trimester of pregnancy, the conflict—political, legal, social, and ethical—has not abated.

Another reason for the intractability of the abortion issue is that the views held by critics and defenders of abortion often occupy extremes. At one extreme, abortion opponents defend an absolute prohibition on abortion, calling abortion nothing less than the murder of an innocent person. At the other extreme are those who defend a woman's absolute right to abortion on demand at any time during pregnancy. Both sides engage in rhetoric and hyperbole; abortion opponents call themselves "pro-life," implying that their opponents are anti-life, while abortion rights supporters call themselves "pro-choice," suggesting that anti-abortionists oppose personal freedom and choice. When the battle lines are largely ideological, as they are in the abortion conflict, there is little room for rational argument. The result is that rather than search for a middle ground, both sides of the conflict have simply dug their heels in deeper.

An additional source of difficulty in reaching agreement about abortion is that the anti-abortion movement in the United States has been led primarily by the Roman Catholic church and fundamentalist Protestants, who base their opposition to abortion on fundamental religious convictions. If it is impossible to argue rationally for or against such convictions, it is no less difficult to argue about an ethical position that is deeply rooted in them.

Finally, the abortion problem is unusually difficult because the fetus is significantly unlike other entities of moral concern, and because the relationship between a fetus and a pregnant woman is unique, in many ways, among human relationships. The moral status of the fetus is itself a highly contested matter, such that the general moral principles that can be appealed to in other areas of human conduct and conflict do not fit cleanly into the abortion picture. Additionally, because the status of the fetus is at issue, abortion can be as much a metaphysical problem as a moral one.

The contemporary moral controversy over abortion focuses on three central issues: the moral status of the embryo or fetus, which many ethicists contend hinges on the ontological status of embryonic and fetal life; the rights conflict between pregnant women and their fetuses; and consequentialist arguments that weigh the potential for harm to women as a result of restricting or abolishing abortion against the negative consequences of terminating fetal or embryonic life.

## Ontological and Moral Status of the Fetus

The question of the ontological status of the fetus can be teased apart from the question of moral status, but in the abortion debate, fetal personhood and the possession of moral rights are often assumed to go hand in hand. The term *person,* however, is ambiguous, having a legal, a descriptive, and a normative sense. To be a legal person is simply to possess legal rights. In *Roe v. Wade* (1973), the Supreme Court held that fetuses are not persons as defined by the 14th Amendment of the Constitution, but declined to offer a positive thesis on personhood, acknowledging the difficulty of doing so. "We need not resolve the difficult question of when life begins. When those trained in the respective disciplines of medicine, philosophy, and theology are unable to arrive at any consensus, the judiciary, at this point in the development of man's knowledge, is not in a position to speculate as to the answer" (*Roe v. Wade,* 1973). To say that

something is a descriptive person is just to say that it satisfies certain criteria of personhood, such as species membership. The claim that a fetus is a person in this sense does nothing to justify the claim that killing a fetus is morally wrong unless the fetus also qualifies as a person in the normative sense. Being a person normatively speaking means being a bearer of moral rights, including the right to life. The crucial question of fetal or embryonic personhood, as it relates to abortion, then, is whether and when the genetically human, living entity resulting from the fertilization of an ovum by a spermatozoon is a normative person, a possessor of rights. There is, however, no more consensus on the proper criteria for personhood, and whether or not fetuses can satisfy these criteria, than there is on abortion.

At one extreme of the personhood debate is the position that personhood begins at fertilization, so even very early embryos, composed of only a few cells, are persons. At the other extreme is the view that personhood does not begin until birth or even later, and so no fetus, and perhaps no infant, qualifies as a person. Between the two extremes, there are a multitude of possibilities.

One approach to personhood is the developmental view, which denies that a bright line can be drawn at any particular point in natural development when the fetus acquires moral standing. The developmental view hinges on the continuity of fetal development, and the difficulty of non-arbitrarily picking out properties that qualify some fetuses, but not others, as persons. Since infants are generally regarded as persons with a right to life, and the difference between a late term fetus and a neonate—particularly in the case of viable premature infants—is merely a matter of location, it appears that in the continuous process of embryonic and fetal development, there is no non-arbitrary place to draw a line where personhood begins. This view is in line with the intuition, shared by many on both sides of the abortion conflict, that fetal life becomes increasingly important as gestation continues, but that it is impossible to say with certainty when, exactly, a fetus becomes a person. The inherent vagueness of the developmental view is an obstacle to translating it into practical moral guidelines or public policies, however.

The potentiality view advances conception or fertilization as the beginning of personhood because it is the fertilized ovum, not its constituent gametes, that is considered to have the potential to develop into a human being with full moral status. This can be criticized in two ways. First, it may be argued that even gametes do have the potential to become human persons. Second, as a number of critics of the potentiality criterion have observed, having the potential to become a person is not the same as being one, and it is being a person that confers moral status and rights.

As Judith Jarvis Thomson noted, "A newly fertilized ovum, a newly implanted clump of cells, is no more a person than an acorn is an oak tree" (Thomson, 1971, p. 199). In *Roe v. Wade*, the Court located fetal viability as a line of demarcation, the point after which the state may have a compelling interest in protecting fetal life. Although viability is not a specific moment in the continuum of fetal development, it occurs at approximately twenty-four to twenty-eight weeks gestation, when a number of other significant developmental markers have been achieved, and is the point at which, given proper support, a fetus can potentially survive outside the womb, independently of its mother. It has taken on significance as a convenient, relatively identifiable and verifiable turning point in fetal development, when personhood plausibly begins. Fetal viability is to some extent dependent on technology—premature neonates often need considerable medical support to survive. As technological advances in neonatal care occur, it is possible that the point at which a fetus is viable may change. Some critics of the viability standard claim that personhood ought not be contingent on external facts about the state of medical technology, and therefore cannot stand as a proper criterion for personhood.

As technology has provided a better understanding of the different stages of embryonic and fetal development, criteria such as implantation (when the conceptus becomes imbedded in the uterine lining), the appearance of external human form, and the presence of detectable brainwave activity have all been advanced as criteria for personhood and rights. Traditional criteria for fetal personhood include *animation,* when fetal movement first occurs, and *quickening,* the time at which a pregnant woman first feels fetal movement. Early Christian authors talked about *ensoulment,* the time at which the embryo or fetus is imbued with a soul.

Species membership, or genetic humanity, is the most lenient criterion for personhood, and the most easily verifiable. According to this definition of personhood, any entity conceived of human parents is a member of the human species, and is therefore a person. John T. Noonan, writing from a Catholic perspective, argues that the fetus acquires personhood at the moment of conception, when it receives from its parents the human genetic code (Noonan). The genetic humanity standard can be regarded as both too broad and too restrictive, however. It is too broad because it implies that any living entity with the human genetic code qualifies as a human life worthy of protection. Cancer cells, sperm, and ova all have a human genetic code, and on the least restrictive definition of genetic humanity, such cells would have a right to life, implying that if abortion is impermissible, then so is contraception and chemotherapy. Ethicists who advance a genetic humanity view generally exclude from personhood cells that lack the potential to become human beings, combining a genetic humanity standard with a potentiality principle. The genetic humanity standard can also be regarded as too restrictive because it excludes from the possibility of personhood all nonhuman beings, including some that may warrant the moral status of rights-bearers.

The philosopher Mary Anne Warren argues for a very strict psychological standard of personhood, defining a person as "a full-fledged member of the moral community" (Warren, 1973, p. 347). Genetic humanity alone isn't sufficient for personhood, according to Warren, so not all human beings are members of the moral community. Warren proposes a set of cognitive criteria that, it is claimed, everyone can and does agree are central to the concept of personhood: consciousness, the developed capacity for reasoning and problem-solving, self-motivated activity, the capacity to communicate, and self-awareness. Beings that satisfy some or all of these criteria are people with a moral claim on us, whether they are human or not, for just as some human beings are not people, "there may well be people who are not human beings" (Warren, 1973, p. 348). Membership in the moral community requires the capacity for moral participation, in Warren's view; it would be absurd to ascribe moral obligations and responsibilities to an entity that cannot satisfy any of the cognitive or psychological criteria for moral personhood, and it is equally absurd to ascribe full moral rights to such a being. It is obvious that no fetus can satisfy any of these criteria, and it is equally obvious, Warren argues, that anything that fails to satisfy any of these criteria cannot be a person. A fully developed fetus is no more like a person than a newborn guppy, and cannot have a right to life sufficient to override a woman's right to have an abortion at any stage of pregnancy.

Critics were quick to point out that Warren's standard of personhood could not be met by infants, nor many children and adults with serious cognitive deficits, and thus would problematically justify not only abortion, but infanticide and nonvoluntary euthanasia as well. Warren responded to such criticism by allowing that although a newborn infant is not a person with a right to life, and infanticide is not murder, there are other, utilitarian reasons for the impermissibility of infanticide. Infanticide is wrong for the same reason it is wrong to destroy great works of art or natural resources, because destroying these things deprives people of a great deal of pleasure. Moreover, most people value infants, even if their own parents do not, and would prefer that they not be destroyed. These considerations are not sufficient to override a pregnant woman's right to freedom, happiness, and self-determination, nor her right to an abortion at any stage of pregnancy, Warren claims, but the moment of birth marks the point at which the infant's continued life no longer violates any of its mother's rights, and is thus the point at which its mother no longer has the right to determine its fate. Birth is also morally significant "because it permits the establishment of direct social relationships between the infant and other members of society" (Warren, 1985, p. 6). Thus, although an infant may lack the intrinsic properties that ground a right to life, "its emergence into the social world makes it appropriate to treat it as if it had such a right" (Warren, 1989, p. 56).

While Warren has been accused of offering an ad hoc solution to the problem of infanticide, Michael Tooley argues that neither abortion nor infanticide is intrinsically wrong or undesirable, and indeed, "in the vast majority of cases in which infanticide is desirable … there is excellent reason to believe that infanticide is morally permissible" (Tooley, 1985, p. 14). Tooley's argument is that personhood requires nothing less than self-consciousness, and "An organism possesses a serious right to life only if it possesses the concept of a self as a continuing subject of experiences and other mental states, and believes that it is itself such a continuing entity" (Tooley, 1972, p. 315). Tooley and Warren both explicitly reject the view that the mere potential to become a person gives the fetus any moral standing.

Philosopher Don Marquis attempts to resolve the personhood standoff by starting with an unproblematic assumption: It is seriously morally wrong to kill an adult human being. Marquis then identifies the natural property that adults have that makes killing them wrong. If the same property is found to belong to fetuses, Marquis argues, it must follow that abortion is also seriously morally wrong. Marquis concludes that what makes killing wrong is that murder deprives its victim of a life and future that is valuable. The victim of a murder is deprived of all the experiences, activities, projects, and enjoyments that would have constituted his or her future, deprived of all that he or she values, or would have come to value, in life. The loss of that valuable future, of what Marquis calls a "future like ours," is ultimately what makes killing wrong. It is also what makes abortion morally wrong, Marquis argues, because fetuses have futures of value. "The future of a standard fetus includes a set of experiences, projects, activities, and such which are identical with the futures of adult human beings and are identical with the futures of young children" (Marquis, p. 192).

Marquis's future-like-ours account implies that it is seriously wrong to kill any being with a future of value—it is non-speciesist in that it does not claim that only human life has value or worth. Rather, like some personhood theories, Marquis's theory leaves open the possibility that other species, if they share the property of having a valuable future, have the same right to life that a human being has, and that killing members of other species would therefore be seriously morally wrong. Marquis offers no account of what a future like ours must look like, or what shared properties of an adult human future make it valuable. This point has been a focus of attack for critics, like David Boonin (see below), Jeffrey Reiman, and Peter K. McInerney, who claim that fetuses do not, indeed cannot, have futures like ours.

Marquis's future-like-ours theory, in opposition to other pro-life accounts, is compatible with the permissibility of euthanasia because it is only the loss of a *valuable* future—not merely the loss of a life—that makes killing wrong. The future-like-ours theory also accounts for the basic intuition that it is seriously wrong to kill young children and infants, for it is presumed they have futures of value. Personhood theories that advance psychological criteria do not straightforwardly account for the intuition or belief that killing infants and children is morally wrong, and must make appeal to other principles, such as social utility, to account for its wrongness. Appeals to social utility, however, cannot explain the wrongness of killing those who are unwanted or unnecessary.

Marquis's critics point out that he fails to provide an argument for why a fetus that is incapable of valuing its own future should count as a being that can suffer a morally relevant loss of its future. The philosopher David Boonin develops an alternative future-like-ours theory that refutes the claim that every fetus has a right to life, and that abortion is in typical cases morally impermissible, on terms that critics of abortion, like Marquis, can and do accept. Boonin argues that a fetus acquires a right to life only at the point in fetal development when organized cortical brain activity is present. The "cortical criterion" is the only morally relevant criterion for moral standing and a right to life, Boonin argues, because organized cortical activity is what makes it possible to have a future like ours. "We have a future-like-ours only because we have a brain which will enable us to enjoy, in the future, the kinds of conscious experiences that make our lives distinctively valuable to us" (Boonin, p. 126). Boonin's theory, like Marquis's, identifies a natural property that fetuses possess that makes killing them morally wrong. But while Marquis's future-like-ours property broadly applies equally to all fetuses and embryos, Boonin's cortical criterion narrows the category of beings with a right to life to those with a developed capacity for conscious desires. "It is because these individuals currently have desires about their futures that our desires about how to behave are not the only ones that are morally relevant" (p. 73). Thus, Boonin's theory does not claim, as some personhood theories do, that no fetus ever has a right to life, but only that this right does not exist from the moment of conception, and he concludes that if, as Marquis proposes, depriving a fetus of a future like ours is the wrong-making feature of abortion, then "abortion in typical circumstances is permissible," because the typically aborted fetus lacks a future like ours (p. 129).

Marquis contends that a desire-based account of the wrongness of killing cannot explain why it is morally wrong to kill individuals who have no desire to live, such as suicidal teenagers, the sleeping, and the unconscious. Any theory in which having a valuable future depends upon actually desiring that one's life continue fails to adequately account for the basic intuition that killing beings who do not occurrently value their own futures is seriously morally wrong. The value of life, Marquis argues, is not secondary to our desire for it. If it were, a mere reordering of desires could make killing morally right. The fact that a fetus does not desire the continuation of its own life does not imply that its future has no value—its future is ultimately valuable to it because it will be valuable to it in the future.

Boonin proposes a modified future like ours principle that can account for the wrongness of killing in Marquis's counterexamples, however, because it does not depend on occurrent desiring. In Boonin's modified future-like-ours principle, *present ideal dispositional desires*—desires an individual would have, given perfect conditions such as rationality, consciousness, and ideal circumstances—account for that being having a valuable future (p. 73). It is only the possession of *actual* dispositional desires, however, and not the mere capacity for such desires in the future that has moral relevance, Boonin argues. Consequently, a preconscious fetus does not have the same moral standing, or the same right to life, as a conscious late term fetus, an infant, a child, or an adult. If Boonin's cortical criterion is accepted, the vast majority of abortions, which take place well before the point at which fetuses can form conscious desires, are morally permissible.

A looser cognitive criterion for personhood is adopted by Baruch Brody, who appeals to the symmetry between the development of a functioning brain as the beginning of fetal humanity and the cessation of brain function as the definition of death, or the end of humanity. That is, the property whose acquisition confers the right to life in the first place is the same property that, when permanently lost, entails the loss of a right to life. That property is the possession of a functioning brain. If the brain death theory is correct, Brody concludes, a fetus becomes a human being about six weeks after fertilization, when it has a functioning brain. After that point, abortions, except under unusual circumstances, are morally impermissible. Brody's is a significantly looser cognitive criterion than Boonin's "organized cortical activity" criterion because it makes fetal humanity dependent on the presence of early brain function which is not sufficiently organized to support consciousness. A difficulty for Brody's

theory is that determining when brain death has occurred may be nearly as difficult as determining when personhood begins. Brain death has proved notoriously difficult to ascertain because detectable electrical activity can continue in a brain that has ceased meaningful functioning. One study shows that at least 20 percent of "brain dead" patients continued to exhibit electrical activity on electroencephalograms, some of it compatible with function (Truog, p. 161). The symmetry Brody appeals to is thus elusive—it may be no easier to define when personhood ends than it is to define when it begins.

Both proponents and opponents of abortion believe that settling the abortion controversy requires settling the question of personhood. While there is room for agreement in positions like Boonin's, Brody's, and even Marquis's, at either extreme standards of personhood like Noonan's and Warren's are incommensurable, leading some to question the utility of defining personhood as a route to resolving the abortion conflict. So long as the fetus's moral standing is believed to depend on fetal personhood, however, the question of personhood will not disappear from the abortion debate.

## Rights Conflicts and Abortion

Most opposition to abortion is grounded in two assumptions: the first is the moral personhood and right to life of the fetus; the second assumption is that, in a conflict of rights, the right to life must trump a woman's right to privacy, choice, and bodily autonomy. Many pro-choice arguments ignore the second assumption—perhaps because it seems intuitively implausible that any other right could outweigh a right to life—and focus solely on the first assumption, either offering support for the claim that fetal personhood occurs substantially later in fetal development than conception, or arguing that the criteria for moral personhood can never be met by a fetus. Neither proposition is acceptable or defensible to abortion opponents for whom it is an article of faith that a fetus has a right to life. Thomson puts forth an argument that grants, for the sake of argument, fetal personhood from conception, but challenges the second pro-life assumption that the right to life always overrides other rights.

Thomson's argument employs an analogy that has engendered controversy among both defenders and critics of abortion. Imagine, Thomson writes, that you awake one morning to find yourself hooked up to the body of an unconscious violinist who is suffering a fatal kidney ailment. The Society of Music Lovers has kidnapped you and plugged this famous violinist into your circulatory system, so that your kidneys can be used to filter his blood. You are told that in nine months, the famous violinist will have recovered, and can be safely detached, but in the meantime, to unhook him from your body would kill him. The violinist is a person, and so he has a right to life. Your life is not endangered, but you must remain tethered to the violinist against your will for nine months, thus greatly diminishing your freedom. If his right to life guarantees him the use of your body for life support, then it is morally incumbent on you to provide it, regardless of the cost to your personal freedom. The implications for abortion are clear: the violinist is meant to be analogous to a fetus, and you and your kidneys are analogous to a pregnant woman providing life support to a fetus. If, Thomson argues, it is implausible that you are morally obligated to sustain the violinist's life at such a cost to your personal freedom, then it ought to be equally implausible that a fetus's right to life guarantees it the right to continued use of a woman's body (Thomson). Thus, the fetus's right to life doesn't make abortion morally impermissible, for "having a right to life does not guarantee having either a right to be given the use of or a right to be allowed continued use of another person's body—even if one needs it for life itself" (Thomson, p. 336).

If Thomson's analogy is accepted, there are serious grounds for questioning the assumption that abortion is morally impermissible if a fetus has a right to life. However, both opponents and proponents of the right to abortion have argued against the soundness of Thomson's analogy. Abortion critics claim that there is a deep, even grotesque disanalogy between a fetus and the violinist, and that Thomson fails to attend to the moral distinction between intentionally killing and letting die. Abortion, it is argued, intentionally kills a fetus, but detaching oneself from the violinist only allows the violinist to die from his kidney ailment, an act with a very different moral status than murder. Abortion proponents and opponents alike raise a responsibility objection to Thomson's argument, claiming that her conclusion only holds in cases where pregnancy results from an involuntary act. Warren criticizes Thomson's analogy on those grounds, arguing that it is too weak to provide a thorough defense of a right to abortion, allowing it only in cases of rape (Warren, 1973). Since the majority of unwanted pregnancies are not the result of rape, Thomson's argument would permit abortion in only a small fraction of unwanted pregnancies. Thomson acknowledges that her argument leaves open the possibility that there may be some cases in which the unborn person acquires, tacitly or by consent, a right to the use of the mother's body, and in which abortion would be an unjust killing. But this possibility does not force the conclusion that all abortions are unjust killings. "Except in such cases as the unborn person has a right to demand it … nobody is morally *required* to make

large sacrifices, of health, of all other interests and concerns, of all other duties and commitments, for nine years, or even for nine months, in order to keep another person alive" (Thomson, p. 338).

It is difficult to consistently maintain the position that a fetus's right to life trumps all other rights or considerations. In cases where the life of a pregnant woman is endangered by pregnancy, only the most extreme opponents of abortion claim that because abortion is the intentional killing of an innocent person, it is still morally wrong and the mother must be allowed to die. More moderate opposition to abortion allows exceptions for the life or health of the mother, and also for cases where pregnancy results from rape or incest. There is a clear inconsistency in the rape and incest exception, however, since it makes the unborn fetus's right to life contingent on the actions of its father. Abortion opponents who grant exceptions in cases of rape and incest must, if they are consistent, explain why those fetuses have a different moral status, or less of a right to life, than other fetuses, or why the right to life loses its priority to a woman's rights in those cases.

Pro-choice feminist arguments charge that most discussions of abortion place undue emphasis on fetal rights and too little emphasis on the contexts in which decisions about abortion take place. Susan Sherwin argues that traditional, nonfeminist approaches to the abortion controversy are too simplistic, considering the permissibility of abortion in isolation from the social and sexual subordination of women, and the struggle of women for control over their bodies and reproduction. Nonfeminist arguments thus mistakenly claim that the moral status of abortion turns exclusively on the moral status of the fetus (Sherwin). The central moral feature of pregnancy, Sherwin argues, is that it takes place in women's bodies and profoundly affects their lives. Because fetuses have a unique physical status of dependence on particular women, they have a unique social status as well—the value of a fetus, Sherwin claims, is determined solely by the nature of its primary relationship to the woman who carries it, and "no absolute value attaches to fetuses apart from their relational status" (p. 111). The focus on the fetus as an independent, rights-bearing entity denies pregnant women their proper roles as independent moral agents who, alone, have "the responsibility and privilege of determining a fetus's specific social status and value" (p. 110).

Some pro-life feminists attempt to sidestep the rights controversy and argue instead that abortion is inconsistent with the goals and ideals of feminism, such as opposition to violence, and the promulgation of an ethic of caring, nurturing, and interconnectedness. Others, like Sidney Callahan, argue that feminist goals cannot be achieved in a society that permits abortion (Callahan). The exclusion of the unborn from the sphere of rights and protection, Callahan argues, is analogous to the exclusion of women in unjust, patriarchal systems where "lesser orders of human life are granted rights only when wanted, chosen, or invested with value by the powerful" (Callahan, p. 368). Moreover, to grant a right to abortion in the name of women's privacy or autonomy validates the view that pregnancy and child-rearing are the sole responsibility of individual women, relieving men and the community from any responsibility. Thus "women will never climb to equality and social empowerment over mounds of dead fetuses …" (Callahan, p. 371). To exercise moral autonomy, Callahan argues, requires responsiveness and responsibility not only to what is wanted or chosen, but to what is unwanted and unchosen as well. Callahan makes no exceptions for pregnancy due to rape, arguing that even the involuntarily pregnant woman has "a moral obligation to the now-existing, dependent fetus whether she explicitly consented to its existence or not" (Callahan, p. 370).

Margaret Olivia Little argues that the literature on abortion deeply undersells the moral complexity of abortion, focusing too much on a thin moral assessment of its permissibility. She proposes that what is needed in the moral discussion of abortion is an ethics of gestation that addresses questions of "what it means to play a role in *creating* a person, how to assess responsibilities that involve *sharing,* not just risking, one's body and life, what follows from the fact that the entity in question is or would be *one's child."* (Little, p. 493). A more complex moral interpretation must move beyond questions of metaphysical and moral status and permissibility to consider abortion's "placement on the scales of *decency, respectfulness,* and *responsibility"* (Little, p. 492).

If fetuses are not persons, Little argues, they are nonetheless respect-worthy because they are burgeoning human lives, and abortion remains a serious matter because it involves the loss of something significant and valuable. Even if we allow that fetuses are persons, however, the important moral question is what positive duties and responsibilities, if any, pregnant women have to continue gestational assistance. Both liberal and conservative positions on the duties of parenthood assume that it is an all or nothing affair, and that pregnant women either have the same obligations and responsibilities to fetuses that they do to children, or that they owe nothing beyond general beneficence. But parenthood, Little claims, is more than a social role—it is, more crucially, a relationship that develops through time, interaction, and emotional intertwinement. Regardless of the view one takes on the personhood of fetuses, gestation uniquely changes the relationship a woman has to her self, bringing with it a new identity and an impending relationship with another that is not always welcome or sustainable. Thus, "assessing the moral status of abortion … is not just about assessing the contours of generic respect owed to burgeoning human life, it's about assessing the salience of *impending relationship"* (Little, p. 498).

The fetus's status becomes progressively weightier as pregnancy continues, Little suggests, but until the fetus is a person, there is a moral prerogative to decline parenthood and end pregnancy because it "so thoroughly changes what we might call one's fundamental practical identity …. As profound as the respect we should have for burgeoning human life, we should acknowledge moral prerogatives over identity-constituting commitments and enterprises as profound as motherhood" (Little, p. 498).

## The Selective Abortion Controversy

The development of tests to prenatally diagnose genetic diseases and disorders has greatly outpaced the development of effective treatments and therapies. The Human Genome Project promises to accelerate the development of prenatal diagnostic tests. Through procedures like chorionic villus sampling (CVS), which can be performed at ten weeks gestation, and amniocentesis, available at fourteen to sixteen weeks, numerous genetic abnormalities in the fetus can be detected in utero. The tests are routinely administered to women at risk for fetal abnormalities, such as older mothers and those with a family history of genetic disorder. Ultrasound, which is routinely performed throughout most pregnancies, can detect a number of abnormalities as well, including neural tube defects that can result in severe physical and cognitive disability and death. In rare instances, fetal therapy, including surgery, can correct the problems, but the overwhelming majority of pregnant women whose fetuses are found to have abnormalities are currently faced with only two options: abort the defective fetus, or risk giving birth to a child that will potentially face a lifetime of disability and hardship. In cases where the fetus's condition will result in severe physical or mental impairment, or where it will lead to inevitable death and a short, painful life, only the most extreme opponents of abortion maintain that it is wrong to abort. Abortion moderates and supporters see those as clear cases where abortion is not only morally permissible, but in some situations, morally required. Less agreement exists regarding the abortion of fetuses with minor abnormalities, genetic predispositions to disease, and genetic diseases that are eventually lethal, but compatible with more or less normal life for many years.

Disabilities rights advocates oppose the routine administration of prenatal screening and the selective abortion of fetuses found to have abnormalities. Although many disabilities rights scholars are pro-choice, and defend a woman's right to choose abortion, they object to the use of selective abortion for fetal indications, which they argue discriminates against existing people with disabilities, and sends the message to those living with disabilities that they should never have been born. This so-called Expressivist Argument claims that selective abortion expresses discriminatory attitudes towards the disabled and undermines efforts to create a more just, inclusive society (Asch, 2000). The disability critique of abortion is novel because it is concerned only with the abortion of otherwise wanted fetuses that possess a single undesirable trait, a disability.

There is profound disagreement about the use of prenatal screening and selective abortion to select fetuses for gender, either for purposes of family "balancing" or because of personal or cultural preferences for children of a particular sex—typically male. Throughout many parts of Asia, where female infanticide was once common, it has been to some extent replaced by the use of ultrasound to prenatally determine the sex of a child, followed by selective abortion of female fetuses. Analysis of census data and predicted sex ratios shows that, by a conservative estimate, more than 100 million females are missing worldwide. In China alone, where selective abortion of females is illegal, it is estimated that there are 30 million missing females, about five percent of the national total; in India and Pakistan, the number exceeds 24 million (Kristof). The criminalization of female infanticide and abortion in China and India has done little to change the deeply ingrained cultural preferences that lead to the practices, and there is good reason to believe that in societies where male offspring are overwhelmingly preferred, missing females who are not aborted are the victims of infanticide, abandonment, or fatal neglect. For consequentialist reasons, many would regard abortion as preferable in those circumstances. Little observes that in cultures that openly discriminate against women and girls, giving birth to a daughter who will face rejection and disrespect can do violence to a woman's ideals of creating and parenthood: "A woman living in a country marked by poverty and gender apartheid wants to abort because she decides it would be *wrong* for her to bear a daughter whose life, like hers, would be filled with hardship" (Little, p. 499). In Western countries where gender equality is avowed, however, the use of abortion for sex selection leaves many abortion rights defenders uneasy with the prospect of justifying a morally serious practice done for reasons regarded as trivial or patently discriminatory.

There is growing controversy over the use of fertility treatments like in vitro fertilization (IVF) and superovulatory drugs, which pose a fairly high risk of multiple gestations and births. Numerous complications affecting both the pregnant woman and her offspring are associated with multiple pregnancies. The high cost and low success rate of fertility treatments contributes to the problem—with IVF, it is typical practice to implant more than the desired number of embryos in order to increase the odds of success; superovulatory drugs, which stimulate a woman's ovaries to produce dozens of ova, afford little control over the number that will ultimately be fertilized and implanted. It is more than a little ironic that the effort to assist couples in achieving pregnancy has led to an abortion controversy over the use of selective reduction, the practice of removing some fetuses in multiple pregnancies in order to increase the chances of a healthy pregnancy and birth for the remaining fetuses. Although the procedure is not without risks—miscarriage, fetal death, and disability are known complications of selective reduction—some commentators question whether in pregnancies with a large number of fetuses—more than two or three—there is a moral imperative to reduce in order to decrease the risks to the surviving offspring. In 1997, twenty-eight-year-old Bobbi McCaughey made history when she gave birth to seven live babies—born eight weeks premature—after using fertility drugs to stimulate ovulation. While the McCaughey septuplets were widely reported as a medical "miracle," some medical ethicists questioned the wisdom of the parents who, as devout Christians, refused the option of selective reduction, thus placing their offspring at increased risk for prematurity, low birth weight, cognitive and physical disability, and death (Steinbock, p. 377). In addition to serious ethical concerns about the risks of fertility treatments and multiple pregnancies, there are consequentialist and social justice concerns about the multimillion dollar cost of neonatal care associated with multiple births, and, in a climate of medical cost-cutting, the responsible use of limited healthcare dollars.

## Partial Birth Abortion

Partial birth abortion is a nonmedical term coined by anti-abortionists to describe an abortion procedure known technically as intact dilation and extraction (D&X). D&X is used primarily in second trimester abortions, and the procedure involves partially delivering a living fetus into the birth canal, then collapsing the skull and completing delivery of a dead but otherwise intact fetus. In an *amici* brief to the Supreme Court, the American College of Obstetricians and Gynecologists noted that D&X involves substantially less risk of complication than other methods of abortion used during the same gestational period (*Stenberg v. Carhart*, 2000). Fewer than five percent of abortions performed in the United States occur in the second trimester, with the vast majority taking place in the first trimester, but when the D&X procedure was widely publicized by abortion opponents in the mid-1990s, it created immediate controversy. President Bill Clinton twice vetoed federal bills to ban partial birth abortions, but a number of state laws were passed prohibiting the procedure. A Nebraska statute that made the performance of D&X a felony was challenged in a case brought to the U.S. Supreme Court in *Stenberg v. Carhart* (2000). The Court held that the Nebraska statute violated the Constitution because it lacked any exemption for the preservation of the health of the mother, and because the law's vagueness imposed an undue burden on a woman's ability to choose the more common dilation and evacuation (D&E) abortion procedure, which sometimes involves partial delivery prior to fetal dismemberment. In striking down the Nebraska ban, the Court invalidated the nearly identical laws of thirty other states.

From a consistent pro-life perspective, there can be no moral difference between partial birth abortions and abortions performed using other methods. Because a second-term fetus more closely resembles an infant than does an embryo or very early fetus, publicizing graphic and often gruesome descriptions of the D&X procedure helped the pro-life cause politically, but aside from its inflammatory aspect, it contributed little to the abortion debate. Many pro-choice ethicists, however, regard later abortions of healthy fetuses as more morally serious than early abortions. When the moral permissibility of abortion depends on the criteria used to determine fetal moral status, there is an unsettled empirical question that becomes more urgent as pregnancy continues. In second trimester abortions, cognitive criteria for fetal personhood or rights, such as sentience or cortical activity, may, by conservative estimates, be satisfied, but it remains an open question whether certainty can be achieved in this substantial gray area of fetal development.

## Consequentialism and Abortion

The abortion debate in the United States has almost exclusively focused on questions of rights, to the exclusion of all other considerations. A consequentialist approach that assesses the morality of abortion in light of its good and bad consequences has the potential to resolve the rights standoff, and a number of consequentialist considerations have bearing on the abortion debate. Abortion critics have long raised fears of a slippery slope, charging that permissiveness about abortion will inevitably lead to the devaluation of human life, and a "culture of death" in which attitudes about other forms of killing, such as infanticide and euthanasia, will

become more permissive. The argument depends on the assumption that the killing of a fetus is regarded as just as serious as the killing of an infant, child, or adult, and that the permissibility of one entails the permissibility of all. The culture of death argument, like other slippery slope arguments, also makes an empirical claim that the evidence to date fails to support. Since abortion was legalized in the United States in 1973, there has been no slide toward permissiveness about other forms of killing. Only one state, Oregon, has legalized physician-assisted suicide, under strict regulation. In all other states that have considered physician-assisted suicide or euthanasia, voters have declined to endorse it. Neither is there evidence to suggest that the killing of newborns is more common in the United States than it was before abortion was legalized, but in parts of the world where infanticide has historically been an acceptable means of eliminating unwanted offspring, the availability of abortion has not increased the incidence of infanticide, but reduced it (Kristof).

The coat hanger has been a powerful symbol of the abortion rights movement, a reminder of the dangerous, sometimes deadly abortions women endured before *Roe v. Wade*. Proponents of abortion rights have substantial evidence to support the claim that legal prohibitions on abortion lead to the deaths of women through self-induced abortions or illegal, unsafe abortions performed by untrained providers. Legal abortion performed under safe and sanitary conditions is generally safer than pregnancy, but in countries where abortion is prohibited, or access is severely limited, the negative consequences of unsafe and self-induced abortions include serious complications such as sepsis, hemorrhage, genital and abdominal trauma, perforated uterus, gangrene, secondary infertility, permanent disability, and death (World Health Organization [WHO]). Treatment of complications from unsafe abortions places a serious strain on the medical infrastructure of developing countries, where a disproportionate share—up to 50 percent—of scarce hospital resources are expended treating abortion complications. Unsafe abortions thus compromise other maternity and emergency health services in poor countries where healthcare is already inadequately resourced (WHO). Statistics on abortion-related mortality are especially telling: In Paraguay, illegal abortions are responsible for an astonishing 23 out of every 100 deaths of young women (United Nations). In Romania, abortion-related deaths increased sharply after 1966, when the government restricted abortion. The maternal death rate rose from 20 per 100,000 live births in 1965 to 150 per 100,000 in 1983. Abortion-related deaths decreased by more than 50 percent in the year after abortion was again legalized in 1989 (WHO). Statistics on abortion-related mortality in the United States tell a very different story about safe, legal abortion: the death rate is 0.6 per 100,000 procedures, making it as safe as a penicillin injection (WHO).

## Social Justice and Access to Abortion

Decades after *Roe v. Wade,* state and federal courts and legislatures continue to address the abortion issue, and government agencies have adopted numerous regulations that affect access and funding for abortion. The practical effect of much of this activity has been the erosion of abortion rights.

Women seeking abortions currently face difficulties that are not encountered in any other area of medical care. The consolidation of the healthcare industry has reduced the number of hospitals that perform abortion, and the majority of abortions in the early twenty-first century take place in free-standing clinics that are often besieged by anti-abortion protesters who block entry to clinics and harass patients. Abortion clinics have been bombed, and doctors who provide abortion murdered. This use or threat of violence by anti-abortion extremists has had a profound effect on access to safe abortion by contributing to a decline in the number of doctors willing to perform abortion. A 1997 study shows that the percentage of obstetrics-gynecology providers willing to perform abortions dropped from 42 to 33 percent between 1983 and 1995 (*Washington Post,* 1998). A 1998 study published by the National Abortion and Reproductive Rights Action League showed that 86 percent of U.S. counties—with nearly one-third of the female American population—had no abortion provider (Michelman).

In such an atmosphere, concerns about equality and social justice arise because limited access to abortion disproportionately affects poor women (Schulman). The deeply divisive moral controversy over abortion has engendered a secondary political conflict over who should pay for abortions. Federal restrictions limit Medicaid funding for abortions to those necessary to preserve a woman's life, or for pregnancies that result from rape and incest. At the same time, state and federal welfare reform initiatives have resulted in many women and children losing welfare benefits, putting a further strain on the ability of the poorest women to procure abortions that are available to financially better-off women, and compounding the economic injustice of a healthcare system already rife with inequalities. When access to safe abortion depends on the ability to pay, the right to abortion exists in principle, but not practice.

Equally problematic from the standpoint of justice are government policies that deny financial assistance to family-planning clinics that provide information to clients about

abortion. The global gag rule imposed on international family planning groups—which sometimes provide the only healthcare available to poor women and their children in developing countries—prohibits those organizations from receiving funds from the U.S. government if they discuss abortion. It is incompatible with principles of justice and equality to deny women access to information about the option and availability of abortions if it means they will be denied healthcare services that are available to women who are wealthier or better educated.

Medical abortion, or the use of the abortion drug RU-486, also known as Mifeprex, was once viewed as a solution to the problem of limited or inconvenient access to surgical abortion, but it has not proven to be an option for most women in the United States. The drug has been widely used in Europe, and was approved by the Food and Drug Administration (FDA) in 2000 despite considerable protest by anti-abortion forces. But recent surveys show that only 6 percent of obstetrician-gynecologists and 1 percent of family doctors provide RU-486 to their patients. There are a number of reasons: RU-486 is expensive, it requires three visits to a doctor—which is particularly difficult for women who must travel substantial distances to see a provider—and it must also be administered early in pregnancy. FDA regulations also require that doctors who administer RU-486 be able to perform surgical abortion, or be affiliated with a hospital that can, which limits the number of doctors who can prescribe the drug (*Washington Post,* 2002).

## Can the Abortion Conflict Be Resolved?

The reasons women choose abortion are as varied as the reasons they often choose not to abort. In countries where abortion is legal, and countries where it is not, millions of women make individual moral choices to end pregnancies. Some seek abortion after contraceptive failure, others because it is the only contraceptive option available to them; some choose to end their pregnancies for financial or emotional reasons, or for the well-being of their families; still others make the tragic decision to terminate a desired pregnancy because of an unwelcome prenatal diagnosis, or because their child is the wrong sex, or because their own health is in jeopardy. Regardless of what courts and politicians, ethicists and church leaders decide about abortion, there will always be unwanted pregnancies, and there will always be women willing to risk their lives and health to have abortions. Those are the facts of the matter.

The moral picture is characterized by far less clarity. Few reasonable people would argue that abortion is not a morally weighty issue, but just how serious it is, or is not, are questions that remain unsettled. Abortion may be an insoluble political problem in a pluralistic society where incommensurable moral and religious convictions hold sway and admit of little compromise. That does not necessarily make it an insoluble moral problem. All sides can agree that the stakes are high in abortion, and the difficulty of resolving the moral conflict should not be understated. Equally reasonable and thoughtful moral theories about abortion have produced greatly divergent conclusions. If none of these theories has yet proved immune to counterargument and criticism, if none has yet prompted a collective sigh of relief that the debate is at last over, they have all contributed to the unavoidable conclusion that the abortion controversy defies simplification, and, in its uniqueness, defies easy assimilation to familiar moral principles.

L. SYD M. JOHNSON

**SEE ALSO:** *Adoption; Autonomy; Conscience; Conscience, Rights of; Double Effect, Principle or Doctrine of; Embryo and Fetus; Genetic Testing and Screening: Reproductive Genetic Testing; Harm; Human Dignity; Infanticide; Life; Maternal-Fetal Relationship; Moral Status; Population Policies; Women, Historical and Cross-Cultural Perspectives;* and other *Abortion* subentries

### BIBLIOGRAPHY

Asch, Adrienne. 2000. "Why I Haven't Changed My Mind about Prenatal Diagnosis: Reflections and Refinements." In *Prenatal Testing and Disability Rights,* ed. Erik Parens and Adrienne Asch. Washington, D.C.: Georgetown University Press.

Boonin, David. 2003. *A Defense of Abortion.* Cambridge, Eng.: Cambridge University Press.

Brody, Baruch. 1975. "The Morality of Abortion." In *Contemporary Issues in Bioethics,* 5th edition, ed. Tom L. Beauchamp and LeRoy Walters. Belmont, CA: Wadsworth Publishing Company.

Callahan, Sidney. 1986. "A Case for Pro-Life Feminism." In *Ethical Issues in Modern Medicine,* 5th edition, ed. Bonnie Steinbock and John D. Arras. Mountain View, CA: Mayfield Publishing Company.

Kristof, Nicholas D. "Stark Data on Women: 100 Million Are Missing." *The New York Times* November 5, 1991: C1.

Little, Margaret Olivia. 2002. "The Morality of Abortion." In *Ethical Issues in Modern Medicine,* 6th edition, ed. Bonnie Steinbock, John D. Arras, and Alex John London. New York: McGraw-Hill Publishing Company.

Marquis, Don. 1989. "Why Abortion Is Immoral." *The Journal of Philosophy* 86(4): 183–202.

McInerney, Peter K. 1990. "Does a Fetus Already Have a Future Like Ours?" *The Journal of Philosophy* 87(5): 264–268.

Michelman, Kate. 1999. "26 Years Later, Abortion Debate Still Raging; Right to Choose Undermined by Limited Access." *The Plain Dealer* January 22: 9B.

Noonan, John T., Jr. 1970. "An Almost Absolute Value in History." In *Moral Problems in Medicine,* ed. Samuel Gorovitz, Ruth Macklin, Andrew L. Jameton, et al. Englewood Cliffs, NJ: Prentice-Hall.

Reiman, Jeffrey. 1998. "Abortion, Infanticide, and the Changing Grounds of the Wrongness of Killing: Reply to Don Marquis's 'Reiman on Abortion.'" *Journal of Social Philosophy* 29(2).

*Roe v. Wade.* 410 U.S. 113; 159 (1973).

"RU-486 Report Card." *Washington Post,* May 5, 2002: B06.

Schulman, Susan. 1998. "Poorer Women Affected Most as Abortion Providers Dwindle." *The Buffalo News* November 15: 1A.

Sherwin, Susan. 1992. *Patient No More.* Philadelphia: Temple University Press.

Steinbock, Bonnie. 1999. "The McCaughey Septuplets: Medical Miracle or Gambling with Fertility Drugs?" In *Ethical Issues in Modern Medicine,* 5th edition, ed. Bonnie Steinbock and John D. Arras. Mountain View, CA: Mayfield Publishing Company.

*Stenberg v. Carhart.* 530 U.S. 914; 120 (2000).

"The Shooting of Dr. Slepian." *Washington Post* October 27, 1998: A22.

Thomson, Judith Jarvis. 1971. "A Defense of Abortion." In *Ethical Issues in Modern Medicine,* 5th edition, ed. Bonnie Steinbock and John D. Arras. Mountain View, CA: Mayfield Publishing Company.

Tooley, Michael. 1972. "Abortion and Infanticide." In *Moral Problems in Medicine,* ed. Samuel Gorovitz, Ruth Macklin, Andrew L. Jameton, et al. Englewood Cliffs, NJ: Prentice-Hall.

Tooley, Michael. 1985. "Response to Mary Anne Warren." *Philosophical Books* XXVI(1): 9–14.

Truog, Robert D. 1997. "Is It Time to Abandon Brain Death?" In *Ethical Issues in Modern Medicine,* 5th edition, ed. Bonnie Steinbock and John D. Arras. Mountain View, CA: Mayfield Publishing Company.

Warren, Mary Anne. 1973. "On the Moral and Legal Status of Abortion." In *Ethical Issues in Modern Medicine,* 5th edition, ed. Bonnie Steinbock and John D. Arras. Mountain View, CA: Mayfield Publishing Company.

Warren, Mary Anne. 1985. "Reconsidering the Ethics of Infanticide." *Philosophical Books* XXVI(1): 1–9.

Warren, Mary Anne. 1989. "The Moral Significance of Birth." *Hypatia* 4(3): 46–65.

### INTERNET RESOURCES

United Nations. "Maternal Mortality Figures Substantially Underestimated, New WHO/UNICEF Study Says." Available from <http://www.un.org>.

World Health Organization. "Unsafe Abortion: Global and Regional Estimates of Incidence of All Mortality Due to

Unsafe Abortion with a Listing of Available Country Data." Available from <http://www.who.int>.

## II. CONTEMPORARY ETHICAL AND LEGAL ASPECTS: B. LEGAL AND REGULATORY ISSUES

Most contemporary legal systems regulate the practice of induced abortion. Governments around the world regulate whether, when, why, and how the estimated 46 million annual abortions occur. In some countries, abortion is governed primarily by national laws; in others, abortion is governed mainly by state or regional laws. Belief that abortion is unsafe, irreligious, immoral, unjust, or genocidal has tended to push regulation in the direction of laws that expressly prohibit some or all abortions. Convictions that abortion can alleviate overpopulation, avert economic hardship, protect women's health, promote sex equality, or eliminate undesirable progeny have tended to produce laws that permit, guarantee, or even compel abortion. More than 75 percent of the world's population live in countries in which abortion is legal, even when the life of pregnant woman is not at stake (Center for Reproductive Law and Policy).

An international survey of existing law reveals four basic patterns or models of express abortion regulation:

1. a model of prohibition;
2. a model of permission;
3. a model of prescription; and
4. a model of privacy.

Under the model of prohibition, the laws of a jurisdiction punish most or all abortions as criminal offenses, as in Ireland, Nigeria, Brazil, and Indonesia. In these countries, abortions are banned other than to save the life of the mother. Under the model of permission, laws permit abortions that meet criteria and conditions established by government, as in Sweden, Germany, England, India, and Zambia. For example, in Sweden abortions are readily available, subject to the approval of a National Health Board. In Germany, women face counseling and waiting period requirements for otherwise permitted early abortions. In the United Kingdom excluding Ireland, abortion for health and disability reasons is lawful up to 24 weeks, but a woman must obtain the approval of two physicians. Under the model of prescription, laws specifically require or encourage the termination of pregnancies falling into certain specific categories, as in The People's Republic of China. Finally, under the model of privacy, laws restrain government from enactments that criminalize or severely restrict

access to medically safe abortions, as in the United States and Canada. The model of privacy treats abortion decisions as substantially a matter of private choice rather than public law. In some countries using models of permission, prescription, and privacy, including the United States, China, France, the Russian Federation, and South Africa, women are not required by law to provide officials or physicians with a state-approved reason for routine legal abortions (Center for Reproductive Law and Policy). In Russia, whose per capita abortion rate was second in the world after Romania's in 2002, 60 percent of all pregnancies end in abortion.

Abortion law is subject to change from one era to the next. Countries under the sway of the model of prohibition in one generation have moved toward the models of permission or privacy in subsequent generations. For example, when the Supreme Court of the United States declared in *Roe v. Wade* (1973) that the nation's constitution bars statutes categorically criminalizing all abortions, it announced a national standard for state and federal law that ushered out the model of prohibition and ushered in the model of privacy. Abortion law can also change from liberal to restrictive and back again, in response to political developments and judicial interpretations of constitutional principle. Thus, Poland adopted more restrictive abortion laws after democratic elections in 1989; greatly liberalized its law in 1996; and then, in response to an adverse constitutional court ruling overturning the permissive 1996 law, quickly revised its law in 1997. Under a 1997 act of Parliament, Poland permits abortion to protect the pregnant woman's life or health, or to terminate pregnancies resulting from criminal acts or in cases of fetal abnormality.

## The Model of Prohibition

The model of prohibition governs official abortion policy in many African, Latin American, South Asian, and Middle Eastern countries. For example, Brazil and Sri Lanka permit abortion only to save the life of the woman. Most jurisdictions in Europe and North America reject the model of prohibition, permitting abortion on request, where pregnancy results from rape or incest, or where the continuation of pregnancy threatens the physical, mental or social well-being of the woman or her fetus. Ireland, a largely Roman Catholic nation, is one of the few European countries whose laws continued to criminalize abortions either absolutely or subject to a strictly limited number of exceptions beyond the 1970s. Under a 1983 amendment to the Irish constitution, Irish law permits abortion only to save the life of the woman. Overturning a ruling that a teenage rape victim who credibly threatened suicide could not travel to England for an abortion, the Irish Supreme Court found in 1992 that abortion would be permissible "if it is established as a matter of probability that there is a real and substantial risk to the life as distinct from the health of the mother, which can only be avoided by the termination of her pregnancy."

Jurisdictions whose laws reflect the model of prohibition often assert a strong religious or humanitarian policy interest in protecting what are thought to be the rights and interests of unborn children. However, other objectives have also prompted strict abortion prohibition. For example, during the nineteenth and twentieth centuries, abortion opponents in the United States cited the need to protect pregnant women from the medical and psychological risks of abortion. There can be no doubt that unskilled, unsanitary abortion procedures are a health risk, and that some women who obtain abortion services experience medical complications and emotional anguish. However, some lawyers and judges doubt that medical abortion performed during the first three months of pregnancy is less safe than pregnancy and childbirth (Tribe; Rhode). They similarly doubt that elective medical abortion poses a serious risk of psychological harm. Although one writer has concluded that "every woman pays a psychological price for abortion" (Reardon, p. 141), the American Psychological Association has concluded that serious emotional problems rarely result from abortion.

Countries whose populations have been ravaged by war and genocide have sometimes proscribed abortion in an effort to increase the birth rate. Strict abortion prohibition has had the additional, if only implicit, goal of reinforcing social roles. The cultural assumption that motherhood is the appropriate social role for women buttressed Joseph Stalin's 1936 abortion prohibitions, enacted to furnish the former Soviet Union with "a new group of heroes" (Sachdev). The belief that bearing children is women's natural destiny may lead some to assume that birth control and abortion are both immoral and unhealthful. After 1933, Adolf Hitler prohibited contraception and declared abortion a capital offense on the belief that birth control was unhealthful. On the other hand, abortion prohibitions adopted in Germany in 1943 aimed at the "vitality of the German people" and excluded from criminality abortions performed on "racially" undesirable women (Sachdev).

The reach of laws prohibiting abortion can be broad. Obtaining an abortion has been subject to criminal penalty in some instances, and so too has distributing abortion information. Provisions of the famous Comstock Law enacted by the Congress of the United States in 1873 —later rescinded—outlawed abortion-related implements and information as "obscene" and "immoral" (Garrow; Rhode). Offenders of the Comstock Law faced imprisonment with hard labor and monetary fines. Jurisdictions prohibiting

abortion generally aim at the conduct of third-party abortion providers. However, some abortion statutes also criminalize pregnant women's own conduct, making it a punishable offense to obtain or seek abortions from third parties. Legal systems rarely punish medical abortion as the full equivalent of felonious unjustified murder.

Criminalizing non-surgical and self-induced abortion poses special problems of detection and law enforcement. Pharmaceuticals approved for other purposes, like the cancer drug methotrexate, can be used to induce abortion. Self-induced abortion has often involved risky procedures, such as inserting knitting needles, wire coat hangers, or other foreign objects through the cervix. Many self-induced abortions are detected because they end tragically in medical and police emergencies. In 1989, a healthcare group in California promulgated a videotape demonstrating "menstrual extraction," a nonmedical abortion technique trainers say women can learn to perform safely at home with the help of a friend. To the extent that they are workable, abortion procedures that can be performed without professional assistance fall beyond the practical reach of law.

Prohibitive abortion law requires lawmakers to define what counts as abortion, and therefore what is subject to criminal penalties. The surgical and medical procedures generally in use by physicians in licensed hospitals and clinics in Europe and the United States plainly qualify as abortion. However, certain forms of birth control not viewed as abortion could conceivably fall under the scope of strict abortion prohibitions. Popularly viewed as a form of contraception, the intrauterine device (IUD) may function as a kind of abortifacient, blocking implantation of a fertilized egg, rather than preventing ovulation or fertilization. Étienne-Émile Baulieu's drug, RU-486, named for its French manufacturer, Roussel Uclaf, poses a related difficulty of definition. Described by French Minister of Health Claude Levin as "the moral property of women, not just the property of the drug company," RU-486 (mifepristone) arrived on the European scene in the 1980s and in the United States in 2000. Unlike pharmaceutical contraceptives that prevent fertilization or ovulation, RU-486 acts to block the successful implantation of a fertilized egg. Rejecting the popular "abortion pill" label, Baulieu has suggested that RU-486 is neither contraception nor abortion but something new—"contragestation." Still, it seems unlikely that a jurisdiction that strictly prohibits abortion would view "contragestation" as anything other than early abortion.

Abortion flourishes under regimes of prohibitive abortion law (Sachdev). In fact, about half of the estimated 46 million abortions that take place each year are illegal in the jurisdictions in which they occur. The criminal code of Bangladesh strictly prohibits most abortions, but physicians commonly induce abortion by performing a uterine evacuation procedure known as "menstrual regulation" on women who are many weeks pregnant. Prohibitive abortion laws commonly fall short of their stated goals and public expectations because governments are unwilling or unable to enforce the letter of the law. The prohibitive laws that governed abortion in the United States prior to *Roe v. Wade* were enacted to preserve unborn life and women's physical and mental health (Garrow). It has been argued that the aim of fetal preservation was at least partly undermined by the large number of clandestine abortions performed, notwithstanding prohibitive laws (Tribe). Although most abortions were illegal in much of the United States prior to 1973, American women obtained an estimated 200,000 to 1.2 million abortions each year in the 1960s and early 1970s (Tietze, Forrest, and Henshaw), compared to about 1.5 million each year throughout the 1980s and early 1990s, and 1.3 million in 1997. David Reardon puts the number of abortions pre-*Roe* at merely 100,000 to 200,000 per year. The aim of preserving women's health may have been frustrated under the regime of prohibition because clandestine abortions were commonplace but were not always performed by skilled practitioners in hygienic settings. This was especially true of the illegal abortions obtained by African-American women, who accounted for a disproportionate number of the victims of illegal procedures. (Twenty percent of the deaths related to pregnancy and childbirth in the United States in 1965 were attributed to illegal abortions.) Legalization of abortion probably resulted in a small-to-moderate increase in the number of abortions, but it appears to have greatly decreased the incidence of abortion-related infertility and death.

## Model of Permission

The model of permission became the pervasive one around the world in the final quarter of the twentieth century. Under the model of permission, abortion is legally available, but only with the approval of government officials or officially-designated decision makers, such as administrative boards, committees, physicians, or judges. In some permission-model jurisdictions, officials grant permission pro forma in nearly every case. In Norway, prior to 1975 reforms that liberalized abortion, as many as 94 percent of the requests for abortions made to Abortion Boards were routinely granted (Olsnes). Official decision makers in permissive jurisdictions rely upon a handful of factors to determine which abortions to permit and which abortions to prohibit (Petersen; Glendon).

The stage of pregnancy is very frequently a factor. Officials called upon to implement legal norms or exercise discretion often permit "early" abortions and prohibit "late" ones. This no doubt helps to explain the statistic that 90 percent of reported abortions take place within the first three months of pregnancy. Another factor decision makers commonly consider is the woman's medical or social status. Restrictive laws require that officials deny permission to abort for reasons other than medical hardship. Liberal laws often require that officials allow abortions because pregnancy or childbirth would involve social or economic hardship for the woman. In many jurisdictions, grounds for social hardship include rape, incest, or the age and marital status of the woman. The health or condition of the fetus can be a third factor in permitting or prohibiting abortion. The law may premise access to abortion on evidence that a child would be born with serious physical or mental abnormalities.

Genetic testing for the purpose of enabling parents to abort fetuses born with undesirable traits is already practiced in the United States. Healthcare providers in some states even face "wrongful life" and "wrongful birth" lawsuits for negligent failure to offer women information needed to prevent or abort an unwanted pregnancy. With advances in prenatal testing that enable detection of the sex of a fetus, it is possible for a pregnant woman to abort selectively unwanted male or female offspring. In some instances, abortion for sex selection may be tied to a desire to avoid giving birth to a child with a gender-related genetic disease. Jurisdictions that permit abortion without regard to reason presumably permit abortion for sex selection.

For most of the twentieth century, a number of countries governed abortion under highly bureaucratic versions of the model of permission (Sachdev). For a time in the eastern European countries of Hungary, Romania, Poland, and Bulgaria, abortion was lawful only if approved by a state board or committee. These countries reportedly permitted abortion in almost every case through the fourth month of pregnancy. Romania reverted to a prohibitive policy in 1966 in response to concerns about underpopulation and the health effects of multiple abortions. It prohibited most contraception and abortion for women who did not have at least four, and eventually five, children. Abortion prohibition was accompanied by a significant incidence of mortality related to illegal abortion. In the mid-1980s, 86 percent of the women in Romania who died as a consequence of pregnancy or childbirth died as a result of illegal abortions, compared with, for example, 29 percent in the former Soviet Union and 13 percent in Sri Lanka.

Other historical instances of the bureaucratic model of permission are the laws and administrative regulations in force in Denmark from 1939 to 1973, and in Sweden from 1939 to 1974. In Denmark, local and national committees consisting of teams of social workers, physicians, and psychiatrists evaluated the applications of women seeking legal abortions. Scandinavian officials on boards or committees charged with decision making typically assessed the impact of childbirth and child care on the mental or physical health of the woman, and the woman's living conditions. Israeli Ministry of Health regulations enacted in 1978 permitted hospitals and clinics to form committees consisting of two physicians and a social worker to decide whether to grant women's abortion requests. Although living conditions, such as other children and economic hardship, were initially an authorized basis for granting abortion requests, Israel amended the law in 1980 under pressure from religious groups and in response to concerns about a declining population rate.

At the beginning of the twenty-first century, a number of countries in Asia, South America, Europe, and North America make a woman's obtaining an abortion dependent upon the approval of one or more physicians, a judge, or one or both parents. Great Britain and countries whose abortion law was modeled on Great Britain's—Hong Kong, Zambia, and Australia—are examples of countries whose laws place decision making in the hands of physicians. The law of Great Britain was transformed over a great many centuries from a model of prohibition, to a model of permission, and even a model of privacy. Early English common law embodied the model of prohibition, at least for abortions taking place after the first few months of pregnancy. The common law proscribed abortion after *quickening*, about the fourth month of pregnancy, when fetal *animation* or *ensoulment* was deemed to have taken place. In 1861 the statutory abortion law of Great Britain defined as a felony any act intended to cause abortion, whether induced by the woman herself, if she were pregnant, or by others, whether or not she was in fact pregnant. The Abortion Act of 1967 abolished the nineteenth-century felony. The act's liberal provisions permit an abortion where any two medical practitioners certify in good faith that pregnancy "would involve risk to the life of the pregnant woman, or of injury to the physical or mental health of the pregnant woman or any existing children of her family, greater than if the pregnancy were terminated." Under this rule, qualifying for abortion poses no practical difficulty for women with the money to pay private physicians. As English law illustrates, the model of permission can have the distinct effect of empowering the medical and psychiatric professions to govern reproduction in accordance with their profession's internal standards of judgment.

Abortion is common in Australia, where abortion rights vary significantly from state to state and are governed both by common law and criminal statute. A liberalizing trend has been observed since the mid-1990s, when only South Australia and the Northern Territory had statutes specifically permitting some abortions. In 1998 controversy erupted over Australian abortion law, when two physicians were arrested in Western Australia for violating a moribund nineteenth-century criminal statute. The doctors had performed a consensual abortion in 1996 on a Maori woman who stored the aborted fetus in her refrigerator, planning to take it to New Zealand for burial in accordance with Maori traditions. Following reforms, early abortion is available virtually on demand in some Australian states, and is subject to enforced restrictions in others.

In India, the Medical Termination Pregnancy law enacted in 1971 permitted abortions that one or, if the woman is more than twelve weeks pregnant, two physicians certify. Grounds for certification are liberal. Abortion may be obtained to preclude a risk to the pregnant woman's mental or physical health, or a risk of the birth of a child with serious mental or physical abnormalities. No abortions after twenty weeks are legal under the law. A woman's mental health is considered at risk in cases of economic hardship and where pregnancy resulted from failed contraception. The 1975 Abortion and Sterilization Act made many abortions lawful in the Republic of South Africa, on the certification of two physicians that statutory requirements are met. The law required that where abortion was sought on grounds of risk to mental health, one of two certifying physicians be a psychiatrist willing to attest to danger of permanent mental harm. South Africa has subsequently liberalized its abortion law, making early abortion available on demand.

French law permits women to make their own judgments (early in pregnancy) about whether they are entitled to abortion on grounds of hardship. In this respect, French law resembles the federal law of the United States under *Roe v. Wade*. French regulations enacted in 1975 are representative of international responses to the judicial transformation of United States law with *Roe v. Wade* in 1973. Reflecting the aspirations of both the model of permission and the model of privacy, the French enactment begins with a declaration that the law guarantees respect for every human being from the beginning of life, and that this principle is to be sacrificed only in case of necessity and according to specific conditions. But the law authorizes any woman who is ten weeks pregnant or less to request a physician for an abortion if she believes pregnancy or childbirth will create hardship. Moreover, at any stage of pregnancy, right up to the moment of birth, abortion is lawful if two physicians, one of them from an official list, certify that continuation of pregnancy would put the woman's health gravely in peril, or that there is a strong possibility that the child would suffer from an incurable condition.

The French abortion law imposes numerous conditions on all abortions. Attending physicians must inform women of the medical risks of abortion and give them an official guide to the forms of assistance available to families, mothers, and children, and to relevant social service organizations. Women then must consult one of the listed social services. Women wishing to proceed with abortion must confirm their request in writing, after a one-week waiting period. Abortions must be performed by physicians in a public or recognized private hospital and must be reported to the regional health authorities. Hospitals must provide women who have obtained abortions with birth control information.

The model of privacy may best describe the overall aspiration of *Roe v. Wade.* However, the model of permission is arguably more descriptive of United States abortion law pertaining to unemancipated minors. The Supreme Court has taken the position that minors have a constitutional right to privacy and may terminate their pregnancies without parental consent, but that minors may not object on constitutional grounds to parental notification requirements and waiting periods. Individual justices on the Court have argued that requiring pregnant minors to notify family members of pregnancy and abortion, in effect, gives veto powers to third parties in a way that is inconsistent with the spirit of *Roe v. Wade.* Yet, a majority held in *Hodgson v. Minnesota* (1990) that states providing a "judicial by-pass procedure" may attempt to involve one or both parents in minors' abortion decision making by requiring minors or their physicians to contact parents in advance of abortion. In judicial bypass procedures, minors must be permitted to ask a judge to waive parental notification requirements. The judge is expected to waive the requirement if he or she determines that the minor is mature or that notification is not in the minor's best interests. Justices in the minority have objected that bypass procedures are unwarranted, since most minors notify parents or other responsible adults of pregnancy and abortion, and most minors seeking judicial waiver obtain it. In addition, the practical effect of mandatory notification is that some teens will delay abortion, increasing costs and medical risks. Some justices have argued that laws requiring parental involvement place minors with abusive parents or broken homes at a disadvantage and even at mortal risk.

## Model of Prescription

Under the models of permission and privacy, a government permits some or all of the abortions women want. Under the model of prescription, a government compels or virtually compels women to obtain abortions the government wants. Far-reaching compulsory abortion laws have been rare in the modern world. In the West, policymakers frown upon official and unofficial policies of mandatory abortion for poor and mentally incompetent women. Although healthcare providers reportedly recommend abortion in some instances—for example, when a pregnant woman is addicted to cocaine or infected with the AIDS virus—the United States government does not officially recommend or mandate abortion for any class of pregnancy. Under a penal code adopted in 1979, Cuban law proscribes abortion performed without the permission of the woman.

In an effort to control overpopulation and protect its economy, China began adopting "planned birth" family-planning measures in 1953. These measures aggressively encourage abortion through a system of penalties and rewards. Under the Chinese constitution, both the government and individuals are responsible for the planned-birth policy. In 1974, couples were limited to two children. Since 1979 couples wishing to bear children have been authorized to have only one child, and then only after securing a government permit. To encourage compliance, abortion is offered at no cost and may entitle the woman to a two-week paid leave of absence; women who have an IUD inserted or a tubal ligation along with abortion may receive additional paid leave. The effect of the planned-birth policy on the abortion rate in China is not known in the West. However, female infanticide and abortion for sex selection are reported. Chinese families have reportedly resorted to infanticide and selective abortion to ensure that their one-child quota is filled by a child of the culturally preferred male sex.

## Model of Privacy

Under the model of privacy, the law rarely compels abortion and permits all or virtually all abortions, as long as they are performed by medically qualified persons in clinics, hospitals, or other qualified facilities. Safety is a frequent goal of legal systems characterized by the model of privacy, although safety is not necessarily suggested by "privacy" nomenclature. The former Soviet Union adopted the model of privacy on safety and privacy grounds in 1920, more than a half century before the model came to dominate understandings of U.S. law. The goal of the Soviet decree legalizing any abortion performed by a physician in a state hospital was both to keep women safe from unskilled abortionists and to secure women's freedom and equality in work, education, and marriage. In 1936, the decree was rescinded in favor of a law prohibiting abortion other than to spare the life or health of the woman or prevent transmission of an inheritable disease. The shift back to the models of prohibition and permission seems to have been motivated by concern about declining birthrates, health effects of medical abortions, and diminished regard for marriage and child-bearing. But in 1955, the Soviet law moved back toward the model of privacy, again to protect women from unskilled abortionists and to give women themselves an opportunity to decide whether to become mothers (Sachdev).

In Japan, abortion has been legal since the government passed Eugenic Protection Laws in 1948 to protect women's health and deter the birth of what were considered undesirable offspring. In practice, abortion is available to women in Japan upon request. The law does limit abortion, but the limitations are extremely liberal: Abortion is permitted when performed by designated physicians to avert mental and physical disease or abnormalities; when pregnancy results from violence; or when the woman's health would be impaired for physical or economic reasons. Functionally, one can view Japan as a model of privacy jurisdiction; yet women's autonomy and equality are not the express policy objectives of its liberal abortion law. Japan follows the model of permission insofar as laws restrict abortion and have not been designed specifically to promote autonomous, private decision making. For nearly thirty years after they had been approved for use in North America and Europe, low-dose birth control pills were banned in Japan out of concerns about safety. The end of the ban in 1999 could mean that abortion will no longer function as a major form of birth control in Japan.

In the United States, abortion policy since the early 1970s has been directed to women's rights. During the early 1970s, the United States and a number of other countries adopted laws approximating the model of privacy. The theory that during the first trimester abortion ought to be available without any restrictions gained popularity. In effect, this approach was adopted in the former East Germany in 1972, Denmark in 1973, Sweden in 1974, France in 1975, and Norway in 1978 (Sachdev; Olsnes). "Fetal viability," the point at which, in some of these countries, the interests of the woman cease to be accorded overriding weight, is variously fixed between twenty weeks and twenty-eight weeks. In Norway, under 1978 amendments to a 1975 law, a woman "shall herself make the final decision concerning termination of pregnancy provided that it is possible to perform the operation before the twelfth week of pregnancy has elapsed." After the twelfth week, abortion sought for a number of medical or social indications is available upon successful application to an "Abortion Board" (Olsnes).

In *Morgentaler et al. v. The Queen* (1988), the Supreme Court of Canada found by a margin of five to two that provisions of the Criminal Code infringed Section 7 of the Canadian Charter of Rights and Freedoms promising "life, liberty and security of the person." The Canadian justices argued that "personal security," and with it "bodily integrity," "human dignity," and "self-respect," were threatened by interference with reproductive choices (Morton). The Canadian legislature remains free to regulate abortion consistent with the *Morgentaler* decision. However, in 1990 a bill to restrict abortion access to women whose physicians certified a health-related need for the procedure failed. The government thereafter announced that it would not seek new abortion legislation.

In Canada, the United States, and other privacy-model jurisdictions, liberal abortion law permits autonomous choices about matters that profoundly affect women's bodies, lifestyles, and equality. However, it is generally recognized that laws that decriminalize and deregulate abortion do not guarantee that every woman who desires an abortion will get one. Abortion is costly, and may or may not be covered by the health insurance of women who have insurance. The U.S. Supreme Court has repeatedly held that state and federal governments may encourage childbirth over abortion by refusing to include abortion among Medicaid and other entitlements awarded the poor. As a consequence, public funding for abortion is not available as a matter of right; publicly funded civilian and military hospitals are not required to perform abortion services; and states may prohibit physicians employed by public hospitals from performing abortions.

## Focus: The United States

The Constitution of the United States does not mention "abortion" by name. However, the Supreme Court has consistently held since *Roe v. Wade* (1973) and *Doe v. Bolton* (1973) that the due process clause of the Fourteenth Amendment guarantees American women a fundamental right to obtain medically safe abortions. States may not categorically ban abortion or unduly burden women's fundamental constitutional right to terminate pregnancy.

The state of Connecticut passed the first American legislation against abortion in 1821 (Garrow). At first, American law did not penalize early (pre-quickening) abortion. However, between 1827 and 1860, twenty states or territories passed statutes against abortion at all stages of pregnancy. By 1868, thirty-six states or territories had antiabortion statutes in place, enforcement of which was often lax. In 1965, all fifty states treated abortion and attempted abortion at all stages of pregnancy as felonies, subject to certain exceptions. In forty-six states and the District of Columbia, the relevant statutes explicitly permitted abortion to save the mother's life, while in two of the other four states a similar exception was recognized by the courts.

Between 1967 and early 1973, a dozen jurisdictions in the United States adopted somewhat permissive abortion laws patterned on the model legislation suggested in 1962 by the influential American Law Institute. These laws permitted abortion when performed by a licensed physician who determined that there was a substantial risk that pregnancy would seriously injure the physical or mental health of the mother; that the child would be born with grave physical or mental defect; or that the pregnancy resulted from rape or incest. Almost all of the other reforming jurisdictions nevertheless sought to strengthen the institutionalization of abortion practice by stipulating that an abortion would be lawful only if performed in an accredited hospital after approval by a committee established in the hospital for that purpose.

The decriminalization of abortion on the national level lagged behind the decriminalization of contraception. In 1965 the Supreme Court decided *Griswold v. Connecticut*, holding that states may not outlaw a married woman's use of birth control. The Court based its ruling on an unenumerated constitutional "right to privacy" implicit in the Bill of Rights and the Fourteenth Amendment. This same right to privacy was invoked in 1973 in *Roe v. Wade* to limit government interference with abortion. The right to privacy was, and is, controversial among lawyers and judges reluctant to recognize novel unenumerated rights. However, both the American Medical Association and the American College of Obstetricians and Gynecologists favored legalization of abortion. The immediate effect of *Roe v. Wade* and *Doe v. Bolton*, its simultaneously decided, lesser-known companion case, was to invalidate the laws regulating abortion in every state, except perhaps the already very permissive laws adopted in 1969 and 1970 in New York, Alaska, Hawaii, and Washington.

*Roe* and *Doe* established that:

1. no law can restrict the right of a woman to have a physician abort her pregnancy during the first three months, or first trimester, of her pregnancy;

2. during the second trimester, the abortion procedure may be regulated by law only to the extent that the regulation reasonably relates to the preservation and protection of maternal health;

3. at the point at which the fetus becomes "viable," a law may prohibit abortion, but only subject to an exception permitting abortion whenever necessary to protect the woman's life or health (including any aspects of her physical or mental health); and

4. no law may require that all abortions be performed in a hospital, or that abortions be approved by a hospital committee or by a second medical opinion, or that abortions be performed only on women resident in the state concerned.

The Court in *Roe* and *Doe* concluded that the Constitution does not accord legal personhood status to the fetus. Critics of this conclusion point out that the unborn are implicitly treated as legal persons in several other areas of the law. The unborn are taken into account in the allocation of property rights and the attribution of criminal and civil responsibility. For example, the unborn can inherit property. Negligently killing or injuring a fetus can give rise to civil liability for wrongful death, wrongful birth, battery, and other torts.

*Roe* made clear that women were not to be ascribed a right to exclusive control over their bodies during pregnancy. Yet the case signaled that the Constitution limits the role government may play in abortion decisions. In the first decade and a half after *Roe*, the Court struck down numerous state abortion restrictions. States unsuccessfully attempted to control abortion through advertising restrictions; zoning restrictions; record-keeping and reporting requirements; elaborate "informed consent" and physician-counseling requirements; mandatory waiting periods; bans on abortions for sex selection; the requirement of the presence of a second physician during the abortion procedure; the requirement that physicians employ methods of abortion calculated to save the lives of viable fetuses; the oversight requirement that physicians send all tissue removed during an abortion to a laboratory for analysis by a certified pathologist; the requirement that insurance companies offer at a lower cost insurance that does not cover most elective abortion; legislating a statewide information campaign to communicate an official state policy against abortion; legislating criminal sanctions for physicians who knowingly abort viable fetuses; and requirements that some or all abortions after the first trimester be performed in a hospital. However, the Supreme Court has repeatedly validated state and federal government policies that prefer childbirth to abortion by declining to pay for the abortions of poor women entitled to welfare benefits for prenatal care and childbirth (Solinger).

A major reaffirmation of *Roe*, *Thornburgh v. American College of Obstetricians and Gynecologists* (1986), held that states were not permitted to indirectly prohibit abortion by encumbering the decision to seek abortion with unnecessary regulations. A series of highly publicized Court decisions handed down since 1989 appear to permit more extensive regulation of first- and second-trimester abortions than *Roe* and *Doe* seemed to contemplate. *Webster v. Reproductive Services* (1989) permitted legislation requiring viability testing and limits on publicly funded physician care. The Court declined in *Webster* to decide the constitutionality of the declaration in the preamble of a Missouri statute that "[the] life of each human being begins at conception," and that "unborn children have protectable interests in life, health and well being" because the state had not yet sought to limit abortion by appeal to it. Encouraged by the *Webster* decision, several states and the territory of Guam sought between 1989 and 1992 to ban or discourage abortion through aggressive new regulation and enforcement. Anticipating that the Supreme Court would welcome an opportunity to overrule *Roe* in the 1990s, Guam enacted legislation prohibiting most abortion and its advocacy. A federal judge quickly declared Guam's law unenforceable under *Roe*.

In two 1990 cases critical of *Roe*, *Hodgson v. Minnesota* and *Ohio v. Akron Center for Reproductive Health*, the Court upheld parental notification requirements for minors. *Rust v. Sullivan* (1991) upheld a federal "gag rule" statute, subsequently eliminated by Congress, prohibiting abortion counseling by physicians in federally supported facilities. *Planned Parenthood v. Casey* (1992) affirmed *Roe v. Wade* as the law of the land and invalidated spousal notification. However, the case upheld a twenty-four-hour waiting period as part of a state's "informed consent" procedures. *Casey* shed the trimester framework of *Roe*, opening the door to regulation at any stage of pregnancy. *Casey* also announced a weaker standard of review in abortion cases that promised to permit more state regulation. Under *Roe*, abortion statutes were to be struck down if they did not further a "compelling" state interest. Under *Casey*, statutes "rationally related" to a "legitimate" state interest are to be upheld, assuming they do not "unduly burden" the abortion right.

Many Americans favor some restrictions on abortion, although a 2000 Gallup poll showed more than 80 percent of Americans approved some or all abortions. A national poll conducted in 1994 by Barna Research Groups showed that 78 percent of the adults surveyed approved the legalization of some (49%) or all (29%) abortions. In a 1994 survey conducted by Yankelovich Partners, Inc., 85 percent said a woman should be able to obtain an abortion no matter what the reason (46%) or in certain circumstances (39%). A CBS News/*New York Times* poll conducted in 1998 found that 61 percent of those surveyed favored legal abortion in the first trimester, 15 percent favored legal abortion also in the second trimester, and 7 percent favored legality in the third trimester. The same poll showed about 45 percent of those surveyed favored more restrictions on abortion, and 22 percent favored blanket prohibition.

The weakening of the standard of review in abortion cases after the *Casey* decision underscores that constitutional abortion law in the United States hovers uneasily between the models of permission and privacy. For this reason, it seems likely that the Supreme Court will be asked again and again to clarify the extent to which the state and federal government may restrict abortion rights. Proposed state and federal statutes such as the Partial Birth Abortion Ban Act of 2000 and the Born Alive Infant Protection Act of 2002 would extend legal protections to viable fetuses and curb certain abortion practices. Yet in *Stenberg v. Carhart* (2000), the Court declared unconstitutional a Nebraska statute outlawing so-called "partial birth" abortions. The Court reasoned that the broadly drafted statute lacked a constitutionally necessary exception for abortions to save the life of the mother, and could be construed to rule out *dilation and evacuation* as well as the more controversial *dilation and extraction* or *partial birth* procedure.

The U.S. Food and Drug Administration approved the controversial drug RU-486 (mifepristone) in 2000. The long awaited "abortion pill" has not become the elected method of abortion for a majority of American patients and providers. Notwithstanding the limited popularity of mifepristone as an abortifacient, state and federal lawmakers who oppose its use acted quickly but unsuccessfully to propose legislation outlawing the drug or limiting the types of physicians authorized to prescribe it. Because of *Roe v. Wade* and possible nonabortion uses of the medication, it is unlikely that blanket legislative bans on mifepristone would be found constitutional.

As long as they stand, *Roe v. Wade* and *Casey* will serve to provide a national abortion law standard for the United States. Since *Roe* in 1973, several attempts have been made in both houses of the U.S. Congress to undercut the judicial decision through legislation. One attempt, premised on the idea of "states' rights," involved legislation which, if adopted, would have established that no right to an abortion is secured by the Constitution and, therefore, that the fifty states are free to adopt restrictions on abortions. A second attempt, premised on "fetal personhood," would have expanded the definition of "person" under the due process and equal protection clauses of the Fifth and Fourteenth Amendments. The fetal personhood legislation would have declared that the right to personhood attaches from the moment of conception.

Supporters of *Roe* in Congress have attempted to legislate the holding of Roe through a federal statute. The Freedom of Choice Act was introduced into Congress several times after *Webster*, beginning in November 1989. Its passage by Congress would prohibit states from enacting restrictions on the right to abortion before fetal viability. A 1994 survey conducted by the Hickman-Brown Research Company found that 56 percent of those polled "strongly" or "somewhat" favored passage of a Freedom of Choice Act, while 38 percent somewhat or strongly opposed such a law. Initiatives to amend the federal constitution to include pro-life or pro-choice strictures have not advanced far beyond the drafting table. State statutes and state constitutions are an increasingly significant source of protection for abortion rights.

With *In re T.W.* (1989), the Florida Supreme Court invalidated that state's parental consent requirement, relying upon the state constitution. As a result of this decision, Florida recognized a fundamental abortion right independent of *Roe v. Wade.* A Maryland referendum endorsed by voters in 1992 similarly established state abortion rights not tied to the fate of *Roe v. Wade* in the Supreme Court.

## The Implications of Abortion Law

The liberalization of abortion law establishes rights for women who wish to terminate their pregnancies. The full implications of those rights are unclear for

1. the use and disposal of fertilized eggs, embryos, and fetal remains;
2. the enforceability of surrogate mother and surrogate gestator contracts granting third parties a legal interest in a woman's pregnancy;
3. the criminalization of pregnant women's conduct;
4. the tort liability of healthcare providers for wrongful birth and wrongful life; and
5. organized protest at abortion facilities (Purdy).

One legal concern is whether women who elect to abort have a familial, proprietary, or other interest in routinely aborted embryos or fetuses. State statutes typically require that abortion providers dispose of fetal remains in the way physicians dispose of other excised tissues. Yet some effort has been made to treat abortion tissues and fetuses differently, either because of their possible commercial value for research into the treatment of diabetes, leukemia, Alzheimer's disease, and Parkinson's disease; or because of their possible value as deceased "children." In 1984 a federal judge in Louisiana held that a statute requiring abortion providers to present patients with the option of burial or cremation was an unconstitutional burden on freedom of choice. About 90 percent of all abortions performed in the United States, and in other countries, are performed during the first trimester. The court implied that women might be discouraged from first-trimester abortions on the mistaken belief that extracted tissue would resemble a baby. Another legal concern is whether aborted embryos and fetuses may be sold for research purposes. American courts and legislators are unlikely to permit outright sales of abortion tissues for research purposes. Indeed, federal agency policies adopted in the 1980s declared a moratorium on the use of abortion tissues derived from elective abortions partly out of concern that women might be encouraged to abort for gain. Signaling a change in policy, in 1993, Democratic President William

Jefferson Clinton issued an executive order lifting the moratorium on fetal tissue research. President George W. Bush reversed this move, with his announcement of new federal restrictions on human embryo-derived stem cell research in 2001.

Hundreds of men and women have been parties to commercial surrogate motherhood contracts in recent decades. Commercial surrogacy agreements commonly obtain provisions in which the would-be surrogate mother or gestator undertakes that she will not obtain an abortion should she become pregnant as a result of the surrogacy transactions. In the celebrated 1988 *Baby M* case, MaryBeth Whitehead agreed in writing that she would "not abort the child once conceived" unless a physician determined it necessary to protect her health or "the child has been determined … to be physiologically abnormal." Although the Supreme Court of New Jersey refused to enforce the surrogacy contract in *Baby M,* other jurisdictions have not done so and face questions about the commercial alienability of constitutional abortion rights.

Another set of issues relates to the extent to which abortion rights may prevent government from intervening to enjoin or punish risky behavior by pregnant women who, for example, smoke cigarettes, consume alcohol, abuse drugs, and fail to heed medical advice. In a number of isolated cases in the United States, judges have jailed pregnant women they feared would abuse or neglect their fetuses. In *Ferguson v. City of Charleston* (2001), the United States Supreme Court struck down a program under which a hospital tested pregnant patients for illegal narcotics use without their informed consent and reported patients who refused prescribed rehabilitation to law enforcement authorities. A somewhat different concern is the legal implications of government intervention in the event that a pregnant woman refuses a blood transfusion needed to save her life, or a cesarean delivery physicians believe to be in the best medical interest of the unborn. Some view *Roe v. Wade* as holding by implication that women have a broad right to control—and even abuse—their own bodies without regard to fetal well-being. Yet a plausible counterview is that *Roe* does nothing more than immunize women from prosecution for early abortions, if they choose to have them.

Abortion is controversial in many countries. Violence aimed at abortion providers has occurred both in Canada and the United States. In May 1992 a bomb blast blamed on antiabortion radicals destroyed the Morgentaler abortion clinic in Toronto. Rare in Canada, dozens of abortion clinic bombings and fires have occurred in the United States. Antiabortion activists throughout the United States have demonstrated at abortion sites to focus attention on their concerns. Generally peaceful, these demonstrations have sometimes become blockades that interfere with the ability of patients and staff to utilize facilities where abortions are believed to take place. Demonstrators have sometimes resorted to harassment, noise nuisance, property damage, and murder. The shooting deaths of two Florida physicians outside abortion facilities in 1993 and 1994 dramatized the conflict between protesters and clinics. The United States Congress passed the Freedom of Access to Clinic Entrances Act of 1994 in an effort to assure freedom of access to reproduction services. The act makes acts of obstruction and interference at places providing reproductive services a federal offense punishable by fines and imprisonment.

The right to abortion has been held by some state courts to provide a rationale for permitting "wrongful birth" or "wrongful life" lawsuits. In wrongful birth actions, parents sue healthcare providers to recover from emotional distress and expenses connected with raising children with congenital abnormalities. In wrongful life actions, disabled offspring sue healthcare providers alleging that professional negligence caused their births into lives of pain, suffering, and extraordinary expenses. Citing *Roe v. Wade,* in *Berman v. Allan,* 80 N.J. 421, 404 A2D 8 (1979), the New Jersey Supreme Court allowed a wrongful life lawsuit for professional negligence to go forward against the obstetricians of a woman who alleged that she was not offered amniocentesis and, as a consequence, was denied an opportunity to exercise her legal right to abort a fetus affected by down's syndrome. Pennsylvania and several other states have refused to permit wrongful birth or wrongful life suits. Permissive jurisdictions stress the fairness of compelling negligent physicians to share the economic burdens borne by the families of the disabled. However, some policy makers believe such suits imply disrespect for the human life and for the right to life of disabled persons.

Abortion rights and free-speech rights clash in the context of conflicts over abortion clinic protests. Women have a legal right to seek abortion without highly offensive intrusion, physical assault, and violence. These rights come into play where, for example, protesters block access to clinics, or broadcast video of clinic patrons over the Internet or on public access television. But antiabortion protesters have a First Amendment right to freedom of speech, expression, and assembly. Citing the First Amendment in *Schenck v. Pro-Choice Network of Western N.Y.* (1997), the Supreme Court refused to uphold an injunction that created a "floating buffer zone" with a 15-foot radius around persons utilizing abortion facilities. Seeking to balance the rights of clinic users and protestors, in *Hill v. Colorado* (2000), the Court upheld a statute creating a narrow, 8-foot "bubble zone" around abortion clinics as a reasonable restriction of protestors' free speech. Following the murders of physicians

who performed abortions, a federal appeals court in *Planned Parenthood of the Colom./Willamette, Inc. v. Am. Coalition of Life Activists* (2002) held that the federal Freedom of Access to Clinics Act's definition of a violent threat extended to the circulation by antiabortion activists of "guilty posters" targeting specific abortion providers. Some federal courts have been reluctant to enjoin abortion protestors accused of actual or threatened violence on the basis of state or federal statutes, such as the Ku Klux Klan Act, not clearly enacted for that purpose. In *National Organization for Women v. Scheidler* (1994), however, the Supreme Court determined that the federal Racketeer Influences and Corrupt Organizations (RICO) statute could apply to a coalition of antiabortion groups alleged to be members of a nationwide conspiracy to close abortion clinics. The alleged conspirators unsuccessfully argued that RICO applies only to conspiracies in which the alleged racketeers act for the sake of economic gain rather than out of religious, moral, or political conviction. The Court found that acts that did not generate income for alleged racketeers but that adversely affected businesses such as abortion clinics were potentially conspiratorial under the RICO statute. The victory for proabortion rights groups was undercut by a later Supreme Court decision, *Scheidler v. National Organization of Women* (2003), which held that antiabortion protesters interfering with the property right of lawful abortion did not amount to racketeering acts of extortion required by the RICO statute.

In sum, the practice of abortion raises numerous legal issues in the jurisdictions that permit it. Because so many oppose abortion on religious and moral grounds, abortion-related questions of legal policy will remain especially complex in the United States and other pluralistic societies. In addition, should reproductive technologies for creating, preserving, and terminating gametes and fetuses continue to proliferate, the number of legal concerns about reproductive rights and responsibilities is as likely to expand as to contract.

ANITA L. ALLEN (1995)
REVISED BY AUTHOR

**SEE ALSO:** *Adoption; Autonomy; Conscience; Conscience, Rights of; Double Effect, Principle or Doctrine of; Embryo and Fetus; Genetic Testing and Screening: Reproductive Genetic Testing; Harm; Human Dignity; Infanticide; Life; Maternal-Fetal Relationship; Moral Status; Population Policies; Women, Historical and Cross-Cultural Perspectives;* and other *Abortion* subentries

## BIBLIOGRAPHY

*Baby M, In re.* 109 N. J. 396, 537 A.2d 1227 (1988).

Callahan, Joan C. 1995. *Reproduction, Ethics, and the Law.* Bloomington and Indianapolis: Indiana University Press.

Center for Reproductive Law and Policy. 2000. *Reproductive Rights 2000: Moving Forward.* Washington, D.C.: Author.

*Doe v. Bolton.* 410 U.S. 179 (1973).

*Ferguson v. City of Charleston.* 121 S. Ct. 1281 (2001).

Garfield, Jay L., and Hennessey, Patricia. 1984. *Abortion: Moral and Legal Perspectives.* Amherst: University of Massachusetts Press.

Garrow, David J. 1994. *Liberty and Sexuality: The Right to Privacy and the Making of Roe v. Wade.* New York: Macmillan.

Glendon, Mary Ann. 1987. *Abortion and Divorce in Western Law.* Cambridge, MA: Harvard University Press.

*Griswold v. Connecticut.* 381 U.S. 479, 483 (1965).

*Hill v. Colorado.* 530 U.S. 703 (2000).

*Hodgson v. Minnesota.* 497 U.S. 417 (1990).

Johnsen, Dawn E. 1986. "The Creation of Fetal Rights: Conflicts with Women's Constitutional Rights to Liberty, Privacy, and Equal Protection." *Yale Law Journal* 95(3): 599–625.

Luker, Kristin. 1984. *Abortion and the Politics of Motherhood.* Berkeley: University of California Press.

Maschke, Karen, ed. 1997. *Reproduction, Sexuality, and the Family (Gender and American Law: The Impact of the Law on the Lives of Women).* New York: Garland Publishing.

McDonagh, Eileen L. 1997. *Breaking the Abortion Deadlock: From Choice to Consent.* New York: Oxford University Press.

Michel, Aaron E. 1981–1982. "Abortion and International Law: The Status and Possible Extension of Women's Right to Privacy." *Journal of Family Law* 20(2): 241–261.

Mohr, James C. 1979. *Abortion in America: The Origins and Evolution of National Policy, 1800–1900.* New York: Routledge.

Morton, Frederick. 1993. *Pro-Choice vs. Pro-Life: Abortion and the Courts in Canada.* Norman: University of Oklahoma Press.

*Ohio Akron Center for Reproductive Health.* 497 U.S. 502 (1990).

Olsnes, Ragnhild. 1993. "The Right to Self Determined Abortion." In *Birth Law,* ed. Anne Hellum. Oslo: Scandinavian University Press.

Petchesky, Rosalind P. 1990. *Abortion and Women's Choice: The State, Sexuality and Reproductive Freedom,* rev. edition. Boston: Northeastern University Press.

Petersen, Kerry A. 1993. *Abortion Regimes.* Brookville, VT: Dartmouth.

*Planned Parenthood of the Colom./Willamette, Inc. v. Am. Coalition of Life Activists.* U.S. App. LEXIS 9314 (9th Cir. 2002).

*Planned Parenthood v. Casey.* 505 U.S. 833 (1992).

Purdy, Laura. 1996. *Reproducing Persons: Issues in Feminist Bioethics.* Ithaca, NY: Cornell University Press.

Reagan, Leslie. 1998. *When Abortion Was a Crime: Women, Medicine, and Law in the United States, 1867–1973.* Berkeley: University of California Press.

Reardon, David C. 1987. *Aborted Women: Silent No More.* Chicago: Loyola University Press.

Rhode, Deborah L. 1989. *Justice and Gender: Sex Discrimination and the Law.* Cambridge, MA: Harvard University Press.

Richards, David A. J. 1986. *Toleration and the Constitution.* New York: Oxford University Press.

Robertson, John A. 1983. "Procreative Liberty and the Control of Contraception, Pregnancy, and Childbirth." *Virginia Law Review* 69(3): 405–464.

*Roe v. Wade.* 410 U.S. 113 (1973).

*Rust v. Sullivan.* 570. U.S. 173 (1991).

Sachdev, Paul, ed. 1988. *International Handbook on Abortion.* New York: Greenwood.

*Schenck v. Pro Choice Network of Western New York, et al.* 519 U.S. 357 (1997).

Siegel, Reva. 1992. "Reasoning from the Body: A Historical Perspective on Abortion Regulation and (2000) Questions of Equal Protection." *Stanford Law Review* 44 (January): 261–381.

Simon Rita James. 1998. *Abortion: Statutes, Policies, and Public Attitudes the World Over.* New York: Praeger.

*Stenberg v. Carhart.* 530 U.S. 914 (2000).

Solinger, Ricki, ed. 1998. *Abortion Wars: A Half Century of Struggle, 1950–2000.* Berkeley: University of California Press.

Solomons, Michael. 1992. *Pro Life? The Irish Question.* Dublin: Lilliput.

*Thornburgh v. American College of Obstetricians and Gynecologists.* 476 U.S. 747 (1986).

Tietze, Christopher; Forrest, Jacqueline Darroch; and Henshaw, Stanley K. 1988. "United States of America." In *International Handbook on Abortion,* ed. Paul Sachdev. New York: Greenwood Press.

Tribe, Laurence H. 1990. *Abortion, the Clash of Absolutes.* New York: W. W. Norton.

*T. W., In re.* 551 S. 2d. 1186 (Fla. 1989).

*Webster v. Reproductive Services.* 492 U.S. 490 (1989).

Weddington, Sarah R. 1992. *A Question of Choice.* New York: Putnam.

## III. RELIGIOUS TRADITIONS: A. JEWISH PERSPECTIVES

The Jewish discussion of abortion is a multi-vocal one that crosses several centuries of text and tradition. However, for a tradition in which much is in contention, the legal and ethical norms surrounding abortion are relatively less controversial. The tradition, in general, takes a clear middle path—allowing some abortions, in certain circumstances, for specific rational moral appeals. For Jews who are not close followers of Talmudic law, the cultural and economic realities of modernity affect religious practice, social justice and ethical norms, but these norms themselves have been shaped by this largely permissive tradition. In Jewish ethics, one considers both the whole of human activity and the whole of the community as well: Women as well as men are moral agents. This argument is primarily contained in the extensive debate and exegesis of the rabbinic literature, a discourse of contention and casuistic narrative ethics that both determines and discusses the 613 commanded acts named as *the mitzvot* by the Rabbis of the Talmudic period (200 B.C.E.–500 C.E.)

Jewish law has developed, in the 1,500 years since the redaction of the Talmud, by an ongoing series of *responsa* to questions about the legal code discussed in the Talmud, called *halacha.* Difficult cases of social crisis of all types are brought before arbiters and scholars who rule on the facts of the cases, on the methodological principles of logical argument, and on certain key principles of relationships in familial, ritual, civic, and commercial spheres. Each commentator is intellectually tied to those who came previously, and is confronted by changes in context: politics, cultural shifts, and scientific understandings that were not available to previous generations. Nowhere is this more evident than in the rapidly changing field of reproductive health.

Nearly all commentators would agree that it is clear that the concerns of the tradition are specific and protective of four principles:

1. to assure that women are not required to have children, since childbirth was seen in the Talmudic period as potentially life-threatening;

2. to assure that the temptation to immerse oneself in a life of study is avoided and that every man is married and in a family with children;

3. that sexuality after reproduction of two children—the required number—could be enjoyed without reproductive consequence; and

4. to allow both women and men to pursue, within limits, options for family planning based on a complex assessment of personal needs and social context.

The discursive method of Jewish ethical reasoning follows from close analysis of key texts—but it is never a history of unanimity—rather, it is a centuries-long argument with sharply disagreeing authorities making definitive and, in some cases, contradictory statements. A review of the development of the internal argument of the classic texts illustrates both the mutability of the tradition and the argumentative nature of the normative debate.

Abortion as such does not appear as an option for women in the Biblical text. There is only one direct reference to the interruption of a pregnancy, and it is a sort of collateral damage: when a woman is hurt as she stands near a fight.

> And if men strive, and hurt a woman with child, so that her fruit depart and yet no harm follows, he shall be surely punished, according as the woman's husband will lay upon him; and he shall pay as the judges determine. But if any harm follows, you shall give life for life…. (Exodus 21:22–23)

The Biblical text assumes the following conditions:

> that the event described—an induced abortion—is an accidental occurrence;
>
> that it is not in woman's control, that the being lost is of value since it is, perhaps, the property of the husband;
>
> that the being that is *departed* is not a life in the way that the woman is a human life;
>
> that a crime of some sort has been committed, but that it is not a capital crime.

What is at stake is whether the woman herself is hurt—the child's loss is explicitly not the loss of a life.

Later texts then address the question of when an abortion is sought. Is this permitted without direct mention in the Biblical scripture? The response is found in the earliest sources of the Mishneh. Clearly seen as an emergency option, it was nevertheless clearly available under several circumstances.

Two later commentaries interpret the Bible text, and they do so with different types of arguments that allow abortion in some circumstances. The first argument follows the general line of thinking that the fetus is in some ways a danger to the woman, and can be aborted because of the more general rule of self defense: This becomes articulated as the argument called the *Rodef* (pursuer). This is evident in the following proof text:

> If a woman suffer hard labor in travail, the child must be cut up in her womb and brought out piecemeal, for her life takes precedence over its life; if its greater part has [already] come forth, it must not be touched, for the [claim of one] life can not supersede [that of another] life. (Mishneh 6)

Here the text assumes three things: Abortion is deliberate; the decision to abort is a conjoint one and somewhat in woman's hands (she is the sufferer, so it is her suffering that calls the question, and it must have something to do with her stated limits); and that all can agree that a *child* is in her womb, but not a child who counts as a *nefesh* (fully ensouled human person) until its head is out.

This first argument is further developed centuries later, by Maimonides:

This, too, is a mitzvah: not to take pity on the life of a pursuer (*Rodef*). Therefore the Sages have ruled that when a woman has difficulty in giving birth one may cut up the child within her womb, either by drugs or by surgery, because he is like a pursuer seeking to kill her. Once his head has emerged he may not be touched for we do not set aside one life for another; this is the natural course of the world. (Maimonides 1:9)

Maimonides assumes three things: that the fetus is in fact a *nefesh;* that it is a *pursuing nefesh* (*Rodef*); and that a life must be at stake to allow the killing of the *Rodef.* The reason for the opinion of Maimonides here, namely, that the fetus is like a pursuer pursuing the mother in order to kill her, is that he believed that a fetus falls into the general law of *pikuah nefesh* (avoiding hazard to life) in the Torah since a fetus, too, is considered a *nefesh* and is not put aside for the life of others (*Hiddushei Rabbi Hayyim Soloveitchik to Mishneh Torah,* Hilkhot Rotze'ah 1:9). Ben Zion Uziel, in the early modern period, then extended this argument to include not just the mother's life, but her health.

We learn in this matter that according to the doctors, the fetus will cause its mother deafness for the rest of her life, and there is no greater disgrace than that, for it will ruin the rest of her life, make her miserable all her … Therefore, it is my humble opinion that she should be permitted to abort her fetus through highly qualified doctors who will guarantee ahead of time that her life will be preserved.… (Ben Zion Uziel, *Mishpetei Uziel,* Hoshen Mishpat 3:46)

Finally, Rabbi Eliezer Waldenberg in the mid-twentieth century interprets the text to include protection of not just physical health, but mental health, allowing abortions in the case of a diagnosis of Tay Sachs in the child:

One should permit … abortion as soon as it becomes evident without doubt from the test that, indeed, such a baby [Tay-Sachs baby] shall be born, even until the seventh month of her pregnancy … If, indeed, we may permit an abortion according to the Halacha because of *great need* and because of pain and suffering, it seems that this is the classic case for such permission. And it is irrelevant in what way the pain and suffering is expressed, whether it is physical or psychological. Indeed, psychological suffering is in many ways much greater than the suffering of the flesh. (Eliezer Waldenberg, *Responsa Tzitz Eliezer,* Part 13, no. 102)

A second line of argument is largely based on developmental moral status, a principle that gains ground via rabbinical medical science. All discharges from the body present a problem to be adjudicated by the rabbis, since persons with discharges need to participate in purification rituals before they can rejoin the larger community. Since examination of the contents of the womb after a miscarriage for the first forty days after conception did not seem to show a fetus, the rabbinic authorities deemed that during this period, the fetus had the status of *mere water.* Abortions during this period, went the reasoning, then could not be opposed.

A third line of justification develops in entirely another tractate of the Mishneh (Arakin) that abortion is permitted as a health procedure since a fetus is not an ensouled person. Not only are the first forty days of conception considered *like water* but even in the last trimester, the fetus has an lesser moral status—more akin to a part of a woman's body, than like a separate being.

Gemara: But that is self-evident, for it is her body! It is necessary to teach it, for one might have assumed since Scripture says "according as the woman's husband shall lay upon him" that it [the woman's child] is the husband's property, of which he should not be deprived. Therefore, we are informed [that it is not so].… (Exodus)

This proof text is the introduction of an argument that the fetus is simply not a *nefesh* and therefore, is seen as a part of a women's body. A later authority, Rashi, assumes this is valid because the fetus is not a separate being until the head is born.

This argument continues in later *responsa* and it is clear that, even after birth, whether the child is fully independent, with it own, separate being and body, is still an issue: For some, the status of the infant remains uncertain for thirty days.

Because when a child dies within thirty days (being then considered a stillborn and not mourned like a person who had died) it becomes evident only in retrospect that it was a stillborn (*nefel*) and that the period of its life was only a continuation of the vitality of its mother that remained in him. (Ben Zion Uziel 3:46)

In the post-Holocaust period, a new and contradictory tradition is developing as some commentators have voiced concern that an overly liberal abortion practice is inappropriate in the face of declining numbers of Jews, and urge a more strongly pro-natalist stand. As Moshe Tendler and Elliot Dorff argue, Jews are "a people are in deep demographic trouble. We lost one-third of our numbers during the Holocaust … the current Jewish reproductive rate among American Jews is between 1.6 and 1.7.… This social imperative has made propagation arguably the most important mitzvah of our time." While this position does not come from classic halachic sources, it has nevertheless, gained some ground in the contemporary period.

Religion for Jews is not a set of external institutional events visited on occasions of crisis or celebration—religion is a binding to a commanded life, in which every single daily act of practice and attention is a part of the being of the faithful person. It is the totality of life that Jewish belief is after—the inescapable call of the stranger, the constancy of the demand for justice in every interaction, and the mattering of minute details of daily life. The commanded life is a matrix of competing and complementary and contentious strands. There is both a temporal aspect to the matrix, in that interpretations are the result of more than 2,000 years of discourse, and an analytic aspect in that any act can be judged in a variety of ways. An act can be prohibited but unpunished, prohibited and punished, permitted but not approved of, permitted and accepted, obligatory but with many exceptions, or obligatory in all cases. Hence, much of our understanding about abortion comes not from these texts that describe variations and exceptions, but from the far broader range of normative texts that support a pronatalist family life.

LAURIE ZOLOTH

**SEE ALSO:** *Authority in Religious Traditions; Judaism, Bioethics in; Population Ethics: Religious Traditions, Jewish Perspectives;* and other *Abortion* subentries

### BIBLIOGRAPHY

Abraham, Abraham. 1984. *Medical Halachah for Everyone.* New York: Feldheim Publishers.

Abrams, Daniel, and Elqayam, Avraham, eds. 2000. *Kabbalah. Journal for the Study of Jewish Mystical Texts.* Los Angeles: Cherub Press.

Abrams, Judith. 1998. *Judaism and Disability.* Washington, D.C.: Gallaudet University Press.

Adler, Rachel. 1998. *Engendering Judaism: An Inclusive Theology and Ethics.* Philadelphia: The Jewish Publications Society.

Baruch, Brody. 1988. *Life and Death Decision Making.* New York: Oxford University Press.

Bleich, David. 1983. *Contemporary Halakhic Problems,* vol. II. New York: KTAV Publishing House, Inc., Yeshiva University Press.

Cohen, Arthur, and Mendes-Flohr, Paul, eds. 1988. *Contemporary Jewish Religious Thought: Original Essays on Critical Concepts, Movements, and Beliefs.* New York: The Free Press.

Dorff, Elliot. 1998. *Matters of Life and Death: A Jewish Approach to Modern Medical Ethics.* Philadelphia: The Jewish Publications Society.

Frank, Daniel, ed. 1992. *Autonomy and Judaism.* Albany: State University of New York Press.

Freedman, Benjamin. 1999. *Duty and Healing. Foundations of a Jewish Bioethic.* New York: Routledge.

Gibbs, Robert. 2000. *Why Ethics? Signs of Responsibilities.* Princeton, NJ: Princeton University Press.

Halevi Spero, Moshe. 1986. *Handbook of Psychotherapy and Jewish Ethics.* Jerusalem: Feldeim Publishers Ltd.

Hand, Sean, ed. 1989. *The Levinas Reader.* Oxford: Basil Blackwell Ltd.

Herring, Basil. 1984. *Jewish and Halakhah for Our Time: Sources and Commentary.* New York: KTAV Publishing House, Inc., Yeshiva University Press.

Jakobovits, Immmanuel. 1962. *Jewish Medical Ethics: A Comparative and Historical Study of the Jewish Religious Attitude and Its Practice.* New York: Bloch Publishing Co.

Kennedy Institute of Ethics. *Ethics Journal,* II (4) December 2001. Baltimore, MD: John Hopkins University Press.

Levinas, Emmanuel. 1987. *Outside the Subject.* Stanford, CA: Stanford University Press.

Mackler, Aaron, ed. 2000. *Life and Death Responsabilities in Jewish Biomedical Ethics.* New York: G & H Soho, Inc.

Meier, Levi, ed. 1986. *Jewish Values in Bioethics.* New York: Human Sciences Press, Inc.

Pence, Gregory, ed. 1998. *Classic Works in Medical Ethics: Core Philosophical Reading.* New York: McGraw-Hill.

Preuss, Julius. 1978. *Biblical and Talmudic Medicine.* New York: Sanhedrin Press.

Rosner, Fred. 1997. *Medicine in the Bible and the Talmud.* New York: KTAV Publishing House, Inc., Yeshiva University Press.

Rosner, Fred, ed. 1990. *Medicine and Jewish Law.* Northvale, NJ: Jacson Aroson Inc.

Shatz, David, and Wolowelsky, Joel, eds. 2001. *The Torah U-Madda Journal.* New York: Yeshiva University.

Zohar, Noam. 1997. *Alterations with Jewish Bioethics.* Albany: State University of New York.

## III. RELIGIOUS TRADITIONS: B. ROMAN CATHOLIC PERSPECTIVES

The following is a revision and update of the first edition entry "Abortion: Roman Catholic Perspectives" by John R. Connery. The Roman Catholic tradition has always treated abortion as a serious sin. Yet Catholic teaching on abortion has not always centered on the "right to life" of the individual fetus, nor has it always viewed all abortion as homicide. For several centuries, early abortion in particular was characterized more as a sexual sin than as killing, and was condemned as an interference in the natural outcome of the reproductive process, often assuming as its context an illicit sexual liaison.

The fact that Catholic views of the precise status of the fetus as human life have changed over time and that the church's position has a philosophical rather than a religious basis are key to late-twentieth-century church teaching on abortion. That teaching is that the fetus must be given the benefit of the doubt, and be treated as if it were a person from conception onward. This teaching is not stated as a sectarian religious proposition, but as a humanistic and philosophical truth to be recognized in civil laws guaranteeing appropriate protection to fetal life. Although exhortations to protect life in the womb have often been supported with religious allusions (for instance, to the will of the Creator or to the image of God in humanity), the duties to continue pregnancy and to sustain infants have been grounded primarily in the "natural law," understood as a shared human morality innate to all persons and knowable by reason.

In examining the foundations and development of the Catholic position, it is important to place modern teaching in the context of changing views of women's roles in family and society. Other factors influencing debates about Roman Catholicism and abortion are the relation of scientific knowledge about the beginnings of human life to the moral status of life; the relation among civil law, morality, and the church as an institutional actor; and contraception and population, especially in international perspective.

## Historical Development

Although Catholic claims about abortion are not narrowly religious, certain biblical and early Christian characterizations of life in the womb no doubt have contributed to an ethos in which abortion is viewed negatively. The Hebrew Scriptures (Old Testament) did not treat the killing of a fetus as the killing of an infant (Exod. 21:22), although the Greek Septuagint translation of the Hebrew (early third century B.C.E.) adds a distinction between the formed and the unformed fetus, and presents abortion of the former as homicide. This distinction reflects the ancient Greek view (Aristotle) that the matter and form of any being must be mutually appropriate (the *hylomorphic theory*), and that the embryo or fetus could not have a human soul (*form*) until the body (*matter*) was sufficiently developed. Often quoting the Septuagint, patristic and medieval theologians maintained this distinction, which remained a key component of Roman Catholic discussion of abortion until at least the eighteenth century.

The Gospels do not address abortion explicitly, though the infancy narratives manifest interest in the importance of the individual before birth, at least in respect of God's will for him or her in the future (Matt. 1:18–25; Luke 1:5–45). In Paul's Letter to the Galatians (5:20) and in Revelation (9:21), condemnations of magical drugs (*pharmakeia*) associated with various forms of immorality, including promiscuity and lechery, may very likely extend to abortifacients. The connection is made clear in two early Christian texts, the Didache and the Epistle to Barnabas. "'You shall not kill. You shall not commit adultery. You shall not corrupt boys. You shall not fornicate. You shall not steal. You shall not make magic. You shall not practice medicine (*pharmakeia*). You shall not slay the child by abortions (*phthora*). You shall not kill what is generated. You shall not desire your neighbor's wife' (Didache 2.2)" (Noonan, p. 9).

Contraceptive and abortifacient drugs, as well as infanticide, were certainly used widely in the ancient world, not only to conceal sexual crimes but also to limit family size and conserve property. Early Christian authors such as Tertullian, Jerome, and Augustine in the Western church, and Clement of Alexandria, John Chrysostom, and Basil in the Eastern church, repudiated these practices. They did not, however, challenge their patriarchal social context, with its requirement that female sexuality serve the good of the family and its assumption that women seeking to avoid pregnancy were usually guilty of sexual infidelity. Local councils tended to support this stand. In 303 C.E., on the Iberian Peninsula, the Council of Elvira excluded from the church for the rest of her life any woman who had obtained an abortion after adultery. In 314, the Eastern church, at the Council of Ancyra (Ankara), reduced the period of penance to ten years, although it retained the lifetime ban for voluntary homicide. Such church laws made no distinction between the formed and the unformed fetus, but Tertullian, Jerome, and Augustine considered that the sin of abortion might not be homicide until after ensoulment. (The fetus was considered by many ancient writers to receive a soul only after the body had "formed," or reached an appropriate level of development, at about three months.)

Formation of the fetus became a consideration in assigning penance in private confession during the seventh century, but it was not universally recognized in church law until the decree *Sicut ex* of Innocent III in 1211. The decree dealt with irregularity, which could be incurred for homicide. An irregularity is a canonical impediment that bars a man from receiving or exercising holy orders. Irregularities are based on defects (such as mental or physical illness) or crimes (including attempted suicide, murder, and abortion). According to the decree, irregularity would not be incurred for abortion unless the fetus was animated. Since the time of animation was identified with formation, the decree implied that only abortion of the formed fetus was considered homicide. Following Aristotle, forty and ninety days were accepted as the time of animation for the male and the female fetus, respectively. Confusion arose, however, from a parallel tradition that extended the notion of homicide not only to the abortion of the unformed fetus but also to sterilization. Both traditions claimed a factual base, the one in the premise that the "man" is contained in miniature in the male seed, and the other in Aristotle's reported observation of aborted fetuses. During the Middle Ages, the distinction between formed and unformed was generally accepted, notably by Thomas Aquinas, and only the abortion of the formed fetus was classified as homicide, even in reference to sacramental penances. Earlier abortions were not murder, but they were still forbidden as serious sins because they interfered with the procreative outcome of sexual acts.

In the early fourteenth century, the Dominican John of Naples introduced an exception, subsequently accepted by several others: It would be permissible to abort the unformed fetus in order to save the life of the mother. Later theologians, particularly Thomas Sánchez (sixteenth century), used the argument of self-defense against an unjust aggressor (so characterizing the fetus) or the principle of totality (looking on the fetus as part of the mother). In 1588, Sixtus V reaffirmed a more rigid position, classifying even sterilization as homicide, and (in the decree Effraenatam) making excommunication a penalty of the universal church for the sin of abortion. A modification in 1591 again limited the provision to the case of the animated fetus, at either forty or ninety days. This legislation remained in effect until 1869, when Pius IX extended it to all direct abortion. Twenty years later, the Holy Office of the Vatican declared that neither craniotomy nor any other action to destroy the fetus directly would be permitted, even if without it both mother and child would die. Until that point, the exception to save maternal life had been debated by the theologians without receiving official condemnation. While theologians sought a balance of the value of the fetus with other values, especially the life of the mother, papal legislation moved toward a reinforcement of the abortion prohibition.

A moderating influence that continues today was exerted via the *principle of double effect*. This principle, pertaining to acts that have both good and evil effects, permits a moral distinction between direct and indirect abortion. Only direct abortions are absolutely prohibited in official Roman Catholic teaching. Indirect (permitted) abortions are those operations that have as their primary effect the saving of the mother's life, with the death of the fetus a foreseen but not directly intended secondary effect. The classic example is the removal of the cancerous uterus of a woman who is pregnant. In this case, the death of the fetus is neither in itself the desired outcome of the intervention, nor even willed and caused as the means by which the woman's life is saved. The removal of the cancer, not the fetus, heals. Double effect may also be applied to the removal of a

fallopian tube in the case of an ectopic pregnancy. The premise behind the justification of indirect abortion is that while the direct killing of an innocent human being is immoral, the woman's life is at least equal in value to that of her unborn offspring, so that she has no duty to assume serious risk to her own life in order to sustain the child.

## Contemporary Teaching

In his 1930 encyclical on marriage, *Casti connubii,* Pius XI affirmed the equal sacredness of mother and fetus, but condemned the destruction of the "innocent child" in the womb, who can in no way be considered an "unjust assailant." (The sticking point here, of continuing interest to moralists, is whether it is necessary to have an unjust intention to qualify as an unjust aggressor, or whether unintentionally posing an unjust danger to another is sufficient. Soldiers in war, for instance, may have noble personal intentions, yet validly be viewed by their opponents as unjust attackers.) The Second Vatican Council (*Gaudium et spes,* no. 51) referred to abortion and infanticide as "unspeakable crimes." The complex agenda of and challenges to current church teaching are well focused by the 1974 Vatican "Declaration on Abortion."

This document is a response to changed Western abortion laws, as well as to population measures in developing nations. Even as it resists these pressures, it adapts its message on abortion to cultural and legal contexts characterized by the emancipation of women and the need to control births. The document responds to the Western political value of free choice by asserting that "freedom of opinion" does not extend further than the rights of others, especially the right to life. It observes that while ensoulment has been debated historically, abortion has always been condemned. Most important, the document insists that human reason can and should recognize respect for human life as the most fundamental of all goods, and the condition of their realization. It sees modern science as confirming that human life begins with fertilization, though allowing that science can never definitively settle what is properly a philosophical question. Still, "it is objectively a grave sin to dare to risk murder" if there is doubt as to whether the fetus is fully a human person.

The "Declaration on Abortion" recognizes that pregnancy can pose serious burdens for the health and welfare of women, families, and children themselves. It advocates that individuals and nations exercise "responsible parenthood" by natural means of avoiding conception. It also exhorts "all those who are able to do so to lighten the burdens still crushing so many men and women, families and children, who are placed in situations to which in human terms there is no solution" (no. 23). It excludes abortion as an answer but also concludes that what is necessary "above all" is to "combat its causes" through "political action" (no. 26). The "Declaration" anticipates later efforts, notably by the U.S. episcopacy, to advocate moral consistency on killing, in that it contrasts growing protests against war and the death penalty with the social vindication of abortion. From the standpoint of both the Vatican and the U.S. bishops, the unborn should be included within a greater respect for life in general, and be protected by more stringent social limits on killing of all kinds.

## Critical Debates

Among the debated questions regarding the Roman Catholic tradition on abortion are certainly the following. First, is it reasonable and scientifically sound to urge that the fetus be treated as a "person" from conception onward, especially if to do so will have dire consequences for the woman who bears it? While most Roman Catholic theologians assume a conservative attitude toward the value of prenatal life, not all accept that full value is present at the outset; rather, it increases in some developmental fashion, at least through the earlier stages. Several authors (Tauer; McCormick; Shannon and Wolter) have pointed to the time of implantation, at about fourteen days, as a "line" after which individuality appears more settled (the possibility of "twinning" being past) and the chance of survival greatly magnified (for a discussion, see Cahill).

Second, is the equality of women, and the substantive legal, social, and material support for women and families enjoined by the "Declaration," really as high on the practical pro-life agenda of Roman Catholicism as is the enactment of punitive sanctions for abortion? A deep skepticism about whether this is so gives the "abortion rights" cry of many feminists its immense symbolic value in the struggle for gender and sexual equality. While some Catholic feminists believe that sexual self-determination and effective birth control is a better way to ensure women's liberation than recourse to a form of killing, other Catholic feminists insist that the choice to terminate pregnancy must be available to women as long as a patriarchal church and society identify women's roles as reproductive and domestic in order to constrain women's moral agency and to exclude women from the range of social participation available to men.

Third, even granted that the fetus has significant value, can and should restrictive abortion laws be kept in place—or reenacted in nations that have moved toward liberalization? John Courtney Murray (ch. 7) distinguishes between law

and morality. Morality in principle governs all human conduct, while law pertains to the "public order," the minimum moral requirements of healthy social functioning. Modern nations vary in the degree of restraint on abortion choice they see public order as requiring (see Glendon). Abortion policy debates, especially in more lenient systems like that of the United States, challenge Roman Catholicism to reshape the social consensus about the value of the unborn. Any legislation not backed by a consensus favoring enforcement will lead both to disrespect for the law and to the proliferation of unregulated extralegal alternatives. A precondition for a less permissive abortion consensus is the creation both of avenues other than "abortion rights" for the exercise of women's social and personal freedoms, and of social supports encouraging women and families to raise children.

A major point of debate within Roman Catholicism is the level of legal compromise acceptable to those who would accord the fetus more value than does the current consensus. Following the principle that law and morality are not coterminous, some argue that a policy that encourages early abortion and restricts it to "hard cases" (e.g., threat to life or health, rape, incest, serious birth defects) could command enough broad support to justify it as a practical advance in the limitation of abortion. Advocates of a more stringent position insist that the full weight of the church's moral authority be marshaled behind a policy that would outlaw abortion altogether.

Finally, can the church credibly defend its antiabortion position while disallowing the most effective forms of birth control? It is relevant to this question that many nations' aspirations to economic and cultural prosperity are plagued by limited freedom for women in marriage and family, and by increasing overpopulation. In the industrialized countries, the abortion controversy tends to focus on individual rights, either of the fetus or of the mother, with Roman Catholic proponents framing the issue in terms of a legally protectable right to life. In such nations, the church tends to address itself to the absolutization of private choice over what it sees as human life, and the trivialization of the abortion decision as it becomes a substitute for sexual responsibility and contraception.

However, the Roman Catholic church is an international organization, with a substantial or growing membership in, for example, Latin America, the Philippines, and Africa. In many nations, the question of women's freedom to combine family with public vocation as the context for the abortion debate is overshadowed by dire poverty; the inaccessibility of education, adequate employment, and healthcare; the ambiguous economic implications of a large family in rural, agricultural settings; and the radically disadvantaged position of girls and women within the family in some traditional cultures. Especially in the absence of ready access to contraception, abortion may appear to such women, to families, and even to government agencies to be a desperate but necessary means of controlling fertility. As the 1974 "Declaration on Abortion" indicates, the global Roman Catholic position on abortion must go beyond the condemnation of abortion as murder to address personal and social situations in which abortion appears as the only viable answer to deprivation or oppression.

LISA SOWLE CAHILL (1995)

SEE ALSO: *Authority in Religious Traditions; Christianity, Bioethics in; Conscience, Rights of; Embryo and Fetus: Religious Perspectives; Feminism; Genetic Testing and Screening: Reproductive Genetic Testing; Human Dignity; Moral Status; Natural Law; Population Ethics: Religious Traditions, Roman Catholic Perspectives;* and other *Abortion* subentries

### BIBLIOGRAPHY

Abbott, Walter M., ed. 1966. *The Documents of Vatican II: All Sixteen Texts Promulgated by the Ecumenical Council, 1962–1965.* New York: America Press.

Ashley, Benedict, and O'Rourke, Kevin D. 1978. *Health Care Ethics: A Theological Analysis.* St. Louis: Catholic Hospital Association.

Cahill, Lisa Sowle. 1993. "The Embryo and the Fetus: New Moral Contexts." *Theological Studies* 54(1): 124–142.

Connery, John R. 1977. *Abortion: The Development of the Roman Catholic Perspective.* Chicago: Loyola University Press.

Glendon, Mary Ann. 1987. *Abortion and Divorce in Western Law: American Failures, European Challenges.* Cambridge, MA: Harvard University Press.

Grisez, Germain G. 1970. *Abortion: The Myths, the Realities, and the Arguments.* New York: Corpus.

Jung, Patricia Beattie, and Shannon, Thomas A., eds. 1988. *Abortion and Catholicism: The American Debate.* New York: Crossroad.

McCormick, Richard A. 1984. *Health and Medicine in the Catholic Tradition: Tradition in Transition.* New York: Crossroad.

Murray, John Courtney. 1960. *We Hold These Truths: Catholic Reflections on the American Proposition.* New York: Sheed and Ward.

Noonan, John T., Jr., ed. 1970. *The Morality of Abortion: Legal and Historical Perspectives.* Cambridge, MA: Harvard University Press.

Pius XI, Pope. 1930. *Casti Connubii. In Matrimony,* pp. 219–291, tr. Michael J. Byrnes. Papal Teachings Series. Selected and arranged by the Benedictine monks of Abbaye Saint-Pierre de Solesmes. Boston: St. Paul Editions, 1963.

Shannon, Thomas A., and Wolter, Allan B. 1990. "Reflections on the Moral Status of the Pre-Embryo." *Theological Studies* 51(4): 603–626.

Tauer, Carol A. 1984. "The Tradition of Probabilism and the Moral Status of the Early Embryo." *Theological Studies* 45(1): 3–33.

Vatican Congregation for the Doctrine of the Faith. 1974. "Declaration on Abortion." *Origins* 4: 386–392.

## III. RELIGIOUS TRADITIONS: C. PROTESTANT PERSPECTIVES

Reviews of the history of Protestant teaching on abortion focus most often upon specific comments regarding abortion in the writings of leaders of the various church reform movements in European Christianity beginning in the sixteenth century. Several of the most effectual Reformation leaders, including Martin Luther (1483–1546) and John Calvin (1509–1564), were powerful both in reconceiving church practice and in articulating reformulations of Christian theological and ethical teaching. Consequently, for many of their followers and spiritual heirs, their teaching has remained uniquely authoritative in discerning Protestant truth claims. The formal criteria for discerning Christian truth proposed by these reformers, however, is best characterized as privileging the role of Christian scripture (usually referred to by Protestants as the Old and New Testaments) in adjudicating doctrinal and moral disputes. This primacy of scripture as theological and moral norm also characterized the teaching of most other sixteenth-century reformers, including the theological leaders of the many Anabaptist movements.

Since the sixteenth century, all dissent from authoritative Roman Catholic teaching and practice, including newly emergent Christian movements, receives the label "Protestant." The rapidly growing Pentecostal movements in Latin America, indigenous Christian movements in Asia, and the African indigenous churches that have become numerically preponderant among Christians on that continent all fall under this rubric. As a result, extreme caution needs to be exercised in characterizing "Protestant" moral teaching in any contemporary moral dilemma. Even when interpreters are familiar with very diverse Protestant cultural traditions, those who identify themselves as Protestants interpret the meaning of conformity to scriptural norms in a wide variety of ways, and reveal wide differences in biblical "hermeneutics," or principles of interpretation, of sacred texts. The diversity of hermeneutical options available accounts in part for the complexity of Protestant voices on abortion today.

Before identifying contemporary Protestant hermeneutical diversity and therefore the range of existing contemporary Protestant viewpoints on abortion, it is important to clarify the cultural roots of Protestantism that shape them.

## Early Protestant Views of Abortion

Martin Luther's and John Calvin's theological and moral reforms were shaped by their reconceptions of both the meaning of Christian life and Christian ritual practice. Neither could be said to have proposed shifts in the foundational notions of human nature embedded in late medieval Christianity. Traditional notions of human nature, including gender and human species reproduction, were not in dispute and did not shift at the time of the Reformation. What is notable among Protestant reformers is the paucity of comment on any questions about human sexuality and reproduction, including abortion. Martin Luther, a prolific preacher and writer, did not mention abortion at all. Had he done so, he likely would have presumed its moral wrongness because he was educated as an Augustinian monk and was learned in the available theological texts of the period, including especially *Sentences* by the twelfth-century theologian Peter Lombard, which contained collations of opinions on abortion by earlier theologians. The lists included the judgments of many who associated abortion with sexual immorality, especially with adultery, and condemned the practice.

John Calvin also knew this authoritative tradition that explicitly condemned abortion, as his commentaries on Genesis 38:10 make clear. His remarks on Exodus 21:22 further attest that he believed abortion to be wrong morally. Modern critical biblical exegetes agree that Exodus 22:21 is the only text in Christian scripture that explicitly refers to abortion, albeit to abortion that occurs because of injury to a pregnant woman. The issue in this passage was not elective abortion. Even so, Calvin used the occasion of comment on this text to make known his view that the fetus is already a person, a matter the text does not address.

On gender, sexuality, and reproduction, these reformers maintained continuity with earlier traditions. Both Luther and Calvin also followed what they took to be early Christian theological consensus, that divine ensoulment (i.e., the point of spiritual animation of human beings by God) of human life occurs at conception, though not all the Protestant theologians who followed them agreed. Modern conservative historical interpreters construe Calvin and Luther's views on this point as confirming their own current

belief that Protestant teaching agrees with modern papal teaching, namely, that full human life occurs at conception. Caution needs to be exercised here, however. Although the majority of Protestant theologians followed the view that ensoulment occurred when the "seed" was planted in utero, their perspectives were not developed in relation to questions about human gestation. To argue that these views speak to the value of fetal life is misleading, since their opinions were developed as aspects of the theological debate about sin and salvation, and not in relation to modern embryological understanding. In any case, Protestant ritual practice suggests that commonsense norms were in fact applied to actual fetuses. Protestants, like Roman Catholics, did not practice baptism in relation to miscarriages or aborted fetuses.

## Modern Protestant Views on Abortion

Specific comment on abortion is rare in most Reformation traditions until the twentieth century. Perhaps in deference to the lack of biblical discussion, most reformers considered matters regarding the morality of abortion, like matters governing all sexual and reproductive behavior, to be ordered by human rational discernment. They were issues of "natural morality" rather than of revealed truth. Despite emphasis on recovering the meaning of Christian biblical tradition, Lutherans, Calvinists, and Anglicans (post-Roman Church of England adherents) maintained the view, longstanding in western Christianity, that much moral knowledge, including the order of human sexuality and reproduction, falls within the purview of "natural" human knowledge, that is, they are matters for rational deliberation and discernment. Contrary to the trend of modern Protestant fundamentalist biblicism in discussions of abortion, most Protestant traditions tended to embrace a type of reasoning that accepted human rational (and therefore "scientific") data as relevant to these moral judgments on these issues. The Anabaptists were often exceptions methodologically, however. They sought guidance on moral issues exclusively from scripture without reference to other sources. However, Anabaptists also stressed freedom of conscience in deliberating moral dilemmas, and often resisted fixed ecclesiastical standards on questions such as abortion. Not surprisingly, contemporary Anabaptist heirs often oppose with great adamance state-prescribed policies making abortion illegal.

It is not too much to say that Protestantism possessed neither an explicitly developed tradition of moral reasoning about abortion nor any elaborated body of teaching on the ethics of so-called medical practice until well into the nineteenth century. Reproduction in Protestant communities, as in all premodern communities, was shaped by female cultural practice and midwifery until at least the very late nineteenth century. Contemporary cultural historians agree that nearly all female subcultures encouraged some means of fertility control, and that most took recourse to abortifacients (substances that induce abortions) in extreme cases. Such methods were primitive and dangerous, however, and documentation regarding the range and scope of their use is all but nonexistent. The fact that women, and not men, both comprised and knew the culture of reproduction probably limited public awareness in prevailing practices. Knowledge about available interventions in pregnancies may not have been widely shared, and such knowledge may have been quite rare among male theologians until the "medicalizing" of pregnancy and reproduction in the twentieth century. In the nineteenth century, male medical practitioners increasingly attempted to discredit midwifery, frequently on the grounds that midwives practiced abortion, but Protestant clergy in the United States showed great reluctance to support such efforts.

The major impact of the Reformation in shaping Protestant attitudes on abortion is rarely mentioned in traditional historiography. The most important influence of Protestantism in the abortion debate arose from the changes in spiritual practice initiated by Reformation Christianity; these changes in turn led to a powerful shift in how socialization into Christian faith took place. Initiation into Christianity moved from a locus in the church-based penitential system to the Christian family, which gradually became the basic social unit of Christian piety. Protestant spirituality was pervasively formed by this embrace of the family as the proper site for transmission of both faith and morals. The change engendered by the Reformation overturned celibacy not only as the proper norm for clerical life but also as the norm of optimal Christian piety. The Reformation movements made the sexually monogamous, procreation-centered family both the center of their basic community and their strongest metaphor for divine blessing. For Calvinists, explicitly from the outset, and for Lutherans, Anglicans, and Anabaptists more slowly, adherence to this form of social practice came to be taught as a Christian duty. Parents were to oversee their children's successful entrance into procreative-centered marriage literally as a mandate of faith.

This shift in the structure of Christian sociology, more than any change in explicit moral teaching, shaped subsequent moral sensibilities toward abortion among Protestants. This new emphasis on the sacerdotal character of the family reinforced the appeal of Protestant Christianity in traditionalist non-European cultures as well. Both ancient Hebraic and Jewish and pre-Protestant Christian sources had at times equated procreation and biological fertility or fruitfulness as signs of divine blessing, and such pronatalist sentiments had had some influence in earlier Christian attitudes toward abortion. However, the rise of Protestantism made such sensibilities powerful in European cultures and central to modern Christian moral sensibility about reproduction. This portended a deep suspicion regarding elective abortion when the practice became widespread and safe.

Many modern Protestants arrive at their judgments about the morality of abortion from a deep-seated sense that any pregnancy is intrinsically a sign of divine blessing and that to deny this is impious. So deep does the equation of fertility and divine blessing run in Protestant cultures that western Christianity itself has strongly reinforced traditional patriarchal norms that female "nature" is centered in and fulfilled only through maternity. Traditional Protestant cultures (those untouched by religious pluralism) tend to experience any weighing of questions about the status of fetal life as expressing a "secular" or "antireligious" mindset.

Despite the strong pronatalist disposition of traditional Protestant spirituality, however, critical historians have also noted a certain tension between Protestant teaching on abortion and Protestant pastoral practice. Even in traditionalist Protestant cultures, where moral and theological discourse is unequivocal in condemning abortion, pastoral practice is frequently far less censorious. Scattered evidence exists that Protestant priests, pastors, and elders often treated those who had abortions or administered them with a surprising degree of compassion or even leniency. There is no evidence that the practice of abortion was deemed "an unforgivable sin," as some ancient church canons insisted, or that abortion was equated with "murder" or "unjustified killing." Even among contemporary Protestant fundamentalists, historians have observed this tension between formal moral condemnation and more permissive ecclesiastical practice. Theological and moral condemnation notwithstanding, noncelibate clergy may be in touch with many of the concrete conditions and dilemmas of pregnancy and reproduction that shape women's lives. In any case, the general stance of Protestant traditionalism and of the newer, postmodernist biblical hermeneutics is toward a degree of pastoral compassion, even if abortion is starkly condemned at the formal level. All current available data suggest that the rate of recourse to abortion among women who are part of Christian communities that formally condemn abortion—Protestant traditionalist, Protestant fundamentalist, or Roman Catholic—is at least as great as it is among women who come from liberal Protestant and Jewish communities or who are nonpracticing with regard to religion.

The most typical contemporary Protestant attitude toward abortion remains a traditionalist, pronatalist negativity toward the practice, with a reluctant recognition that abortions do occur frequently, even within the Protestant communities of faith. Such cautious negativity is maintained without strong, elaborated moral justification, chiefly because the strong cultural ethos of the existing family-centered sociology of the Protestant churches gives this view such plausibility. Traditionalist consensus tends to break down, however, whenever Protestant communities are confronted with debates shaped by conflicts within the wider culture or from newly articulate dissent within these Protestant communities themselves. Such debate is now ongoing in all churches rooted in the continental Reformation. For the most part the debate reflects the divisions in biblical hermeneutics already mentioned.

Three newer hermeneutical positions appear in the abortion debate. First, there is a quite unprecedented biblical fundamentalist hermeneutic asserting itself in many Protestant cultural contexts. This new fundamentalism is developed particularly to resist change in issues involving gender, sexuality, family, and reproduction. On all of these issues, restoration of a premodern interpretation of sex/gender and the reproductive system is the primary goal. Human gender and sexual identity, this approach insists, are rooted in "nature" and in "divine decree" central to the presumed "biblical" message. Using both the language of natural law and tradition of the mandate of divine revelation as synonymous and as equally legitimated by scripture, the new fundamentalists contend that the essence of the biblical witness is the biological-religious "givenness" of male/female nature and the revealing of the proper "telos," or end, of human sexuality. Abortion is unthinkable, a violation of all of the norms of faith and morals. This hermeneutic aims to make even the discussion of abortion taboo in Protestant theological and moral discourses, to make it literally unthinkable. This approach tends to drive from the field several generations of historical-critical study by Protestant theological liberals. Previously, liberal biblical scholarship had successfully persuaded interpreters of the Bible within mainline Protestantism that interpretation of scriptural texts had to be guided by awareness of different historical times and variations among cultures. Liberals recognized that biblical worldviews do not presuppose modern ideas about the origin and nature of the universe and its inhabitants. Such considerations undergirding previous Protestant biblical interpretation, once widely accepted, are often forgotten in the wake of the force of the new fundamentalist hermeneutic.

Second, although the new fundamentalism gains force in Protestant communities, most "oldline" Protestant denominations (rooted in Europe) remain informed by historical-critical methods of scriptural interpretation and continue to speak in a voice consistent with conclusions of the earlier liberal biblical hermeneutic. Broadly speaking, these churches acknowledge that biogenetic and other scientific knowledge must be given its due in deliberating the morality of abortion. Most concede that decisions to have abortions are justified in some cases and can be consistent with biblical faithfulness. This casts several major Protestant denominations on the side of the public policy debate that supports limited legality of abortions. Although several of the "old line" denominations have been strongly pressed by fundamentalists and traditionalists in their ranks to shift to antiabortion public-policy positions, Lutherans, Anglicans, Methodists, Presbyterians, and United Church of Christ denominations, among others, have maintained their public positions. Discussion of what may constitute "justifiable reasons" for choosing abortion is decidedly underdeveloped in such Protestant communions. A strong consensus prevails that supports abortions in cases of pregnancies due to sexual violence (rape and incest); in cases where the life or physical health of the mother is at stake; and, perhaps, in cases where prospective parents lack the spiritual and physical resources to rear an additional child. There are also important historical reasons why old-line liberal Protestant communities place a strong emphasis on "responsible parenthood," but that story is outside the scope of this entry. This too is an important and largely unexamined chapter in understanding Protestant views on both family planning and abortion.

Finally, in nearly all contemporary Protestant communities/cultures, another hermeneutic for interpreting the Christian abortion tradition is emerging. It may be called a *liberationist* or even a *profeminist liberationist* principle of interpretation. Although it is still a decided minority position within formalized Protestant theological-moral discourse, this hermeneutic is influencing many, especially women. It calls upon Protestant theology and ethics to reformulate moral and religious judgments with special attention to concerns for women's well-being and in recognition that Christian teaching on gender, sexuality, and reproduction is embedded in a wider system of social control of women's lives. Acknowledging internal contradictions within scripture, a liberation hermeneutic refuses authority to culturally repressive male-supremacist readings of biblical texts and postscriptural theological interpretations. Like liberals, proponents of the emerging liberation hermeneutic represent a spectrum of convictions about what reasons might justify specific acts of abortion, but strongly concur that the Protestant Christian moral voice must actively advocate broad-based social change to enable women to shape their reproductive capacity. They contend that the moral evaluation of abortion must not be predicated on discourse that obscures women's full standing as moral agents or that fails to include realism about the historical pressures surrounding biological reproduction in women's lives. Among Protestants, only Unitarian/Universalists have adopted such a hermeneutic officially.

The contesting voices characterized here are most visible and most intense within Protestant Christian communities in the United States. However, analogous dynamics are at work in Protestant communities in other areas of the globe, as they are within Roman Catholic, Orthodox, and other religious communities. The struggle over which hermeneutical voice shall prevail in Protestant teaching on abortion remains unresolved.

BEVERLY WILDUNG HARRISON (1995)

SEE ALSO: *Christianity, Bioethics in; Embryo and Fetus: Religious Perspectives; Feminism; Genetic Testing and Screening, Reproductive Genetic Testing; Human Dignity; Moral Status; Population Ethics: Religious Traditions, Protestant Perspectives;* and other *Abortion* subentries

### BIBLIOGRAPHY

Brown, Peter R. L. 1988. *The Body and Society: Men, Women, and Sexual Renunciation in Early Christianity.* New York: Columbia University Press.

Cohen, Sherrill, and Taub, Nadine, eds. 1989. *Reproductive Laws for the 1990s.* Clifton, NJ: Humana.

Connery, John R. 1977. *Abortion: The Development of the Roman Catholic Perspective.* Chicago: Loyola University.

Gordon, Linda. 1976. *Woman's Body, Woman's Right: A Social History of Birth Control in America.* New York: Grossman.

Grobstein, Clifford. 1988. *Science and the Unborn: Choosing Human Futures.* New York: Basic Books.

Harrison, Beverly Wildung. 1983. *Our Right to Choose: Toward a New Ethic of Abortion.* Boston: Beacon Press.

Jones, Jacqueline. 1986. *Labor of Love, Labor of Sorrow: Black Women, Work, and the Family. From Slavery to the Present.* New York: Vintage.

Kennedy, David M. 1970. *Birth Control in America: The Career of Margaret Sanger.* New Haven, CT: Yale University Press.

McLaren, Angus. 1990. *A History of Contraception from Antiquity to the Present Day.* Oxford: Basil Blackwell.

Mohr, James. 1979. *Abortion in America: The Origins and Evolution of Public Policy: 1800–1900.* Cambridge, MA: Harvard University Press.

Noonan, John T., Jr., ed. 1970. *The Morality of Abortion: Legal and Historical Perspectives.* Cambridge, MA: Harvard University Press.

Olasky, Marvin. 1992. *Abortion Rites: A Social History of Abortion in America.* Wheaton, IL: Crossways.

Rapp, Rayna, and Schneider, Jane, eds. 1995. *Articulating Hidden Histories: Exploring the Influence of Eric R. Wolf.* Berkeley: University of California Press.

Rich, Adrienne C. 1976. *Of Woman Born: Motherhood as Experience and Institution.* New York: W. W. Norton.

Rousselle, Aline. 1988. *Porneia: On Desire and the Body in Antiquity.* New York: Basil Blackwell.

## III. RELIGIOUS TRADITIONS: D. ISLAMIC PERSPECTIVES

Since ancient times every human society has dealt with the issue of abortion. The way each treats the issue has depended on the way each views fundamental questions of individual and societal life, such as the meaning and sanctity of human life, sexuality and gender relations, the role of marriage and family, the meaning of human freedom, and the related issues of rights and responsibilities of the individual.

### The Roles of Medicine and Law in the Islamic Debate on Abortion

Islam's response to abortion during the fourteen centuries of its existence has been documented mostly in the jurisprudential works of its doctors of law and the medical writings of its physicians. Islamic perspectives on abortion have been shaped directly by both its theology and its revealed law (*Shari'a*). Because of the centrality of the latter as a practical guide in the religious and spiritual life of Muslims, however, they depend heavily on the deliberations and ethico-legal decrees (*fatwās*) of experts whenever practical problems arise in society. The main practical role of theology is to provide the necessary spiritual and intellectual framework within which ethico-legal debates are pursued.

Since the Divine Law of Islam refuses to make a separation between law and ethics, the traditional Muslim jurist (*faqih*) is at once an ethicist and a legal expert. The physician's duty in matters concerning abortion is to provide medical advice and recommendations befitting each individual case, as Islamic law generally permits abortion on medical and health grounds up to a certain stage of pregnancy. Close collaboration between medicine and law in Islam has generated a well-developed branch of Islamic jurisprudence that deals with many biomedical issues, including contraception and abortion.

In all cases of abortion, the physician is an important witness. The idea of the testimony of a trustworthy physician is well known in Islam, since Islamic law puts great emphasis on the idea of a trustworthy witness, whom it always defines in terms of believing in God and having a good moral character. The close rapport between medicine and law in Islam is further strengthened by the fact that this religion has produced a sizeable number of jurists who either practiced medicine or at least possessed a sound general knowledge of the subject. Ibn Rushd (known by the Latin name Averröes, d. 1198), Ibn al-Nafīs (d. 1288), the discoverer of the minor circulation of the blood, Ibn Ḥazm (d. 1064), Fakhr al-Dīn Rāzī (d. 1209), and in more recent times, Ḥasan al-ʿAṭṭar al-Khalwatī (d. 1835), a rector of the prestigious al-Azhar University in Cairo, were some of the most famous jurists–medical practitioners. Al-Shāfiʿī (d. 820), the founder of one of the four Sunni schools of law, is credited in traditional sources with knowledge of medicine.

Conversely, there have been many Muslim physicians who were well versed with the philosophy of the Shariʿa and the ethical teachings of the Qurʾan and *hadiths* (i.e., recorded sayings, behavior, and actions attributed to the Prophet, and in the case of the Shiʾite branch of Islam, also to the Imams, their foremost spiritual leaders), but who were never recognized as jurists in the technical sense of the term. The most famous of these was Ibn Sīnā (d. 1037). These physicians were generally knowledgeable in embryology. As scholars of natural philosophy, of which psychology is a part, many of these physicians also developed a comprehensive theory of the soul that includes a treatment of the problem of identifying the stage of pregnancy when the ensoulment of the body takes place in the womb. The connection between embryology and psychology is therefore of great practical interest to Islamic law.

At ensoulment a fetus attains the legal status of a human being, with all the rights accorded by the Shariʿa. Although Muslim jurists rely substantially on the Qurʾan and prophetic medicine for their knowledge of embryology, they also demonstrate a positive attitude toward the scientific embryology of the philosopher–physicians, since they do not see any basic contradiction between the two sources.

## The Theological Context

The abortion debate in Islam takes place in a particular religious environment created by the divinely revealed teachings of the religion. These teachings are accepted by Muslims as sacred and immutable and have remained unquestioned in the debate over the centuries. The most important of these teachings concerns the meaning and purpose of human life.

Islam teaches that human life is sacred because its origin is none other than God, who is the Sacred and the ultimate source of all that is sacred. Human beings are God's noblest creatures by virtue of the fact that he has breathed his spirit into every human body, male and female, at a certain stage of its embryological development. This breathing of the divine spirit into the human fetus is called its ensoulment; it confers on the human species the status of theomorphic beings. Islam shares with Judaism and Christianity the teaching that God has created humans in his own image.

Islam teaches that a human is not just a mind–body or soul–body entity that has come into existence through an entirely physical, historical, or evolutionary process. He or she is also a spirit whose reality transcends the physical space–time complex and even the realm of the mind. This spiritual substance present in each human individual, to which Muslim philosophers and scientists refer as the most excellent part of the rational soul and which has cognitive powers to the extent of being able to know itself, God, and the spiritual realm in general, is what distinguishes humans from the rest of earthly creatures.

The Qurʾan refers more than once to the ensoulment of the human body, almost always in the context both of describing God's creation of Adam, the first ancestor of the human race, and of affirming the superiority of humans over the rest of creation, including the angels (for example, at 15:28–30). There is also a more specific reference to the ensoulment of the human fetus that is made as part of its description of the process of pregnancy and birth. The Qurʾanic passage quoted perhaps most often in the abortion debate is, "We [i.e., God and his cosmic agents] have created man out of an extraction of clay [the origin of semen]; then we turn it into semen and settle it in a firm receptacle. We then turn semen into a clot [literally, something which clings] which we then fashion into a lump of chewed flesh. Then we fashion the chewed flesh into bones and we clothe the bones with intact flesh. Then we develop out of it another creature. So blessed be God, the best of creators" (23:12–14).

Both ancient and modern commentators on the Qurʾan generally agree that the last stage in the formation of the human fetus as indicated by the phrase "develop out of it another creature" mentioned in this Qurʾanic passage refers to the ensoulment of the fetus, resulting in its transformation from animal into human life. As to exactly when the ensoulment of the fetus takes place, the Qurʾan does not provide any information. The prophetic hadiths contain a detailed periodization of each of the different stages of fetal growth mentioned in the Qurʾan. In theology as in law, matters on which the Qurʾan is either silent or held to be less explicit than the hadith, the latter takes a decisive role. Thus it is the testimony of the hadith concerning the ensoulment of the fetus that has proved decisive in the formulation of Islamic theological doctrine concerning abortion.

According to one hadith, organ differentiation in the fetus does not begin to take place until six weeks after the time of fertilization. According to another, an angel who is a divine agent of ensoulment of the fetus is sent to breathe a distinctively human soul into it after 120 days of conception have passed. In his commentary on the Qur'anic verse on human reproduction cited above, basing his views on hadiths as well as on the findings of physicians, Jalāl al-Dīn al-Suyūtī (d. 1505), an encyclopedist and author of a popular work on prophetic medicine, declared, "All wise men are agreed that no soul is breathed in until after the fourth month" (Elgood, 1962, p. 240).

If God has given a theomorphic nature to human persons and has created them in the best of molds (Qur'an, 95:4), having unique faculties not enjoyed by creatures of other species, it is not without a noble purpose. According to the Qur'an, human beings have been created to know God and to be God's servants and representatives on Earth in accordance with his own wishes as revealed to all branches of the human family through his prophets and messengers. One of the six fundamental articles of the Islamic creed is belief in a future life—not in this world of sensual experience and mental images, but in another world whose space–time complex is entirely different from the one we presently experience.

In the Qur'anic view, human life does not end with death. In reality, death is only a passage between two parts of a continuous life, namely the present and the posthumous. How we fare in that future life depends on how we conduct ourselves in this present life. By leading a spiritually, ethically, and morally healthy life in this world, we will attain salvation and prosperity in the after-death life. The previously cited verse on human conception and birth is immediately preceded by a reference to life in paradise and immediately followed by a statement on the certainty of death and resurrection. Muslims understand from this and other verses that there is a grand divine scheme for humans that they have no right to disturb. On the contrary, they are to participate fully in this cosmic scheme as helpers of God in both their capacities as his servants and representatives.

Human reproduction, birth, and death are part of this grand divine scheme. Indeed, the Qur'anic view is that there is even a preconception phase of human existence. The Qur'an refers to a covenant between God and all the human souls in the spiritual world before the creation of this world. God addressed the souls collectively, asking them "Am I not your Lord?" Without hesitation they all bore witness to his Lordship, thus implying that God-consciousness is in the very nature of the human soul.

The general implication of the Islamic teachings on the meaning and purpose of life for reproduction and abortion is

clear. Although reproduction is not explicitly commanded in the Qur'an, it does appear to be encouraged. A few hadiths are explicit in their encouragement of procreation. The most popular is the hadith that says that, on the Day of Resurrection, the Prophet would be proud of the numbers of his community compared with other communities and that he admonishes his followers to reproduce and increase in number.

One can say with certainty that the general religious climate that prevailed in Muslim societies throughout the ages even until modern times is one in which procreation is encouraged and abortion very much discouraged. Cyril Elgood observes that "in Islamic countries moral approval of the practice of abortion was not readily given" (Elgood, 1970) although procurement of abortion, of which there were many cases, was not necessarily considered a criminal act. When he further says that "it is almost universally recognized by civilized nations that abortion is to be practiced only on the rarest of occasions" (Elgood, 1970, p. 240), the majority of Muslims would make the spontaneous response that this is precisely the Islamic view of abortion.

If Islam encourages the propagation of the human species, then it also insists that every human life be given due protection. (Abortion, however, is not considered the ending of a human life unless ensoulment of the fetus has occurred.) One of the fundamental goals of Islamic law is the protection of human life. Islam takes a serious view of the taking of human lives (except in cases that have been legitimized by the Divine Law itself) and of all acts injurious to life. One of the five basic human rights enshrined in the Shari'a is the protection by the state of every human life. The Qur'an asserts that "whosoever kills a [single] human for other than murder or other than the corruption of the earth [i.e., war], it is as though he has killed all humankind and whosoever has saved one human, it is as though he has saved all humankind" (5:35). The phrase "other than murder" in this verse refers to justifiable homicide, like self-defense and capital punishment as prescribed under the Islamic law of equality (qisas).

The Islamic view of marriage and sexuality also casts a long shadow on the abortion debate. Human reproduction should take place within the framework of the sacred institution of marriage. Islam describes marriage as "half of religion" and strongly condemns sexual relations outside of marriage. The main purpose of the institution of marriage is the preservation of the human species, although Islam also recognizes the spiritual, psychological, and socioeconomic functions of marriage. That there is indeed much more to marriage than just procreation or sexual fulfillment has been amply clarified by many classical Muslim thinkers.

One of the best treatises on the wisdom of marriage in all its dimensions was composed by the prominent jurist, theologian, and Sufi, al-Ghazzālī (d. 1111). This highly influential religious scholar and critic of Aristotelian philosophy defends the permissibility of married couples' practicing contraception on the ground of their need to secure a happy marriage. He goes so far as to hold that a man who fears that his wife's bearing children might affect her health or good looks, and that he might therefore begin to dislike her, should refrain from having children (Rahman). Al-Ghazzālī's view clearly suggests that procreation is not the sole purpose of marriage.

Islamic discussion of abortion is always related to the question of the rights and responsibilities of both the husband and the wife. One of the major issues in contemporary debate on abortion in the West concerns the rights of women to procure abortion. Islam answers the question not only by appealing to its theological doctrines on the meaning and scope of human rights and responsibilities, but also to its religious theory of conception based on revealed data and hadith teachings. The Qur'an stresses the idea that everything in the heavens and on earth belongs to God. Metaphysically speaking, humans do not own anything, not even their own bodies. It is God who has apportioned rights and responsibilities to males and females, husbands and wives, fathers and mothers. Men and women in Islam obtain their mutual rights through the arbitration of the Divine Law.

In general, Muslim jurists pay great attention to women's rights in the practice of contraception and the procurement of abortion. In the words of Basim F. Musallam, "One can speak of a classical Islamic opinion on contraception generally and consistently adopted in Islamic jurisprudence, regardless of school. This classical opinion was the sanction of coitus interruptus with a free woman provided she gave her permission" (Musallam). A "free woman" is a nonslave and married. Islamic jurisprudence treats coitus interruptus under three categories, namely (1) with a wife who is a free woman; (2) with a wife who is a slave of another party; and (3) with a man's own slave or concubine. All schools of Islamic law consider coitus interruptus permissible. The majority of them insist on the woman's consent only if she belongs to the first category, since Islamic law recognizes her basic rights to children and sexual fulfillment. No permission is needed from a slave woman. In the case of abortion, the Hanafis granted the pregnant woman the right to abort even without her husband's permission provided she has a valid reason in the eyes of the Shari'a. (The Hanafis are followers of the Islamic school of law founded by the prominent jurist Abu Hanifah and are mainly found in Turkey and the Indian subcontinent.) The Qur'anic teaching that children are not created of the man's semen alone, but of both parents together, has a bearing also on Muslim discussion of the mutual rights of husband and wife in the permissibility of abortion.

## Islamic Law and Abortion

The Islamic view of fetal development based on the Qur'an and hadith is central to the Muslim arguments on abortion. All Muslim jurists believe that the fetus becomes a human being after the fourth month of pregnancy. Consequently, abortion is prohibited after that stage (Musallam). However, the jurists differ in their views concerning the permissibility of abortion during the first four months of pregnancy, that is, the period prior to the ensoulment of the fetus.

Jurists of the Hanafi school of law allowed abortion to be performed at any time during the four-month period. A special document compiled by five hundred Hanafi *ulamā* (religious scholars) decrees that "the woman has the right to adopt some method of obtaining abortion if quickening of the fetus has not occurred, which happens after 120 days of conception" (Abedin, p. 121).

Most Maliki jurists, by contrast, prohibit abortion absolutely. Their main argument is that although the fetus does not become a human until after its ensoulment, one should not tamper with the natural process of conception once the semen has settled in the womb, since the semen is destined for ensoulment. A minority of Maliki jurists, however, allow abortion of a fetus up to forty days old. Other schools of Islamic jurisprudence, among both Sunnis and Shi'ites, agree with the Hanafis in their tolerance of abortion, although again they differ on the specifics.

It is important to emphasize the fact that there is a specific theological and ethico-legal context in which abortion has been permitted in Islam. Muslim jurists classify all human acts into five categories, namely (1) the obligatory (*wājib*), (2) the recommended (*mandūb*), (3) the allowable or the indifferent (*mubāh*), (4) the blameworthy or the discouraged (*makrūh*), and (5) the forbidden (*harām*). Abortion, at the most liberal level, has been placed by jurists in the third category, that of the allowable. Jurists have deliberated on the special conditions under which abortion is permitted, apart from the biological factor of ensoulment. They have also discussed cases of criminal abortion and types of penalties to be imposed on convicted wrongdoers.

Muslim jurists permit abortion mostly on medical and health grounds. One of the valid reasons often mentioned is the presence of a nursing infant. It is feared that a new pregnancy would put an upper limit on lactation. The jurists believe that if the mother could not be replaced by a wet nurse, the infant would suffer, if not die.

Contemporary Muslim society is faced with the reality that the practice of abortion is on the rise. In a number of Muslim countries, many unwanted pregnancies result from illicit sexual relations as well as from rapes. There are also related issues of birth control or family planning as a national policy, easy access to modern contraceptives, and the challenge to traditional Islamic doctrines on abortion and contraception arising from advances in genetics and biomedical technology. A well-defined Islamic response to these contemporary challenges has not yet emerged, but interest in these subjects is gaining momentum. As contemporary Muslim intellectuals and religious scholars debate these problems, traditional sources on contraception and abortion will be of immense value.

OSMAN BAKAR (1995)

SEE ALSO: *Authority in Religious Traditions; Islam, Bioethics in; Medical Ethics, History of: Near and Middle East; Population Ethics: Religious Traditions, Islamic Perspectives;* and other *Abortion* subentries

### BIBLIOGRAPHY

Abedin, Saleha Mahmood. 1977. "Islam and Muslim Fertility: Sociological Dimensions of a Demographic Dilemma." Ph.D. thesis, University of Pennsylvania.

Anees, Munawar Ahmad. 1989. *Islam and Biological Futures: Ethics, Gender and Technology.* London: Mansell.

Bakar, Osman. 1991. *Tawhid and Science: Essays on the History and Philosophy of Islamic Science.* Penang-Kuala Lumpur: Secretariat for Islamic Philosophy and Science.

Bouhdiba, Abdelwahab. 1985. *Sexuality in Islam,* tr. Alan Sheridan. London: Routledge & Kegan Paul.

Ebrahim, Abul Fadl Mohsin. 1988. *Biomedical Issues: Islamic Perspective.* Mobeni: Islamic Medical Association of South Africa.

Elgood, Cyril. 1962. "Tibb-ul-Nabbi or Medicine of the Prophet: Being a Translation of Two Works of the Same Name." *Osiris* 14: 33–192.

Elgood, Cyril. 1970. *Safavid Medical Practice; or, The Practice of Medicine, Surgery and Gynaecology in Persia between 1500 A.D. and 1750 A.D.* London: Luzac.

Maudoodi, Abul A'la. 1968. *Birth Control: Its Social, Political, Economic, Moral, and Religious Aspects.* 3rd ed. Lahore, Pakistan: Islamic Publications.

Musallam, Basim. 1983. *Sex and Society in Islam: Birth Control before the Nineteenth Century.* Cambridge, Eng.: Cambridge University Press.

Rahman, Fazlur. 1987. *Health and Medicine in the Islamic Tradition: Change and Identity.* New York: Crossroad.

Sayyid-Marsot, Afaf Lutfi, ed. 1979. *Society and the Sexes in Medieval Islam.* Malibu, CA: Undena.

# ABUSE, INTERPERSONAL

• • •

## I. CHILD ABUSE

Current pediatrics and social-work textbooks generally include chapters on child abuse that describe the epidemiology, clinical manifestations, differential diagnosis, and treatment of abused children. They usually discuss the legal requirement to notify state child-protection agencies of suspected abuse, and may describe the investigations such reports trigger. It is accepted by most pediatricians, social workers, and laymen that investigations may result in legal actions against parents and other responsible adults. Children may be removed from their homes. Parents may have their custodial rights terminated, and may face criminal charges. The entire process of diagnosis and intervention for child abuse is presented as both necessary and morally compelling.

### Changing Attitudes on Child Abuse

However, within this seeming consensus of moral sentiment lies a mystery. Until the twentieth century, much of what we now consider to be child abuse was regarded as morally acceptable and legally permissible. In fact, people generally argued not only that it was permissible to oppress and punish children to the point of physical abuse, but also that such abuse was necessary for the children's moral edification (Radbill). Thus, "Spare the rod and spoil the child." Parents and teachers had absolute authority over children's lives. They could, and did, physically and sexually abuse children with an impunity so complete that such acts were seldom recognized or acknowledged.

Our current approaches to child abuse reflect a radical change in our moral view of the family. Until the twentieth century, families were usually seen as small, autocratic moral universes. Parents (in most cases, fathers) could use children (and wives) as they saw fit. Children had no independent moral rights. The movement to recognize and prevent child abuse, and to punish abusers, reflects a partial empowerment of the child. Such a sea change in moral sentiment raises important questions about the timelessness of moral principles affecting the care of children. Either child abuse was always wrong but not recognized as wrong, suggesting that our moral sensitivities are improving over time, or child abuse became wrong only recently, suggesting that moral values are not timeless and immutable but transient and constantly evolving.

Whether moral principles, such as those designed to guide the care of children, have changed over time or whether people have gradually become more or less virtuous in the treatment of children will be debated elsewhere in this work. Currently, attempts to formulate standards for appropriate ethical and legal responses to child abuse can be seen as efforts to craft social and legal policies that reflect our views of how children should be cared for and reared. But parents and other caregivers receive conflicting messages from current social policies; whereas our society restricts child abuse, its institutions and laws condone other activities—such as sexual activity during early teenage years and exposure to violence in television, films, and daily life—that would have been regarded as morally problematic in societies of previous eras and are so regarded in non–U.S. societies in the early twenty-first century. From one perspective, these conflicting efforts can be seen as experiments in social policy; from another perspective, selective legal interventions in the area of child abuse are viewed as justified by the legal doctrine of *parens patriae*. In this doctrine the state claims an interest in protecting the lives and well-being of children, even if this means limiting parental autonomy and infringing on family privacy.

Nevertheless, physical and sexual abuse of children is still common; in most instances, abuse is never reported or discovered.

## Defining Child Abuse

Definitions of abuse are notoriously variable, circular, or designed to leave room for interpretation on a case-by-case basis. In the United States, the Child Abuse Prevention and Treatment Act of 1974 (PL93–247) defines abuse and neglect as:

> the physical and mental injury, sexual abuse, negligent treatment or maltreatment of a child under the age of 18 by a person who is responsible for the child's welfare under circumstances which indicate that the child's health and welfare is harmed or threatened thereby....

State definitions based on this law vary. Arguments about whether a particular act constitutes abuse under such a definition may focus on the nature of the act itself, whether

the act caused harm, whether there was or should have been prior recognition that the act would cause harm, and whether the caretaker might have prevented the harm.

In both physical and sexual abuse, different individuals or communities distinguish acceptable from unacceptable behaviors using different criteria. In physical abuse, a distinction must be made between acceptable forms of discipline or punishment and abuse. As Kim Oates (1982) points out, definitions must specify whether abuse should be defined in terms of particular actions or particular effects. He describes two children who are pushed roughly to the ground by their fathers. One falls against a carpeted floor, the other hits a protruding cupboard door. The second sustains a skull fracture, the first is uninjured. If an act must cause harm to be abuse, then the second child was clearly abused, while the first may not have been. Acts that leave no physical marks are harder to classify as abuse, and it is generally harder to sustain criminal convictions or obtain civil sanctions in such cases, even though an unmarked child may sustain as much or more psychological harm as from actions that cause physical signs of abuse.

In sexual abuse, definitional problems also arise. Child sexual abuse is generally intrafamilial, and falls under the rubric of incest. While prohibitions against incest are universal, different cultures define incest to include, or exclude, different activities. "Parent-child nudity, communal sleeping arrangements, and tolerance for masturbation and peer sex play in children coexist with stringent incest taboos.... (M)others in many cultures use genital manipulation to soothe and pleasure infants. Some cultures prescribe the deflowering of pubertal girls by an adult male or by the father" (Goodwin, p. 33). Exotic cultural differences may be mirrored by different beliefs in our own culture. Some parents may sleep with their children, bathe with them, or take pictures of the children naked on the beach. In some jurisdictions, these activities may be defined as illegal or morally inappropriate.

Cultural or religious differences may also play a role in evaluating what constitutes medical neglect. Christian Scientists, for example, may claim that it is appropriate not to take their sick children to a doctor, while courts may determine that such behavior constitutes neglect. Some Native Americans believe that organ transplantation is prohibited, and so may refuse lifesustaining treatment for their children in liver failure. Similarly, Jehovah's Witnesses may, on the basis of their belief, seek to refuse consent for blood transfusions for their children, even if transfusions would preserve life. In situations like these, judgments must be made about the relative importance of respecting religious and cultural diversity, on the one hand, and protecting the interests of vulnerable children, on the other.

In addition to cultural differences in defining what behaviors are or are not permissible, serious moral problems arise when we attempt to determine whether, in any particular case, a behavior that is clearly not permissible in fact occurred. Court cases may turn on the rules governing the collecting and presentation of evidence. Even in adult rape cases, victims have difficulty convincing juries that they have been raped. Such difficulties are compounded in child-abuse cases, where young children often cannot testify convincingly on their own behalf.

In summary, both physical abuse and sexual abuse of children exist along a spectrum, from obvious cruelty and exploitation to grayer areas of corporal punishment or sexual game playing. The strong moral arguments against egregious abuse of children often lose strength as the definition of abuse expands along a spectrum including activities that may be considered morally praiseworthy, morally acceptable, morally forgivable, or immoral but noncriminal.

## Reporting Child Abuse

Most laws are vague in defining the reporting requirements for child abuse. Generally, they require reporting if someone "has reasons to believe that a child has been subjected to abuse." Such laws do not attempt to quantify the degree of suspicion, the quality of the evidence, or the likelihood of abuse that must be present to compel a report. In the crafting of such laws, it seems that the goal was to protect people who report abuse by allowing broad latitude to individuals in defining what they mean by a "suspicion" of abuse. A utilitarian calculus seems to be at work—that it would be better to have reports made that prove to be groundless than to allow subtle cases of abuse to go unreported. Even with such vague and permissive requirements, evidence suggests that abuse is underreported rather than overreported.

There are a number of reasons why people might not report child abuse even though they believe it to be wrong. Child abuse may be ignored because people have difficulty defining and recognizing it (Besharov; Zellman, 1992). It may go undiscovered because adults who are aware that a child is being abused are reticent to get involved and do not report it (Dhooper et al.). Or professionals may feel reticent to threaten what they perceive as a therapeutic relationship with the adult or adults involved. When abuse is reported, health professionals and legal agencies need to weigh the relative risks and benefits of preserving the family against those of removing the child from it (Zellman, 1990).

Reticence to report suspected child abuse may be based on the sociology of healthcare delivery, on respect for confidentiality in the doctor-parent relationship, on unwillingness to stigmatize parents when there is doubt about the actual occurrence of abuse, or on a desire to preserve a therapeutic relationship or avoid the perception that professionals are enemies.

Pediatricians in private practice are paid by the parents or other adults responsible for the children to whom they provide care, and often develop long-term relationships with these adults and the children. In such situations, relationships must be based on mutual trust. Pediatricians may give adults the benefit of the doubt regarding injuries that may be associated with abuse. They may also be fearful that child-abuse reports will be bad for business. These factors may partially explain why reports of abuse are more likely to come from hospital emergency rooms than from private doctors' offices (Badger).

In addition to economic considerations, moral aspects of the doctor–parent (or other adult) relationship may impede reporting. Generally, doctors promise confidentiality, and the moral reasons for confidentiality are compelling. Adults must confide in doctors, and may need to tell them information that would be embarrassing or damaging were it known by others. However, this promise of confidentiality may conflict with a pediatrician's concern about the child's best interest. Although the law requires doctors to report suspected child abuse, reporting is quite sporadic and inconsistent (Dhooper et al.; Zellman, 1990; Oates). Studies of pediatricians reveal that older doctors are less likely to report child abuse than are younger doctors, and males are less likely to report it than females (Kean and Dukes). None of the studies that document inconsistent reporting disentangle the economic, moral, and legal considerations that lead doctors and other child-welfare professionals to report or not to report abuse.

Reticence to report may also result from a lack of faith in the efficacy of interventions. Many child-protection agencies are underfunded and understaffed. In times of tight budgets, they may not receive the highest legislative priority. As a result, they may be unable to provide counseling and supervision services to every child or family reported to them. In some states, child-protection agencies operate under court supervision because they have been found to neglect the children in their custody. While such agencies clearly provide excellent services to most children, highly publicized cases in which they have failed to provide adequate protection may lead to skepticism about the efficacy of reporting.

## Risks and Benefits of Intervention

Because society only recently recognized the problem of child abuse, there has been little time to evaluate the effects of different responses to abuse. Three types of responses have been attempted: (1) those designed to prevent abuse; (2) those designed to deal with the psychological consequences of abuse; and (3) those designed to punish offenders.

Preventive programs are difficult to evaluate because of almost insurmountable ethical and methodological problems (Conte). Abuse is a hidden problem. Assessing whether heightened awareness of the problem leads to increased reporting or decreased occurrence would require intrusive evaluation and follow-up for enormous numbers of people (Reppucci and Haugaard; Fink and McCloskey). Generally, studies focus on surrogate outcome measures, such as "ability to discriminate safe from unsafe situations," rather than on actual decreases in the incidence of sexual abuse (Hazzard et al., p. 134).

Intervention for children who have suffered abuse requires a delicate balance between trying to protect the child, trying to help the parents, and trying to preserve the family. Parents who abuse children often have been abused themselves, and may have a higher incidence of psychiatric problems (Steele and Pollack). Many parents regret their actions, desire psychiatric help, and comply with treatment programs. However, 5 to 30 percent of abused children who stay in their family are subject to further episodes of abuse (Jellinek et al.). At present, there are no reliable indicators of which parents will continue to abuse their children and which are likely to respond to therapy. Furthermore, any data that might address this issue will necessarily be probabilistic. Thus, decisions about the value of such data in an individual case will incorporate normative values about the degree of risk appropriate for a particular child facing a particular custody decision.

Programs designed to punish child abusers are driven less by considerations of the risks and benefits of interventions and more by the dictates of the legal system. Evidence against alleged abusers seldom establishes guilt beyond a reasonable doubt. As a result, criminal prosecution is rare, and conviction even rarer (Peters). Furthermore, it is unclear whether stricter laws or harsher punishments decrease the incidence of child abuse. As in other areas of criminal law, the justification for criminal prosecution seems to derive more from a notion of punitive justice than from a calculation of the degree to which punishment of offenders deters potential future offenders. Debate about this issue must take place in the context of more general debates about the morality of incarceration or the potential for rehabilitation in any criminal situation.

## Conclusion

An apparent consensus about child abuse masks profound disagreements about the proper boundaries of family privacy, the obligations of parents and health professionals, and governmental responsibility to oversee the care and nurturing of children. These disagreements are reflected in difficulties in defining child abuse, difficulties in enforcing compliance with mandatory reporting requirements, and difficulties in evaluating the effects of interventions. Thus, while the law requires that child abuse be reported if it is suspected, health professionals can create their own index of suspicion. Some providers may report ambiguous cases, while others rarely report suspected abuse at all.

Individuals who work with children must balance their legal and ethical obligations to children, to their parents or caretakers, and to society. Professionals who have a higher regard for familial privacy and parental authority may develop a stricter standard or a higher threshold for suspecting abuse, and thus may be less likely to report it. Professionals who believe more strongly in the independent rights of children may develop a lower threshold for suspecting abuse, and may thus be more likely to report it. Current legal and moral approaches, while theoretically compelling, are quite recent, and have not been thoroughly evaluated. The principle that children deserve protection and nurturance is generally accepted, but the means by which the principle is to be brought to fruition remain uncertain.

JOHN D. LANTOS (1995)
BIBLIOGRAPHY REVISED

SEE ALSO: *Children: History of Childhood; Circumcision, Female; Harm; Homicide; Social Work in Healthcare;* and other *Abuse, Interpersonal* subentries

### BIBLIOGRAPHY

American Academy of Pediatrics, American Academy of Pediatrics Committee on Bioethics. 1997. "Religious Objections to Medical Care." *Pediatrics* 99(2): 279–81.

Badger, Lee W. 1989. "Reporting of Child Abuse: Influence of Characteristics of Physician, Practice, and Community." *Southern Medical Journal* 82(3): 281–286.

Besharov, Douglas J. 1981. "Toward Better Research on Child Abuse and Neglect: Making Definitional Issues an Explicit Methodological Concern." *Child Abuse and Neglect* 5(4): 383–390.

Conte, Jon R. 1987. "Ethical Issues in Evaluation of Prevention Programs." *Child Abuse and Neglect* 11(2): 171–172.

Dhooper, Surjit S.; Royse, David D.; and Wolfe, L. C. 1991. "A Statewide Study of the Public Attitudes toward Child Abuse." *Child Abuse and Neglect* 15(1–2): 37–44.

Fink, Arlene, and McCloskey, Lois. 1990. "Moving Child Abuse and Neglect Prevention Programs Forward: Improving Program Evaluations." *Child Abuse and Neglect* 14(2): 187–206.

Gilbert, Neil, ed. 1997. *Combating Child Abuse: International Perspectives and Trends (Child Welfare).* New York: Oxford University Press.

Goodwin, Jean M. 1988. "Obstacles to Policymaking About Incest: Some Cautionary Folktales." In *Lasting Effects of Child Sexual Abuse,* pp. 21–37, ed. Gail Elizabeth Wyatt and Gloria Johnson Powell. Newbury Park, CA: Sage.

Greipp, M. E. 1997. "Ethical Decision Making and Mandatory Reporting in Cases of Suspected Child Abuse." *Journal of Pediatric Health Care* 11(6): 258–65.

Hazzard, Ann; Webb, Carol; Kleemeier, Carol; Angert, Lisa; and Pohl, Judy. 1991. "Child Sexual Abuse Prevention: Evaluation and One-Year Follow-up." *Child Abuse and Neglect* 15(1–2): 123–138.

Jellinek, Michael S.; Murphy, J. Michael; Poitrast, Francis; Quinn, Dorothy; Bishop, Sandra J.; and Goshko, Marilyn. 1992. "Serious Child Mistreatment in Massachusetts: The Course of 206 Children through the Courts." *Child Abuse and Neglect* 16(2): 179–185.

Kalichman, S. C. 1999. *Mandated Reporting of Suspected Child Abuse: Ethics, Law, and Policy,* 2nd edition. Washington, D.C.: American Psychological Association.

Kean, Robert B., and Dukes, Richard L. 1991. "Effects of Witness Characteristics on the Perception and Reportage of Child Abuse." *Child Abuse and Neglect* 15(4): 423–435.

Lutzker, J. R., ed. 1998. *Handbook of Child Abuse Research and Treatment.* New York: Plenum Publishing.

Oates, Kim. 1982. "Child Abuse: A Community Concern." *In Child Abuse—A Community Concern,* pp. 1–12, ed. Kim Oates. London: Butterworths.

Peters, James M. 1989. "Criminal Prosecution of Child Abuse: Recent Trends." *Pediatric Annals* 18(8): 505–506, 508–509.

Radbill, Samuel X. 1974. "A History of Child Abuse and Infanticide." In *The Battered Child,* 2nd edition, pp. 3–21, ed. Ray E. Helfer and C. Henry Kempe. Chicago: University of Chicago Press.

Reppucci, N. Dickon, and Haugarrd, Jeffrey J. 1989. "Prevention of Child Sexual Abuse: Myth or Reality." *American Psychologist* 44(10): 1266–1275.

Steele, Brandt F., and Pollack, Carl. 1974. "A Psychiatric Study of Parents Who Abuse Infants and Small Children." In *The Battered Child,* 2nd edition, pp. 89–133, ed. Ray E. Helfer and C. Henry Kempe. Chicago: University of Chicago Press.

Steinberg, A. M.; Pynoos, R. S.; Goenjian, A. K.; et al. 1999. "Are Researchers Bound By Child Abuse Reporting Laws?" *Child Abuse and Neglect* 23(8): 771–777.

Zellman, Gail L. 1990. "Report on Decision-Making Patterns among Mandated Child Abuse Reporters." *Child Abuse and Neglect* 14(3): 325–336.

Zellman, Gail L. 1992. "The Impact of Case Characteristics on Child Abuse Reporting Decisions." *Child Abuse and Neglect* 16(1): 57–74.

## II. ABUSE BETWEEN DOMESTIC PARTNERS

Common sense suggests that abuse between domestic partners is "just plain wrong." Nonetheless, domestic violence began to be recognized as an ethical issue only because of the advocacy work of grassroots battered-women's movements and of feminist and liberationist movements in theology, ethics, and the social sciences. This entry defines domestic violence, explores some of the reasons it is difficult for women to escape abuse, and outlines some of the underlying social and ethical issues.

### Definition of Domestic Violence and Its Broader Social Context

The term *domestic partners* implies some serious bond, such as marriage, a child in common, cohabitation, or financial ties. It also usually implies emotional and sexual connections between people who have chosen to be with each other. Emotional, legal, and material connections make it difficult to end the relationship once abuse occurs. Police officers, lawmakers, medical professionals, and the general public have found it difficult to acknowledge the prevalence of domestic violence or act to prevent it because of the voluntary, emotional nature of a relationship based in the private rather than the public sphere and because of patriarchal assumptions about women and marriage.

In any intimate relationship people may hurt each other, but abuse occurs when one person systematically hurts, threatens, rapes, manipulates, tries to kill, or kills the other, and when fear replaces trust and respect as the basis of the relationship. Physical violence, with the intent of one spouse to cause harm to the other, is the accepted definition of spouse abuse in all countries where spouse abuse has been studied (Gelles and Cornell). Consistent insults, criticism, disregard for one partner's needs, isolation, damage to property and pets, and withholding money, food, or other necessities are other ways abusers try to dominate and control the relationship. The overwhelming majority of spousal abuse throughout the world is by men against women (Gelles and Cornell; Levinson), suggesting the pervasive influence of patriarchal family and social structures on abuse.

It is hard to document the extent of domestic abuse for several reasons. First, until recently, very few countries have kept records of it—violence has to be reported to some authority in order to be recorded (Gelles and Cornell). Many countries lack the bureaucratic infrastructure to maintain centralized records about domestic violence even if they desired to do so. Second, domestic violence incidents are consistently underreported, because of the shame of the abused, the desire to protect the abuser, and the failure of many agencies where women seek help to ask for and record many kinds of evidence of abuse. Third, the information kept (e.g., percentage of police calls related to family disputes, homicide statistics, number of women served by shelters, percentage of people reporting violence in surveys) varies widely. Research about domestic abuse against women tends to lag behind research about child abuse. Most research studies have analyzed family violence in a single country, using approaches that provide no basis for crosscultural comparison (Gelles and Cornell).

Domestic violence is an international problem. The World Bank reports that gender-based violence accounts for as much death and ill-health in women between the ages of fifteen and forty-four as cancer, and more death and illhealth than malaria and car accidents combined (Venis and Horton). The World Health Organization (WHO) initiated a multi-country study on women's health and domestic violence in 1997 in response to the recommendation of an Expert Consultation on violence against women and the Beijing Platform for Action. Its objectives are to obtain reliable estimates of the prevalence of different forms of violence against women, to document the consequences of domestic violence on women's reproductive health, mental health, injuries, and general use of health services; to identify and compare risk and protective factors for domestic violence; and to identify strategies and services used by battered women. Research began in seven countries in 1999 and is expected to continue through 2002 (World Health Organization Multi-Country Study on Women's Health and Domestic Violence, Progress Report).

In the United States on average each year from 1992 to 1996 approximately 8 in 1,000 women and 1 in 1,000 men age twelve or older were violently victimized by a current or former spouse, boyfriend, or girlfriend (Henderson, 2000). In 1995, 26 percent of all female murder victims were slain by their husbands or boyfriends (FBI, 1996).

Despite the lack of statistical information and survey data, awareness of domestic abuse is increasing. In 1993 the United Nations (UN) General Assembly adopted the Declaration on the Elimination of Violence against Women and established a Special Rapporteur on Violence Against Women (U.S. Department of State). The UN designated November 25 as an International Day for the Elimination of Violence against Women in 1999. The U.S. Department of State highlighted the problem of rampant discrimination against women for the first time in 1993 in its annual report on human rights abuses. Examples cited included physical abuse against women in all countries; "honor killings" for alleged adultery by wives, especially in South America; denial in many countries of political, civil, or legal rights in voting, marriage, travel, testifying in court, inheriting and owning property, and obtaining custody of children; forced prostitution and the refusal to recognize marital rape as a crime on several continents; genital mutilation in many African countries; sexual and economic exploitation of domestic servants in Southeast Asia; and dowry deaths (murder of a bride when her family cannot give her husband's family the expected dowry) in Bangladesh and India. The Violence Against Women Act of 1994 set federal guidelines for intervention, arrest, prosecution, and treatment of battered women in the United States.

## The Psychological and Social Context of Domestic Abuse

The changes that occur in a battered woman's sense of selfesteem and competence are often more lasting and more damaging to the woman than the actual physical abuse. Battered women learn to pay attention to their partner's needs instead of their own in hopes of reducing the violence. They begin to distrust their own judgment and their own abilities to provide for themselves and their children (if they have children). They may eventually come to believe that they deserve the abuse they receive. When family, friends, religious leaders, police officers, and helping professionals disbelieve, blame, or trivialize battered women's experiences and do not respond to their appeals for help, women feel even more trapped and convinced that abuse is inevitable. Chances to escape abusive relationships or find a loving relationship begin to seem impossible (Moore).

Another psychological dynamic first described by Lenore E. Walker in her 1979 book, *The Battered Woman*, also helps to explain why it is so difficult for battered women to decide to leave an abusive relationship. Walker documented a three-part cycle of (1) a violent episode; (2) regret by the abuser, love, attention, reparation, and promises never to be abusive again (the "honeymoon period"); and (3) cessation of loving attention and a period of escalating tension between partners, leading to another violent episode. Battered women yearn for the honeymoon period of love and attention that reinforces their initial hopes for the relationship. Unfortunately, over time, the honeymoons become shorter and the severity and frequency of abuse increase, sometimes resulting in death. Walker also described the "learned helplessness syndrome," where women lose faith in their ability to act effectively because batterers respond so unpredictably and illogically to so many of their actions.

The emotional, psychological, and physical consequences of abuse must be understood in their larger context of sexism, patriarchy, and paternalistic dominance (Lerner). Gerda Lerner defined sexism as "the ideology of male supremacy, of male superiority, and of beliefs that support and sustain it" (Lerner, p. 240). Sexism undergirds patriarchy, "the institutionalization of male dominance over women and children in the family and the extension of male dominance over women in society in general" (Lerner, p. 239). A sociological study of domestic abuse in Scotland documented the connection between domestic violence and patriarchal marriage. The researchers concluded that the law, the church, economic opportunities, appeals to science or to "the natural order," and social customs all promote women's subordinate status in marriage. Women find their struggle to resist domination, including violence, within marriage labeled "wrong, immoral, and a violation of the respect and loyalty a wife is supposed to give her husband" (Dobash and Dobash, p. ix). A study of ninety small-scale societies found that economic inequality, inequality of domestic decision-making authority, and restrictions on women's freedom to divorce were the strongest predictors of wife beating (Levinson). The major religious faiths have traditionally taught male superiority, the duty of women to obey men, and the sin of divorce even in the case of extreme abuse, which only exacerbates religious women's difficulties in escaping abuse.

Women's subordination is ostensibly mitigated by the unwritten contract for exchange of services in marriage, which Lerner called "paternalistic dominance": Men are expected to provide economic support and protection from harm in exchange for obedience, sexual service, and unpaid domestic service, including care of dependent family members (Lerner). These expectations are built into marriage and divorce laws (Weitzman) and help define women's roles, opportunities, and sense of self (Degler). The perception and public rhetoric that women's subordination is "normal," "necessary," and even desirable for women may contradict women's lived experiences. Yet without language and communities in which women may define their own experience, subordination often goes unchallenged.

In a 1990 article in the *Annual of the Society of Christian Ethics,* Karen Lebacqz offered a powerful analysis of the role conditioning of men and women that contributes to domestic abuse in marital and nonmarital relationships. She argued that "'normal' patterns of male–female sexual relating in U.S. culture are defined by patterns of male dominance over women," so that women come to expect male domination and the possibility of violence in heterosexual relations (Lebacqz, p. 3). Many recent studies (Fortune; *Against Her*

*Will*) find that women have often experienced undesired forced sexual relations with male acquaintances that neither women nor men considered to be rape. Male power over women is eroticized in mainstream media and pornography and comes to be perceived as sexually desirable, even when women know their experiences of abuse are not desirable (Lebacqz).

Expectations of male dominance in private heterosexual relations are reinforced by men's greater access to economic, political, religious, and cultural power in public life. In a 1992 contribution to the *Annual of the Society of Christian Ethics,* Christine Firer Hinze analyzed how the creation and maintenance of distinct public and private realms tends to keep women dependent on male earning power and status. "A 'feminized' private realm confers indirect status and informal power in childbearing, homemaking, and other personalized nurturing, caretaking and consumption tasks … a separate, 'masculinized' public arena disperses public status and formal power in cultural, political, and economic matters" (Hinze, p. 283). Even within the public realm, women are most frequently employed in domestic service and in technical service and sales occupations with lower status and salaries than male-dominated occupations. In the United States, women of color are disproportionately represented in the lowest-paid positions in domestic service compared with white women (U.S. Department of Labor). Delores S. Williams, in her contribution to the 1994 book, *Violence against Women,* offered a nuanced analysis of violence in the United States against women of color. She insisted that the analytic context of violence against African-American women must include attention to three levels: (1) the national level, the history of national violence against African-American people; (2) the work level, including the violence African-American women experience working in the homes of white employers; and (3) the home level, violence experienced in their own homes. The differences between male and female access to power and between women of different ethnic groups become especially apparent when women who decide to leave abusive partners try to find adequate jobs, housing, medical care, child care, and education for their children.

## Emerging Awareness of Domestic Violence as a Social and Clinical Problem

The understanding of the *paterfamilias* (male head of a household) with life and death control over wife (wives), children, slaves, and property is found in most every culture throughout the world: in ancient Greek and Roman society; in the Middle Eastern cultures represented in Christian,

Jewish, and Muslim scriptures; and in Confucian understandings of the family, to name a few examples. Religious values have played an ambiguous role, sometimes perpetuating, sometimes condemning domestic abuse. For instance, trends in Christian history that attribute to women responsibility for the presence of evil in creation also sanctioned public torture and murder of women accused of being witches or heretics (Brown and Bohn; Fortune). Yet ideals in all religions, such as the intrinsic worth of all people in Christianity or of special obligations of husbands toward wives and vice versa in Christianity and Judaism, have also condemned domestic abuse. The emergence of religious and secular movements to prevent child abuse and violence against women could not occur until women and children began to be seen as individuals in their own right. In her 1999 book, *Wounds of the Spirit,* Traci West offered a model of how churches can support African-American women in their resistance to violence based on the obligation of congregations to be agents of healing in their families and communities.

The gradual shift in attention from silent acceptance of abuse to its recognition as a problem can be illustrated by examining the history of changing laws in the United States. Until the late nineteenth century, the assumptions underlying laws and social policy in the United States came from English common law, where the husband was considered the head of the house with absolute control over his wife and children. The term *rule of thumb* comes from a modification of English common law that gives husbands the right to beat wives "provided that he used a switch no bigger than his thumb" (Martin, p. 32). From 1874 until the 1970s, the prevailing U.S. court precedents held that although husbands do not have the legal right to chastise their wives, the courts should not interfere in domestic affairs except when permanent injury, malice, cruelty, or dangerous violence can be proven (Martin). In the 1970s, growing recognition of the severity of abuse against women, due largely to the "women's liberation movement," led most states to offer women legal protection against abuse by their husbands or by the fathers of their children. In many states, however, access to information about legal options, advocates to clarify procedures and support women, and affordable remedies are still hard to find.

The first battered women's shelters were established in the 1970s in England and the United States when women who had suffered abuse came to newly formed women's support groups asking for a place to stay (Schechter). In her 1992 book, *Trauma and Recovery,* Judith Lewis Herman described the interaction of consciousness-raising groups, increased public awareness, and changes in social policy and

the treatment of female victims of rape and domestic violence by medical and psychological professionals in the United States, beginning in the 1970s. Public discussion of domestic violence gave its victims the language, the courage, and the end to isolation that enabled them to decide that abuse against them was wrong even when prevailing social norms had led them to accept abuse as normal and justifiable (Herman; Schechter; Russell).

"Why don't women just leave?" is a frequent query. Unlike children or the elderly, adult women are expected to be able to protect themselves, so women who "choose" to remain with an abuser are often blamed for their situation. Men and women are—in theory—peers in a relationship of mutual equality and need, although the reality of male privilege undermines genuine equality. The long-term effects of abuse by a chosen lover, the economic, social, and legal barriers faced by women living independently or with children, the fear of even greater violence or death for the woman or for other family members if she leaves, and the pressure on women to sustain intimate relationships with men reduce the options available to women who want abuse to end. These same factors also reduce battered women's ability to recognize and act on existing options. According to the National Clearinghouse on Domestic Violence, more than 79 percent of all violent attacks occur after a woman leaves her abuser.

## Legislative Issues

Increasing awareness of the extent and severity of violence against women in the United States led to the passage of the federal Violence Against Women Act in 1994. This act made orders of protection enforceable, recommended mandatory arrest laws, and granted federal money for battered women's shelters and legal services. It also allowed battered women who were not legal residents to petition for immigration privileges without the help of their abusive spouse. Twenty-nine states recognize domestic violence as a factor in custody disputes, and "battered women's defense" is legally recognized under federal and state law. Mandatory arrest policies have become central to most states' strategies to protect women, punish offenders, deter future violence and convey the new social norm that battering is wrong (Sontag). Perhaps in partial response, the number of violent victimizations of women by an intimate partner declined from 1993 to 1996, from 1.1 million reported incidents to 840,000 incidents (Greenfield et al.).

Yet some people are beginning to question the effectiveness of mandatory arrest policies because they undermine women's right to self-determination, their complicity in the violence, and their ability to negotiate safety for themselves and their children without police intervention (Mills). Is a male-dominated and racially biased judicial system revictimizing women by forcing them to share intimate and often shameful accounts of their lives in front of court authorities and to subject the men they still love to a legal system whose racial and economic fairness they question? Mandatory arrest policies also disproportionately affect low-income batterers, perhaps because more affluent batterers and victims have more access to private lawyers, doctors, escape places, and treatment options before the police are called. In their 1997 report, *Preventing Crime,* Lawrence W. Sherman and colleagues found a correlation between men's social status and increased violence: Arrests seem to deter employed men but make unemployed men more violent. Advocates for battered women counter that though the laws are imperfect they are at present the best way to protect battered women and ensure that domestic violence is treated as the crime that it is.

## Medical Care

Questions about the possibility of domestic violence should be part of all regular medical histories for all women in all settings where women come for medical care. Domestic violence affects women of all economic groups, educational levels, ethnic groups, religions, and ages. Routinely asking about violence and childhood sexual abuse may help abused women recognize that they are not alone and that help is available. Questions should be posed so that they do not impute blame to women. Women who are abused may well deny their abuse out of fear, shame, or distrust. This is far more likely when their partners accompany them to doctors' offices or emergency rooms: Women need to be asked about abuse when they are alone, or at least when their partners are not able to hear their responses. Information about resources for battered women should be prominently displayed and easily available for women to take without their asking.

Battered women who have left their abusers are also likely to return more than once before they are ready to leave permanently. This can be frustrating to medical professionals who treat a particular woman's injuries repeatedly and can lead them to blame the woman, who needs to take her own time to decide how she can live in safety. Accurate medical records, including clinical reasons for suspecting abuse, are essential evidence for women who may eventually press criminal or civil charges against their abusers. Suspicious bruises should be noted on medical charts for an accurate history and evidence for possible future use. No laws require reporting suspected abuse against women

(whereas there are such laws for suspected child abuse), because women are not "dependent." Nonetheless, if medical professionals incorporate questions and information about domestic violence into their routine treatment of women, they will address some of the social barriers that keep battered women from finding safety.

Ignorance about domestic violence and childhood sexual abuse also plagues psychotherapists, psychiatrists, and clergy who do not understand the emotional or material barriers that make leaving difficult. Often, they either blame women for remaining in dangerous relationships or they consistently ignore signs of abuse and refuse to pay serious attention to women who talk about abuse. Couples therapy often tries to assign responsibility for problems equally to each partner in the relationship, which ignores the reality of violence and the fear of the abuser that makes abusive relationships inherently unequal. Attributing responsibility for the violence to the offender, and specific treatment for the batterer in individual therapy or groups, is essential if abuse is to end. Fear of retaliation by the abuser can also prevent counseling professionals from intervening in situations of domestic abuse.

Treatment resources for male abusers are still scarce. Most abusers deny they have a problem. Most batterers participate in treatment groups for batterers only when they are ordered to do so by a judicial authority. Inconsistent prosecution, enforcement, and sentencing often reinforce abusers' beliefs that their abuse is not a serious problem. Mandated treatment programs are often predominantly attended by low-income men, men on welfare, or men with prior criminal records. They are likely to conclude that learning to avoid arrest is more important than changing their abusive behaviors. Treatment programs take several different approaches: Some are primarily didactic (designed to teach), some use cognitive and behavioral approaches, and some include attention to a batterer's psychological history and psychodynamic issues and the circumstances of the abuse. There is no definitive study that has proved the effectiveness of any treatment approach (see Sherman et al.).

## Conclusion

Ethical issues raised by abuse between domestic partners fall into categories of treatment and prevention. Treatment includes breaking the silence that surrounds domestic violence; holding abusers legally accountable for their actions and requiring them to cease their violence; listening to victims; helping victims recognize their strengths and believe they are worthy to live in safety; and helping victims navigate through social, economic, legal, and religious barriers to safety (NiCarthy). The balance between active intervention to keep women from being hurt or killed, and respecting their need to decide how and when to end an abusive relationship, is difficult to find.

Nuancing the caricature of completely violent man and wholly submissive victimized woman is also essential in prevention, treatment, and ethical analysis. Unpacking the complicated dynamics of love, anger, and violence in particular relationships may reduce incidences of violence in those relationships. Some men are battered by women, and abuse occurs in same-sex relationships. Yet it is vital to remember the context of unequal power within which men and women learn to love, fight, attack, and seek safety. No woman will be safe until social, political, and economic institutions ensure her access to the material resources she needs to support herself and her children.

Laws alone are not enough, in the United States or any other country, to prevent abuse. In Bangladesh, a nation with very strong laws against battering, violence against women continues to rise sharply (Venis and Horton). Prevention includes challenging the prevailing social norms of sexism and patriarchy, the cultural definitions of masculinity and femininity, and the assumption that violence is a legitimate way of resolving conflict between people or groups of people. Broad economic and educational empowerment of women is ultimately the only way to end violence against women.

ALLISON W. MOORE (1995)
REVISED BY ALLISON W. MOORE
LAURA A. RUSSELL

SEE ALSO: *Family and Family Medicine; Feminism; Harm; Human Rights; Sexual Ethics; Women, Historical and Cross-Cultural Perspectives;* and other *Abuse, Interpersonal* subentries

### BIBLIOGRAPHY

*Against Her Will: Rape on Campus.* 1989. Directed by Jorn Winther. Lifetime Productions. Cited in Karen Lebacqz, "Love Your Enemy: Sex, Power, and Christian Ethics," *Annual of the Society of Christian Ethics* 1990: 3–26.

American Medical Association. Council on Ethical and Judicial Affairs. 1992. "Physicians and Domestic Violence: Ethical Considerations." *Journal of the American Medical Association* 267(23): 3190–3193.

Brown, Joanne Carlson, and Bohn, Carole R., eds. 1989. *Christianity, Patriarchy, and Abuse: A Feminist Critique.* New York: Pilgrim.

Browne, Angela. 1987. *When Battered Women Kill.* New York: Free Press.

Degler, Carl N. 1980. *At Odds: Women and the Family in America from the Revolution to the Present.* New York: Oxford University Press.

Dobash, R. Emerson, and Dobash, Russell. 1979. *Violence against Wives: A Case against the Patriarchy.* New York: Free Press.

Fortune, Marie M. 1983. *Sexual Violence: The Unmentionable Sin.* New York: Pilgrim.

Gelles, Richard J., and Cornell, Claire Pedrick, eds. 1983. *International Perspectives on Family Violence.* Lexington, MA: Lexington Books.

Gondolf, Edward W. 1985. *Men Who Batter: An Integrated Approach for Stopping Wife Abuse.* Holmes Beach, FL: Learning Publications.

Greenfeld, Lawrence A.; Rand, Michael R.; Craven, Diane; et al., eds. 1998. *Violence by Intimates: Analysis of Data on Crimes by Current or Former Spouses, Boyfriends, and Girlfriends.* Washington, D.C.: U.S. Department of Justice, Office of Justice Programs, Bureau of Justice Statistics. Cited in Helene Henderson, *Domestic Violence and Child Abuse Sourcebook.* Detroit, MI: Omnigraphics, 2000.

Henderson, Helene. 2000. *Domestic Violence and Child Abuse Sourcebook.* Detroit, MI: Omnigraphics.

Herman, Judith Lewis. 1992. *Trauma and Recovery.* New York: Basic.

Hinze, Christine Firer. 1992. "Power in Christian Ethics: Resources and Frontiers for Scholarly Exploration." *Annual of the Society of Christian Ethics,* pp. 277–290.

Kumari, Ranjana. 1989. *Brides Are Not for Burning.* New Delhi: Radiant.

Lebacqz, Karen. 1990. "Love Your Enemy: Sex, Power, and Christian Ethics." *Annual of the Society of Christian Ethics* 1990: 3–26.

Lerner, Gerda. 1986. *The Creation of Patriarchy.* New York: Oxford University Press.

Levinson, David. 1989. *Family Violence in Cross-Cultural Perspective.* Newbury Park, CA: Sage.

Martin, Del. 1983. *Battered Wives,* rev. edition. New York: Pocket Books.

Mills, Linda G. 1999. "Killing Her Softly: Intimate Abuse and the Violence of State Intervention." *Harvard Law Review* 113(2): 550–613.

Moore, Allison. 1990. "Moral Agency of Women in a Battered Women's Shelter." *Annual of the Society of Christian Ethics* 1990: 131–148.

NiCarthy, Ginny. 1982. *Getting Free: A Handbook for Women in Abusive Relationships.* Seattle, WA: Seal.

Pizzey, Erin. 1974. *Scream Quietly or the Neighbors Will Hear.* London: If Books.

Roy, Maria. 1988. *Children in the Crossfire.* Deerfield, FL: Health Communications.

Russell, Diana E. H. 1984. *Sexual Exploitation: Rape, Child Sexual Abuse, and Workplace Harassment.* Beverly Hills, CA: Sage.

Schechter, Susan. 1982. *Women and Male Violence: The Visions and Struggles of the Battered Women's Movement.* Boston: South End.

Sherman, Lawrence W.; Gottfredson, Denise C.; MacKenzie; et al. 1997. *Preventing Crime: What Works, What Doesn't, What's Promising: A Report to the United States Congress.* Washington, D.C.: U.S. Department of Justice, Office of Justice Programs.

Sontag, Deborah. 2002. "Fierce Entanglements." *New York Times Magazine,* November 17, pp. 52–57, 62, 84.

"Special Report: Everyday Violence against Women." 1990. *Ms.* September–October, 33–56.

United Nations. General Assembly. 1979. Thirty-Fourth Session. Official Records. Supplement (no. 46) at 193. *Convention on the Elimination of All Forms of Discrimination against Women.* UN General Assembly Resolution 34/180.

United Nations. General Assembly. 1993. Forty-Eighth Session. Official Records. Supplement (no. 49) at 217. *Declaration on the Elimination of Violence against Women.* UN General Assembly Resolution 48/104.

U.S. Department of Justice. Federal Bureau of Investigation (FBI). 1996. *Crime in the United States, 1995.* Washington, D.C.: Government Printing Office. Cited in Helene Henderson, *Domestic Violence and Child Abuse Sourcebook.* Detroit, MI: Omnigraphics, 2000.

U.S. Department of Labor. Women's Bureau. 1986. "Twenty Facts about Women Workers." Washington, D.C.: Government Printing Office.

U.S. Department of State. 1994. *Country Reports on Human Rights Practices for 1993: Report Submitted to the Committee on Foreign Affairs.* Washington, D.C.: Government Printing Office.

Venis, Sarah, and Horton, Richard. 2002. "Violence against Women: A Global Burden." *Lancet* 359(9313): 1172.

Walker, Lenore E. 1979. *The Battered Woman.* New York: Harper and Row.

Weitzman, Lenore J. 1981. *The Marriage Contract: Spouses, Lovers, and the Law.* New York: Free Press.

West, Traci. 1999. *Wounds of the Spirit.* New York: New York University Press.

Wetzel, Janice Wood. 1992. *The World of Women: In Pursuit of Human Rights.* New York: New York University Press.

Williams, Delores S. 1994. "African-American Women in Three Contexts of Domestic Violence." In *Violence against Women,* ed. Elisabeth Schüssler Fiorenza and M. Shawn Copeland. Maryknoll, NY: Orbis Books.

INTERNET RESOURCE

World Health Organization Multi-Country Study on Women's Health and Domestic Violence, Progress Report, May, 2001. Available from <http://www.who.int/mipfiles/2255/FinalVAWprogressreportforwebpagewithoutcover.pdf>.

## III. ELDER ABUSE

The phenomenon known as elder abuse first appeared in the British scientific literature in 1975 (Burston) to describe the physical abuse of an elderly dependent person by a caregiving family member. In the years that followed, the definition expanded to include acts of commission (physical, psychological, and financial abuse) and omission (neglect) that result in harm to a person sixty-five years (in some states, sixty years) or older by a relative or a person with whom the elder has a trusting relationship. Self-neglect and self-abuse typically are included under broad conceptualizations of elder abuse. They refer to neglectful or abusive behaviors of older persons directed at themselves that threaten their own health or safety.

Beginning in the mid-1980s the meaning attached to elder abuse expanded further to reflect a criminalization of the phenomenon. Accordingly, there evolved interest in such areas as sexual assault in later life, battered older women, and fraud and scams (e.g., Ramsey-Klawsnik; Harris; Tueth). Likewise, since the 1990s there has been a resurgence of attention given to elder abuse in institutions, particularly nursing facilities. Exposure of fires and inadequate care in these settings during the 1970s fueled the enactment of federal legislation to protect residents. Investigations of resident conditions led to the identification of additional institutional elder abuse forms, like violation of rights, thefts, and examples of covert abuse (e.g., Meddaugh; Payne and Kovic; Harris and Benson). Finally, international perspectives on elder abuse resulted in the United Nations (2002) World Assembly on Aging's delineation of still more abuse forms. Included among them are variations emanating out of social conditions in individual countries, like systemic abuse as well as political violence and armed conflict.

Throughout this thirty-year period of problem recognition and definition expansion, there has been concern about the lack of universally accepted definitions and forms of elder abuse evident in either research or state laws. The most notable attempts to standardize both are found in research conducted by Margaret Hudson and her associates (Hudson, 1991; Hudson and Carlson, 1999; Hudson et al., 2000). Using a national panel of elder abuse experts, Hudson developed a five-level elder abuse taxonomy with eleven related definitions. Subsequent work compared the experts' perceptions to public perceptions across cultures, the results suggesting differences between cultural groups in defining and responding to elder abuse. Other studies have yielded similar findings (Tatara, 1997, 1999). For example, Georgia Anetzberger, Jill Korbin, and Susan Tomita (1996) focused on four ethnic groups in Ohio and Washington and discovered that the worst thing family members could do to an elderly person was psychological neglect, according to European-American and Puerto Rican subjects, and psychological abuse, according to Japanese-American and African-American subjects. Only African Americans listed financial abuse or exploitation among the worst things. Moreover, response to elder abuse varied by ethnic group. European-Americans and African Americans typically would contact an agency serving elders, Japanese Americans would talk to family or friends, and Puerto Ricans would contact the proper authorities.

## Policy Development

In the United States interest in elder abuse was sparked by testimony on battering of parents before a U.S. House of Representatives subcommittee investigating family violence in 1978. The growing numbers of elderly persons in society, the rising political power of the older population, and the existing state bureaucracies for delivering protective services lent legitimacy to making elder abuse a public issue. Despite the efforts of a few representatives to pass national legislation throughout the 1980s, no action was taken by the Congress. Nevertheless, federal agencies did incorporate elder abuse into their agendas, but not at the funding level of the U.S. Children's Bureau program for child abuse.

Without a national focus, a knowledge base, or model statutes, the states developed their own laws, definitions, and reporting procedures. Some used existing adult protective legislation; others, domestic violence acts. Still others passed specific elder abuse laws. By the late 1980s, each of the fifty states had a system in place for receiving reports and investigating, assessing, and monitoring cases. Four-fifths of the states adopted the child-abuse approach, making it mandatory for health and social-service professionals and others who work with older persons to report suspected cases of abuse and neglect, subject to a fine or imprisonment or both. In the other states, reporting is voluntary.

Despite the widespread enactment of mandatory reporting laws, most elder abuse is not reported to authorities charged with investigating the problem. It is estimated that only one in eight (or fewer) abuse situations are reported (Pillemer and Finkelhor; U.S. House Select Committee on Aging). Still, elder abuse reporting has increased over time. From 1986 to 1996 the number of reports nationwide grew 150 percent (i.e., 117,000 to 293,000). During this period reports of neglect and self-neglect increased; those of sexual abuse remained constant; and reports of physical, financial, and psychological abuse decreased (Tatara and Kuzmeskus).

Since the 1980s all states have made revisions to their protective or elder abuse laws, often to clarify definitions, increase penalties for perpetrators, or criminalize certain abuse types. Much recent policy activity seems centered at the federal level. This includes convening the first National Policy Summit on Elder Abuse in 2001. More than eighty individuals and agencies from across the country identified priority recommendations to address elder abuse at multiple levels of responsibility. Some of these recommendations are evident in the first comprehensive legislation to address elder abuse—the Elder Justice Act, introduced in the U.S. Senate in 2002. Among its many provisions, the Act seeks to create Offices of Elder Justice in the Departments of Health and Human Services and Justice, develop forensic capacity in abuse detection, establish safe havens and other programs for elderly victims, and increase efforts to address abuse in long-term care.

## Theoretical Considerations

Early attempts to understand the nature of elder abuse were influenced by the child-abuse model. Victims were viewed as very dependent older women mistreated by well-meaning but overburdened adult daughters. Later findings suggested that spouse abuse might be a more useful framework for study, since the individuals involved were legally independent adults. To some health researchers, however, using the family violence paradigm, with its emphasis on harm, intentionality, and responsibility, was counterproductive, particularly in cases that involved elders with unmet needs (Phillips, 1986; Fulmer and O'Malley). They recommended that elder abuse be considered from the perspective of family caregiving. None of these interpretations are sufficient in and of themselves. Neither the child abuse nor the spouse abuse model takes into consideration the impact of the aging process, while the family caregiving theory cannot explain abusive situations in which the victim has no unmet physical needs. It has been suggested that the concept of elder abuse may be too complex to be encompassed in one unifying theoretical model (Stein).

## Risk Factors and Characteristics

Although early studies were useful in documenting the existence of the problem and promoting state elder abuse policies, they were generally based on data collected from agency files, used small, unrepresentative samples, and lumped together the various types of abuse. Karl Pillemer (1986) sought to overcome some of these methodological weaknesses by interviewing victims directly, adding a nonabused comparison group, and limiting the investigation to physical abuse. His results showed that the abusers were much more likely than the comparison group of caregivers to have mental, emotional, and/or alcohol problems and to be dependent on the victims. Conversely, the abused elders were less functionally dependent than the control group in carrying out their activities of daily living. The families in which abuse occurred also tended to have fewer outside contacts and were less satisfied with them than were their nonabuse counterparts. Similar results have been reported by other researchers (Phillips, 1988; Bristowe and Collins; Anetzberger; Lachs et al., 1997).

A comparison of 328 cases by abuse type revealed three distinct profiles (Wolf et al.). Perpetrators of physical/ psychological abuse were more likely than perpetrators of neglect to have a history of mental illness and alcohol abuse, and to be dependent on the victim for financial resources. The victims were apt to be in poor emotional health but relatively independent in the activities of daily living. In contrast, those cases involving neglect appeared to be very much related to the dependency needs of the victim. Neither psychological problems nor financial dependency was a significant factor in the lives of these perpetrators; instead, the victims were a source of stress. Financial abuse represented still another profile. The victims were generally widowed and had few social supports. The perpetrators had financial problems and histories of substance abuse. Rather than interpersonal pathology or victim dependency, the salient factor in explaining these cases was the desire for money.

Few studies have examined the consequences of elder abuse. Those that have suggest that the effects of abuse infliction may have physical, behavioral, psychological, or social dimensions. In particular, victims of elder abuse seem to experience higher levels of depression than non-victims (Pillemer and Prescott; Harris). Furthermore, they are three times as likely to die sooner (Lachs et al., 1998).

## Prevalence and Incidence

Although knowledge about the extent of elder abuse is sorely needed to guide policy and planning activities, no national prevalence study has been conducted in the United States. Among localized studies, the best known used a methodology that had been validated in two national family violence surveys. Karl Pillemer and David Finkelhor (1988) surveyed 2,020 noninstitutionalized elders living in the metropolitan Boston area and found that 3.2 percent had experienced physical abuse, verbal aggression, and/or neglect in the period since they reached sixty-five years. Spouse abuse was more prevalent (58%) than abuse by adult children (24%), the proportion of victims was roughly equally divided between males and females, and economic status and age

were not related to the risk of abuse. Using comparable methodologies, but typically including financial abuse among forms to be investigated, national prevalence studies in Canada, Great Britain, Finland, and the Netherlands found that between 4 and 6 percent of older people surveyed were elder abuse victims (Podnieks; Ogg and Bennett; Kivelä et al.; Comijs et al.).

In 1998 the National Center on Elder Abuse completed the first national incidence study on elder abuse in the United States. Using a representative sample of twenty counties in fifteen states, two data sources were examined to identify the number of unduplicated new cases of elder abuse in a single year. The data sources were reports to Adult Protective Services and reports from sentinels, namely, specially trained community agency personnel having frequent contact with older people. The results for 1996 suggested a national incidence rate of 551,011, with self-neglect and neglect comprising over two-thirds of all elder abuse reported.

## Treatment and Ethical Issues

A number of potential conflicts face practitioners who are handling elder abuse cases. While tangible proof may be obtainable in situations involving physical and financial abuse, psychological abuse and neglect are far more difficult to verify. Symptoms of sexual abuse may elude the investigator who is not aware that old people can be so victimized. Cultural biases and lack of full knowledge about the circumstances involved in a case may lead a worker to conclude, falsely, that abuse has occurred. The instability of the mental and physical status of the victim and/or the perpetrator and the dynamics of their relationship may add to case uncertainty. The issue of competency can be particularly troublesome. There may be resistance on the part of the victim to undergo medical assessment, or of the perpetrator to allow it, or even of the medical profession to make a decision.

An individual who under the law is mandated to report a case of suspected abuse may hesitate because the details of the situation have not been fully documented. Whether the problem is civil or criminal may be unclear. Certainly, the unwillingness of the victim to press charges has been a major hindrance to intervention efforts. Even though the law may require an investigation, the older person may not wish to cooperate or to accept the services that are offered. This negative response brings the worker face to face with a dilemma: the interest of the state, professionals, and society in protecting vulnerable persons versus the individual's right to self-determination; in terms of ethical principles, the tension between autonomy and beneficence.

## Conclusion

Advances in understanding the nature of elder abuse will necessitate examining the problem from many perspectives. Not only must distinctions be made among the various types of elder abuse, but more attention must be paid to differences based on gender, race, culture, relationships, and circumstances. The growing interest in the problem among social scientists and medical personnel all over the world is important. The results of their efforts should be very constructive in building the theoretical and empirical base for successful treatment and prevention programs.

ROSALIE S. WOLF (1995)
REVISED BY GEORGIA J. ANETZBERGER

SEE ALSO: *Aging and the Aged: Old Age; Dementia; Harm; Long-Term Care;* and other *Abuse, Interpersonal* subentries

### BIBLIOGRAPHY

Anetzberger, Georgia J. 1987. *The Etiology of Elder Abuse by Adult Offspring.* Springfield, IL: Charles C. Thomas.

Anetzberger, Georgia J.; Korbin, Jill E.; and Tomita, Susan K. 1996. "Defining Elder Mistreatment in Four Ethnic Groups across Two Generations." *Journal of Cross-Cultural Gerontology* 11: 187–212.

Bristowe, Elizabeth, and Collins, John B. 1989. "Family Mediated Abuse of Non-Institutionalized Frail Elderly Men and Women Living in British Columbia." *Journal of Elder Abuse and Neglect* 1(1): 45–64.

Burston, G. R. 1975. "Granny-Battering." *British Medical Journal* 3(5983): 592.

Comijs, Hannie C.; Pot, Anne M.; Smit, Johannes H.; Bouter, Lex H.; and Jonker, Cees. 1998. "Elder Abuse in the Community: Prevalence and Consequences." *Journal of the American Geriatrics Society* 46: 885–888.

Fulmer, Terry, and O'Malley, Terrence. 1987. *Inadequate Care of the Elderly: A Health Care Perspective on Abuse and Neglect.* New York: Springer.

Harris, Diana K., and Benson, Michael L. 1998. "Nursing Home Theft: The Hidden Problem." *Journal of Aging Studies* 12(1): 57–67.

Harris, Sarah B. 1996. "For Better or for Worse: Spouse Abuse Grown Old." *Journal of Elder Abuse and Neglect* 8(1): 1–33.

Hudson, Margaret F. 1991. "Elder Mistreatment: A Taxonomy with Definitions by Delphi." *Journal of Elder Abuse and Neglect* 3(2): 1–20.

Hudson, Margaret F.; Beasley, Cherry; Benedict, Ruth H.; et al. 2000. "Elderly Abuse: Some Caucasian-American Views." *Journal of Elder Abuse and Neglect* 12(1): 89–114.

Hudson, Margaret F., and Carlson, John R. 1999. "Elder Abuse: Its Meaning to Caucasians, African Americans, and Native Americans." In *Understanding Elder Abuse in Minority Populations,* pp. 187–204, ed. Toshio Tatara. Philadelphia: Brunner/Mazel.

Kivelä, Sirkka-Liisa; Köngäs-Saviaro, Päivi; Kesti, Erkki; Pahkal, Kimmo; and Ijäs, Maija-Liisa. 1992. "Abuse in Old Age—Epidemiological Data from Finland." *Journal of Elder Abuse and Neglect* 4(3):1–12.

Lachs, Mark S.; Williams, Christianna; O'Brien, Shelley; Hurst, Leslie; and Horwitz, Ralph. 1997. "Risk Factors for Reported Elder Abuse and Neglect: A Nine-Year Observational Cohort Study." *The Gerontologist* 37(4): 469–474.

Lachs, Mark S.; Williams, Christianna S.; O'Brien, Shelley; Pillemer, Karl A.; and Charlson, Mary E. 1998. "The Mortality of Elder Mistreatment." *Journal of the American Medical Association* 280(5): 428–432.

Meddaugh, Dorothy I. 1993. "Covert Elder Abuse in the Nursing Home." *Journal of Elder Abuse and Neglect* 5(3): 21–38.

National Center on Elder Abuse. 1998. *The National Elder Abuse Incidence Study.* Washington, D.C.: Author.

Ogg, Jim, and Bennett, Gerry C. J. 1992. "Elder Abuse in Britain." *British Medical Journal* 305: 998–999.

Payne, Brian K., and Kovic, Richard. 1995. "An Empirical Examination of the Characteristics, Consequences, and Causes of Elder Abuse in Nursing Homes." *Journal of Elder Abuse and Neglect* 7(4): 61–74.

Phillips, Linda R. 1986. "Theoretical Explanations of Elder Abuse: Competing Hypotheses and Unresolved Issues." In *Elder Abuse: Conflict in the Family,* pp. 197–217, ed. Karl A. Pillemer and Rosalie S. Wolf. Dover, MA: Auburn House.

Phillips, Linda R. 1988. "The Fit of Elder Abuse with the Family Violence Paradigm and the Implications of a Paradigm Shift for Clinical Practice." *Public Health Nursing* 5(4): 222–229.

Pillemer, Karl A. 1986. "Risk Factors in Elder Abuse: Results from a Case-Control Study." In *Elder Abuse: Conflict in the Family,* pp. 239–264, ed. Karl A. Pillemer and Rosalie S. Wolf. Dover, MA: Auburn House.

Pillemer, Karl A., and Finkelhor, David. 1988. "The Prevalence of Elder Abuse: A Random Sample Survey." *Gerontologist* 28: 51–57.

Pillemer, Karl, and Prescott, Denise. 1989. "Psychological Effects of Elder Abuse: A Research Note." *Journal of Elder Abuse and Neglect* 1(1): 65–74.

Podnieks, Elizabeth. 1992. "A National Survey on the Abuse of the Elderly in Canada." *Journal of Elder Abuse and Neglect* 4(1/2): 1–25.

Ramsey-Klawsnik, Holly. 1991. "Elder Sexual Abuse: Preliminary Findings." *Journal of Elder Abuse and Neglect* 3(3): 73–90.

Stein, Karen. 1991. "A National Agenda for Elder Abuse and Neglect Research: Issues and Recommendations." *Journal of Elder Abuse and Neglect* 3(3): 91–108.

Tatara, Toshio, ed. 1997. "Elder Abuse in Minority Populations." *Journal of Elder Abuse and Neglect* 9(2).

Tatara, Toshio, ed. 1999. *Understanding Elder Abuse in Minority Populations.* Philadelphia: Brunner/Mazel.

Tatara, Toshio, and Kuzmeskus, L. M. 1997. *Summaries of Statistical Data on Elder Abuse in Domestic Settings for FY 95 and FY 96.* Washington, D.C.: National Center on Elder Abuse.

Tueth, Michael J. 2000. "Exposing Financial Exploitation of Impaired Elderly Persons." *American Journal of Geriatric Psychiatry* 8(2): 104–111.

United Nations, Economic and Social Council. 2002. *Abuse of Older Persons: Recognizing and Responding to Abuse of Older Persons in a Global Context: Report of the Secretary-General.* New York: Author.

U.S. House Select Committee on Aging. 1990. *Elder Abuse: A Decade of Shame and Inaction.* Washington, D.C.: U.S. Government Printing Office.

Wolf, Rosalie S.; Godkin, Michael A.; and Pillemer, Karl A. 1986. "Maltreatment of the Elderly: A Comparative Analysis." *Pride Institute Journal of Long Term Home Health Care* 5(4): 10–17.

# ACCESS TO HEALTHCARE

• • •

The question of access occupies a curious position in the complex ethos of healthcare. On the one hand, it would seem to be the most basic of all ethics issues, for if people do not have access to care, all the other problems that providers and ethicists worry about are more or less moot. If there were no patients, it would be impossible to provide healthcare, at least to human beings.

On the other hand, despite all the rights that have been addressed (and, in some cases, created) by modern bioethics—including, but not limited to, the right to refuse treatment, the right to informed consent, the right to protection as a human subject of research, and the right to die on one's own terms—no right of access to care has been formally established. It is not addressed in the Declaration of Independence. Its only association with the U.S. Constitution is the 1976 Supreme Court ruling in *Estelle v. Gamble,* which held that deliberate indifference to an inmate's serious illness or injury on the part of prison officials violates the Eighth Amendment prohibition against cruel and unusual punishment.

Access is not addressed in the Nuremberg Code or the Universal Declaration of Human Rights. Even the World Health Organization's (WHO) oft-cited definition of health, set out in the preamble to its constitution (1946), as "a state of complete physical, mental, and social well-being and not merely the absence of disease or infirmity" does not specifically address the issue of access, although the same preamble states that "the extension to all peoples of the benefits of medical, psychological, and related knowledge is essential to the fullest attainment of health."

Perhaps the closest the United States has come to a formal policy statement is the language in the 1983 report of the President's Commission for the Study of Ethical Problems in Medicine and Biomedical and Behavioral Research. The commission concluded that "society has an ethical obligation to ensure equitable access to healthcare for all" and that "equitable access to care requires that all citizens be able to secure an adequate level of care without excessive burdens" (p. 4). Despite these recommendations, no policy initiatives were undertaken.

Yet, in both charitable tradition and public policy, there is a history of implicit acknowledgement that the sick and injured should be able to obtain the care they need. Most major religions have, to one degree or another, adopted the provision of care as a ministry, usually in the form of hospitals. Most developed nations (and some others) have formally committed themselves to access to care for most or all of their residents. Public funds support hospitals, nursing homes, clinics, and other sources of care, and in some nations (the United States and Australia being prominent examples), these funds are also used to subsidize insurance coverage, which is usually public but sometimes private.

In the United States, federal law requires that any person seeking care in a hospital emergency department must receive an examination and evaluation, and if the person is at grave risk of death or severe debility, or is a pregnant woman in labor, the hospital may not transfer that patient unless it is clinically necessary. Many states have similar laws. There are also civil penalties for providers who are perceived to have refused care if the need was dire (and sometimes, even if it was not). Furthermore, public opinion surveys conducted by a wide range of opinion research organizations have found that most Americans support universal access to needed care, even if definitions of what that means vary considerably.

In the twentieth century, the United States also passed laws providing public funding for many healthcare services for people sixty-five or older (Medicare); for some of the poor, including some pregnant women and young children and the disabled (Medicaid); and for other low-income children (State Children's Health Insurance Program). Many states have also enacted programs subsidizing the care of low-income individuals.

## Philosophy Versus Practice

Despite both rhetoric and law, access to care is hardly universal in the United States. To be fair, access to care is undoubtedly compromised, to one degree or another, in every nation on earth, because of lack of facilities, difficult terrain, poor transportation, poverty, weather, and other factors. The United States is no exception.

However, at least three factors make the United States unique with regard to access. First, unlike those of other developed nations, its federal government has never made a political commitment to universal access. Second, the key to access, generally speaking, is insurance coverage—and with few exceptions, the provision and acquisition of insurance is voluntary on the part of employers and individuals. Third, there is no political or societal consensus that access to care should be a right.

The most obvious evidence of resultant access problems is that a significant portion of the population lacks coverage. As of 2001 (the last year for which complete data were available), 16 percent of non-elderly Americans were uninsured; that represents 40.9 million people (U.S. Bureau of the Census, 2002b). Among them were 8.5 million children younger than eighteen and 272,000 people over sixty-five. Furthermore, members of minority groups were far more likely to lack coverage: Although 13.6 percent of whites were uninsured, 19 percent of African Americans and 33.2 percent of Latinos were uninsured (U.S. Bureau of the Census, 2002a).

There were also significant variations in the rate of lack of coverage among states, ranging from 23.5 percent in Texas and 20.7 percent in New Mexico to 7.5 percent in Iowa and 7.7 percent in Rhode Island and Wisconsin (U.S. Bureau of the Census, 2002c).

It is often argued that coverage is not equivalent to care, and that although it might be less convenient and will likely consume more time, the uninsured are usually able to obtain care when they need it. Some proponents of this position cite the system of public hospitals, operated by counties and cities and occasionally by states and even the federal government; the legal obligation of non-public hospitals to treat the seriously ill and injured; and hundreds (if not thousands) of subsidized clinics, public and private. Millions of people receive care through these avenues every year.

However, the network of public hospitals has contracted in recent years, and often those that remain are severely stressed financially, leading to long waiting times and delays in preventive and nonemergency care. Voluntary and for-profit hospitals vary significantly in terms of how much free care they can and do provide, and many limit what they do beyond the requirements of law. And although clinics often provide excellent and timely primary care, they are unable to offer the technology and specialty care that are available in hospitals.

Seeking to explore the validity of the argument that coverage does not determine access, in 1999 the Institute of Medicine of the National Academy of Sciences undertook a study of the interrelationship of coverage, access, and health status; the results were released in May 2002. The report estimated that 18,000 or more people die prematurely each year because of lack of coverage and a resultant lack of care.

The report concluded, "As a society, we have tolerated substantial populations of uninsured persons as a residual of employment-based and public coverage since the introduction of Medicare and Medicaid more than three and a half decades ago. Regardless of whether this is by design or default, the consequences of our policy choices are becoming more apparent and cannot be ignored" (Institute of Medicine, p. 15–16). But the United States has demonstrated on many occasions that for the most part, it can and will ignore them, at least as a matter of policy. Indeed, even when there was widespread awareness of the coverage crisis on the part of policy makers in the late 1990s, as well as a federal budget surplus, they focused most of their efforts on improving access to care for members of health maintenance organizations—who were already insured.

## The Ethics Issues

Policy decisions (or the lack thereof) do not occur in a vacuum; there are always guiding philosophies at work. And with regard to access, the philosophical and ethical issues are exceedingly complex. They include:

- Is there a right of access to care?
- To what should a person have access?
- Should there be a standard of merit or *deservedness*?
- Are two or more tiers of care acceptable?
- If there must be denial or harm, to whom should it apply?

RIGHT OF ACCESS. Virtually all of the rights that patients and families have been able to claim, at least in the early twenty-first century, are individual in nature and involve the protection and honoring of a single person's (or a single family's) decisions. The idea of a right of access to care involves a great deal more than that. In order for such a right to be acknowledged, it must be agreed to by patients, the general public, providers, and whoever will pay for the care that is provided. Furthermore, at least in healthcare, there do not appear to be many endemic, universally supported rights that have consequences as profound as those that a right to healthcare would entail. The sudden enfranchisement of more than 40 million people would have profound consequences for the healthcare system as a whole—and for the society as a whole, if public money were to fund that enfranchisement, as it likely would.

It is impossible to state unequivocally that rights exist unless they are acknowledged to exist and are honored in practice. Americans may have a right to "life, liberty, and the pursuit of happiness," but unless conditions are created that allow these rights to be real, they are only abstractions. Even a general religious and moral consensus that people should be able to obtain the care they need does not constitute a right, if that access is not present in fact. Thus, as a practical matter, there is little evidence that a general right of access to care exists. What can be stated is that a person at grave risk of immediate or imminent death, or a woman who is in the process of giving birth, has a right of access to care, because both a general consensus and the presence of law and penalties make it so. No overall right of access exists except as a moral desirability; if access is granted, it is largely a voluntary act.

**TO WHAT SHOULD A PERSON HAVE ACCESS?** The general abstraction of a right of access becomes more real when the question is what a person should have access to. The ethical standard here is usually thought to be necessity—that is, a person should be able to obtain the care that he or she needs. As for what constitutes necessity, there are certain broad agreements: Purely cosmetic surgery is hardly ever necessary, whereas treatment for a serious bullet wound is almost always necessary.

At that point, however, any further consensus evaporates, because the standard becomes almost totally subjective. Many services, from breast reduction (or enlargement) to chiropractic to acupuncture to preventive colonoscopy, are seen as necessary for one and as frills for another. Those who provide these services believe (or at least profess to believe) that they are necessary for good health; those who seek them believe the same. Those who pay for them (if they are not the patients) and those who do not seek them have a different opinion. The difficulties that the state of Oregon encountered when it sought (successfully) to reduce the scope of services covered by its Medicaid program attest to this.

Yet it is possible that an ethically acceptable consensus could be achieved in terms of what a person should have access to, if it fulfilled four requirements: First, that it would satisfy most people, which is necessary in a democracy; second, that those services deemed necessary were seen to be so by objective experts; third, that the people who were most likely to be affected were part of the decision making process; and fourth, that some form of exception was provided for in unusual cases (for example, even if organ transplants were limited to one for any patient, retransplantation might be allowed if the donor organ proved unusable or the operation had been bungled and if there were a reasonable possibility of success). The obstacles to such a consensus are largely financial and political in nature, and not ethical.

**SHOULD THERE BE A STANDARD OF MERIT OR DESERVEDNESS?** One of the most widespread means of allocating resources is on the basis of merit, one of six principles of social justice often used in healthcare (Fox, Swazey, and Cameron, 1984). This *meritarian* principle has been used in situations as widely varied as allocation of kidney dialysis machines when they were scarce to determination of eligibility for Medicaid to pricing of health insurance. It has been argued that access to care should be governed by the same principle, that is, those who do not work for a living by choice, or who practice poor health habits, or who live socially irresponsible lives, should not have access to care, or at least not the same access that more *deserving* individuals merit. Certainly this principle has been applied elsewhere in U.S. social policy and practice, notably in what is colloquially known as the welfare system.

The problem here is threefold. First, if the goal being pursued is universal access to some level of care, then the core of that goal is *universality*. Determining the eligibility for access of individuals on the basis of any criteria, no matter how persuasive, negates the primary principle. However repugnant some individuals are to society—convicted mass murderers (who, as mentioned earlier, have a legal right of access, however spottily honored), child molesters, terrorists, obese fast-food addicts, smokers—their inclusion is necessary if there is to be universality. On the other hand, if the system is allowed to be selective on the basis of meritarian criteria, history suggests that it is quite likely that the same people excluded under the old system would be excluded under the new, and that many of them would probably be poor, powerless, and nonwhite.

Second, what constitutes merit? In public policy debates, much is made of tax monies being used to subsidize those who are *undeserving* because they do not work. Yet leaving the work force in order to raise a child is considered perfectly acceptable if the family has the financial means. The association of racial and ethnic minorities with welfare (and because the two programs were tied until recently, with

Medicaid) led to a widespread stereotypic belief that nonwhites were less deserving of public largesse. In general, society condemns obesity, use of tobacco products, overuse of alcohol, use of illegal drugs, and lack of exercise. Yet exercise-induced injuries, stress from overwork, misuse of prescription drugs, and anorexia are all excused, and insurance will usually pay for treatment.

It is extremely difficult to establish an ethical standard that will be generally accepted when the criteria appear to be random, or, worse yet, when the criteria appear to follow a pattern of racial, gender, age, or income discrimination. Nonetheless, these patterns are evident in the making of other social policy, and thus can be expected in healthcare.

Third, because access to care appears to have a direct effect on longevity, the denial of care based on a person's current character and behavior may effectively deny the possibility of redemption, a concept that is important in most ethical thought. Were society to deny access to care on the basis of irresponsible behavior, millions of young people under the age of thirty would likely be barred. Were society to deny access to care on the basis of poor health habits, many people who changed their behaviors after a health scare would never have the opportunity to do so. And, however unfortunate it is that the criterion is used, there are those who were born into poverty who went on to become successful, who might not have lived long enough to change their lives if they had not had access (if they did). A standard that denies the possibility of redemption seems exceedingly harsh.

**ARE TWO OR MORE TIERS OF CARE ACCEPTABLE?** Part of the debate over access, and to what one should have access, is the question of whether one standard of care should be applied to all patients, or whether tiers of care should be allowed, largely determined on the basis of either income and location.

For example, should someone living in a remote part of Alaska expect the same access as someone living a block away from a renowned teaching hospital? More germane is the question of whether a person of significant means should be able to buy coverage or services that are not fiscally available to most others, or, conversely, whether someone who is unable to pay for coverage or care should receive the same services that others must pay for, directly or indirectly.

There are both philosophical and practical responses. The philosophical responses are sharply divided. On the one hand, those who believe that healthcare is a public common that belongs to everyone would argue that one standard must apply to all, in order to preserve both quality of care

and equality of opportunity. As former U.S. Surgeon General David Satcher said in 1999, "Bioethical principles call for one standard of health for all Americans" (Friedman, p. 5). Indeed, the nation of Canada has gone to great lengths, in policy and practice, to ensure such a standard by refusing to allow private insurance to cover any service that is also covered by the national health program.

On the other hand, in a market-capital society such as the United States, having more money usually means that one can buy more or better—a larger house, a fancier car, gourmet food. That is part of the reason wealth is sought after. Why should this principle not extend to healthcare? If one wishes to purchase more lavish insurance, or more personal healthcare attention, or services that are not available to lower-income people, why should that be denied?

Both arguments have merit. Perhaps a middle ground can be found in a compromise and a reality. The compromise is that tiers of care may be allowed to exist as long as the bottom tier offers acceptable access, quality and outcomes—a criterion that the U.S. healthcare system has so far failed to meet. The reality is that tiers of care exist in every healthcare system on earth, including those of Canada and the United Kingdom, because of the existence of a private sector willing to fulfill the demands of those willing to pay more, and because of the existence of national and international air transportation.

The purest ethical standard would demand absolute equality of access, of opportunity, and of care. Yet no nation on earth has been able to achieve this. That is not to say that this standard should be abandoned, but rather that the measure should be how close a society comes to meeting that standard, and what the consequences are when it does not. Lack of access to *frill* healthcare services may not be harmful, clinically or ethically, especially in light of the dangers posed by hospital-induced infections, insufficient nurse staffing, and substandard care. Lack of access to desperately needed care, based on ability to pay, is not ethically acceptable. The problems, as is usual in ethics, lie in the gray area between these two extremes.

"Two tiers of healthcare services will by right exist: those provided as part of the minimal social guarantee to all and those provided in addition through the funds of those with an advantage in the social lottery who are interested in investing those resources in healthcare," argues H. Tristram Engelhardt (Engelhart, p. 69). Others would disagree, arguing that wealth should not be able to buy health when it is denied to others. But whether they exist by right, by policy, or by accident, tiers exist, and the ethical imperative is to protect those at the bottom, rather than engaging in a fruitless effort to constrain those at the top.

**IF THERE MUST BE DENIAL OR HARM, TO WHOM SHOULD IT APPLY?** With respect to this question, it is instructive to consider who is harmed or denied under the system in the early twenty-first century: the uninsured, especially the uninsured poor; patients with certain diagnoses such as AIDS; racial and ethnic minorities; the chronically ill; and, in some cases, the dying (whether in this case the harm comes from overtreatment or undertreatment). Traditionally in U.S. society, those with less power and money are more vulnerable, because being poor, powerless, or politically irrelevant is equivalent to failure, and, as Roger Evans has written, "While the lives of the uninsured are clearly worth less than those of the insured, their plight reflects the unwillingness of our sociopolitical system to reward failure" (Evans, p. 17). The question is whether such failure should be punished by denial of access to care.

There is a reason that so many other societies have made a commitment to universal access to care, no matter how imperfect their efforts to implement it. That commitment is rooted in a communitarian ideal, an ethics precept that states that everyone is involved in what is happening and everyone is equally vulnerable to the consequences. This is not based only on theoretical ideals—however appealing they might be—but also on practicality: If only some individuals are protected, then some individuals are at more risk than others, although one's level of risk can change very quickly indeed. If all are protected, either none are at risk, or else all are. The strength of purpose that such an arrangement engenders leads to a stronger commitment to access, because it affects everyone. As the late Joseph Cardinal Bernadin wrote, "It is best to situate the need for healthcare reform in the context of the common good—that combination of spiritual, temporal, and material conditions needed if each person is to have the opportunity for full human development" (Bernadin, p. 65).

## Conclusion

As an ethics issue, access to care will continue to be challenging, not so much on its merits as in the inability of the United States to act on the challenge. Norman Daniels has written, "If the glaring inequalities in access in the United States are justifiable, it must be because acceptable general moral principles provide justification for them" (p. 4). No such principles provide that justification, at least when it comes to denial of all but the most critically needed care, which is often halfheartedly provided. Thus there is no moral or ethical justification for the continued denial of access to care, whether intended or not. In the absence of any ethical defense of this ongoing denial, the explanation must be found in a lack of political and social will—and in the failure to find a workable communitarian ideal in a highly individualistic society.

EMILY FRIEDMAN

**SEE ALSO:** *Healthcare Systems; Health Insurance; Health Policy in the United States; Hospital, Modern History of; Human Rights; Immigration, Ethical and Health Issues of; International Health; Justice; Medicaid; Medicare*

### BIBLIOGRAPHY

Bernadin, Joseph Cardinal. 1999. *Celebrating the Ministry of Healing: Joseph Cardinal Bernadin's Reflections on Healthcare.* St. Louis, MO: Catholic Health Association of the United States.

Daniels, Norman. 1985. *Just Health Care.* Cambridge, Eng.: Cambridge University Press.

Engelhardt, H. Tristram, Jr. 1984. "Shattuck Lecture—Allocating Scarce Medical Resources and the Availability of Organ Transplantation: Some Moral Presuppositions." *New England Journal of Medicine* 311(1): 66–71.

Evans, Roger W. 1992. "Rationale for Rationing." *Health Management Quarterly* 14(2): 14–17.

*Estelle v. Gamble,* 429 U.S. 97 (1976).

Fox, Renée C.; Swazey, Judith P.; and Cameron, Elizabeth M. 1984. "Social and Ethical Problems in the Treatment of End-Stage Renal Disease Patients." In: *Controversies in Nephrology and Hypertension,* ed. Robert G. Narins. New York: Churchill Livingstone.

Friedman, Emily. 2002. "Separate and Unequal." *Health Forum Journal* 45(5): 5.

Institute of Medicine. 2002. *Care without Coverage: Too Little, Too Late.* Washington, D.C.: National Academy Press.

Institute of Medicine. 2002. *Coverage Matters: Insurance and Health Care.* Washington, D.C.: National Academy Press.

President's Commission for the Study of Ethical Problems in Medicine and Biomedical and Behavioral Research. 1983. *Securing Access to Health Care: The Ethical Implications of Differences in the Availability of Health Services,* vol. I. Washington, D.C.: Author.

World Health Organization Constitution, Preamble. 1946.

### INTERNET RESOURCES

U.S. Bureau of the Census. 2002a. "Health Insurance Coverage: 2001, Table 1: People Without Health Insurance for the Entire Year by Selected Characteristics, 2000 and 2001." Available from <http://www.census.gov/prod/2002pubs/p60–220.pdf>.

U.S. Bureau of the Census. 2002b. "Current Population Survey, March Supplement, Table H101: Health Insurance Coverage Status and Type of Coverage by Selected Characteristics, 2001." Available from <http://ferret.bls.census.gov/macro/032002/health/h01_000.htm>.

U.S. Bureau of the Census. 2002c. "Current Population Survey, March Supplement, Table H106: Health Insurance Coverage Status by State for All People: 2001." Available from <http://ferret.bls.census.gov/macro/032002/health/h06_000.htm>.

# ADDICTION AND DEPENDENCE

• • •

While addiction has been called a *victimless crime,* nothing could be further from the truth. Research consistently demonstrates that acts of violence against self and others, accidents, decreased productivity, health problems, and a number of other social ills have links to alcohol and drug abuse and addiction. Every day we read about, hear about, or know someone who is a victim of a crime caused by those who use or seek drugs. For some, it is tempting to ignore the ravages of addiction by rationalizing their lack of substance use. However, much like recent findings on secondhand smoke, researchers are identifying other deleterious second-hand effects of substance abuse and dependence. These events include dealing with noise from intoxicated partiers, assault from intoxicated persons, and encountering intoxicated drivers (Wechsler, Lee, Nelson et al.).

Few people disagree that substance abuse and dependence are destructive health behaviors, yet there seems to be a vast sea of confusion surrounding these behaviors. The facts are clear: Addiction to and dependence on tobacco, alcohol, illicit and legal drugs, and possibly biologically driven behaviors such as sex and eating, and social activities such as gambling, are widespread and very destructive.

Addiction has wide-ranging consequences. In 1998 over 500,000 full-time college students were unintentionally injured under the influence of alcohol and over 600,000 were hit or assaulted by another student who had been drinking (Hingson, et al.). Over 1,400 students died from unintentional alcohol injuries (Hingson, et al.), 42 percent of adolescents admitted to a trauma center tested positive for drugs or alcohol and 72 percent of adolescents who were victims of gunshot wounds tested positive for substance use (Madan, et al.). Young persons are not the only ones affected by drug and alcohol abuse. For example, almost half of patients over 65 years old who were treated at trauma centers tested positive for alcohol (Zautcke et al.).

As can be seen from the above data, drug and alcohol abuse puts an extreme burden on the healthcare system. Over the past eighteen years, persons admitted to level I trauma centers testing positive for alcohol has declined by about one-third. However, during this same period, the number of patients testing positive for cocaine has increased 212 percent and for opioids, 543 percent. (Soderstrom et al.)

Drug and alcohol abuse and dependence cut across all geographic, ethnic, and social boundaries although some groups have rates higher than other ethnic groups (National Household Survey on Drug Abuse, 2000). According to the Drug Enforcement Agency (DEA), the total sales of illicit drugs in the United States in 1993 amounted to $100 billion. This makes the sale of illicit drugs as large a business as a top ten company on the Fortune 500 list.

Despite concerted efforts at education and interdiction, drug use is still commonplace in the United States. For example, National Household Survey on Drug Abuse data indicate that 14 million Americans (6.3% of the population age twelve and older) used an illicit drug in the month prior to the survey. Marijuana was the most commonly used drug (4.8%). National rates for other drugs were as follows: cocaine (0.5%), hallucinogens (0.4%), and inhalants (0.3%). Approximately 130,000 Americans (0.1%) are heroin users. MDMA (Ecstasy) use between 1999 and 2000 increased by almost 25 percent to 6.4 million persons (National Household Survey on Drug Abuse, 2000). This statistic is particularly alarming given the propensity of Ecstasy to cause permanent brain damage in its users.

The business community is so concerned about substance abuse and dependence that pre-employment drug screening of prospective employees has become commonplace. The majority of Fortune 500 companies have some sort of drug-testing program. Drug testing is the norm in the U.S. armed forces, and many court cases in the early twenty-first century are examining if and when the government has the right to test its employees. In 2002 the U.S. Supreme Court, in *Board of Education of Independent School District No. 92 of Pottawatomie County et al. v. Earls et al.,* held that drug testing of students is a reasonable means of preventing and deterring drug use among school children and is not a violation of Fourth Amendment rights.

The death toll from health problems caused by smoking is staggering. A study published in the *Journal of the American Medical Association* (JAMA) in 2000, estimated that almost 400,000 Americans die each year from smoking related illnesses (Thun, et al.).

Beyond the health consequences for adults, smoking is a serious threat to young people on several levels. Despite widespread antismoking programs, 14.9 percent of teenagers smoke on a regular basis. Unfortunately, many youth perceive low risk of dangers from smoking and others start smoking tobacco cigarettes after smoking *safe* marijuana.

Smoking is not the only potential threat from addictive substances to young people. The National Household Survey on Drug Abuse estimates that 27.5 percent of twelve- to twenty-year-olds have used alcohol in the past month. The 2000 Household Survey found that 6.6 percent of the household population, ages twelve to seventeen, had used marijuana in the preceding month while 9.8 percent reported using some illicit drug during the same period.

Why would anyone engage in such behavior in the face of such obvious and dire consequences? What are the root causes of such behavior? Why is there any debate about drug use when the frightening consequences are known? Part of the answer comes from exploring the question of what addiction really means.

## What Is Addiction?

The concept of addiction—whether to alcohol, cigarettes, heroin, or sexual behavior—is widely misunderstood. Although there is room for debate about the *levels* of addiction caused by different substances, and perhaps about the *rights* of people to use addictive substances, there is no debate about what constitutes addiction. Addictive disease is defined by compulsion, loss of control, and continued, repeated use despite adverse consequences. Even though a person knows what will happen, he or she will use the addictive substance again. Thus, addiction is a disease characterized by repetitive and destructive use of one or more substances, and stems from a biological vulnerability exposed or induced by environmental factors such as drug taking.

Until scientists learned how popular *recreational* drugs such as cocaine affected the brain, it was thought that addiction required a physical withdrawal syndrome. That is not necessarily true. While a mild withdrawal has been described, positive effects drive compulsive use of cocaine. This information has contributed to research that clearly indicates there is no valid distinction between physical and psychological addiction.

Anyone who uses any chemical in the way described above is suffering from addictive disease. Users are distinguished by the type of drug, genetic vulnerabilities, individual predisposition to addiction, and the setting in which the drug is used.

Addiction includes preoccupation with the acquisition of a drug. In general, when obtaining a drug plays a central role in a person's life, addiction is present or near. Many studies have shown that addicts rank finding and using their drug above work, family, religion, hunger, sex, and survival. Even when the high is no longer achieved, the drug and its use are paramount. Drug taking fools the brain, giving the user a false sense of accomplishment that is at odds with reality, to the point that denial is common.

Since drugs cause a chronic disease in an otherwise healthy person, staying clean, or straight, becomes a daily problem. Relapse, therefore, is another significant and expected part of addictive disease. It is common for addicts to have relatively long periods of abstinence intermingled with drug-use binges. Chemical addiction does not happen overnight. Addicts are not moral failures but victims of a disease.

If addiction is understood as defined above, it is easy to see why it can be called a process: Use leads to brain changes; tolerance leads to abuse, which leads to loss of control, chemical dependence, and addiction.

## Who Becomes Addicted?

Who becomes addicted is a complex disease process that is best understood in a biopsychosocial model where biological, environmental, and social influences create this brain disease (Tsung et al.). While research in this area is ongoing, several findings are clear. First, genetics plays a powerful role in who becomes addicted and to what. For example, approximately 10 percent of the population has a preexisting biological, or genetic, predisposition to drug and alcohol dependency. This genetic relationship is supported by the higher concordance rates (likelihood of one twin having the condition if the other has) of substance dependence among identical twins (those who share the same genetic material), compared to fraternal twins (those with non-identical genetic material). Genetic factors underlie neurotransmitter receptor patterns in the brain that predispose a person to addiction (Rose et al.). Genetic factors are important in explaining why one person can have a drink and walk away and another person cannot stop drinking until he or she passes out.

Second, there is clearly a drug effect. That is, while all drugs impact upon similar reward properties of the brain, the pharmacological properties of some drugs are more addictive than others. Some substances such as cocaine or narcotics can cause addiction in almost anyone, regardless of genetic predisposition, if they are used frequently for a long enough time.

Third, environmental factors and drug use expectancies (i.e., motivation and intent) also play a role in the addiction process (Jang et al.). For example, rarely do cancer patients become addicts despite taking powerful doses of narcotic pain medication. Similarly, while an estimated 20 percent of American soldiers in Vietnam developed heroin addiction, 90 percent were able to give up heroin once they returned from Vietnam. An outcome rate much higher than typically seen among heroin users. Finally, as Russian physiologist Ivan Pavlov (1849–1936) proved, whether it is food and a bell or a drug and a bell, salivation is salivation. Drugs are powerful conditioners shaping behavior and responses.

Despite all of this evidence of addiction, the fields of psychiatry in particular and medicine in general have been slow to respond to the medical and societal challenges posed by addiction. Even the 2000 Diagnostic and Statistical Manual of Mental Disorders (DSM-IV-R), the bible of psychiatric diagnosis, does not mention addiction, per se, but instead discusses dependence.

## What Is Dependence?

What is meant by *dependence*? Is there a real distinction between dependence and addiction or is the difference only semantic? Examination of the DSM-IV-TR criteria for Substance Dependence reveals that the above criteria cited for addiction (e.g., compulsive use, loss of control, and continued use despite adverse consequences) are included in the Dependence criteria. However, the Substance Dependence criteria also include the additional factors of tolerance and withdrawal. Thus, traditional distinctions that viewed dependence as a stage below addiction, where the choice to continue taking drugs or alcohol or to continue certain behaviors can be stopped if the person really wants to stop, may be of reduced utility (Kleiman).

In any event, once a person's drug use progresses from abuse to dependence, the capacity for voluntary control is significantly reduced. The addicted brain becomes an impaired brain because the original drug free condition has been replaced by a drug present new normality. As drug policy expert Mark A. R. Kleiman explains, people act and make decisions differently when they are intoxicated than when they are sober. Making decisions such as having another round, Kleiman points out, may lead to further bad choices. The nature of the drug—to reduce inhibition when intoxicated—brings about *drugged choices*.

## Is Addiction a Real Disease?

In addition to genetics, addiction as a disease is supported by the common signs and symptoms among the homeless and physician drug addicts. The target for drugs of abuse is the brain and changes in the neuroanatomy of the brain occur in all addicts and underlie the disease of addiction. Recent research in neuroscience has identified a specific area of the brain described as the *reward center*. This area of the brain makes essential survival behaviors such as eating, drinking

and sex pleasurable, reinforcing, and thus likely to reoccur. It has become evident that virtually all drugs of abuse target this same area of the brain and result in neurotransmitter brain reward. The problem is that the neurotransmitter changes caused by these drugs far exceed those produced by the natural reinforcers. Animals will press a lever for a drug injection or a puff of cocaine. Once they learn that pressing the lever gives them cocaine, they press and press and press, frequently at the expense of eating, drinking, and ultimately their lives. Unfortunately, the same is true in humans where it is not uncommon to see addicts lose family, careers, and even their lives because of their addiction.

This same area has connections to the emotional areas of the brain (i.e., limbic system). Thus, drug use and addiction can be seen as a disease of brain reward with significant physical and psychological consequences. To truly understand the concept of addiction, one must look at issues of both positive and negative reinforcement. The pleasure effects of the drugs obviously result in positive reinforcement. However, continued drug use ultimately leads to changes in neurotransmitter levels and a host of negative states and emotions (e.g., depression, anxiety, fatigue, etc.). In these cases, continued use of the drug leads to a decrease in these unpleasant effects and results in what is called *negative reinforcement* (e.g., removal of unpleasant feelings) and the subsequent return to a *normal* (in this case, drugged brain) state. Research has led to a new understanding of addiction that is not based solely on withdrawal effects.

To understand this process in more detail let us examine the drug cocaine. Drugs like cocaine trick the limbic system by triggering the reward response through the release of neurotransmitters. Neurotransmitters are chemical messengers between nerve cells that are intricately involved in regulating moods. Cocaine use, for example, acutely leads to the increased availability of the neurotransmitter dopamine. Dopamine causes specific nerve cells to fire, and the result is endogenous brain reward or euphoria. Since cocaine uses brain systems normally reserved for species survival reward, the user feels as if he or she has just accomplished something important. The euphoria and brain reward produced by cocaine make the brain view the drug as a substance critical for survival. Hence the brain asks for more cocaine and excessive amounts of dopamine are released. Normally, any surplus dopamine released by the nerve cells is reabsorbed by them; however, cocaine interferes with this reabsorption. Finally, the brain's store of dopamine is depleted. With their supply of neurotransmitters depleted, cocaine users experience intense depression and cravings for more cocaine. In addition, the limbic system remembers cocaine's pleasurable response, a memory that can be triggered by talking about the drug, or smelling it, or even a visual stimulus such as talcum powder. It is believed that the action of drugs in a section of the brain called the nucleus accumbens is primarily responsible for the feelings of positive reinforcement that result from use of virtually all substances of abuse.

Other factors besides the pharmacological effects of drugs may lead to positive reinforcement. For example, drug use may enhance a person's social standing, encourage approval by drug-using friends, and convey a special status to the user. Recent research has shown that environmental factors can account for a considerable amount of the variance attributed to whether teens decide to use or abstain from alcohol (Rose et al.).

Given enough repetitions, drug and alcohol use become as entrenched as the desire for food, water, or sex. Furthermore, the dopamine pathways have many other influences, from the hypothalamus and hormones to the frontal lobe of the brain—the area responsible for judgment and insight. Not only do drugs cause the addict's brain to demand more drugs; the addict's ability to handle this demand rationally in the context of other everyday demands (such as work, family responsibilities, health and safety concerns) is distorted. Tormented by the acquired drive for the drug, memory of euphoria, and denial of obvious consequences, the addict becomes out of control.

Obviously, the complexity of the body and the brain means that no simple answer for the cause of addiction will be found. However, researchers are using sophisticated diagnostic examinations to uncover more information in an attempt to understand better the effects of drugs upon the brain. While it is doubtful that these procedures will provide a definitive, simple answer to the cause of addiction, the information gleaned from them may result in more effective treatment and prevention strategies.

## What Is Tolerance?

Tolerance may occur when the brain environment redefines normal and resets that level of feeling due to continued drug use. If drugs are taken to seek pleasure, they develop a life of their own as the brain redefines normal to require their presence in expected quantities. In other words, it takes more and more just to feel normal.

Interestingly, the emphasis on drug reward in the addiction process paves the way for other conditions, such as eating disorders and even sexual or gambling disorders, to be considered addictions. Eating disorders, in particular, share common behavioral symptoms, biological reward pathways, high relapse rates, and treatment strategies with other forms of substance abuse. More research is necessary to establish

the legitimate inclusion of sexual and gambling behaviors with other expressions of addiction.

## Drug Triggers: The Brain Learns

Drug use provides a quick and powerful means of changing one's moods and sensations. In a cost-benefit analysis, the user seeks the immediately gratifying effects as a benefit that outweighs the long-term cost of drug use. Other users may be influenced by physical or psychological states such as depression, pain, or stress that may be temporarily relieved by drug consumption. Drug use is such a powerful reinforcer and shaper of behavior that drug paraphernalia and virtually all of the events associated with finding and using drugs become reinforcers.

A variety of nondrug factors, including psychological states such as depression or anxiety, and/or environmental factors (such as drug paraphernalia and drug-using locations or friends) can become so associated with drug taking that merely being depressed or seeing drug paraphernalia may trigger the urge to use drugs.

WITHDRAWAL. While significant evidence supports the role of dopamine in the reward process, the neuroanatomy of withdrawal is not as clearly defined. However, a wide variety of abused drugs, with apparently little in common pharmacologically, have common withdrawal effects in certain areas of the brain. Opiates, benzodiazepines, nicotine, and alcohol have all had their withdrawal symptoms treated effectively with clonidine, a medication that works in an area of the brain called the locus coeruleus.

Unlike opiate and alcohol withdrawal, symptoms of cocaine withdrawal are relatively mild and disappear relatively quickly. This dearth of withdrawal symptoms helps to explain the episodic pattern of use reported by many cocaine addicts: Periods of intense bingeing alternate with intervals of abstinence. The intense craving and high relapse rate associated with cocaine use appear to derive more from a desire to repeat a pleasurable experience than to avoid the discomfort of withdrawal.

In fact, for all drugs, reward may be more important than withdrawal in the persistence of addiction and relapse, in that successful treatment of withdrawal has not generally improved recovery.

TREATMENT IMPLICATIONS. The disease model of addiction is supported by the high degree of addiction that various substances of abuse cause and the likelihood that someone addicted to one drug often will be using more than one drug. This multiple addiction is a major factor and plays a significant role in the treatment of addiction. Treatment strategies aimed at eliminating one specific form of addiction, such as cocaine abuse, without addressing other mood-altering substances, have usually failed. The addict who abuses only one drug is very rare. The Epidemiologic Catchment Area study of over 20,000 respondents found that 16 percent of the general population experienced alcoholism at some point during their lifetime—with 30 percent of these alcoholics also abusing other drugs. Alcoholics were 3.9 times more likely than nonalcoholics to have comorbid drug abuse. Similarly, the rates of alcohol abuse among other drug addicts were high: 36 percent of cannabis addicts, 62 percent of amphetamine addicts, 67 percent of opiate addicts, and 84 percent of cocaine addicts were also alcoholics. These studies, combined with clinical observations regarding the concurrent use of multiple substances, suggest common biological determinants for all addiction (Miller and Gold).

The success of Alcoholics Anonymous, with its broad ban of all mood-altering substances, lends further support to the unified disease concept of addiction. Similarly, naltrexone, a medication known previously for its efficacy in helping opiate addicts to recover, has been used successfully to treat alcoholism, cocaine addiction, and eating disorders. Although naltrexone can block the effects only of opiates, it appears to be effective against other drugs of abuse primarily because of the involvement of the opiate system in reward. According to this theory, naltrexone's opiate inhibition makes other drug use less reinforcing and ultimately prevents full-blown relapse to drug use as the addict's body learns not to associate drug use with reward. However, even with the use of Alcoholics Anonymous and viable pharmacological therapies like naltrexone, addiction remains difficult to treat primarily because drug use is so intertwined with the biological reward system.

For an addict, drug use becomes an acquired drive state that permeates all aspects of life. Withdrawal from drug use activates separate neural pathways that cause withdrawal events to be perceived as life threatening, and the subsequent physiological and psychological reactions often lead to renewed drug consumption. The treatment research consensus is that time in treatment and/or abstinence is the greatest predictor of treatment success and may reflect the time required to reinstate predrug neural homeostasis, fading of memory of euphoria and conditioned cues, and the reemergence of endogenous reinforcement for work, friends, shelter, food, water, and sex.

Drug reinforcement is so powerful that even when it is eliminated by pharmacological blockade (e.g., naltrexone), humans quickly identify themselves as opiate available or unavailable and change their behavior without changing their attachment to the drug and its effects. Once pharmacological intervention is discontinued, the addict will often resume self-administration.

Moods and other mental states, such as drug craving and anxiety, can become conditioned stimuli that may lead to drug use. Clinicians have used relaxation training, in which patients are taught relaxation and breathing techniques, to use in the presence of drug-related stimuli or the mental states they would normally associate with the need to use drugs.

Clearly, relapse prevention and successful treatment of addiction require much more than the alleviation of withdrawal symptoms. It is well known that patients with higher pretreatment levels of social support, employment, and productivity have a better prognosis for successful response to initial treatment and long-term abstinence. Treatment outcomes for these patients may improve because they perceive the long-term cost of drug use (loss of family or job) as outweighing the short-term benefit of drug use. Educational efforts that stress the risks associated with drug abuse help individuals to avoid drug use. No pharmacological or nonpharmacological treatment strategy can match the success of prevention. Research has shown that treatment efforts and relapse prevention are especially effective in impaired professionals (i.e., healthcare and other professionals whose licenses are controlled by state agencies). It appears as though these individuals have access to necessary inpatient and residential care to reverse the patterns of this devastating disease. These programs use a carrot and stick approach and rely on abstinence verification through objective urinalysis testing. Lessons from treatment of these patients can be used to improve the treatment of all patients with addiction.

The disease model of addiction should not be used to excuse the addict's responsibility; abuse has to begin somewhere. The addict remains culpable for the initial decision to use the drug and for continuing to use it despite adverse consequences. Nevertheless, an understanding of addiction and the addiction process allows us to comprehend the existence of addiction as well as why abstinence in treatment is difficult to achieve.

## Summary

All abuse-prone drugs are used, at least initially, for their positive effects and because the user believes the short-term benefits of this experience surpass the long-term costs. Once initiated, drug use permits access to the reinforcement reward system, which is believed to be anatomically distinct from the negative/withdrawal system in the brain. This positive reward system provides the user with an experience that the brain equates with profoundly important events like eating, drinking, and sex.

While studies have confirmed an encouraging decline in the number of illicit drug users, substance abuse continues to be a national problem. National Household Survey suggests that over 14 million Americans are users of illicit drugs (National Household Survey, 2000). Estimates of the presence of drugs like cocaine and opiates in trauma victims has increased several hundredfold from less than two decades before. Ecstasy use among adolescents jumped almost 25 percent between 1999 and 2000. In 2001, 5.2 percent of 8th graders, 8.0 percent of 10th graders, and 11.7 percent of high school seniors had used Ecstasy in their lifetimes (NIDA Infofax). Increased use has resulted in a dramatic increase in emergency room visits. According to data from the Substance Abuse and Mental Health Services Administration's Drug Abuse Warning Network, Ecstasy-related hospital emergency room incidents increased from 253 in 1994 to over 4,500 in 2000. The number of MDMA related deaths has also been increasing. (Goldberger and Gold).

Better news is increased understanding of the role that genetics and inheritance play in possible predisposition to addiction. And the best news of all is the widespread acceptance of the biological nature of drug addiction and the disease model, which brings hope to millions of people who think they are at fault because they cannot overcome their body's desires. The future will bring greater understanding of the biological pathways and, with that, cures for addiction and dependence.

MARK S. GOLD (1995)
REVISED BY MARK S. GOLD
MICHAEL J. HERKOV

**SEE ALSO:** *Alcoholism; Freedom and Free Will; Harmful Substances, Legal Control of; Health and Disease: History of Concepts; Impaired Professionals; Maternal-Fetal Relationship; Organ Transplants; Smoking*

### BIBLIOGRAPHY

American Psychiatric Association. 2000. *Diagnostic and Statistical Manual of Mental Disorders (DSM-IV-R)*. Chicago: Author.

*Board of Education of Independent School District No. 92 of Pottawatomie County et al. v. Earls et al.* #01–332 (2002).

Dackis, Charles A., and Gold, Mark S. 1988. "Psychopharmacology of Cocaine." *Psychiatric Annals* 19(9): 528–530.

Elders, M. Joycelyn; Perry, Cheryl L.; Eriksen, Michale P.; et al. 1994. "Report of the Surgeon General: Preventing Tobacco Use Among Young People." *American Journal of Public Health* 84(4): 543–547.

Gawin, Frank H. 1991. "Cocaine Addiction: Psychology and Neurophysiology." *Science* 251: 1580–1586.

Gold, Mark S. 1991. *The Good News about Drugs and Alcohol: Curing, Treating, and Preventing Substance Abuse in the New Age of Biopsychiatry.* New York: Villard.

Gold, Mark S. 1994. *The Facts about Drugs and Alcohol,* 4th edition. New York: Bantam.

Goldberger, Bruce A., and Gold, Mark S. 2002. "Ecstasy Deaths in the State of Florida: A Post-Mortem Analysis." *Biological Psychiatry* V51(8S): 192S.

Griffiths, Roland R.; Bigelow, George E.; and Henningfield, Jack E. 1980. "Similarities in Animal and Human Drug Taking Behavior." *Advances in Substance Abuse: Behavioral and Biological Research* 1: 1–90.

Helzer, John E., and Burnam, M. Audrey. 1991. "Epidemiology of Alcohol Addiction: United States." In *Comprehensive Handbook of Drug and Alcohol Addiction,* ed. Norman S. Miller. New York: Marcel Dekker.

Hingson, Ralph; Heeren, Timothy; Zakocs, Rhonda C.; et al. 2002. "Magnitude of Alcohol-Related Mortality and Morbidity among U.S. College Students Ages 18–24." *Journal of Studies on Alcohol* 63: 136–144.

Jang, Kerry L.; Vernon, Phillip A.; Livesley, W. John; et al. 2001. "Intra- and Extra-Familial Influences on Alcohol and Drug Misuse: A Twin Study of Gene-Environment Correlation." *Addiction* 96: 1307–1318.

Johnston, Lloyd; O'Malley, Patrick M.; and Bachman, Jerald G. 1993. *National Survey Results on Drug Use from the Monitoring the Future Study, 1975–1992.* 2 vols. Washington, D.C.: National Institute on Drug Abuse.

Killam, Keith F., and Olds, J. Sinclair. 1957. "Further Studies on the Effects of Centrally Acting Drugs on Self-Stimulation." (Abstract of a paper given at the Fall Meeting of the American Society for Pharmacology and Experimental Ethics, November 8–10, 1956). *Journal of Pharmacology and Experimental Therapy* 119: 157.

Kleiman, Mark A. R. 1992. *Against Excess: Drug Polity for Results.* New York: Basic Books.

Madan, Atul; Beech, Derrick J.; and Flint, Lyle. 2001. "Drugs, Guns, and Kids: The Association between Substance Use and Injury Caused by Interpersonal Violence." *Journal of Pediatric Surgery* 36: 440–442.

McLellan, A. Thomas; Luborsky, Lester; Woody, George E.; et al. 1983. "Predicting Response to Alcohol and Drug Abuse Treatments." *Archives of General Psychiatry* 40(6): 620–625.

Miller, Norman S., and Gold, Mark S. 1991. *Alcohol.* New York: Plenum Medical.

*National Household Survey on Drug Abuse.* 1991. Rockville, MD: U.S. Department of Health and Human Services, Public Health Administration.

National Household Survey on Drug Abuse. 2000. Substance Abuse and Mental Health Services Administration. *Summary of Findings from the 2000 National Household Survey on Drug Abuse.* Office of Applied Studies, NHSDA Series H–13, DHHS Publication No. (SMA) 01–3549. Rockville, MD, 2001.

Novello, Antonia C. 1993. "From the Surgeon General, U.S. Public Health Service." *Journal of the American Medical Association* 270(7): 806.

Prochaska, James O.; DiClemente, Carlo C.; and Norcross, John C. 1992. "In Search of How People Change: Applications to Addictive Behaviors." *American Psychologist* 47(9): 1102–1114.

Robins, Lee N.; Helzer, John E.; Przybeck, Thomas R.; et al. 1988. "Alcohol Disorders in the Community: A Report from the Epidemiologic Catchment Area," In *Alcoholism: Origins and Outcome,* ed. Robert M. Bose and James E. Barrett. New York: Raven.

Rose, Richard J.; Dick, Danielle M.; Viken, Richard J.; and Kaprio, Jaakko. 2001a. "Gene-Environment Interaction in Patterns of Adolescent Drinking: Regional Residency Moderates Longitudinal Influences on Alcohol Use." *Alcoholism, Clinical and Experimental Research* 25: 637–643.

Rose, Richard J.; Dick, Danielle M.; Viken, Richard J.; Pulkkinen, Lea; and Kaprio, Jaakko. 2001b. "Drinking or Abstaining at Age 14? A Genetic Epidemiological Study." *Alcoholism, Clinical and Experimental Research* 25: 1594–1604.

Soderstrom, Carl A.; Dischinger, Patricia C.; Kerns, Timothy J.; Kufera, Joseph A.; Mitchell, Kimberly A.; and Scalea, Thomas M. 2001. "Epidemic Increases in Cocaine and Opiate Use by Trauma Center Patients: Documentation with a Large Clinical Toxicology Database." *The Journal of Trauma* 51: 557–564.

*Substance Abuse: The Nation's Number One Health Problem: Key Indicators for Policy Update.* 2001. Prepared by the Schneider Institute for Health Policy, Brandeis University. Princeton, NJ: Robert Wood Johnson Foundation.

Thun, Michael J.; Apicella, Lewis F.; and Henley, S. Jane. 2000. "Smoking vs Other Risk Factors as the Cause of Smoking-Attributable Deaths." *Journal of the American Medical Association* 284: 706–712.

Tsuang, Ming T.; Bar, Jessica L.; Harley, Rebecca M.; et al. 2001. "The Harvard Twin Study of Substance Abuse: What We Have Learned." *Harvard Review of Psychiatry* 9: 267–279.

Wechsler, Henry; Lee, Jae E.; Nelson, Toben F.; et al. 2001. "Drinking Levels, Alcohol Problems and Secondhand Effects in Substance-Free College Residences: Results of a National Study." *Journal of Studies on Alcohol* 62: 23–31.

Wikler, Abraham. 1973. "Dynamics of Drug Dependence: Implications of a Conditioning Theory for Research and Treatment." *Archives of General Psychiatry* 28(5): 611–619.

Zautcke, John L.; Coker, Steven; Morris, Ralph W.; et al. 2002. "Geriatric Trauma in the State of Illinois: Substance Use and Injury Patterns." *American Journal of Emergency Medicine* 20: 14–17.

INTERNET RESOURCES

NIDA Infofax. Available from <http://www.nida.nih.gov/Infofax/HSYouthtrends.html>.

Substance Abuse and Mental Health Services Administration's Drug Abuse Warning Network. July 2001. Available from <http://www.samhsa.gov/oas/dawn.htm>.

## ADOLESCENTS

**SEE** *Pediatrics, Adolescents*

# ADOPTION

• • •

Adoption is an institution as old as civilization. It may be defined as a social transaction through which a person belonging by birth to one family or kinship group acquires, through legal means, a new family or new kinship ties.

## Historical Background

In its broadest sense, the term "adoption" may be used to describe the taking in, nurturing, and rearing of biologically unrelated children in need of protection and care. The terms "adoption" and "fostering" are used interchangeably in some countries, but in the United States adoption, in contrast to temporary foster arrangements, is a legal and permanent transaction.

Shaped by the laws and cultures of each society, adoption was seldom concerned primarily with rescuing abandoned children but rather with the transfer of a child or adult from one set of parents to another in order to ensure property rights or family continuity. Yet the perception of adoption has always wavered between the legal fiction that a child is reborn into the adoptive family and the folk belief that blood is thicker than water. The Egyptians and the Hebrews practiced adoption; the Old Testament chronicles the story of Moses, who was adopted by the daughter of the Pharaoh but later returned to his people and led them out of bondage.

Roman law, the foundation of institutionalized legal adoption, was concerned primarily with property and inheritance rights but permitted birth parents to reclaim their abandoned children if they paid expenses incurred by the adoptive parents (Boswell). The Code of Napoleon, enacted in 1804, which was the beginning of modern adoption legislation and is still a major influence in French and Latin American law, allowed adoptees to have knowledge of family background and the option to retain their original name.

The modern French government social security system provides for both "simple" (open) adoption and "complete" (closed) adoption.

English common law, the basis for U.S. law, stressed blood lineage and did not legalize stranger adoption, the total legal transfer of the child to nonrelatives, until 1926. Until then, a form of apprenticeship existed in which children lived with and worked under the master training them. Orphans were sent as indentured servants to the American colonies to help with the labor shortage. Economic considerations superseded any concern for the welfare of the individual child.

From the mid-nineteenth century until the beginning of the twentieth century, New York City street urchins were routinely rounded up and loaded into boxcars on "orphan trains" that carried them to "God-fearing" farm families in the West. There were no legal contracts or protections for the children who, once severed from their families, were regarded as orphans and forced into a life of domestic or manual labor thousands of miles away.

The transition from apprenticeship and indenture to present-day adoption was gradual in the United States, but by 1929 every state had some form of statutory adoption. Licensed adoption agencies established in the 1920s investigated prospective adoptive families to try to ensure the well-being of adopted children. Adoption records were open, but in the late 1930s a few states began to close them.

After World War II, U.S. adoption shifted its focus from the needs of homeless children to the desires of infertile couples to adopt healthy white newborns. Adoption became the means for the childless to create a family. As state after state closed their records, the adopted child's birth certificate was sealed and replaced with an amended document that named the adoptive parents as the birth parents. The original intent was to spare the child the stigma of illegitimacy, not to cut him or her off from the birth heritage. Over the years the rationale of protecting the confidentiality of the birth mother was added, but an even greater concern was the protection of the adoptive parents, who feared the birth parents might reappear to reclaim their biological, though no longer legal, child. By 2003 all but six states had sealed records.

## Adoption Practice in the United States in the Mid- to Late Twentieth Century

The social upheavals of the 1960s and 1970s had a major impact on adoption practice. The legalization of abortion, along with the widespread use of contraceptives and the increased tendency of unmarried mothers to keep their children, led to a shortage of white, adoptable newborns. At the same time, there was a rise in infertility among couples who delayed having children.

The states regulate adoption practice; most states permit both independent and agency adoption. As the shortage of white, adoptable babies grew more acute, adoption became a commercial enterprise. Lawyers and "baby brokers" took over most infant adoptions from the agencies, frequently using newspaper advertisements to entice pregnant women and couples to give up their children with offers of money and other benefits.

Without regulation by the child-welfare field, there is little protection for the baby and both sets of parents. Prospective adopters may spend a great deal of money for medical, living, and legal costs only to have the pregnant woman change her mind and keep the baby or choose another family. Conversely, a birth mother who has been promised open communication with the adoptive parents and the child may find herself cut off once the adoption is finalized. Or the birth mother may break her promise to stay in touch with the family if she finds visits too difficult to continue. Safeguards for the baby are lacking when the investigation of the family by an agency occurs after the infant is already in the home and petition has been filed for legal adoption.

## Special Needs and Biracial Adoption

In the 1990s adoption agencies, both private and public, focused primarily on finding families for "hard to place" children, a category that includes older children, sibling groups, disabled children, and biracial or minority-racial children. The U.S. Department of Human Services estimated in 1998 that 520,000 children lived in foster care in the United States, a sizable increase from 1992. About 110,000 children were reported to be legally free for adoption. Many child-welfare specialists believe that if sufficient effort were expended, homes could be found for them. Some states offer subsidies to families who are willing to adopt and raise disabled children. Single persons and gay and lesbian couples, not generally approved for newborn babies, are often considered acceptable for placement of children who otherwise might not find permanent homes. This remains a controversial issue in some parts of the United States, as a number of individuals and groups question the ability of these nontraditional adoptive parents to raise healthy, normal children.

In 1972 the National Association of Black Social Workers (NABSW) launched a campaign against allowing white families to adopt black or biracial children. The NABSW called this practice genocide. They maintained that, with enough effort and focus, black families could be found for these children. Proponents of interracial adoption argue that the benefits children gain from having permanent and loving homes outweigh the social and psychological difficulties they may face because of society's prejudice toward mixed-race families. Mental-health professionals generally agree that permanency, whether with legal adoption or long-term placement, is a paramount need for all children; they believe that growing up without roots and a stable home is a primary cause of lifelong problems. Many child advocates prefer that a child be placed with his or her extended family or within his or her community of race or religion, but accept the fact that biracial placement is preferable to no permanency as long as the families are sensitive to biracial issues and seek integrated communities in which to raise their children.

Adoption of Native American children is a related and equally controversial issue. Many Native Americans believe that adoption by Caucasians robs them of their children and robs the children of their native heritage. When Congress enacted the Indian Child Welfare Act of 1978, giving tribal courts exclusive jurisdiction over adoption proceedings involving Native American children, each tribe developed its own guidelines concerning the Native American lineage a child needed to qualify as a member. Children identified as members of a particular tribe must be placed for adoption with a family of that tribe.

## Intercountry Adoption

The shortage of desirable adoptable babies in the United States has led many who wish to adopt to seek children in other countries. The first international adoptions generally involved Amerasian children, that is, those fathered by GIs in Japan during and after World War II, in Korea during and after the Korean War, and in Vietnam during the U.S. involvement there. These adoptions were first sponsored by church groups and then by licensed adoption agencies (Lifton, 1994).

Since the middle of the 1980s, international adoption has shifted from the rescue of war orphans to the legal or (in some cases) illegal trafficking of children. Most of the children are drawn from Korea, China, Russia, Eastern Europe, and Latin America because these countries have made the emigration of children more accessible. Human-rights organizations report that many children are taken away from their families without formal relinquishments (Mantaphon). Studies of intercountry adoptions suggest that children cut off from their own culture and transplanted into a totally foreign environment may be more vulnerable to emotional problems (Verhulst et al., 1990a, 1990b).

Many have difficulty in attaching to their new family or feeling part of the community, where they may not find full acceptance because of racial differences.

The 1989 U.N. Convention on the Rights of the Child addressed the rights of the adopted child along with the rights of all children. According to the convention, each child has a right to receive a name, to acquire a nationality, and, as far as possible, to know and be cared for by his or her parents. A child placed outside of his or her family of origin has the right to maintain contact with his or her birth parents.

## The Sealed-Record Controversy

For over half a century, closed adoption (i.e., with sealed records) was viewed by U.S. society as beneficial to everyone: The homeless child born out of wedlock was given a second chance in a new family, the infertile couple was able to become "real" parents, and the birth mother was free to go on with her life as if she had never had a child. Yet research conducted since the mid-1970s has consistently indicated that the secrecy in the closed-adoption system can often create lifelong psychological problems for everyone involved (Sorosky et al.).

Although adopted children comprise less than 5 percent of the population, the percentage of adopted children in mental-health facilities and residential treatment centers has been reported to be as high as 30 percent. Some researchers have found that adopted children score lower in academic achievement and social skills than the nonadopted, have a high incidence of learning disabilities, and display behavior characterized as impulsive, aggressive, and antisocial (Schecter et al.; Brodzinsky and Schecter; Brinich). Psychotherapists have postulated that an adopted child's perception of rejection and abandonment by the birth mother can cause low self-esteem. Ignorance of origins ("genealogical bewilderment") can lead a child to rebellion against the adoptive parents and society, and eventually to delinquency (Wellisch; Sants; Kirschner and Nagel).

Women who relinquish their infants often suffer a profound loss and experience lifelong difficulties. Like the child, they are encouraged by society to deny and repress the feelings that accompanied giving up their children for adoption. Some studies indicate that these women never forgive themselves. Some may feel they have no right to a happy marriage and other children, while others may try without success to have other children as replacements for the one that they relinquished (Deykin et al.; Millen and Roll).

The closed-adoption system also encourages adoptive parents to deny their grief at not being able to produce a child that will carry on their lineage. They are expected to conceal their unresolved conflicts over infertility as they pretend that adopting a child is the same as giving birth (Blum). Adoptive parents who are able to acknowledge the differences between an adoptive and birth family, instead of denying them, have been shown to have better communication and closer relationships with their children (Kirk).

The closed-adoption system tends to pit the right of the adopted child to know the identity of his or her birth parents against the right of the birth mother to confidentiality, and against the right of the adoptive parents to maintain exclusive parental roles. The National Council for Adoption (NCFA), a lobbying organization representing traditional adoption agencies, contends that sealed records protect the privacy of the birth mother, who was promised confidentiality (Caplan). A national birth-parent group, Concerned United Birth Parents (CUB), argues that the majority of birth mothers did not ask for confidentiality and in fact want to have knowledge of or some contact with the children they gave birth to. Until 1976, birth fathers had no rights, only responsibilities. At that time, the U.S. Supreme Court gave birth fathers equal right of consent with birth mothers in adoption arrangements.

## Search and Reunion

One of the effects of the civil-rights movement of the 1960s was the emergence of an adoption-reform movement led by adult adoptees. Its rallying cry was that the civil rights of the adopted had been violated when their original birth records were sealed, denying them access to information available to nonadopted people. Adoption support groups have been established across the United States to provide emotional support, lobby for open records, and facilitate the search for birth parents.

Some states, rather than open their previously sealed adoption records, have established "reunion registries" that will connect adoptees with their birth parents if both register and indicate their mutual desire. In other jurisdictions, there is an intermediary system, in which the court, or an adoption agency is empowered to search for the birth mother if an adoptee requests a reunion. The birth mother retains the right of refusal of contact. Adopted activists believe that both registries and intermediaries violate their right to information and the ability to make direct contact with birth relatives.

More adopted women search for their birth parents than adopted men. The quest to find the birth mother is usually stronger than the need to locate the birth father. Adoptees tend to begin their search when they become aware of formerly repressed feelings that often surface at times of life transitions, such as impending marriage, parenthood, or death of adoptive parents (Sorosky et al.; Lifton, 1988).

The secrets inherent in the closed-adoption system make reunion difficult for both birth mother and adoptee. To return to each other is to return to their earlier traumas. The adoptee experiences grief, anger, and divided loyalties; the birth mother relives the unresolved sadness, guilt, and humiliation she felt at the time of pregnancy, birth, and relinquishment (Lifton, 1994).

No matter whom adoptees find—a loving, a withholding, or even a deceased parent—the opportunity to heal arises when they can integrate the past with the present. Adoptees' relationship to their adoptive parents is usually strengthened once they have resolved their identity issues. Reality replaces their fantasies, and they are able to recognize the important role of their adoptive parents (Gonyo and Watson; Sorosky et al.; Lifton, 1994). Birth parents also enter a healing process after reunion because they have the opportunity to explain to their child why they relinquished him or her and to forgive themselves and be forgiven (Gediman and Brown).

Some adoptees and birth parents develop close, ongoing kinship ties. Others maintain a more distant relationship that may involve little more than exchanging holiday cards. A few, after one or two meetings, close off contact. Whatever follows the reunion, however, the individuals involved have been able to take control of this important aspect of their lives.

## Open versus Closed Adoption

Since the early 1980s there has been a trend toward openness in adoption. In the placement of older children, good adoption practice dictates providing each child with a "life book" that has information and photographs about their history. Often these children are encouraged to maintain contact with the previous foster mother and with relatives, such as grandparents, in the extended birth family.

In infant adoption, a birth mother may choose the parents for her baby, but completely open arrangements— where there is an ongoing relationship between birth and adoptive families—are still rare. Semi-open adoption is more usual. It may vary from little more than a single meeting between the birth mother and adoptive parents, with no disclosure of names or discussion of future contact, to annual exchanges of photographs and information and the promise of more contact when the child grows up (McRoy et al.). Professionals describe open-adoption arrangements as a process in which all parties move at their own pace over the years (Silber and Dorner).

Opponents of open adoption argue that it makes it difficult for the birth mother to accept that she has given up a child, that it hinders adoptive parents in forming secure ties with an infant, and that it deprives the child of a sense of permanence with the adoptive family (Caplan). Proponents of open adoption believe that birth mothers who take an active part in the placement process can resolve their guilt and grief about giving up their baby; that it obviates adoptive parents' fantasies about the child's background because they have facts; that it permits adopted children to know that their birth parents are real persons, not ghosts; and that they were not given up because there was something wrong with them (Silber and Dorner).

### Court Battles between Birth Parents and Adoptive Parents

Since the mid-1980s the number of contested adoption cases has multiplied. Many have been brought by birth mothers (and increasingly by birth fathers) who feel that they did not receive proper counseling or enough time, or were coerced into signing relinquishment papers. When the birth mother seeks the return of the child, lawyers for the adoptive parents may delay action in order to prolong the child's presence in the adoptive home. The longer that period, the stronger the argument that it is in the best interests of the child to stay in the only home he or she has ever known. Adoptive-parent lobbies seek to limit the time that birth parents may have to revoke their consent or relinquishment. There is also a strong movement to develop uniform state laws that would limit the problems of interstate placements and decrease the legal conflicts of different jurisdictions.

### Conclusion

The adoption field is betwixt and between stasis and change. The records remain sealed in most states, but the traditional closed system is gradually giving way to a more open one that allows birth parents and adoptive parents to meet and even maintain contact over the years for the sake of the child.

Adoption practice is no longer exclusively concerned with healthy white newborns. Adoptees include transracial and biracial children and older handicapped children with special needs. Standards for adoptive parents, once modeled on white, middle-class, heterosexual couples, have changed to include single parents, homosexual couples, and minority and biracial couples of any age.

Uniform state laws are necessary to regulate adoption practice, but there is much disagreement about the relative importance of birth-parent versus adoptive parent rights.

The term "best interests of the child" has come to mean whatever people want it to mean. Prospective adoptive parents and birth parents find themselves in adversarial roles where their own best interests may conflict with the best interests of the child.

Adoption-reform activists believe it is in the best interests of the child to have adoption practice limited to nonprofit agencies and child-welfare specialists. They stress the need for adequate legal and psychological counseling for both birth parents and adoptive parents before and after the birth of the baby and especially before finalizing relinquishment plans.

Reformers would like to see adoption records unsealed so that adopted children can integrate their dual heritage and avoid many of the psychological problems that are caused by secrecy. They advocate a nationwide program that would promote sex education, pregnancy prevention, family preservation, and legally enforced open-adoption arrangements when relinquishment and placement are necessary.

## POSTSCRIPT

### Twenty-First Century Adoption Practices

During the late 1990s, laws erasing the secrecy and anonymity of the last century of adoption practice have been enacted in a number of states. Adopted adults are gaining access to their original birth certificates through legislative acts and voter referendums, despite the fact that there is still resistance to opening adoption records in most states. However, even in states where the records remain sealed, there has been an increase in reunions between birth parents and adoptees relinquished in infancy or childhood.

The Internet has revolutionized the adoption field. Searches for identifying information have become easier than in previous decades due to the nation's fascination with genealogy and the growth of databases on the Internet. Potential adopters and pregnant women considering relinquishment are also using the Internet to make contact. Families with special-needs children can turn to a variety of websites, help lines, chat rooms, and referral sources. There are also special websites on international adoption that lay out the unique problems one can encounter in the various countries where children are available.

The lucrative business of adoption in the marketplace continues to grow as attorneys, private agencies, and intermediaries use the Internet for networking in both domestic and international placements. International adoption is increasing as the number of adoptable healthy newborn Caucasian infants born in the United States decreases. Most women, married or single, choose to raise, rather than relinquish, their babies. Potential adoptive couples fear that even those women who initially choose to relinquish their babies will change their minds, or that the birth father will challenge the legality of the adoption. The publicity around and pain caused by contested adoptions has resulted in the introduction of new codes and procedures in many states to act as safeguards.

At the same time, open arrangements between birth and adoptive families in the United States are becoming the accepted practice with both infants and older children. The degree of openness varies and may be modified over the years, but all parties generally have identifying knowledge of each other. Agencies and other adoption practitioners can no longer offer guarantees of confidentiality or anonymity. In fact, many agencies offer post-adoption services in which they act as intermediaries in reunions, conduct support groups, and do counseling with all members of the triad.

By the beginning of the twenty-first century, private and public adoption agencies served different communities. The private agency or practitioner deals primarily with Caucasian infants born in the United States and with international adoptions of infants and toddlers. Public agencies, connected to the welfare system, place special-needs children. These children are usually older, part of a sibling group, non-Caucasian, racially mixed, or with medical or developmental problems. The federal government has enacted special programs, with financial incentives to local public agencies, to increase the numbers of children moving from foster home placement into permanent or adoptive homes. In both public and private agencies, there is greater acceptance of adoptions by single persons and gay and lesbian couples.

Those couples or individuals who prefer international adoption discover that the availability of children and the cost involved shifts from country to country, depending on political, economic, and legal issues. Regulations in the United States as well as in the country of the child's origin and in international umbrella agencies all contribute to the complicated procedures facing those applying to adopt. Nevertheless, a growing number of children are adopted through these routes. Those who choose international adoption to avoid the risk of legal challenges or interference from the birth parents overlook the psychological need of adopted children to know their heritage. Many young adults adopted from Asia, Europe, and South America have returned to seek their biological families in an attempt to resolve their ethnic, racial, and cultural identity.

Another revolutionary development in the adoption field is its connection with alternative reproductive techniques. Adult children who have learned they were conceived by donor insemination have organized a world wide movement, still small in number, to gain the right to have identifying information about their fathers. They refer to themselves as "in utero adoptees." Their initiative has brought about a growing acceptance of the right to access of identifying information in both egg and sperm donations. The American Adoption Congress recognizes donor offspring as adoptees, and advocates opening their records, as well as promoting future openness in all alternative family building methods. Embryo adoptions are being seriously considered as an alternative, due to the surplus of fertilized embryos no longer needed by couples. Rather than defrost and destroy them, a few agencies are encouraging donation of these embryos to infertile couples.

Researchers have not yet determined what the psychological effects will be on children born to parents to whom they are not genetically related when they learn of their high tech origins. One thing is certain: that they will ask the same question that legions of adoptees since Oedipus have struggled with: "Who Am I?"

ANNETTE BARAN
BETTY JEAN LIFTON (1995)
REVISED BY AUTHORS

SEE ALSO: *Abortion; Children: History of Childhood; Embryo and Fetus: Religious Perspectives; Infanticide; International Health; Natural Law; Sexism*

## BIBLIOGRAPHY

Baran, Annette, and Pannor, Reuben. 1990. "Open Adoption." In *The Psychology of Adoption,* ed. by David M. Brodzinsky and Marshall D. Schechter. New York: Oxford University Press.

Blum, Harold P. 1983. "Adoptive Parents: Generative Conflict and Generational Continuity." *Psychoanalytic Study of the Child* 38: 141–163.

Boswell, John. 1988. *The Kindness of Strangers: The Abandonment of Children in Western Europe from Late Antiquity to the Renaissance.* New York: Pantheon.

Bowlby, John. 1982. *Attachment and Loss,* 2nd edition. New York: Basic Books.

Brinich, Paul. 1989. "Psychoanalytic Psychotherapy with Adoptees." Paper presented at the 36th Annual Meeting of the American Academy of Child and Adolescent Psychiatry, New York, October 13.

Brodzinsky, David M., and Schechter, Marshall D. 1992. *Being Adopted: The Lifelong Search for Self.* New York: Doubleday.

Caplan, Lincoln. 1990. *An Open Adoption.* New York: Farrar Straus Giroux.

Deykin, Eva Y.; Campbell, Lee; and Patti, Patricia. 1984. "The Postadoption Experience of Surrendering Parents." *American Journal of Orthopsychiatry* 54(2): 271–280.

Erikson, Erik H. 1980. *Identity and the Life Cycle: Selected Papers.* New York: W. W. Norton.

Gaylord, C. Lester. 1976. "The Adoptive Child's Right to Know." *Case and Comment* 81(2): 38–44.

Gediman, Judith S., and Brown, Linda P. 1989. *Birthbond: Reunions between Birthparents and Adoptees—What Happens After.* Far Hills, NJ: New Horizon.

Gonyo, Barbara, and Watson, Kenneth W. 1988. "Searching in Adoption." *Public Welfare* 46(1): 14–22.

Kingsolver, Barbara. 1993. *Pigs in Heaven: A Novel.* New York: HarperCollins.

Kirk, H. David. 1964. *Shared Fate: A Theory of Adoption and Mental Health.* New York: Free Press.

Kirschner, David, and Nagel, Linda S. 1988. "Antisocial Behavior in Adoptees: Patterns and Dynamics." *Child and Adolescent Social Work* 5(4): 300–314.

Lifton, Betty Jean. 1988. *Lost and Found: The Adoption Experience.* New York: Perennial Library.

Lifton, Betty Jean. 1994. *Journey of the Adopted Self: A Quest for Wholeness.* New York: Basic Books.

Mantaphon, Withit. 1993. "Sale of Children: Report." Geneva: U.N. Economic and Social Council.

McKenzie, Judith K. 1993. "Adoption of Children with Special Needs." *Future of Children* 3(1): 62–76.

McRoy, Ruth G.; Grotevant, Harold D.; and White, Kerry L. 1988. *Openness in Adoption: New Practices, New Issues.* New York: Praeger.

Millen, Leverett, and Roll, Samuel. 1985. "Solomon's Mothers: A Special Case of Pathological Bereavement." *American Journal of Orthopsychiatry* 55(3): 411–418.

Rynearson, Edward K. 1982. "Relinquishment and Its Maternal Complications: A Preliminary Study." *American Journal of Psychiatry* 139(3): 338–340.

Sants, H. J. 1964. "Genealogical Bewilderment in Children with Substitute Parents." *British Journal of Medical Psychology* 37: 131–141.

Schecter, Marshall D.; Carlson, Paul V.; Simmons, James Q., III; and Work, Henry H. 1964. "Emotional Problems in the Adoptee." *Archives of General Psychiatry* 10(2): 109–118.

Silber, Kathleen, and Dorner, Patricia. 1990. *Children of Open Adoption and Their Families.* San Antonio, TX: Corona.

Sorosky, Arthur D.; Baran, Annette; and Pannor, Reuben. 1978. *The Adoption Triangle: The Effects of the Sealed Record on Adoptees, Birth Parents, and Adoptive Parents.* New York: Anchor.

Verhulst, Frank C.; Althaus, Monika; and Versluis-Den Bieman, Herma J. 1990a. "Problem Behavior in International Adoptees: I. An Epidemiological Study." *Journal of the American Academy of Child and Adolescent Psychiatry* 29(1): 94–103.

Verhulst, Frank C.; Althaus, Monika; and Versluis-Den Bieman, Herma J. 1990b. "Problem Behavior in International Adoptees: II. Age of Placement." *Journal of the American Academy of Child and Adolescent Psychiatry* 29(1): 104–111.

Wellisch, Erich. 1952. "Children without Genealogy: A Problem of Adoption." *Mental Health* 13: 41–42.

Winnicott, Donald W. 1955. "Adopted Children in Adolescence." In Report of the Residential Conference Held at Roehampton, July 8–11, 1953, pp. 33–41. Roehampton, Eng.: A. Rampton.

# ADVANCE DIRECTIVES AND ADVANCE CARE PLANNING

• • •

Advance directives are oral or written statements in which people declare their treatment preferences in the event that they lose decision-making capacity. Advance directives may allow patients to prevent unwanted and burdensome treatments when struck by terminal illness, permanent unconsciousness, or profound mental disability. Advance directives are only one part of a process known as advance care planning, in which patients, ideally in consultation with physicians and loved ones, plan in a thoughtful and reflective manner for medical care in the event of future incapacity.

This entry discusses the various types of advance directives along with the goals of and the ethical basis for advance care planning. It explores practical problems associated with advance care planning and concludes with discussions of how advance directives are used in clinical practice, and how decision makers ought to proceed in the absence of a clear advance directive.

## Goals of Advance Care Planning

Advance care planning refers to any planning by patients for decision making in the event of future decisional incapacity. Although it could refer simply to signing a form in a lawyer's or doctor's office, ideally it creates an opportunity for patients to explore their own values, beliefs, and attitudes regarding quality of life and medical interventions, particularly as they think about the end of their lives. Patients may speak with loved ones, physicians, spiritual advisers, and others during the process. This reflective work can help patients make important decisions about issues that may come up even when they still have the capacity to make decisions. When a patient loses decision-making capacity, physicians and loved ones who have been involved in the advance care planning process may feel that they know the patient's goals and values better. This allows them to make medical decisions that are likely to be consistent with the patient's values and preferences.

Advance care planning accomplishes a variety of goals for patients and families. First, patients may use the process to clarify their own values and to consider how these affect their feelings about care at the end of life. Second, patients can learn more about what they can expect as they face the end of life and about various options for life-sustaining treatment and palliative care. Third, they can gain a sense of control over their medical care and their future, obtaining reassurance that they will die in a manner that is consistent with their preferences. Finally, patients may increase the probability that loved ones and healthcare providers will make decisions in accordance with their values and goals.

Advance care planning may serve other goals, not directly related to medical treatments. Patients may wish to relieve loved ones of the burden of decision making and to protect loved ones from having to watch a drawn-out dying process. Patients also may use the process to prepare themselves for death. Advance care planning may help one reflect more deeply about one's life—its meaning and its goals. Patients may reflect on relationships with loved ones, "unfinished business," and fears about future disability and loss of independence. In this way, advance care planning may improve patients' feelings of life completion and satisfaction with their treatment in their final days.

Many people engage in advance care planning through conversations with their lawyers or loved ones. Peter A. Singer and colleagues reported in 1998 that among the HIV patients that they had studied, many had engaged in serious discussions with loved ones but had not seen any reason to involve their doctors. Nevertheless, physicians, physician extenders, nurses, chaplains, and medical social workers can play an important role in assisting patients in advance care planning.

Healthcare providers have their own reasons for wanting to engage their patients in advance care planning. First, providers may use these discussions to reassure patients that their wishes will be respected. This can enhance a sense of trust. Second, providers may hope that advance directives will help to decrease conflict among family members and between family members and the healthcare team when the patient is seriously ill. Finally, they may hope that advance directives will assist them in making difficult decisions when the patient has lost decision-making capacity.

Advance care planning discussions vary depending on a patient's state of health. Patients who are in good health may benefit from selecting a healthcare proxy and thinking about whether there are any situations so intolerable that they would not want their lives prolonged. When patients are older or have more serious chronic illnesses, physicians may wish to begin a discussion that is broader in scope. Although many view advance care planning as an opportunity for patients to make known their "preferences" for treatment, many patients do not have well-formed treatment preferences. By careful exploration of patients' values, healthcare providers can help patients discover these preferences. Patients can be asked to talk about their goals for life, their fears about disability, their hopes for what the end of their life will look like, and their ideas about states worse than death. This expanded view of advance care planning allows people to think about their mortality and legacy. From such discussions, healthcare providers can help patients consider specifically whether there are certain treatments that they might wish to forgo, and to think about the circumstances under which they might forgo them.

When the patient's illness has progressed to its final stages, healthcare providers can use the groundwork from these earlier discussions to make specific plans about what is to be done when the inevitable worsening occurs. Among other things, the patient and the healthcare providers can decide the following: Should an ambulance be called? Should the patient come to the hospital? Which life-prolonging treatments should be employed and which should be forgone? Are there particular treatments aimed at symptomatic relief that should be employed?

## Types of Advance Directives

Advance care planning may lead to written documentation of the patient's wishes. Although this documentation can take the form of a physician's note documenting a discussion, patients often complete written advance directives. These are particularly important in states with formal requirements about the level of evidence surrogates need to forgo treatments or in situations in which conflicts are likely.

There are two types of advance directives: proxy directives and instructional directives. Both proxy and instructional directives are invoked only if the patient has lost decision-making capacity. Proxy directives, often referred to as *durable powers of attorney for healthcare,* allow patients to specify a person or persons to make decisions. They are relatively easy for physicians and other healthcare providers to discuss with patients and are straightforward for patients to understand. Proxy directives, however, do not indicate the patient's wishes, preferences, or values, and used alone they do not provide any information to the decision makers about what treatments the patient might have wanted under the circumstances at hand.

Instructional directives attempt to fill this gap. These directives, often referred to as *living wills,* identify situations in which the patient would or would not want specified treatments. For example, a patient's directive might state that "if I am permanently unconscious or terminally ill, I would not want to undergo cardiopulmonary resuscitation." Documents vary in terms of the scenarios described and the specificity of the different treatments. Some documents use general terms such as "heroic measures" or "aggressive care," whereas others list the specific interventions in detail.

Instructional directives apply only under the circumstances specified in the document. If a patient has a directive relating to treatment in the event of permanent unconsciousness, the directive will not help in decision making if that patient has suffered a devastating stroke. Although advance directives often focus on situations in which the patient would want to forgo treatment, they sometimes state circumstances under which a patient would want aggressive treatment. Finally, on some forms, people have the opportunity to provide more comprehensive information about their values and goals in relation both to their lives generally and to medical care specifically.

## Philosophical Issues

The ethical argument that advance directives should be honored is based on the principle of patient autonomy and is a logical extension of the doctrine of informed consent. Patients with decision-making capacity have the right to refuse treatment, even if the treatment would extend their lives. Advance directives are a means for patients to continue to exercise this right, even if they lose decision-making capacity, by making thoughtful and informed decisions in advance. This approach allows patients to direct that medical care be given in a way that they feel best reflects their values and goals. Because physicians generally feel that they have an ethical obligation to work to preserve life, advance directives most commonly give patients a way to tell physicians caring for them the circumstances under which they would not want to be kept alive. On the other hand, some patients might use advance directives to indicate that they would want life-sustaining treatment, even under conditions in which most patients would choose to decline these measures.

Advance directives also serve ethical principles other than autonomy, such as beneficence. Physicians often feel duty-bound to preserve life under almost all circumstances, regardless of quality, even if they are uncertain that this serves the patient's best interests. Encouraging a patient to engage in advance care planning is a means for a physician to safeguard the patient's best interests.

A number of objections to the use of advance directives have been proposed in the literature. In a 1991 article, Alan S. Brett argued that an advance directive form cannot possibly direct the care that is to be given in a real clinical situation. If a patient writes a very general form, stating, for example, that "if I have no reasonable chance of recovery, I direct that no life-sustaining treatment be used," decision makers will have to determine how much of a chance of recovery is "reasonable," how much of a recovery would be worth trying for, and what precisely are "life-sustaining" interventions. Even if one specifies a list of treatments to be forgone in a number of detailed scenarios, this, too, creates problems. First of all, no matter how specific the document, it is unlikely to capture the circumstances of a real clinical situation exactly. Also, patients might not truly understand the specific treatments that they are listing in the document, running the risk of erroneously requesting or forgoing a treatment.

This objection is sound as far as it applies to advance directive documents, and it illustrates the need for a rich advance care planning process. Documents are inherently limited for the reasons Brett suggested. While they provide some insight into the patient's wishes, they nearly always require interpretation. If, however, the patient had engaged in discussions with doctors and proxies about his values, beliefs, and wishes, then decision makers will be in a better position to interpret a document and to make medical decisions with the patient's values in mind.

A related objection is the concern that patients can never know what they would want under conditions that they have not experienced or that they may change their minds. There is certainly reason to be cautious in this matter. Nevertheless, advance directives apply when patients have lost decision-making capacity, often for what is anticipated to be an indefinite period of time. Because these patients can no longer express their preferences, the choice is either to listen to their previous wishes about the situation or to apply some standard external to the patient (the provider's opinion or some societal consensus). Given these alternatives, it would seem most respectful to patients to rely on their previously stated wishes to make treatment decisions, unless there is good reason to believe that the patient did not understand what was written in the directive. Patients also should be told that they may change their advance directive at any time.

In a 1989 article, Rebecca Dresser and John A. Robertson raised another objection regarding whether advance directives should determine the medical care of a patient who has become demented. They believe that when one becomes severely demented, that individual may, in a sense, become a new person, no longer having the thoughts, memories, attitudes, values, and beliefs of one's "former self," who wrote the advance directive.

Now, imagine a moderately demented patient who has pneumonia. Until she developed pneumonia, she had appeared content and comfortable, chatting socially with the staff even though she is unable to recognize anyone, has severe memory loss, and needs assistance with daily activities. This woman has an advance directive stating that if she ever became moderately demented, she would not want lifesaving antibiotics for pneumonia. When she wrote the directive, she said that she would find such a life intolerable. Dresser and Robertson contended that the advance directive would have no moral authority over the new person, who now has pneumonia. Instead of relying on the values and beliefs of a person who no longer exists, a decision should be made based on what is in the best interests of the demented person in her current state. If she appears content and able to enjoy life, Dresser and Robertson argued, she ought to be treated with the antibiotics.

There is significant controversy over what to do in this instance. Accepting Dresser and Robertson's argument would mean frustrating the desires of many people who would not want the final chapter of their lives to involve being kept alive in a demented state. After all, the demented individual is not treated as a new person in any other way. She continues to have ownership of the property that she acquired when she was healthier. She continues to be responsible for any debts that she incurred previously. When she dies, the will that she wrote when she was of sound mind will be operative.

## Practical Problems with Advance Directives

There are practical barriers to the use of advance directives. Although this entry describes an ideal of advance care planning in which patients first consult with loved ones and physicians, and then document their wishes, most advance directives are not products of this sort of process. Patients often write advance directives when they create an estate will. They may leave the document in a safe-deposit box or with their lawyer. Occasionally, they will give it to a family member. All too often, they will not take it to their doctors. Advance directives created in this manner might not be

available when needed for decision making. Because there has been no discussion with physicians about life goals and values and how medicine fits into these, the physicians are deprived of critical information that is needed in interpreting the advance directives. Patients, meanwhile, might have signed documents that they do not completely understand and that are not truly in keeping with their values. The same is true for documents created in the hospital in the midst of a medical crisis. To overcome this problem, physicians need to routinely ask their patients if they have advance directives.

Furthermore, advance directives may not be available when needed. They often do not accompany patients transferred to the hospital from a nursing home. Patients may not be under the care of their regular doctor when they are hospitalized, and the hospital staff may not know about the existence of an advance directive. In addition to the federal regulations requiring hospitals to ask about advance directives, electronic medical records and registries of advance directives may also help with this problem.

Another problem is that physicians are often reluctant to raise the subject with their patients. They may be under overwhelming time constraints. They may have never been trained to discuss this issue and are not sure how to introduce the topic. They may be worried that they will give patients the impression that they are "giving up" on them or that they think they will die soon. If they have focused in past discussions on interventions rather than patient values and goals, they may have found these discussions frustrating and unhelpful.

Time constraints are difficult to overcome. Physicians could dedicate visits to discussing advance directives; but insurance companies may not pay for such a visit, and many patients may not wish to make a separate trip to the doctor for this purpose. The use of booklets and other tools to introduce the concepts involved in advance care planning may help physicians efficiently use their time to answer specific questions patients may have and to guide patients through the process. Enlisting nurses and social workers to help patients with the advance care planning process may also help.

Although physicians are often worried that patients will be put off by a discussion about advance care plans, surveys show that most patients want to discuss these issues, early in the course of their disease, and that they think that the doctor should bring up the topic. Nevertheless, there will be some patients who are not ready to discuss advance directives. Healthcare providers must be sensitive to these patients. Advance care planning is a process that should be offered to patients, not forced upon them.

The root cause of much of physicians' reluctance stems from lack of training in how to have these discussions. With training, physicians can feel more comfortable having these discussions, can learn how to deal with patients' emotional responses, and can have effective discussions that the physician will find truly helpful in caring for patients.

## Clinical Use of Advance Directives

Rarely do advance directives clearly dictate the care that should be given to a patient who lacks decision-making capacity. Generally, some interpretation of the document is required, a responsibility left to the named surrogate decision maker, other family members, and the healthcare team.

When a patient who has an advance directive lacks decision-making capacity and is seriously ill, the healthcare providers should discuss the situation with the named surrogate and other appropriate loved ones. Reviewing the advance directive, those involved should decide what they think the patient would have wanted under the current circumstances. People who are not used to working with advance directives often misunderstand them. For example, an advance directive may state that life-sustaining treatment should be forgone but mention only the scenario of permanent unconsciousness. If the patient under discussion has had a devastating stroke but is not permanently unconscious, the document itself may not provide much evidence of the patient's wishes. In this case, it will be necessary to proceed almost as if there were no advance directive. In such situations, prior discussions involving the patient, his loved ones, and physicians about the patient's values regarding prolongation of life would be extremely useful. For example, when the patient under discussion expressed the preference to forgo treatment in the case of permanent unconsciousness, he might have given reasons for this that can shed light on his likely preferences in the circumstances of the stroke.

Even when there seems to be an applicable advance directive, there may be disagreement among family members or between family members and the healthcare team regarding the patient's care. These disagreements can occur even when everyone agrees that the advance directive applies to the current circumstances. Loved ones may disagree with the content of the advance directive, believe that the patient changed her mind, or believe that the patient made an error. In these situations, it helps to focus the decision makers on what the patient would have wanted and why the advance directive was written in the first place. Healthcare providers should, however, listen carefully to evidence that the patient changed her mind. This is a realistic possibility, and patients do not always remember to destroy the advance directive or issue a written revocation.

Other times, disagreements may occur because of differing interpretations of the document. Loved ones or healthcare providers may disagree on the meaning of a "reasonable chance of recovery," for example. In this case as well, it is helpful to try to focus decision makers on what they think the patient would have wanted.

Although it is best to gain a consensus of all the interested parties, especially about forgoing life-sustaining treatment, ultimately a named proxy has the final decision. Healthcare providers who wish to override proxies based on a patient's written advance directive should be wary. It is not clear that all patients would want their proxy's or loved one's wishes overruled. Because people often write advance directives to relieve family members of the burden of decision making, the patient may not have wanted it followed if doing so would cause tremendous anguish. In a 1992 study, Ashwini Sehgal and colleagues found that over half of a group of dialysis patients thought their doctors or proxies should have at least some leeway to interpret their advance directive. Rather than taking unilateral actions against the wishes of proxies, healthcare providers might be best off consulting with the hospital ethics committee.

When no advance directive is present, decision making often proceeds in a similar fashion. Generally, the physician will initiate a discussion with those who seem closest to the patient to discuss the patient's medical situation. Physicians should then focus the family on discussing whether the patient had ever discussed similar situations and what he or she would want under the current situation. Some states have laws regarding who is the surrogate decision maker in the absence of a written durable power of attorney. In other cases, the healthcare providers should try to determine who was closest to the patient or may find it best to reach a consensus decision. Advance directives do not change this process much but are a mechanism for the patient to provide evidence about his own wishes.

## Conclusion

Advance directives provide documentation of patients' wishes for medical care in the event of future incompetence. Healthcare providers can assist patients in developing useful advance directives through the process of advance care planning. The goals of advance care planning will be different for patients at different stages of life and health, but the aim in all cases is to help patients articulate health-related values in a manner that can assist decision makers when the patients can no longer speak for themselves. In this manner, patients' autonomy and uniqueness as individuals can be respected.

GARY S. FISCHER
JAMES A. TULSKY
ROBERT M. ARNOLD

SEE ALSO: *Autonomy; Beneficence; Cancer, Ethical Issues Related to Diagnosis and Treatment; Competence; Conscience, Rights of; Dementia; Death, Professional Education; DNR; Ethics Committees and Ethics Consultation; Informed Consent; Life Sustaining Treatment and Euthanasia; Medical Futility; Nursing Ethics; Pain and Suffering; Palliative Care and Hospice; Right to Die; Surrogate Decision-Making*

## BIBLIOGRAPHY

Brett, Alan S. 1991. "Limitations of Listing Specific Medical Interventions in Advance Directives." *Journal of the American Medical Association* 266(6): 825–828.

Buchanan, Alan E., and Brock, Dan W. 1990. *Deciding for Others: The Ethics of Surrogate Decision-Making.* New York: Cambridge University Press.

Doukas, David J., and McCullough, Larry B. 1991. "The Values History: The Evaluation of the Patient's Values and Advance Directives." *Journal of Family Practice* 32(2): 145–153.

Dresser, Rebecca, and Robertson, John A. 1989. "Quality of Life and Non-Treatment Decisions for Incompetent Patients: A Critique of the Orthodox Approach." *Law, Medicine, and Health Care* 17(3): 234–244.

Emanuel, Linda L.; Barry, Michael J.; Stoeckle, John D.; et al. 1991. "Advance Directives: A Case for Greater Use." *New England Journal of Medicine* 324(13): 889–895.

Fischer, Gary S.; Tulsky, James A.; Rose, Mary R.; et al. 1998. "Patient Knowledge and Physician Prediction of Treatment Preferences after Discussion of Advance Directives." *Journal of General Internal Medicine* 13(7): 447–454.

Hofmann, Jan C.; Wenger, Neil S.; Davis, Roger B.; et al. 1997. "Patient Preferences for Communication with Physicians about End-of-Life Decisions." *Annals of Internal Medicine* 127(1): 1–12.

Johnston, Sarah Coate; Pfeifer, Mark P; and McNutt, Robert. 1995. "The Discussion about Advance Directives: Patient and Physician Opinions regarding When and How It Should Be Conducted." *Archives of Internal Medicine* 155(10): 1025–1030.

Kolarik, Russ C.; Arnold, Robert M.; Fischer, Gary S.; et al. 2002. "Objectives for Advance Care Planning." *Journal of Palliative Medicine* 5(5): 697–704.

Pearlman, Robert A.; Cain, Kevin C.; Patrick, Donald L.; et al. 1993. "Insights Pertaining to Patient Assessments of States Worse than Death." *Journal of Clinical Ethics* 4(1): 33–41.

Sehgal, Ashwini; Galbraith, Anne; Chesney, Margaret; et al. 1992. "How Strictly Do Dialysis Patients Want Their Advance Directives Followed?" *Journal of the American Medical Association* 267(1): 59–63.

Singer, Peter A.; Martin, Douglas K.; Lavery, James V.; et al. 1998. "Reconceptionalizing Advance Care Planning from the Patient's Perspective." *Archives of Internal Medicine* 158(8): 879–884.

The SUPPORT Principle Investigators. 1995. "A Controlled Trial to Improve Care for Seriously Ill Hospitalized Patients: The Study to Understand Prognoses and Preferences for Outcomes and Risks of Treatments (SUPPORT)." *Journal of the American Medical Association* 274(20): 1591–1598.

Tulsky, James A.; Fischer, Gary S; Rose, Mary R.; et al. 1998. "Opening the Black Box: How Do Physicians Communicate about Advance Directives?" *Annals of Internal Medicine* 129(6): 441–449.

# ADVERTISING

• • •

As the cost of healthcare becomes an increasing focus of attention, advertising becomes an increasing object of concern. At its best, advertising can provide information to help consumers make informed choices. Conversely, it can also inflate expectations, create demand, manipulate desire, transform wants into perceived needs, and increase the use and cost of healthcare services. In the not too distant past, healthcare was understood as medical care. The activities of physicians were regulated by standards of ethics that eschewed commercialism. Though there has always been an economic aspect (usually a fee) associated with the physician–patient encounter, the revolution in the financing of healthcare delivery is transforming the personal doctor–patient relationship into a socially complex interaction in which physicians are cast among a multitude of providers, and patients are transformed into consumers. The focus on the economics of healthcare underscores the commercial aspects of healthcare delivery both by physicians and other providers. Though physicians and not-for-profit institutions should be responsive to a service ethic, they compete in the same economic arena as for-profit organizations and often behave similarly. Furthermore, in some cases the patients are not the direct consumers; services may be purchased by employers, alliances, the state, or other contracting entities, whose interests may not entirely coincide with those of patients.

Advertising may be judged by the standards of business ethics: truthfulness, nondeceitfulness, nonexploitativeness, and profitability. But healthcare is not strictly a commodity to be sold effectively with profit to the public. The care of health is also a fundamental human endeavor binding the caregiver and the care-seeker in mutually reciprocal ways. Otto E. Guttentag, noting the essential human quality of healthcare, defined medicine as "the care of health of human beings by human beings." Lawrence J. Nelson and colleagues argued in a 1989 article that several key features distinguish caring for the sick from other commercial products: (1) Patients are in a distinctive position of vulnerability and dependency on those providing the services; (2) their own self and destiny—even life—are at stake in the encounter with the provider; and (3) the relationship with the provider may become an important aspect of the healing encounter. All of these elements suggest that there are special obligations incumbent on healthcare providers that go beyond the usual obligations of the seller to the buyer of most commodities.

Traditional prohibitions against advertising attempted to orient professionals to their service obligations by minimizing the commercialization of the encounter (Relman). According to the traditional view, physicians and other professionals should obtain business by developing a reputation for quality service, getting referrals from satisfied patients/clients or from others who know their work, not through any kind of self-promotion.

The major ethical issue in advertising in a market economy is truthfulness. If given adequate information, the consumer should make appropriate choices: what kind of healthcare, where, when, provided by whom, at what cost. A larger question concerns the justice of a market system of choice based on individual self-interest. Proponents view advertising in healthcare as a way to promote competition and thus reduce cost in a highly regulated industry. Opponents criticize advertising for inflating expectations and thus increasing cost. Others suggest that the quality of care has been lowered by making cost rather than quality the focus of allocation decisions (Rodning and Dacso).

The high cost of healthcare in the United States has prompted a search for ways of reducing both the cost of medical services and the percentage of gross national product devoted to healthcare without appreciably lowering quality of care. Advertising is located at the crossroads between cost and quality, between regulated markets with an emphasis on quality and free markets with an emphasis on cost and choice. Regulations that provide standards for training, licensure, specialty certification, and hospital accreditation have resulted in high-quality, but expensive, healthcare. Market solutions, such as encouraging advertising to promote competition, have been seen as a way of reducing cost.

## Historical Background

Physicians participate in markets, but traditionally orient themselves by ethical standards that go beyond economic behavior.

THE ORIGINS OF PROFESSIONALISM. Modern professional organizations, defined by their codes of ethics and regulating themselves by ethical principles, take their origin from the Aesculapian societies of the fourth century B.C.E. and in particular from the oath of the Greek physician Hippocrates, which bound its members to ethical standards that did not apply to society as a whole. The Hippocratic oath emphasized the principle of patient benefit, placing the patient at the center of the physician's attention.

By the nineteenth century, when the British Medical Association (BMA) and the American Medical Association (AMA) were founded, the concept of a profession organized around explicit standards of ethics was well established. Prohibitions against advertising were among the first professional standards because treatments based on scientific knowledge distinguished physicians from their main competitors, itinerant nostrum salesmen promoting often dubious products with even more dubious promotional claims. Advertising was expressly prohibited as unprofessional and undignified in virtually all countries in which physicians had established their professional identity through professional associations such as the BMA and AMA, which were organized around a code of ethics (Havighurst; Dyer, 1985). Although the actual license to practice is granted and regulated by the state, the task of enforcing the ethics codes falls to the professional associations or the specialty societies.

THE ANTITRUST CHALLENGE TO THE PROFESSIONS. The professions have always maintained a delicate balance between altruism and economic self-interest (Jonsen, 1990). As the medical profession became more scientifically effective and better organized, it enjoyed regulations (licensure, specialty certification, and accreditation) that guaranteed a virtual monopoly on healthcare delivery. Healthcare became synonymous with medical care. Although the Sherman Antitrust Act of 1890 banned monopolies, the learned professions were considered exempt from the act, which applied only to businesses. Late in the twentieth century, however, the business aspects of medicine began receiving increased attention, and the learned professions exemption ended in 1975 with the U.S. Supreme Court's *Goldfarb v. Virginia State Bar* decision, in which Virginia lawyers were found liable to charges of price-fixing the fees charged for title searches. The *Goldfarb* decision heralded a flurry of antitrust activity in the professional arena, most notably the 1975 suit by the Federal Trade Commission (FTC) against the American Medical Association, holding that the AMA was in restraint of trade because its code of ethics prohibited advertising. The AMA Principles of Medical Ethics then in effect (1957 version) said simply, "[A physician] shall not solicit patients," meaning that a physician should not attempt to obtain patients by deception. The 1980 revision eliminated all reference to advertising. Nonetheless, in the 1982 case *Federal Trade Commission v. American Medical Association,* the U.S. Supreme Court decided in favor of the FTC, barring the AMA from making any reference to advertising and the solicitation of patients, and further prohibiting the AMA from "formulating, adopting and disseminating" any ethical guidelines without first obtaining "permission from and approval of the guidelines by the Federal Trade Commission."

The FTC suit hinged on the questions of cost, advertising, and the mercantile aspects of medical practice. The position of the FTC was that costs were high because doctors had a monopoly on healthcare delivery and could thus maintain artificially high costs for their own profit. If doctors were not prohibited from advertising, it was argued, prices would come down because patients could shop for the best prices. In other words, medicine could better be controlled if it were regulated as a business rather than as a profession (Pertschuk).

## The Ethics and Goals of Advertising

Advertising serves two very distinct and divergent objectives: (1) dissemination of information, and (2) product differentiation, which economists define as public perception of differences between two products, even though such differences may not in fact exist.

Dissemination of information provides the facts on which rational consumers can make informed choices. In healthcare, information about the services provided, location, hours of service, fees charged, and languages spoken are examples of services that might be advertised. Arguments in favor of advertising in healthcare are based on an understanding of advertising as dissemination of information.

Advertising also serves to differentiate products, and the methods for doing so are more ethically problematic. How can the claim be made and justified that one product is better than another? The FTC requires that any claims of product differentiation be empirically measurable. For example, in order to claim that a particular mouthwash "kills germs on contact by millions," it is necessary to be able to count killed germs. Usually advertisers attempt to differentiate products not on the basis of objective criteria about the product but by manipulating unconscious wishes and fantasies (such as

youth, power, beauty, sex, and affluence), associating the product with images of attractive people in beautiful surroundings. The consumer is left to feel tremendous anxiety about the possible consequences of making the wrong choice of detergent, antiperspirant, or health plan.

Though many physicians have shown reluctance (or an aversion) to advertising their services, healthcare institutions have readily accepted the imperative to advertise in an attempt to create markets, capture market share, and find niches in the marketplace. Notable in this regard is advertising directed at target populations, for example, women, cancer patients, and those needing psychiatric and substance abuse services.

Truth in advertising was the concern when the field of advertising itself attempted to follow the course of professionalism in the early part of the twentieth century. At issue were the values that distinguished professional advertisers from retail-space merchants. The American Marketing Association established university training programs and codes of ethics that promoted the scientific ideal of detachment and statistical analysis. The scientific vision of community and definition of people as consumers replaced the older, empathic, and value-laden world in which a merchant understood what customers (not consumers) wanted and needed based on living in the same community (Christians, Schultze, and Simms; Schultze).

Professional advertising is illustrative because medicine's traditions of professionalism are derived from an era in which physicians participated in the life of the community in which they practiced. Knowledge of the patient as a person, as well as the patient's life history and social situation, has traditionally been deemed essential to quality care. At issue in 2003 for medicine is whether it will be possible to preserve the values of personal care that characterized the ideals of an earlier era.

## The Commodification and Commercialization of Medicine and Medical Technology

Some aspects of healthcare are unquestionably commercial. The pills that only a doctor can prescribe are things, and a price must be attached to their acquisition. Hospital overhead becomes part of healthcare costs. Physicians' services (either for procedures or for time spent with a patient) involve a commercial aspect, though they are not just commercial. The locus of ethical decision-making shifts as the mechanism for financing shifts. Whereas physicians once made decisions on behalf of patients or with patients (according to principles of beneficence or autonomy), decisions are being made by corporations on behalf of populations or in the interest of reducing costs to populations. As this happens marketing of goods and services becomes an investment opportunity, not necessarily in the interest of conserving resources, but in the interest of creating capital for investors.

Medicine and medical technologies are increasingly considered in economic terms as commodities. It is fashionable to think of healthcare as an "industry," and as such the activities of the players—doctors and patients, providers and consumers, hospitals and healthcare organizations, equipment manufacturers and pharmaceutical suppliers—are seen in terms of market value rather than values deriving from a personal healing encounter. Value becomes a matter of money rather than a matter of conscience. It is the job of a market economy to distribute goods and services, bringing together consumers and products. Markets may be trusted to be free (laissez-faire) to the extent they do not violate their own frame of reference. Markets must be valued and controlled on their own terms, such as in the admonition, *caveat emptor* (let the buyer beware). But when vast public resources are involved, public oversight is also required. Deceptive or coercive marketing practices cannot be tolerated and require regulatory restraints on market freedoms.

DIRECT-TO-CONSUMER MARKETING. The growing trend of direct-to-consumer marketing needs to be evaluated in terms of the integrity of the information provided and the nature of the appeals made. Informed consumers make good partners in the healing relationships. Advertisements whose message is "Ask your doctor if this pill is right for you" provide little or no information about the product being promoted. Hair loss, impotence (erectile dysfunction), unhappiness, and sleeplessness are all subjects to be discussed with physicians and for which pharmacologic remedies may be expected. Once the expectation is created, it may be harder for the physician to assess risks (such as addiction liability) or side effects versus benefits, especially if a drug company has already courted the physician with gifts ranging from pens and notepads (bearing the name of a drug) to dinners (where "information" about products is offered) to vacations in expensive resorts.

The traditional way of mediating such claims is through scientific research, published in peer-reviewed journals. Consumers have access via the Internet to all sorts of information that does not receive such academic scrutiny. In the United States, federal regulatory agencies, such as the Food and Drug Administration (FDA) and the FTC, are charged with evaluating the research on which such claims are made. Yet much of the research is performed or funded by product manufacturers, and results that are unfavorable to the product may be suppressed, resulting in a publication bias in which only positive results are published and leading to a false (unscientific, but commercially advantageous) impression of the efficacy of a particular product (Otto et al.). Expensive high-technology screening tests (such as computed tomography scans for heart disease and cancer) are similarly promoted as educational information directly to consumers even though these tests' lack of specificity (resulting in false positives and negatives) causes physicians to question their value (Lee and Brennan). The ethical standard for judging such advertisements would be the truthfulness of the claims made. But presenting such appeals as informational when they are in fact promotional is a manipulation of demand, especially when the research on which such claims are made is not presented or, even worse, when it is skewed (Wolfe).

Several dramatic examples bring into mind the ethical constraints that might be necessary on advertising designed to create markets. Cosmetic surgery to improve a person's subjective sense of one's own beauty, for example, is medical in a way that is different from reconstructive surgery to repair a face damaged by an accident, although both involve similar skills and may be performed by the same plastic surgeon. Similarly (in an economic sense) assisted reproductive technologies, such as in vitro fertilization, may like other medical treatments relieve the distress of a childless couple, although the availability of such services is based more on the ability to pay than on need. The assisted reproduction industry commodifies the product, a human pregnancy, in ways that are more ambiguous ethically than they are commercially (Macklin and White). Technologies such as assisted reproduction along with the emerging genetic technologies, as well as more established technologies such as safe abortion, intensive care, and organ transplantation, help one to imagine limits on commercialization, advertising, and marketing (Dyer, 1997). As Allen Verhey noted in a 1997 article, "There are some boundaries and limits to the sphere of the marketplace. We do not want a market in which body parts are profitable; we prohibit the sale of organs, even those of the dead. We do not want babies sold at auction. Some things are not to be commodified and commercialized" (p. 135).

## Conclusion

It could be debated whether advertising that goes beyond dissemination of information is ever ethical, though it is an accepted feature of market economies. The ethical issue for advertising is whether advertising is truthful and whether there can be objectively measurable standards for judging the truthfulness of advertising claims. A more problematic concern is the way in which advertising plays upon people's unconscious wishes and fantasies: sex, greed, and the quest for power, status, and perfection. The scientific basis for advertising rests on the ability to identify and manipulate such longings and fears. When one speaks of "the market" or "market forces" or "demand," one is generally talking about human wants and wishes.

Key questions facing the ethics of advertising in healthcare include:

- What standards or regulations should be in place concerning the placement of advertisements?

- Is any appeal legitimate so long as it does not mislead, make false claims, or actually harm?

- Is the negative portrayal of women in, for example, the promotion of unhealthful products such as tobacco or alcohol so morally offensive as to persuade the government to extend the scope of regulation of what is permissible in advertising, such as limiting advertising to dissemination of information?

- Is the effectiveness of the psychology of persuasion sufficient to justify advertisements, or can some higher principle be brought to bear?

Perhaps advertising itself should be subjected to the first principle of Hippocratic ethics, *primum non nocere* (first do no harm). Or to echo the caveat of President Dwight D. Eisenhower about the "military-industrial complex," beware the medical-industrial complex. Advertising that promotes consumer choice by providing information is consistent with the ethical ideal to promote patient autonomy. Advertising that deceptively promotes the interest of the provider at the expense of the consumer could not be ethically condoned, especially when the consumer is a patient.

ALLEN R. DYER (1995)
REVISED BY AUTHOR

SEE ALSO: *Harmful Substances, Legal Control of; Lifestyles and Public Health; Medicine, Profession of; Pharmaceutical Industry; Professional-Patient Relationship; Profit and Commercialism*

## BIBLIOGRAPHY

Christians, Clifford G.; Schultze, Quentin J.; and Simms, Norman H. 1978. "Community, Epistemology, and Mass Media Ethics." *Journalism History* 5(2): 38–41, 65–67.

Colman, Richard D. 1989. "The Ethics of General Practice and Advertising." *Journal of Medical Ethics* 15(2): 86–89, 93.

Dyer, Allen R. 1985. "Ethics, Advertising, and the Definition of a Profession." *Journal of Medical Ethics* 11(2): 72–78.

Dyer, Allen R. 1988. *Ethics and Psychiatry: Toward Professional Definition.* Washington, D.C.: American Psychiatric Press.

Dyer, Allen R. 1997. "Ethics, Advertising, and Assisted Reproduction: The Goals and Methods of Advertising." *Women's Health Issues* 7(3): 143–148.

*Federal Trade Commission v. American Medical Association.* 638 F.2d 443 (1982).

Gillon, Raanan. 1989. "Advertising and Medical Ethics." *Journal of Medical Ethics* 15(2): 59–60, 85.

*Goldfarb v. Virginia State Bar.* 421 U.S. 773; 44 L.Ed.2d 572; 92 Sup. Ct. 2004 (1975).

Guttentag, Otto E. 1963. Personal communication. See also "On Defining Medicine." *Christian Scholar* 46: 200–211.

Jonsen, Albert R. 1990. *The New Medicine and the Old Ethics.* Cambridge, MA: Harvard University Press.

Lee, Thomas H., and Brennan, Troyen A. 2002. "Direct-to-Consumer Marketing of High-Technology Screening Tests." *New England Journal of Medicine* 346(7): 529–531.

Macklin, Ruth, and White, Gladys B. 1997. "Art, Ads, and Ethics." *Women's Health Issues* 7(3): 127–131.

Morreim, E. Haavi. 1988. "A Moral Examination of Medical Advertising." *Business and Society Review* 64(1): 4–6.

Nelson, Lawrence J.; Clark, H. Westley; Goldman, Robert L.; et al. 1989. "Taking the Train to a World of Strangers: Health Care Marketing and Ethics." *Hastings Center Report* 19(5): 36–43.

Otto, Michael W.; Tuby, Kimberly S.; Gould, Robert A.; et al. 2001. "An Effect-Size Analysis of the Relative Efficacy and Tolerability of Serotonin Selective Reuptake Inhibitors for Panic Disorder." *American Journal of Psychiatry* 158(12): 1989–1992.

Pertschuk, Michael. 1977. "FTC Conference." Quoted in Rosoff, A. F. "Antitrust Laws and the Health Care Industry: New Warriors into an Old Battle." *Saint Louis University Law Journal* 23: 478.

Relman, Arnold S. 1978. "Professional Directories—but Not Commercial Advertising—as a Public Service." *New England Journal of Medicine* 299(9): 476–478.

Rodning, Charles B., and Dacso, Clifford C. 1987. "A Physician/Advertiser Ethos." *American Journal of Medicine* 82(6): 1209–1212.

Schultze, Quentin J. 1981. "Professionalism in Advertising: The Origin of Ethical Codes." *Journal of Communication* 31(2): 64–71.

Verhey, Allen. 1997. "Commodification, Commercialization, and Embodiment." *Women's Health Issues* 7(3): 132–142.

Wolfe, Sidney M. 2002. "Direct-to-Consumer Advertising: Education or Emotion Promotion?" *New England Journal of Medicine* 346(7): 524–526.

# AFRICAN RELIGIONS

• • •

This entry presents a brief, general picture of Africa's traditional religious heritage, focusing on the major beliefs because these underlie the general attitudes of individuals and society and shape their worldview. Various terms are used to refer to the indigenous religious heritage, including African religion, African traditional religions, African indigenous religions, and African religious traditions. This entry makes use of the most current term, "African religion." It is clear that in such a vast continent, there are diversities of religious life and concepts, but there are also similarities that make it possible to give a general picture.

After a brief word on the origin of African religion, this entry considers it in terms of belief in God and other spiritual beings, mystical power, and the continuation of human life after death. It describes how human beings are seen to be at the center of the world, and traces the journey of individual life from birth to death and beyond. Moral and ethical values are shown to regulate people's relationships with one another, nature, and God. African peoples give health and related problems much attention, for both their physical and their spiritual welfare. Religions originating outside of Africa, together with the influences of "modern" life, also have an impact upon the traditional religious heritage.

## Origin and Sources of African Religion

African Religion evolved gradually as people experienced different life situations, raising questions and reflecting on such mysteries of life as birth and death, joy and suffering, the forces of nature, and the purpose of life. Its history is bound up with the history of each people or tribe, and goes back to prehistoric times. Some elements distinguish it from Christianity and Islam, the other major religions of Africa, while other elements resemble them. African religion is practiced in the early twenty-first century mostly in the southern two-thirds of Africa, including Madagascar, where Christianity is statistically dominant. In the northern one-third, dominated by Islam, African religion exists beneath the surface, among indigenous peoples, despite their having been subjugated and dominated by Arab immigrants for many centuries.

African religion is found primarily in oral sources, including stories, myths, proverbs, prayers, ritual incantations, songs, names of people and places, and the specialized and carefully guarded knowledge of religious personages. Other sources are art and language; ceremonies and rituals; religious objects and places like shrines, altars, and ceremonial symbols; and magical objects and practices. It also emerges among Christians and Muslims in times of crisis like severe illness or death, disputes, political and sports competitions, examinations, and the search for employment. Since the nineteenth century these sources have increasingly been recorded in writing, and since the second half of the twentieth century, on film and on audiotapes and videotapes.

African religion spread to the western hemisphere through African peoples who were forcibly transplanted to the West Indies and the Americas by the slave trade. It settled there and survived in a mixture with Christianity, despite the influence of other cultures and environments. For example, the spirit possessions that abound among people of African descent in Brazil and the West Indies have their origins in Africa. Voodoo in the Caribbean and macumba in Brazil are remnants of African religion that have been modified to suit local practice. Some names of people in Jamaica, like Cudjoe, Acheampong, Kwaku, and Obi are originally African, but these are said to be disappearing. After careful study of the American scene, Gayraud Wilmore concludes that "an essential ingredient of Afro-American Christianity prior to the Civil War was the creative residuum of the African Religions," characterized by a spirituality of response to the reality of the spirit world and its reaction with objective reality (1983, p. 26).

## Major Beliefs in African Religion

As an all-embracing worldview, African religion has a number of beliefs held in common by the community. Individuals cannot reject a particular belief, since beliefs are part and parcel of the wider community. The term "community" is used here to refer to a grouping of persons in a particular area who lead a fairly similar cultural life, within a given people or in a town.

**BELIEF IN GOD.** Belief in God is found among all African peoples. The Creator and Preserver of all things, God is invisible, but the ongoing work of creation points to God's existence and involvement in the world. There are no atheists in African traditional society; belief in God is part of the common knowledge of everyone, including children. There are no pictorial or other representations of God by African peoples. Oral appellations of God include Father,

Mother, Parent, Friend, Savior, Protector, Giver of Children, Giver of Rain, the Shining One, the Kind One, and the Everlasting One. God is good, compassionate, just, and loving to all people. The overall picture of God is of one who is above gender classification, neither male nor female, since God is Spirit. To grasp some aspects of God, people find anthropomorphic concepts useful and, according to the situation, may speak of God in male or female terms for that purpose. Furthermore, many African languages do not distinguish gender grammatically. People express their belief in and awareness of God through prayers, invocations, sacrifices and offerings, praise songs, and dedication of children to God. In some areas priests and priestesses officiate at religious ceremonies, pray on behalf of their communities, and pass on the theological, philosophical, and practical knowledge of their religion. They are, or should be, morally upright. In Nigeria and Uganda, priestesses regard themselves as "married" (i.e., wholly dedicated) to God for a given period of time in their life, but later marry human husbands.

**BELIEF IN OTHER SPIRITUAL BEINGS.** There is widespread belief in the existence of other spiritual beings created by and subject to God. The spirits can be considered in two categories: those associated with nature and those that are remnants of human beings after death. Nature spirits are personifications of heavenly or earthly objects and phenomena: the stars, the sun, thunder, rain and storms, mountains, earthquakes, lakes, waterfalls, and caves.

Some communities, especially in West Africa, have "divinities," spirit functionaries prominent in the life of the community. This particularly reflects the political structure, with the queen or king at the top and various chieftains or ministers below. Some "divinities" are said to have assisted God in the ordering of the world; others, to be in charge of aspects of nature like the weather, earthquakes, and epidemics. But many African peoples do not have divinities in their cosmology.

Most of the human spirits are those of people who died more than five generations ago; the others are of persons who are remembered by name and known collectively as the "living dead," since they are regarded as part of the family. When they "appear" to the living, either directly or through a medium, they are recognized by name, and what they communicate, in the form of requests, instructions, or warnings, is taken very seriously by their families. However, the spirits of the departed generally have little or no place in the beliefs of nomadic peoples, probably because they do not remain for years on the land where they bury their dead.

Spirits of the unknown dead are sometimes called upon or otherwise used in divination and medical practice, but otherwise they have no personal family ties to the living. They are said to possess people or animals, and are often featured in folk stories in which they perform great feats, although sometimes they are depicted as stupid or as fearful of the living. Many stories are told about spirits, resulting in an integration of their world into the world of living human beings.

**HUMANITY AT THE CENTER OF THE WORLD.** African religion places humans at the center of the world. It is believed throughout Africa that God created human beings, and thousands of stories and myths visualize how this happened. According to some, humans were created at the end of the primal creation, formed from clay as husband and wife (or as two pairs), or created in heaven (sky) and lowered to the earth. Others say that husband and wife were created in a vessel, in water, or in the fruit of a tree. Creation stories relate that the original state of humanity was one of bliss, in which people were endowed with immortality, rejuvenation (if they became old), or resurrection (if they died). The earth was directly linked to heaven (the sky); God and humans lived close to each other, as a family. For various reasons these gifts were lost; death, disease, and suffering appeared, as well as the separation between heaven and earth, between God and humans. However, God did not abandon humans, but he endowed them with various abilities and knowledge, so that they could survive. Through sacrifices and prayers humans still have access to God at any time. Through prayers people praise and thank God, and solicit God's help in the fight against disease, suffering, danger, and death.

A strong feature of African cosmology is the recognition of the world as comprising two interlinked realities: the visible and the invisible, the physical and the spiritual. Both are bound together in a primordial unity. They interact, and Africans do not make a strong distinction between the two. This helps to explain African awareness of and insights into the spiritual realm, an awareness at both shallow and deep levels ranging from visions, dreams involving spiritual objects or beings or messages, contact with the living dead and spirits, and divination to concepts about and experiences of God.

The life journey of the individual is marked with rites, particularly at birth, initiation, marriage, and death. Birth and name-giving ceremonies express joy in the family and gratitude to God for the child. Children are the symbol and actualization of immortality; they counteract death with new life, and old age with rejuvenation. At adolescence, initiation ceremonies are performed, often followed by a period of seclusion for the initiated, during which they learn matters pertaining to adult life. Initiation ceremonies serve, among other things, to give the individual an identity as a member of the community to which he or she is thereby mystically bound. The most dramatic involve circumcision for boys and clitoridectomy for girls. The personal shedding of blood forges mystical links to the ground, to the land.

Marriage is a religious duty that, under normal circumstances, everyone is obliged or expected to fulfill. The bearing of children is the central part of marriage, and no efforts are spared to ensure that there are children in each marriage; otherwise, the couple fails to become a family. In effect the family never dies; only its members do. If, for example, the husband is impotent, his "brother" (in the wider sense of kinship ties) will (must) sleep with his wife so that she will bear him children. If the wife is barren, her husband will marry another wife, who will be expected to bear children for both wives. Polygamy is an accepted and respected form of marriage in about 15 percent of African families. Children knit the community into a vast network of relationships: brothers, sisters, cousins, parents, grandparents, uncles, aunts, and many distant relatives. The basic philosophy says "I am because we are, and since we are therefore I am."

Burial and funeral rites serve, among other things, to send the departed in peace to the spirit world, and to express condolences to the bereaved. Various symbols and acts speak of death and the continuation of life: normal activities are stopped for a day following a death or funeral; hair on the head is shaved; the house of the departed is closed or even abandoned; clothes of colors that symbolize bereavement (white, black, or red) are worn; the bodies of surviving members of the family are smeared with mud or white chalk; cattle are driven away from the homestead of the departed; people fast; and fires in the home are extinguished. Some societies bury a few personal belongings with the dead, such as spears, cooking pots, ornaments, money, and clothes. Among other groups the property of the deceased is distributed—by force if need be—among relatives or clan members.

**LIFE AFTER DEATH.** Belief in the continuation of life after death is held all over Africa. The next world is pictured as being like the present one, inhabited by spirits and located in thick forests, desert places, underground, or on mountains. There is neither reward for a good life on earth nor punishment for an evil life. The departed retain their human characteristics and the living dead are still part of their earthly families, to whom they appear in dreams, in waking, or through divination, particularly if there is a major family event.

The living show remembrance of the departed through such acts of affection as naming new children after them, taking care of their graves, and pouring libations of beer, wine, milk, or tea and placing bits of food on the floor, on the graves, or in a family altar. People who die without children are considered most unfortunate, since they have no descendants to "remember" them, something that the extended family only rarely does. In some societies people invoke departed members of the family, especially parents and grandparents, and ask them to relay their requests further, until they reach God. There is thus a unity and a line of communication between the living, the departed, and God. Harmony is necessary to maintain this unity in a healthy spiritual condition.

**BELIEF IN MYSTICAL POWER.** There is a deeply rooted belief in a mystical power or force in the universe that derives from God. This power is used in medical practice, divination, protecting people and property, predicting where to find lost articles, and foretelling the outcome of an undertaking. It is also employed in the practice of magic, sorcery, and witchcraft. Diviners, traditional doctors, and witches know better than others how to employ it. The belief in and practice of magic causes much fear in African life, which leads to accusations, quarrels, fights, and countermeasures in families and communities. The positive use of this mystical power is cherished and plays a major role in regulating ethical relations in the community and in supplying answers to questions about the causes of good luck and misfortune.

**SACRED PLACES AND OBJECTS.** Sacred places and objects—including mountains, caves, waterfalls, rocks, trees, rainmaking stones, and certain animals, as well as altars, sacrificial pots, masks, drums, and colors—are set aside for religious activities. Some places are kept as sanctuaries in which no human beings or animals may be killed, and where no trees may be felled. Some homesteads have family altars or graves that serve as sacred spots where prayers, offerings, and small sacrifices are made. Nature is often personalized in order that humans may communicate and live in harmony with it. If humans hurt nature, nature hurts them. Humans are the priests of nature, indeed of the universe; this is a sacred trust given to them by God, who endowed them with more abilities than other creatures on earth.

**ETHICS AND MORALS.** The ethics and morals of African religion are embedded in values, customs, traditional laws, and taboos. God is ultimately the giver of morality. Moral offenses include disrespect toward elderly people, sexual transgressions (incest, rape, intercourse with children, adultery, and homosexual intercourse), murder, stealing, robbery, telling lies, deliberately causing bodily harm, and the use of sorcery and witchcraft. Such acts are punished by making the offender and his or her family feel shame or ostracism, or pay a fine; sometimes the offender is beaten or stoned to death.

On the other hand, kindness, friendliness, truthfulness, politeness, generosity, hospitality, hard work, caring for elderly parents, respect for elderly people and the weak and retarded, and protection of children and women are virtues that earn praise and admiration in the community. Women are regarded and treated as full moral agents; they are also protected against maltreatment by men, since they are considered to be less able or equipped to defend themselves physically, especially when they are pregnant or aged. Society rewards the good and punishes the evil. The spirits of the living dead maintain interest in the morals of their descendants, and may punish offenders by causing failure in undertakings, sickness, and bad dreams as warnings or deterrents. God is ultimately watching over the moral life of the community, society, and humankind. From time to time, if moral order is severely broken, God may punish the wider society or give warnings through calamities, epidemics, drought, war, and famine.

The home and the community convey moral teaching, generally from the older to the younger members, through word and example. Initiation ceremonies (some of which may last several years) are the formal communal occasions for instilling moral values in young people. Stories, proverbs, and taboos are employed in the teaching of morals. Where the basic philosophy of life is "I am because we are," it is extremely important that the two dimensions of "I am" and "We are" be carefully observed and maintained for the survival of all, through moral values. The individual is very much exposed to the community, and anonymity is virtually out of the question.

African religion affirms and celebrates life. Laughter is heard even in the most difficult situations. Communal festivals filled with rejoicing—laughter, eating, dancing, singing, and drumming—renew and strengthen community ties. Even sad occasions like funerals are communal events that bring many people together to share in mourning, and thus lighten the burden of bereavement.

## Health and Medicine

Life in African communities is often a struggle against forces of destruction: illness, disease, accidents, childlessness, suffering, misfortune, spirit possession, quarrels, war, and death. Natural threats such as drought, earthquakes, epidemics, famines, and locust invasions affect the whole community. When these forces of destruction strike the individual or the family, people ask "who" has caused it to happen. Even if there are physical explanations of how an accident has occurred, or how a disease like malaria or AIDS

is caused, human agents are believed to be behind it. These agents are said to use mystical power—magic, witchcraft, sorcery, the spell, the curse, or broken taboos—following quarrels, acting out of jealousy, hatred, greed, or evil intentions. Health is seen as a fundamentally ethical question pointing to relationships in the family, in the community, and between people and nature.

Medicine women and men (traditional doctors) are found in every village. Their work is highly appreciated and in constant demand. They undergo long training and apprenticeship to acquire knowledge of herbs, roots, fruits, shells, insects, and juices, especially of their medicinal properties. They learn to diagnose illnesses and complaints that affect not only human beings but also animals and fields. They use divination to communicate with the invisible world at the psychic level of consciousness. They perform healing rituals and invocations. Their "medicine" is directed not only against the disease or misfortune in question but also to the removal and prevention of its mystical cause, such as witchcraft. The human or spirit agent "behind" the problem is usually named, and part of the healing process involves coming to terms with the "diagnosed offender." The process of diagnosis, cure, and preventive measures is often carried out in the presence of the family or community, which thus participates in the healing.

African society generally shows great care toward handicapped and retarded people. Part of this special treatment comes from the fear that if you mistreat or fail to help the handicapped, you or members of your family will become similarly handicapped. Likewise, the issue of abortion is partly undergirded by the fear that a major misfortune, such as the failure to bear more children, will befall the family of a woman who has an abortion. Furthermore, the high rate of infant mortality has probably contributed to the great value that people attach to children and their consequent abhorrence of abortion. There are extremely few written references to abortion, and in some societies a woman who has had one is killed by the community or a curse is placed on her. There are, however, areas where twins were traditionally considered to bring misfortune, and consequently one or both children would be killed for the protection of the community. On the other hand, in certain areas twins were (and still are) considered to be special people, bearers of blessings or extraordinary abilities, and even called "children of God." Written information on so-called mercy killing is scanty, but suicide and homicide occur in many areas. From time to time the community is provoked beyond endurance and a mob kills by stoning, beating, or burning an offender, such as someone accused of stealing and robbery (nearly always men), practicing witchcraft (nearly always women), or committing sexual offenses like incest, intercourse with children, or rape (only men). In such cases the community undergoes a healing process, physically and ethically. The life and dignity of the community are thereby placed above the lives of individual members who do not maintain its values and order.

"Medicine" is also used to bring good fortune (health, success, loving relations, protection against danger). In their practice, traditional doctors hold that it is God who heals or brings about good results, and some of them regularly invoke God for healing and the welfare of the individuals and community. These doctors are upright, trustworthy, and respected members of their community, the symbols of its welfare and health. Through them, folk medical knowledge and practice have been passed on through many generations. Since modern or Western medicine and its wonders are too expensive for most Africans, the traditional doctors continue to respond to the health needs of many people, and complement or even replace the services of modern medicine. As in other spheres of religious life, women are very active in health matters and are believed to show deeper sensitivities than men, especially since they carry human life in their own bodies and are more attuned to the spiritual dimension of health. In many communities female traditional doctors outnumber their male counterparts, and nearly all mediums are women.

## Conclusion

African religion has encountered other religions, notably Christianity and Islam, and other cultures, especially Western. Many of its adherents convert to Christianity or Islam. But conversion does not mean abandoning the world of traditional religiosity. On the contrary, many Christians derive rich spirituality from African religion. Translations of the Bible into some seven hundred African languages (as of 1992) use religious terms and concepts of African religion. But while it seems to find ways of surviving and of accommodating to contemporary life, there are changes in social, political, educational, technological, and scientific life for which it has not prepared itself.

In the nineteenth century African religion was studied almost exclusively by foreigners: missionaries, anthropologists, colonial rulers, and self-styled African experts. On the whole it was presented negatively, often interpreted falsely, and ridiculed by those with racist attitudes. However, since about the middle of the twentieth century, a more objective approach has gained ground not only in Africa but also in the New World, where peoples of African descent find in it a meaningful part of their heritage. The African religious heritage in North America provided the cultural, social, and spiritual setting for modeling Christianity among African

Americans—for example, the place of the church as a focal point of community life, the dynamic worship tradition, and the assimilation of African cultural traits. In Latin America, especially in Brazil, African religion has blended firmly with Roman Catholicism, so much so that many people do not know where to draw the line (if need be). Some of the healing practices called *folk medicine* are traceable to those of traditional doctors in Africa. Gayraud Wilmore (1983), Roger Bastide (1978), and Leonard Barrett (1976), among others, have documented the survival and strong impact of African religion in the New World.

We are in a much better position to understand African religion academically at the beginning of the twenty-first century than at the beginning of the twentieth century. Just as it has survived since prehistoric times and has done so in new social and cultural environments across the oceans, we may presume that it will survive in new forms in the coming generations.

JOHN S. MBITI (1995)

**SEE ALSO:** *Circumcision; Islam, Bioethics in; Environmental Ethics; Medical Ethics, History of: Africa; Medicine, Anthropology of; Minorities as Research Subjects; Population Ethics: Religious Traditions, Islamic Perspectives*

### BIBLIOGRAPHY

Awolalu, J. Omosade, and Dopamu, P. Adelumo. 1979. *West African Traditional Religion.* Ibadan, Nigeria: Onibonoje Press.

Barrett, Leonard E. 1976. *The Sun and the Drum: African Roots in Jamaican Folk Tradition.* Kingston, Jamaica: Santer's.

Bastide, Roger. 1978. *The African Religions of Brazil: Toward a Sociology of the Interpenetration of Civilizations,* tr. Helen Sebba. Baltimore: Johns Hopkins University Press.

Harjula, Raimo. 1980. *Mirau and His Practice: A Study of the Ethnomedical Repertoire of a Tanzanian Herbalist.* London: Tri-Medi.

Idowu, E. Bolaji. 1973. *African Traditional Religion. A Definition.* London: SCM Press.

Mbiti, John S. 1990. *African Religions and Philosophy,* 2nd edition. Oxford: Heinemann.

Mbiti, John S. 1991. *Introduction to African Religion,* 2nd edition. Oxford: Heinemann.

Mulago, Gwa Cikata. 1980. *La religion traditionelle des Bantu et leur vision du monde,* 2nd edition. Kinshasa, Zaire: University of Kinshasa.

Obbo, Christine. 1980. *African Women: Their Struggle for Economic Independence.* London: Zed Press.

Olupona, Jacob K., ed. 1991. *African Traditional Religions in Contemporary Society.* New York: International Religious Foundation.

Opoku, Kofi A. 1978. *West African Traditional Religion.* Accra, Ghana: Far Eastern Publishers.

Parrinder, E. Geoffrey. 1962. *African Traditional Religion,* 2nd edition. London: SPCK.

Ranger, Terence O., and Kimambo, Isaiah, eds. 1972. *The Historical Study of African Religion: With Special Reference to East and Central Africa.* London: Heinemann.

Sempebwa, Joshua W. 1983. *African Traditional Moral Norms and Their Implications for Christianity: A Case Study of Ganda Ethics.* St. Augustin, Germany: Steyler.

Setiloane, Gabriel M. 1976. *The Image of God among the Sotho-Tswana.* Rotterdam: A. A. Balkema.

Wilmore, Gayraud S. 1983. *Black Religion and Black Radicalism: An Interpretation of the Religious History of Afro-American People,* 2nd edition. Maryknoll, NY: Orbis.

# AGING AND THE AGED

• • •

## I. THEORIES OF AGING AND LIFE EXTENSION

Theory without fact is fantasy, but fact without theory is chaos. C. O. Whitman (1894)

An old adage says that nothing is certain except death and taxes. That is true, but it does not say anything about four score being the absolute measure of a person's years. That is good because knowledge about the biology of aging is changing, and with it people's expectations of what they can do about it. This new knowledge and the likely uses people will make of it will challenge perceptions of what constitutes a full human life as well as force people to rethink the increasing ability to alter aging. However, it is necessary here to define what is being talked about. What exactly do people mean when they talk about aging and senescence, and what is known about how aging comes about?

One goal of the material that follows is to answer the first question briefly in modern biological terms. Another goal is to describe the current understanding of the biological mechanisms that underlie aging. The final goal is to review successful cases of longevity intervention in laboratory animals and discuss their implications for humans. More extensive details and references on these general topics can be found in Arking (1998), Masoro and Austad (2001), and the Science of Aging-Knowledge Environment website.

The twenty-first century is forecast to be "the century of biology." Not only has the genome of many organisms been sequenced, scientific understanding of the way in which a fertilized egg transforms itself into a complex multicellular organism has taken giant strides to the point where developmental biology in the twenty-first century is taught as a complex series of gene-environment interactions. An outcome of these investigations has been the realization that there are few truly different developmental mechanisms. Apparently disparate organisms such as flies and humans use the same basic mechanisms in somewhat different ways. The modular nature of living organisms makes it possible to translate findings obtained with one species (e.g., flies or worms) to another species (e.g., humans). However, the adult that arises from this developmental process goes on to age and senesce and die. Somehow the sophisticated interactions fail to keep working. This seems paradoxical. As the Nobel laureate Francois Jacob wrote, "It is truly amazing that a complex organism, formed through an extraordinarily intricate process of morphogenesis, should be unable to perform the much simpler task of merely maintaining what already exists" (1982, p. 50).

Jacob's paradox contains two different questions. The first is the longtime philosophical poser: Why do people age? The second is the mechanistic consideration: How do people age? In the terminology of Ernest Mayr, the first component addresses the nature of the ultimate processes and the second addresses the details of the proximate mechanisms. Therefore, the answer to Jacob's paradox must be bipartite because the understanding of the mechanistic processes of aging depends crucially on an understanding of the evolutionary rationale for aging.

### Definition of Aging

Aging is not a single biological event but a process in which multiple biological events accumulate in different tissues over time. Despite the complexity of this process, a workable operational definition is that "aging is the time-independent series of cumulative, progressive, intrinsic, and deleterious (CPID) functional and structural changes that usually begin to manifest themselves at reproductive maturity and eventually culminate in death" (Arking, p. 12).

Although *senescence* often is used interchangably with *aging,* here it will be used to refer specifically to the changes that underlie the loss of biological function that are characteristic of aging. Studies at the cellular level have shown that the inability of cells to continue dividing in vitro is accompanied by substantial alterations in patterns of gene expression. These SAGE (i.e., senescence-associated gene expression) patterns are objective although complex indicators of a phenotype that differs from that of a normal (i.e., "young") cell primarily in its altered repertoire of expressed functions. It is the author's belief that the term *senescence* soon will gain a more precise meaning as these SAGE patterns are cataloged and those associated with a loss of function are identified. Tissue-specific manifestations of age-related disease, such as congestive heart failure, are being characterized in terms of their own particular SAGE patterns. Aging was defined above as being time-independent, for which there is strong theoretical support, but this has been demonstrated empirically in only a few instances (e.g., Finch). The existence of tissue-specific changes in SAGE patterns supports this concept by providing a mechanism by which functional loss can occur independently of time.

Aging thus should be viewed as being composed of a series of such patterns of gene expression, certain of which when induced by a variety of internal or external stimuli result in (or inhibit) a SAGE cascade, leading to the alteration of cellular and tissue functions. The large differences in life span between mice and humans, for example, can be ascribed in part to the greater efficiency of the cellular anticancer defenses in humans and thus their gene expression patterns, not to the circular observation that mouse cells live "faster" than do human cells. Also, the differences in life spans between individuals in one species, such as humans, can be ascribed to the genetic and contingent factors that collaborate to confer some extraordinary stability (in the case of centenarians) or instability (in the case of premature mortality) of their SAGE patterns. Time is, for a number of technical and conceptual reasons, a poor measure of age; and researchers will likely use SAGE patterns and other biomarkers of aging in the future. The candles on the physiologically correct (P.C.) birthday cakes of the future might be based on gene expression patterns.

## The Ultimate Explanation: Evolutionary Considerations

"Nothing in biology makes sense except in the light of evolution." This statement by the well-known geneticist Theodosius Dobzhansky has been verified by the study of aging. The operation of natural selection means that some genetic variants of any population will be more successful (i.e., leave more copies of their genes in the next generation) than will other variants, and the first variant will be favored.

Most known populations are structured by age; that is, the population is composed of individuals of different age classes, each of which represent a different proportion of the population. The high mortality rates resulting from predation, illness, and accidents that are common among wild populations indicate that only a few, if any, individuals live long enough to show signs of aging and senescence. Thus, in any wild population there are many more young breeding adults than old adults, and in each generation the genetic contributions to the next generation come predominantly from young adults. One consequence of this age structure is that deleterious genetic variants that act late in life are not selected against because their carriers probably will have died from environmental hazards before they reach old age or will have survived, but as postreproductive adults. In either case they are invisible to the operations of natural selection. Another consequence is that long-lived genetic variants will not be selected because they are expressed only in those few surviving postreproductive individuals.

From an evolutionary point of view, the "name of the game is to play again"; that is, the whole point of being a reproductive adult is to pass copies of one's genes to the next generation. This is a game that no one can win but anyone can lose simply by not transmitting sufficient copies of his or her genes to the next generation. There is no evolutionary value (i.e., Darwinian fitness) in any trait, including extended longevity, if that trait does not materially assist one in playing the game. There is evolutionary value in living long enough to reproduce, but there usually is no increased fitness associated with living so long that an individual is postreproductive (see Rose for review and references).

However, because people live so long already, why are they not capable of reproducing and living indefinitely or at least much longer than they do now? The answer to this question involves energy. Organisms must channel and apportion their energies into reproductive activities as well as into the maintenance and repair of the soma. Although the energy cost of making an egg or sperm probably stays more or less constant over time and is therefore the same for both young and old, this is not the only energy cost incurred in reproduction. The energy costs of courtship, pregnancy, and child rearing are high and represent a significant investment of energy by an organism. In addition, some energy must be devoted to the repair and maintenance of the soma if an organism is to survive reproduction. It is reasonable to assume that even a well-fed organism has only a limited amount of energy available to it. Thus, the problem facing the organism is how best to allocate its finite metabolic energy to maximize both reproduction and repair.

A theoretical analysis by Kirkwood (1987) showed that increasing the amount of energy expended on somatic repair results in increased survivorship but decreased fecundity, and vice versa. A choice must be made. Reproduction requires less energy than does repair. Therefore, allocating sufficient energy to maximize somatic repair will reduce fecundity and thus decrease an organism's Darwinian fitness. In contrast, increasing fecundity will decrease the energy available for repair and thus probably result in shortened longevity. In most cases decreased fecundity over a longer life span yields fewer copies of an individual's genes in the next generation than does higher fecundity over a shorter lifetime. Thus, fitness is maximized at a repair level lower than that required for indefinite somatic repair. Hence, people die. It is easy to see how this theory came to be known as the disposable soma theory. This process is nothing more than the cost-benefit analysis most people make when faced with the decision whether to continue to invest their hard-earned money in repairs to the old car or invest it in purchasing a new car. At some point the cost of repairs exceeds the cost of purchase, and so the old car is junked and a new one is obtained.

Because modern humans have a very low and culturally controlled rate of reproduction, it is reasonable to question whether the disposable soma theory still applies to human beings. It does, for people evolved under its aegis and the control mechanisms of the body that set fitness and repair levels are not reversed by one or two centuries of nonheritable demographic change. This concept provides a plausible mechanism by which evolution can act and has made people what they are today. Shakespeare foresaw this relationship in Sonnet 12:

> When I do count the clock that tells the time,
> and see the brave day sunk in hideous night; …
> Then of thy beauty do I question make,
> That thou among the wastes of time must go, …
> And nothing 'gainst Time's scythe can make defence
> Save breed, to brave him when he takes thee hence.

Therefore, people age not because of a philosophically satisfying cosmic reason that requires senescence and death but simply because the body's energy allocations are such that failure to repair ensures that there is no reason not to age. This biological conclusion may seem dark:. Who, after all, wants to believe that his or her death serves no larger purpose? The major religions of the world are based on the opposite premise (but see Holliday). Some people, however, find it liberating. Jacob compared embryonic development to adult aging and saw a paradox. What biogerontologists see in the early twenty-first century is the fact that there is no evidence for the existence of a genetically based aging program. People do not have an organismal death program

built into their genes. *Human beings are not required to age.* It follows that if people age only because there is no biological reason for them not to age, this clearly implies that people need not age (or at least not age so quickly) if they can supply their bodies with a relevant biological reason not to age. It is the business of biogerontologists, then, to provide those reasons (de Grey, 2002).

## Penultimate Explanations: Mechanisms of Aging

How good are those reasons? The categorization of the reasons leads to the different mechanisms that are known to be involved in the aging process. There are several methods by which one can organize the different theories of aging. None of these systems is fully satisfactory, but the origins of the change and its level of action both appear to be reasonable and logical pegs from which to hang these descriptions. Here a dual classification scheme is employed in which one considers whether the theories suggest that their particular effects are exerted within all or most cells (intracellular theories) or whether they are exerted mostly on the structural components and/or regulatory mechanisms that link groups of different cells (intercellular theories). In addition, the following paragraphs will consider simultaneously whether the effects postulated by each theory are conjectured to take place accidentally (stochastic theories) or are the result of the hierarchical feedback cascades characteristic of the species (systemic theories). Table 1 lists fourteen major theories sorted out by this dual classification scheme, and Table 2 offers a very brief summary of each theory. The highlighted terms in both tables indicate those theories for which the empirical data support their playing a central and important role.

The experimental data also show that certain aging phenomena are observed in almost all species. For example, experimental organisms extend their life spans significantly if those organisms are maintained under a reduced food intake regime but under conditions that maintain good nutrition. This method, called caloric restriction (CR), has worked in almost all species tested. It also is generally accepted that longevity is inversely related to early adult fecundity or reproduction. Elevated resistance to oxidative stress is observed commonly in many longevity mutants.

Interestingly, all these phenomena appear to be interrelated. For example, experimental organisms maintained under CR conditions have higher levels of antioxidant defense system (ADS) activities and lower levels of fecundity compared with controls. In addition, the mild dwarfism noted in CR-raised animals also is observed in mutants screened for longevity. Finally, it has been demonstrated

**TABLE 1**

**A Classification of Aging Theories**

| Level at Which Effect of Change Is Executed | Origin of the Change | |
|---|---|---|
| | Stochastic | Systemic |
| Intracellular | Altered Proteins | Metabolic Theories |
| | Somatic Mutations | **Genetic Theories** |
| | DNA Damage and Repair | Selective Death |
| | Error Catastrophe | |
| | Dysdifferentiation | |
| | **Free Radicals** | |
| | Waste Accumulation | |
| Intercellular | Cross-linkage | **Neuroendocrine** |
| | Wear and Tear | Immunological |

SOURCE: Arking, 1998, Tables 8.1 and 8.2.

that the stimuli used to extend longevity experimentally are not maximally effective (i.e., do not induce a delayed onset of senescence) unless those stimuli are capable of bringing about a particular type of metabolic reorganization and energy economy in the organism. Thus, metabolic profiles, caloric intake, growth, stress resistance, fecundity, and longevity are all empirically intertwined (see Arking et al., 2002a, or Tatar et al., 2003 for references).

This observation is important, for it demonstrates that the theories listed in Tables 1 and 2 are not the discrete entities presented there but involve different facets of the same process. What is needed are much wider and more inclusive theories of the biology of aging that emphasize the interactions between these different components. One such integrative theory addressing the relationships at the organismal level among metabolism, stress resistance, and longevity has been put forth by Arking et al. (2002a). Another integrative theory that addresses the relationships at the cellular level of the roles of DNA damage, cell division, genomic stability, and longevity was put forth by Guarente et al. (2001) and Hasty et al. (2003).

Perhaps the most successful integrative theory that has been propounded is that involving the insulinlike signaling system (ISS) (Braeckman et al.; Tatar et al.). Insulin is a protein hormone that plays a vital role in regulating a cell's response to glucose. Insulin and the subcellular signaling system associated with it are not unique to humans but are widespread in animals, being found even in species in which molecules different from but similar to insulin are used for this purpose. It is an example of the modular organization of living organisms.

This ISS is thought to play a major role in an organism's response to CR because decreasing the intake of calories has the effect of partially repressing the activity of the ISS. If one uses mutations to inactivate components of the ISS and thus bring about a genetically based repression of the ISS, one finds that the mutated flies and worms live long and express a delayed onset of senescence. The molecular basis for the apparent ability of the ISS to bring about a shift in the body's emphasis from growth to repair lies in the fact that the subcellular signaling system controlled by the insulin molecule eventually results in the activation or repression of two diametrically opposed sets of genes. One set includes the ADS genes discussed above, and the other set includes genes that bring about the rapid bodily growth and high reproductive rate of the organism. When the ISS is activated by high amounts of insulin in the blood (as a result of a high-calorie diet), the ADS genes are repressed and the pro-growth genes are activated. When the ISS is repressed because there are low amounts of insulin in the blood (as a result of caloric restriction), the ADS genes are activated and the growth genes are repressed. It seems that the ISS may be one of the body's conserved molecular switches that bring about the change in energy allocations and reproduction predicted by evolutionary theory.

## Laboratory Interventions into the Aging Process

An obvious limitation of the laboratory record is that there are few human data: One cannot experiment on humans for both ethical and practical reasons. There are four species of multicellular animals that account for most of the recent research into longevity extension. Two of those "model systems," the mouse and the rat, are mammals commonly used in biomedical research. The other two are invertebrates beloved of geneticists: the fruit fly and the worm. Also, some laboratories focus on the use of *in vitro* cell cultures with which to investigate the biology of the individual cells of the mammalian organism. Modular organization and common descent ensures that the genes each of these organisms carries are homologous to the genes humans carry and often have similar if not identical functions. For example, some 62 percent of the genes that are recognized to cause human diseases are known to exist in flies and to give rise to similar disorders when mutated. By investigating these model organisms, human beings investigate themselves by proxy.

**PATTERNS OF AGING.** When people intervene in the aging process, how can they tell if they are successful? Obviously, by extending longevity, but it turns out that there are at least three different manners of extending longevity, and only one of them is likely to be useful (Arking et al., 2002b). Compared with their normal-lived controls, experimental animals can live long by (1) increasing their early survival

**TABLE 2**

## An Overview of Some Theories of Aging

| Theory | Major Theoretical Premise and Current Status |
|---|---|
| Altered Proteins | Time-dependent, post-translational change in molecule which brings about conformational change and alters enzyme activity. This affects cell's efficiency or nature of the extracellular matrix. |
| | Proven. |
| Somatic Mutation | Somatic mutations alter genetic information and decrease cell's efficiency to ubvital level. |
| | Disproven in a few cases, but the occurrence of age-related neoplasms at least is apparently due in part to somatic mutation. |
| DNA Damage and DNA Repair | Cell contains various mechanisms which repair constantly occurring DNA damage. The repair efficiency is positively correlated with life span and decreases with age. |
| | Proven but exact role not clear. |
| Error Catastrophe | Faulty transcriptional and/or translational processes decrease cell's efficiency to subvital level. |
| | Disproven but modern reformulation has empirical support. |
| Dysdifferentiation | Faulty gene activation-repression mechanisms result in cell's synthesizing unnecessary proteins and thus decreasing cell's efficiency to subvital level. |
| | Proven. Modern reformulation based on SAGE patterns is likely to be a conceptually powerful approach. |
| **Free Radicals** | Longevity is inversely proportional to extent of oxidative damage and directly proportional to antioxidant defense activity. Damage likely originates in mitochondria and spreads out from there. |
| | Proven. Appears to be widespread damage mechanism. |
| Waste Accumulation | Waste products of metabolism accumulate in cell and depress cell's efficiency to subvital level if not removed from cell or diluted by cell division. |
| | Possible but unlikely. |
| Post-translational Protein Changes | Time dependent chemical cross-linking of important macromolecules (e.g., collagen) impairs tissue function and decreases organism's efficiency to subvital level. Related to altered protein theory. |
| | Proven. |
| Wear and Tear | Ordinary insults and injuries of daily living accumulate and decrease organism's efficiency to subvital level. |
| | Proven in restricted examples (e.g., loss of teeth leading to starvation) but modern reformulations are part of other theories. |
| **Metabolic Theories** | Longevity is inversely proportional to metabolic rate. |
| | Disproven in orginal form but reformulated into a form of the free radical theory and that reformulation appears to be correct. |
| **Genetic Theories** | Changes in gene expression cause senescent changes in cells. Multiple mechanisms suggested. May be general or specific changes. May function at intracellular or intercellular level. Analysis of changes in gene expression may be a powerful tool with which to understand the progressive loss of function in a cell or organism. |
| | Proven. |
| Apoptosis | Programmed suicide of particular cells induced by extracellular signals. |
| | Proven. Failure to induce or repress apoptosis probably is responsible for a variety of diseases. Role in non-pathological aging changes not clear. |
| Phagocytosis | Senescent cells have particular membrane proteins which identify them and mark them for destruction by other cells such as macrophages. |
| | Proven but only in restricted cases. |
| **Neuroendocrine** | Failure of cells with specific integrative functions brings about homeostatic failure of the organism, leading to senescence and death. |
| | Proven for female reproductive aging and other specialized cases. Probably involved in many other cases. Exact role needs to be ascertained as a general case. |
| Immunological | Life span is dependent on types of particular immune system genes present, certain alleles extending and others shortening longevity. These genes are thought to regulate a wide variety of basic processes, including regulation of neuroendocrine system. Failure of these feedback mechanisms decrease organism's efficiency to subvital level. |
| | Probable. |

SOURCE: Arking, 1998, Tables 8.1 and 8.2.

rate, (2) increasing their late survival rate, or (3) delaying the onset of senescence. The first two longevity patterns are conceptually interesting but have no practical application because neither affects the basic aging rate. The organisms age normally but seem to be somewhat more resistant to the various stresses that kill off their normal comrades. For example, exercising humans have a higher early and midlife survival and a lower level of morbidity. They age, however, in a normal fashion and show no real decrease in mortality later in life. Centenarians, in contrast, seem to have a higher late-life survival rate, but although they have a lower rate of morbidity and mortality, no one would mistake a centenarian for a middle-aged person. They have aged in a normal fashion but are simply a bit healthier than their normal fellows. Their health span is not affected, only their late-life mortality. These two extended longevity patterns are not useful clues to the attainment of people's longevity goals.

The most interesting alteration involves the third type: the delay in the onset of senescence. There are many examples of this pattern in animals but none in humans, yet this is the one people want. Figure 1 shows the survival curves of normal-lived and long-lived fruit flies created in the author's laboratory by means of artificial selection for increased longevity. It is clear that both the mean and maximum life span values are shifted to the right. If one assumes that the flies' health span covers the period of time from birth until 10 percent of the initial population has died, the low mortality and high survival characteristic of the first thirty days of the normal-lived animals' life span has been extended so that it now spans the first sixty days of the long-lived animals' life span. The health span has been doubled, but the senescent period occupies the same length of time (approximately thirty-five days) in both strains and thus represents a smaller proportion of the maximum life span in the long-lived flies.

These data demonstrate that the health span and the senescent span are two separate phases of the life span and that longevity extension through a doubling of the health span is possible. The fact that each of the model organisms can express this "delayed-onset extended-longevity phenotype" strongly suggests that the potential to double the health span is built into each species, including mammals. The task is not to introduce alien mechanisms into organisms but instead to discover how to activate the already existing longevity mechanisms effectively and safely. In this sense, what is being done is "natural."

What would be the outcome if this knowledge was applied to humans? If one projects a survival curve for contemporary U.S. females on the simplifying assumption that they would follow the same survival and mortality kinetics as do long-lived fruit flies, there would be no real decrease in survival (and therefore no increase in age-related mortality) until the age of about 102 years. The 82-year health span in this projected population is double that of the 40 years (i.e., 20 to 60 years) characteristic of contemporary normal-lived humans. If it is possible to understand the mechanisms in the fly that delay the onset of senescence and make them happen in humans, the goal will have been achieved.

Is it realistic to believe that the extension of longevity in laboratory organisms foretells a comparable achievement in humans? All the genes known to be involved in delaying the onset of senescence in the author's laboratory model systems are known to have homologues in humans. This implies that the relevant mechanisms are in place. In light of this fact, it seems reasonable to conclude that the failure to induce the delayed-senescence extended-longevity phenotype in humans represents a transient limitation of knowledge rather than a permanent limitation imposed by human biology. Thus, the question becomes one of understanding the biological mechanisms that regulate this pattern and deciphering the cellular signals that control its expression by the organism.

EXAMPLES OF PROVEN LABORATORY INTERVENTIONS. The delayed-senescence extended-longevity phenotype has been induced successfully in laboratory animals as a result of genetic interventions designed to decrease oxidative stress and/or alter the energy metabolism of the organism.

*Decreasing oxidative stress.* People need oxygen. Without it, human beings cannot generate enough energy to live and quickly die. However, the oxygen that keeps people alive is a double-edged sword, for it also can break down within the cell to yield highly chemically reactive molecules of various kinds that are termed collectively reactive oxygen species (ROS) or, less accurately, free radicals. These ROS chemically combine with any of the cell's components and transform them into oxygen-based damage products, a process referred to as oxidative stress. In lay terms, one might envision the cell undergoing something akin to self-perpetuating rusting.

Organisms have within them a very elaborate system with which to defend themselves against the depredations of oxidative stress. That system seems to be reasonably effective at getting rid of most (but not all) of the ROS molecules that are generated in young animals and thus keeping the level of oxidative stress to a low (but measurable) level. But even this low level of oxidative stress causes some damage, which accumulates. Eventually the failure to repair completely causes increasing inefficiencies in the body's ADS. This then allows the rate of oxidative stress and cell damage to increase at a compound rate, and the age-related loss of function soon

**FIGURE 1**

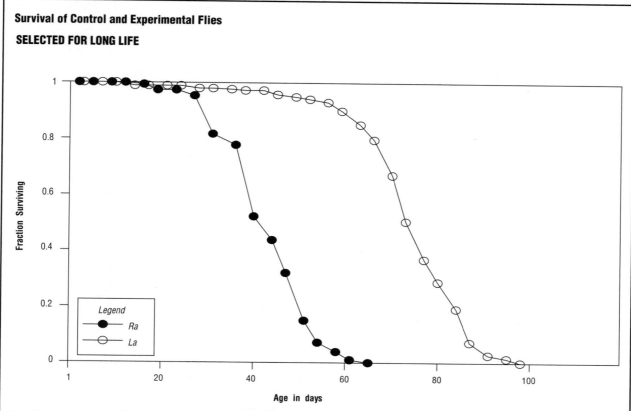

**Survival of Control and Experimental Flies**

**SELECTED FOR LONG LIFE**

Note: Survival curves of normal-lived control flies (Ra) and of the long-lived experimental flies (La) derived from them by artificial selection for extended longevity. Note the "health-span" portion of the life cycle is increased significantly in the La flies whereas the length of the "senescent span" is about the same in both strains.

SOURCE: Redrawn from Arking and Colleagues, 2002.

becomes apparent. This process is sped up in mutant flies and in worms and mice in which the ADS genes have been made inactive. In the laboratory such mutant organisms aged and died very quickly. The mice exhibit systemic failures similar to those observed in various age-related diseases.

It occurred to many investigators that perhaps one could extend an organism's health span by increasing the level of its ADS mechanisms. Genetic engineering techniques were used independently in several laboratories to introduce extra copies of certain ADS genes into otherwise normal flies. The flies then lived longer, displaying a delayed-senescence extended-longevity pattern (Parkes et al.). Equally interesting was the observation derived from the author's selection experiments, in which a normal-lived population gave rise eventually to long-lived descendants because only the longer-lived flies of each generation were bred. After some twenty-two generations the descendants had a much higher level of ADS activities, a lower level of oxidative

damage, and a significantly delayed onset of senescence, as is shown in Figure 1. Other experiments showed that certain mutants in the nematode worms also up-regulate (i.e., turn on to a higher degree) certain ADS genes—the same ones that are operative in the fly—and the resulting worms also live long because of a delayed onset of senescence (Honda and Honda). The ISS-based interventions mentioned above bring about the delayed onset of senescence inevitably coupled with an enhanced resistance to oxidative stress and an altered metabolism; this finding may well identify an evolutionarily conserved regulatory mechanism (Tatar et al.).

*Altering energy allocations.* The first intervention known to delay the onset of senescence in mammals and increase the health span significantly was reported in 1934. Reducing the amount of calories in an animal's diet by about 40 percent while keeping the different nutrients at normal levels results in healthy and long-lived mice and rats (and flies and worms as well). These findings have been replicated literally hundreds of times and are probably the most robust experimental findings in the field. However, it has also been noted that these long-lived animals cannot withstand as much stress as can their normally fed littermates (Hopkins). Similar experiments are under way in primates such as macaque monkeys; although these long-term experiments are still in progress and thus incomplete, the available data suggest that a similar response may be happening in primates. The limited human data that are available lead to the same conclusion (Walford et al.).

CR radically changes an animal's metabolism and SAGE patterns so that the animal becomes a physiologically different organism than is its normally fed sib. Many, perhaps all, of these differences can be attributed to a shift in the animals' functions from growth and reproduction to repair, possibly as a result of altering the output signals of the ISS, as was described above.

## Pharmaceutical Interventions into the Aging Process

The genetic manipulations used in the laboratory are not likely to be well received as therapeutic tools. Once the longevity extension mechanisms described above were identified, many scientists independently tried to develop pharmaceutical interventions by feeding various drugs suspected of regulating those two processes to their laboratory animals. Five of those experiments have shown signs of success. Although those independent experiments used different intervention strategies and administered different molecules to the laboratory animals, they all recorded significant increases in the animals' health span (comparable to those in Figure 1) and/or a significant extension of the animals' functional and mental abilities.

A recent experiment done by Kang et al. (2002) may serve as an example of this category of data. Those researchers fed a drug called 4-phenylbutyrate to fruit flies throughout all or part of their lives. This dietary pharmaceutical intervention resulted in a delayed onset of senescence in the treated flies, with survival curves similar to those shown in Figure 1. It turns out that this drug alters the manner in which DNA normally wraps itself around certain chromosomal proteins, in what appears to be an evolutionarily conserved manner (Hekimi and Guarente), and this alteration significantly changes the pattern of gene expression in the animal. Some genes are repressed, and others are enhanced. One of the genes most significantly enhanced is an ADS gene identical to that found to be highly effective in extending longevity in genetically engineered flies and worms. Thus, it is possible, although not yet proved, that this drug can bring about its longevity extension effects because it increases an animal's resistance to oxidative stress. Another interesting observation from this experiment is the fact that different strains of flies needed different drug doses to yield the same result. This implies the existence of genetically based individual differences in the response to drug-based longevity interventions. No reports are available regarding the existence of various side effects or trade-offs in any of these experiments.

## Is a Complete Understanding of Aging Needed Before Intervening in the Process?

There are other mechanisms that the laboratory data suggest also may be involved in regulating the aging rate. Perhaps the most persuasive is the cell senescence/telomere theory. Except for stem cells, body cells either divide very rarely (i.e., nerve cells, muscle cells) or divide either continuously (i.e., blood cells, skin cells) or when stimulated (i.e., liver cells). Those cells that divide seem to have an upper limit on the number of divisions they can undergo. There is some evidence that the telomerase enzyme may play a still not quite understood role in regulating this process. The failure to maintain cell numbers in different tissues probably underlies some aspects of age-related loss of function. The operative part of the cell senescence theory may not be the actual number of divisions cells undergo but the probability that nondividing senescent cells alter their SAGE pattern from one that inhibits oxidative damage and permits division to one that permits oxidative damage and inhibits both cell repair and cell division. If this is the case, one could merge the cell senescence/telomerase theory, the oxidative damage theory, and the metabolic change theory into a single general aging theory based on harmful changes in gene expression that shift the cell from a "youthful" preventive stance to an "older" damage-permitting stance. Such a general theory of aging is reasonable although still under construction, and a persuasive data-based account of it can be found in Fossel.

However, the fact that researchers have accomplished successful interventions into the aging process in the absence of a complete understanding suggests that total comprehension is dispensable: It is desirable but not required. How can this be? The evolutionary considerations discussed above make clear that organisms usually are geared toward reproduction as opposed to repair. This means that any population of animals will contain very few, if any, individuals that are optimally configured for repair. Most, if not all, individuals will have one or more physiological processes that are less than optimal. Tweaking any one of them—oxidative stress resistance, metabolic change, for example—will have the effect of making that organism better in that one respect. Other physiological processes not directly affected by the intervention will show no change or a secondary and dependent change induced by the initial perturbation. The animal will have some measurable improvement in at least one of the several aging processes that operate in its body and as a result will age more slowly and live healthier and longer.

This is in effect what has been done with the flies, worms, and mice. The very specific interventions used appear to have brought about a global effect on the organism. The animals live longer despite the researchers' ignorance about exactly what kind of a control cascade brought this about.

An interesting implication comes out of this observation. The more complex an organism is, the greater the number it will possess of different regulatory and control processes that affect aging mechanisms. More complex organisms, which are organized in a hierarchical modular manner, should have more potential sites where intervention could take place. In principle, mammalian aging should be subject to alteration by more interventions than will work in flies and worms (see de Grey et al.). The greater role that cell division, for example, plays in mammalian aging relative to the invertebrates and the probable relationship between cell division and altered gene expression patterns bolster this point. However, having a greater number of potential drug targets is not an unmitigated blessing. The trade-off is that the mammalian interventions probably need to be very biologically specific in order to be effective. There have been interventions that work in flies and worms but so far have failed in mice, possibly because they were not specific enough to coax the mammalian regulatory systems into altering the organism's SAGE patterns. It is likely that deciphering these specificities will constitute much of the research necessary for the development of a successful mammalian pharmaceutical intervention.

The gap between the predicted and actual effects of extended longevity on human society is likely to be huge. All the writing in the world will not define the texture of that future society. Many people would not go forward without detailed knowledge of the consequences. In the twentieth century people faced the question of whether society should permit human flight. It is necessary to ask if people really wish the Wright brothers had failed (or, worse, that their success was suppressed) and that this was still a flightless society.

ROBERT ARKING

SEE ALSO: *Dementia; Genetic Engineering, Human; Health and Disease: History of the Concepts; Human Dignity;* *Justice; Long-Term Care; Medicare; Natural Law; Population Ethics; Transhumanism and Posthumanism;* and other *Aging and the Aged* subentries

### BIBLIOGRAPHY

Arking, R. 1998. *Biology of Aging: Observations and Principles,* 2nd edition. Sunderland, MA: Sinauer Associates.

Arking, R.; Buck, S.; Novoseltsev, V. N.; Hwangbo, D.-S.; and Lane, M. 2002a. "Genomic Plasticity, Energy Allocations, and the Extended Longevity Phenotypes of Drosophila." *Aging Research Review* 1: 209–228.

Arking, R.; Novoseltsev, J.; Hwangbo, D.-S.; Novoseltsev, V.; and Lane, M. 2002b. "Different Age-Specific Demographic Profiles Are Generated in the Same Normal-Lived Drosophila Strain by Different Longevity Stimuli." *Journal of Gerontology: Series A: Biological Sciences and Medical Sciences* 57(11): B390–B398.

Braeckman, P. P.; Houthoofd, K; and Vanfleteren, J. R. 2001. "Insulin-Like Signaling, Metabolism, Stress Resistance and Aging in Caenorhabiditis elegans." *Mechanisms of Aging and Development* 122: 673–693.

Buck, S., and Arking, R. 2002. "Metabolic Alterations in Genetically Selected Drosophila Strains with Different Longevities." *Journal of the American Aging Association* 24: 151–162.

de Grey, A. D. N. J.; Ames, B. N.; Andersen, J. K.; Bartke, A.; Campisi, J.; Heward, C. B.; McCarter, R. J.; and Stock, G. 2002. "Time to Talk SENS: Critiquing the Immutability of Human Aging." *Annals of the New York Academy of Science* 959: 452–462.

Dobzhansky, T. 1973. "Nothing in Biology Makes Sense Unless in the Light of Evolution." *American Biology Teacher* 35: 125–129.

Finch, C. E. 1988. "Neural and Endocrine Approaches to the Resolution of Time as a Dependent Variable in the Aging Processes of Mammals." *The Gerontologist* 28: 29–42.

Fossel, M. 2003. *Cell Senescence and Aging.* New York: Oxford University Press.

Guarente, L. 2000. "Sir2 Links Chromatin Silencing, Metabolism, and Aging." *Genes and Development* 14: 1021–1026.

Hasty, P.; Campisi, J.; Hoeijmakers, J.; van Steeg, H.; and Vijg, J. 2003. "Aging and Genome Maintenance: Lessons from the Mouse?" *Science* 299: 1355–1359.

Hekimi, S., and Guarente, L. 2003. "Genetics and the Specificity of the Aging Process." *Science* 299: 1351–1354.

Holliday, R. 2001. "Human Ageing and the Origins of Religion." *Biogerontology* 2: 73–77.

Honda, Y., and Honda, S. 2002. "Life Span Extensions Associated with Upregualtion of Gene Expression of Antioxidant Enzymes in Caenorhabditis elegans: Studies of Mutations in the Age-1, PI3 Kinase Homologue and Short-term Exposure to Hyperoxia." *Journal of American Aging Association* 25: 21–28.

Jacob, F. 1982. *The Possible and the Actual.* New York: Pantheon.

Kang, H.-L., Benzer, S., and Lim, K.-.T. 2002. "Life Extension in Drosophila by Feeding a Drug." *Proceedings of the National Academy of Sciences of the United States of America* 99: 838–843.

Kirkwood, T. B. L. 1987. "Immortality of the Germ-Line versus Disposability of the Soma." In *Evolution of Longevity in Animals: A Comparative Approach,* ed. A. D. Woodhead and K. H. Thompson. New York: Plenum Press.

Masoro, E. J., and Austad, S. N. 2001. *Handbook of theBiology of Aging,* 5th edition. San Diego: Academic Press.

Mayr, E. 1961. "Cause and Effect in Biology." *Science* 134: 1,501–1,506.

Parkes, T. L.; Elia, A. J.; Dickinson, D.; Hilliker, A. J.; Phillips, J. P.; and G. L. Boulianne. 1998. "Extension of Drosophila Lifespan by Overexpression of Human SOD1 in Motorneurons." *Nature Genetics* 19: 171–174.

Rose, M. R. 1991. *Evolutionary Biology of Aging.* New York: Oxford University Press.

Tatar, M.; Bartke, A.; and Antebi, A. 2003. "The Endocrine Regulation of Aging by Insulin-Like Signals." *Science* (February): 1346–1351.

Walford, R. L.; Mack, D.; Verdery, R.; and MacCallum, T. 2002. "Caloric Restriction in Biosphere 2: Alterations in Physiologic, Hematologic, Hormonal, and Biochemical Parameters in Humans Restricted for a Two-Year Period." *Journal of Gerontology: Series A: Biological Sciences and Medical Sciences* 57A: B211–B224.

Whitman, C.O. 1894. "Evolution and Epigenesis." Biol. Lect. (Woods Hole) 3: 205–224.

INTERNET RESOURCES

de Grey, A. N. D. J. 2003. Strategies for Engineered Negligible Senescence. Available from <http://www.gen.cam.ac.uk/sens/index.html>.

Hopkins, K. 2003. "Dietary Drawbacks." Available from the Science of Aging Knowledge Environment website. Available from <http://sageke.sciencemag.org/cgi/content/full/sageke;2003/8/ns4>.

Science of Aging Knowledge Environment (SAGE-KE) website. 2003. Available from <http://sageke.sciencemag.org>.

## II. LIFE EXPECTANCY AND LIFE SPAN

In the United States in 1900, the average life expectancy (also referred to as longevity) of a newborn baby was 47.7 years—46.4 for males and 49.0 for females. By 1990 the average life expectancy increased to 75.4 years—78.8 for females and 72.0 for males. Why did life expectancy increase so rapidly in the twentieth century, and what are the prospects for increasing it further? Perhaps more important, has the overall health of the population improved or worsened during this transition, and what are the health consequences of further increases in life expectancy?

The measure of life expectancy at birth is a statistic that represents the expected duration of life for babies born during a given time period, usually one calendar year. Calculated from death rates observed at every age, it is based on the critical assumption that the age-specific risks of death observed during a given year will prevail for all babies born in that year, for the remainder of their lives. In contrast, life span is the theoretical upper limit to life that would be observed if everyone in the population adopted ideal lifestyles from birth to death and if external threats to life were eliminated. Some researchers believe that there is no biologically determined life span per se (Carey et al.), but rather a series of time-dependent physiological declines that may eventually be subject to modification.

Life expectancy in the developed nations increased rapidly during the twentieth century because of rapid declines in death rates (usually expressed as the number of deaths per 100,000 population over one year) at younger and middle ages. This transformation in death rates, which has occurred to some extent in every nation, is referred to as the epidemiologic transition (Omran). During this transition, death rates from infectious and parasitic diseases, which tend to kill at younger ages, decline rapidly and the saved population lives to older ages, at which they are exposed to aging-related disorders such as vascular diseases and cancer. Although a small fraction of the population has always survived to older ages, the epidemiologic transition allows over 90 percent of all babies born to survive past the age of sixty-five. The redistribution of death from younger and middle ages to older ages is a general characteristic of the epidemiologic transition, although varying degrees of decline in death rates are experienced by different nations and subgroups of populations within nations.

## Mortality Transition Patterns

There are two interesting patterns in the epidemiologic transition of the United States. In 1900 the average life expectancy for women was 2.6 years greater than that of men. By 1990 this difference had increased to 6.8 years. Although the increasing gender gap in longevity is attributable to more rapid declines in death rates for women at every age and for most causes of death, it is unclear why the mortality transition of women has proceeded at a faster pace than that of men. The prevailing explanation for the widening gender gap in life expectancy in the twentieth century is a combination of lifestyle characteristics among men that make them more prone to vascular diseases and cancer, and, with extended longevity, the increased expression of genetic differences.

Another interesting pattern in the U.S. mortality transition is the difference observed in historical trends in longevity between blacks and whites. In the early part of the twentieth century, the expectation of life at birth was lower for blacks than for whites by about ten years because blacks had higher death rates than whites. The difference in death rates between blacks and whites is thought to be due to a combination of biological, social, and environmental factors, but scientific studies to date have not adequately determined the relative importance of these factors. In the later twentieth century the racial gap in longevity was reduced to seven years. This indicates that the mortality transition for blacks was faster than that of whites—particularly for black females. However, it is important to remember that because blacks had considerably higher mortality at most ages than whites early in the century, larger reductions in death rates were required for blacks to close the racial gap in longevity.

An interesting aspect of racial trends in longevity is that at older ages (i.e., at ages seventy and older), the death rates for blacks in 1995 were lower than those of whites. This is caused either by poor data quality, resulting in an underestimation of old-age mortality for blacks, or by selective survival, in which only the most robust segment of the black population survives to older ages. Also interesting is the trend since 1984 toward declining life expectancy for blacks, while life expectancy for the rest of the population continues to increase. This unexpected trend is a direct result of increasing death rates for blacks between the ages of fifteen and forty-four—a product of higher mortality from accidents, homicides, and AIDS.

## Extending Life Expectancy

The prospect for increasing life expectancy further is a subject of intense scientific debate. Projections of life expectancy can have a significant influence on anticipated changes in social programs, such as Social Security and Medicare, that are influenced by the future size and health status of the older population. Some scientists have argued that life expectancy at birth for humans cannot practically exceed about eighty-five years (Olshansky et al., 1990). This conclusion is based on the facts that (1) survival up to and beyond the age of 110 is as rare in the early twenty-first century as it has always been; (2) the rapid increase in death rates from aging-related diseases that begins in the second decade of life has not changed in recorded history—instead, death rates have shifted down at comparable rates for most age groups; (3) the reduction in death rates required at every age to increase average life expectancy at birth to eighty-five years is extremely large—in fact, larger than what would

occur with the elimination of cancer and heart disease; and (4) life expectancy has been shown to be a demographic statistic that becomes less sensitive to declining death rates as it approaches higher levels. Taken together, these facts point clearly to the difficulty in achieving the reduction in death rates required to increase life expectancy past eighty-five years.

Other researchers have argued that theoretically, average life expectancy at birth could reach 100 years (Manton et al.; Ahlburg and Vaupel). Several conditions are required for this to occur. Under one scenario, everyone in the population would have to adopt an "optimal" risk-factor profile, maintain their physical functioning throughout life, retain the risk-factor status of a thirty-year-old for the duration of life, and respond in the same beneficial way to a fixed regime of risk-factor modifications (Manton et al.). This means that everyone would have to eliminate behaviors such as smoking, drinking, and overeating, and somehow avoid the health problems, such as arthritis and sensory impairments, that now tend to compromise physical functioning in older ages.

In a second scenario, a life expectancy of 100 could be achieved if death rates declined by 2 percent at every age for every year for the next century (Ahlburg and Vaupel). Recent evidence indicates that mortality declines of this magnitude have been rare in the historical record of the United States (Olshansky and Carnes), and that such models lead to death rates that are inconsistent with evolutionary theories about the onset and progression of death rates from aging-related causes (Carnes and Olshansky). It is doubtful that either of these scenarios is practicably achievable, although they do represent laudable goals for healthcare planners.

## Effects of Extended Life Expectancy on General Population

Observing historical trends in mortality, and anticipating future improvements, raises the question of how the overall health of the population is influenced by these trends. From a historical perspective, there is little doubt that the thirty-year increase in life expectancy in the twentieth century was a result of trading one set of diseases and causes of death for another. The epidemiologic transition allowed much larger proportions of each birth cohort to survive to older ages, something that had never before been experienced by the human population. There is little doubt this was a worthwhile trade. Now that the focus of modern medicine is to attack the causes of death that were traded for earlier in the century, we are faced with the same sort of question: What do we get in return for reducing the risk of death from vascular diseases and cancer? This is a particularly interesting question, since successful efforts to reduce the death rate from fatal diseases will produce much smaller gains in life expectancy than those achieved in the twentieth century, when primarily the younger population was saved from early death.

This question of how future declines in old-age mortality will influence the health status of the population is also an area of intense scientific debate. The debate is framed around what is generally referred to as the expansion versus compression of morbidity hypotheses. Those who follow the *compression-of-morbidity* hypothesis believe that improved lifestyles and advances in medical technology will postpone the onset of disease to older ages, thus compressing the period of disease and disability into a shorter time before death (Fries). With this hypothesis the critical assumption is that both fatal diseases, and nonfatal but highly disabling age-dependent diseases, will simultaneously be postponed and compressed against a biologically fixed and immutable upper limit to life.

The *expansion-of-morbidity* hypothesis, however, points out that factors that are known to reduce the risk of death from fatal diseases do not alter the age at onset or progression of the most debilitating diseases of old age, such as Alzheimer's disease and hearing and vision loss. Further reductions in old-age mortality from present levels are therefore hypothesized to allow much larger segments of the population to survive to the oldest ages (over eighty-five), where the risk of age-related disabling diseases is particularly high and currently immutable (Verbrugge; Olshansky et al., 1991). The empirical data used to test these competing hypotheses indicate that morbidity and disability may in fact be declining for those under the age of eighty-five, but after that age the risk of disability and its duration appear to be increasing. However, it is not yet possible to draw definitive conclusions about these hypotheses because of deficiencies in the available data.

Is it possible to extend the human life span beyond early twenty-first century practical limits and achieve an increase in the duration of healthy life among the older population? Answers to these questions may be found in work under way in molecular biology. Based on a current understanding of the process of senescence, extending the human life span would require slowing down the aging rate itself. There is no definitive evidence at this time to indicate that the life span of humans can be modified by any means. However, there is suggestive evidence to indicate that dietary restriction could postpone many of the physiological decrements associated with aging—including those associated with both fatal and nonfatal diseases of aging (Weindruch and Walford). Although it is not practical to expect that human experiments will be conducted on the longevity benefits associated with dietary restriction, or that enough people will actually restrict their diets to influence national statistics, research in this area may eventually reveal the underlying physiological mechanisms that link dietary restriction to increased longevity. In this way it may eventually become possible to imitate the effects of dietary restriction without actually altering diet.

Scientists debate these issues on scientific grounds, but there are important moral issues close to the surface in the discussions. For example, we know that a lower life expectancy observed among subgroups of the population is linked to poverty and minority status. If we are interested in preventing premature death, then social conditions may be a more direct target than efforts to manipulate the basic rate of aging. Also, the definition of "premature death" is no longer obvious, and raises questions about the value of length of life compared with quality of life when extreme longevity is also associated with the expression of frailty and disability.

Since societies do not have homogeneous views on these competing values, whose values should prevail? Further, societies almost always provide public support for infirm elderly people. How shall we value policies in the context of increasing life expectancy when many other social goods and needs are unfulfilled? This question is stated most clearly in the intergenerational equity debate. That is, should we be donating so much of our resources to the old when so many children live in poverty, when public schools are so needy? Some would argue that increasing longevity is a triumph of modern society, and if we work hard enough on prevention, we can eliminate old-age disability. But even for those who believe this is theoretically possible, it does not seem likely in the foreseeable future. Finally, the push toward increasing life expectancy raises fundamental resource-allocation questions for those concerned about the problems posed by global population growth. For example, it is inescapable that in the long run (i.e., beyond the middle of the twenty-first century), gains in longevity beyond those already expected will accelerate growth rates that, even at early twenty-first century rates of increase, will inevitably lead to a doubling of the size of the human population by the year 2050.

## The Impact of Science on Life Expectancy

Population aging also has implications in the context of human evolution. Scientists in the field of evolution biology have hypothesized, in nonhuman species, a link between reproduction and the rate of senescence (Finch). Although it is unlikely that the physiological mechanisms regulating human reproduction will be altered intentionally to postpone senescence, it may eventually become possible to manipulate the genome to achieve the same effect. In fact, the mapping of the human genome may eventually reveal these and other aging-related genes that could be manipulated by methods being developed in molecular biology. There is reason to believe that breakthroughs in this area are forthcoming and that by controlling genes that influence diseases of aging, it may become possible to allow more people to survive longer and healthier than is currently the case. Just how much longer and healthier people can survive through manipulating the genome is the subject of intense debate. It may also become possible to achieve increases in longevity by introducing pharmaceuticals that alter the environment in which the genome operates. One example is the effort to introduce into the human diet natural and artificial antioxidants (i.e., substances that reduce the amount of damage caused by the presence of free radicals, products of normal metabolism implicated in the aging process). The result may be a general deceleration of the entire aging process.

If methods of increasing human longevity are realized by manipulating the genome or introducing pharmaceuticals, then a new set of questions will arise: How would such developments influence the age structure of the human population and the social and economic institutions that have been developed under the assumption that human longevity is limited? These may prove to be a much more difficult set of problems than those we face today.

S. JAY OLSHANSKY (1995)
BIBLIOGRAPHY REVISED

SEE ALSO: *Autonomy; Death; Future Generations, Reproductive Technologies and Obligations to; Harmful Substances, Legal Control of; Human Dignity; International Health; Justice; Life, Quality of; Natural Law; Population Ethics; Right to Die, Policy and Law;* and other *Aging and the Aged* subentries

### BIBLIOGRAPHY

Ahlburg, Dennis A., and Vaupel, James W. 1990. "Alternative Projections of the U.S. Population." *Demography* 27(4): 639–652.

Carey, James R.; Liedo, Pablo; Orozco, Dina; and Vaupel, James W. 1992. "Slowing of Mortality Rates at Older Ages in Large Medfly Cohorts." *Science* 258(5081): 457–461.

Carnes, Bruce A., and Olshansky, S. Jay. 1993. "Evolutionary Perspectives on Human Senescence." *Population and Development Review* 19(4): 793–806.

DeGray, A. D., Ames B. N., Anderson, J. K.; et al. 2002. "Time to Talk SENS: Critiquing the Immutability of Human Aging." *Annals of the New York Academy of Sciences* 959: 452–462.

Finch, Caleb E. 1990. *Longevity, Senescence, and the Genome.* Chicago: University of Chicago Press.

Fries, James F. 1980. "Aging, Natural Death, and the Compression of Morbidity." *New England Journal of Medicine* 303(3): 130–135.

Manton, Kenneth G.; Stallard, Eric; and Tolley, H. Dennis. 1991. "Limits to Human Life Expectancy: Evidence, Prospects and Implications." *Population and Development Review* 17(4): 603–637.

Moody, Harry R. 1996. *Ethics in an Aging Society.* Baltimore, MD: Johns Hopkins University Press; Reprint edition.

Olshansky, S. Jay, and Carnes, Bruce A. 1994. "Demographic Perspectives on Human Senescence." *Population and Development Review* 20(1): 57–80.

Olshansky, S. Jay, and Carnes, Bruce A. 2001. *The Quest for Immortality: Science at the Frontiers of Aging.* New York: W. W. Norton.

Olshansky, S. Jay; Carnes, Bruce A.; and Cassel, Christine K. 1990. "In Search of Methuselah: Estimating the Upper Limits to Human Longevity." *Science* 250(4981): 634–640.

Olshansky, S. Jay; Carnes, Bruce A; and Cassel, Christine K. 1998. "The Future of Long Life." *Science* 281(5383): 1612–1613; discussion 1613–1615.

Olshansky, S. Jay; Carnes, Bruce A; and Desesquelles, A. 2001. "Demography. Prospects for Human Longevity." *Science* 291(5508): 1491–1492.

Olshansky, S. Jay; Haflick, L.; and Carnes, Bruce A. 2002. "No Truth to the Fountain of Youth." *Scientific American* 286: 92–95.

Olshansky, S. Jay; Rudberg, Mark A.; Carnes, Bruce A.; Cassel, Christine K.; and Brody, Jacob A. 1991. "Trading Off Longer Life for Worsening Health: The Expansion of Morbidity Hypothesis." *Journal of Aging and Health* 3(2): 194–216.

Omran, Abdel R. 1971. "The Epidemiologic Transition: A Theory of the Epidemiology of Population Change." *Milbank Memorial Fund Quarterly* 49(4): 509–538.

Parens, Erik, ed. 2000. *Enhancing Human Traits: Ethical and Social Implications* Washington, D.C.: Georgetown University Press.

Rose, M. R. 1999. "Can Human Aging Be Postponed?" *Scientific American* 281(6): 106–111.

Verbrugge, Lois M. 1984. "Longer Life but Worsening Health? Trends in Health and Mortality of Middle-Aged and Older Persons." *Milbank Memorial Fund Quarterly Health and Society* 62(3): 475–519.

Weindruch, Richard, and Walford, Roy L. 1988. *The Retardation of Aging and Disease by Dietary Restriction.* Springfield, IL: Charles C. Thomas.

## III. SOCIETAL AGING

A society is said to age when its number of older members increases relative to its number of younger members. The societies of the United States and of many other industrialized nations have been aging since at least 1800. In 1800 the demographic makeup of developed countries was similar to that of many Third World countries in the early 1990s, with roughly half the population under the age of sixteen and very few people living beyond age sixty. Since that time, increases in life expectancy, combined with declines in fertility rates, have dramatically increased the proportion of older persons in developed nations. By contrast, the age profile in many Third World countries is still heavily weighted toward younger age groups, even though the increase in actual numbers of old people is even greater in many developing countries than it is in the developed world. What future societies will regard as distinct about population aging in the twentieth and twenty-first centuries is the rapid pace at which it is occurring. Since 1900 the percentage of Americans sixty-five and over has become eleven times more numerous (from 3.1 million in 1900 to 35.0 million in 2000). The fastest growth has occurred among the oldest old. Thus, in 2000, the group aged sixty-five to eighty-four (18.4 million) was eight times larger than in 1900, but the seventy-five to eighty-four age group (12.4 million) was sixteen times larger, and those over the age of eight-five (4.2 million) were thirty-four times larger (Administration on Aging).

During the last century or more that population records have been kept, women's life expectancy has always exceeded men's (Cassel and Neugarten). Although at younger ages there are more men than women, by old age women far outnumber men (Cassel and Neugarten). In 2000 there were 143 women for every 100 men sixty-five and over. Sex-based disparities increase with age. The ratio of older women to older men ranges from a low of 117 to 100 for persons sixty-five to sixty-nine, to a high of 245 to 100 for those eighty-five and older (Administration on Aging). Although demographic predictions have sometimes been proven wrong by subsequent facts, demographers in the early twenty-first century predict this sex differential will increase until the year 2050, at which time it will level off; but before it does, there will be only 38.8 men per 100 women aged eighty-five and over.

## Ethical Implications

The rapid increase in the number of older persons relative to younger ones carries important implications for society. In the area of healthcare, societal aging will increase costs and exert greater pressure to ration services. It will thus bring to the fore questions regarding a just distribution of healthcare between young and old. The population's aging will also alter the nature of health services by increasing the number of patients who have chronic and disabling conditions that are not life threatening. This, in turn, will change the face of bioethical debate, from a focus on acute life-and-death medical decisions made at a particular instant in time, to an emphasis on ongoing and often relatively mundane problems spanning many years. Finally, societal aging portends changes for family life. Already, the imbalance between young and old is placing strains on offspring who undertake care-giving responsibilities and is prompting questions about the scope and limits of filial duties. To the extent that family members play an increasing role in elder care, their role in healthcare decision making is a significant and vigorously debated question.

HEALTHCARE RATIONING. The aging of society will increase healthcare expenditures simply because persons over the age of sixty-five consume far more healthcare than other age groups do. In the United States, persons sixty-five and over account for roughly 12 percent of the population but utilize one-third of the country's total personal healthcare expenditures (exclusive of research costs). In an era of fiscal constraints, this makes the elderly an obvious target for healthcare rationing. The financial savings that would accrue if the elderly were disfranchised from various forms of healthcare is disproportionately high, because the elderly are more frequent utilizers of healthcare. According to one estimate, if those over the age of fifty-five were excluded from treatment for renal disease in the United States, 45 percent of the costs of the renal-disease program would be saved. In many other areas a large financial saving could be achieved through excluding elderly persons.

Arguments supporting age-based rationing and the shifting of scarce resources from old to young groups have been advanced by Daniel Callahan, Norman Daniels, Richard Lamm, and Samuel Preston, among others. Callahan, for example, proposes rationing publicly funded life-extending care based on old age. Such a proposal might be implemented once society comes to accept the idea that "government has a duty, based on our collective social obligation, to help people live out a natural life span, but not actively to help extend life beyond that point" (Callahan, p. 137). Both Lamm and Preston favor directing fewer resources to older age groups and more to younger persons as a necessary condition of meeting duties to younger and future generations. They maintain that unless society limits healthcare expenditures for the old, it will eventually impoverish health services and other social goods for the young. Finally, Daniels urges one to think about justice between the young and old from a first-person point of view. According to him, when we succeed in viewing our lives as a whole, rather than from a particular point in time, it will sometimes be prudent for us to prefer a healthcare plan that distributes fewer services to our old age in exchange for more services earlier in life.

Critics of age-based rationing object, for example, to the implications of age-based rationing for women (Jecker, 1991); to the violation that age-based rationing implies of the moral thrust of both Judaism and Christianity (Post); and to the message that age-based rationing conveys about the meaning and worth of the lives of aged persons (Murray). Finally, critics cast doubt on the prediction that age-based rationing would yield large financial savings in healthcare expenditures. They point out that the amount of money that would be saved by old age-based rationing would be negligible if these dollars were simply spent elsewhere in the healthcare system.

LONG-TERM CARE. In addition to increasing healthcare expenditures, societal aging will increase the number of disabled persons and the need for long-term care, including adult day care, in-home services, and care in resident facilities, convalescent homes, and intermediate and skilled nursing facilities. Several factors will contribute to a greater need for long-term care. First, the ratio of older women to older men is expected to increase, and older women experience a greater incidence of morbidity and disability than older men. Second, the population over age eighty-five constitutes the fastest-growing age group in the population, and this group is also the heaviest users of long-term care. More than 70 percent of those eighty-five and over require some kind of assistance with one or more activities of daily living. Finally, fewer offspring will be available to serve as informal caregivers for future generations of elderly persons. This is because individuals are having fewer children than previous generations did, and greater numbers of women are joining the paid labor force.

The growing need for long-term care raises social and policy questions concerning the just allocation of funds between acute hospital care and *low technology* supportive services for chronic disabling conditions. In addition, it alters the nature of clinical ethical cases by changing the sorts of decisions faced and the age, gender, and health profile of the affected population. According to Harry R. Moody, bioethical analysis has tended to emphasize a principle of individual autonomy and respect for persons' self-determination. Yet this principle begins to break down as the patient population becomes increasingly geriatric, increasingly dependent, and increasingly disabled. In this environment, it is argued, the ideals of human dignity and self-respect, ideals that are intimately linked to human relationship and community, will assume greater significance. Yet others suggest, to the contrary, that the values of autonomy and privacy must retain their central importance because such values are inextricably linked to assuring a good quality of life in old age.

FAMILY RELATIONSHIPS. The rapid aging of society will reshape relationships within the family as parent-child relationships extend over many more years and pose new challenges in later life. Although most agree that parents undertake special duties toward offspring, there are different opinions as to whether grown children have corresponding duties toward aging parents. For example, Jane English denies that adult offspring owe their parents anything by virtue of being their offspring. Instead, she defends the idea that "the duties of grown children are those of friends, and result from love between them and their parent, rather than being things owed in repayment for the parents' earlier sacrifices" (English, p. 147). Others object to special duties of any form, whether founded on friendship, filial status, citizenship, or other bases. The favoritism implied by special duties is sometimes considered logically or psychologically at odds with the ethical requirements of impartiality and equal respect for persons. Still others object, on justice grounds, to the disproportionate share of caregiving borne by women.

On the other side of this debate are those who defend special duties. Various underpinnings for adult children's responsibilities toward aging parents have been offered, including gratitude, reciprocity, and duties to the vulnerable.

## Historical and Cultural Perspectives

An aging society, defined as a society in which the population of older individuals is increasing relative to the population of younger individuals, presupposes that individuals can be separated into meaningful categories of old and young. Although contemporary Western society tends to conceive of youth, adolescence, middle age, and old age as unique life stages with distinct sets of problems, this perspective is hardly universal. Indeed, present conceptions of the life course are a relatively recent phenomenon. Thomas Cole traces the metaphor of life's stages to the cities of northern Europe in the sixteenth and seventeenth centuries, where the current life-stage metaphor first emerged. Picturing life as a series of ordered stages represents the life course as in conformity with the order of the universe and makes it possible for every individual to "step outside of his own life experiences and view it as a whole" (Cole, p. 25).

Just as society's recognition of aging reflects historical and cultural traditions, so society's beliefs about the meaning and value of old age bespeak historical and cultural heritage. The social rank of elderly persons varies during different historical and culture periods, depending upon the perceived cost of supporting older age groups and the contribution they are thought to make (Amoss and Harrell). For example, the Akamba people of Africa believe that "the older a person becomes, the more intricately interwoven that person becomes in the lives of others, and the greater the damage done if that person is removed. At the same time, the older person has wisdom—a perspective on life that comes only with age—which is considered to be a particularly important social resource" (Kilner, p. 19). By contrast, U.S. society has traditionally valued "pragmatism, action, power, and the vigor of youth over contemplation, reflection, experience and the wisdom of age" (Butler, p. 243); hence, ageism (age discrimination) is especially evident in U.S. society.

Despite different cultural conceptions of aged persons and their role in society, anthropologists identify common biological and cultural features of aging. Thus, every known society has "a named category of people who are old— chronologically, physiologically, or generationally. In every case these people have different rights, duties, privileges, and burdens from those enjoyed or suffered by their juniors" (Amoss and Harrell, p. 3). This suggests that people in culturally distinct societies may face similar ethical questions concerning relationships among people of different ages.

NANCY S. JECKER (1995)
REVISED BY AUTHOR

SEE ALSO: *Chronic Illness and Chronic Care; Future Generations, Reproductive Technologies and Obligations to; Healthcare Resources, Allocation of; Human Dignity; International Health; Justice; Life, Quality of; Long-Term Care; Natural Law; Population Ethics; Right to Die, Policy and Law; Women, Historical and Cross-Cultural Perspectives;* and other *Aging and the Aged* subentries

### BIBLIOGRAPHY

Administration on Aging. 2001. *A Profile of Older Americans: 2001: The Older Population.* Washington, D.C.: U.S. Department of Health and Human Services.

Amoss, Pamela T., and Harrell, Stevan, eds. 1981. *Other Ways of Growing Old: Anthropological Perspectives.* Stanford, CA: Stanford University Press.

Butler, Robert N. 1969. "Age-Ism: Another Form of Bigotry." *Gerontologist* 9(3): 243–246.

Callahan, Daniel. 1987. *Setting Limits.* New York: Simon and Schuster.

Cassel, Christine K., and Neugarten, Bernice L. 1988. "A Forecast of Women's Health and Longevity: Implications for an Aging America." *Western Journal of Medicine* 149(6): 712–717.

Cole, Thomas R. 1992. *The Journey of Life: A Cultural History of Aging in America.* New York: Cambridge University Press.

Daniels, Norman. 1988. *Am I My Parents' Keeper? An Essay on Justice between the Young and the Old.* New York: Oxford University Press.

English, Jane. 1991. "What Do Grown Children Owe Their Parents?" In *Aging and Ethics: Philosophical Problems in Gerontology,* ed. Nancy S. Jecker. Clifton, NJ: Humana.

Foner, Nancy. 1984. *Ages in Conflict: A Cross-Cultural Perspective on Inequality between Old and Young.* New York: Columbia University Press.

Jecker, Nancy S. 1991. "Age-Based Rationing and Women." *Journal of the American Medical Association* 266(25): 3012–3015.

Jecker, Nancy S. 2002. "Taking Care of One's Own: Justice and Family Caregiving." *Theoretical Medicine* 23: 117–133.

Kane, Rosalie A., and Caplan, Arthur L., eds. 1990. *Everyday Ethics: Resolving Dilemmas in Nursing Home Life.* New York: Springer.

Kilner, John F. 1984. "Who Shall Be Saved? An African Answer." *Hastings Center Report* 14(3): 18–22.

Lamm, Richard D. 1987. "Ethical Care for the Elderly: Are We Cheating Our Children?" In *Should Medical Care Be Rationed by Age?,* ed. Timothy M. Smeeding, Margaret P. Battin, Leslie P. Francis, et al. Totowa, NJ: Rowman & Littlefield.

Meyers, Diana T.; Kipnis, Kenneth; and Murphy, Cornelius F., eds. 1993. *Kindred Matters: Rethinking the Philosophy of the Family.* Ithaca, NY: Cornell University Press.

Moody, Harry R. 1992. *Ethics in an Aging Society.* Baltimore, MD: Johns Hopkins University Press.

Murray, Thomas. 1991. "Meaning, Aging, and Public Policy." In *Too Old for Health Care? Controversies in Medicine, Law, Economics, and Ethics,* ed. Robert H. Binstock and Stephen G. Post. Baltimore, MD: Johns Hopkins University Press.

Post, Stephen. 1991. "Justice for Elderly People in Jewish and Christian Thought." In *Too Old for Health Care?,* ed. Robert H. Binstock and Stephen G. Post. Baltimore, MD: Johns Hopkins University Press.

Preston, Samuel H. 1984. "Children and the Elderly in the U.S." *Scientific American* 251(6): 44–57.

Smeeding, Timothy M.; Bettin, Margaret P.; Francis, Leslie P.; et al., eds. 1987. *Should Medical Care Be Rationed by Age?* Totowa, NJ: Rowman & Littlefield.

## IV. HEALTHCARE AND RESEARCH ISSUES

What is so different about the ethics of healthcare and research in older people that would render a general discussion of these topics insufficient? Basic principles, such as autonomy, beneficence, and justice, are no different and no less important because the individuals involved in healthcare or research are older. Many factors associated with aging, however, do alter substantially the facts of clinical and research encounters with older people.

## Healthcare of Older People

The nature of illness in older people greatly influences the ethical issues in their healthcare. Older people have a higher burden of illness than younger people. On average, they are likely to have several chronic medical conditions, be on multiple medications, and have frequent encounters with the healthcare system, including more hospitalizations. Because older people are closer to the end of their life expectancy, they have a greater chance of being involved in situations where difficult healthcare decisions must be made. Decisions about the appropriate use of life-sustaining medical treatment for older patients are commonplace. These range from Do-Not-Resuscitate (DNR) orders, to decisions to discontinue dialysis, to decisions about withholding or withdrawing artificial nutrition and hydration. Many, if not most, deaths in healthcare institutions in the United States are preceded by explicit decisions to limit treatment. These treatment limitation decisions, more properly viewed as decisions to change to a palliative care plan from life-sustaining or death-delaying efforts, are generally more common in the care of older people.

While any individual may become incompetent during a critical illness, older people are at greater risk of impaired decision-making capacity because of either a transient delirium or a chronic dementing illness, such as Alzheimer's disease, which results in permanent cognitive impairment. Thus, older people are not only at risk of having end-of-life decisions made in the healthcare setting; they frequently are not capable of making those decisions themselves at the time required. In such situations, physicians routinely turn to the family of an older person to serve as a surrogate decision maker or proxy. Several studies of the treatment preferences of older patients and their potential proxies (spouses, children, and physicians), like that of Allison Seckler and her colleagues in 1991, have uncovered serious discord between the choices that would be made by patients and by their proxies. While this raises concerns about the validity of proxy decision making vis-à-vis its accuracy as a substituted judgment, one can argue that family members are still appropriate surrogates and that many older people care more about who makes decisions for them than about the exact decisions being made.

The foreseeability of both serious illness and the loss of competency for older people, as well as questions about proxy decision making, have created a strong interest in the use of advance directives in the care of older people. Advance directives include instructional documents, such as living wills, and proxy appointment documents, such as the durable power of attorney for healthcare. Interestingly, most of the empirical studies done on both proxy decision making and advance directives have focused on older people. Advance directives have received increasing attention in the United States with the 1991 enactment of the Patient Self-Determination Act, a federal law requiring healthcare institutions to educate patients about the availability and use of these instruments. While it is hoped that these efforts will increase the number of older people giving advance instructions for their healthcare, it remains to be seen if older people will execute advance directives in significant numbers, and if physicians will respect the preferences outlined in these documents. Data from the 1997 SUPPORT study cast doubt on the effectiveness of advance directives.

Because of its effects on the competency of older individuals, dementia occasions significant ethical dilemmas as discussed by Greg Sachs and Christine Cassel in their article on the subject. Dementia affects perhaps as high a proportion as 10.3 percent of individuals over age sixty-five and 47 percent of those over age eighty-five, and raises ethical concerns for several reasons. First, rather than presuming competence and working within the bounds of confidentiality, truth telling, and patient autonomy expected in the normal doctor-patient dyad, when the patient has dementia, the doctor-patient relationship is altered in a fundamental fashion. A physician caring for an older person with dementia must reassess decision-making capacity frequently, carefully evaluate what the patient says for useful information, weigh what can be shared with the patient, and rely on others for information and assistance in executing a care plan. Second, the progressive and irreversible nature of the most prevalent kinds of dementia alters the goals of medical care of the patient with dementia. While promising research on dementia continues, existing treatments provide only modest benefits and there are no therapies that will either arrest or cure progressive dementias. As with hospice care or rehabilitation medicine, many, including Nicholas Rango, argue that the medical care of a patient with dementia properly focuses on maximizing function, including socialization, palliation of symptoms, maintaining hygiene, and preserving dignity. Third, the family members of an older person with dementia are not only proxies for decision making, they also usually provide the bulk of their relative's daily care needs. The great burden of caregiving places family members at risk of depression and other illness, causing health professionals to consider the psychosocial needs of the family as well as the patient.

While only about 5 percent of people over the age of sixty-five are in a nursing home at any one time, in 1991 Peter Kemper and Christopher Murtaugh estimated that the lifetime risk of spending time in a nursing home in the United States is as high as 40 percent. Thus, many older people do receive medical care in a nursing home for some portion of their lives and it is the location of death for an increasing number of older Americans, as noted by Joan Teno in 2002. At least in the United States, nursing home care frequently has been cited more for its deficiencies: unwarranted mechanical restraint of residents, inattention to treatable conditions such as urinary incontinence, and inappropriate and excessive use of psychotropic medications. At least part of the problem of poor nursing home care has been the lack of continuity in medical care of older people once they enter a nursing home. A minority of physicians in the United States visits their older patients once the patients enter a nursing home (as few as 28% in one U.S. nationwide study), according to research by Janet Mitchell and Helene Hewes. Subspecialty care, including psychiatry, is even less available to older people residing in nursing homes. On a more positive note, in 1997 Catherine Hawes and her colleagues noted that changes in nursing home regulations do appear to be having beneficial effects on many aspects of the quality of nursing home care.

Problems with access to good medical care for nursing home residents are actually a subset of the larger problem of the level of expertise in the medical care of all older people. While geriatrics is an established specialty in the United Kingdom, a subspecialty certifying exam in geriatric medicine in the United States was offered for the first time only in 1988. Very few physicians enter fellowship programs that provide postresidency training in geriatric medicine. In his study of these programs, David Reuben contends that the shortage of fellowship-trained geriatricians remains a significant challenge despite changes made in the late 1990s to shorten the duration of training required for certification (Reuben).

## Research on Older People

As with the relationship between healthcare of older people and healthcare in general, research involving older people emphasizes different ethical issues because of the history of research on older people and specific healthcare attributes of older populations. As geriatrics has been late in being recognized as a specialty in American medicine, so too has serious research on older people been a relatively recent phenomenon in the United States. The National Institute on Aging (NIA) was established within the National Institutes of Health (NIH) in 1974 to promote research on aging. That the creation of NIA was necessary is supported by the dearth of research on the problems of older people in earlier years. People over the age of sixty-five were frequently excluded from clinical studies, even from trials examining cancer, heart disease, diabetes, and hypertension, all conditions more prevalent in older populations. Older people have remained under represented in clinical trials even after

investigators stopped employing arbitrary age cutoffs as documented in a 1999 study by Laura Hutchins and her fellow researchers.

While it is not clear why older people were excluded from research in the past, conducting research on older people is more difficult than working with younger subjects. Surveys have shown that older people tend to be less willing than younger people to become research subjects. As noted earlier, they are likely to have multiple medical conditions and to be taking several medications, factors that may cause them to be excluded from research projects that are trying to study single illnesses and the unadulterated effects of single medications. Because of these factors, older people also have a higher attrition rate, necessitating larger numbers of older subjects when the study begins in order to compensate for dropouts over time. Impairments in vision, hearing, or cognition may make efforts to obtain informed consent and enroll older subjects more time consuming and labor intensive. These factors together may make research on older people more expensive to complete. For all of the above reasons, it is clear that under representation of older people in clinical research will remain a persistent challenge. Specific, targeted initiatives from funding agencies and clinical trial consortia, however, can facilitate important studies with adequate numbers of older subjects.

Two additional attributes of older people that most affect research ethics were mentioned in discussing their healthcare: the prevalence of dementia and the frequent use of nursing homes. Dementing illnesses fundamentally change the investigator-subject relationship, as well as the doctor-patient relationship. Far less is known empirically about issues in the research setting, such as the ability of subjects with dementia to give informed consent, the reliability of proxies in giving consent for experiments, or the practices of investigators in safeguarding vulnerable, cognitively impaired subjects. The assessment of decision-making capacity for research consent, for example, is best characterized as a growing but still quite immature field. Serious concerns were raised by a 1991 study, conducted by John Warren and others, of relatives who gave proxy consent for their cognitively impaired older family members residing in nursing homes. Many of these proxies gave consent for a study on urinary catheters despite saying that they thought the older person would not have wanted to participate and that they themselves would not want to be in such a study.

Over the 1980s and 1990s, various organizations and authorities have published guidelines for research involving subjects with dementia. In the first decade of the twenty-first century, the National Bioethics Advisory Commission (NBAC) and state commissions in New York and Maryland weighed in on these issues. Most authorities endorse the practice of proxy consent, as long as the subject assents when the particular study commences. Some explicitly prohibit the participation of subjects with dementia if it is known that the older person would not have wanted to participate in a study. Others worry, however, that excessive safeguards may end up serving as barriers to research that might benefit people with dementia.

The ethics of research on older people in nursing homes also focuses on consent issues because of the high prevalence of dementia in nursing homes, but there are other ethical concerns as discussed in an article edited by Brian Hofland in *Gerontologist.* On the one hand, access to research may mean access to improved care and increased socialization for an older nursing home resident. On the other hand, limited freedom and the existence of less than optimal care in many nursing homes may create a coercive environment for enrolling subjects. Another concern is that although much nursing home research is conducted in large, academically affiliated, well-staffed nursing homes, these conditions do not exist in many nursing homes, raising the question of how much one can generalize the research findings to more typical nursing homes.

Finally, all of these research ethics issues regarding older people have been playing out on a background that changed significantly in the United States in the late 1990s. Articles in the *New York Times* and *Washington Post* have reported on the concerns about safety and research oversight, prompted by deaths of research subjects, which led to the temporary suspension of clinical research at many prestigious academic centers. Clinical research is under greater scrutiny. In addition, serious questions have been raised about the relationship between academic investigators and industry.

## Additional Ethical Issues

Unfortunately, many of the issues that affect younger individuals with regard to access to healthcare and research do not disappear when people get older. While this is not a great concern in countries with a national health service or national health insurance, it remains a major issue in the United States. Many people, including a surprising number of older people, assume that Medicare, the federal health insurance program for older people, covers most healthcare needs. While Medicare pays a substantial portion of hospital and physician fees for acute care, it does not cover the cost of medications, many preventive services, and important items for older people such as eyeglasses and hearing aids; most important, Medicare pays for very few long-term care services. Older people who are poor, female, or minority,

especially African Americans, are disproportionately affected by problems with access to care. In the United States, as noted by David Barton Smith, the difference between African Americans and whites in terms of access to hospitals and nursing homes narrowed from the 1960s to the 1980s. However, studies in the late 1980s and 1990s, such as that by Kenneth Goldberg and others, continued to uncover less utilization of aggressive and expensive treatments for cardiac disease, for example, in African Americans and women compared with white men, even when insurance status was taken into account.

GREG A. SACHS (1995)
REVISED BY AUTHOR

**SEE ALSO:** *Access to Healthcare; Dementia; Grief and Bereavement; Life Sustaining Treatment and Euthanasia; Long-Term Care; Medicaid; Medicare; Research, Human; Research Policy;* and other *Aging and the Aged* subentries

### BIBLIOGRAPHY

American College of Physicians. 1989. "Cognitively Impaired Subjects [Position Paper]." *Annals of Internal Medicine* 111(10): 843–848.

Angell, Marcia. 2000. "Is Academic Medicine for Sale?" *New England Journal of Medicine* 342: 1516–1518.

Attorney General's Working Group. 1998. *Final Report on Research Involving Decisionally Incapacitated Subjects.* Baltimore, MD: Office of the Maryland Attorney General.

Berg, Joseph; Karlinsky, Harry; and Lowy, Frederick, eds. 1991. *Alzheimer's Disease Research: Ethical and Legal Issues.* Toronto: Carswell.

Coiffier, Bertrand; Lepage, Eric; Brière, Josette; et al. 2002. "CHOP Chemotherapy plus Rituximab Compared with CHOP Alone in Elderly Patients with Diffuse Large-B-Cell Lymphoma." *New England Journal of Medicine* 346: 235–242.

Danis, Marion; Southerland, Leslie I.; Garret, Joanne M.; et al. 1991. "A Prospective Study of Advance Directives for Life-Sustaining Care." *New England Journal of Medicine* 324(13): 882–888.

Emanuel, Linda L.; Barry, Michael J.; Stoeckle, John D.; et al. 1991. "Advance Directives for Medical Care—A Case for Greater Use." *New England Journal of Medicine* 324(17): 889–895.

Goldberg, Kenneth C.; Hartz, Arthur J.; Jacobsen, Steven J.; Krakauer, Henry; et al. 1992. "Racial and Community Factors Influencing Coronary Artery Bypass Graft Surgery Rates for All 1986 Medicare Patients." *Journal of the American Medical Association* 267(11): 1473–1477.

Hawes, Catherine; Mor, Vincent; Phillips, Charles D.; et al. 1997. "The OBRA–87 Nursing Home Regulations and Implementation of the Resident Assessment Instrument: Effects on

Process Quality." *Journal of the American Geriatrics Society* 45(8): 977–985.

High, Dallas M. 1991. "A New Myth about Families of Older People?" *Gerontologist* 31: 611–618.

Hofland, Brian, ed. 1988. "Autonomy and Long Term Care." *Gerontologist,* suppl. 28: 2–96.

Hutchins, Laura F.; Unger, Joseph M.; Crowley, John J.; et al. 1999. "Underrepresentation of Patients 65 Years of Age or Older in Cancer-Treatment Trials." *New England Journal of Medicine* 341: 2061–2067.

Jonas, Hans. 1970. "Philosophical Reflections on Experimenting with Human Subjects." In *Experimentation with Human Subjects,* ed. Paul A. Freund. New York: George Braziller.

Kane, Rosalie A., and Caplan, Arthur L., eds. 1990. *Everyday Ethics: Resolving Dilemmas in Nursing Home Life.* New York: Springer.

Kelch, Robert P. 2002. "Maintaining the Public Trust in Clinical Research." *New England Journal of Medicine* 346: 285–287.

Kemper, Peter, and Murtaugh, Christopher M. 1991. "Lifetime Use of Nursing Home Care." *New England Journal of Medicine* 324(9): 595–600.

Kim, Scott Y. H.; Karlawish, Jason H. T.; and Caine, Eric D. 2002. "Current State of Research on Decision-Making Competence of Cognitively Impaired Elderly Persons." *American Journal of Geriatric Psychiatry* 10(2): 151–165.

Melnick, Vijaya L., and Dubler, Nancy N., eds. 1985. *Alzheimer's Dementia: Dilemmas in Clinical Research.* Clifton, NJ: Humana.

Mitchell, Janet B., and Hewes, Helene T. 1986. "Why Won't Physicians Make Nursing Home Visits?" *Gerontologist* 26: 650–654.

New York State Advisory Work Group. 1998. "Recommendations on the Oversight of Human Subjects Research Involving the Protected Classes." Albany: State of New York Department of Health.

Rango, Nicholas. 1985. "The Nursing Home Resident with Dementia: Clinical Care, Ethics, and Policy Implications." *Annals of Internal Medicine* 102(6): 835–841.

Reuben, David B. 1997. "A Report Card on Geriatrics Fellowship Training Programs." *Journal of the American Geriatrics Society* 45(1): 112–113.

Sachs, Greg A., and Cassel, Christine K. 1989. "Ethical Aspects of Dementia." *Neurologic Clinics* 7(4): 845–858.

Sachs, Greg A., and Cassel, Christine K. 1990. "Biomedical Research Involving Older Human Subjects." *Law, Medicine, and Health Care* 18(3): 234–243.

Seckler, Allison B.; Meier, Diane E.; Mulvihill, Michael; et al. 1991. "Substituted Judgment: How Accurate Are Proxy Predictions?" *Annals of Internal Medicine* 115(2): 92–98.

Smith, David Barton. 1990. "Population Ecology and the Racial Integration of Hospitals and Nursing Homes in the United States." *Milbank Quarterly* 68(4): 561–596.

Stotberg, Sheryl Gay. 1999. "The Biotech Death of Jesse Gelsinger." *New York Times Sunday Magazine,* November 28, 1999.

Teno, Joan M; Licks, Sandra; Lynn, Joanne; et al. for the SUPPORT Investigators. 1997. "Do Advance Directives Provide Instructions That Direct Care? SUPPORT Investigators. Study to Understand Prognoses and Preferences for Outcomes and Risks of Treatment." *Journal of the American Geriatrics Society* 45(4): 508–512.

Warren, John W.; Sobal, Jeffrey; Tenney, James H.; et al. 1986. "Informed Consent by Proxy: An Issue in Research with Elderly Patients." *New England Journal of Medicine* 315(12): 1124–1128.

Weiss, Rick. 1999. "U.S. Halts Research on Humans at Duke University: Can't Ensure Safety, Probers Find." *Washington Post,* May 12, 1999; p. A1.

Wendler, Dave, and Prasad, Kiran. 2001. "Core Safeguards for Clinical Research with Adults Who Are Unable to Consent." *Annals of Internal Medicine* 135: 514–523.

Zimmer, Anne Wilder; Calkins, Evan; Hadley, Evan; et al. 1985. "Conducting Clinical Research in Geriatric Populations." *Annals of Internal Medicine* 103(2): 276–283.

INTERNET RESOURCES

National Bioethics Advisory Commission. "Ethical and Policy Issues in Research Involving Human Participants. Final Recommendations, May 18, 2001." Available from <http://bioethics.gov/pubs.html#final>.

Teno, Joan M. "Facts on Dying: Policy Relevant Data on Care at the End of Life." Available from <http://www.chcr.brown.edu/dying/factsondying.htm>.

## V. OLD AGE

Every generation seems to yearn for some glorious era in a mythic past when older people were honored and suffered little from material deprivation, derision, or debility. In the late twentieth century, the aging society of the United States has many reasons to seek such comforting ideas about the experience of old age in Western history. Growing alarm about the "graying" of an unbalanced federal budget, concern about allocating expensive medical resources, fears of intergenerational conflict, anxiety about prolonged technological dying and medical indigence, all give a strikingly contemporary, secular resonance to the Psalmist's plea: "Do not cast me off in old age, when my strength fails me and my hairs are gray, forsake me not, O God."

Recent historical scholarship (Cole et al.) reveals no grand narrative, and certainly no "golden age," capable of unifying the diverse experiences of aging and old people in the past. Of all previously silenced groups, the elderly—"clothed as they were with official respect and buried, as they often were, in reality"—may prove the greatest challenge to historians (Stearns, p. 2). Despite the difficulty of generalizing about the historical experience of older people, we can follow the evolution of life in Western history. This entry will sketch these themes. It will also highlight research findings about aging and the life course in ancient, medieval, early modern, and modern Western societies and conclude with the problems posed by the end of modernity.

Every society creates symbols, images, and rituals that help people live meaningfully within the limits of human existence. Cultural meanings of aging and old age are linked to these symbolic forms. Western culture has traditionally relied on two archetypal images to represent the wholeness, unity, or meaning of human experience in time: the division of life into ages (or stages), and the metaphor of life as a journey. Classical antiquity first connected the ages of life and the journey of life, weaving them into its beliefs about the nature of human existence and the cosmos to which human life was intimately linked. In the Middle Ages, Christian writers adopted Greco-Roman ideas about the ages of life and conceived the journey of life as a sacred pilgrimage. Between the sixteenth and the twentieth centuries, secular, scientific, and individualistic tendencies steadily eroded ancient and medieval understandings that aging was a mysterious part of the eternal order of things. Instead it became an individual experience that was best explained scientifically and divorced from larger communal rituals and cosmic meanings. In the early twenty-first century, we are living through the search for ideals adequate to contemporary culture, in which the recovery of cosmic and collective sources of meaning may stimulate appreciation of the spiritual and moral aspects of aging without devaluing individual development (Cole).

All traditions that preceded the modern, scientific effort to master old age share an appreciation of its mystery and complexity. The resulting tendency to view old age as both a blessing and a curse is therefore prominent in Hebrew, Greco-Roman, and Christian writings, each with its own variation.

## Ancient Societies

Ancient Hebrew religious literature contained an ambiguous vision of old age. It commanded the young to honor their parents and respect the old for their wisdom, yet it also described the old as "apelike … and childlike," loathed by their children and household (Isenberg, p. 149). Despite the special place Jewish biblical culture reserved for the old, the ancient Hebrews acknowledged that not all old people would be wise, nor would all children support their elders in time of need. The Book of Job specifically challenges the view that old age brings wisdom and asks why God grants long life to the wicked. Later rabbinic law translated the Biblical injunction to honor one's parents as requiring

children to provide care, a task that belonged primarily to women.

Greco-Roman literature on old age shares three common themes: the "relationship between wisdom and age; the social and political authority of the elderly; and the care of the aged" (Falkner and de Luce, pp. 4–5). While the Greeks of the classical era generally portrayed old people more harshly than did the Romans, they also viewed old age as one of life's great mysteries. Plato considered virtue a possibility, rather than a necessary by-product, of old age. Aristotle saw middle age as the peak of human life and considered old men unfit for political office. Weakness and poor judgment rendered them objects of pity or scorn.

Greek representations of old age also revealed practical worries. In ancient Greece, a son's coming of age did not absolve him of legally enforced filial duties. Greek drama emphasized that every hero's death deprived his father of *threpteria,* or support in old age. "Sons formed the only pension plan available to the elderly" (Falkner and de Luce, p. 15). While care of older family members also fell to Roman children, the absolute power of the Roman *paterfamilias,* who retained authority over his children as long as he lived, intensified the fires of intergenerational conflict (Bertman). Roman comedy, which openly flaunted rules of respect for elders, mercilessly portrayed old men as weak fools or aging lovers as objects of ridicule.

The evidence on attitudes toward and conditions of older women in Greco-Roman antiquity is scanty yet suggestive. Greek idealization of young men and emphasis on female fertility weighed against cultural appreciation for older women. Yet, postmenopausal women of substance may have experienced unusual freedom in a male-dominated, hierarchical society. Despite the literary contempt that older Roman women received, those with the necessary resources and relations apparently achieved a measure of personal freedom after the constraints of spousal roles and motherhood were removed (Falkner and de Luce). Roman custom accorded respect and authority to aging women and expected sons to support their older mothers (Banner). Even prior to menopause, Roman women did not experience the same exclusion from education or power that Greek women suffered.

The ancients divided the cycle of human life into ages or stages, each corresponding to a generation, each possessing its own set of natural characteristics. Aristotle formalized this threefold division in the *Rhetoric.* Hippocrates' four physiologically determined ages was the most common scheme until the late Middle Ages, when Ptolemy's astrologically based system of seven ages was translated into the vernacular and eventually immortalized by Shakespeare's cynical Jaques:

> All the world's a stage,
> And all the men and women merely players.
> They have their exits and entrances;
> And one man in his time plays many parts,
> His acts being seven ages. (*As You Like It*,
>   Act II, vii)

In *De Senectute* (On Old Age), Cicero identified the philosophical bedrock beneath these ages-of-life schemes, that is, the belief that despite the diversity of size, appearance, ability, and behavior that characterizes the different stages, the human life span constitutes a single natural order. "Life's racecourse is fixed," he wrote, "nature has only a single path and that path is run but once, and to each stage of existence has been allotted its appropriate quality" (cited in Burrow, p. 1).

Ancient writers such as Aristotle, Galen, Hippocrates, and Cicero also sought to explain the nature and causes of aging. Associating old age with "dryness" and "coldness," they saw aging as a process of diminution of vital heat or fluids.

## Medieval Societies

In the Middle Ages, Christian writers took up these explanations and added a supernatural cause—the Fall of Man. According to Saint Augustine, sickness, aging, and death were unknown in the Garden of Eden; they entered the world after the sin of Adam (Post). While Christian theology considered aging a punishment for original sin, medieval writers also envisioned the journey of life as a sacred pilgrimage to God and eternal judgment. Thus Christian writers fashioned a vision encompassing both physical decline and the possibility of spiritual ascent (Cole).

For the period after the decline of the Roman Empire and the emergence of a decentralized feudal society in Europe, generalizations about the material conditions of older people become even more perilous. The practical experiences of growing old in the chaotic and often violent Middle Ages are difficult to isolate. Early wills reveal the practice of notarizing contracts by which middle-aged peasants agreed to maintain their parents. This was a sign that loss of property or physical vitality rendered older people vulnerable. Such negotiated retirement practices were apparently most common among urban artisans and merchants (Troyansky). To date, there is little evidence on the socioeconomic status of older women in the Middle Ages. While old women and widows were cruelly attacked in both high and popular culture, older widows of substance may have often maintained the authority of their late husbands, while poor, single women and widows became even more vulnerable.

## Early Modern Society

Early modern Europe—the age of Montaigne and Shakespeare, of Petrarch and the revival of Ciceronian Stoicism, and later of the Protestant Reformation—was an age of widely disparate images of old age (Troyansky). It was also the period when quintessentially modern ideas and images of the human lifetime were born (Cole). During the Reformation, the traditionally circular representations of life's stages were recast iconographically into a rising and falling staircase, a visual map of the life course, complete with virtues and vices for each stage of life. This new iconography encouraged urban burghers to envision life as a career, a sequence of events over which individuals had some control. Long before longevity became a realistic expectation, Protestant writers and artists urged people to seek a long, orderly, and stable life. They wove together qualifications for salvation with requirements for longevity, thus drawing the cultural cognitive maps for the secular, institutionalized life course of the modern era.

Historians no longer identify the transition to modernity as the key to understanding changes in the lives of older people. In the shift from rural, communal, preindustrial to urban, individualist, industrial society, old people did not simply lose venerated positions of power or security and become scorned outcasts of the past (Stearns). While historians have spilled considerable ink debating the power and status of older people in North America since the colonial period, we still lack sufficient empirical data to justify strong generalizations (Achenbaum; Fischer; Haber).

It is clear, however, that the experience of growing old in modernizing Western societies was shaped by basic changes in the structure of the life course conceptualized not simply as an aggregate of individuals, but as "a pattern of rules ordering a key dimension of life" (Kohli, p. 271). Beginning in the late eighteenth century, shifts in demography and family life, as well as the growth of age-stratified systems of public rights and duties, forged the modern life course. Demographically, age at death was transformed from a pattern of relative randomness to one of predictability (Imhoff). Average life expectancy rose dramatically, especially after 1900. By the mid-twentieth century, death struck primarily in old age, and with much less variance than in the past. (The AIDS [acquired immunodeficiency syndrome] epidemic that began in the 1980s altered this trend.)

Meanwhile, the experience of a modern family cycle (including marriage, children, survival of both spouses to age fifty-five, "empty nest," and widowhood) became increasingly common and standardized (Hareven and Adams).

## Modern Society

In the century roughly between 1870 and 1970, the social transition to adulthood (end of school, first job, first marriage) became more abrupt and uniform for a growing segment of the population. At the same time, the spread of universal, age-homogeneous public school and chronologically triggered public pension systems divided the life course into three "boxes": education, work, and retirement. In the modern life course, old age was transformed from a cultural category and a negotiated phase of work and family life into a separate, bureaucratically defined segment of the life course.

The rise of the welfare state facilitated the creation of old age as the capstone of the institutionalized life course. Following the example of Germany (in 1889) and other industrial democracies (e.g., Great Britain, 1908; Austria, 1909; France, 1910; the Netherlands, 1913), the United States instituted a national pension system in 1935 through its Social Security Act (Quadagno). In linking retirement benefits to a specific age, public pension systems provided the economic basis for a chronologically defined phase of life beyond gainful employment. During the middle third of the twentieth century, this "new" phase of life became a mass phenomenon. Increasing life expectancy, the dramatic growth of the elderly population, the spread of retirement benefits, the emergence (in 1965) of Medicare and Medicaid to help defray medical costs, a booming nursing-home industry, and the rise of gerontology as an area of scientific research and professional service transformed old age into the final stage of the institutionalized life course.

By the mid-1970s, increasing longevity, economic security, and medical care available to most older people testified to the success of welfare-state policies. Shortly thereafter, however, economic troubles, initially provoked by the 1973 oil crisis, helped undermine the political legitimacy of old age (Minkler). To a number of critics, an aging society threatened the welfare of other age groups. These critics, who focused on Social Security and Medicare, blamed the deteriorating condition of children and families on the graying of the federal budget, and raised questions of generational equity (Longman). Heightened awareness of an aging population blended silently with fears of nuclear holocaust, environmental deterioration, economic decline, social conflict, and cultural decadence.

Fears about the economic consequences of an aging society framed in terms of generational equity seemed especially troubling, because modern U.S. culture offered no convincing answers to questions of meaning or purpose in old age. During the long period between the Reformation and the modern welfare state, old age was removed from its ambiguous place in life's journey, rationalized, and redefined as a scientific problem. The triumph of mass longevity was not accompanied by culturally rich notions of what old age could or should mean for individuals or society. Instead, modern old age became a permanent threshold, marked by exit but devoid of entry into a world of shared ideals, a season without a purpose.

In the early twenty-first century, which coincides with the end of the modern era, we are living through a search for ideals and roles in later life—a search involving renewed concern about the moral and spiritual dimensions of growing old (Cole). The outcome of this search, which attempts to integrate the ancient value of submission to natural limits with the modern value of unlimited individual development, will influence the answers to many pressing ethical questions in our aging society (Moody).

THOMAS R. COLE
MARTHA HOLSTEIN (1995)
BIBLIOGRAPHY REVISED

SEE ALSO: *Autonomy; Death; Future Generations, Reproductive Technologies and Obligations to; Harmful Substances, Legal Control of; Human Dignity; International Health; Justice; Life, Quality of; Natural Law; Population Ethics; Right to Die, Policy and Law;* and other *Aging and the Aged* subentries

### BIBLIOGRAPHY

Achenbaum, W. Andrew. 1978. *Old Age in the New Land: The American Experience since 1790.* Baltimore: Johns Hopkins University Press.

Aristotle. 1924. *Rhetoric,* tr. W. Rhys Roberts. London: Oxford University Press.

Banner, Lois W. 1992. *In Full Flower: Aging, Women, Power, and Sexuality: A History.* New York: Alfred A. Knopf.

Bayer, R. 1997. "Costs of Health Care for the Elderly." *New England Journal of Medicine* 336(9): 663.

Bertman, Stephen. 1976. "The Generation Gap in the Fifth Book of Vergil's Aeneid." In *The Conflict of Generations in Ancient Greece and Rome,* pp. 205–210, ed. Stephen Bertman. Amsterdam: Grüner.

Burrow, John A. 1986. *The Ages of Man: A Study in Medieval Writing and Thought.* Oxford: Clarendon Press.

Callahan, Dan. 1996. "Must the Young and Old Struggle over Health Care Resources?" *Journal of Long Term Home Health Care* 15(4): 4–14

Cole, Thomas. 1992. *The Journey of Life: A Cultural History of Aging in America.* Cambridge, Eng.: Cambridge University Press.

Cole, Thomas; Van Tassel, David; and Kastenbaum, Robert, eds. 2000. *The Handbook of the Humanities and Aging,* 2nd edition. New York: Springer.

Evans J. G. 1996. "Health Care for Older People. A Look across a Frontier." *Journal of the American Medical Association* 275(18): 1449–1450.

Falkner, Thomas, and de Luce, Judith. 1992. "A View from Antiquity." In *The Handbook of the Humanities and Aging,* pp. 3–39, ed. Thomas Cole, David Van Tassel, and Robert Kastenbaum. New York: Springer.

Fischer, David Hackett. 1977. *Growing Old in America.* New York: Oxford University Press.

Gillick, M. R., and Mendes, M. L. 1996. "Medical Care in Old Age: What Do Nurses in Long-term Care Consider Appropriate?" *Journal of the American Geriatrics Society* 44(11): 1322–1325.

Haber, Carole. 1983. *Beyond Sixty-Five: The Dilemma of Old Age in America's Past.* New York: Cambridge University Press.

Hareven, Tamara K., and Adams, Kathleen, eds. 1982. *Aging and Life Course Transitions: An Interdisciplinary Perspective.* New York: Guilford.

Imhoff, Arthur E. 1986. "Life-Course Patterns of Women and Their Husbands: The 16th to the 20th Century." In *Human Development and the Life Course: Multidisciplinary Perspectives,* ed. Aage Sorensen, Franz Weinert, and Lonnie Sherrod. Hillsdale, NJ: Erlbaum.

Isenberg, Sheldon. 1992. "Aging in Judaism: 'Crown of Glory' and 'Days of Sorrow.'" 1: 147–174, ed. Thomas Cole, David Van Tassel, and Robert Kastenbaum. New York: Springer.

Kapp, Marshall B., ed. *Ethics, Law and Aging Review: Liability Issues and Risk Management in Caring for Older Persons* (Springer Series on Ethics, Law, and Aging), Springer Pub. Co. (October 2001).

Kohli, Martin. 1986. "The World We Forgot: A Historical Review of the Life Course." In *Later Life: The Social Psychology of Aging,* pp. 271–303, ed. Victor Marshall. Beverly Hills, CA: Sage.

Longman, Philip. 1987. *Born to Pay: The New Politics of Aging in America.* Boston: Houghton Mifflin.

Minkler, Meredith. 1990. "Generational Equity and the Public Policy Debate: Quagmire or Opportunity?" In *A Good Old Age? The Paradox of Setting Limits,* pp. 222–239, ed. Paul Homer and Martha Holstein. New York: Simon & Schuster.

Moody, Harry R. 1992. *Ethics in an Aging Society.* Baltimore: Johns Hopkins University Press.

Plato. 1968. *The Republic,* tr. Francis MacDonald Cornford. London: Oxford University Press.

Post, Stephen. 1992. "Aging and Meaning: The Christian Tradition." In *The Handbook of the Humanities and Aging,* pp. 127–146, ed. Thomas Cole, David Van Tassel, and Robert Kastenbaum. New York: Springer.

Quadagno, Jill S. 1988. *The Transformation of Old Age Security: Class and Politics in the American Welfare State.* Chicago: University of Chicago Press.

Stearns, Peter N. 1982. *Old Age in Preindustrial Society.* New York: Holmes & Meier.

ter Meulen R. 1994. "Are There Limits to Solidarity with the Elderly?" *Hastings Cent Report* 24(5): 36–38.

Troyansky, David. 1992. "The Older Person in the Western World: From the Middle Ages to the Industrial Revolution." In *The Handbook of the Humanities and Aging,* pp. 40–61, ed. Thomas Cole, David Van Tassel, and David Kastenbaum. New York: Springer.

## VI. ANTI-AGING INTERVENTIONS: ETHICAL AND SOCIAL ISSUES

An estimated 2,500 physicians in the United States had established specialty practices devoted to "longevity medicine" by 2003, and the American Academy of Anti-Aging Medicine (A4M) boasted 11,000 members in that year. The goal of this clinical community is to extend the time their patients can live without the morbidities of the aging process; namely "memory loss, muscle loss, visual impairment, slowed gait and speech, wrinkling of the skin, hardening of the arteries, and all the other maladies we call aging" (Shelton). At the beginning of the twenty-first century, however, there was little the practitioners of anti-aging medicine could prescribe that had any scientific validation (Olshansky, Hayflick, and Carnes; Butler et al.). But the scientists who study the biology of human aging, known as *biogerontologists,* are slowly making headway, and a central research agenda for this community is to provide clinicians with the tools they require to make anti-aging medicine a reality (Kirkwood; Olshansky and Carnes).

Biogerontologists pursue a wide array of scientific strategies, based on a variety of different theories about the biological process of aging. However, their research programs generally fall into one of three basic types, depending on their goals. The most conservative model is commonly described as seeking *compressed morbidity* (Fries). The goal of biogerontological research under this paradigm is to forestall the chronic ailments of old age so that humans will be able to live long, healthy, and vigorous lives within the limits of the maximum life span for the human species. Its approach, however, is to prevent age-associated maladies by intervening in the underlying aging processes that make people vulnerable to them, rather than attack them piecemeal (Kirkland). In this model, biogerontologists are actively seeking increases in the average human life expectancy, but not increases in the maximum human life span. The successful realization of this paradigm will result in a society with many more very old people playing active social roles right up until their death.

A second, more ambitious paradigm seeks to produce *decelerated aging*. Here, the research goal is to develop ways to slow the fundamental processes of aging to the extent that both average life expectancy and maximum life span are increased beyond the species' prior experience. Under this model, people would continue to move through the same stages of senescence (decline) as they age, but the process would take place against an elongated timescale, providing more years of vigorous life before the declines of old age. One prominent biogerontologist suggests, for example, that it may be possible to produce ninety-year-old individuals who are as healthy and active as today's fifty-year-olds, as well as to achieve a mean life expectancy of about 112 years for Caucasian American and Japanese women, with an "occasional outlier" reaching an age of about 140 years (Miller).

The most radical paradigm being subscribed to by biogerontologists is arrested aging. Here the hope is to develop the ability to continously reverse the processes of aging as they occur in adults, in order to maintain vitality and function indefinitely (Fossel; De Grey et al.). Some scientists envision that "negligible senescence" could be accomplished by finding ways of removing the damage inevitably caused by basic metabolic processes, and thereby attaining an indefinite postponement of aging. They expect that substantive progress toward this objective will be feasible by the second decade of the twenty-first century (De Grey et al.).

## Should Scientists Attempt to Control Aging?

The fundamental philosophical and cultural challenge of anti-aging research is the blow that it could deal to aging's historical role as a constant in human affairs. If it is not necessary to assume the universality of aging in the ordering of society, new choices present themselves. From the point of view of the public good, is aging, as it is now known, a human experience to be encouraged or discouraged? Both biomedicine and American culture reinforce the inclination to interpret the biological changes that accompany human aging as losses that harm those who experience them (Cole and Gadow). Society in general and health professionals in particular have a fundamental obligation to do what they can to protect people from the harms to which they are vulnerable, whether those harms originate with terrorists, epidemic disease, the accumulated insults of the environment, or genes. Though not everyone would choose to avoid

the "harms" of aging, should those who wish to use these interventions be discouraged from doing so?

It is clear that there is a powerful psychological dynamic at work behind the bioethical debates over anti-aging research. Against the mythic power of rejuvenation, almost any form of social and personal risks involved in pursing the mastery of aging fade away. This is because it has so often been rejuvenation—in the forms of resurrection, reincarnation, renewal, or rebirth—that defeat deterioration and death in human belief systems (Gruman).

Critics of anti-aging medicine suggest that cultural and medical assumptions about the biological changes of late adulthood might be different if society were not so pervasively influenced by the perspective of those who have not yet undergone them (Callahan, 1993). Perhaps, when seen from the other side, not all the changes that young adults view as the harmful losses of aging are harms at all. One familiar example of this is menopause—this loss of reproductive capacity, though fraught with physical and emotional turbulence, is one that many women come to celebrate as opening new opportunities and life pleasures (Martin; Logothetis). Similarly, in many societies the loss of physical strength and endurance that comes with aging allows the individual to relinquish responsibility for the labor of survival and move into an even more important role as an elder for his or her community (Moody, 1986).

Traditionally, even the health challenges of aging (e.g., failing senses, vulnerability to disease and accident) have been seen as contributing to the life experiences of older adults in a way that gives them a level of equanimity and insight difficult to achieve at earlier stages in life (Post). The psychologist Erik Erikson has looked to old age as a crucial source of generativity in the human life cycle, and the philosophers Daniel Callahan and Leon Kass have argued that growing old provides special opportunities for teaching, wisdom, and altruism. This does not mean that the major diseases that threaten human health in late adulthood are not a cause of concern, but it does suggest that attempting to intervene in the aging process itself, for all its attendant complaints, may be shortsighted and harmful because it would deny adults the wider benefits of growing old.

On the other hand, advocates of anti-aging medicine claim that, at best, this argument leads to the position that it would be wrong to deny people the right to "grow old gracefully" if they value the benefits of doing so (Stock). The physical burdens that accompany aging can be very serious, and modern society is not designed to optimize the role of the elderly. Given the social realities of aging in modern Western culture, many adults would consider the price of the late stages of human development high enough to warrant attempts to postpone and compress them as much as possible. Advocates of anti-aging research point out that respecting that human ability to project and pursue a life plan is at the heart of what it means to respect self-determination and personal autonomy.

### Is There a Natural Life Cycle?

In reply, the critics of anti-aging medicine ask us to imagine our reactions to a hypothetical biomedical intervention that would interrupt the development of a child and extend childhood by delaying puberty (Hayflick). What is worrisome about that is not simply the psychological harm such a developmental distortion might produce. Nor is it just a matter of violating the child's rights to self-determination—those rights are not yet in full flower and it is their parents' role to protect, and to some extent define, the child's best interests. If interrupted, the child's bodily development is no longer progressing on its own schedule, nor is it being driven by the complex, automatic interplay of genes and their reactions to the environment. Such a disruption of the child's "developmental autonomy" alienates his or her life story from the temporal narrative that characterizes the human species.

Postponing the normal biological changes of aging, the critics argue, constitutes a similar disruption. Whether or not the biological changes of aging are beneficial or harmful, they are meaningful: They and their natural timing constitute part of the normal life cycle for human beings, and thus part of what it means to be human (Kass, 2001). Intentionally distorting that cycle alienates the elderly from the definitive human life story, and dehumanizes them in the process. In this view, adults should be taught to seek the meaning of the later stages of human development, and biomedical research should focus on making the experience of that part of life as healthy and pleasant as possible, but not interfere in its essential rhythm (Callahan, 2000).

Of course, arguing that the traditional human life cycle is normative for human beings requires a good bit of philosophical work if it is not be reduced to a statement of religious faith or accused of making a virtue of necessity (Overall). Just because human beings have always lived their lives within a traditional time frame is not necessarily a reason to continue doing so. In fact, the social and technological dimensions of the "typical human life story" have been rewritten continuously during human history, without diminishing the moral status of those people whose lives are made possible by that evolution (Gruman). Given this history of pushing back the natural limits of human life through science and technology, the burden of proof, the

advocates argue, is on the critics to complete their philosophical project convincingly. Until then, theirs is one ideology among many, which autonomous adults (and researchers) in a free society should have the right to assess, adopt, or reject as they will.

### The Limits of Medicine

Interestingly, one sector of medicine that is strongly wed to a naturalist ideology is biomedicine. Human health is usually understood by biomedicine not merely as the absence of diagnosable disease, but as functioning within a range that is typical for human beings of one's age and gender (Boorse). For functionalists in biomedicine, the statistically "normal" is morally normative; that is, it represents the state of health that is supposed to be the goal of research and the priority of practice. This is why biomedical professionals strive to draw a line between their work devoted to addressing health problems and the use of their work for cosmetic, aesthetic, athletic, or social enhancements (Juengst). The use of medical tools for enhancement might be tolerated in a free society, but to the extent that they do not address *bona fide* health needs, they should not be given a high priority by health professionals and researchers. On what side of this professional boundary line should human growth hormone (HGH) replacement fall? If there is nothing pathological about the aging process itself, critics argue, all the current efforts that health professionals are mounting to combat it seem wrong-headed and wasteful (Callahan, 2000).

From this perspective, it becomes crucial for the ethical debate over anti-aging research to answer the question of whether or not intervening in human aging is a legitimate form of healthcare. Part of the problem, of course, is the current limited knowledge of the fundamental causes and dynamics of the aging process. In this debate, the scientific contest between the theories of aging that rely on accumulated insults and those that look to genetics is crucial. If the aging process turns out to be a confluence of conditions that would individually be considered health problems, and that vary between individuals and across populations, it would be plausible to conceptualize the process as ultimately accidental, and thus to medicalize the causal cofactors as individual health problems (Caplan).

On the other hand, if aging is a natural and inevitable consequence of normal physiology, then the process itself is normal, and therefore healthy. This is a matter of scientific interpretation, but to the extent that cellular, metabolic, and organismic senescence is inherent in the human species, the less legitimate anti-aging research appears as a field of health science. This in itself does not mean that there is anything intrinsically wrong with anti-aging research, of course, any more than research into advanced tattoo techniques is wrong. It only means that anti-aging researchers must give up their claims to be promoting human health—and the measure of public support that mantle provides (Murphy).

It is unlikely that anti-aging researchers will be able to offer any intervention that could address the genetically programmed aspects of the aging process in the foreseeable future. Instead, partial interventions, such as HGH replacement, will be developed in response to genuine health concerns. Almost any intervention that would postpone specific milestones of normal aging would also help prevent the health problems common to those milestones. Would successful HGH replacement prolong the vitality of the musculature or prevent the onset of aged-related weakness? As long as these are two sides of the same coin, the anti-aging effects of such interventions will always be eclipsed by the medical obligation to prevent disease, effectively deciding the question of the intervention's appropriateness and the need for its development (Juengst). Against this conceptual backdrop, anti-aging researchers might insist, it would be better to embrace the anti-aging goals of the patients and researchers interested in these interventions, rather than foster increased off-label (unapproved) use of interventions without appropriate safety and efficacy testing. A well-regulated and thoughtful program of anti-aging research, they could argue, will ultimately do more to protect the public welfare than relegating the effort to the margins of biomedicine (Mehlman).

## Fairness in Anti-Aging Medicine

Critics might reply that appeals to the public welfare change the terms of the debate once again. At the level of social policy, the dangers of the off-label use of medical interventions for anti-aging purposes dim in comparison to the injustices that might be facilitated if anti-aging interventions are treated as elective enhancements. Public attitudes toward the enhancement technologies already available suggest that the demand for truly effective anti-aging interventions will be so substantial that legal prohibition would simply produce a robust black market in these interventions. On the other hand, if the interventions are seen as "elective" or "cosmetic" enhancements, they are likely to be left to the market to distribute, according to the ability of consumers to pay.

If anti-aging interventions are, like other cosmetic uses of medical tools, available only to those who can afford them, society would see the disparities between the haves and the have nots exacerbated in a particularly insidious way. For example, if wealthier older adults can maintain their youthful features, they may come to have more interests in

common with young adults than with the poor elderly population, and this may lead to a shift in political allegiances. If they were to continue to identify with their age cohort, a larger population of youthful elderly might benefit the interests of the aging elderly. If other interests realign allegiances, however, the poorer aging elderly could find themselves increasingly marginalized. If anti-aging medicine ultimately stigmatizes the aging process as a pathology of the poor, this political disadvantage could be compounded even further by social intolerance (Seltzer).

One alternative, of course, is for the government to play a role in financing and distributing these interventions. For candidates of equal age, should the previously treated or the untreated have the highest priority? For candidates of equal health status, should the chronologically younger or older take precedence? Finally, how should the benefits of these interventions be measured in order to determine the amount of public funds that should be spent on making them widely available?

These are critical public-policy questions that will have to be addressed as anti-aging interventions become available. On the other hand, they are not problems that should guide the progress of scientific work. In practice, medicine is not likely to police anti-aging interventions for social policy reasons unless it becomes clear that the social problems created by their availability as elective medical services are severe enough to compare with public health emergencies. According to some critics, such crises are not unforeseeable in a long-lived society (Hayflick). But until it is clearer that medicine should steer by social justice as well as patient welfare, the advocates argue complicity that with these social problems is not likely to stand in the way of anti-aging medicine.

## Conclusion

The prospect of anti-aging interventions raises searching questions for individual families, biomedical professionals, and public policy. Most of the issues described here are questions that need to be addressed at all three levels, and they call for both social-scientific research and deep cultural reflection on the meaning of aging. Nevertheless, it not too early for anticipatory public discussions of these questions to begin.

ERIC T. JUENGST

SEE ALSO: *Enhancement Uses of Medical Technology; Human Dignity; Transhumanism and Posthumanism;* and other *Aging and the Aged* subentries

**BIBLIOGRAPHY**

Binstock, Robert. 1998. "Public Policies on Aging in the 21st Century." *Stanford Law and Policy Review* 9: 2311–2328.

Boorse, Christopher. 1977. "Health as a Theoretical Concept." *Philosophy of Science* 44: 542–573.

Butler, Robert, et al. 2002. "Is There an Anti-Aging Medicine?" *Journal of Gerontology: Biological Sciences* 57A(9): B333–B338.

Callahan, Daniel. 1993. *The Troubled Dream of Life: Living with Mortality.* New York: Simon & Schuster.

Callahan, Daniel. 2000. "Death and the Research Imperative." *New England Journal of Medicine* 342: 654–656.

Caplan, Arthur. 1981. "The Unnaturalness of Aging: A Sickness unto Death?" In *Concepts of Health and Disease,* ed. A. Caplan, H. T. Engelhardt, and J. McCartney. Reading, MA: Addison Wesley.

Cole, Thomas, and Gadow, Sally, eds. 1986. *What Does It Mean to Grow Old? Reflections from the Humanities.* Durham, NC: Duke University Press.

De Grey, Aubrey; Ames, B. N.; and Andersen, J. K.; et al. 2002. "Time to Talk SENS: Critiquing the Immutability of Human Aging." *Annals of the New York Academy of Sciences* 959: 452–462.

Erikson, Erik. 1982. *The Life Cycle Completed: A Review.* New York: Norton.

Fossel, Michael. 1996. *Reversing Human Aging.* New York: William Morrow.

Fries, J. 1988. "Aging, Illness, and Health Policy: Implications of the Compression of Morbidity." *Perspectives in Biology and Medicine* 31(3): 407–428.

Gruman, Gerald. 1966. "A History of Ideas about the Prolongation of Life." *Transactions of the American Philosophical Society, New Series* 56: 5–97.

Hackler, Chris. 2001–2002. "Troubling Implications of Doubling the Human Lifespan." *Generations* 25:15–19.

Hayflick, Leonard. 2001–2002. "Anti-aging Medicine: Hype, Hope, and Reality." *Generations* 25: 20–26.

Juengst, Eric. 1988. "What Does Enhancement Mean?" In *Enhancing Human Traits: Ethical and Social Implications,* ed. E. Parens. Washington, D.C.: Georgetown University Press.

Kass, Leon. 1983. "The Case for Mortality." *American Scholar* 52: 173–191.

Kass, Leon. 2001. "L'Chaim and Its Limits: Why Not Immortality?" *First Things* 113(May): 17–25.

Kirkland, J. L. 2002. "The Biology of Senescence: Potential for Prevention of Disease." *Clinics in Geriatric Medicine* 18: 383–340.

Kirkwood, Thomas. 1999. *Time of Our Lives: The Science of Human Aging.* New York: Oxford University Press.

Logothetis, M. L. 1993. "Disease or Development: Women's Perceptions of Menopause." In *Menopause: A Midlife Passage,* ed. Joan Callahan. Bloomington: Indiana University Press.

Martin, M. 1985. "Malady and Menopause." *Journal of Medicine and Philosophy* 10: 329–339.

Mehlman, Maxwell. 1999. "How Will We Regulate Genetic Enhancement?" *Wake Forest Law Review* 34: 671–715.

Miller, Richard. 2002. "Extending Life: Scientific Prospects and Political Obstacles." *Milbank Quarterly* 80: 155–174.

Moody, Henry. 1986. "The Meaning of Life and the Meaning of Old Age." In *What Does It Mean to Grow Old? Reflections from the Humanities,* ed. T. Cole and S. Gadow. Durham, NC: Duke University Press.

Moody, Henry. 2001–2002. "Who's Afraid of Life Extension?" *Generations* 25: 33–37.

Murphy, Timothy. 1986. "A Cure for Aging?" *Journal of Medicine and Philosophy* 11: 237–257.

Olshansky, Stephen J., and Carnes, Bruce. 2001. *The Quest for Immortality: Science at the Frontiers of Aging.* New York: Norton.

Olshansky, S. J.; Hayflick, L.; and Carnes, B. 2002. "Position Statement on Human Aging." *Journal of Gerontology: Biological Sciences* 57A(8): B292–B297.

Overall, Christine. 2003. *Aging, Death, and Human Longevity: A Philosophical Inquiry.* Berkeley: University of California Press.

Post, Stephen. 2000. "The Concept of Alzheimer Disease in an Hypercognitive Society." In *Concepts of Alzheimer Disease: Biological, Clinical and Cultural Perspectives,* ed. Peter Whitehouse, K. Maurer, and J. Ballenger. Baltimore, MD: Johns Hopkins University Press.

Seltzer, M., ed. 1995. *The Impact of Increased Life Expectancy: Beyond the Gray Horizon.* New York: Springer.

Shelton, D. 2000. "Dipping into the Fountain of Youth." *AMA News* December 4: 25.

Stock, Gregory. 2002. *Redesigning Humans: Our Inevitable Genetic Future.* New York: Houghton Mifflin.

# AGRICULTURE AND BIOTECHNOLOGY

• • •

Among approximately 80,000 types of plants that are known to be edible, only about 100 are cultivated intensively worldwide, and of that number fewer than 20, such as rice, maize, wheat, and rapeseed, provide 90 percent of food crops. This handful of species has been subjected to genetic manipulation for millennia so that even before the advent of gene splicing, they diverged dramatically in genotype and phenotype from their wild ancestors.

## The Distinction between Conventional Breeding and Genetic Engineering

For thousands of years human beings have altered the genomes of all major crops radically and constantly to change growth and ripening characteristics, speed maturity, eliminate grain shattering, improve taste and reduce toxins, increase size, and even get rid of seeds, as in grapes and bananas. Pictures comparing the wild and cultivated types of any crop invite incredulity because the differences are so sweeping.

Crops that are very different from each other, such as Brussels sprouts, cabbage, cauliflower, and broccoli, derive from the same ancestral stock, whereas other crops, such as bread wheat and canola, are artifacts. Wheat used for bread was created when technologists about 4,000 years ago hybridized tetraploid durum wheat with an inedible goat grass. Canola (Canada oil) was fabricated in the twentieth century by Canadian biologists who assaulted and pummeled by heat, radiation, and other means the genome of an inedible rape (mustard) plant. They selected for mutations that eliminated toxic acids and smelly glucosinolates that had made the plentiful rapeseed oil unpalatable. Every cultivar has a story of genetic manipulation and hybridization that explains its stark differences from its wild ancestors. Some of those stories, such as those of kiwi fruit, strawberry, and tomato, suggest that one can make the agronomic equivalent of a silk purse out of a sow's ear.

To assess ethical objections to agricultural biotechnology one must distinguish concerns that apply to forced mutation, hybridization, and artificial selection generally from those that apply only to the changes—often small by comparison—associated with genetic manipulation (GM). Because conventional breeding techniques have become more sophisticated and in principle may be able to achieve (although more arduously) the same mutations that GM accomplishes easily, the boundary between old and new biotechnologies may be hard to draw. The principal difference may be this: GM performs "outcrosses" that take advantage of the apparent fact that all life has the same origin, whereas conventional techniques cross species that are more closely related or apply pressure to a genome to induce hoped-for changes.

## Health Risks and Benefits of GM Food

Critics of GM food present three kinds of arguments to suggest that it may not be good to eat (Thompson, p. 76). First, GM foods may produce allergic reactions because known or unknown allergens could be introduced into products people believe are safe. The food industry should and does take this problem seriously; the liability issues alone are sobering. For example, because many people are allergic to peanuts, it would be risky to introduce into other crops genes that code for a protein unique to the peanut. The fact that GM foods should be tested or screened for allergens— and this may be true of all foods—seems incontrovertible.

Second, critics contend that GM foods are not more nutritious or tasty or otherwise better for the consumer than the foods that traditionally have been available (Kneen). This is largely correct. Although all kinds of crops that promise benefits to the consumer are said to be on the horizon, few have materialized; even the highly touted vitamin A–rich "golden" rice may not be better—or cheaper or more acceptable to target consumers—than simple vitamin pills. As things stand, the benefits of GM crops go principally to farmers; those benefits will be considered below. Time will tell whether GM foods will offer significant benefits to consumers.

Third, critics invoke the precautionary principle to argue that GM is novel and untested: How can one be sure it is safe? (Pence, ch. 5). Defenders of the technology answer that GM crops are hardly new; hybridization, including distant outcrossing, has been the basis of agriculture for millennia (Prakash). The genetic alterations GM achieves are more precise and therefore less extensive than are those associated with conventional breeding. There is no evidence that suggests that genetic material introduced into a plant from more distant relatives is more dangerous than that introduced from closer cousins. The food product, moreover, will not be any less safe because of the placement of a few nucleotides in its DNA. The oil from GM soy or canola, indeed, will not contain in principle any DNA or protein (there could be traces) and thus will be chemically identical to that from the non-GM plant, which is itself an artifact of conventional breeding. Those who study the extent to which genomes of plant crops have been manipulated over the millennia see no reason to think that twenty-first century techniques produce food that is inherently more dangerous (IFT).

Those who make this reply do not contend that forced mutation and artificial selection—whether by conventional methods of breeding, more advanced techniques of hybridization, or genetic recombination—are always or necessarily safe. Instead, they contend that the risks are the same across all these ways of re-creating plant genomes. Techniques of embryo rescue, mutation-forcing irradiation, and wide crosses that transformed varieties of nightshade into the tomato, for example, dwarf twenty-first century's molecular methods in scope and effect.

As expert panels typically find, "Crops modified by modern molecular and cellular methods pose risks no different from those modified by earlier genetic methods…"

(IFT, p. 23). Similarly, a FAO/WHO (1991) report stated: "Biotechnology has a long history of use in food production and processing. It represents a continuum embracing both traditional breeding techniques and the latest techniques based on molecular biology. The newer biotechnological techniques, in particular, open up very great possibilities of rapidly improving the quantity and quality of food available. The use of these techniques does not result in food that is inherently less safe than that produced by conventional ones."

## GM and the Farmer

Farmers eagerly adopt GM varieties, especially herbicide-resistant soybean and insect-resistant cotton and corn, for several economic reasons. Farmers like to rotate soy with corn, for example, because soy, a legume, nourishes the soil corn depletes. However, soy is sensitive to the residues of glyphosphate herbicide that control weeds in corn. A glyphosphate-tolerant (Roundup-Ready) soy allows rotation; an insect-resistant corn goes far toward eliminating that risk. As farmers produce a more predictable crop—and are able to plant more closely because they do not have to cultivate it—their harvests increase. This is a mixed blessing, however, because the resulting surpluses drive down prices. As the risks decrease, moreover, farms become a target for vertical integration by agribusiness.

In the developed world GM crops represent the latest turn in the technological treadmill, with the usual consequence: glut. According to the pure theory of the treadmill, as overproduction causes crop prices to fall, farmers adopt new technology to increase yields and lower cost. The early adopters of the new technology eke out a profit by underpricing the competition, thus driving farm prices down farther. Those who are late to adopt the technology go broke and sell their land to those who still operate, leading to ever-greater concentration in the industry. The survivors must adopt increasingly more efficient technology, and so the cycle continues (Cochrane, p. 429).

In the twenty-first century, although about 593,000 Americans identify farming as their principal occupation, most of those farmers produce less than $100,000 in annual sales; only about 172,000 farmers produce the bulk of American crops. Demographers expect these numbers to continue to fall; for every full-time farmer under age thirty-five, three are over sixty-five years old. The majority of the nation's crops, many experts predict, will in a few decades be fabricated by computer-run systems overseen by engineers and other technologists directing huge machines over a vast unpeopled landscape covered with grain (Berardi and Geisler).

Whatever services are not automated will be provided by contract labor, as is presently with hogs and chickens.

Farming in the traditional sense may become a "cottage" industry like glassblowing, or there may be two different kinds of agriculture: one method utterly industrialized and efficient and the other a "craft" system responsive to aesthetic, cultural, landscape, and noneconomic concerns. Large corporations may integrate food production vertically by absorbing farms. Those companies also may make and market "craft" food products, as General Mills manufactures organic foods through its subsidiary, Cascadian Farms.

Critics protest with good reason that industrial farming by megacorporations—genetic manipulation of seed is only one aspect of the industrialization of agriculture—undermines the cultural, aesthetic, ethical, ecological, and landscape values and commitments that are associated with pastoralism or with the traditional farming of the agrarian past (Comstock). These critics contend that the products of industrial agriculture, even if they are technically safe, are so manipulated, artificial, and unnatural that they are inherently disgusting, distasteful, demoralizing, and repellent. Even if food safety is not the issue, one can argue that food is more than nourishment; it is part of a way of life and has symbolic and aesthetic value. GM undermines nature and, with it, the value of food.

These are credible criticisms, but there is a rub. The people who make these charges generally are unwilling to grow their own food. They expect other people, such as farmers, to do it for them. Farmers do the best they can against nearly impossible economic odds. They find that they cannot provide the variety, quality, and abundance of food people demand at anything close to the prices people pay unless they take advantage of the efficiencies offered by technology. Farmers will absorb the relatively higher costs of raising GM-free crops, however, if people are willing to pay a large enough premium for them. Just as members of religious communities—Jews who keep kosher, for example—pay a little more for food that meets their requirements, so too may people who prefer non-GM foods. Consumers should have an "exit" option with respect to GM foods; presumably, the market for "organic" food provides that option.

## Labeling

Critics of GM foods may agree that they have to send a message not only through political advocacy but also through the consumer choices they make. For consumers to send a message through their choices, they must know which foods contain GM ingredients. No one questions the right of the consumer to make informed choices. Why not require that GM food be labeled to guide consumer choice?

Industry representatives offer three responses to this question. First, they observe that any manufacturer can state on a label or in advertising that its product is GM-free as long as this is true; indeed, the "organic" label implies as much. If the label does not say that a product is "GM-free" or "organic," the consumer can assume that it is not. The label "May Contain GM Ingredients," if stamped on food products, would add no information. In international forums U.S. representatives have appeared to be ready to accept this type of universal label or symbol. The label would underscore the fact that a product not labeled as being GM-free may contain at least some amount of an ingredient from a GM plant (USDS).

Second, to segregate commodity flows would be enormously costly. If a drop of soy oil from an engineered plant is mixed into a tank of oil—chemically identical to it—from conventional soy, would that taint the whole lot? How well would the tanker have to be cleaned to remove the taint? Those who observe religious restrictions have over the centuries worked out rules to determine, for example, how milk and meat are to be separated and how plates are to be washed. Are the resources available to segregate and trace through the entire food industry flows of commodities, such as canola oil, to segregate by source substances that are nearly indistinguishable chemically? No one objects if those who wish to observe aesthetic, ceremonial, or religious distinctions do so, but this must be done at their own expense. At present purveyors of "organic" food pay to assure its identity and history. Those who produce, sell, and buy ordinary products do not want the burden of that expense (IFT, pp. 124–136).

Third, so many methods of genetic manipulation enter into the production of food at so many levels—bacteria that produce enzymes that catalyze fermentation are genetically engineered but are not found in the cheese, for example— that it would be a nightmare to write regulations that determine what is or is not manipulated. By comparison, to set up rules to define "organic" food was an exercise as difficult as squaring the circle; in a literal, biological sense all food is organic. Virtually all foods are genetically manipulated as the products of artificial selection; to say which ones are not manipulated in a relevant sense is not easy. Worse, megacorporations design for the label; lawyers and engineers find ways to make the products of industrial processes comply with any set of regulations. This is the way the food industry works. This situation frustrates those who want to get food from Mother Nature rather than from Consolidated Agribusiness (Pollan).

## Biotechnology and the Developing World

From a global perspective, increased production of food, however efficient, will not relieve the principal causes of famine and hunger, for these forces involve powerlessness, destitution, civil war, and oppression. The road to food security lies in making governments less corrupt, reducing ethnic and racial rivalries and hatreds, ending civil wars, improving education, providing employment, and halting gender discrimination. Food security is a function of social justice. With or without the latest advances in genetic engineering, a peaceful and just world could feed its people easily.

Farmers can and will plant and harvest as much as they can sell. As the economist Amartya Sen has written, "food output is being held back by a lack of effective demand in the marketplace" rather than by ecological constraints on production. In other words, food is not scarce but demand is because many people are too poor or powerless to purchase food even at the twenty-first century's historically low prices. As Gordon Conway of the Rockefeller Foundation points out, however, even if global production is ample, "there could still be nearly a billion people who lie outside the market and are chronically undernourished." Conway believes that agricultural biotechnology can benefit peasants who depend on local, subsistence farming. In Kenya, for example, scientists funded by Monsanto have developed a recombinant sweet potato that resists a devastating virus. Edible vaccines may be engineered into crops such as bananas. A rust-resistant cassava could make a huge difference in Africa. There is no general economic theory that shows why or how biotechnology can benefit people in developing countries. A long list of examples can be supplied, however, of the nearly miraculous potential of genetic engineering to relieve malnutrition and hunger on a crop-by-crop, problem-by-problem basis.

However, as an article in *Foreign Policy* observed, biotechnological innovations that create "substitutes for everything from vanilla to cocoa and coffee threaten to eliminate the livelihood of millions of Third World agricultural workers." Vanilla cultured in laboratories costs a fifth as much as vanilla extracted from beans and thus jeopardizes the livelihood of tens of thousands of vanilla farmers in Madagascar. A rapeseed (canola) engineered to express high levels of laurate, an ingredient in soaps and shampoos, allows growers in Canada to take markets away from producers of palm oil in developing countries. In general, genetic engineering of crops leads to biosubstitution, biorelocation, and bioreplication, enabling industrialized countries to produce the equivalent of traditionally tropical products and thus cease importing those commodities from developing countries. Developing nations by virtue of the same technology may flood world markets. The technological treadmill is poised to increase commodity surpluses, especially of commodities, such as cocoa and coffee, which sustain the developing world, and therefore, ironically, result in further impoverishment and further declines in demand. Rather than tending by its logic to make everyone better off, biotechnology may make wealthy countries more wealthy while taking from poor countries the monopoly on the few export commodities that once were exclusively theirs.

## The Ecological Implications of Biotechnology

Critics contend that GM crops are likely to have deleterious environmental effects. For example, they will lead to greater pesticide resistance among weeds and insects because genetic material from GM organisms will drift into wild varieties; plant leaves and pollen that contain Bt or other insecticides will kill nontarget species; drought tolerance, salt tolerance, cold-hardiness, and other feats of genetic engineering will permit farms to expand into wild areas that formerly were not arable; and animals, particularly fish such as salmon, will hybridize with wild stocks, domesticating all of nature (Graziano). Nothing will evolve free of human influence.

Although all these concerns are credible, defenders of biotechnology respond that these objections are not specific to genetic engineering but apply to agriculture and aquaculture generally. Indeed, GM technologies may only increase slightly—or indeed decrease slightly—the relentless, total, and overwhelming impact of agriculture on the natural world. Even before the discovery of the structure of DNA, the entire midsection of the United States had been turned from prairie or savanna ecosystems to amber waves of grain. To restore the prairie, ecologists searched for native species in abandoned cemeteries and railroad rights-of-way. Modern agriculture roots out nature literally and figuratively and replaces it with monocultures that cover millions of acres. Nature is equally devastated whether those monocultures consist of conventional hybrids or GM plants.

Insecticides promote resistance whether they are sprayed on or bred into a plant. When they are sprayed from airplanes over large areas, these chemicals may kill nontarget species more extensively than they would if they were engineered into the leaves of crops. Weeds subjected to dousings of glyphosate eventually must evolve to withstand the herbicide; the addition of herbicide resistance in crops may hasten this inevitable process somewhat. Crops that are the products of conventional breeding are no more "natural" than GM crops are; indeed, human-caused mutation and selection have just taken longer to achieve the desired properties. These conventional hybrids—both crops

and animals, including fish—can intermingle their genes with wild types if and when wild types are found.

The effect of farming on nature can be seen best in Europe, where agriculture counts as "nature," with the alternative being urban or suburban development. Americans think of nature as wilderness, although the wilderness that remains is managed, designated wilderness—a kind of botanical garden maintained in national parks. To estimate the extent to which GM plants threaten nature, one must ask what "nature" is, whether it is more than the smile of the Cheshire cat. Environmental historians such as William Cronon state that agriculture and industry have transformed the landscape so thoroughly so many times over that it is hard to say what people are trying to protect. Also, the pressure of *Homo sapiens* on other organisms has directed their evolution for millennia; humans are the "keystone" species that structures the natural environment that people consider wild (McKibben).

## Human Biotechnology

Many of the most controversial technologies bioethicists study in medicine—artificial fertilization and cloning are obvious examples—originated in the barnyard. The genetic manipulation of animals will be the proving ground for the genetic manipulation and enhancement of human beings. What may be most interesting in the ethical study of agricultural biotechnology, therefore, may lie in its effort to identify something "natural"—some essence, condition, history, or pedigree—that makes an animal characteristically itself and that can be lost as a result of genetic engineering. If this essence proves elusive in the agricultural context or if it turns out that everything physically possible is equally natural, by analogy, it may not be possible to identify any limits in the nature of humans (e.g., mortality) that people may not try to transcend. Human beings may be tempted, then, to improve human qualities through germ cell engineering just as they have improved the qualities of plants and animals.

The distinction between the "natural" and the "artificial" may not survive the advance of biotechnology because everything, including the human genome, may become both. This makes the human species responsible for everything, or it greatly diminishes the "given" or contingent in nature. The ability to manipulate the human genome—as people have manipulated the genomes, say, of salmon and chickens—for many technical reasons is a long way off. Indeed, it still may be considered science fiction. Someday human beings may cultivate themselves as they do other organisms. The idea that people eventually may apply to the human genome the same techniques by which they have changed crops and livestock could be the ultimate irony of agricultural biotechnology.

MARK SAGOFF

SEE ALSO: *Animal Research; Animal Welfare and Rights; Cloning; Environmental Ethics; Environmental Policy and Law; Technology*

### BIBLIOGRAPHY

Bailey, Britt, and Lappe, Marc, eds. 2002. *Engineering the Farm: Social and Ethical Aspects of Agricultural Biotechnology.* Washington, D.C.: Island Press.

Berardi, G. M., and Geisler, C.C. 1984. *The Social Consequences and Challenges of New Agricultural Technologies* Boulder, CO: Westview Press.

Cochrane, Williard. 1993. *The Development of American Agriculture: A Historical Analysis,* 2nd edition. Minneapolis: University of Minnesota Press.

Comstock, Gary, ed. 1988. *Is There a Moral Obligation to Save the Family Farm?* Ames: Iowa State University Press.

Conway, G. 2000. "Genetically Modified Crops: Risks and Promise." *Conservation Ecology* 4(1): 2.

Cronon, William. 1983. *Changes in the Land: Indians, Colonists, and the Ecology of New England.* New York: Hill and Wang.

Food and Agriculture Organization and World Health Organization (FAO/WHO). 1991. "Strategies for Assessing the Safety of Foods Produced by Biotechnology." Report of a Joint FAO/WHO Consultation. Food and Agriculture Organization / World Health Organization. Geneva: World Health Organization.

Graziano, Karen. 1996. "Comment, Biosafety Protocol: Recommendations to Ensure the Safety of the Environment, Colorado." *Journal of International Environmental Law and Policy* 7: 179–196.

Institute of Food Technologists. 2000. "FT Expert Report on Biotechnology and Foods." *Food Technology* 54(8): 124–136.

Kneen, Brewster. 1999. *Farmageddon: Food and the Culture of Biotechnology.* Gabriola Island, British Columbia: New Society Publishers.

McKibben, Bill. 1989. *The End of Nature.* New York: Random House.

National Academy of Sciences. 2000. *Genetically-Modified Pest-Protected Plants: Science and Regulation.* Washington, D.C.: National Academies Press.

Paarlberg, Robert. 2000. "The Global Food Fight." *Foreign Affairs* 79(3): 24–38.

Pollan, Michael. "Behind the Organic-Industrial Complex," *New York Times Magazine* May 13, 2001.

Pence, Gregory. 2002. *Designer Food: Mutant Harvest or Breadbasket for the World.* Lanham, MD: Rowman & Littlefield.

Prakash, Channapatna S. 2000. "The Genetically Modified Crop Debate in the Context of Agricultural Evolution," *Plant Physiology* 126(May): 8–15.

Sen, Amartya. "Population: Dulsion and Reality," *New York Review of Books* September 22, 1994.

Thompson, Paul B. 1995 (reprint 1997). *Food Biotechnology in Ethical Perspective* London: Blackie Academic.

### INTERNET RESOURCES

AgBioForum. Available from <http://www.agbioforum.org/>.

National Agricultural Biotechnology Council. Available from <http://www.cals.cornell.edu/extension/nabc/>.

Pew Initiatiave on Food and Biotechnology. Available from <http://pewagbiotech.org/>.

Union of Concerned Scientists. Available from <http://www.ucsusa.org/agriculture/>.

U.S.D.A. Agricultural Biotechnology Home Page. Available from <http://www.usda.gov/agencies/biotech/>.

USDS. 2000. Fact sheet: The Cartagena Protocol on Biosafety. Office of the Spokesman, U.S. Dept. of State, Washington, D.C., Feb. 16. Available from <www.state.gov/www/global/oes/montreal_2000–01_index.html>.

# AIDS

• • •

I. Public Health Issues

II. Healthcare and Research Issues

## I. PUBLIC HEALTH ISSUES

At the conclusion of *Plagues and People,* a magisterial account of epidemics and their impact on history, William McNeill asserts, "Infectious disease, which antedates the emergence of humankind, will last as long as humanity itself and will surely remain, as it has been hitherto, one of the fundamental parameters and determinants of human history" (McNeill, p. 291). In the mid-1970s, this observation seemed overdrawn, especially in relation to economically advanced societies, where chronic diseases had displaced infectious threats to communal well-being. Yet just five years later, McNeill's comment seemed prescient.

In June 1981, the first cases of what would ultimately be called acquired immunodeficiency syndrome (AIDS) were reported by the U. S. Centers for Disease Control

(CDC). Within three years of the first CDC report, human immunodeficiency virus (HIV), the viral agent responsible for AIDS, was identified. Although those who were infected could experience a long disease-free state—50 percent remained symptom-free for up to ten years—in the end the virus attacked the immune system, resulting in a series of ultimately fatal opportunistic disorders. By the beginning of the twenty-first century, it was estimated that approximately 900,000 Americans and more than 42 million people worldwide were infected. Although found on every continent, AIDS had made its most stunning impact on Africa. Projections by the World Health Organization (WHO) forecast a grim picture, with catastrophic spread of HIV in Asia and the former Soviet Union.

## Exceptionalism and the Ethics of Testing, Reporting, and Partner Notification

In the early and mid-1980s, at the outset of the American encounter with AIDS, it was necessary to face a set of fundamental questions: Did the history of responses to lethal infectious diseases provide lessons about how best to contain the spread of HIV? Should the policies developed to control sexually transmitted diseases or other communicable conditions be applied to AIDS? If AIDS were not to be so treated, what would justify such differential policies?

To understand the importance of these questions, it is necessary to recall that conventional approaches to public health threats typically provided a warrant, when deemed appropriate, for mandating compulsory examination and screening, breaching the confidentiality of the clinical relationship by reporting to public health registries the names of those diagnosed with "dangerous diseases," imposing treatment, and in the most extreme cases, confining persons through the power of quarantine. To be sure, many aspects of this public health tradition, forged at the outset of the twentieth century, had been modulated over the decades, in part because of changes in the patterns of morbidity and mortality.

Nevertheless, it was the specter of the historically coercive aspects of the public health tradition that most concerned proponents of civil liberties and advocates of gay rights and bioethics as they considered the potential direction of public health policy in the presence of AIDS, a disease that so disproportionately affected disfavored groups—gay men, drug users, the poor in minority communities. In place of the conventional approach to public health threats, there emerged an alternative view—broadly defined as exceptionalism (Bayer, 1991)—that took as its starting point the need to craft policies that were persuasive rather than coercive, which viewed the protection of the rights of

those who were infected as integral rather than as antagonistic to the goals of disease prevention. For those who advanced this new perspective, privacy and confidentiality were to be accorded great importance. In all, the goal was to avoid measures and practices that might be counterproductive, which might "drive the epidemic underground" by inspiring fear and distrust rather than fostering engagement between public health officials and those most at risk. How the exceptionalist perspective with its commitment to noncoercive approaches to HIV affected policy is most clearly illustrated in the debates over HIV testing, reporting of HIV, and partner notification efforts.

HIV TESTING. From the moment of its introduction in 1985, the HIV test became the subject of intense debate. Fear that those identified as having HIV might be subject to discrimination and stigma; concern about how the diagnosis of HIV infection, in the absence of effective therapy, could produce unbearable psychological burdens; and a belief that testing had little to do with behavioral change led AIDS activists generally, and gay leaders specifically, to adopt a posture of hostility and/or skepticism regarding the test. On the other hand, many public health officials believed that the identification of infected persons could play a crucial role in fostering behavioral change. Out of their confrontations emerged a broad consensus that, except in a very few well-defined circumstances, people should be tested only with their informed, voluntary, and specific consent (Bayer, 1989).

Much of the early discussion of HIV testing occurred in the context of extreme therapeutic limits. And indeed in the epidemic's early years the primary function of testing was as an adjunct to prevention efforts. By 1990, as a result of clinical developments—the belief that treatment with zidovudine (also known as azidothymidine, or AZT) could delay the onset of symptomatic AIDS and the recognition of the importance of primary prophylaxis against Pneumocystis carinii pneumonia—the medical significance of identifying those with early HIV disease had become clear. Consequently, the clinical and political context—involving a wide range of constituencies—of the debate about testing underwent a fundamental change (Bayer, Levine, and Wolf). Gay organizations began to urge homosexual and bisexual men to have their antibody status determined under confidential or anonymous conditions. Physicians pressed for AIDS to be incorporated into the medical mainstream and for the HIV-antibody test to be treated like other blood tests—that is, given with the presumed consent of the patient.

Pressure to shift the paradigm of testing away from the exacting standard of informed consent was especially pronounced in the case of pregnant women and newborns (Bayer, 1995). Diagnostic progress was to make it possible to determine whether HIV-positive newborns were truly infected soon after birth, and the improved prospects of clinical management were to make such determinations for infected infants appear all the more critical. So it is not surprising that pediatricians became increasingly impatient with the strict regimen of explicit and specific consent that surrounded the testing of newborns for HIV (Hegearty and Abrams)—all the more so because routine and unconsented testing of newborns for inborn errors of metabolism such as phenylketonuria was mandated in virtually every state and had provoked little ethical objection.

In 1994 a research study discovered that the administration of zidovudine during pregnancy could reduce the rate of maternal–fetal HIV transmission by two-thirds (to about 8%) (Connor, Sperling, and Gelber). In the aftermath of that finding, pressure mounted to ensure that infected women were identified early in pregnancy. In 1996 the American Medical Association's House of Delegates passed a resolution calling for mandatory testing of pregnant women (Shelton). Even the Institute of Medicine, which early in the epidemic had opposed testing policies that abrogated the privacy rights of pregnant women, was by the end of the 1990s to endorse routine testing on the basis of an informed right of refusal, a much less exacting standard than specific informed consent (Institute of Medicine).

In other contexts as well, the retreat from the exacting standard of specific informed consent with pretest counseling has taken the form of efforts to integrate HIV testing into clinical practice where standards of presumed consent prevail.

REPORTING OF HIV. A course similar to that which occurred with testing characterized the debate surrounding case reporting for HIV infection. Given the profound stigma that surrounded AIDS in the epidemic's first years, and the extent to which individuals with or at risk for HIV feared the social consequences of having their diagnoses made public, it is not surprising that confidentiality of AIDS-related information assumed great salience. From the pragmatic perspective of the public health officials, it was crucial to preserve confidentiality as a way of assuring that those at risk would come forward for testing and counseling (Institute of Medicine). Others objected on grounds of principle. Privacy was a value that should not be lightly set aside.

But however central were the claims of privacy and the duty to protect confidentiality, they were not absolutes. One of the conventionally accepted limits to those claims occurred when individuals with infectious diseases were reported by name to confidential public health registries. It was thus not surprising that despite concerns about privacy,

little opposition existed in the epidemic's first years to making AIDS cases reportable by name (Bayer, 1989). The acceptance of AIDS case reporting requirements was facilitated by the well-established record of state health departments in protecting such records from unwarranted disclosure.

With the inception of HIV testing, however, debate emerged about whether the names of all infected persons, regardless of whether they had received an AIDS diagnosis, should be reported. Activists who accepted AIDS case reporting opposed HIV reporting because of heightened concerns about privacy, confidentiality, and discrimination. For them the potential public health benefits of reporting were too limited and the burden on those who would be the subject of reporting too great to justify an abrogation of privacy.

While many public health officials, especially those who came from states with large AIDS caseloads, opposed HIV reporting because of its potential effect on the willingness of people to seek testing and counseling, some public health officials did become strong advocates of such reporting. In their arguments in favor of such reporting, they sought to underscore the extent to which the public health benefits of HIV reporting would be similar to those that followed from more broadly conceived reporting requirements, such as those that applied to syphilis, tuberculosis, and AIDS itself (Vernon).

As therapeutic advances began to emerge in the late 1980s, and as the logic of distinguishing between HIV and AIDS became increasingly difficult to sustain, fissures began to appear in the relatively broad and solid alliance against named HIV reporting. At the end of November 1990, the CDC declared its support for HIV reporting, which it asserted could "enhance the ability of local, state and national agencies to project the level of required resources" for care and prevention services (CDC, 1990, p. 861). The House of Delegates of the American Medical Association also endorsed the reporting of names (Bayer, 1999).

Central to the argument for HIV name reporting was the assertion that AIDS case reporting captured an epidemic that was as much as a decade old and that an accurate picture of the incidence and prevalence of HIV infection—especially in light of the impact of treatment—required a surveillance system based on HIV case reporting.

At the end of 1999, in the face of lingering opposition from most AIDS activists, the CDC finally proposed that all states put in place an HIV reporting system. And while it left open the possibility of reliance on unique identifiers that met strict performance criteria, it was clear that the use of names was viewed as preferable (CDC, 1999). Remarkably, of those states that adopted HIV case surveillance after the publication of the CDC's recommendations, virtually all adopted coded systems. By 2002 only one state—Georgia—had not adopted some form of HIV reporting.

PARTNER NOTIFICATION. In the controversy over partner notification the limits of privacy were also encountered. What emerged as a source of contention in the first decade of the epidemic was the extent to which the protection of identifiable third parties who had been or were currently placed at risk for HIV by already infected individuals provided a warrant for public health interventions. This was not a new issue; it had been confronted in the context of psychiatry in the so-called *Tarasoff* doctrine (from the mid-1970s court case, *Tarasoff v. Regents of the University of California*), which held that physicians who knew that their patients were about to inflict serious harm on other identifiable individuals had a duty to act to warn or protect. While opinions differed about the wisdom of such efforts, there was little principled objection to breaching confidentiality under such circumstances.

Thus in the mid- to late 1980s, when many AIDS activists argued that the principle of confidentiality had to be inviolable, and when public health officials were loath to endorse legislative mandates requiring third party notification, many ethicists suggested that protection of unsuspecting sexual partners took precedence over privacy. In 1988 the American Medical Association's House of Delegates embraced the duty to warn.

Some states sought to meet the challenge of endangered third parties by enacting statutes that secured a "privilege to disclose." Under such laws physicians could, if they chose, breach confidentiality to warn unsuspecting individuals but would not be held liable if they failed to do so.

The depth of antagonism to public health interventions in matters of sexual intimacy was further demonstrated by the deep suspicion of contact tracing programs, under which public health officials would notify those who had been placed at risk without divulging the identity of the individual who had imposed the risk. Such efforts were typically voluntary and relied on the willingness of index patients to provide the names of their contacts.

Despite the four decades of experience with contact tracing, efforts to undertake such public health interventions in the context of AIDS met with fierce resistance in the first years of the epidemic. Opposition by gay leaders and civil liberties groups had a profound impact on the response of public health officials, especially in states with relatively large numbers of AIDS cases, where contact tracing efforts remained all but moribund (Bayer, 1989). In part the opposition was fueled by the fact that throughout most of the 1980s, no therapy could be offered to asymptomatic infected individuals. Thus, the role of contact tracing in the context of HIV infection differed radically from its role in the context of other sexually transmitted diseases. In the latter case, effective treatments could be offered to notified partners. Once cured, such individuals would no longer pose a threat of transmission. In the case of HIV, nothing could be offered other than information about possible exposure.

Public health officials saw in such information an opportunity to target efforts to foster behavioral changes among individuals still engaging in high-risk behavior—behavior that could place both the individual contacted and future partners at risk; for such officials, this was reason enough to undertake the process. For opponents of contact tracing, the very effort to reach out to such individuals represented a profound intrusion on privacy with little or no compensating benefit. The task of behavioral change, they asserted, could be achieved more effectively and efficiently through community-based HIV prevention efforts (Bayer and Toomey).

Early misapprehensions about the extent to which public health officials typically relied on overt coercion in the process of contact tracing, and the degree to which confidentiality might be compromised, had by the end of the 1980s all but vanished. With such concerns allayed, many gay leaders had come to recognize that partner notification, in fact, could be a "useful tool" in efforts to control AIDS (Schram). The debate began to shift to one centered on relative efficacy (APHA). That dispute was informed by questions that had already surfaced about the usefulness of contact tracing in the control of syphilis in populations where individuals had large numbers of sexual partners, many of whom were anonymous (Andrus et al.).

In short, by the early 1990s the exceptionalism of the first years of the AIDS epidemic began to fade and a process of normalization had set in.

## Public Health and Clinical Research

The HIV epidemic provided the circumstances for the emergence of a broad and potent political movement that sought to reshape radically the conditions under which research was undertaken. Brought into question were the role of the randomized clinical trial, the importance of placebo controls, the centrality of academic research institutions, the dominance of scientists over subjects, the sharp distinction between research and therapy, and the protectionist ethos of *The Belmont Report* (the landmark formulation of research ethics published in 1979 by the U.S. National

Commission for the Protection of Human Subjects of Biomedical and Behavioral Research). Although scholars concerned with the methodological demands of sound research and ethicists committed to the protection of research subjects played a crucial role in the ensuing discussions, both as defenders of the received wisdom and as critics, the debate was largely driven by the articulate demands of those most threatened by AIDS (Epstein). Most prominent were groups such as the People with AIDS Coalition and ACT UP, organizations made up primarily of white, gay men. They were joined by community-based physicians who identified closely with the plight of their patients.

What was so stunning—disconcertingly so to some, exciting to others—was the rhythm of challenge and response. Rather than the careful exchange of academic arguments, there was the mobilization of disruptive and effective political protest. Most remarkable was the core demand. As Carol Levine noted in 1988, "The shortage of proven therapeutic alternatives for AIDS and the belief that trials are, in and of themselves, beneficial have led to the claim that people have a right *to be* research subjects. This is the exact opposite of the tradition started with Nuremberg—that people have a right *not to be* research subjects" (Levine, p. 172). That striking reversal resulted in a rejection of the model of research conducted at remote academic centers, with restrictive (protective) standards of access and strict adherence to the "gold standard" of the randomized clinical trial.

Having blurred the distinction between research and treatment—expressed forcefully through the slogan "A Drug Trial Is Health Care Too"—those insistent on radical reform sought to open wide the points of entry to new "therapeutic" agents both within and outside of clinical trials; they demanded that the paternalistic ethical warrant for the protection of the vulnerable from research be replaced by an ethical regime informed by respect for the autonomous choice of potential subjects who could weigh, for themselves, the potential risks and benefits of new treatments for HIV infection. Moreover, the revisionists demanded a basic reconceptualization of the relationship between researchers and subjects. In place of protocols imposed from above, they proposed a more egalitarian and democratic model in which negotiation would replace a scientific authority. Indeed, research "subjects" were now thought of as "participants." Furthermore, the role of the carefully controlled clinical trial as providing protection against the wide-scale use of drugs whose safety and efficacy had not been proven no longer commanded unquestioned respect (Bayer, 1990).

The new perspective did not go without challenge, of course. Some were concerned that the proposed regime would make all but impossible the conduct of research so crucial to the needs of those with HIV/AIDS ("Parallel Track," 1989), while others feared that desperate individuals would, in the absence of the now discredited (paternalistic) ethos, be subject to deception (Annas).

The AIDS-inspired challenge to the ethics of research was not restricted to issues within the United States. Just as the protective regime surrounding research in the United States was a product of a history of abuse, efforts to enunciate ethical standards for the conduct of research in Third World nations was shaped by a history of exploitation, a history characterized by investigations on the poor designed to serve the interests of the privileged. Central to those efforts was the belief that the ethical principles first encountered in industrialized nations had direct bearing on the norms that should govern research in very different settings (IJsselmuiden and Faden). Such universalism took as a given the need to assume that insights regarding cultural differences not serve as the basis for moral relativism.

Just as individual informed consent was the first principle of the ethics of research in advanced industrial nations, it was at the heart of the codes designed to guide research in the poorest nations. To preclude exploitation, international consensus also existed on the extent to which it was critical that research be responsive to the health needs and priorities of the community in which it is to be carried out (CIOMS). What would remain a matter of uncertainty, however, was whether the needs of the poorest and the requirement of responsiveness could justify research that would be unacceptable in the richest nations—whether the principle of universalism could accommodate research in Burundi that would be prohibited in Brooklyn.

That was the issue that would animate a furious international debate occasioned by the 1994 finding that AZT administered to infected women in the second and third trimesters and to their infants for six weeks could reduce by two-thirds the rate of mother-to-child HIV transmission (Connor, Sperling, and Gelber). Although superficially a conflict over a technical matter involving research design—the role of placebos—the dispute touched on the deepest questions of what ethical conduct meant in a world characterized by great inequalities and profound inequities.

Given the burden of pediatric AIDS in Africa and Asia, it was a matter of some urgency that trials begin to determine whether radically cheaper alternatives to the standard regimen could achieve at least some measure of reduced maternal–fetal HIV transmission. In June 1994 a special consultation of the World Health Organization (WHO) considered the challenge and called for the launching of studies to achieve that goal. The consultation made clear its conclusion that placebo-controlled trials—trials in which a comparison is made between an inert substance and the potentially active agent—"offer the best option for obtaining rapid and scientifically valid results."

There was no question that a placebo-controlled trial would have been considered unethical in the United States or any other advanced industrial nation. No trial that denied access to the effective standard, or to an intervention thought to hold the promise of being at least as effective as, if not more effective than, the prevailing standard of care, would have satisfied the requirements of ethical review. The question posed by the furious controversy that unfolded was whether it was ethical to conduct such a trial in a poor country. In 1997 the *New England Journal of Medicine* gave its answer unambiguously: "Only when there is no known effective treatment is it ethical to compare a potential new treatment with a placebo. When effective treatment exists, a placebo may not be used. Instead, subjects in the control group of the study must receive the best known treatment" (Angell, p. 847).

Given this premise, the *Journal* rejected as irrelevant the fact that healthcare available in most Third World countries provided nothing like healthcare available in industrialized countries. Citing for authority the Declaration of Helsinki— the international code of research ethics adapted by the World Medical Association in 1964—the editorial noted that control groups had to be provided with the best current therapy, not simply that which was available locally. "The shift in wording between 'best' and 'local' may be slight, but the implications are profound. Acceptance of this ethical relativism could result in widespread exploitation of vulnerable Third World populations for research programs that could not be carried out in the sponsor country" (Angell, p. 848).

Those who rejected the *Journal*'s viewpoint made clear that placebo-controlled trials were dictated by the urgency of the situation. Only placebo-controlled trials could provide "definitive," "clear," "firm" answers about which interventions worked, thus allowing governments to make "A sound judgment about the appropriateness and financial feasibility of providing the intervention" (Varmus and Satcher, p. 1004). The failure to employ a placebo would have made it difficult to clearly determine whether the affordable but less effective intervention was better than no intervention at all. In short, they concluded that placebos were crucial to policymakers required to make relatively costly decisions under conditions marked by profound poverty and scarce public health resources (Varmus and Satcher).

Paralleling the debates over maternal–fetal transmission of HIV were those that surfaced over the ethics of AIDS vaccine trials. In this case the focus was on those research participants who might become infected with HIV during a trial. On the one hand there were those who argued that such individuals be provided with optimal care—the retroviral therapy available in the developed countries. On the other hand there were those who asserted that care should reflect that which was consistent with what was available in the host nation (Bayer, 2000). So divisive was this controversy that the Joint United Nations Programme on HIV/AIDS (UNAIDS) could not come to an agreement on the appropriate ethical norm and indeed had to settle for a procedural rather than substantive solution, a solution that focused on how to reach acceptable agreement rather than one that put forth a standard to guide such deliberations (UNAIDS).

Thus were the issues joined. These controversies ultimately provoked an international effort to consider ethical standards of research in the Third World. The World Medical Association undertook a series of consultations on the revision of the Declaration of Helsinki; the Council for International Organizations of Medical Sciences (CIOMS) did so as well. Finally, within the United States, which funded much of the international research that had been subject to scrutiny, the National Bioethics Advisory Commission took up the issue of studies in poor nations.

Whereas those who saw in any effort to craft "flexible" standards that reflected the uniquely pressing context of international poverty and inequality the treacherous embrace of moral relativism, their opponents persisted in arguing that a failure to consider the context of investigation was a failure of moral understanding. Principles could be universal; their application could not be rigid. (Singer and Benatar; Benatar and Singer).

## Securing Access to Care

In the first years of the epidemic there was little that medicine could offer those with HIV. Indeed, that was the context within which AIDS activists struggled to increase access to experimental trials. As the prospects for clinical intervention improved, first with the use of prophylactic treatment to prevent Pneumocystis carinii pneumonia and other opportunistic infections and then with AZT, the first widely prescribed antiretroviral agent, it was inevitable that the inequities of the U.S. healthcare system would be encountered.

Some who needed treatment had private insurance— although they frequently faced efforts on the part of their insurers to deny them coverage for their HIV-related conditions; those who were poor or who became impoverished because of their disease could qualify for Medicaid; but many remained unprotected (Green and Arno). To meet the needs of the latter group, special programs were developed. The federal government, through the Ryan White Comprehensive AIDS Resources Emergency Act of 1990, directed significant sums to localities to provide medical services. Among the initiatives under the act was the AIDS Drug Assistance Program (ADAP), designed to pay for AIDS-related medicines. Like the End Stage Renal Disease Program that assured access to dialysis and transplantation regardless of the ability to pay, these AIDS programs left untouched the basic patterns of medical inequality.

When the protease inhibitors emerged in the mid-1990s and combination antiretroviral therapy became the standard of care, the system was strained to the limits. Medication costs alone for those receiving care could range from $10,000 to $15,000 per year (Deeks et al.). A 1996 review of dramatically improved therapeutic prospects added the caveat that the new achievements were important "at least for those socioeconomically privileged" (Richman, p. 1887). ADAP experienced persistent shortfalls in funding. When that was the case, it was necessary to resort to a host of rationing strategies (Henry J. Kaiser Family Foundation). At one point, nearly half of the ADAP programs limited access to protease inhibitors (Carton).

The remarkable advances in therapeutics have provided a critical element in the argument that the exceptionalism of the epidemic's early years is no longer appropriate. It is therefore a remarkable paradox that the very same achievements have set the stage for challenging the exceptionalist programs that seek to ensure—however inadequately—access to those same treatments. These expressions of disquiet must be understood, at least in part, as a reflection of concern that the American AIDS epidemic may no longer be seen as immediately threatening, that the unique services for those with HIV would be vulnerable unless they were embedded in a broader system of a just healthcare system.

On an international plane the prospect of effective antiretroviral treatment would pose challenges vaster by many orders of magnitude. What justification was there for a system of pricing that made the cost of drugs beyond the reach of the desperate? Could markets ever respond to need where effective demand was nil? Could the monopoly confirmed by patent rights be compatible with a response dictated by claims of the dying? Was the treaty on intellectual property rights, incorporated into the World Trade Organization's international regime, a barrier to survival in

context of the AIDS epidemic? What moral obligation did the wealthiest nations have to the poorest to provide the resources necessary to purchase the new lifesaving agents and build the medical infrastructure necessary for their appropriate administration? Was there any reason to believe that a global community that permitted millions to die each year from treatable and preventable diseases such as tuberculosis and malaria would respond differently in the face of AIDS?

AIDS activists ultimately seized on this issue and began an international campaign to confront the pharmaceutical industry. What might have seemed an utterly quixotic undertaking would ultimately, however, take on worldwide dimensions linking protesters in the United States, France, and South Africa (Berkman), institutional proponents of global health such as the World Health Organization, and a sympathetic public. By the end of the 1990s the pharmaceutical industry was placed on the defensive, perceived as protecting narrow self-interest when the lives of millions were at stake. Against the claims that high prices were necessary to fuel the engine of research, and that patent protections were crucial to spurring investments in drug investigations, those who sought to turn the terms of discourse asserted that urgency demanded that the barriers to drug access tumble.

Ultimately, under pressure from generic drug manufacturers, prices began to fall, and pharmaceutical firms began to accept the notion of differential or equity pricing.

As prices began to fall, it became ever more apparent that even if drugs were to be provided at cost, even if the principle of equity pricing were to guide sales, even if nations pursued the option of compulsory licensing and parallel imports, the cost of providing antiretroviral therapy was simply beyond the reach of the poorest and most HIV-burdened nations. And even if drugs could be paid for, the necessity of a medical infrastructure that could offer and monitor the use of drugs in a way that was attentive to the needs of individual patients and the risks to public health from drug resistance would require huge investments. This was the context within which a remarkable movement would take shape to create a massive funding effort to respond to the threat of AIDS.

The moral urgency of AIDS treatment was amplified by United Nations Secretary General Kofi Annan, who called for a global trust fund that would spend $7 to $10 billion a year over an extended period to face the threat to the world's poorest people. Most striking was his assertion that the care that had for so long eluded men, women, and children in the less-developed nations was a matter of moral right. Everyone who was infected should have access to medicine and medical care. That was a moral imperative. What was the unfortunate had become the unfair; inequality had become inequity (Bayer, 2002).

## Conclusion

This discussion began with an analysis of ethical and policy issues that emerged in the United States as it confronted the AIDS epidemic. These issues were commonly addressed in other economically advanced nations bounded by the liberal tradition, even when the resolution of the controversies that surfaced took on divergent forms.

No ethical analysis of the challenges posed by AIDS will ever again be sufficient if it is restricted to the challenges faced in wealthy developed nations. Indeed, increasingly the analysis will need to be driven by the complexities of an epidemic in the world's poorest nations. Older concerns rooted in a focus on the need to protect the privacy rights of individuals will inevitably be overshadowed by new concerns about global equity.

RONALD BAYER (1995)
REVISED BY AUTHOR

SEE ALSO: *Confidentiality; Epidemics; Healthcare Resources, Allocation of; Homosexuality; Human Dignity; Human Rights; Life, Quality of; Public Health; Sexual Identity;* and other *AIDS* subentries

### BIBLIOGRAPHY

American Public Health Association (APHA). 1988. *Contact Tracing and Partner Notification.* Washington, D.C.: Author.

Andrus, Jon K.; Fleming, David W.; Harger, Douglas R.; et al. 1990. "Partner Notification: Can It Control Syphilis?" *Annals of Internal Medicine* 112 (7): 539–543.

Angell, Marcia. 1997. "The Ethics of Clinical Research in the Third World." *New England Journal of Medicine* 337(12): 847–849.

Annas, George J. 1989. "Faith (Healing), Hope, and Charity at the FDA: The Politics of AIDS Drug Trials." *Villanova Law Review* 34: 771–797.

Bayer, Ronald. 1989. *Private Acts, Social Consequences: AIDS and the Politics of Public Health.* New Brunswick, NJ: Rutgers University Press.

Bayer, Ronald. 1990. "Beyond the Burdens of Protection: AIDS and the Ethics of Research." *Evaluation Review* 14(5): 443–446.

Bayer, Ronald. 1991. "Public Health Policy and the AIDS Epidemic: An End to HIV Exceptionalism?" *New England Journal of Medicine* 324(21): 1500–1504.

Bayer, Ronald. 1995. "Women's Rights, Babies' Interests: Ethics, Politics, and Science in the Debate of Newborn HIV Screening." In *HIV Infection in Women,* ed. Howard L. Minkoff, Jack A. DeHovitz, and Ann Duerr. New York: Raven Press.

Bayer, Ronald. 1999. "Clinical Progress and the Future of HIV Exceptionalism." *Archives of Internal Medicine* 159: 1042–1048.

Bayer, Ronald. 2000. "Ethical Challenges of HIV Vaccine Trials in Less Developed Nations: Conflict and Consensus in the International Arena." *AIDS* 14(8): 1051–1057.

Bayer, Ronald. 2002. "From the Bowels of an Epidemic: AIDS, Human Rights, and International Equity." *Macalester International* 11: 201–232.

Bayer, Ronald; Levine, Carol; and Wolf, Susan M. 1986. "HIV Antibody Screening: An Ethical Framework for Evaluation Proposed Programs." *Journal of the American Medical Association* 256(13): 1768–1774.

Bayer, Ronald, and Toomey, Kathleen E. 1992. "HIV Prevention and the Two Faces of Partner Notification." *American Journal of Public Health* 82(8): 1158–1164.

Benatar, Solomon R., and Singer, Peter A. 2000. "A New Look at International Research Ethics." *British Medical Journal* 321(7,264): 824–826.

Berkman, Allan. 2001. "Confronting Global AIDS: Prevention and Treatment." *American Journal of Public Health* 91(9): 1348–1349.

Carton, Barbara. 1996. "New AIDS Drugs Bring Hope to Provincetown, but Unexpected Woes." *Wall Street Journal* (October).

Centers for Disease Control and Prevention. 1990. "Current Trends Update: Public Health Surveillance for HIV Infection: United States, 1989 and 1990." *Morbidity and Mortality Weekly Report* 39(47): 853, 859–861.

Centers for Disease Control and Prevention. 1999. "Guidelines for National Human Immunodeficiency Virus Case Surveillance, Including Monitoring for Human Immunodeficiency Virus Infection and Acquired Immunodeficiency Syndrome." *Morbidity and Mortality Weekly Report* 48(13): 1–28.

Connor, Edward M.; Sperling, Rhoda S.; Gelber, Richard; et al. 1994. "Reduction in Maternal–Infant Transmission of HIV Type 1 with Zidovudine Treatment." *New England Journal of Medicine* 331(18): 1173–1180.

Council for International Organizations of Medical Sciences (CIOMS), in collaboration with the World Health Organization. 1993. *International Ethical Guidelines for Biomedical Research Involving Human Subjects.* Geneva, Switzerland: Author.

Deeks, Steven G.; Smith, Mark; Holodniy, Mark; et al. 1997. "HIV-1 Protease Inhibitors: A Review for Clinicians." *Journal of the American Medical Association* 277(2): 145–153.

Epstein, Stephen. 1996. *Impure Science: AIDS, Activism, and the Politics of Knowledge.* Berkeley: University of California Press.

Green, Jesse, and Arno, Peter S. 1990. "The 'Medicaidization' of AIDS: Trends in the Financing of HIV-Related Medical

Care." *Journal of the American Medical Association* 264(10): 1261–1266.

Hegearty, Margaret, and Abrams, Elaine. 1992. "Caring for HIV-Infected Women and Children." *New England Journal of Medicine* 326(13): 887–888.

Henry J. Kaiser Family Foundation. 1998. "National ADAP Monitoring Project: Interim Technical Report." Menlo Park, CA: Author.

IJsselmuiden, Carel B., and Faden, Ruth R. 1996. "Medical Research and the Principle of Respect for Persons in Non-Western Cultures." In *The Ethics of Research Involving Human Subjects: Facing the Twenty-First Century,* ed. Harold Y. Vanderpool. Frederick, MD: University Publishing Group.

Joint United Nations Programme on HIV/AIDS (UNAIDS). 2000. *Ethical Considerations in HIV Preventive Vaccine Research: UNAIDS Guidance Document.* Geneva, Switzerland: Author.

Levine, Carol. 1988. "Has AIDS Changed the Ethics of Human Subjects Research?" *Law, Medicine, and Health Care* 16(3/4): 167–173.

McNeill, William. 1976. *Plagues and Peoples.* Garden City, NY: Anchor Press.

"Parallel Track System Defended." 1989. *CDC AIDS Weekly* (December 11).

Richman, David D. 1996. "HIV Therapeutics." *Science* 272(5,270): 1886–1888.

Schram, Neil. 1988. "Partner Notification Can Be Useful Tool against AIDS Spread." *Los Angeles Times* (June 28).

Shelton, D. L. 1996. "Delegates Push Mandatory HIV Testing for Pregnant Women: American Medical Association House of Delegates Vote: Annual Meeting News." *American Medical News* 31: 1.

Singer, Peter A., and Benatar, Solomon R. "Beyond Helsinki: A Vision for Global Health Ethics." *British Medical Journal* 322(7,289): 747–748.

*Tarasoff v. Regents of the University of California.* 118 Cal. Rptr. 129 (Cal. Sup. Ct. 1974).

U.S. Institute of Medicine. 1986. *Confronting AIDS: Directions for Public Health, Health Care, and Research.* Washington, D.C.: National Academy Press.

U.S. Institute of Medicine. Committee on Perinatal Transmission of HIV; and U.S. National Research Council. Board on Children, Youth, and Families. 1999. *Reducing the Odds: Preventing Perinatal Transmission of HIV in the United States,* ed. Michael A. Stoto, Donna A. Almario, and Marie C. McCormick. Washington, D.C.: National Academy Press.

U.S. National Commission for the Protection of Human Subjects of Biomedical and Behavioral Research. 1979. *The Belmont Report: Ethical Principles and Guidelines for the Protection of Human Subjects of Research.* Washington, D.C.: Government Printing Office.

Varmus, Harold, and Satcher, David. 1997. "Ethical Complexities of Conducting Research in Developing Countries." *New England Journal of Medicine* 337(14): 1003–1005.

Vernon, Thomas. 1986. "Remarks." In *AIDS: Impact on Public Policy,* ed. Robert Hummell, W. Leavy, R. Rampola, et al. New York: Plenum.

World Health Organization (WHO). 1994. "Recommendations from the Meeting on Mother to Infant Transmission of HIV, Geneva, Switzerland, June 23–25." Geneva, Switzerland: Author.

## II. HEALTHCARE AND RESEARCH ISSUES

The early ethical debates regarding the AIDS epidemic were largely driven by the concerns of the politically active, primarily white, homosexual or bisexual men in the United States in whom the disease was first identified. Because of severe discrimination against HIV/AIDS patients, early activists argued for special confidentiality protections for HIV information. Because infection at that time was almost always fatal, patients also demanded access to experimental treatments, which offered the only chance of survival. Over the 1980s and 1990s, however, the epidemic changed, as did many of the ethical issues.

The global impact of HIV/AIDS in the twenty-first century dominates ethical and policy debates. In late 2001 an estimated 40 million people worldwide were HIV infected, with approximately 5 million new infections and 3 million deaths that year. More than 95 percent of new infections are in developing countries. AIDS is the leading cause of death in sub-Saharan Africa and the fourth leading cause of death worldwide. Although Africa has been particularly hard hit by the AIDS epidemic, with about 70 percent of HIV-infected persons and new infections, the looming epidemic in other developing areas, particularly China and India, may surpass it. Failure of governments to acknowledge the threat of HIV may be exacerbating the epidemic.

In the United States, HIV/AIDS remains a serious public health problem. Spread primarily through sexual transmission and injection drug use, the epidemic in the United States increasingly affects poor people of color. In 2001 an estimated 800,000 to 900,000 people in the United States were HIV-infected, with over 300,000 diagnosed with AIDS. But as a result of the introduction of highly active antiretroviral therapy, as well as prevention and education efforts, the number of AIDS deaths in the United States has fallen dramatically.

This entry discusses ethical issues regarding HIV testing, confidentiality of HIV information, HIV infection in women and children, end-of-life issues for HIV-infected patients, and access to healthcare for HIV disease. This entry also discusses clinical research issues, with particular attention to international HIV research and HIV vaccine research.

## Healthcare Issues

Fear and social stigma may be barriers to seeking HIV testing or care. In the United States, special procedures, protections, and programs have been developed to encourage testing and to provide care.

TRANSMISSION AND PREVENTION. HIV is transmitted by direct contact with bodily fluids that contain the virus. The major modes of transmission are sexual contact and injection drug use (through sharing needles and drug paraphernalia). HIV can also be transmitted from mother to infant during pregnancy or through breast-feeding. Prevention measures, such as safer sex education, condoms, needle exchange, and methadone maintenance, have proven effective at preventing HIV transmission.

Nevertheless, these prevention efforts often meet with strong resistance. Some object that providing condoms and discussing safer sex techniques inappropriately encourage sexual behaviors outside of heterosexual marriage. Similarly, some object that providing clean needles fosters illegal and harmful injection drug use. From a population perspective, however, such preventive measures reduce the incidence of a serious, often fatal illness. Empirical studies do not demonstrate an increase in high-risk behaviors after these preventive interventions.

HIV TESTING. Because of the sensitivity surrounding HIV, testing for the disease is treated differently from most other medical tests.

*Special procedures for HIV testing.* Because the physical risks are minimal, in the United States, blood tests typically do not require extensive informed-consent discussions, and consent often is implied rather than explicit. Early in the AIDS epidemic, however, HIV testing was recognized as different from other blood tests because it presented serious psychosocial risks, such as familial rejection, employment discrimination, and/or loss of healthcare, insurance, and housing. Moreover, because there was no proven treatment at that time, the benefits of early diagnosis to individual patients were uncertain. In recognition of these circumstances and to encourage voluntary testing, special procedures were adopted for obtaining consent for an HIV test, such as pretest counseling and specific informed consent. Special protections for confidentiality of HIV test results also were enacted. For the most part, these special requirements

remain in effect. Numerous states require pretest counseling, and the majority of states require specific (often written) informed consent to HIV testing.

*Availability of anonymous testing.* Because of the serious stigma and potential psychosocial risks associated with HIV testing and to further encourage voluntary testing, most states offer anonymous HIV testing. At special, anonymous test sites, individuals are not required to provide their names or other identifying information. Upon testing, they are given a unique code to use to obtain results. People identified as HIV-infected at these sites are not reported to public health officials.

*Exceptions to informed consent.* States may permit HIV testing without informed consent under limited circumstances. For example, many states permit testing of patients without their permission after emergency response workers or healthcare workers are exposed to their blood or other fluids. Nevertheless, the patient's permission must be requested even though it is not required. In addition, some states permit the testing of prisoners and persons accused of sex crimes without their consent. Two states also require HIV testing of newborns, which indirectly reveals maternal HIV status.

*Conventional versus rapid testing.* Conventional HIV test results typically are not available for one to two weeks because initial positive tests must be confirmed with more sophisticated and accurate tests. In the United States, such testing is required to avoid mistakenly informing someone that they are HIV-infected based on a falsely positive test. However, this approach can be problematic when there is time urgency, such as when women first seek medical care when in labor and without a previous HIV test, or when people are unlikely to return for results, such as in clinics for sexually transmitted diseases. Effective interventions cannot be implemented without timely test results.

Rapid HIV tests are available that provide test results within hours of testing. Rapid testing is commonly used in developing countries. Because of the high prevalence of HIV in this setting, the risk of false positive results is lower than in the United States. In addition, several different rapid tests can be used to improve accuracy. In this setting, the benefits of identifying an infected individual using a rapid test are considered to outweigh the risks of false positive results.

CONFIDENTIALITY. Although medical information generally is considered confidential, there are additional requirements that apply to HIV-related information.

*Protections.* In the United States, physicians and healthcare organizations have ethical and legal obligations to preserve the confidentiality of all medical information. Because of the sensitivity of HIV-related information, many states in the United States have adopted laws that provide additional protection to HIV-related medical information. For example, many states require specific authorization from patients to disclose HIV-related information to third parties. Such protections are particularly important where stigma associated with HIV infection is high. Although the U.S. Supreme Court determined that HIV infection can be a disability under the Americans with Disabilities Act of 1990 (*Bragdon v. Abbott,* 1998), HIV-infected individuals still experience negative effects, such as ineligibility for certain governmental jobs (e.g., Peace Corps, foreign service, Job Corps, and the military) and limitations on international travel.

*Exceptions.* There are a number of exceptions to the legal and ethical rules of HIV-related confidentiality. First, healthcare providers in the United States have a duty to report AIDS cases and, in most states, HIV infections to public health authorities. The public health benefits of this reporting justify overriding the duty to maintain confidentiality. Reporting of AIDS cases includes the patient's name and other identifying information. Although reporting of HIV infections initially was not done by name, there has been a recent and controversial movement in the United States toward confidential name-based reporting of HIV infection. Supporters of name-based reporting argue that because antiretroviral therapies successfully delay progression to AIDS, the reporting of names is needed for more accurate epidemiological information. This information can be used for better planning and funding of HIV-related programs. Other proponents support name-based reporting because it would facilitate partner notification. Opponents of name-based reporting argue that it will deter testing and increase the risk of discrimination. Opponents contend that reporting of HIV infection can be effectively accomplished using codes, rather than names. Because of the potential psychosocial consequences associated with HIV infection, anonymous testing continues to be offered in states that require name-based reporting.

Second, healthcare providers may be permitted to inform an infected patient's sexual or drug-sharing partner of the patient's HIV infection. In some states, such as California, a healthcare provider must first inform the patient of the intended disclosure. Such a breach of confidentiality is justified on the grounds that it is the only means of preventing serious harm to an identifiable person and that the breach of confidentiality is minimized. Public health officials may also carry out partner notification. Although notification is typically conducted confidentially, it may inadvertently reveal the identity of the source patient.

Third, U.S. policy recommends that an expert panel review the cases of any HIV-infected healthcare workers who perform invasive procedures that might lead to transmission of HIV/AIDS. The panelists have to decide if an HIV-infected healthcare worker should be permitted to continue to perform such procedures, or if doing so would constitute too great a risk to the patients to be permitted. Additionally, the panel should decide if it is necessary to inform the healthcare worker's patients of any risk of infection, so that the patients can make an informed decision about whether they wish to continue in the healthcare worker's care. There is wide variation in state law and not all states require disclosure of HIV infection.

HIV INFECTION IN WOMEN AND CHILDREN. Worldwide, mother-to-child transmission is a major public health crisis. In parts of Africa, 45 percent of pregnant women are HIV-infected. Their children contract HIV in 25 to 45 percent of cases, resulting in some 540,000 perinatal cases annually. In the United States, the introduction of antiretroviral therapy has significantly reduced mother-to-child HIV transmission in the United States; by the early 2000s there were fewer than 300 perinatal HIV cases annually.

*United States.* To take advantage of the proven effectiveness of antiretroviral therapy for preventing perinatal HIV transmission, women must know that they are HIV-infected. U.S. policy strongly encourages HIV testing of all pregnant women, but at the same time U.S. policy embraces the state-based requirements for specific informed consent. Because many women are not offered and do not receive HIV testing during pregnancy, several consensus guidelines from professional societies have recommended that HIV testing should be made a routine part of prenatal care for all pregnant women. Notification that an HIV test will be performed, along with other prenatal blood tests, would be required, but specific consent to the HIV test would not. This proposal raises several concerns. First, women may not have enough information to know that they may refuse testing. Second, routine HIV testing in the prenatal context may undermine pretest counseling and informed consent for HIV testing in other clinical contexts. Third, because it forgoes certain opportunities for education and counseling, routine testing may undermine prevention efforts. Despite these concerns, the clear benefits of prenatal antiretroviral therapy in reducing the risk of mother-to-child HIV transmission may justify routine universal prenatal HIV testing.

*Developing world.* In developing countries, to date, the high cost of antiretroviral therapy to reduce the risk of mother-to-child HIV transmission has prevented the vast majority of women from receiving it. Even if antiretroviral therapy were to become affordable, the full protocol followed in the United States, which includes administration of antiretrovirals to the woman during the third trimester of pregnancy and during labor and delivery and administration to the infant after birth, may not be achievable because many women in the developing world do not receive prenatal care or deliver their babies in the hospital. Nevertheless, a single dose of nevirapine to the woman during labor and the infant after delivery has proven effective at significantly reducing mother–child HIV transmission. This simpler preventative regimen is more feasible, and some governments have committed to providing it.

Transmission from mother to child may also occur after birth through breast-feeding. A randomized clinical trial has shown that bottle-feeding instead of breast-feeding reduces the risk of transmission. Nevertheless, bottle-feeding is not a feasible option in many countries because of lack of access to clean water and cost. Moreover, some women may resist bottle-feeding, even if it were safe, because, unlike in the United States, breast-feeding is the norm in many developing countries and may play an important symbolic role in conveying social status to mothers. In such cultures, failure to breast-feed may indirectly reveal HIV status, which could subject women to risk of physical harm or loss of housing and support, particularly when there is a history of domestic violence. Women need to know about the steps they can take to reduce the risk of HIV transmission to their infants so that they can assess the risks and benefits in light of their own circumstances and make informed decisions.

**END-OF-LIFE ISSUES.** Early in the U.S. epidemic, before antiretroviral therapy was available, HIV infection often quickly progressed to a terminal illness. In many cases, AIDS patients were unable to make medical decisions for their care as a result of complications from their disease. There was uncertainty, however, as to who should serve as a patient's surrogate decision-maker. In the absence of a written advance directive from the patient, the law and physicians typically look to family members for surrogate decision-makers. But many homosexual men with AIDS were estranged from their family. These patients often would have preferred to give decision-making authority to committed partners or friends with whom the patient had discussed his wishes. Because the availability of highly active antiretroviral therapy has prolonged survival, end-of-life care in HIV infection has become a less prominent issue in the United States.

In the developing world, where antiretroviral therapy is generally not available, palliative care, which focuses on relief of suffering, is often the only tenable goal. Severe resource constraints may make it difficult to provide palliative measures such as opioids for pain control or dyspnea (difficult breathing). Under these circumstances, care may be limited to psychosocial support and helping patients make plans for such practical issues such as burial or child custody and support.

**ACCESS TO HEALTHCARE FOR HIV DISEASE.** Access to healthcare for HIV disease remains an important issue both domestically and internationally.

*United States.* In the United States, the average annual cost of care for an HIV-infected individual is between $10,000 and $15,000 annually. For those in the "advanced stages" of AIDS, the average annual cost of care is $34,000. In delving further into access to healthcare in the United States, it is necessary to discuss two areas: private coverage of HIV infection and coverage of HIV infection by public programs.

HIV-infected individuals may face several difficulties with private healthcare insurance. Most individuals in the United States with healthcare coverage receive it through their employers. Employers and insurers may seek to control the soaring cost of health insurance by limiting coverage for HIV infection. A 1990 federal appeals court case affirmed employers' "freedom to amend or eliminate employee benefits" in health insurance and allowed self-insured employers to reduce or eliminate benefits for any particular illness, even if all other medical conditions are covered (*McGann v. H & H Music Company,* 1991). A 2000 federal appeals court decision concluded that such limits do not violate the Americans with Disabilities Act (*Doe v. Mutual of Omaha Insurance Co.,* 2000). Those who do not receive healthcare coverage through their employers may find it impossible to obtain private coverage for their HIV infection because, if coverage for individual applicants with HIV infection is available at all, it is very expensive or provides limited coverage.

As their disease progresses, previously employed persons cease working and lose their employment-based health insurance. About half of HIV-infected adults and 90 percent of HIV-infected children receiving medical care are covered through publicly funded sources. There are several ways to receive such coverage. First, patients may be insured through Medicaid. To be eligible for Medicaid, patients must either have AIDS or HIV-related disability *and* meet (low) income eligibility requirements. Second, state AIDS drug assistance programs (ADAP), which are funded through the federal Ryan White Comprehensive AIDS Resources Emergency

(CARE) Act of 1990, make HIV medications available to low-income and uninsured persons. Because each state receives different funding and determines eligibility and benefits packages, Medicaid coverage and access to medications vary widely from state to state. In addition, because, unlike Medicaid, the drug assistance programs are not entitlement programs (i.e., programs in which all those who meet the eligibility criteria are entitled to receive the benefits), they are funded through annual appropriations, which may vary year to year. Finally, the CARE Act provides funding for HIV/AIDS services that are not covered by Medicaid or state or local government funds. Although the majority of the CARE Act funds are used for medical care (including the ADAP programs), they also provide funding for HIV/AIDS-related support services. These services include counseling, emergency housing assistance, training for clinicians who treat HIV-infected patients, and developing programs to improve treatment. States and other local governments receive CARE Act funds based, in part, on the prevalence of HIV/AIDS in their populations. Because of shifts in the epidemic and the effectiveness of antiretroviral therapies in delaying progression to AIDS, using AIDS cases to allocate funds may not accurately reflect the burden of HIV disease in the population. Reporting of HIV infection can provide essential information to ensure that funds are appropriately distributed to meet the needs of HIV-infected patients.

The shift to Medicaid and other public funding causes several problems. Because of low reimbursement levels, many physicians do not accept Medicaid patients. Thus, patients who lose private insurance may also lose access to care. As a result, emergency departments and public hospitals bear a greater burden of care. In addition, because of large budget deficits, many states and counties are finding it increasingly difficult to pay for such care.

Specific funding that provides for HIV care, but not for other fatal illnesses whose treatments are expensive, such as cancer, raises issues about equitable allocation of resources. AIDS activists exerted considerable political pressure to obtain this funding and to continue the programs supported by it. There are public policy reasons for providing special funding for HIV care. First, HIV is an infectious disease. Providing care and access to antiretroviral medications slows the progress of disease, which may decrease transmissibility and, therefore, help control the spread of the epidemic. In addition, because AIDS patients are categorically eligible for Medicaid and the overall cost of antiretroviral therapy is less than caring for a patient with AIDS, it may be more cost effective for the government to provide antiretroviral therapy to delay progression to AIDS.

*Developing world.* There have been many efforts to make HIV medications more available to the developing world by pressuring pharmaceutical manufacturers to reduce prices, permitting production of generic versions of effective therapies, and providing funds for drug purchases. Even though the annual cost of antiretroviral therapy has been reduced to between $500 and $1,350 for the developing world, this cost is beyond the means of many developing nations. In 2001 the United Nations secretary general, Kofi Annan, proposed a $7 billion to $10 billion fund to combat AIDS globally, although, as of 2003, funding has fallen well short of this goal. The obligation of developed nations to address the AIDS epidemic in the developing world can be justified on several grounds. First, compassion may motivate developed nations to help alleviate the suffering caused by the AIDS epidemic. Second, to the extent that good health and healthcare are basic human rights, nations who are able are obligated to contribute resources to guarantee these rights. Third, because the wealth (and health) disparities between the developed and developing world are largely a legacy of colonialism, the developed nations have an obligation to address those problems to which they contributed. Finally, it is in the self-interest of developed nations to assist the developing world. If the AIDS epidemic is not controlled in the developing world, the resulting economic and political instability will threaten the security of all nations.

Even if antiretroviral therapy can be made affordable, there are challenges in providing treatment in developing countries that have little healthcare infrastructure. Because failure to adhere to the treatment regimen may lead to drug resistance, it is important to develop treatment protocols that can be implemented effectively using existing infrastructure. Once-a-day regimens are being developed that could facilitate implementation of antiretroviral treatments in the developing world. Also being studied are programs for providing care when intensive laboratory monitoring is not available. To successfully maintain HIV treatment programs in the developing world, host-country personnel must be trained to provide and monitor the treatments.

## Clinical Research Issues

Activists and the scope of the HIV epidemic forced society and scientists to reconsider fundamental questions about clinical trials of promising new therapies (Lo, 2000b).

**WHAT IS THE GOAL OF THE CLINICAL TRIAL?** To most scientists and to the U.S. Food and Drug Administration (FDA), the goal of clinical trials is to determine the safety and effectiveness of new drugs. Historically, clinical research has been considered dangerous for subjects. The HIV epidemic, however, caused many patients to consider clinical trials beneficial rather than risky, because they offer access to promising new treatments, closer medical follow-up, and more sophisticated laboratory monitoring than does standard care.

## WHO SHOULD PARTICIPATE IN CLINICAL TRIALS?

Historically, women, children, and people of color have been underrepresented in clinical trials. Usually, children are restricted from clinical trials to protect them from the risks of unproven therapies. Unlike adults, children cannot give informed consent. The rationale for excluding women of childbearing age, particularly women who are pregnant, is to protect their developing and future children from possible long-term side effects of unproven drugs. But restricting women and children from clinical trials also harms them. Unless they participate in clinical trials, the effectiveness and safety of therapies cannot be rigorously established. For example, the trials of the effect of zidovudine (also known as azidothymidine, or AZT) on mother-to-child transmission provided important information that has dramatically reduced perinatal HIV transmission. Without the participation of pregnant women in clinical trials, the effectiveness of antiretroviral therapy in preventing mother-to-child transmission of HIV would not be proven. What is more, there would be no evidence basis for enhanced public health measures and increased funding to prevent mother-to-child transmission. Similarly, the increased inclusion of minorities in trials has provided information on the efficacy and adverse effects in these populations. In addition, it is problematic to take away women's decision-making about research participation simply because they are pregnant.

## INTERNATIONAL RESEARCH.

Because of the great disparities of wealth between the developed and the developing world and a history of exploitation, research conducted in the developing world has been controversial. There are concerns that research that will never benefit the host country is being conducted in developing countries solely because costs are lower and the local ethical requirements are not as onerous as those in the sponsoring nation. Moreover, there are concerns that people will participate in research, regardless of the level of risk, because research participation represents the only opportunity to receive medical care. Nevertheless, unlike research associated with many other conditions, HIV-related research in developing countries typically does not involve privately sponsored trials of new drugs that are unlikely to become available to the host country. Rather, such research generally is publicly funded and designed to assess efficacy of affordable treatment regimens or behavioral interventions. Government involvement and sponsorship may result in research addressing health policy issues that are more salient to the host countries.

*Controversy over perinatal trials.* Placebo-controlled trials testing interventions to reduce perinatal HIV transmission conducted by U.S. researchers in Africa and Asia sparked extensive debate over research in developing countries. Relying on the World Medical Association's (WMA) Declaration of Helsinki (first adopted in 1964), which stated that "[i]n any medical study, every patient—including those of a control group, if any—should be assured the best proven diagnostic and therapeutic methods" (World Medical Association, 2000), some argued that the placebo-controlled trials were unethical because zidovudine was a proven effective treatment, even though it generally was not available in the countries in which the trials were taking place because of cost, poor health infrastructure, and lack of prenatal care. Others argued that such placebo-controlled trials can be ethically justified because they provide information that responds to local needs. A developing country needs to know whether a simpler, cheaper therapeutic regimen is superior to what is currently available in the country (generally no therapy) rather than whether a simpler, cheaper treatment is comparable to the best proven treatment, which the country cannot afford.

*Appropriate comparison group.* The controversy over the perinatal HIV transmission trials influenced the larger debate regarding international research, particularly as the WMA revised the Declaration of Helsinki in 2000. After considerable debate about the role of placebo-controlled trials, the final version reads: "[t]he benefits, risks, burdens and effectiveness of a new method should be tested against those of the best current prophylactic, diagnostic, and therapeutic methods. This does not exclude the use of placebo, or no treatment, in studies where no proven prophylactic, diagnostic or therapeutic methods exists" (World Medical Association, 2000). There is a growing recognition, however, that it may be ethically permissible to compare an inexpensive, simple regimen to a current practice of no therapy in developing countries when the regimen used in developed countries is not feasible. For example, the WMA issued a clarification after the 2000 revision of the Declaration of Helsinki that "a placebo-controlled trial may be ethically acceptable, even if proven therapy is available … where for compelling and scientifically sound methodological reasons its use is necessary to determine the efficacy or safety of a prophylactic, diagnostic or therapeutic method" (World Medical Association, 2001).

In its 2001 report, *Ethical and Policy Issues in International Research,* the U.S. National Bioethics Advisory Commission (NBAC) concluded that members of any control group should be provided with an established effective treatment, whether or not such treatment is available in the host country. NBAC also declared, however, that a placebo-controlled design may be permissible based on the health needs of the host country, but that such a design requires strong justification.

*Post-trial access to treatment.* There is general agreement that research in a developing country should not go forward unless there is a realistic chance that its inhabitants will gain access to the treatment after the trial. For example, HIV vaccine trials would be permissible in a developing country only if the vaccine candidate, if successful, would be made available within the host country. There is, however, disagreement regarding how far researchers' obligations extend toward assuring access and to whom the obligation is owed (i.e., trial participants only or others within the community or nation). NBAC points out that researchers are not in control of government policy and funding for clinical care. It therefore would be unfair to hold them responsible for ensuring post-trial access to therapies. NBAC suggests instead that researchers should be obligated only to make good faith efforts to make therapies available after completing a trial. Moreover, the successful results in a well-designed clinical trial may cause resources to become available to provide a new therapy, even though such resources were not available before the trial commenced.

*Informed consent.* U.S. federal regulations, the Declaration of Helsinki, and other international ethics guidelines all require individual consent for research participation. However, U.S. requirements regarding informed consent may present challenges for research in developing countries. Informed consent is often not the norm for clinical care in many developing nations. People may therefore be uncomfortable or even scared by being asked to provide consent. In addition, most people assume that the doctor is giving them something that is known to work. It may be difficult to overcome this presumption and to get them to appreciate the risks involved in participating in the research. In addition, women may be used to deferring decisions to husbands, fathers, or other family members. In some communities, it may not be possible to approach individuals without the community leader's permission. In such cases, although assent from the authority figure may be needed to approach people regarding the research, voluntary consent must be obtained from individual participants. Finally, in some communities, documentation of consent may be difficult because of illiteracy or because people fear that a signed document may be used against them. In such cases, it may be necessary to seek approval of the institutional review board to modify the documentation of consent to accommodate these local conditions.

*Vulnerable participants.* Vulnerability is particularly important in the context of HIV-related research. Those infected with HIV may be medically vulnerable from their infection. In addition, homosexuals, injection drug users, minorities, and women, who, for various reasons, may be at higher risk of HIV infection, are more likely to be socially and economically vulnerable because of historical attitudes and discrimination. This may be particularly true in the international setting, and the degree of vulnerability for these groups may vary from country to country. Accordingly, investigators conducting HIV-related research, especially internationally, must pay particular attention to vulnerability and take steps to protect potentially vulnerable research participants.

SPECIAL ISSUES IN HIV VACCINE RESEARCH. HIV vaccine trials present special ethical concerns. First, HIV vaccine trials must go forward with less preclinical evidence of efficacy than other interventions. This is because a good animal model does not exist, HIV is highly variable and undergoes rapid mutation, and there is little information about how to build protection against HIV. Nevertheless, because of the enormous suffering caused by HIV, such trials are ethically appropriate if there are credible scientific reasons to believe the candidate vaccine may be effective.

Second, vaccine trial participants may mistakenly believe that they will receive protection from the vaccine and, therefore, may increase risky behaviors. This issue is a particular concern because, unlike most vaccines, HIV vaccines are unlikely to confer full immunity. While researchers need outcomes (i.e., seroconversions—positive HIV tests in persons who previously tested negative for HIV) to evaluate the efficacy of the vaccine candidate, they also have an obligation to protect research participants. Accordingly, researchers must provide high-quality risk-reduction counseling and emphasize the uncertainty about the effectiveness of the candidate vaccine to all participants, even though, if such counseling were totally effective, the clinical trial would be undermined. To avoid this potential conflict, it may be necessary to have separate staff for the counseling and research aspects of the trial.

Finally, HIV vaccine trials pose unique risks to participants. Participants may be prevented from participating in future vaccine trials, and subsequently developed vaccines may be less effective for them. In addition, because participants may react positively to certain HIV antibody tests, they may be excluded from certain professions and activities, even if their seroconversion does not represent a true infection. Subjects may also face stigmatization from family or friends to whom they disclose information. Mere participation in some trials may identify the subject as someone at high risk of contracting HIV. Because of the high stakes if confidentiality is breached, researchers should take extra steps to protect the confidentiality of the information they collect in HIV vaccine trials.

## Conclusion

In summary, the HIV epidemic has raised new ethical and policy dilemmas and has forced reconsideration of established guidelines and policies that apply to a much broader range of issues. In the future, controversies will likely continue to focus on addressing the global impact of HIV/AIDS and what justice requires in healthcare access and research.

BERNARD LO (1995)
REVISED BY LESLIE E. WOLF
BERNARD LO

SEE ALSO: *Children: Healthcare and Research Issues; Confidentiality; Epidemics; Healthcare Resources, Allocation of; Homosexuality; Human Dignity; Human Rights; Life, Quality of; Public Health; Research Policy;* and other *AIDS* subentries

### BIBLIOGRAPHY

Angell, Marcia. 1997. "The Ethics of Clinical Research in the Third World." *New England Journal of Medicine* 337(12): 847–849.

Bayer, Ronald. 1991. "Public Health Policy and the AIDS Epidemic: An End to HIV Exceptionalism?" *New England Journal of Medicine* 324(21): 1500–1504.

Bozzette, Samuel A.; Berry, Sandra H.; Duan, Naihua; et al. 1998. "The Care of HIV-Infected Adults in the United States." *New England Journal of Medicine* 339(26): 1897–1904.

*Bragdon v. Abbott.* 524 U.S. 624 (1998).

Centers for Disease Control and Prevention. 2001. "HIV and AIDS: United States, 1981–2000." *Morbidity and Mortality Weekly Report* 50(21): 430–434.

Centers for Disease Control and Prevention. 2001. "Revised Guidelines for HIV Counseling, Testing, and Referral." *Morbidity and Mortality Weekly Report* 50(19): 1–58.

Centers for Disease Control and Prevention. 2001. "Revised Recommendations for HIV Screening of Pregnant Women." *Morbidity and Mortality Weekly Report* 50(19): 59–86.

Chesney, Margaret A.; Lurie, Peter; and Coates, Thomas J. 1995. "Strategies for Addressing the Social and Behavioral Challenges of Prophylactic HIV Vaccine Trials." *Journal of Acquired Immune Deficiency Syndromes and Human Retrovirology* 9(1): 30–35.

De Cock, Kevin, and Janssen, Robert. 2002. "An Unequal Epidemic in an Unequal World." *Journal of the American Medical Association* 288(2): 236–238.

*Doe v. Mutual of Omaha Insurance Co.* 179 F.3d 557 (7th Cir. 1999), cert. denied 528 U.S. 1106 (2000).

Farmer, Paul; Leandre, Fernet; Mukherjee, Joia S.; et al. 2001. "Community-Based Approaches to HIV Treatment in Resource-Poor Settings." *Lancet* 358(9279): 404–409.

Ferriman, Annabel. 2001. "Doctors Demand Immediate Access to Antiretroviral Drugs in Africa." *British Medical Journal* 322(7293): 1012.

Gostin, Lawrence O. 2000. "A Proposed National Policy on Health Care Workers Living with HIV/AIDS and Other Blood-Borne Pathogens." *Journal of the American Medical Association* 284(15): 1965–1970.

Gostin, Lawrence O.; Ward, John W.; and Baker, A. Cornelius. 1997. "National HIV Case Reporting for the United States: A Defining Moment in the History of the Epidemic." *New England Journal of Medicine* 337(16): 1162–1167.

Guay, Laura A.; Musoke, Philippa; Fleming, Thomas; et al. 1999. "Intrapartum and Neonatal Single-Dose Nevirapine Compared with Zidovudine for Prevention of Mother-to-Child Transmission of HIV-1 in Kampala, Uganda: HIVNET 012 Randomised Trial." *Lancet* 354(9181): 795–802.

Joint United Nations Programme on HIV/AIDS (UNAIDS). 2000. *AIDS Epidemic Update, December 1, 2001.* Geneva, Switzerland: Author.

Joint United Nations Programme on HIV/AIDS (UNAIDS). 2000. *Ethical Considerations in HIV Preventive Vaccine Research: UNAIDS Guidance Document.* Geneva, Switzerland: Author.

Kallings, Lars, and Vella, Stefano. 2001. "Access to HIV/AIDS Care and Treatment in the South of the World." *AIDS* 15: IAS1–IAS3.

Langan, Michael, and Collins, Chris. 1998. "Paving the Road to an HIV Vaccine: Employing Tools of Public Policy to Overcome Scientific, Economic, Social, and Ethical Obstacles." San Francisco: Center for AIDS Prevention Studies, AIDS Research Institute, University of California, San Francisco.

Levine, Carol; Dubler, Nancy N.; and Levine, Robert J. 1991. "Building a New Consensus: Ethical Principles and Policies for Clinical Research on HIV/AIDS." *IRB: A Review of Human Subjects Research* 13(1): 1–17.

Levine, Robert J. 1999. "The Need to Revise the Declaration of Helsinki." *New England Journal of Medicine* 341(7): 531–534.

Lo, Bernard. 2000a. "Confidentiality." In *Resolving Ethical Dilemmas: A Guide for Clinicians,* 2nd edition. Philadelphia: Lippincott Williams & Wilkins.

Lo, Bernard. 2000b. "Ethical Issues in Clinical Research." In *Designing Clinical Research,* 2nd edition, ed. Stephen Hulley. Philadelphia: Lippincott Williams & Wilkins.

Lo, Bernard, and Steinbrook, Robert. 1992. "Health Care Workers Infected with the Human Immunodeficiency Virus: The Next Steps." *Journal of the American Medical Association* 267(8): 1100–1105.

Lurie, Peter, and Wolfe, Sidney M. 1997. "Unethical Trials of Interventions to Reduce Perinatal Transmission of the Human Immunodeficiency Virus in Developing Countries." *New England Journal of Medicine* 337(12): 853–856.

*McGann v. H & H Music Company.* 946 F.2d 401 (5th Cir. 1991).

Nduati, Ruth; John, Grace; Mbori-Ngacha, Dorothy; et al. 2000. "Effect of Breastfeeding and Formula Feeding on Transmission of HIV-1: A Randomized Clinical Trial." *Journal of the American Medical Association* 283(9): 1167–1174.

Steinbrook, Robert. 1998. "Caring for People with Human Immunodeficiency Virus Infection." *New England Journal of Medicine* 339(26): 1926–1928.

Steinbrook, Robert. 2002. "Beyond Barcelona: The Global Response to HIV." *New England Journal of Medicine* 347(8): 553–554.

U.S. Institute of Medicine. Committee on Perinatal Transmission of HIV, and U.S. National Research Council. Board on Children, Youth, and Families. 1999. *Reducing the Odds: Preventing Perinatal Transmission of HIV in the United States,* ed. Michael A. Stoto, Donna A. Almario, and Marie C. McCormick. Washington, D.C.: National Academy Press.

U.S. National Bioethics Advisory Commission (NBAC). 2001. *Ethical and Policy Issues in International Research: Clinical Trials in Developing Countries,* Vol. 1: *Report and Recommendations of the National Bioethics Advisory Commission.* Bethesda, MD: Author.

U.S. National Bioethics Advisory Commission (NBAC). 2001. *Ethical and Policy Issues in Research Involving Human Participants.* Rockville, MD: Government Printing Office.

Varmus, Harold, and Satcher, David. 1997. "Ethical Complexities of Conducting Research in Developing Countries." *New England Journal of Medicine* 337(12): 1003–1005.

Wolf, Leslie E., and Lo, Bernard. 1999. "What about the Ethics? [HIV Vaccine Trials]" *Western Journal of Medicine* 171(5–6): 365–366.

Wolf, Leslie E.; Lo, Bernard; Beckerman, Karen P.; et al. 2001. "When Parents Reject Interventions to Reduce Perinatal Transmission of HIV." *Archives of Pediatrics and Adolescent Medicine* 155: 927–933.

World Medical Association (WMA). 2000. "Declaration of Helsinki: Ethical Principles for Medical Research Involving Human Subjects." Ferney-Voltaire, France: Author.

World Medical Association (WMA). 2001. "Declaration of Helsinki: Note of Clarification on Placebo-Controlled Trials." Ferney-Voltaire, France: Author.

INTERNET RESOURCES

Global HIV Prevention Working Group. 2002. "Global Mobilization for HIV Prevention: A Blueprint for Action." Available from <http://www.gatesfoundation.org/connectedpostings/hivprevreport_final.pdf>.

Joint United Nations Programme on HIV/AIDS (UNAIDS). 2000. *AIDS Epidemic Update, December 2001.* Available from <http://www.unaids.org/epidemic_update/report_dec01/index.html>.

Joint United Nations Programme on HIV/AIDS (UNAIDS). 2000. *Ethical Considerations in HIV Preventive Vaccine Research: UNAIDS Guidance Document.* Available from <http://www.unaids.org/publications/documents/vaccines/>.

Joint United Nations Programme on HIV/AIDS (UNAIDS). 2001. *Children and Young People in a World of AIDS.* Available from <http://www.unaids.org/youngpeople/index.html>.

# ALCOHOL AND OTHER DRUGS IN A PUBLIC HEALTH CONTEXT

• • •

Psychoactive drugs are substances that alter the mental state of humans after ingestion. There are a wide variety of those substances, both naturally occurring and synthesized, including tobacco, alcoholic beverages, coffee, tea, chocolate, and some spices, as well as substances that are legally available only through medical channels, such as benzodiazepides, cannabinols, opiates, and cocaine. Such substances often have other use values along with their psychoactive properties. Users may like the taste or the image of themselves that the use of those substances conveys. Substance use may be a medium of sociability (Partanen) or part of a religious ritual. Some substances have other useful properties; alcohol, for example, is a source of calories and is used as a solvent in many tinctures.

Psychoactive drugs differ in their metabolic pathways and mechanisms of action in the human body, the strength of their effects, and the states of mind and feelings they induce. However, the effects of drug use also are highly dependent on the pattern of use and on the set and setting, that is, the expectations of the user and of others who are present and the context of use (Zinberg). Although the psychoactive effect of tobacco may not register in the consciousness of a habituated cigarette smoker, in other circumstances the effect of tobacco use may be so strong that the user is rendered unconscious, as early Spanish observers reported in describing tobacco use among native South Americans (Robicsek).

Psychoactive substances frequently are valued by potential consumers well above the cost of production. On the one hand, this means that taxes on alcohol, tobacco, and other drugs have long been an important fiscal resource for the state. On the other hand, it means that there are substantial incentives for an illicit market to emerge in places where the sale of drugs is forbidden or stringently restricted.

A consideration of drugs in a public health context may start with an examination of general cultural patternings and understandings of drug use. This entry continues by discussing the major approaches to limiting harm from drug use. The entry concludes with a characterization of the major directions in the development of drug policies in the United States and other industrialized countries.

## General Cultural Framings of Drug Abuse

Three social patternings of psychoactive drug use can be distinguished as prototypical: medicinal use, customary regular use, and intermittent use. In many traditional societies some drugs or formulations have been confined to medicinal use, that is, use under the supervision of a healer to alleviate mental or physical illness or distress. For several centuries after the technique for distilling alcoholic spirits had diffused from China through the Arab world to Europe, for instance, spirits-based drinks were regarded primarily as medicines (Wasson). This way of framing drug use has been routinized in the modern state through a prescription system, with physicians writing the prescriptions and pharmacists filling them. Drugs included in the prescription system usually are forbidden for nonmedicinal use.

When a drug becomes a regular accompaniment of everyday life, its psychoactivity often is muted and even unnoticed, as is often the case for a habitual cigarette smoker. Similarly, in southern European wine cultures wine is differentiated from intoxicating "alcohol"; wine drinkers are expected to maintain their original comportment after drinking. This may be called a pattern of *banalized use*: A potentially powerful psychoactive agent is domesticated into a mundane article of daily life that is available relatively freely in the consumer market.

Intermittent use—for instance, on sacred occasions, at festivals, or only on weekends—minimizes the buildup of tolerance to a drug. It is in the context of those patterns that the greatest attention is likely to be paid to a drug's psychoactive properties. The drug may be understood by both the user and others as having taken control of the user's behavior and thus to explain otherwise unexpected behavior, whether bad or good (see the "disinhibition hypothesis" in Pernanen; see also Room, 2001b). As in Robert Louis Stevenson's fable of Jekyll and Hyde, normal self-control is expected to return when the effects of the drug wear off. In

light of the power attributed to the substance, access to it may be limited: in traditional societies by sumptuary rules keyed to social differentiations and in industrial societies by other forms of market restriction.

In industrial societies a fourth pattern of use is commonly recognized for certain drugs: addicted or dependent use that is marked by regular use, often of large doses. Because the pattern of use of a particular drug is not defined in the society as banalized, addiction is defined as an individual failing rather than a social pattern. Although attention is paid to physical factors that sustain regular use, such as use to relieve withdrawal symptoms, most formulations of addiction focus on psychological aspects, including an apparent commitment to drug use to the exclusion of other activities and despite default in performing major social roles. An addiction concept thus also focuses on the loss of normal self-control, but the emphasis is not so much on the immediate effects of the drug as it is on a repeated or continuing pattern of an apparent inability to control or refrain from use despite the adverse consequences.

## Addiction as a Modern Governing Image

The concept of addiction as an affliction of habituated drug users first arose in its modern form for alcohol as heavy drinking lost its banalized status in the United States and some other countries under the influence of the temperance movement of the nineteenth century (Levine; Valverde). Habitual drunkenness had been viewed since the Middle Ages as a subclass of gluttony; now abstinence from alcohol was singled out as a separate virtue and an important sign of the key virtue in a democracy of autonomous citizens: self-control. Along with other mental disorders, *chronic inebriety,* as alcohol addiction usually was termed, was reinterpreted as a disease suitable for medical intervention, although without losing all of its negative moral loading.

In nineteenth-century formulations addictiveness was seen as an inherent property of alcohol no matter who used it, and that perception justified efforts to prohibit its sale. By the late nineteenth century such addiction concepts were being applied also to opiates and other drugs, and this formulation has remained the governing image (Room, 2001a) for those drugs to the present day. However, as temperance became unpopular with the repeal of national alcohol prohibition in the United States in 1933, for alcohol the concept was reformulated to be a property of the individual "alcoholic," who was mysteriously unable to drink like a normal drinker. This "disease concept of alcoholism" received its classic scholarly formulation by Jellinek (1952), although that author (1960) later retreated to a broader formulation of alcohol problems.

In popular thinking and often in official definitions addiction has remained a property of the drug for illicit drugs but of the person for alcohol (Christie and Bruun). The inherent addictiveness attributed to illicit drugs is the primary rationale for their prohibition. The extent of the anathema imposed in U.S. cultural politics by labeling a substance as addictive can be gauged from the unanimous testimony of cigarette company executives to the U.S. Congress in 1994 that they did not believe that cigarettes are addictive despite the evidence of their own corporate research (Hilts).

In recent years philosophers and cultural analysts have begun to question and rethink the meaning of addiction concepts (Szasz; Fingarette; Keane) and consider the implications for drug policy (Husak). In a related initiative economists have begun propounding and testing theories of *rational addiction* (Elster and Skog). By the early 2000s that critical thinking had had no discernible influence on the American political consensus in favor of an addiction-based policy for illicit drugs.

## Approaches to Limiting the Problems from Drug Use

Most human societies have known of and used psychoactive drugs, and most also have made efforts to limit the use of one or more drugs, customarily if not legislatively. Historically, the main aim of those restrictions was to diminish threats to the social order or to increase the labor supply. Public health concerns sometimes were expressed in attempts to justify restrictions—for instance, in the efforts of James I of England to stem tobacco smoking (Austin)—but such concerns were rarely decisive. The restrictions on the spirits market adopted in Britain as a response to the extreme alcoholization of eighteenth-century London (depicted in Hogarth's famous print of "Gin Lane") are an early example of limits substantially motivated by concern about public health (Warner; Dillon). Only in recent decades have public health concerns become a major element in discussions of drug policies, although those concerns often are subordinated in the case of legal drugs to fiscal and economic considerations and in the case of illicit drugs to moral and lifestyle issues.

Health hazards from psychoactive drugs occur in two main ways: in connection with particular occasions of use and in connection with the patterning of use over time. Thus, an overdose from barbiturates, a traffic casualty from drunk driving, and an HIV infection from sharing a needle to inject heroin are all consequences associated with a particular occasion of use, whereas lung cancer from tobacco smoking, liver cirrhosis from alcohol use, and (by definition) addiction all reflect a history of heavy use (Room, 1985). As

is discussed below, measures to prevent event-related problems often differ from and even conflict with measures to prevent cumulative, condition-related problems. For alcohol the ethical situation with regard to public health measures is complicated by the possibility of a protective effect of drinking on heart disease that must be balanced against the undoubted negative health effects (Room, 2001c; Rehm et al.).

Efforts to limit problems from drug use can be seen as oriented to controlling whether a drug is used at all; influencing the amount, context, and pattern of use; or preventing harmful consequences of use (Bruun; Moore and Gerstein).

**PROHIBITING USE TO ALL OR SOME.** Efforts to impose a general prohibition on the use of a drug for all the members of a society have a lengthy history, although those efforts frequently have failed (Austin). Perhaps the most sustained effort has been the prohibition on alcoholic beverages in Islamic societies. In general, religious taboos on drug use tend to have had more lasting effect than have state prohibitions. Prohibiting the sale or use of a drug that some might choose to use and enjoy involves a degree of intervention in the marketplace and in private behavior that is unusual in modern democratic states. If there are people who use a drug without problems, the prohibition on their use of that drug must be justified as benefiting others who would have or would cause problems if they used it. In societies with a strong tradition of individual liberties and consumer sovereignty discomfort with the use of this line of argument to support prohibition commonly is resolved by presumptions that users sooner or later will become addicted and that users without problems do not really exist.

A common form of prohibition of use in village and tribal societies has been sumptuary rules restricting use to particular status groups, most commonly the most powerful segments of the society. Depending on the culture, a variety of arguments are offered for the inability of lower-status groups to handle drug use appropriately. Because psychoactive drugs offer visions of an alternative reality (Stauffer) and may be associated with disinhibition, dominant groups may fear challenges to their power if subordinates have access to drugs (Morgan). The universalist ethic of modern states has made explicit sumptuary restrictions untenable, with the substantial exception of prohibitions on use by children. Even the provisions, still common in U.S. state laws, that the names of habitual drunkards be posted and that those listed be refused service of alcoholic drinks are largely unenforced because of their perceived interference with individual liberties.

A third form of modified prohibition of use that often is employed in modern societies is limitation to medicinal use. The individual's supply of such medications is controlled by state-licensed professionals who are backed up by a state system of market controls. National controls on psychopharmaceuticals are backed up by an unusual and elaborate international control structure (Bruun et al.; Room and Paglia). In principle, prescription and use of these drugs are limited to therapeutic purposes. For psychoactive drugs, which commonly are prescribed to relieve negative affective states or mental distress, the definition of therapeutic use often is quite wide, and a substantial proportion of the resources of the health system in industrial societies is absorbed in superintending the provision of psychoactive drugs.

Except for methadone as a remedy for heroin addiction and nicotine as a remedy for tobacco smoking, it generally is considered illegitimate to prescribe a drug to help a person maintain a habitual pattern of use without withdrawal or other distress. Use for pleasure or for the sake of the psychoactive experience is considered nontherapeutic, and so the functions of drugs that are considered psychopharmaceuticals always are described in terms of the relief of distress rather than the provision of pleasure. To some extent the medical prescription system in a modern state serves as a covert form of control by status differentiation, according to the prejudices of the prescriber; for instance, older and more respectable adults find it easier than do the younger and more disreputable to obtain a prescription for a psychopharmaceutical.

INFLUENCING THE PATTERN OF USE. An enormous variety of formal and informal strategies have been used to influence the amount, pattern, and context of the use of drugs. Among the potential aims of those strategies is the public health goal of reducing the prevalence of hazardous use.

*Controlling availability.* One class of such strategies attempts to reduce drug-related problems by controlling the market in drugs by means of taxes, general restrictions on availability, or user-specific restrictions (Room, 2000; Babor et al.). Public health considerations are one reason among several that governments tax legally available drugs such as alcohol and tobacco. Those taxes often constitute a substantial portion of the price to the consumer. Raising taxes does diminish levels of use among heavier as well as lighter users, although demand usually diminishes proportionately less than the increase in price; that is, demand is relatively inelastic. Thus, short of levels that create an opening for a substantial illicit market, raising taxes on drugs tends both to have positive public health effects and to increase government revenues.

Governments often also control the conditions of availability, particularly for alcohol. Through a system of retail licenses or a government monopoly of sales, limits are placed on the hours and conditions of sale. Changes in those limits sometimes have been found to affect patterns of consumption and of alcohol-related problems (Babor et al.). However, with the strengthening of the ideology of consumer sovereignty—legal goods should be readily available, with purchases limited only by the consumer's means—controls on availability tend to have been loosened in the contemporary period (Mäkelä et al.).

A generally stronger and more direct effect on hazardous alcohol consumption has been found to result from measures that ration or restrict the availability of alcohol for specific purchasers (Babor et al.). A general ration limit for all purchasers restricts heavy consumption or at least raises the effective price, but such measures strongly conflict with the ideology of consumer sovereignty and are thus politically impracticable nearly everywhere. As was noted above, proscriptions or limits on sales to named heavy users also have fallen out of favor because they are considered infringements on individual liberty.

*Controlling the circumstances of use.* Another class of strategies aims to deter drinking or drug use in particularly hazardous circumstances, usually through the use of criminal sanctions. The prototypical situation is driving after drinking. Because alcohol consumption impairs the ability to drive a vehicle, most countries treat driving with a blood-alcohol level above a set limit as a criminal offense, and enforcement of those laws often absorbs a substantial proportion of the criminal justice system's resources. Popular movements as well as policy makers have expended much energy, particularly in the United States and other Anglophone and Scandinavian countries, in seeking a redefinition of drunk driving as a serious crime rather than a "folk crime" (Gusfield). This type of situational limit or prohibition has been extended to other skill-related tasks and also has been applied to driving after using other psychoactive drugs, particularly illicit drugs. A related development has sought to eliminate illicit drug use in working populations and alcohol use in the workplace by means of random urine testing of workers, with job loss as the sanction (Zimmer and Jacobs).

The ethics of this measure, which was pushed strongly by the U.S. government in the 1980s, are controversial, particularly because the tests detect illicit drug use that has not necessarily affected work performance (Macdonald and Roman). Random blood-alcohol tests of drivers to deter drinking before driving also have proved controversial: They are effective, well accepted, and widely applied in Australia (Homel et al.; Peek-Asa); legally permissible but not intensively applied in the United States; and viewed as an impermissible infringement on individual liberty and privacy in many countries.

*Education and persuasion about use.* A third class of strategies seeks to educate people or persuade them not to engage in hazardous drug use. Because such strategies are seen as the least coercive, at least for those beyond school age, they are used very widely and commonly despite the frequent lack of clear evidence on their effectiveness (Paglia and Room). Education of schoolchildren about the hazards of drug use is very widespread, indeed nearly ubiquitous, in the United States. Most countries also have made at least a token effort at public information campaigns about the hazards of tobacco smoking, and poster and slogan campaigns against drinking before driving and illicit drug use are also widespread. Other public information campaigns on alcohol have promoted limits on drinking (e.g., suggestions of safe levels in Britain and Australia) or campaigned against drinking in various hazardous circumstances.

Often these public information campaigns compete for attention in a media environment saturated with advertising on behalf of use from tobacco or alcohol companies. In the last two decades of the twentieth century some governments imposed substantial restrictions on tobacco and, to a lesser extent, alcohol advertising, for example, banning advertisements on electronic media, and mandated warning labels in advertisements or on product packages. These restrictions often have precipitated court fights about the constitutional permissibility of restrictions on the freedom of "commercial speech."

**REDUCING THE HARM FROM USE.** The strategies considered above are directed primarily at influencing the fact or pattern of use. They thus fall into the category of either supply reduction or demand reduction, to use terminology commonly applied to the use of illicit drugs. Since the late 1980s substantial attention has been directed toward a third option: harm reduction, or strategies that reduce the problems associated with drug use without necessarily reducing drug use (O'Hare et al.; Heather et al.). Attention to this class of strategies has a somewhat longer history for alcohol (Room, 1975). Usually these strategies focus on the physical or social environment of drug use, seeking physical, temporal, or cultural insulation of the drug use from harm. Thus, needle exchanges are intended to remove the risk of HIV infection from injection drug use, and seat belts and air bags insulate drivers who drink and those around them from the possibility of becoming casualties.

The debate over harm reduction strategies for illicit drugs has raised classic ethical issues for public health. Some argue that insulating the behavior from harm will encourage and thus increase the prevalence of the undesirable behavior.

A further consideration is the effectiveness of the insulation provided. Thus, efforts to provide a safer tobacco cigarette largely have been undercut by compensatory changes in puffing and inhaling by smokers. At an empirical level it seems that insulating drug use from harm does not necessarily increase the prevalence of drug use (Yoast et al.). Even if it did, an old public health tradition that is epitomized by the operation of venereal disease clinics would argue that reducing the immediate risk of harm has a higher ethical priority than affecting the prevalence of disapproved behaviors.

## The Political Reality in the Early 2000s: Lopsided Policies

The United States and many other countries have experienced recurring "moral panics" in recent decades concerning illicit drug use and have invested substantial resources in efforts to prevent such use. These resources have been invested largely in two areas: a particular preventive strategy—interdicting the illicit market—and the provision of treatment. The first strategy has received the greatest investment of government resources. There was a substantial decrease in illicit drug use in North America in the late 1980s and early 1990s, but it was followed by a rise in the 1990s.

Governments often are blamed for these ebbs and flows, but they may have more to do with cyclical patterns in youth fashions and social mores. The illicit market remains strong, and drug-related imprisonments have helped propel the United States to having the highest rate of incarceration among industrial societies. Meanwhile, the highest rates of health and social harm come from legal drugs. For instance, the World Health Organization (WHO) estimates that 13.3 percent of the net disability and death (in disability-adjusted life-years) in the subregion consisting of the United States, Canada, and Cuba is attributable to tobacco, 7.8 percent to alcohol, and 2.6 percent to illicit drugs (Ezzati et al.), yet alcohol and tobacco have received a much lower priority. In government policy making on these licit substances public health considerations often have been subordinated to economic concerns. In recent years, for example, the United States has successfully attacked control structures and forced a greater availability of both alcohol and tobacco in other countries through lawsuits under the General Agreement on Tariffs and Trade (Ferris et al.).

A substantial emphasis on the treatment of addiction has accompanied the attention paid to prevention. However, in this mixed policy environment the role of treatment has been highly differentiated by the type of drug. To a large extent tobacco smoking has continued to be defined as a health problem rather than a social problem, with the emphasis on the health consequences of smoking rather than the physical dependence of smokers on tobacco. Thus, there has been very little public provision of treatment for smoking addiction; most of those who have quit have done it by themselves or by using nicotine substitutes.

At the other extreme the goals for an illicit drug treatment system have been highly ambitious: In theory, in the mid-1970s and again in the late 1980s, the United States aspired to provide treatment to every unincarcerated addict. Quite explicitly, treatment for illicit drug use has been seen as a form of social control, and a high degree of coercion has been taken for granted (Gerstein and Harwood). On occasion U.S. drug strategies have argued for the provision of treatment as a means to encourage courts to be tougher on those who choose not to accept it (Strategy Council on Drug Abuse), and drug treatment agencies have argued routinely for maintaining jail sentences for drug use in order to force users into treatment as an alternative.

In the case of alcohol there also has been substantial growth in treatment provision, and not only in the United States (Klingemann et al.). However, in the United States alcohol treatment until recently was only an adjunct of the criminal justice system, and it remains quite separate in many countries. The growth of alcohol treatment provision, it has been argued, accompanied and served as a "cultural alibi" for the dismantling of the alcohol control structure left behind by the temperance era (Mäkelä et al.). Although there is an increasing contradiction between the demands for sobriety in a technological environment and the increased market availability of alcohol, managing that contradiction is seen as a character test for the individual consumer, with treatment for alcoholism provided for those deemed to have failed the test.

These policy trends for alcohol and tobacco apply in broad terms to other industrial countries, although high-tax strategies have been applied more commonly outside the United States, particularly for tobacco. For illicit drugs the U.S. "drug war" ideology has been exerted internationally as well as at home (Traver and Gaylord). Through mechanisms such as the international narcotics control conventions and through active multilateral and bilateral diplomacy the United States has been relatively successful in maintaining and often strengthening legal prohibitions. Nevertheless, the international illicit market continues to grow. In debates about drug policies in the 1990s and early 2000s the practical relevance and the ethics of U.S. policies have been questioned increasingly by scholars (Bertram et al.; MacCoun and Reuter).

ROBIN ROOM (1995)
REVISED BY AUTHOR

SEE ALSO: *Addiction and Dependence; Alcoholism; Public Health; Smoking*

## BIBLIOGRAPHY

Austin, Gregory. 1979. "Perspectives on the History of Psychoactive Substance Use." In *Research Issues,* vol. 24. National Institute on Drug Abuse, DHEW Publication No. (ADM) 79–810. Washington, D.C.: U.S. Government Printing Office.

Babor, Thomas; Caetano, Raul; Casswell, Sally; et al. 2003. *Alcohol—No Ordinary Commodity: Research and Public Policy.* Oxford: Oxford University Press.

Bertram, Eva; Blachman, Morris; Sharpe, Kenneth; and Andreas, Peter. 1996. *Drug War Politics: The Price of Denial.* Berkeley: University of California Press.

Bruun, Kettil. 1970. "Finland: The Non-Medical Approach." In *Proceedings of the 29th International Congress on Alcoholism and Drug Dependence,* ed. L.G. Kiloh and David S. Bell. Australia: Butterworths.

Bruun, Kettil; Pan, Lynn; and Rexed, Ingemar. 1975. *The Gentlemen's Club: International Control of Drugs and Alcohol.* Chicago and London: University of Chicago Press.

Christie, Nils, and Bruun, Kettil. 1968. "Alcohol Problems: The Conceptual Framework." In *Proceedings of the 28th International Congress on Alcohol and Alcoholism,* vol. 2, ed. Mark Keller and Timothy G. Coffey. Highland Park, NJ: Hillhouse Press.

Dillon, Patrick. 2003. *Gin: The Much-Lamented Death of Madam Geneva: The Eighteenth-Century Gin Craze.* Boston: Justin, Charles & Co.

Elster, Jon, and Skog, Ole-Jørgen, eds. 1999. *Getting Hooked: Rationality and Addiction.* Cambridge, Eng.: Cambridge University Press.

Ezzati, Majid; Lopez, Alan D.; Rodgers, Anthony; Vander Hoorn, Stephen; Murray, Christopher J. L.; and the Comparative Risk Assessment Collaborating Group. 2002. "Selected Major Risk Factors and Global and Regional Burden of Disease." *Lancet* 360: 1347–1360.

Ferris, Jacqueline; Room, Robin; and Giesbrecht, Norman. 1993. "Public Health Interests in Trade Agreements on Alcoholic Beverages in North America." *Alcohol Health and Research World* 17: 235–241.

Fingarette, Herbert. 1988. *Heavy Drinking: The Myth of Alcoholism as a Disease.* Berkeley and Los Angeles: University of California Press.

Gerstein, Dean R., and Harwood, Henrick J., eds. 1990. *Treating Drug Problems: A Study of the Evolution, Effectiveness, and Financing of Public and Private Drug Treatment Systems,* vol. 1. Committee for the Substance Abuse Coverage Study, Institute of Medicine. Washington, D.C.: National Academy Press.

Gusfield, Joseph R. 1981. *The Culture of Public Problems: Drinking-Driving and the Symbolic Order.* Chicago: University of Chicago Press.

Heather, Nick; Wodak, Alex; Nadelmann, Ethan; and O'Hare, Pat, eds. 1993. *Psychoactive Drugs and Harm Reduction: From Faith to Science.* London: Whurr Publishers.

Hilts, Philip J. 1994. "Embattled Tobacco: One Maker's Struggle." *New York Times,* June 16, 17, 18.

Homel, Ross; Carseldine, Don; and Kearns, Ian. 1988. "Drink-Driving Countermeasures in Australia." *Alcohol, Drugs and Driving* 4: 113–144.

Husak, Douglas N. 1992. *Drugs and Rights.* Cambridge, Eng.; New York; and Oakleigh, Victoria, Australia: Cambridge University Press.

Jellinek, Elwyn M. 1952. "Phases of Alcohol Addiction." *Quarterly Journal of Studies on Alcohol* 13: 673–684.

Jellinek, Elwyn M. 1960. *The Disease Concept of Alcoholism.* New Haven, CT: Hillhouse Press.

Keane, Helen. 2002. *What's Wrong with Addiction?* Melbourne: Melbourne University Press.

Klingemann, Harald; Takala, Jukka-Pekka; and Hunt, Geoffrey, eds. 1992. *Cure, Care or Control: Alcoholism Treatment in Fourteen Countries.* Albany: State University of New York Press.

Levine, Harry Gene. 1978. "The Discovery of Addiction: Changing Concepts of Habitual Drunkenness in American History." *Journal of Studies on Alcohol* 39: 143–174.

MacCoun, Robert, and Reuter, Peter. 2001. *Drug War Heresies: Learning from Other Vices, Times and Places.* Cambridge, Eng.: Cambridge University Press.

Macdonald, Scott, and Roman, Paul M., eds. 1994. *Drug Testing in the Workplace: Research Findings and Perspectives,* vol. 11 of *Research Advances in Alcohol and Drug Problems.* New York and London: Plenum.

Mäkelä, Klaus; Room, Robin; Single, Eric; et al. 1981. *Alcohol, Society, and the State: 1. A Comparative Study of Alcohol Control.* Toronto: Addiction Research Foundation.

Moore, Mark, and Gerstein, Dean, eds. 1981. *Alcohol and Public Policy: Beyond the Shadow of Prohibition.* Washington, D.C.: National Academy Press.

Morgan, Patricia. 1983. "Alcohol, Disinhibition, and Domination: A Conceptual Analysis." In *Alcohol and Disinhibition: Nature and Meaning of the Link,* ed. Robin Room and Gary Collins. NIAAA Research Monograph No. 12, DHHS Publication No. (ADM) 83–1246. Washington, D.C.: U.S. Government Printing Office.

O'Hare, Pat A.; Newcombe, Russell; Matthews, Alan; Buning, Ernst C.; and Drucker, Ernest. 1992. *The Reduction of Drug-Related Harm.* London and New York: Routledge.

Paglia, Angela, and Room, Robin. 1999. "Preventing Substance Use Problems among Youth: A Literature Review and Recommendations." *Journal of Primary Prevention* 20: 3–50.

Partanen, Juha. 1991. *Sociability and Intoxication: Alcohol and Drinking in Kenya, Africa, and the Modern World,* vol. 39. Helsinki: Finnish Foundation for Alcohol Studies.

Peek-Asa, Corinne. 1999. "Effect of Random Alcohol Screening in Reducing Motor Vehicle Crash Injuries." *American Journal of Preventive Medicine* suppl. 16(1): 57–67.

Pernanen, Kai. 1976. "Alcohol and Crimes of Violence." In *The Biology of Alcoholism,* vol. 4: *Social Aspects of Alcoholism,* ed. Benjamin Kissin and Henri Begleiter. New York and London: Plenum.

Rehm, Jürgen; Sempos, Christopher T.; and Trevisan, Maurizio. 2003. "Average Volume of Alcohol Consumption, Patterns of Drinking and Risk of Coronary Heart Disease—A Review." *Journal of Cardiovascular Risk* 10: 15–20.

Robicsek, Francis. 1978. *The Smoking Gods: Tobacco in Maya Art, History and Religion.* Norman: University of Oklahoma Press.

Room, Robin. 1975. "Minimizing Alcohol Problems." In *Proceedings of the Fourth Annual Alcoholism Conference of the National Institute on Alcohol Abuse and Alcoholism: Research, Treatment and Prevention,* ed. Morris Chafetz. DHEW Publication No. ADM 76–284. Washington, D.C.: U.S. Government Printing Office.

Room, Robin. 1985. "Alcohol as a Cause: Empirical Links and Social Definitions." In *Currents in Alcohol Research and the Prevention of Alcohol Problems,* ed. Jean-Pierre von Wartburg, Pierre Magnenat, Richard Müller, and Sonja Wyss. Berne, Stuttgart, and Toronto: Hans Huber.

Room, Robin. 2000. "Control Systems for Psychoactive Substances." In *Nicotine and Public Health,* ed. Roberta Ferrence, John Slade, Robin Room, and Marilyn Pope. Washington, D.C.: American Public Health Association.

Room, Robin. 2001a. "Governing Images in Public Discourse about Problematic Drinking." In *International Handbook of Alcohol Dependence and Problems,* ed. Nick Heather, Timothy J. Peters, and Tim Stockwell. Chichester, Eng.: John Wiley.

Room, Robin. 2001b. "Intoxication and Bad Behaviour: Understanding Cultural Differences in the Link." *Social Science and Medicine* 53: 189–198.

Room, Robin. 2001c. "New Findings in Alcohol Epidemiology." In *Alcohol in the European Region: Consumption, Harm and Policies,* by Nina Rehn with Robin Room and Griffith Edwards. Copenhagen: World Health Organization Regional Office for Europe.

Room, Robin, and Paglia, Angela. 1999. "The International Drug Control System in the Post–Cold War Era: Managing Markets or Fighting a War?" *Drug and Alcohol Review* 18: 305–315.

Stauffer, Robert. 1971. *The Role of Drugs in Political Change.* New York: General Learning Press.

Strategy Council on Drug Abuse. 1973. *Federal Strategy for Drug Abuse and Drug Traffic Prevention.* Washington, D.C.: U.S. Government Printing Office.

Szasz, Thomas. 1985. *Ceremonial Chemistry,* rev. edition. Holmes Beach, FL: Learning Publications.

Traver, Harold H., and Gaylord, Mark S., eds. 1992. *Drugs, Law and the State.* New Brunswick, NJ, and London: Transaction Publishers.

Valverde, Mariana. 1998. *Diseases of the Will: Alcohol and the Dilemmas of Freedom.* Cambridge, Eng., and New York: Cambridge University Press.

Warner, Jessica. 2002. *Craze: Gin and Debauchery in an Age of Reason.* New York: Four Walls Eight Windows.

Wasson, R. Gordon. 1984. "Distilled Alcohol Dissemination." *Drinking and Drug Practices Surveyor* 19: 6.

Yoast, Richard; Williams, Michael A.; Deitchman, Scott D.; and Champion, Hunter C. 2001. "Report of the Council on Scientific Affairs: Methadone Maintenance and Needle-Exchange Programs to Reduce the Medical and Public Health Consequences of Drug Abuse." *Journal of Addictive Diseases* 20: 15–40.

Zimmer, Lynn, and Jacobs, James B. 1992. "The Business of Drug Testing: Technological Innovation and Social Control." *Contemporary Drug Problems* 19: 1–26.

Zinberg, Norman E. 1984. *Drug, Set and Setting: The Basis for Controlled Intoxicant Use.* New Haven, CT: Yale University Press.

# ALCOHOLISM

• • •

What are the benefits and problems that attend the use of alcoholic beverages? In what ways may drinking cause harm? Is the use of alcohol hazardous for all individuals or only for some? Who is at risk? Should an intoxicated person be held accountable for his or her actions while "under the influence"? How is excessive drinking like or unlike other self-injurious appetitive behaviors such as overeating, smoking, or other substance abuse? Should society limit or control the use of alcohol, and should it warn consumers of potential risks associated with drinking? Is alcoholism a disease, primarily a medical rather than a moral problem?

Opinion remains divided on many of these issues, reflecting the diversity of beliefs, practices, and emotions surrounding the use of beverage alcohol in various cultures. Historical and cross-cultural investigations indicate that prevailing cultural beliefs about alcohol and alcohol problems play an important role in determining moral attitudes. Research continues to generate new data about the biomedical and behavioral aspects of drinking. An informed consideration of the use of alcohol must attend simultaneously to the implications of new information and the influence of shifting values.

## Alcohol: Blessing or Curse?

A product of natural fermentation, beverage alcohol, or ethanol, is perhaps the oldest known and most universally consumed psychoactive substance. Ancient peoples drank copious amounts of wine, beer, and other naturally fermented alcoholic beverages, praising their ability to lift the spirits, relieve fatigue, and enhance health. In many societies, alcohol was regarded as a divine gift and was incorporated into religious rituals. Early historical records indicate, however, that alcohol also brought problems. The Hebrew Bible, for example, tells how Noah embarrassed his sons by getting drunk (Gen. 9:20–24) and warns of calamity for "those who tarry long over wine" (Prov. 23:29–35).

Ambivalence toward alcohol use has persisted into modern times and is expressed cross-culturally in a wide diversity of attitudes, beliefs, and practices. The French, for example, regard wine as essential to their diet and lifestyle, and tend to view abstainers as deviant. Millions of Muslims, by contrast, forswear all alcohol as evil. Even within a particular society, attitudes may be heterogeneous and historically variable. Seventeenth-century colonial settlers in North America, for example, viewed drink as the Good Creature of God; three centuries later, the United States banned Demon Rum (Rorabaugh).

Empirical evidence suggests that the use of alcohol offers both modest benefits and significant hazards. In moderate amounts, alcohol is a mild relaxant that stimulates appetite and facilitates social interaction. Sociocultural norms play an important role in determining specific contexts in which drinking may normally occur and influence the experience and behavior of the drinker as well. Aside from alcohol's subjective benefits, there is evidence that moderate drinking may reduce the risk of coronary artery disease in some individuals (Klatsky).

## Hazards of Alcohol Use

The potential social and economic costs of alcohol use to society can be staggering. In the United States alone, it is estimated that abuse of alcohol cost $136.3 billion in 1990 for alcohol-related diseases, accidents, lost productivity, and rehabilitation (Harwood et al.). Three aspects of alcohol use may present problems: drinking itself, acute intoxication, and chronic heavy drinking, commonly referred to as alcoholism.

Ethanol is a simple yet highly toxic molecule that is rapidly absorbed throughout the body and brain. While moderate consumption of alcohol (no more than two drinks per day) does not appear to pose significant health risks for most individuals, there are some populations for whom even moderate drinking may be ill-advised. Specifically, there is evidence that drinking by pregnant women may expose the fetus to serious risk of a number of permanent morphological and cognitive defects collectively known as fetal alcohol syndrome (FAS) (U.S. Department of Health and Human

Services). The relatively recent discovery of FAS (and its milder form, fetal alcohol effects [FAE]) has raised vexing ethical questions concerning the moral and legal culpability of women who drink during pregnancy. Acknowledging society's duty to warn consumers about this previously unrecognized hazard, the U.S. government passed legislation in 1988 that requires manufacturers, bottlers, and importers of alcoholic beverages to include a surgeon general's health warning on all containers.

Acute intoxication and chronic heavy use of alcohol pose the greatest hazards and raise the most pressing ethical concerns. Acute intoxication directly impairs a range of perceptual and motor functions, thereby increasing the risk of accidental injury and death by motor vehicle accidents, falls, slips, drownings, and other mishaps. The risk of serious accidental injury is greatly increased in modern technological societies, where alertness is required to safely operate heavy machinery and high-powered vehicles. In recent years, there has been a growing movement in many countries to reduce alcohol-related automobile injuries and fatalities through tougher laws and preventive education aimed at deterring drunk driving. The late twentieth-century legal consensus appears to be that while intoxication undoubtedly affects judgment and competence, the drunk driver should be held accountable for the decision to drive while impaired. Doubts about the ability of some individuals to make this choice when drinking is reflected in the enactment of new laws that hold bartenders, party hosts, and other servers of alcoholic beverages responsible for monitoring consumption and refusing drinks to inebriated individuals.

Intoxication may also lead to harm through its apparent ability to break down inhibitions on sexual and aggressive impulses in some individuals. In the United States, for example, alcohol intoxication has been strongly associated with assault, murder, rape, spousal violence, and other types of violence. It has not been established that intoxication itself is the direct cause of these outcomes, since in some societies drinking and intoxication are not commonly associated with such violence. Personality variables and culturally influenced expectations regarding intoxication may be important in mediating the relationship between alcohol and violence (Anglin).

In addition to the problems directly related to episodes of acute alcohol intoxication, there is widespread recognition of the harm caused by chronic excessive drinking, commonly referred to as alcoholism. At sufficient doses, the daily or frequent drinker may experience increased tolerance and, eventually, physiological dependence and withdrawal symptoms. Prolonged heavy drinking is implicated in a number of serious and potentially fatal health problems, including cirrhosis, pancreatitis, peptic ulcer, hypertension

and cardiovascular disease, and various cancers. Moreover, both the central and the peripheral nervous systems are damaged by chronic alcohol abuse. In addition to well-known complications such as peripheral neuropathy, ataxia, and alcohol-related dementias, researchers have discovered more subtle cognitive deficits resulting from chronic alcoholism (Tarter et al.).

Epidemiological studies indicate that about one person in ten in the United States is a problem drinker. The persistence of excessive drinking in the face of adverse consequences is the primary criterion in the diagnosis of alcohol abuse; alcohol dependence is diagnosed if tolerance and withdrawal symptoms have developed. Sex, age, and ethnicity are significant variables in the distribution of problem drinking. Men are at least four times as likely to be diagnosed with alcohol dependence as women. D.W.I.-related accidents and fatalities are most frequent among the young. In some ethnic groups, such as Chinese Americans and Orthodox Jews, alcohol problems are rare, while in certain Native American tribes alcoholism is a leading cause of death.

Alcoholism is associated with an increased prevalence of psychiatric disorders, although symptoms of anxiety and depression may often abate following detoxification and a period of abstinence. Whether alcoholism is a cause or a consequence of other mental disorders continues to be debated. An important longitudinal study challenges the view that alcoholism is but a symptom of preexisting emotional problems with the finding that the mental health of nonalcoholics and future alcoholics does not differ significantly in childhood (Vaillant).

## Is Alcoholism a Disease?

Beliefs about the cause or causes of alcoholism and the nature of drinking problems exert an important influence on public perceptions, institutional responses, and treatment and prevention, and shape the framework that guides ethical inquiry and response.

The disease concept of alcoholism, first articulated by Elvin M. Jellinek in the 1940s, was actively promoted by a loose coalition of reformers, service providers, and recovering alcoholics. Since then, it has become the official view of the American medical profession and the World Health Organization (WHO), and has gained wide acceptance among the public at large in the United States and many other Western countries. Proponents of the disease concept argue that alcoholism, like diabetes, essential hypertension, and coronary artery disease, is a biologically based disease precipitated by environmental factors and manifested in an irreversible pattern of compulsive, pathological drinking behavior in individuals who are constitutionally vulnerable. Central to the disease model is the belief that the alcoholic effectively loses control over his or her consumption of alcohol and can never safely drink again. The disease model also holds that alcoholism is a progressive disease that may be arrested by abstinence but never cured.

Although subsequent research has provided evidence of a genetic predisposition for some types of alcoholism (Goodwin), attempts to demonstrate empirically a biological basis for alcoholism have yielded inconclusive results. Whatever influence genetics and biology have in the pathogenesis of alcoholism, many authorities agree that psychosocial variables are of equal importance to the onset and course of drinking problems. The current consensus among researchers and scholars is that alcoholism is a complex biopsychosocial disorder in which multiple factors play a role.

Critics of the disease concept argue that empirical research has failed to support its basic tenets. Herbert Fingarette refers to the disease concept as a myth, asserting that "almost everything that the American public believes to be the scientific truth about alcoholism is false" (p. 1). Reviewing research, Fingarette challenges the following tenets of the disease concept of alcoholism: (1) irresistible craving and loss of control after the first drink; (2) inevitable progression; and (3) the impossibility of a return to controlled drinking. More specifically, he cites studies that show alcoholics do not always experience craving and retain a considerable degree of volition in their actual drinking behavior (Mello and Mendelson); epidemiological studies that suggest patterns of alcohol abuse are highly variable and may spontaneously remit without intervention (Cahalan and Room); and, finally, evidence that at least some alcoholics have successfully returned to more moderate drinking (Davies; Polich et al.).

Arguing that the disease concept is pseudoscientific, Fingarette and other critics (Peele, 1989) imply that by lending the legitimizing mantle of medical science to the disease concept—at least as it is currently formulated—proponents deprive the public of accurate information that forms the necessary basis for informed consent regarding treatment. Others (Vaillant), while conceding that alcoholism is not a disease in the strict medical sense, continue to defend the disease model; they argue that its value in destigmatizing alcoholism and legitimizing treatment outweighs issues of epistemological rigor.

The modern disease concept emerged and gained acceptance primarily in response to humanitarian concerns rather than on the basis of scientific evidence. Eager to undo the religious underpinnings and moralistic legacy of the American temperance movement and prohibition, advocates of the disease concept correctly perceived its ability to recast the alcoholic as sick rather than as morally deviant. If the alcoholic is unable to control self-destructive drinking because of an incurable illness, then he or she deserves compassion and treatment rather than blame. Paradoxically, the attempt to reconceive alcoholism in medical rather than moral terms can be seen as fulfilling a moral agenda, that is, a desire to help rather than condemn the problem drinker. This ethical stance can be seen, in turn, as part of a broader movement in modern society to destigmatize deviant behavior of all types by promoting understanding and compassionate intervention. Thus, much of the controversy surrounding the disease model arises out of a tacit conflict between scientific and moral agendas, a confounding of facts and values in society's response to alcohol.

Anthropology offers a possible semantic solution to the disease controversy by distinguishing between *illness* and *disease* (Chrisman). Whereas diseases are defined by objective scientific criteria, social anthropologists view illnesses as cultural constructions defined by subjective distress, loss of normal social functioning, and adoption of the sick role. Within these terms, alcoholism can be seen as a culturally defined illness or *folk disease* for which society has sanctioned the sick role and compassionate intervention.

## The Role of Alcoholics Anonymous

Despite the widespread acceptance of the disease concept, the leading approach to overcoming alcoholism in the United States is, ironically, not a medical treatment but a self-help program based on principles of moral and spiritual renewal. Founded in 1935 by Bill Wilson, an alcoholic stockbroker, Alcoholics Anonymous (AA) borrowed many of its ideas from an evangelical Christian movement known as the Oxford Group. Though it embraces the disease concept as part of its holistic view of alcoholism as a threefold illness (physical, mental, and spiritual), AA's primary emphasis is on achieving sobriety through a process of moral-spiritual renewal as set forth in the Twelve Steps. Central to AA's approach is the alcoholic's decision to abstain from alcohol "one day at a time." Believing alcoholism to be a disease that may be arrested but never cured, AA views "recovery" as a lifelong process requiring constant vigilance and regular attendance at meetings where members "share their experience, strength, and hope." The Twelve Steps encourage AA's members to admit their faults, make amends to those they have hurt, and help other alcoholics achieve sobriety. Members are also encouraged to select sponsors, experienced AA members who are available for advice and support.

How effective is AA? AA's membership, estimated at 1.5 million worldwide (General Service Office), provides impressive evidence of its success in reaching problem drinkers. However, the overwhelming majority of alcoholics remain untreated. Of those who are exposed to AA, many drop out; those who remain may constitute a self-selected group receptive to its message and style. Moreover, because of the methodological difficulties of conducting research on a self-help group of anonymous individuals, few controlled studies exist on AA's effectiveness compared with other treatment approaches (Ogborne and Glaser). Nonetheless, AA has come to exercise a pervasive influence over both inpatient and outpatient treatment programs in the United States, where the primary goal is often to motivate the alcoholic to participate in AA.

Advocates of AA's approach to treatment have been accused of intolerance toward alternative approaches, especially behavior modification therapies that pursue the goal of controlled drinking rather than total abstinence. Despite evidence that not all problem drinking follows a progressive, deteriorating course and that some problem drinkers are able to return to more moderate patterns of consumption, controlled drinking advocates have been criticized as irresponsible for even suggesting an alternative to abstinence (Pendery et al.). AA's success presents a curious dilemma for researchers and clinicians: The very elements that may contribute to its effectiveness as a self-help group—simple beliefs, group loyalty and cohesiveness, and an emphasis on personal experience and testimony—leave it resistant to outside influence and to new information that appears to contradict its core assumptions (Galanter). The employment of large numbers of recovering alcoholics as counselors and administrators in alcohol treatment programs has further complicated the situation as personal loyalty to AA's "one disease, one treatment" approach has come into conflict with the more empirically based, eclectic approach of researchers and of clinicians trained in the mental-health professions. The difficulty of reconciling these two orientations finds expression in a growing trend toward *dual diagnosis* in which alcoholics are assigned an additional psychiatric diagnosis and treated with medication. Wary of all drugs as potentially addictive, many AA-based paraprofessionals have been uneasy with psychiatric diagnosis and medication; in turn, mental-health professionals have viewed alcoholism counselors as insufficiently aware of psychiatric disorders and treatments. Such tensions point to fundamental differences in the assumptive frameworks that each group brings to diagnosis and treatment.

The first of AA's Twelve Steps declares that the alcoholic is powerless over alcohol and must therefore surrender to a "higher power." Believing this to be a self-defeating prescription for helplessness and relapse in the face of a needlessly mystified "disease," Stanton Peele has argued for restoring an explicitly moral model of alcoholism and other addictions that emphasizes the alcoholic's ability rationally to choose sobriety and commit to new values (Peele, 1988). Advocates of AA's approach argue, however, that this is precisely what AA accomplishes: a daily commitment to abstinence and "a new way of life." That alcoholics may regain a sense of control by admitting powerlessness, they say, may simply reflect a spiritual paradox rather than a contradiction.

Medicalization of alcohol problems has yet to resolve the question of what causes alcoholism or to provide satisfactory solutions to the moral problems posed by the use and misuse of alcohol. Motivated by the desire to destigmatize alcoholism in order to promote compassionate treatment, the disease model still has not adequately disposed of the issue of personal responsibility. The drinker makes choices, but these choices are significantly influenced by biological, psychological, and sociocultural forces beyond conscious control. An important element of AA's success may be that it embraces both aspects of this duality: It holds that alcoholics do not choose their condition—they are subject to multiple systemic forces beyond their awareness—yet, with support, they can effectively assume responsibility for their problem and choose to abstain. Meaningful ethical inquiry must embrace both poles of this duality by recognizing the complex interplay of personal choice with the many factors that may influence or limit it.

RICHARD W. OSBORNE (1995)
BIBLIOGRAPHY REVISED

SEE ALSO: *Alcohol and Other Drugs in a Public Health Context; Addiction and Dependence; Behavior Modification Therapies; Freedom and Free Will; Genetics and Human Behavior; Harmful Substances, Legal Control of; Impaired Professionals; Maternal-Fetal Relationship; Mental Health Services; Smoking*

### BIBLIOGRAPHY

Alcoholics Anonymous World Services. 1976. *Alcoholics Anonymous,* 3rd edition. New York: Author.

Ames, Genevieve M. 1985. "American Beliefs about Alcoholism: Historical Perspectives on the Medical-Moral Controversy." In *The American Experience with Alcohol: Contrasting Cultural Perspectives,* pp. 23–39, ed. Linda A. Bennett and Genevieve M. Ames. New York: Plenum.

Anglin, Douglas M. 1982. "Alcohol and Criminality." In *Encyclopedic Handbook of Alcoholism,* pp. 383–394, ed. E. Mansell Pattison and Edward Kaufman. New York: Gardner.

Cahalan, Don, and Room, Robin. 1974. *Problem Drinking among American Men.* New Brunswick, NJ: Rutgers Center of Alcohol Studies.

Chrisman, Noel J. 1985. "Alcoholism: Illness or Disease?" In *The American Experience with Alcohol: Contrasting Cultural Perspectives,* pp. 7–21, ed. Linda A. Bennett and Genevieve M. Ames. New York: Plenum.

Davies, D. L. 1962. "Normal Drinking in Recovered Alcohol Addicts." *Quarterly Journal of Studies on Alcohol* 23: 94–104.

Doweiko, Harold E. 1998. *Concepts of Chemical Dependency,* 4th edition. Belmont, CA: Wadsworth Publishing Company.

Edwards, Rem B., and Shelton, Wayne, eds. 1997. *Values, Ethics and Alcoholism.* JAI Press.

Fingarette, Herbert. 1988. *Heavy Drinking: The Myth of Alcoholism as a Disease.* Berkeley: University of California Press.

Galanter, Marc. 1990. "Cults and Zealous Self-Help Movements: A Psychiatric Perspective." *American Journal of Psychiatry* 147(3): 543–551.

General Service Office of Alcoholics Anonymous. 1987. *World AA Directory.* New York: Alcoholics Anonymous World Services.

Goodwin, Donald W. 1985. "Genetic Determinants of Alcoholism." In *The Diagnosis and Treatment of Alcoholism,* 2nd edition., pp. 65–87, ed. Jack H. Mendelson and Nancy K. Mello. New York: McGraw-Hill.

Harold, J. 2000. "Alcohol, Freedom, and Responsibility." *Journal of Health Politics, Policy, and Law.* (4): 760–9.

Harwood, Henrick J.; Kristiansen, P.; and Rachel, J. V. 1985. *Social and Economic Costs of Alcohol Abuse and Alcoholism.* Issue Report no. 2. Research Triangle Park, NC: Research Triangle Press.

Heath, Dwight B. 1982. "In Other Cultures They Also Drink." In *Alcohol, Science, and Society Revisited,* pp. 63–80, ed. Edith L. Gomberg, Helene R. White, and John A. Carpenter. Ann Arbor: University of Michigan Press.

Helzer, John E., and Pryzbeck, Thomas R. 1988. "The Co-Occurrence of Alcoholism with Other Psychiatric Disorders in the General Population and Its Impact on Treatment." *Journal of Studies on Alcohol* 49(3): 219–224.

Hester, Reid K., and Miller, William R. 1989. *Handbook of Alcoholism Treatment Approaches: Effective Alternatives.* New York: Pergamon.

Jellinek, Elvin M. 1960. *The Disease Concept of Alcoholism.* New Haven, CT: Hillhouse.

Klatsky, Arthur L. 1990. "Alcohol and Coronary Artery Disease." *Alcohol, Health and Research World* 14(4): 289–300.

Kurtz, Ernest. 1979. *Not-God: A History of Alcoholics Anonymous.* Center City, MN: Hazelden, Educational Services.

Marlatt, G. Alan. 1983. "The Controlled Drinking Controversy." *American Psychologist* 38(10): 1097–1110.

Marlatt, G. Alan, and Rohsenow, Damaris J. 1980. "Cognitive Processes in Alcohol Use: Expectancy and the Balanced Placebo Design." *Advances in Substance Abuse: Behavioral and Biological Research* 1: 159–199.

Mello, Nancy K., and Mendelson, Jack H. 1972. "Drinking Patterns during Work-Contingent and Noncontingent Alcohol Acquisition." *Psychosomatic Medicine* 34(2): 139–164.

Miller, William R. ed., Weisner, Constance M. 2002. *Changing Substance Abuse through Health and Social Systems.* New York: Kluwer Academic Publishers.

Ogborne, Alan C., and Glaser, Frederick B. 1985. "Evaluating Alcoholics Anonymous." In *Alcoholism and Substance Abuse: Strategies for Clinical Intervention,* pp. 176–192, ed. Thomas E. Bratter and Gary G. Forrest. New York: Free Press.

Pattison, E. Mansell, and Kaufman, Edward. 1982. *Encyclopedic Handbook of Alcoholism.* New York: Gardner Press.

Peele, Stanton. 1988. "A Moral Vision of Addiction: How People's Values Determine Whether They Become and Remain Addicts." In *Visions of Addiction: Major Contemporary Perspectives on Addiction and Alcoholism,* pp. 201–233, ed. Stanton Peele. Lexington, MA: Lexington Books.

Peele, Stanton. 1989. *The Diseasing of America: Addiction Treatment Out of Control.* Lexington, MA: Lexington Books.

Pendery, Mary L.; Maltzman, Irving M.; and West, L. Joylon. 1982. "Controlled Drinking by Alcoholics? New Findings and a Re-Evaluation of a Major Affirmative Study." *Science* 217(4555): 169–175.

Polich, J. Michael; Armor, David J.; and Braiker, Harriet B. 1980. *The Course of Alcoholism: Four Years after Treatment.* Santa Monica, CA: Rand.

Rorabaugh, W. J. 1979. *The Alcoholic Republic: An American Tradition.* Oxford: Oxford University Press.

Spike, J. 1997. "A Paradox about Capacity, Alcoholism, and Noncompliance." *Journal of Clinical Ethics* 8(3): 303–306

Tarter, Ralph E.; Arria, Ameilia M.; and Van Thiel, David H. 1989. "Neurobehavioral Disorders Associated with Chronic Alcohol Abuse." In *Alcoholism: Biomedical and Genetic Aspects,* pp. 113–129, ed. H. Werner Goedde and Dharam P. Agarwal. New York: Pergamon.

U.S. Department of Health and Human Services. 1990. *Alcohol, Drug Abuse, and Mental Health Administration. National Institute on Alcohol Abuse and Alcoholism.* Seventh Special Report to the U.S. Congress on Alcohol and Health. Rockville, MD: Author.

Vaillant, George E. 1983. *The Natural History of Alcoholism.* Cambridge, MA: Harvard University Press.

Wanck, Bick. 1990. "Mentally Ill Substance Abusers." In *Handbook of Outpatient Treatment of Adults: Nonpsychotic Mental Disorders,* pp. 577–603, ed. Michael E. Thase, Barry A. Edelstein, and Michel Hersen. New York: Plenum.

World Health Organization. 1978. *Mental Disorders: Glossary and Guide to Their Classification in Accordance with the Ninth Revision of the International Classification of Diseases.* Geneva: Author.

# ALTERNATIVE THERAPIES

• • •

I. Social History

II. Ethical and Legal Issues

## I. SOCIAL HISTORY

Healing is a profoundly cultural activity. The very act of labeling a disease and prescribing treatment expresses a healer's commitment to a particular set of assumptions about the nature and structure of reality. These assumptions not only help specify the agents thought to cause disease but also contain implicit understandings of what health optimally or normatively enables humans to do. Because rival medical systems typically subscribe to differing philosophical and cultural outlooks, the notion of orthodoxy pertains to medicine as surely as it does to religion or politics. What makes a therapy "orthodox" is its adherence to a belief system that, for intellectual and sociological reasons, informs the practice of the dominant members of a culture's medical delivery system. A therapy is therefore "unorthodox" to the extent that its diagnoses and treatments are not deemed legitimate by the dominant belief system.

The philosophical and professional differences that separate orthodox and unorthodox therapies give rise to complex ethical questions. How, for example, are we to understand medical "legitimacy," when this notion is the product of ever-changing philosophical, cultural, and social factors? What does it mean for a medical treatment to be unethical? Must it in some way bring about negative results, or is it unethical even if it is—such as vitamin placebo treatment—merely a harmless fraud? What constitutes a therapeutic benefit? Is it an improvement in physical, mental, or spiritual well-being?

First, the sheer diversity of alternative therapies hampers attempts to generalize about the kinds of ethical issues that unorthodox treatments present. There is an almost bewildering array of alternative therapies, ranging from chiropractic, osteopathy, and acupuncture, to shiatsu, herbal medicine, and religious faith healing. Further complicating this task is the fact that these alternative therapies find themselves labeled unorthodox for quite different reasons. Some, for example, are practiced by healers committed to an alternative belief system or worldview that grants reality to causal forces that differ greatly from those specified by medical orthodoxy. Such is the case with various "faith healing" traditions and New Age medical systems. Religious therapies such as these invoke an overtly metaphysical explanation of the causes of physical illness and depict human health in terms of adherence to specific spiritual or ethical outlooks on life.

Second, healing systems may become unorthodox when they employ therapies that, although predicated upon the consensus worldview, have not yet been validated or confirmed as efficacious by orthodox medical standards. Many of the treatments suggested for combating cancer or acquired immunodeficiency syndrome (AIDS) are considered unorthodox for this reason. Third, healers find themselves outside the medical mainstream when they provide services that are typically ignored or deemed of secondary importance by a culture's dominant medical practitioners. This has been the case, for example, with dentists in the nineteenth century, podiatrists in the early twentieth century, and midwives throughout most of modern history. The case of midwifery is instructive. While never as widespread in the United States as in other parts of the world, the use of midwives provided the only obstetrical assistance available to many women until early in the twentieth century. As obstetrics became a recognized medical specialty, primarily under the control of male physicians, hospitals equipped with surgical facilities supplanted the home as the normal site for giving birth. Increasingly the last resort of those who could not afford hospital births, midwifery generally fell into disrepute. Midwifery, then, became an "unorthodox" form of medical care not because it employed an alternative worldview or because it could not be validated as a treatment, but because the dominant providers of medical services decided that the home and the assistance of other women at childbirth were not of primary importance. Interestingly, midwifery has witnessed a modest resurgence in recent decades as part of a general cultural trend toward "natural" medicine and woman-centered healthcare. Nursemidwives perform about 2 percent of all deliveries in the United States, and more than a dozen universities offer certification programs for midwives.

What alternative therapies have in common is economic, legal, and cultural disenfranchisement from the socially empowered institution of scientific medicine. Any attempt to reflect upon the ethical questions raised by these "alternative" approaches to healing requires sensitivity to the historical and philosophical roots of this disenfranchisement. "Regular" physicians coalesced into state and local medical societies during the nineteenth century, securing an institutional power base for what was to become medical orthodoxy in the United States. This emerging corps of physicians shared a more or less common approach to medical practice and were eventually able to "institutionalize" this approach through the influence they exerted over licensure laws enacted by state and federal governments, the accreditation of medical schools, and access to technologically equipped hospitals. The American Medical Association (AMA) (founded in 1847, but lacking strong organization and sufficient membership until the early twentieth century) eventually succeeded in organizing and promoting the interests of the nation's dominant medical practitioners on a national level.

Medical orthodoxy aligned itself with the worldview spawned by the Western scientific tradition. Its approach to therapeutic intervention has been firmly rooted in the evolving body of information that has emerged from advances in physiology, chemistry, and pharmacology. Accompanying this reliance upon the Western scientific tradition has been an implicit endorsement of a secularist and rationalist ontology (i.e., a worldview skeptical of claims concerning the supernatural or other unquantifiable influences). What has given scientific medicine its "public" character is its insistence that theories concerning the etiology and treatment of disease specify physical, as opposed to spiritual or metaphysical, causal forces. Its theories and strategies for therapeutic intervention are thus more susceptible to empirical verification, and disputes can at least potentially be resolved by an appeal to observable and quantifiable sets of data. This is also why scientific medicine found itself more amenable than many of its alternative counterparts to the economic and legal institutions of modern Western governments. Rejecting the "private" claims to truth made in religious arguments, Western democracies have required that all civic discourse be advanced according to rational and public grounds of argumentation.

To the extent that scientific medicine's academic and experimental foundations facilitate such "public" argumentation, it has largely merited its enfranchisement within the legal and economic institutions that make judgments about the allocation of medical resources. Any consideration of the ethical status of these judgments and their effect upon the practice of alternative medical systems must take into account the important role that such rational and public discourse has had in the development of Western culture.

## Nineteenth-Century Alternative Medicine

THE THOMSONIAN SYSTEM. One of the first challenges to the orthodoxy of "regular physicians" occurred in the early 1800s. Samuel Thomson (1769–1843) was a poor New Hampshire farmer whose mother and wife had suffered from the bleedings and mercurial drugs forced upon them by regular physicians. Thomson believed that better treatments must be available, and he began studying the therapeutic value of herbs. He soon developed his own system of botanical medicine predicated upon the assumption that there is only one cause of disease, cold, and one cure, heat. Thomson believed that by restoring heat to his patients' systems, he could cure any ailment. Using botanics such as cayenne pepper, supplemented with steam baths, Thomson sought cures without the incessant bloodletting or mercurial drugs utilized by the era's orthodox physicians.

The Thomsonian system reached the height of its popularity in the 1820s and 1830s. Some estimate that its methods were employed in varying degrees by as many as a million Americans. One obvious reason for its appeal was that its treatments were generally more benign than the aggressive arsenal of bloodletting, alcohol, opium, mercury, arsenic, and strychnine that many regular physicians used to stimulate their patient's systems. Perhaps more important, Thomsonianism could be studied relatively inexpensively (although the official price for the right to use his methods was a substantial $20) and practiced by family members. During the days of medical professionalization in the United States, Thomsonianism strengthened the role of parents, and especially mothers, in caring for family members. Thomsonianism also fit nicely with the period's moral and religious climate, which urged individuals to take responsibility for their own moral and spiritual regeneration. It endeavored "to make every man his own physician" and encouraged individuals to take responsibility for restoring their rightful relationship to the divinely decreed laws of nature. Of lasting significance is the fact that Thomsonianism was the first system to take on the issue of licensing of medical practitioners, and to assert the public's right to free choice of healers. Thomsonians led the successful campaign to repeal medical licensing legislation in the mid-1800s and drew public attention to the somewhat predatory tactics with which orthodox physicians sought to restrict the right of would-be healers to practice whatever system they wanted.

HOMEOPATHY. A second form of sectarian medicine, homeopathy, emerged more or less concurrently with the public's gradual loss of enthusiasm for the Thomsonian system. The homeopathic system of medicine was the creation of the German physician Samuel Christian Hahnemann (1755–1843), who grew increasingly critical of the indiscriminate prescription of drugs by contemporary physicians. He coined the term *allopathic* to refer to orthodox medicine's alleged overreliance upon invasive therapeutic treatments (e.g., bloodletting, surgery, or the administration of strong pharmacological agents). In contrast to allopathic medicine, Hahnemann enunciated a medical theory that he thought relied more upon the body's natural powers to bring about recovery. The first principle of homeopathic medicine is "like cured by like." By this Hahnemann meant that physicians should treat symptoms by prescribing drugs that produce similar symptoms in a healthy individual. The second fundamental principle of homeopathic medicine is the doctrine of infinitesimals. It was Hahnemann's conviction that the greatest therapeutic benefit was to be achieved by administering diluted doses of a drug, sometimes only 1/1,000,000 of a gram. Although homeopathic physicians' use of infinitesimal doses undoubtedly negated any therapeutic value their drugs might have had, at least these small doses had the virtue of not assaulting the patient's recuperative powers. It is thus not surprising that many turned to homeopathy as a viable alternative to orthodox medicine.

Homeopathy spread quite rapidly in the United States. It was introduced by Hans Gram, who opened an office in New York after studying the homeopathic system in Europe. By 1835 a homeopathic college had been formed, and in 1844 the American Institute of Homeopathy was organized. Throughout the 1800s, 10 to 12 percent of the country's medical schools and medical school graduates were adherents to homeopathy. In contrast to Thomsonianism, which was practiced by nonprofessionals, homeopathic practitioners were educated professionals who often came from the ranks of regular physicians. Moreover, while those who received Thomsonian treatment tended to be rural and poor, there is evidence to suggest that homeopathy thrived among the urban upper and middle classes. This latter fact led to direct economic competition with the regular system and proved an important catalyst in the formation and success of the American Medical Association as economic motives joined with scientific ones to rally regular physicians in opposition to their irregular competitors. As the most popular of the century's alternative systems, homeopathy raised a number of important ethical questions. For example, could allopathic physicians consult with "unscientific" practitioners? (The AMA's original code of ethics included a consultation clause that prohibited such interactions.) Or should homeopathic physicians be allowed to practice in publicly supported hospitals or in the military? Even in the late twentieth century there was some debate about whether pharmacies should be required to stock homeopathic medicines.

**HYDROPATHY AND DIETARY REGIMENS.** In the mid-1840s another alternative therapy, hydropathy (water cure), began to attract a following in the United States. Based on the theories of Vincent Priessnitz of Austria, hydropathy was based on enhancing the body's inherent vitality and purity. Priessnitz believed that pure water could be used to flush out bodily impurities and stimulate the body's inherent tendencies toward health. Water-cure treatments emphasized drinking large amounts of water and applying water externally through baths, showers, or wrapping wet sheets around the body. Most American adherents of water cure advocated an eclectic approach to health based on the curative powers of fresh air, diet, sleep, exercise, and proper clothing. The philosophy of water cure also had a decidedly moral tone. As one anonymous American enthusiast put it, "We regard Man, in his primitive and natural condition as the perfect work of God, and consider his present degenerated physical state as only the natural and inevitable result of thousands of years of debauchery and excess, of constant and wilful perversions of his better nature, and the simple penalty of outraged physical law, which is just and more severe than any other" ("Water-Cure World," 1860).

Hydropathy thus equated disregard of the laws of healthful living with defiance of God's will. Systematic efforts to promote healthful living were not only the means to physical well-being but also the key to the spiritual renovation of Earth. The hydropathic cause naturally attracted many of the period's moral and religious reformers. William Alcott, Lucy Stone, Amelia Bloomer, Susan B. Anthony, and Horace Greeley visited major hydropathic retreat centers, where they circulated reformist agendas ranging from vegetarianism to utopian socialism. Critical of the alleged superiority of "official" medical authorities, advocates of hydropathy had a natural affinity with the feminist thought of the time. Hydropathy looked to nature, not credentialed male physicians, as the ultimate source of healing, and in so doing, it provided a vehicle for those seeking to redress what they thought were faulty notions of social and political authority.

Another nineteenth-century forebear of contemporary alternative therapy in the United States was Sylvester Graham (1794–1851), who combined conservative religious beliefs with zealous concern for health reform. An ordained Presbyterian minister and itinerant evangelist, Graham believed that human physical, moral, and spiritual well-being required scrupulous adherence to the natural order established by God. Graham admonished his followers that avoiding alcohol and the overstimulation of the sexual organs could help them maintain moral and physical health. His advice for a healthful diet included a coarse bread, later produced in the form of a cracker that still carries his name. Graham's dietary principles, widely circulated throughout the nineteenth century, served the cause of keeping the soul's "bodily temple" free from impurities.

Ellen White (1827–1915) occasionally visited a hydropathic resort in Dansville, New York, where she became a convert to Graham's dietary gospel. White thereafter had a series of mystical visions in which God revealed to her that he expected humans to follow the divinely given laws governing health and diet as faithfully as his moral laws. The Seventh-Day Adventist denomination founded by White has since then adopted Grahamite principles and a vegetarian diet as essential parts of purifying themselves in expectation of the Second Coming of Christ. Seventh-Day Adventists, one of the largest religious groups to originate in the United States, support a number of health sanatoriums and combine their evangelical religious faith with a strong emphasis on healthy dietary practices. This emphasis upon a healthful diet does not in and of itself constitute an alternative medical practice. Their dietary concerns are, however, closely connected with their belief in the efficacy of petitionary prayer.

## The Rise of Mental Healing Practices

MESMERISM. The introduction of Franz Anton Mesmer's "science of animal magnetism," commonly known as mesmerism, in the 1830s and 1840s popularized a belief in the power of the unconscious mind to draw upon an invisible healing energy. Mesmer (1734–1815), a Viennese physician, believed that he had detected the existence of an almost ethereal fluid that permeates the universe. This fluid, called animal magnetism, flows continuously into, and is evenly distributed throughout, a healthy human body. If for any reason an individual's supply of animal magnetism is thrown out of equilibrium, one or more bodily organs will begin to falter. Mesmer proclaimed, "There is only one illness and one healing." The science of animal magnetism revolved around the identification of techniques for restoring a patient's inner receptivity to this mysterious, life-giving energy.

Mesmer held magnets in his hands and repeatedly passed them over the heads and bodies of his patients in an effort to induce the flow of animal magnetism into their systems. His followers later dispensed with the magnets, finding that verbal suggestions from the healer could induce patients into a trance, ostensibly heightening their receptivity to the influx of this metaphysical healing agent. Mesmerized patients claimed to feel prickly sensations running up and down their bodies that they attributed to the influx and movement of animal magnetism. Awaking from their sleeplike trance, they reported feeling refreshed, invigorated, and healed of such disorders as arthritis, nervousness, digestive problems, liver ailments, stammering, insomnia, and the abuse of coffee, tea, or alcohol. Some patients even claimed

that the mesmerizing process enabled them to open up the mind's latent powers for telepathy, clairvoyance, and precognition. These claims contributed as much, or even more, to mesmerism's growing popularity than its reputation for healing.

A good many of those drawn to mesmerism were middle- and upper-class individuals who styled themselves progressive thinkers and were interested in uniting science and religion in a single philosophical account of human nature. Mesmerism struck them as an important step in this direction. The phenomena surrounding mesmeric trances were thought to provide empirical proof that each human is inwardly connected with higher, metaphysical planes of reality. Adherents of mesmerism believed that under certain conditions of psychological receptivity, humans are able to open themselves to an influx of energy or guidance from these higher realms. American mesmerists borrowed terminology from transcendentalism, spiritualism, and Theosophy to provide their middle-class reading audience with a new vocabulary for understanding the interconnection of their physical, mental, and spiritual natures.

MIND CURE AND CHRISTIAN SCIENCE. A popular philosophy known as the mind-cure or New Thought movement grew out of the mesmerists' healing practices. Mind-cure writers in the United States published books and pamphlets describing how thought controls the extent to which we are able to become inwardly receptive to spiritual energies. From Phineas P. Quimby and Warren Felt Evans in the late 1800s to Norman Vincent Peale, Norman Cousins, and Bernie Siegel in the late 1900s, Americans have displayed a remarkable enthusiasm for this "power of positive thinking" literature. The mind-cure movement gave rise to a novel form of religious piety based on the belief that the deeper powers of our mind control our access to a metaphysical power that can instantly help us to achieve peace of mind, improved health, and a never-ceasing flow of energy. The holistic health movement of the 1960s and 1970s relied heavily upon this cluster of metaphysical ideas.

Mesmerism was also instrumental in the formation of Christian Science. In 1862 Mary Baker Eddy, in great physical and emotional distress, arrived on the doorstep of the famous mesmerist healer Phineas P. Quimby. Quimby's treatments gradually cured her of her ailments; they also gave her a new outlook on life, based upon the principle that our thoughts determine whether we are inwardly open to, or closed off from, the creative activity of a spiritual energy (animal magnetism). Soon after Quimby's death, Eddy transformed his mesmerist teachings into the foundational principles of Christian Science. Her principal text, *Science and Health with Key to the Scriptures* (1875), reveals her intention to shift the science of mental healing away from the categories of mesmerism to those that bear more resemblance to Christian Scripture, albeit her own unique interpretation of it. The basic theological postulate of Christian Science is that God creates all that is, and all that God creates is good. Sickness, pain, and evil are not creations of God, and therefore they do not truly exist. They are simply the delusions produced in an erring, mortal mind that has lost a firm hold on the belief that only those things created by God have true existence. For Christian Scientists the universe is spiritual. What we call matter (e.g., bacteria, viruses, etc.) consequently does not really exist and therefore has no causal power. Christian Science healers, known as practitioners, help individuals to overcome their faulty thinking and to elevate their mental attitudes above the delusions of the senses. Healing occurs as the individual learns to function on a metaphysical, rather than a physical plane. Healings are understood not as miracles or faith healings but as the lawful consequence of exchanging false conceptions for true ones, which center solely on the higher laws of God's spiritual presence.

Both Christian Science and the "holistic health" philosophies that emerged from the mind-cure tradition teach that our thoughts control the degree to which we avail ourselves of the higher spiritual source from which health proceeds. As a consequence, illness or disease is understood as something the sufferer has brought upon himself or herself through failure to sustain a "correct" mental posture toward life. Any ethical analysis of these forms of alternative therapy must take seriously their built-in skepticism about whether a medical system really needs to attend to material causes of illness (bacteria, viruses, etc.). The issue is not quite so acute for holistic healing practices that teach that the mind can draw upon a higher energy capable of invigorating matter but do not teach that matter itself is unreal. In other words, most holistic health systems do not deny that there are physical and material causes of illness. They simply maintain that mental and spiritual factors are entailed in the etiology of most illnesses and must be taken into account in any comprehensive medical system. And thus, although they insist that a patient's mental outlook often is a significant factor in the creation and cure of illness, they do not espouse a medical theory that puts all the "blame" for illness or "credit" for recovery upon the patient.

Christian Science, by contrast, goes much further in challenging the empirical and rational foundations of Western science. By denying the ontological reality of matter, and hence the causal power of viruses or bacteria, Christian Science is clearly at philosophical loggerheads with both medical orthodoxy and the legal systems of most Western, democratic nations. For example, the Christian Scientists'

belief system is opposed to immunization. The courts have understandably become concerned over the medical well-being of the children of Christian Science practitioners, as well as other students with whom they attend school; this has led to legal restrictions on the right of Christian Scientists to practice their form of religious healing. In 1990 the U.S. courts decided that two Christian Science parents were guilty of child neglect when their sole reliance on Christian Science methods was deemed responsible for their child's death (*Hodgeson v. Minnesota*). Such cases draw attention to the important ethical distinction between "private" religious belief and actions that have consequences in the "public" domain regulated by the legal system.

Christian Science healing practices, fundamentalist faith healing, and outright quackery have prompted strong responses from practitioners of orthodox medicine. The American Medical Association, emerging as a powerful national organization early in the twentieth century, set itself the task of prompting state and federal agencies to enact stricter licensing regulations. Its efforts to restrict medical practice to graduates of AMA-accredited medical schools surely furthered the cause of scientific medicine and protected the public from potentially harmful forms of quackery. It also tended, however, to force out of the medical marketplace those whose approaches to healing utilized a nonscientific worldview or whose medical services did not fit with dominant approaches to medical care.

## Chiropractic and Osteopathic Medicine

Osteopathic and chiropractic medicine provide interesting examples of the fate of alternative philosophical, religious, and ethical interpretations of healing in an age dominated by scientific medicine. Osteopathic medicine emerged from the healing philosophy of Andrew Taylor Still (1828–1917). A former spiritualist and mesmeric healer, Still developed techniques for manipulating vertebrae along the spine in ways that he thought removed obstructions to the free flow of "the life-giving current" that promotes health throughout the body. Still explained the healing principles of osteopathy (a term derived from two Greek words meaning "suffering of the bones") in overtly metaphysical terms that described the origin and nature of "the life-giving current" ultimately responsible for human well-being. His followers largely discarded the occult-sounding dimensions of Still's philosophy and instead insisted that osteopathic medical education be grounded in anatomy and scientific physiology. Thus, although osteopaths originally relied only upon manual manipulations of the spine as a means of restoring health, they soon added surgery and eventually drug therapy to their medical practice.

By the 1950s, so few differences existed in the training or practice of osteopaths and M.D.s that their two national organizations agreed to cease the rivalry that had existed for several decades and to cooperate in such matters as access to hospitals, residency programs, and professional recognition. Having jettisoned the alternative worldview of its founder, osteopathy no longer bore any overt signs of unorthodoxy and finally found itself within the medical mainstream. Interestingly, during the 1960s many osteopaths were concerned about being absorbed into allopathic medicine and gave renewed focus to osteopathy's philosophical origins. Their commitment to osteopathy's historical concern with enhancing the body's natural powers for recuperation made them champions of holistic medicine long before the term *holistic* became commonplace among alternative healers. As of 1990, over 24,000 physicians practiced osteopathic medicine, collectively treating over 20 million patients per year.

The case of chiropractic medicine is more complex. Chiropractic originated in the work of Daniel David Palmer (1845–1913), a mesmerism-inspired magnetic healer in Iowa. Palmer, who knew of Still's osteopathic techniques, theorized that dislocations of the spine are able to block the free flow of the life force, which he called Innate (his nomenclature for animal magnetism). Palmer and his son, B. J. Palmer, explained that Innate is a part of the Divine Intelligence that fills the universe, bringing full physical health whenever it flows freely through the human body. Chiropractic medicine represents the Palmers' art and science of adjusting the spine in ways that remove obstructions to the free flow of Innate within the body.

Over the years, chiropractic physicians began downplaying the movement's metaphysical origins and emphasized its scientific approach to the treatment of musculoskeletal disorders. In this way, they minimized their theoretical unorthodoxy and identified an area of medical practice largely ignored by most medical doctors. Chiropractic physicians' sustained attention to this void in the "orthodox" medical system has earned them a viable niche in the medical marketplace; as of 1990, more than 19,000 chiropractic physicians were treating more than 3 million patients annually. Even though most medical insurance companies have come to recognize the medical functions performed by chiropractic medicine, M.D.s are still largely wary of chiropractic medicine because it has failed to elucidate an empirically validated theory that would substantiate its therapeutic claims. This professional tension provides a fascinating example of a continuing theme in the history of alternative medicine: the clash between orthodox medicine's rationalism (its insistence on an acceptable scientific explanation for all methods) and alternative medicine's pragmatism (discovery of therapies that produce results regardless of whether they are "proved" with rational theories).

## Holistic, New Age, and Folk Medicine

During the last few decades of the twentieth century, the holistic healing movement led a surge of popular interest in therapies based on an explicitly religious, or quasi-religious, interpretation of the healing process. The precise meaning of the term *holistic medicine* varies among healing systems. Among its meanings are emphasis upon "natural" therapies, patient education and responsibility, prevention, and treating patients as "whole" people. Also common to holistic healing is the basic assumption that, as one handbook put it, "every human being is a unique, wholistic, interdependent relationship of body, mind, emotions, and spirit." The term *spirit,* alongside *body, mind,* and *emotions,* carries holistic healing beyond psychosomatic medical models; it also represents commitment to a belief in the interpenetration of physical and nonphysical spheres of causality. Even holistic healing's exhortations concerning reliance upon the body's own regenerative and reparative processes are typically laden with references to opening individuals up to the inflow of a divine healing energy. Persons who call themselves holistic health practitioners typically operate according to a worldview that is incompatible with the naturalistic framework of the modern Western scientific heritage.

One example of such a holistically oriented healing movement is Alcoholics Anonymous (AA), and its Twelve-Step program, which has influenced many other "self-regenerative" therapies. Founded in the 1930s, Alcoholics Anonymous has well over one million members, with about 35,000 groups meeting weekly in over ninety countries. The principal founder of the movement, Bill Wilson, was an alcoholic who became acutely aware of his inability to overcome his addiction. A mystical experience of "a great white light" convinced him that a loving Presence surrounds us and is capable of healing our broken inner lives. Wilson maintained that we need only to cease relying upon our own willpower and surrender to this Higher Power. Wilson was extremely wary of institutional religion, especially the moralism associated with biblical religion. From psychologists such as William James and Carl Jung, he pieced together a form of spirituality based upon opening the unconscious mind to a higher metaphysical reality. AA counsels its members that "in order to recover, they must acquire an immediate and overwhelming 'God-consciousness' followed at once by a vast change in feeling and outlook" (Alcoholics Anonymous, p. 569). AA's mystical, nonscriptural approach to personal regeneration sets its doctrines apart from most of America's religious establishment; its denunciation of both material and psychological/attitudinal factors in favor of an overtly spiritual view of healing sets its practices apart from the American medical and psychological establishments. But its open-minded and eclectic sense of the presence of spiritual forces in the determination of human well-being makes it one of the most powerful mediators of wholeness in America in the late twentieth century.

The various religious and healing groups that comprise the New Age movement endorse a holistic approach to health and medicine; they envision every human being as a unique combination of body, mind, emotions, and spirit. Central to New Age piety is the conviction that each person exists simultaneously in both the physical and the metaphysical (i.e., the astral and etheric) planes of reality. New Age therapies such as the use of crystals, therapeutic touch, and psychic healing seek to channel healing energies from higher metaphysical planes into the physical body. New Age crystal healing, for example, maintains that illness in the physical body is frequently caused by a disruption or disharmony of energies in what is called the *etheric body* (the portion of the self that extends into the astral and etheric planes). Healing consequently requires techniques to achieve harmony between the physical and subtle or etheric bodies. Crystals are thought to have unique properties that enable them to serve as receptors and capacitors of energies that emanate from the astral and etheric planes. Used properly, crystals are assumed to be capable of transmitting these energies in ways that bring the individual's physical, moral, and spiritual natures back into harmony. To this extent, New Age adherents do not reject the therapeutic efficacy of established medical science (though they do condemn what they perceive to be an overreliance on drugs and invasive surgical techniques) so much as its secularist and materialistic worldview, which fails to take into account our spiritual nature or potentials. Healing, for New Agers, is a by-product of the more fundamental goal of attaining an expanded spiritual awareness.

New Age healers are especially drawn to Eastern religious systems that involve entering into meditative states that heighten receptivity to the inflow of a higher spiritual energy, variously referred to as *ch'i, prana, kundalini,* animal magnetism, or divine white light. Yoga, t'ai chi ch'uan, Ayurvedic medicine, shiatsu, acupuncture, and various Eastern massage systems are studied for their advocacy of attitudes and lifestyles geared to the renovation of our moral and spiritual lives. Although each of these healing systems has its own philosophical basis and history, Americans tend to approach them with agendas left over from such nineteenth-century movements as mesmerism, spiritualism, and Theosophy. Even acupuncture, whose ability to alleviate pain

and promote healing is more or less recognized—though poorly understood—by medical science, is embraced by many Americans not only for its obvious physical benefits but also for its connections with Eastern mystical philosophies.

A wide variety of folk and ethnic remedies exist alongside medical science. Botanical and herbal remedies, while ordinarily aimed at promoting health rather than curing illness, represent a noninvasive approach to physical well-being. Rural Pennsylvania Dutch still practice variations of *powwow,* an eclectic tradition using charms, prayers, and rituals, to prevent and cure disease. In the American Southwest, *curanderismo* still flourishes in Mexican-American communities, and recent immigration to the continental United States from the Caribbean has rekindled folk medicine practices (e.g., charms, herbs, incantations) peculiar to the African-American heritage. Immigration from Southeast Asia has brought Hindu and Buddhist medical practices like Ayurvedic medicine and prayers to the heavenly saints (bodhisattvas), who reward the faithful with their healing powers. Far East Asian immigrants have included dedicated practitioners of such religiomedical systems as t'ai chi ch'uan, shiatsu, and acupuncture. The continued presence of such folk or ethnic medical treatments may represent a form of preserving cultural identity, economic disenfranchisement from the nation's more expensive established medical system, or the seeds of a new era of genuine medical pluralism. In any case, both legal and economic attitudes toward alternative therapies must be philosophically and culturally nuanced.

## The Challenge to Bioethics

Persons with life-threatening diseases who have not been helped by conventional treatments understandably become interested in pursuing alternative therapeutic strategies. The highly publicized debate over the effectiveness of laetrile for retarding cancer, for example, drew attention to the potential risks of the regulation of medicine by the U.S. Food and Drug Administration (FDA). At stake was the unresolved issue of whether a drug should be restricted only when it is known to cause harm or only when laboratory testing has failed to reveal measurable physical benefits. This debate continues in the controversy over various treatments for AIDS. Persons given a bleak prognosis by medical doctors seek immediate access to experimental drugs that have just entered the slow and laborious regulatory processes mandated by U.S. federal law. Although much has been done to try to speed up the evaluation of experimental AIDS-related treatments, a growing number of persons find themselves barred from access to innovative scientific treatment.

The central ethical question raised by alternative therapies is whether genuine medical treatment can be distinguished from various forms of quackery. Except for isolated instances in which individuals engage in deliberate medical fraud, quackery is difficult to identify or prove. Any reliable definition of therapeutic benefit requires being able to define the factors "known" to affect human well-being and what optimal health consists of. The practitioners of many forms of alternative medicine criticize the assumptions they believe underlie contemporary medical science. They argue that alternative therapies better understand human well-being and are cognizant of mental, moral, and spiritual factors that go well beyond the physiological considerations on which scientific medicine relies. To those who say that their practices or those who utilize them are "irrational," they respond that every therapy is rational insofar as its methods of treatment are logically entailed by its fundamental premises or its assumptions about the nature of disease.

Establishing criteria with which to mediate between competing medical systems is complicated by the fact that the plausibility of the beliefs or assumptions that underlie them are every bit as dependent on sociological factors as on intellectual "proofs." What we consider valid evidence, whom we consider expert authorities, and how we should go about separating relevant from irrelevant information turn not on objective, rational criteria but on the ways we were socialized into one belief system or another. Who, then, is in a position to decide what is an "irrational" medical choice? With what degree of confidence or philosophical integrity can orthodox physicians seek to dissuade persons from seeking alternative treatments? Do persons have a right to what seems to be an utterly ineffective therapy simply because it conforms to their personal belief system?

Alternative therapies may reasonably be expected to demonstrate their benefits to patients and to substantiate the claim that their distinctive healing practices directly cause these therapeutic results. Medical ethics is concerned with protecting persons from intended or inadvertent harm. Well-intentioned tolerance of alternative therapies should not preclude their undergoing rigorous scrutiny. Governmental agencies, healthcare facilities, and insurance companies are forced to allocate limited resources and to ensure the welfare of the general public. They must be prepared to make reasonable assessments of alternative medical systems that are based upon belief systems at considerable variance with modern Western science.

Because of the inherent threat that quackery poses to both personal and public well-being, ethical and policy-related judgments must exercise caution and strive for the unrelenting application of "public" (openly demonstrable and subject to empirical scrutiny) standards of evidence. The scientific study of psychosomatic interaction (e.g., of the role of psychological variables in the etiology of ulcers) promises to help practitioners of alternative therapies justify their practices in ways that are more amenable to these standards of evidence. Because psychosomatic medicine has expanded scientific appreciation of the roles nonmaterial factors play in the etiology of illness, alternative medicines have access to a set of medical categories that will potentially enable them to argue for the therapeutic efficacy of treatments that focus on such nonmaterial factors.

Cases involving patients' desire to be permitted to use drugs before they have received FDA approval testify to the conflict between private needs and the regulation of public well-being. Unlike alternative therapies that are based on different belief systems, unvalidated drug therapies are usually discussed using medically orthodox terms and logic. The ethical concerns here are more frequently about the speed with which regulatory agencies arrive at decisions on potentially lifesaving drugs or the possible collusion of powerful pharmaceutical companies with regulatory agencies to keep competitors from the marketplace. Perhaps the most important consideration in assessing unvalidated therapies is that contemporary medicine differs from its predecessors not because we have become more rational but because we have learned to use the controlled trial to determine the relative merits of competing medical treatments.

Medical systems that are labeled unorthodox because their concerns or treatments are at the periphery of mainstream medicine are reminders that dominant professional groups tend over time to employ predatory tactics to ensure their continued supremacy and keep potential competitors at a distance. These "medically peripheral" systems alert us to the fact that medical science has philosophical and institutional blinders that may close off, rather than open, innovative approaches to human health. The presence of alternative health professionals in the wider system of healthcare helps safeguard against the kinds of complacency and narrowness of vision that frequently creep into economically entrenched professions. By providing a range of services that address both curative and preventive issues typically neglected by allopathic physicians, many of these alternative therapies contribute to a comprehensive understanding of human health and well-being.

ROBERT C. FULLER (1995)
BIBLIOGRAPHY REVISED

SEE ALSO: *Healing; Health and Disease: Anthropological Perspectives; Medicine, Anthropology of; Medicine, Philosophy of; Medical Ethics, History of the Americas;* and other *Alternative Therapies* subentries

## BIBLIOGRAPHY

Alcoholics Anonymous. 1955. *Alcoholics Anonymous,* 2nd edition. New York: Author.

Astin, J. A. 1998. "Why Patients Use Alternative Medicine: Results of a National Study" *Journal of American Medical Association* 279(19): 1548–1553.

Bynum, William Frederick, and Porter, Roy, eds. 1987. *Medical Fringe and Medical Orthodoxy, 1750–1850.* Wolfeboro, NH: Croon Helm.

Callahan, Daniel, ed. 2002. *The Role of Complementary and Alternative Medicine: Accommodating Pluralism.* Washington, D.C.: Georgetown University Press.

Cayleff, Susan E. 1987. *"Wash and Be Healed": The Water-Cure Movement and Women's Health.* Philadelphia: Temple University Press.

Frohock, Fred M. 1992. *Healing Powers: Alternative Medicine, Spiritual Communities and the States.* Chicago: University of Chicago Press.

Fuller, Robert C. 1989. *Alternative Medicine and American Religious Life.* New York: Oxford University Press.

Gevitz, Norman. 1982. *The D.O.s: Osteopathic Medicine in America.* Baltimore: Johns Hopkins University Press.

Gevitz, Norman, ed. 1988. *Other Healers: Unorthodox Medicine in America.* Baltimore: Johns Hopkins University Press.

Gordon, Rena J.; Nienstedt, Barbara Cable; Gesler, Wilbert M. eds. 1998. *Alternative Therapies: Expanding Options in Health Care.* New York: Springer Publisher.

*Hodgeson* v. *Minnesota.* 110 S. Ct. 2926 (1990).

Hufford, David. 1988. "Contemporary Folk Medicine." In *Other Healers: Unorthodox Medicine in America,* pp. 228–264, ed. Norman Gevitz. Baltimore: Johns Hopkins University Press.

Inglis, Brian. 1965. *The Case for Unorthodox Medicine.* New York: G. P. Putnam.

Kaufman, Martin. 1971. *Homeopathy in America: The Rise and Fall of a Medical Heresy.* Baltimore: Johns Hopkins University Press.

Numbers, Ronald L. 1976. *Prophetess of Health: A Study of Ellen G. White.* New York: Harper & Row.

Porter, Roy. 1989. *Health for Sale: Quackery in England, 1680–1850.* Manchester, U. K.: Manchester University Press.

Raboteau, Albert J. 1986. "The Afro-American Traditions." In *Caring and Curing: Health and Medicine in the Western Religious Traditions,* pp. 539–562, ed. Ronald L. Numbers and Darrel W. Amundsen. New York: Macmillan.

Ramsey, M. 1999. "Alternative Medicine in Modern France." *Medical History* 43(3): 286–322.

"Water-Cure World." 1860. Unsigned article. April, no. 5.

Whorton, James C. 1982. *Crusaders for Fitness: The History of American Health Reformers.* Princeton, NJ: Princeton University Press.

Young, James H. 1967. *The Medical Messiahs: A Social History of Health Quackery in Twentieth-Century America.* Princeton, NJ: Princeton University Press.

## II. ETHICAL AND LEGAL ISSUES

*Alternative medicine* covers a dizzyingly heterogeneous group of medical theories and practices. Alternatives range from the different forms of faith healing, Christian Science, and folk medicine to allegedly scientific systems like homeopathy, chiropractic, and visualization therapy. Also included under the term are acupuncture; herbalism; iridology; the traditional medicines of India, China, Japan, the Philippines, and indigenous peoples; holistic medicine; naturopathy (treatment using agents or elements found in nature); shamanism; yoga; radiesthesia (therapy based on detection of natural waves of force emanating from nature); color healing; aromatherapy; transcendental meditation; crystal therapy; thalassotherapy (treatment based on sea bathing, sea voyages, etc.); massage therapy; midwifery; and many others. Certain shared negative elements justify lumping together such diverse medical theories and practices. They include marginal social standing or fringe status; exclusion from mainline professional journals and public funding for research; exemption from mainline licensing requirements; and opposition to conventional medicine. The essential ethical and legal considerations raised by alternative medicine are veracity and nonmaleficence. Because false claims of healing efficiency can cause direct and indirect harm to patients, any such claims violate the essential ethical standards of all medical practice, whether alternative or conventional practice.

### The Meaning of *Alternative* and *Conventional*

"Alternative" implies alternative to orthodox, regular, mainline, or conventional medicine. These latter adjectives refer to a medical theory, based on modern science, that began to emerge in the Renaissance with medical innovators such as Andreas Vesalius (1514–1564) and Paracelsus (1493–1541), and to scientifically validated medical therapies that blossomed in the twentieth century. If alternative medicine is characterized by an enormous variety of different medical theories and practices with little in common either conceptually or culturally, conventional medicine has the appearance of a single powerful system based on a narrowly conceived biology and focused primarily on the organic needs of sick people. Besides being scientific and materialistic, conventional medicine is also rationalistic: a system that relies on hard data, observation, controlled experimentation, logical argument, and a somewhat outdated view of causality. Alternative and conventional medicine actually help to define one another by contrast and opposition.

What is now classified as either *conventional* or *alternative* medicine was not always so designated. Formerly alternative medical theories and practices have moved into conventional standing; for example, the use of antioxidant vitamins and other dietary remedies for both prevention and therapy (Steinberg; Stampfer et al.; Rimm et al.). Formerly conventional medicine is in the alternative category; this includes most nineteenth-century therapies like baths, massage, and purgatives. Between the Renaissance beginnings of modern orthodoxy and its dominance in the twentieth century, conventional medicine was practiced by relatively few university-trained physicians. Most sick people during these centuries got along on remedies developed under older theories. Even university physicians used bleedings and purgings, sweating, and vomiting in addition to quinine and digitalis; not much separated scientific orthodoxy from nonscientific alternative practice when it came to therapeutic interventions. In the nineteenth and twentieth centuries, university-educated physicians established their own medical associations, adopted updated ethical standards, reformed their educational systems, proved that microorganisms cause infectious disease, developed vaccines to control them, employed technologies to improve both diagnosis and therapy, and finally gained legal status for their practice, along with monopolistic control of healthcare institutions. The line between a unified, socially supported, conventional medicine and separate, alternative medical practices became much more clearly drawn.

Differences between conventional and alternative medicine are accentuated by a continuing polemic. The term *alternative* is still used by conventional physicians as synonymous with quackery, falsehood, uselessness, and dishonesty. *Alternative* is frequently used to mean foreign or antiquated, or to emphasize the different cultural origins and ancient practices of alternative medicine. In literature favoring alternative therapies, conventional medicine is characterized by toxic and addictive drugs, high costs, aggressive procedures, impersonalness, unnecessary surgeries, economic monopoly, and iatrogenic (physician-induced) illnesses. For their part, orthodox critics create the impression that alternative medicines are products of prescientific cultures, but that conventional medicine is purely scientific and transcends historical and cultural influence.

What constitutes disease and illness, however, as well as how they are understood and treated by any medical system, is necessarily historical and cultural. Contemporary culture's medical–industrial complex, for example, has as much influence on mainline medicine as the military–industrial complex has on modern warfare. Indeed, the historical and cultural content of conventional and alternative medicines is an important consideration wherever legal and ethical issues are addressed. What is ethically right cannot simply be reduced to what is culturally dominant. Cultural dominance does not equate with ethical correctness; minority status or identification with another culture does not reduce to moral incorrectness. Only when cultural and historical factors are identified on both sides can ethical and legal questions about alternative medicine be clearly addressed. Then dialogue can be substituted for hostility and common ethical standards can be developed for both types of practice.

## Conventional Allopathic Medicine: Justifying Its Preferred Status

Conventional medicine is known as *allopathy*. This term sets it apart from homeopathy, a nineteenth-century theory and practice that treated disease by administration of minute doses of a remedy that would, in healthy persons, produce the same symptoms as the disease being treated (*similis similibus curantur*). Allopathy, in contrast, is a system that counteracts disease by the use of remedies that produce effects different from those produced by the disease (*contraria contrariis curantur*). Allopathic medicine by definition combats, counteracts, and aggressively opposes specified disease entities. Today's conventional allopathic medicine has its own history and is the product of strong cultural influences. The allopathic approach, originating in ancient Greece with the Hippocratics, was reinforced in the nineteenth century by opposition to the homeopathic alternative. Another important historical influence was a high school teacher from Kentucky, Abraham Flexner, who wrote a book on U.S. medical practice that laid the foundations of what we call medical orthodoxy.

The Flexner Report, published in 1910, not only criticized medical education and practice in North America but also held up a model of ethical medicine grounded on hard laboratory science and universal laws. For Flexner, ethical medicine targeted disease objects rather than patient complaints, and like engineering was founded upon hard science. Under his influence, nineteenth-century German medicine came to be orthodox medicine in the United States, and a new medical school at Johns Hopkins University was held up as the model for the way orthodox medicine should be taught and practiced. Doctors William Welch (1850–1934), William Osler (1847–1919), William S. Halsted (1852–1922), and Howard Kelly (1858–1943) at

Johns Hopkins became the architects of mainline orthodoxy, and all four were products of German training (Ackerknecht). Because Flexner applied the images of war to medical practice, orthodox medicine became an aggressive, hands-on science. Engineering and military science shaped mainline medical attitudes and procedures, while biology, histology, embryology, anatomy, physiology, pathology, and bacteriology provided the substance of orthodox medical understanding. For Flexner all other approaches were both unscientific and unethical.

What over several centuries came to be orthodox medicine enjoys great power and prestige in so-called developed societies because it alone of the classic professions (law, medicine, ministry) wrapped itself in the mantle of hard science. Alternative medicine is alternative because it lacks that mantle. If alternative medicine is ethically suspect, it is because hard science became the ethical as well as the epistemological standard in twentieth-century culture. Being unscientific or deficiently scientific amounts to being irresponsible in medicine. All alternative medicines are not the same in this regard, but in general, alternative medicine's moral weakness can be traced to an absent or weak science.

Some alternative medicines claim to use "a different science." They adopt the stand that modern science is just another cultural variable or another historical belief system. Some defenders of alternative medicine argue that one cultural variable or belief system is as good as another. No rational grounds exist, they claim, to prefer one medical system to another or to assign to one a greater social and ethical standing. From the fact that mainline science is itself cultural and historical, radical advocates for alternative medicine make their basic argument for equal legal and ethical status. Patients, they insist, must be totally free to make their own choices about treatment. Their argument is strengthened by calling attention to the theoretical flaws in modern science.

Karl Popper's work, *The Logic of Scientific Discovery* (1939 German edition; 1959 English edition), on the concepts of verifiability and falsifiability undermined claims about what is proved in science. He argued that the best science can do is demonstrate what is false, not prove what it true. Later, Popper's claims about falsifiability were themselves shown to be flawed. Then Thomas Kuhn (*The Structure of Scientific Revolution*, 1962) showed how what he called a *paradigm* defines what counts as admissible evidence in science, and how these paradigms change. The foundations, then, on which modern medical orthodoxy bases its claims to ethical and social superiority are strongly influenced by cultural-historical factors.

Modern science and mathematics may have rational and conceptual flaws, but all flaws are not equal. Despite the flawed epistemological foundations of science and mathematics, they still can be used to build bridges that work and spacecrafts that arrive at their destinations. Modern medical science too has real explanatory power. The rigor of scientific explanation, however, is often absent in alternative medicines. Mainline scientific research is much more credible than unscientific and unsubstantiated claims. Admittedly, alternative medicines lack the government funding to carry out sound research, which is expensive, but many alternative medicines ignore research and have unrigorous standards for subjecting therapeutic claims to critical review. If a medicine is ethical and earns preferential social status because it bases its claims and practices on publicly confirmable evidence and continuing critical review, then orthodox scientific medicine warrants the ethical and legal priority it enjoys.

## Some Alternative Medicines

**CHRISTIAN SCIENCE.** All alternative medicines do not have the same relationship to modern science. Christian Science is an alternative to conventional medicine in the most radical sense: denying the existence of matter as well as disease, illness, pain, and death. Mary Baker Eddy (1821–1910) was a sickly person who had a healing experience in 1866, which she understood as the discovery of Christian Science, a religion centered on healing and health. Her book *Science and Health: With Key to the Scriptures* (1875) is read at all Christian Science services along with the Bible, thereby continuing her healing ministry. It contains her metaphysical beliefs about disease, death, matter, spirit, and God, one famous synopsis of which is as follows:

> *Question.* What is the scientific statement of being?
>
> *Answer.* There is no life, truth, intelligence, nor substance in matter. All is infinite Mind and its infinite manifestation, for God is All-in-all. Spirit is immortal Truth; matter is mortal error. Spirit is the real and eternal; matter is the unreal and temporal. Spirit is God, and man is His image and likeness. Therefore man is not material; he is spiritual. (Eddy, p. 469)

Christian Science healing is not like the "miracle cures" of faith healers. Ministers who claim to heal acknowledge the existence of disease and evil, but Mary Baker Eddy did not. Her religion trains "practitioners," who devote their energies to healing in a different sense. They are called upon by believers just as non-Christian Scientists seek out physicians when they are ill. The practitioner talks to people on the phone, visits them at home, and heals by restoring patients to the spiritual plane of thinking that according to Christian Science is reality. Healing, then, is actually reeducation, in which the patient is brought to exchange mental errors and delusions for God's truth and God's reality, where evil, illness, disease, and death have no place.

Christian Science is a radical alternative because it is founded upon a worldview at odds with the theoretical base of conventional medicine. According to this metaphysical theory, disease, pain, sickness, and death only seem real because people believe them to be so, and practitioners heal by stripping away these false beliefs. Conventional doctors in this view are engaged in "un-Christian and sinful" activities; indeed, they live in an unreal world. And yet a certain civility characterizes the debate between orthodox medicine and Christian Science. The latter belief system may be too bizarre for most mainline physicians to take seriously. Christian Science apologists, however, tend to be middle-class and well educated, and they respond to objections with reasoned discourse.

This civility has been strained by several legal cases involving parents whose children died after being treated by Christian Science practitioners instead of by conventional physicians. Following the court decisions, calls were issued in the *Journal of the American Medical Association* and *New England Journal of Medicine* for stronger child-protection legislation and stronger penalties for "parents who use the pain and anguish of their children to demonstrate the strength of their belief in Christian Science." Conventional physicians warned against child-neglect legislation in Colorado, Texas, and Louisiana that provides religious exemptions for Christian Scientists. In some places Christian Science has become in effect the legal equivalent of conventional medicine. Mainline doctors object to this as well as to the fact that Christian Science practitioners have legal standing comparable to their own. Blue Cross and Blue Shield pay practitioners in some states, as do major insurance companies and Medicare. Practitioners may even sign certificates for sick leave and for disability payments. According to conventional physicians, this policy creates a double standard. Practitioners, they insist, should be required to meet much higher standards if they are to receive comparable medical responsibilities (and benefits).

In 1989 the parents of a seven-year-old girl were convicted of third-degree murder and child abuse in connection with her death from diabetes. A Sarasota, Florida, jury rejected the parents' claim that they had not sought medical treatment for their daughter because of Christian Science belief. This was the first case in the United States since 1967 in which Christian Scientists were held criminally responsible for relying on the practices of their faith alone to cure a child's illness.

In July 1990, a Boston jury convicted Christian Science parents of manslaughter because they relied on the services of practitioners rather than conventional medical care to treat their two-year-old son, who had died of bowel obstruction in 1986. The parents were sentenced to ten years' probation and ordered to take their other children for periodic medical checkups. This case aroused unusual interest because it took place in Boston, the headquarters of the Christian Science Church. Both cases reflect a pattern in U.S. courts, which have ruled that competent adults have a right to refuse treatment—even life-saving treatment—for themselves, but not for their children. The same response was made regarding Jehovah's Witness children whose parents refuse blood for them based on religious belief.

Official Christian Science response to these decisions has been reserved and moderate. In an official publication (First Church of Christ, Scientist), church officials recognize that the state has an interest in and a responsibility to protect children against abuse, including the possibility of their being used by parents to prove the strength of their faith. They acknowledge that the death of a child treated by practitioners alone is a tragedy, but counter with examples of thousands of children cured from certified illnesses by Christian Science practitioners and many deaths resulting from treatment with conventional medicine. They also recognize the distinction between unrestricted First Amendment freedom of belief, on the one hand, and restrictions on behavior or acting on belief, on the other. Still, church officials argue against any law that would radically restrict Christian Science treatment of children. Like advocates of alternative medicine generally, they argue for a right to unrestricted practice on the basis of the patient's right not to be interfered with in private matters. It would, however, be more ethically responsible for Christian Scientists to make explicit the childhood conditions where practitioners can cooperate with physicians, instead of forcing parents to make an either-or choice. This same solution could apply to other alternative practices; it would require increased communication and cooperation between conventional physicians and alternative practitioners.

Cases involving children put at risk because of parents' religious beliefs pose questions that can be addressed either by ethics or by law. In the language of ethics, these cases create a conflict between a negative individual right—not to be interfered with in private matters like religious belief and healthcare decisions—and a positive societal right or obligation: to protect vulnerable people. Put differently, they reflect a conflict between the principle of individual autonomy and the principle of justice. If the principle of autonomy is respected, justice is compromised, and vice versa.

In the history of Western ethics, individual rights and autonomy concerns are late arrivals—dating from the eighteenth-century Enlightenment period. Societal rights to protect life and the duties of citizens to obey societal norms are much older. Dilemmas involving the two types of ethics are worked out by emphasis on the importance of societal rights and justice, but restriction and limitation of their implementation by reference to individual rights and autonomy. Societal rights (justice) in effect are balanced with individual rights (autonomy), and the only justified degree of societal influence is that which is necessary to accomplish basic justice. In ethical language, the state has an interest not only in justice but in the protection of individual autonomy; therefore it has an interest in balancing the two goods. In legal language it is the balancing of negative constitutional rights—founded on the Bill of Rights (freedom of religion)—and a positive legal obligation of *parens patriae*. The particulars of the legal balancing are worked out through common law decisions in Anglo-Saxon systems. Statutory laws and policies that in effect deny a child access to effective treatment for serious illness can be considered both ethically and legally deficient.

**LAETRILE.** Alternative medicine is used by most patients for prevention and as an adjunct to conventional treatments. Alternative medicine, however, also flourishes where conventional medicine is weak, inattentive, or an outright failure. When conventional medicine has nothing more to offer and the patient faces death, many people look to alternatives. Cancer at certain stages of development provides a case in point. Because of devastating side effects associated with conventional cancer treatment (chemotherapy and radiation), alternative approaches are particularly attractive. Ten billion dollars is spent annually on unproven alternative cancer treatments, in many cases by affluent and well-educated patients. One such alternative that generated great public debate, court cases, and then finally involvement by the federal government was laetrile, a controversial drug derived from apricot pits and held up as the last hope for terminal cancer patients.

In the 1970s this drug, which had been around for decades, received wide publicity not only because of claims made about its effectiveness but also because the U.S. Food and Drug Administration (FDA) had banned its interstate shipment and sale. This created another conflict between an individual negative right not to be interfered with in choosing treatment and the positive social right to protect vulnerable people against exploitation. In 1979, the U.S. Supreme Court ruled that the FDA could legally inhibit the distribution of the drug, based on the agency's powers to establish "safe and effective" standards; this ruling validated the agency's positive social right. In *Rutherford v. United States* (1979), the Supreme Court remanded the case to the U.S. Tenth Circuit Court of Appeals for reconsideration of other arguments. The appeals court held that the FDA ban did not violate the individual negative right to privacy of cancer patients.

Responding to public pressure, the FDA on January 3, 1980, gave approval for the National Cancer Institute to initiate scientific trials to study laetrile. First, animal studies would be conducted, then stage-one toxicity trials on six human patients, and finally a clinical trial involving 200 to 300 advanced cancer patients who volunteered for the laetrile treatment. The studies were delayed by debate over the money and time required to test an allegedly ineffective drug and over who would perform the tests. Although some alternative practitioners were board certified in conventional medicine, most conventional physicians and scientists resisted involvement with an "alternative" therapy.

On April 30, 1981, the National Cancer Institute announced that it had found laetrile, or amygdalin, to be ineffective as a cancer treatment. The announcement was made at a meeting of the American Society of Clinical Oncology. Over half the patients given the alternative therapy had died and the rest had not responded to the treatment. Charles G. Moertel, director of cancer treatment at the Mayo Clinic, who gave the report, added that he hoped the study would end "the exploitation of desperate cancer patients" by doctors prescribing the drug in twenty-three states where its use was legal despite the FDA ban on interstate sale and shipment. (This apparent contradiction is rooted in the fact that federal regulations are often imperfectly coordinated with state statutes, which may allow the use of federally banned drugs.) Laetrile advocates claimed that the test was rigged and that a less than optimum form of laetrile was used. The contemporary debate over alternative therapies—especially for cancer—continues, although one hears little about laetrile (Cassileth et al.).

**HOMEOPATHY.** Homeopathy originated in Germany at the end of the 1700s in the work of Samuel Hahnemann. By the end of the next century, one in every seven physicians in the United States was a homeopath. The nineteenth- and twentieth-century successes of allopathic medicine considerably reduced the influence of homeopathy. As the limits of allopathic medicine have become better recognized, homeopathy has begun to make something of a comeback. About 1,500 homeopaths practice in the United States, and medical practitioners use homeopathy in Australia, the United Kingdom, Germany, India, Brazil, and Argentina.

Included under conventional allopathic practices are drug therapies in the process of scientific trial but not yet officially approved (unproven or nonvalidated therapies), and fully approved and scientifically validated drugs being used in novel ways (innovative therapies). Homeopathy uses its own special brand of unproven and innovative "drugs." Homeopathic medicines or remedies are available in many health and natural food stores in the United States. Because mainline pharmacy and professional pharmacists are strongly aligned with the allopathic system and conventional physicians, they have few incentives to become involved with homeopathic practices. Licensed conventional pharmacists would have little understanding of homeopathic preparations and little economic motivation to add these to their stock. Homeopathic pharmacists/practitioners prepare their own medications; a large part of the homeopathic doctors' work involves modifications (dilutions) of these remedies for each individual illness or patient.

If interest in alternative medicine continues, mainline drug stores may begin to carry some over-the-counter homeopathic remedies. Then, presumably, mainline pharmacists will learn about homeopathic background theories in order to explain these preparations to customers. Would doing so compromise the scientifically trained pharmacist's belief system because of the appearance of endorsement? Ordinarily not. Pharmacists as a group learn about natural remedies and understand the importance of patient belief in such products for therapeutic effectiveness. Pharmacists have their own professional code (American Pharmaceutical Association, 1981; see the Appendix) and standards of practice. These would be compromised only if an alternative therapy were known to be harmful.

VISUALIZATION THERAPIES. The biological sciences of orthodox medicine are materialistic (i.e., founded on physical realities and quantifiable data) and are ill-equipped to handle many of the problems listed as disease categories in psychiatry's diagnostic manual (American Psychiatric Association). A narrowly focused conventional psychiatry relies on chemical therapies and restricts practice to drug prescriptions and medication reviews. Beyond this narrow range of orthodoxy, psychological and social theories have added a broad assortment of nonchemical approaches to conventional practice—from classical psychoanalysis (through cognitive, behavioral, and group treatments) to visualization therapies.

Hypnosis, guided imagery, and biofeedback are all forms of visualization therapy often used in orthodox treatment centers. Practitioners may be conventional physicians,

psychologists, social workers, or nurses. The conditions addressed by these techniques include everything from mental and emotional illness to immunological disorders, childhood hyperactivity, and cancer and senility. On the theoretical level, practitioners and advocates work to demonstrate just how the mind controls the brain and immune system (the mechanisms of psycho-neuro-immunology). The effect of biofeedback on psyche (stress reduction) and physiology (temperature, heart rate, blood pressure) is well documented. Advocates of visualization therapies argue that they can enhance the functioning of the immune system. Controversy about this last use of visualization therapies has centered on its scientific status. Whether it will be considered an alternative therapy or an extension of conventional medicine, in the sense that it broadens conventional medicine's positivistic base to include psyche, will depend on whether the visualization techniques can generate satisfactory scientific proof of effectiveness in this important area. Advocates of mainline medicine, such as Norman Cousins, Bernie Siegel, and Andrew Weil, testify to the need for a wider theoretical base for mainline practices, one that includes a place for the mind's influence on bodily healing (Cousins; Siegel; Weil).

CHIROPRACTIC. Chiropractic is probably the best-known alternative medicine in the United States. Practitioners call themselves doctors and complain bitterly about being excluded from mainline medical institutions. The effectiveness of manual manipulations, they insist, is based on scientific studies, but it is difficult for hands-on chiropractic manipulation to eliminate placebo effect and to satisfy double-blind requirements. Back pain could be called the chiropractic specialty, and orthopedic physicians the mainline competition. One double-blind scientific study of the effectiveness of chiropractic versus conventional treatment conducted in 1990 strongly favored chiropractic therapy (Meade et al.). Conventional physicians attacked the study's science, attempting to show that the statistics were unreliable because the study's method was not rigorous enough. Most chiropractors feel discomfort about requiring that any claim of effectiveness satisfy a double-blind requirement, because doing so would throw doubt upon many of their own scientific studies of effectiveness, which are statistical but not double-blind. Some chiropractic medical schools have their own research institutes and are continuously involved in effectiveness or outcome studies; one example is the ongoing research of the Palmer College of Chiropractic Graduate School in Davenport, Iowa. Despite extensive use of chiropractic in certain parts of the United States, serious dialogue and cooperation with mainline practitioners are limited.

## Orthodox Public Health and Alternative Practices

No practice has been more orthodox since the nineteenth century than public-health medicine. When microscopic technologies aided in the discovery of bacterial causes of infectious diseases, public-health physicians began energetic application of laboratory science on behalf of societal health. Public-health physicians were laboratory science's strongest advocates. They insisted upon strict quantitive standards of proof for what they considered ethical medical practice. Only what could be shown quantitatively to be effective (e.g., vaccine) commanded their respect and endorsement. Laboratory science alone was the ground for real medicine. They used the police power associated with public health (health laws and their enforcement) to support the narrow positivistic foundation of conventional medicine. Medicine for them was narrowly focused on microbes and they tended to leave broader cultural and environmental issues out of consideration. We know that an adequate science does not leave ecology out of consideration, and it does not ignore sociocultural influences on behaviors that spread disease.

The new public-health practice requires "cultural competence," that is, an understanding of the culture of the people to whom public-health policies are applied. Ethnic ways, which include particular attitudes and practices related to health and disease, have to be taken into consideration in order to provide the most effective public-health services. Cooperation between conventional physicians and alternative practitioners, we know, may make the difference between compliance and noncompliance in minority populations.

The World Health Organization (WHO) has strongly advocated cooperation between conventional physicians and alternative practitioners because neither one is likely to disappear. In the United Kingdom in 1995, one in seven people visited alternative practitioners. In the Netherlands, a survey of 293 conventional generalists showed that many believe in the efficacy of certain alternative practices: manual therapy, yoga, acupuncture, hot baths, and homeopathy. In Germany, a distinction is made between scientifically supported alternatives such as naturopathy, which stimulates the body's own healing resources, and unscientifically based alternatives. The former are covered by some insurance policies and the state plan pays a subsidy to patients using them. In Norway, a group of conventional physicians and alternative practitioners are meeting to promote closer cooperation (Rankin-Box).

Because the use of alternative treatments continues to increase both in the United States and in Europe, new studies of alternative approaches have been initiated. In 1993, the National Institutes of Health (NIH) created an office of alternative medicine, where alternative approaches are tested; the public will be kept informed of research results. The U.S. Congress mandated the creation of this project and required that NIH spend two million dollars of its annual budget on it. An oversight committee includes both conventional physicians and alternative practice advocates. They have agreed that alternative practices will be evaluated with the same methods and standards as conventional therapies (outcome research, relative efficiency, double-blind where possible). This is an important development because ethical considerations of alternative practices have to start from reliable information about their effectiveness. This project has added ethical importance because the projects funded require cooperation and collaboration between alternative and conventional practitioners wherever possible.

## Ethical Standards and Alternative Practice

Alternative medicine is governed by ethical obligations derived from what medical practitioners of any variety publicly profess and what societies have always required of them: to heal, to relieve pain, to restore function, and to comfort and accompany their dying, when patients are beyond treatment. In the Hippocratic tradition this basic ethical standard was encapsulated in the imperative "to help and not to harm." Early twenty-first century medical ethics talks about the same basic ethical obligation in terms of the principles of beneficence and nonmaleficence.

Alternative or conventional interventions that harm patients without providing offsetting benefits are unethical. Alternative treatments that are harmless may not violate either individual or social ethical standards—especially if patients have strong faith in them or if the illnesses for which they are used are self-limiting and conventional treatments are either expensive, have serious side effects, or have proven ineffective. When diseases being treated are more serious, however, harmlessness is not enough to satisfy individual and social ethical standards. If harmless alternative remedies prevent patients from seeking an effective treatment available from conventional medicine, then individual alternative practitioners would actually be preventing patients from being helped, and just social policy would require that such practice be curtailed. Although alternative remedies are most often adjuvant and complementary to mainline remedies, it remains important to respect the social and professional ethical requirement that treatment actually provide some benefit to patients. Patient benefit is a complicated concept that sometimes involves unquantifiable quality of life considerations, but patient benefit cannot be permitted to slip beyond empirical proof entirely. Societies have to make laws that use rigorous empirical standards for approval of treatment modalities. Anecdotal evidence of therapy effectiveness or claims of effectiveness dependent upon depth of commitment to an alternative belief system are not enough to satisfy basic individual and social medical ethical obligations.

Modern medical-ethical standards add another basic obligation derived from patient rights, that is, that the patient has the right to consent to treatment or to refuse consent. Alternative practitioners, like conventional doctors, are ethically obligated to provide patients with information relevant to their decisions and to protect patients against coercion, fraud, or manipulation. If patients are not competent, informed consent or refusal must be provided by surrogates—either family members or, in their absence, a guardian. Even decisions of competent patients, however, must meet professional standards, so that an irrational choice or insistence upon a treatment that is ineffective or futile or economically devastating might not—perhaps should not—be respected. The modern principle of patient autonomy must be balanced with the ageless principle of beneficence/nonmaleficence, which protects patients against irrational or incompetent decisions that involve harm without offsetting benefit. Care must be exercised, however, in judging irrationality so as not to confuse it with decisions based on value systems different from those of the treating physician or practitioner. Patients have their own values, and these cannot be set aside because they differ from what a scientifically focused specialist may think is organically best for a patient. True patient benefit requires consideration of both personal and scientific interests.

A competent adult may refuse an effective conventional treatment associated with real burden and choose instead an unproven or ineffective alternative therapy. Similar choices, made for children or for incompetent adults without advance directives, however, are neither ethically nor legally acceptable. Justice and autonomy, beneficence and nonmaleficence are broad, abstract ethical standards. Agreement about these standards in their abstract form is possible even in pluralistic and heterogeneous societies. But principles can come into conflict with one another. Respect for patient autonomy may mean not providing patient benefit or violating principles of justice and equality. When such conflict occurs, ethics at a more pragmatic level of discourse is required: concrete norms and rules that attempt to offer compromise, or to effect a balance between the conflicting principles. Working out the relationship between mainline conventional medicine and alternative practices involves just this form of concrete ethics. Appeal to abstract principles only in a situation of conflict between conventional and alternative medicine can turn an ethics discussion into an exchange of slogans. One important test of an ethics that addresses the relationship between alternative and conventional medicine is whether it encourages a needed dialogue between different practitioners and whether it can generate concrete norms and public policies to handle interaction between the two traditions (Eisenberg et al.).

Ethics has been intimately associated with mainline medicine since its beginning in Hippocratic times. Hippocratic physicians were distinguished from other healers not only by their emphasis on science but also by their commitment to patient benefit rather than to selfish goals. Medicine of any variety derives its ethics from obligations generated by a doctor-patient relationship in which a healer commits himself or herself to help someone in need by cure or pain relief or function restoration. Unselfishness and altruism are at the core of medicine's professional ethics. Truthfulness traditionally was not part of medical ethics, but recently it has been added in order to fulfill the obligations associated with patient autonomy. This essential and structural medical ethics is applicable to alternative and conventional medicine alike.

Mainline medicine obliges physicians to high ethical standards but has been weak in policing deviant members and sanctioning ethical failures. Alternative practitioners are not as well organized as conventional physicians, and some lack the strong ethical emphasis of the mainline tradition. Both face a daunting challenge: developing and maintaining the character traits without which concrete moral rules and abstract ethical principles are ineffective, in a new economic climate that encourages profit making more than altruism.

JAMES F. DRANE (1995)
BIBLIOGRAPHY REVISED

SEE ALSO: *Autonomy; Emotions; Healing; Healthcare Professionals, Legal Regulation of; Jehovah's Witness Refusal of Blood Products; Medicine, Philosophy of; Public Health Law;* and other *Alternative Therapies* subentries

### BIBLIOGRAPHY

Ackerknecht, Erwin H. 1982. *A Short History of Medicine,* rev. edition. Baltimore: Johns Hopkins University Press.

American Cancer Society. 2002. *American Cancer Society's Complementary and Alternative Cancer Methods Handbook.* Atlanta, GA: American Cancer Society.

American Psychiatric Association. 1994. *Diagnostic and Statistical Manual of Mental Disorders: DSM-IV.* Washington, D.C.: Author.

Callahan, Daniel., ed. 2002. *The Role of Complementary and Alternative Medicine: Accommodating Pluralism.* Washington, D.C.: Georgetown University Press

Cassileth, Barrie R.; Lusk, Edward J.; Strouse, Thomas B.; and Bodenheimer, Brenda J. 1984. "Contemporary Unorthodox Treatments in Cancer Medicine: A Study of Patients, Treatments, and Practitioners." *Annals of Internal Medicine* 101(1): 105–112.

Clouser, K. Danner, and Hufford, David J. 1993. "Nonorthodox Healing Systems and Their Claims." *Journal of Medicine and Philosophy* 18(2): 101–106.

Clouser, K. Danner; Hufford, David J.; O'Connor, B. B. 1996. "Informed Consent and Alternative Medicine." *Alternative Therapies in Health and Medicine* 2(2): 76–8.

Cohen, M. H.; Eisenberg, David M. 2002. "Potential Physician Malpractice Liability Associated with Complementary and Integrative Medical Therapies." *Annals of Internal Medicine.* 136(8): 596–603.

Cousins, Norman. 1979. *Anatomy of an Illness.* New York: W. W. Norton.

Davidoff, F. 1998. "Weighing the Alternatives: Lessons from the Paradoxes of Alternative Medicine." *Annals of Internal Medicine* 129(12): 1068–1070.

Eddy, Mary Baker. 1903. *Science and Health: With Key to the Scriptures.* Boston: J. Armstrong.

Eisenberg, David M. 1997. "Advising Patients Who Seek Alternative Medical Therapies." *Annals of Internal Medicine* 127(1): 61–9.

Eisenberg, David M.; Kessler, Ronald C.; Foster, Cindy; Norlock, Francis E.; Calkins, David R.; and Delbanco, Thomas L. 1993. "Unconventional Medicine in the United States: Prevalence, Costs and Patterns of Use." *New England Journal of Medicine* 328(4): 246–252.

Ernst E.; Cohen, M. H. 2001. "Informed Consent in Complementary and Alternative Medicine." *Archives of Internal Medicine* 161(19): 2288–2292.

First Church of Christ, Scientist. 1989. *Freedom and Responsibility: Christian Science Healing for Children.* Boston: Author.

Flexner, Abraham. 1910. *Medical Education in the United States and Canada: A Report to the Carnegie Foundation for the Advancement of Teaching.* Birmingham, AL: Classics of Medicine Library.

Frohock, Fred M. 1992. *Healing Powers: Alternative Medicine, Spiritual Communities, and the State.* Chicago: University of Chicago Press.

Fuller, Robert C. 1992. "The Turn to Alternative Medicine." *Second Opinion* 18:11–31.

Gevitz, Norman C. 1991. "Christian Science Healing and the Health Care of Children." *Perspectives in Biology and Medicine* 34(3): 421–438.

Gevitz, Norman C., ed. 1988. *Other Healers: Unorthodox Medicine in America.* Baltimore: Johns Hopkins University Press.

Greenberg, Kurt. 1991. *Challenging Orthodoxy: America's Top Medical Preventives Speak Out!* New Canaan, CT: Keats.

Hufford, David J. 1993. "Epistemologies in Religious Healing." *Journal of Medicine and Philosophy* 18(2): 175–194.

Kottow, Michael H. 1992. "Classical Medicine v. Alternative Medical Practice." *Journal of Medical Ethics* 19(1): 51.

Kuhn, Thomas. 1996 (1962). *The Structure of Scientific Revolution.* Chicago: University of Chicago Press.

Meade, T. W.; Dyer, Sandra; Browne, Wendy; Townsend, Joy; and Frank, A. O. 1990. "Low Back Pain of Mechanical Origin: Randomised Comparison of Chiropractic and Hospital Outpatient Treatment." *British Medical Journal* 300(6737): 1431–1437.

Murray, Raymond H., and Rubel, Arthur J. 1992. "Physicians and Healers—Unwitting Partners in Health Care." *New England Journal of Medicine* 326(1): 61–64.

Patterson, Elizabeth G. 1989. "Health Care Choice and the Constitution: Reconciling Privacy and Public Health." *Rutgers Law Review* 42(1): 1–91.

Popper, Karl R. 1959. *The Logic of Scientific Discovery.* New York: Basic Books.

Rankin-Box, Denise. 1992. "European Developments in Complementary Medicine." *British Journal of Nursing* 1(2): 103–105.

Rimm, Eric B.; Stampfer, Meir J.; Ascherio, Alberto; Giovannucci, Edward; Colditz, Graham A.; and Willett, Walter C. 1993. "Vitamin E Consumption and the Risk of Coronary Heart Disease in Men." *New England Journal of Medicine* 328(20): 1450–1456.

*Rutherford v. United States.* 99 S. Ct. 2470 (1979).

Saks, Mike, ed. 1992. *Alternative Medicine in Britain.* Oxford: Oxford University Press.

Salmon, J. Warren, ed. 1985. *Alternative Medicines: Popular and Policy Perspectives.* London: Tavistock.

Schneiderman, L. J. 2000. "Alternative Medicine or Alternatives to Medicine? A Physician's Perspective." *Cambridge Quarterly of Healthcare Ethics* 9(1): 83–97.

Siegel, Bernie S. 1986. *Love, Medicine, and Miracles: Lessons Learned about Self-Healing from a Surgeon's Experience with Exceptional Patients.* New York: Harper & Row.

Stampfer, Meir J.; Hennekens, Charles H.; Manson, JoAnn E.; Colditz, Graham A.; Rosner, Bernard; and Willett, Walter C. 1993. "Vitamin E Consumption and the Risk of Coronary Heart Disease in Women." *New England Journal of Medicine* 328(20): 1444–1449.

Steinberg, Daniel. 1993. "Antioxidant Vitamins and Coronary Heart Disease." *New England Journal of Medicine* 328(20): 1487–1489.

Stone, Julie. 2002. *An Ethical Framework for Complementary and Alternative Therapists* New York: Routledge.

Studdert, D. M.; Eisenberg, David M.; Miller, F. H.; Curto, D. A.; Kaptchuk, T. J.; Brennan, T. A. 1998. "Medical

Malpractice Implications of Alternative Medicine." *Journal of the American Medical Association* 280(18): 1610–1615.

Sugarman, J.; Burk, L. 1998. "Physicians' Ethical Obligations Regarding Alternative Medicine." *Journal of the American Medical Association.* 280(18): 1623–1625.

Tavolaro, Karen B. 1991. "Effectively and Efficiently Protecting Children in Faith Healing Cases: A Proposed Statutory Revision for State Intervention." *Medicine and Law* 10(4): 311–325.

Weil, Andrew. 1983. *Health and Healing: Understanding Conventional and Alternative Medicine.* Boston: Houghton Mifflin.

Weintraub, M. I. 1999 "Legal Implications of Practicing Alternative Medicine." *Journal of the American Medical Association* 281(18): 1698–1699.

# ANIMAL RESEARCH

• • •

I. Historical Aspects

II. Philosophical Issues

III. Law and Policy

## I. HISTORICAL ASPECTS

The historical background of the discussion of the ethics of animal experimentation will be examined by considering first the rise of medical research (physiology and pharmacology particularly), then the emergence and consolidation of opposition to research using live animals. Both developments were shaped, of course, by the capabilities and goals of science in every era, and were also powerfully influenced by the philosophical and religious environments within which science operated.

### The History of Animal Experimentation

Vivisection—the cutting open of living animals to observe their inner structure and functioning—can be traced to Greek antiquity, but it was Galen (129–c. 210 C.E.), the most celebrated physician of the Roman Empire, who developed vivisection as a tool for methodical physiological investigation. By such procedures as ligation of the ureters to show they channeled urine from the kidneys to the bladder, and sectioning of the spinal cord at different levels to establish the relations between individual nerves and the body regions

they served, Galen demonstrated the power of surgical interventions to produce a deeper understanding of bodily functions (Rupke).

During the early medieval period, animal experimentation fell into the same desuetude as other areas of scientific inquiry. To be sure, ancient scientific traditions were preserved and elaborated upon by Arabic scholars, but not until the late Middle Ages did an experimental spirit revive in the European world. Skepticism about the adequacy of ancient scientific ideas built to a head during the 1500s, culminating for the life sciences in the 1543 publication of *De Humani Corporis Fabrica* by Andreas Vesalius (1514–1564). The first anatomy text based on careful dissection of the human body, Vesalius's work sharply revised the long-accepted anatomical system of Galen (which had been derived entirely from animal dissections), and thus encouraged experimental reevaluation of Galenic theories of physiology as well.

The most significant correction of Galen's physiology was accomplished by the English physician William Harvey (1578–1657), whose demonstration of the circulatory movement of the blood through the body was based on observations of the contractions of the heart, ligation of the aorta and vena cava, and other vivisection procedures performed on more than eighty species. Harvey's *De Motu Cordis* (1628) heightened misgivings about the validity of other Galenic ideas and confirmed animal experimentation as an invaluable technique for physiological discovery. Vivisection became a commonplace scientific activity by the later 1600s; it was used over the next century and a half to investigate such varied phenomena as respiration, pancreatic secretion, and blood pressure (Rupke; Foster).

Yet as late as 1800, experimentation was still only one of several approaches to elucidating physiological processes. Drawing conclusions about function on the basis of structure—deducing physiology from anatomy—remained popular, as did *a priori* theorizing in accord with some physical or chemical model; experimentation might be employed in either of those cases, but only to substantiate the preestablished theory. That overly rationalistic orientation to physiology and medicine was already coming under attack, however, by the *philosophe*-physicians of the "Paris School." Their call for a medicine rooted in empiricism was answered most eagerly and effectively by Francois Magendie (1783–1855), who from 1805 through the 1820s used animal experimentation to clarify such questions as the mode of action of strychnine, the mechanism of emesis, and the functioning of the nervous system. Magendie insisted on analyzing function without being prejudiced by anatomical structure, and thereby established irrevocably the superiority of the experimental method for physiological inquiry. (Contemporaneously, researchers at French veterinary schools were also developing physiology along experimental instead of speculative lines). Magendie's pupil, Claude Bernard (1813–1878), utilized the experimental method even more successfully, discovering the vasomotor nerves, the glycogenic activity of the liver, the digestive role of pancreatic juice, and the mechanism of curare's effects on neuromuscular function. Bernard was equally significant for the philosophical analysis of the necessity of animal experimentation presented in his *Introduction a l'etude de la medecine experimentale* (1865). There he argued that it was unethical to experiment on human beings, no matter how beneficial the findings might prove for others, if the experiment could harm the subject to any extent whatever. Benefit to others did, on the other hand, justify experiments, including painful ones, on animals. The fact that many human lives could be saved by a relatively few animal deaths made the practice of vivisection a "right," he concluded, "entirely and absolutely" (p. 178). Bernard's analysis solidified the recognition of experimental research with animals as an essential practice for medical progress (Lesch; Rupke; Schiller).

At the same time, physiology and other experimental medical sciences were achieving the status of distinct, institutionalized professions. Historically, physiology had been pursued by physicians in whatever time they had left from treating patients or giving university lectures (and also, on occasion, by amateurs of means). The French had taken the lead in making physiology an independent discipline, yet it was in Germany that research physiology bloomed as a new professional field. The nineteenth-century reformation of universities in the German states, with its emphasis on research and the uncovering of new knowledge, led to the establishment of research institutes employing full-time physiologists, along with pharmacologists and other biological experimenters (Coleman and Holmes). The expectation that research would result in practical medical applications useful to humankind attracted both political and philanthropic support, and ultimately expectation was fulfilled with the flowering of medical microbiology and immunology in the 1880s. The germ theory was built upon laboratory experiments on thousands of animals; applications of the theory quickly made surgery far more effective and safe, and sharply refined programs for the prevention of epidemic disease. Louis Pasteur (1822–1895) discovered a vaccine for rabies in 1885 by infecting numerous dogs and rabbits with the disease, while the research leading to the introduction of diphtheria antitoxin in 1891 involved injecting guinea pigs, rats, and other species with diphtheria toxin. Such breakthroughs allowed experimental medicine to grow by feeding

on itself, discovery generating support for more laboratories and scientists, leading to further discovery. By 1900, the German research ethos had established itself throughout the Western hemisphere, even in the United States (Fye). During the course of the twentieth century, moreover, the use of animals in research spread beyond the boundaries of physiology and pharmacology into areas such as psychology, the standardization of drug products, and toxicity testing of cosmetics and other consumer products. The "laboratory animal" has become a universal tool and symbol of medical progress and modern civilization.

## The History of Opposition to Animal Experimentation

The laboratory animal also became, in the later years of the twentieth century, the chief object of attention of an aggressive animal rights movement (Plous). The movement's concentration on the immorality of animal experimentation seems odd on first consideration, since medical research, unlike other uses of animals as means to human ends (for food, clothing, sport, entertainment), has yielded unquestionable and inestimable benefits, and for animals as well as people. When examined historically, however, the focus on medical research becomes understandable, as it was the development of vivisection that most forcefully raised the question, "Do animals deserve the same moral consideration as humans?"

Initially, the answer was no. The rapid expansion of animal experimentation during the 1600s did provoke objections, but complaints were the exception, and were usually an experimenter's personal expression of revulsion rather than the product of a moral philosophy condemning cruel treatment of animals (anesthetics were not introduced into surgery, or research, until the mid-1800s). The absence of significant opposition to animal experimentation in the seventeenth century has often been attributed to the influence of the French philosopher and speculative physiologist René Descartes (1596–1650), who believed animals to be insensitive automata. Yet most experimenters recognized that animals did indeed feel pain; they simply did not regard the infliction of pain in experiments as cruelty. Physiologists accepted, with the rest of society, that humankind had been given dominion over animals to use as they saw fit. As scientists, furthermore, they considered experimentation the noblest of uses, since the unveiling of nature's design was a moral duty whose fulfillment deepened understanding of the Creator (Guerrini; Ritvo; Rupke). Animal research continues to the present to be justified on those two grounds, that it is a practical good—it benefits people; and an intellectual good—it enlarges understanding of the natural world.

Those justifications came under attack with increasing frequency during the second half of the eighteenth century. The humanitarian turn of mind engendered by the philosophical and religious emphases of the Enlightenment included a greatly heightened sensitivity to suffering that was readily extended beyond fellow humans to the higher animals. William Hogarth's print "The Four Stages of Cruelty" (1750–1751), for example, depicted the barbarous treatment of dogs and cats as the first stage of descent into savagery. The revolutionary's declaration of liberty, equality, and fraternity could likewise be interpreted as applicable to the animal creation. To be sure, the great majority of philosophers believed the exercise of natural rights required rational thought and speech, and thus could be granted only to humans. The Enlightenment's abhorrence of pain, however, made sentience a primary consideration for some thinkers. Jeremy Bentham (1748–1832) argued that animals' ability to feel and suffer earned them entrance to the sphere of moral consideration; less well-known writers even insisted that kind handling was a "right" to which animals were entitled. And although the most common criticisms of abuse were directed at the use of animals for food, labor, and sport, explicit attention was occasionally given to experimentation. Samuel Johnson (1709–1784), for one, not only denied that any practical benefits had come from animal research, he maintained that even if there had been a payoff, the gain was ill-gotten, tainted by the torture of innocent creatures. He repudiated obtaining knowledge through torment, in fact, as ultimately hurtful to society as well, for the callous treatment of animals would harden experimenters' hearts toward human suffering. Through assertions of the inutility, immorality, and corrupting influence of experimentation, philosophical argument overtook empathy as the basis of opposition to animal research (Passmore; Stevenson).

Philosophical argument matured into political action during the nineteenth century, hardening that triad of objections into the spearhead of an organized antivivisectionist movement. At first, the protesting of vivisection lacked an independent identity; rather it was subsumed under the broader animal welfare movement, largely because the country where animal protectionist sentiment was strongest—England—was the country where experimental physiology was weakest. Despite Harvey's example of two centuries earlier, English physiologists had come to rely primarily on dissection and anatomical reasoning rather than vivisection. There was too little animal experimentation at home to necessitate a distinct campaign; it seemed sufficient to fire occasional shells at less civilized scientists across the Channel.

By the 1850s, however, English physiologists realized that they had fallen behind their continental counterparts, and that animal experimentation was the key to catching up. Since ether and chloroform had been introduced as anesthetics in the 1840s, vivisection was far less harrowing, and it soon became as common in England as in Europe. Medical experimentation involved any number of species, but dogs and cats were especially common, and since the keeping of domestic pets had assumed an almost sacred place in genteel British culture during the first half of the century, vivisection could be horrifying even with anesthesia. (And not all researchers employed anesthetics, as the drugs sometimes interfered with the experiment.) Animal protectionists could thus still equate vivisection with cruelty, and this invasion of British soil by scientific barbarism incited a counterattack. The redoubtable Frances Power Cobbe (1822–1904) assumed generalship of the antivivisection forces, mobilizing them in 1875 into The Society for the Protection of Animals Liable to Vivisection—the first organization dedicated to overthrowing animal experimentation. Parliament, meanwhile, had appointed a Royal Commission to investigate charges of experimental cruelty, and though the Commission discovered no significant mistreatment of laboratory animals, it did recommend that vivisection be regulated by the state. The Cruelty to Animals Act of 1876 resulted, bringing experimenters and their laboratories into a system of registration and inspection, and requiring the administration of anesthesia (the 1876 Act was replaced in 1986 by the Animals [Scientific Procedures] Act) (French; Ritvo; Turner; Ryder, 1989).

Like so many pieces of legislation, the English Cruelty to Animals Act was a compromise that pleased neither side. Scientists regarded it as an insulting interference with their search for truth, antivivisectionists saw it as a skimpy fig leaf for scientists' arrogance. In truth, many proponents of animal welfare were placated by the requirement of anesthesia, but others noted the law permitted experiments without anesthetics if drugs would interfere with a potentially valuable study, insisted the inspection system was inadequate to insure anesthetics would be used in ordinary experiments, and declared that even when anesthesia was employed, the deprivation of freedom and life suffered by the animals was unacceptable cruelty. The 1876 law actually roused antivivisectionists to more vigorous opposition, because it struck them as official hypocrisy—it claimed to rescue animals from suffering when in fact it gave legal blessing to their confinement and killing.

Objections to animal experimentation now came to be broadcast more loudly than ever, and began to appear in other countries, including the United States, where Henry Bergh launched an antivivisection movement in the 1870s

(Rupke). The arguments raised against vivisection were not essentially new. As in the eighteenth century, the utility of vivisection experiments was denied, corruption of the experimenters' character was alleged, and, most important, the sacrificing of animals' lives for human comfort was condemned as fundamentally immoral. Ultimately, practical benefits from animal experiments were deemed irrelevant, as sinfully earned as if they had been derived from painful experiments on humans.

Yet it was the supposed utility of vivisection that gave experimentation overriding significance in the early formulation of a philosophy of animal rights. If one wished to extend animals the same rights as people, treating them as ends in themselves rather than as means to humans' ends, animal experimentation was the purest test case. The ends supposedly achieved by vivisection—saving human lives and relieving suffering—were clearly far worthier than the ends obtained by hunting, trapping, butchering, or other forms of animal slaughter. If the principle of equal rights for animals could be shown to obtain in the laboratory, it would necessarily obtain everywhere else. It was vitally important as well that experimentation was the one form of animal abuse practiced exclusively by educated and refined people, by an elite who should serve as models of civilized behavior for the rest of society. If scientists could not be made to recognize the moral claims of fellow creatures, what hope was there for educating drovers and butchers? The very nobility of the ends of medical research made (and makes) it the most attractive target for animal rights marksmen. Thus Henry Salt's 1892 treatise—*Animals' Rights Considered in Relation to Social Progress*—attacked every form of animal abuse, but singled out medical research as "the *ne plus ultra* of iniquity" (p. 102).

By 1900, however, the question of the utility of animal experimentation had blown up in the faces of antivivisectionists, for animal research was finally delivering its long-promised benefits. The newfound power over diphtheria, for so long the gruesome slayer of innocent children, was particularly important for eroding public empathy for innocent laboratory animals, and with the advent of the wonder drug era in the 1930s, criticism of animal experimentation effectively disappeared.

There followed several decades of dormancy, but during the last third of the twentieth century opposition to animal research underwent a dramatic resurgence. The extraordinary expansion of government funding of medical research in the post-World War II decades markedly increased the number of animals used in the laboratory; nearly 30 million warm-blooded animals were being used for research annually in the United States by 1980, and the number would reach an estimated 60 million by the early 1990s. During the 1970s and 1980s, furthermore, several instances of scandalous abuse of laboratory animals were brought to light (Fox; Finsen and Finsen). At the same time, studies demonstrating complex social interactions and the use of language within many species strengthened humans' feelings of kinship with higher animals, while heightened awareness of the endangerment of whole species by human activities fostered resentment of all forms of animal mistreatment (Wise; Clark). Finally, just as the political and religious trends of the late eighteenth century generated broad social sympathy for oppressed people, which was then extended to animals, so the late twentieth century's sensitivity to racial and sexual discrimination revived motivation to be just to all creatures; in 1975, the term *speciesism* was introduced to parallel racism and sexism (Ryder, 1975).

Within this environment, the ethics of animal experimentation became the subject of serious philosophical analysis. Particularly influential critiques were provided by Peter Singer, whose 1975 *Animal Liberation* presented a utilitarian argument against speciesism, and Tom Regan, who in 1983 advanced the case for animals' possession of inherent rights to liberty and life. By both analyses, animal research is a morally impermissible way of pursuing science (Singer; Regan). The philosophy of animal rights was translated into practical action by a number of organizations, most notably the Animal Liberation Front (ALF), founded in 1976, and People for the Ethical Treatment of Animals (PETA), established in 1980. The former group, as its name implies, has gone beyond the conventional activities of picketing laboratories and publicizing scientists' violations of animal rights principles, to the invasion of research facilities to free experimental animals and destroy property; estimates of the property damage caused by the ALF are in the millions of dollars (Finsen and Finsen; Petrinovich; Ryder, 1989).

The recent attacks on animal experimentation as unethical have, of course, provoked responses from the medical research community. For the most part, the reaction has been to bluntly assert the primacy of human interests over those of animals, and to emphasize the many medical advances that have come from animal research. There have also, however, been attempts to refute the animal rights position on its own terms, through strict philosophical analysis (Fox). Additionally, a great deal of consideration has been given to the "three Rs": reducing the numbers of animals used in experiments; refining procedures so as to lessen animals' discomfort; and replacing animals when possible with alternatives such as tissue cultures and mathematical models (Russell and Burch; Smyth; Rowan). Beginning in the late 1980s, in fact, several major producers of cosmetic products started abandoning animal testing; the publicity those companies have given to their action is a clear indication of continuing public uneasiness over the morality of animal experimentation (Welsh).

JAMES C. WHORTON (1995)
REVISED BY AUTHOR

**SEE ALSO:** *Cloning: Scientific Background; Harm; Hinduism, Bioethics in; Jainism, Bioethics in; Moral Status; Pain and Suffering; Veterinary Ethics; Xenotransplantation;* and other *Animal Research* subentries

### BIBLIOGRAPHY

Bernard, Claude. 1865. *Introduction a l'etude de la medecine experimentale.* Paris: Balliere.

Clark, Stephen. 1977. *The Moral Status of Animals.* Oxford, Eng.: Clarendon Press.

Coleman, William, and Holmes, Frederic, eds. 1988. *The Investigative Enterprise. Experimental Physiology in Nineteenth-Century Medicine.* Berkeley, CA: University of California Press.

Finsen, Lawrence, and Finsen, Susan. 1994. *The Animal Rights Movement in America: From Compassion to Respect.* New York: Twayne.

Foster, Michael. 1970. *Lectures on the History of Physiology During the Sixteenth, Seventeenth, and Eighteenth Centuries.* New York: Dover.

Fox, Michael. 1986. *The Case for Animal Experimentation: An Evolutionary and Ethical Perspective.* Berkeley: University of California Press.

French, Richard. 1975. *Antivivisection and Medical Science in Victorian Society.* Princeton, NJ: Princeton University Press.

Fye, W. Bruce. 1987. *The Development of American Physiology: Scientific Medicine in the Nineteenth Century.* Baltimore, MD: Johns Hopkins University Press.

Guerrini, Anita. 1989. "The Ethics of Animal Experimentation in Seventeenth-Century England." *Journal of the History of Ideas* 50: 391–407.

Lesch, John. 1984. *Science and Medicine in France: The Emergence of Experimental Physiology, 1790–1855.* Cambridge, MA: Harvard University Press.

Passmore, John. 1975. "The Treatment of Animals." *Journal of the History of Ideas* 36: 195–218.

Petrinovich, Lewis. 1999. *Darwinian Dominion: Animal Welfare and Human Interests.* Cambridge, MA: MIT Press.

Plous, S. 1991. "An Attitude Survey of Animal Rights Activists." *Psychological Science* 2: 194–196.

Regan, Tom. 1983. *The Case for Animal Rights.* Berkeley: University of California Press.

Ritvo, Harriet. 1987. *The Animal Estate: The English and Other Creatures in the Victorian Age.* Cambridge, MA: Harvard University Press.

Rowan, Andrew. 1984. *Of Mice, Models, and Men: A Critical Evaluation of Animal Research.* Albany: State University of New York Press.

Rupke, Nicolaas, ed. 1987. *Vivisection in Historical Perspective.* London: Croom Helm.

Russell, W. M. S., and Burch, R. L. 1959. *The Principles of Humane Experimental Technique.* London: Methuen.

Ryder, Richard. 1975. *Victims of Science: The Use of Animals in Research.* London: Davis-Poynter.

Ryder, Richard. 1989. *Animal Revolution: Changing Attitudes Toward Speciesism.* Oxford, Eng.: Basil Blackwell.

Salt, Henry. 1892. *Animals' Rights Considered in Relation to Social Progress.* London: Bell.

Schiller, Joseph. 1967. "Claude Bernard and Vivisection." *Journal of the History of Medicine and Allied Sciences* 22: 246–260.

Singer, Peter. 1975. *Animal Liberation.* New York: Avon.

Smyth, D. H. 1978. *Alternatives to Animal Experiments.* London: Scolar Press.

Stevenson, Lloyd. 1956. "Religious Elements in the Background of the British Anti-Vivisection Movement." *Yale Journal of Biology and Medicine.* 29: 125–157.

Turner, James. 1980. *Reckoning With the Beast: Animals, Pain, and Humanity in the Victorian Mind.* Baltimore, MD: Johns Hopkins University Press.

Welsh, Heidi. 1990. *Animal Testing and Consumer Products.* Washington, D.C.: Investor Responsibility Research Center.

Wise, Steven. 2000. *Rattling the Cage: Toward Legal Rights for Animals.* Cambridge, MA: Perseus Books.

## II. PHILOSOPHICAL ISSUES

Ethical problems related to research on nonhuman animals are grounded in the assertion that animals have conscious experiences and that their lives can go well or badly. Central to this issue is the belief that nonhuman animals can experience pain and other unpleasant or distressing mental states. The seventeenth-century philosopher René Descartes denied this (Regan and Singer), and one or two contemporary philosophers continue to deny it (Carruthers). On the whole, however, popular opinion and the overwhelming majority of contemporary scientists and philosophers agree that animals, especially vertebrate animals, can suffer (Smith and Boyd; DeGrazia, 1996, 2002). To take a contrary view, one must refute not just the experience of everyday owners of animal companions but also the increasing body of empirical evidence, both physiological and behavioral, suggesting close parallels between animal behavior and human behavior (Dawkins, 1980, 1993; Rollin; Griffin). Moreover, these behavioral parallels are supported by the known similarities among the nervous systems of all vertebrate animals and by the fact of common animal and human evolutionary origin (Rachels).

It is difficult to believe that despite all these similarities the nervous systems of human and nonhuman animals operate in radically different ways. Many codes regulating animal experimentation instruct regulating committees to assume that procedures that would cause pain in humans also will cause pain in vertebrate animals unless there is evidence to the contrary. From this point, therefore, the existence of animal suffering will be taken for granted.

Before considering the ethical questions that arise from the existence of animal suffering, however, it is necessary to provide some further information.

## Nature and Extent of Animal Experimentation

Some governments provide detailed information on the number of animal experiments carried out each year. In the United Kingdom, for instance, the annual report on scientific procedures performed on living animals under the Animals (Scientific Procedures) Act 1986 for the year 2000 showed that 2.71 million animals were used in that year, a significant decrease from the 1980s, when the figure topped 5 million, although the decline appears to have leveled out. An estimated 12 million animals are used in the fifteen member nations of the European Union, which includes the United Kingdom. An incomplete Japanese survey published in 1988 reported a total in excess of 8 million. There are no accurate figures for the United States because the official figures compiled by the U.S. Department of Agriculture do not include rats, mice, and birds, the species used most commonly in research. In 1986 the U.S. Congress, Office of Technology Assessment, estimated that "at least 17 million to 22 million" animals are used in research annually (U.S. Congress, Office of Technology Assessment). Many think that this figure is very conservative, and several unofficial estimates indicate a higher figure. In addition to rats and mice, dogs, cats, primates, guinea pigs, and rabbits are used widely (Singer, 1990 [1975]; Orlans).

Opponents of animal experiments have focused on examples such as those discussed below (Singer, 1990 [1975]).

TOXICITY TESTING. From about 1950 until the late 1980s the standard method for assessing the toxicity of any product was the $LD_{50}$ (lethal dose 50%) test. The object of this test is to find the dose level that will fatally poison 50 percent of a sample of animals. Often more than one species of animal is used. In the process of stepping up the dose until half the experimental animals die, all of them are likely to become ill, experiencing symptoms such as nausea, thirst, diarrhea, stomach cramps, and fever. The $LD_{50}$ test was carried out routinely on most household products, including food colorings, household cleaners, shampoos, and cosmetics.

After campaigns against the test by the animal rights movement, most U.S. government agencies began to discourage the use of the classical $LD_{50}$ test, and the Center for Laboratory Animal Welfare estimates that its use has fallen by as much as 90 percent (Center for Laboratory Animal Welfare). In 2000 the Organization for Economic Cooperation and Development announced that it was planning to delete the $LD_{50}$ test from its testing guidelines in favor of three alternative methods. Nevertheless, the $LD_{50}$ test still is used in some circumstances, and even if only 10 percent as many animals are subjected to it, that still amounts to hundreds of thousands of animals every year. The replacement for that test, the limit test, still uses animals but does not require doses sufficient to kill them. Instead, other signs of toxicity are used. In addition to undergoing toxicity testing, many products, especially cosmetics and shampoos, used to be placed in the eyes of conscious, unanesthetized rabbits in what is known as the Draize eye test, which was designed to assess the likelihood that a product would cause eye damage. In the late 1980s, after a decade of campaigning against that test, some leading cosmetic companies developed an alternative to the Draize test and stopped conducting tests on animals.

MILITARY TESTING. It is often difficult to find out exactly what happens to animals who undergo military experimentation, but in the United States, in experiments carried out in 1984, monkeys were trained with electric shock to run for hours on a treadmill and then were exposed to lethal doses of radiation to see how long the sick and dying animals could keep running (when they stopped, they received more electric shocks). At Brooks Air Force Base, in Texas, research that involves observation of the effect of radiation on the behavior of monkeys is, according to the most recent information available, still being funded. So too is research in which monkeys are trained to "fly" a device called a "primate equilibrium platform" which simulates some of the tasks that a pilot has to perform when flying a plane. They are then exposed to radiation, to see how this affects their ability to perform. This research was first carried out in the 1960s by Donald Barnes, a psychologist who later came to consider it cruel and pointless (Barnes). Nevertheless, the U.S. Department of Defense continues to fund the training of monkeys to operate the primate equilibrium platform before being exposed to "degradation in the functioning of the central nervous system."

PSYCHOLOGY EXPERIMENTS. In a psychology experiment performed at the University of Pennsylvania in 1968 dogs were placed in cages with wire floors that could be electrified. Subjected to repeated, inescapable electric shock, the dogs at first jumped, ran, attacked the cage, howled, defecated, and urinated, but the shocks continued until the dogs stopped attempting to escape. The experiment was designed to demonstrate the existence of a state known as "learned helplessness" in the belief that such research might throw light on some forms of depression in human beings. From 1984 to 1986 researchers at Temple University used rats in similar experiments with inescapable electric shock; at the same time researchers at the University of Tennessee at Martin were trying to apply inescapable electric shock to goldfish. Learned helplessness experiments on animals are continuing at various centers in the United States, including the University of Colorado at Boulder, where research of this kind has been carried out since 1993 (National Institutes of Health). Experiments in maternal deprivation in monkeys and other animals have been going on in American universities since the 1960s and are continuing. In research at the University of California, Davis, published in 2000, researchers carried out experiments over a five-year period to discover whether there are differences in the problem-solving abilities of monkeys reared with inanimate "surrogate mothers," as compared with the problem-solving abilities of monkeys reared by dogs (Capitanio and Mason).

STUDENT USE OF ANIMALS. Although it has been estimated that more than 5 million animals are used for dissection annually in the United States alone, there has been a move away from the use of living animals for practice surgery in medical schools. Only a minority of U.S. and Canadian medical schools still require the use of live animals, and in almost all those schools students may choose not to participate. In 2000 the Tufts University School of Veterinary Medicine became the first veterinary school in the United States to eliminate the use of healthy dogs for surgical training (Tufts). A number of valuable alternatives to the use of live animals in education have been developed (Smith and Boyd).

## Guidelines and Codes

Many countries have national, legally enforceable guidelines, for the protection of animals in research. Among the more advanced are those developed by the Australian National Health and Medical Research Council and the Swedish regulations. Both require experiments to be approved by ethics committees. In Australia the ethics committee must include a lay member and, in addition, a person from an animal welfare organization (National Health and Medical Research Council). In Sweden the ethics committees consist of six scientists and six lay members and are chaired by a judge (European Science Foundation). Both the European Union and the Council of Europe have their own codes, dating from the mid-1980s. From the same period comes the most frequently cited international code, the International Guiding Principles for Biomedical Research Involving Animals developed by the Council for International Organizations of Medical Sciences (CIOMS). The CIOMS code is, however, much weaker than the relatively more advanced codes in specific countries, such as the European nations and Australia. Instead of mandatory review by committees that include lay members, for example, the CIOMS code allows "voluntary self-regulation by the biomedical community."

## In Defense of Current Animal Experimentation

Defenders of animal experimentation emphasize the use of animals in medical experimentation, particularly in areas such as diabetes and hypertension research, where the use of animals is claimed to have led to important medical breakthroughs (Paton; U.S. Congress, Office of Technology Assessment). They assert that statistics on the large numbers of animals used can be misleading because a great deal of animal experimentation is of a relatively harmless nature, for example, running a rat through a maze with a reward of food as encouragement for good performance rather than an electric shock as punishment for poor performance. They argue that animal experimentation is the only way to advance basic knowledge of human anatomy and physiology and that it offers the best hope of finding cures for diseases such as cancer and AIDS. They also may point out that a considerable amount of animal experimentation is carried out in schools of veterinary medicine to find ways to treat diseases that affect animals. The majority of this work is concerned with farm animals, but some is directed toward companion animals and wild animals.

If experiments now being carried out inflict substantial suffering on animals, how can this practice be defended? The usual justification offered is that the suffering of animals is outweighed by the benefits to humans of discoveries that can be made only through the use of animals. Sometimes, however, it is said that the goal of increasing scientific knowledge is an overriding one and thus provides sufficient justification for whatever suffering might be inflicted on animals in the process of advancing toward that goal. Because this goal is not said to justify inflicting substantial suffering on nonconsenting human experimental subjects, however, further justification is needed to account for the alleged difference in moral status of human beings and other animals.

Behind such arguments lie a variety of philosophical positions. For instance, it may be said that, as related in Genesis 1:26, God has given human beings "dominion" over the other animals, to use them as we please. Combined with other theological notions, such as the idea that humans, alone of all animals, have immortal souls, this idea has been influential throughout the Christian world. But it can be turned the other way: As long ago as 1713 Alexander Pope argued against cruel experiments on the grounds that dominion requires us to play the role of the good shepherd, caring for our flock (Turner). More recently a number of Christians have suggested that the gift of dominion should be interpreted as one of "stewardship," which makes us responsible for the care of the nonhuman creation (Attfield; Linzey). It remains unclear, however, precisely what follows from this reinterpretation. In particular, does it imply that humans are not entitled to use animals in harmful experiments or only that there must be a strong reason for doing so?

It also has been said by writers as diverse as Thomas Aquinas and Immanuel Kant that animals are not "ends in themselves" or that they have no rights (Regan and Singer). In support of this idea it is alleged that the status of a being who is an "end in itself" or has rights belongs only to a being who is rational, is capable of autonomous action, or is a moral agent. This position attempts to equate the universe of moral agents—those *to whom* moral judgments or prescriptions can sensibly be addressed—with the universe of moral patients—those *about whom* it matters, morally, what people do. One possible justification for this equation would be a social contract model of ethics: We have a moral obligation to respect the rights or interests only of those who can reciprocate respect for their rights or interests (Gauthier; Carruthers). This position, however, does not provide any grounds for distinguishing between nonhuman animals, on the one hand, and infants and the profoundly intellectually disabled, on the other. It may be true that many people care more about members of their own species and hence wish to give infants and the intellectually disabled "courtesy status" as members of the moral community. But what if they do not? A social contract theory of morality, then, offers no footing for insisting on equal consideration for the interests of those human beings.

A second justification claims that all human beings form a moral community not because of an implicit contract but because of people's natural feelings for members of the human species. Those natural feelings, it is argued, resemble the natural affection of parents for their own children, which people take as a basis for the special moral obligation they think parents have to give preference to the interests of their own children over the greater interests of the children of strangers. The natural ties between members of a species should, the argument continues, serve as the basis for holding that humans have a greater obligation to other humans than they do to members of other species (Midgley; Gray, 1991a, 1991b).

If this argument were valid, it is not clear how much experimentation on animals it would justify because people do not think that parents are justified in causing serious harm to the children of strangers in order to benefit their own children. But is this argument valid? Understandably, those who use these arguments are silent about the obvious case that lies between the family and the species: preference for the interests of the members of one's own ethnic group or race over the greater interests of members of other ethnic groups or races. It would seem that if the argument works for both the narrower circle of the family and the wider sphere of the species, it also should work for the middle case. If we reject the extension from families to ethnic groups, the further extension to the whole of the human species looks very dubious (Singer, 1991).

A utilitarian defense of the current practice might be based on the idea that the benefits produced outweigh the harm done to the animals (Paton; U.S. Congress, Office of Technology Assessment). Prominent among the claimed benefits is a considerable extension of the human life span. The first question raised by this defense is how much animal experimentation has helped extend human longevity. In polemical debates dramatic claims often are made, but the consensus among those who have studied trends in human health from a historical point of view is that almost all of the increase in human longevity that has occurred over the last century has been due to improved sanitation, diet, and living conditions rather than to medical research of any kind, whether on animals or not (McKeown; McKinlay et al.).

It is possible to accept this verdict but to maintain that medical research, including research on animals, has benefited humans. For example, defenders of the value of animal research often point to the development of coronary artery bypass graft surgery as an achievement that was facilitated by research on animals. The contribution of this form of surgery to the prolongation of life is not clear, but the surgery is more effective than conventional medication in relieving angina, a painful condition that results from coronary artery disease (U.S. Congress, Office of Technology Assessment). Thus, it may contribute to a better quality of life rather than to a greater quantity of life. Against this it might be claimed that the funds spent on this research as well as on the surgery itself would have been more effective if they had been directed toward reducing the cause of the disease by promoting healthier diets and lifestyles. It also has been argued that misleading animal models sometimes have slowed the development of a cure for major diseases, such as polio (LaFollette and Shanks).

A second point in considering a genuinely utilitarian defense of current practice in animal research is that the classical utilitarian tradition has steadfastly required people to take *all* suffering—that of humans and that of nonhuman animals—into consideration. The leading nineteenth-century utilitarians—Jeremy Bentham, John Stuart Mill, and Henry Sidgwick—were unwavering on this point (Bentham; Mill; Sidgwick). Modern utilitarians who cast their views in terms of the satisfaction of preferences rather than in terms of pleasure and pain are equally comprehensive in the scope of their theories (Singer, 1993 [1979]; Hare). This makes it more difficult to claim that a genuinely utilitarian approach favors animal experimentation in general or as an institution. Nevertheless, some individual experiments—those which do not involve any or very much suffering for the animals and promise major benefits for humans or animals—may be defensible on utilitarian grounds.

Some seek to justify what researchers do to animals by appealing to a human-centered version of utilitarianism. In the extreme version of this view the conscious experiences of beings who are not members of our own species do not matter at all. In the more moderate version those experiences do matter, but they do not matter as much as the similar experiences of members of our own species. Both positions frankly endorse an ethic that is limited to, or biased toward, our own species. Once such an ethic is accepted, of course, the justification for animal experimentation becomes much easier. The difficulty of this position lies in defending such a *speciesist* ethic (see below).

Finally, defenders of current practice often accuse their opponents of a lack of consistency in objecting to the deaths of animals in laboratories while continuing to participate in the practice of rearing and killing animals for food. The rise of the animal rights movement in the 1980s has made this accusation less effective because most of those actively involved in that movement have been vegetarians as well as opponents of animal experimentation. In any case, the issue of whether animal experimentation is justified cannot be resolved by reference to the character of some individuals who object to animal experimentation.

## Objections to Current Animal Experimentation

Critics of the current practice of experimenting on animals tend to fall into two groups: abolitionists and reformers. Abolitionists usually rely on the principle that the end does not justify the means. To inflict pain and death on an innocent being is, they maintain, always wrong. They point out that people do not think that the possibility of advancing scientific knowledge justifies taking healthy human beings and inflicting painful deaths on them; similarly, they say, the infliction of suffering on animals cannot be justified by reference to future benefits either for humans or for other animals (Ryder; Regan).

A weakness of the abolitionist position is that when the end is sufficiently important, most people think that otherwise unacceptable means are justifiable if there is no other way of achieving the end. People do not approve of telling lies, but most people accept the idea that politicians should tell lies to mislead the enemy when their country is fighting a war that they believe is right. Similarly, if the prospects of finding a cure for cancer depended on a single experiment, most people probably would think that the experiment should be carried out.

In response to objections along these lines, some abolitionists argue that although a single experiment, taken in isolation, may appear justifiable, the benefits of such experiments do not outweigh the suffering inflicted by the institution of animal experimentation as a whole. One also must take into account, these abolitionists would say, two other factors: First, a large (if uncertain) proportion of experiments are worthless; second, even if no pain or distress is caused by the experiments, experimental animals typically have been raised in conditions that constitute severe deprivation for beings of their species. The common laboratory rat, for instance, is a highly intelligent animal with a strong urge to explore new surroundings. Rats also like to get into small, dark spaces, yet in most laboratories they are kept in bare plastic buckets with a bit of sawdust at the bottom. Such treatment indicates the lack of consideration for the interests of animals that prevails in the world of animal experimentation, and abolitionists doubt that this will ever change as long as people continue to regard laboratory animals primarily as tools for research.

Reformers believe that a changed practice of experimenting on animals could be defensible. They demand that any benefits that are believed to be likely to arise from the experimentation should be sufficiently probable and sufficiently great to offset the costs to the animal subjects; they urge that every experiment should come under close and impartial scrutiny to determine whether this is the case.

Reformers point out that although during the 1980s and 1990s several countries (for example, Australia, Sweden, Switzerland, and the United Kingdom) developed legally obligatory systems of review based on an institutional ethics committee's review of proposals to carry out experiments on animals, experimenters usually are well represented on such committees, whereas animal welfare advocates either are not represented or are heavily outnumbered by experimenters. An impartial committee that weighed the cost to the animal in the same way that people would weigh a comparable cost to a human would, the reformers maintain, approve at most a small fraction of the experiments now performed. In other countries, such as the United States, institutional ethics committees exist but are not legally required for corporations or other institutions that do not receive federal funds, and their coverage of animal experimentation is incomplete. Moreover, in the United States these committees do not always have the authority to prevent experimenters from going ahead with painful experiments if the experimenters assert that alleviating the animals' pain would interfere with the purpose of the experiment (U.S. Congress, Office of Technology Assessment; Dresser; Smith and Boyd; Gavaghan; Orlans).

Among opponents of current practices of animal experimentation the line between reformers and abolitionists is not clear-cut because questions of long-term goals and short-term strategy intervene. A threefold division might be more appropriate: In the first category one could place those whose long-term goals do not extend beyond better regulation and control of animal experiments to eliminate the most painful and trivial experiments. In the next category would be those who have the long-term goal of abolishing all or virtually all animal experiments but who consider this an ideal rather than a realistic objective for the immediate future. This group therefore seeks reforms in the interim period, and its short-term goals do not differ significantly from those of members of the first category. The third category consists of those who aim at abolition and are not interested in advocating anything less.

Although members of these three categories disagree sharply among themselves, they all agree that the current situation is indefensible. They also agree on promoting the use of alternatives to animal experimentation. The use of such alternatives by cosmetic companies to replace the Draize eye test was mentioned above. Opponents of animal experimentation suggest that alternative methods would be developed more rapidly if they received more substantial government support (Ryder; Rowan; Balls).

The ethical stance of those in the first category, who seek only limited reforms, is often of a relatively conventional type: They can be thought of as following an "animal welfare" line rather than accepting an ethic of "animal rights" or "animal liberation." They accept the idea that animals may be used for human purposes but want safeguards to ensure that the purposes are serious ones and that no more suffering occurs than is necessary for the purpose to be realized. Those who take an animal rights or animal liberation stance want to narrow the ethical gulf that separates humans from other animals in regard to conventional morality. They thus raise a philosophically deep question with implications that go beyond experimentation, extending to the treatment of animals in general.

## The Moral Status of Animals

In examining the case for current practices, this entry examined some attempts to justify in ethical terms the sharp distinction that is made currently between the treatment of members of the human species and the treatment of members of other species. The problems noted in this entry bedevil all attempts to make the boundary of the human species coincide with the boundary of human moral obligations. Although it is said frequently that humans are superior to other animals in such respects as rationality, self-awareness, the ability to communicate with others, and a sense of justice, human infants and humans with severe intellectual disabilities fall below many nonhuman animals on any objective test of abilities that could mark humans as superior to other animals. Yet surely these less capable human beings are also "ends in themselves," and it would not be legitimate to experiment on them in the ways in which people experiment on animals. For a contrary view that accepts the moral possibility of harmful experimentation on both nonhuman animals and humans at a similar mental level, see Frey.

Ryder, Singer, Regan, and other critics of current practices claim that respect for the interests of those humans and comparative neglect of the interests of members of other species with equal or superior capacities constitutes *speciesism*, a prejudice in favor of "our own kind" that is analogous to and no more justifiable than racism. This argument has been seen by many people as the most difficult for defenders of animal experimentation to counter, so much so that a leading philosopher has referred to it as a "won argument" (McGinn).

Certainly the view that species is in itself a reason for giving more weight to the interests of one being than to the interests of another is more often assumed than explicitly defended. Some writers who have claimed to be defending *speciesism* have in fact been defending a very different position: that the morally relevant differences between species—such as differences in mental capacities—entitle people to give more weight to the interests of members of the species with the superior mental capacities (Cohen; Leahy). If this argument were successful, it would not justify speciesism because the claim would not be that species in itself is a reason for giving more weight to the interests of one being than to those of another. The real reason would be the difference in mental capacities, which happens to coincide with the difference in species. However, in view of the overlap in mental capacities between some members of the species *Homo sapiens* and some members of other species, it is difficult to see how this argument can be used to defend current practices. In other contexts people insist on treating beings as moral individuals rather than lumping them together as members of a group; it is precisely those who practice racism and sexism who treat all members of a group in the same way (for instance, assuming that women cannot perform heavy physical labor as well as men can) without recognizing individual variation.

Defenders of animal experimentation sometimes have portrayed the animal rights position in an extreme form, for example, as implying that it is as wrong to kill a mosquito as it is to kill a normal human adult. This is, however, a caricature. Animal advocates do not claim that all animals have the *same* interests, only that interests are not to be given less consideration solely on the grounds of species. Thus, it is compatible with the animal liberation view to say that the interests of beings with different mental capacities vary and that these variations are morally significant (DeGrazia, 1996, 2002). If people are forced to choose between saving the life of a being who understands the meaning of death and wants to go on living and saving the life of a being who is not capable of having desires for the future because that being's mental capacities do not enable it to grasp that it is a "self," a mental entity existing over time, it is entirely justifiable to choose in favor of the being who wants to go on living. This is a choice that is based on mental capacity and not on species membership, as one can see by considering that the former being may be a chimpanzee and the latter being a human with profound brain damage (Singer, 1990 [1975]).

At least one scientist who experiments on animals has attempted to sweep aside such issues by denying that animal experimentation raises a moral issue at all. Robert J. White, whose work has involved keeping severed monkeys' heads alive and apparently conscious for as long as possible, has written that "the inclusion of lower animals in our ethical system is philosophically meaningless" (p. 507). Unfortunately, White does not explain why, to take only one example, the clear proposal of utilitarian writers—that pain as such is evil regardless of the species of the being that suffers it—is devoid of meaning. It may be difficult to compare the suffering of a human and that of, say, a rabbit, but sometimes rough comparisons can be made. It seems undeniable that to put into the eye of a rabbit a chemical that causes the eye to blister or become ulcerated is to do more harm to the rabbit than people would do to any number of human beings by denying them the possibility of using a new type of shampoo that could be marketed only if the chemical was tested in this way. When such rough comparisons can be made, the mere fact that rabbits are "lower animals" is no reason to give less weight to their suffering.

Seen in this light, the argument that restricting experiments on animals interferes with scientific freedom and medical progress appears less conclusive. People do not grant scientists the freedom to experiment at will on humans, although such experiments would do more to advance knowledge of human physiology and be more likely to find cures for diseases such as AIDS than would animal experiments. It would seem, therefore, to be incumbent on the defenders of experiments on animals to show that there is a relevant difference between all humans and other animals that justifies experiments on the latter but not on the former. Success at this task, however, still eludes defenders of animal experimentation.

## Conclusion

Controversy over experiments on animals often has been polarized, and, especially in the United States, public exchanges between those who carry out animal experiments and those who oppose them often generate more heat than light. There has been a more serious discussion of the status of animals in philosophical journals and in books by philosophers, and it can be hoped that this level of discussion eventually will influence popular debate on the use of animals in research.

PETER SINGER (1995)
REVISED BY AUTHOR

**SEE ALSO:** *Animal Welfare and Rights: Ethical Perspectives on the Treatment and Status of Animals; Conscience, Rights of; Holocaust; Moral Status; Research Policy; Utilitarianism* *and Bioethics; Veterinary Ethics; Xenotransplantation;* and other *Animal Research* subentries

## BIBLIOGRAPHY

Attfield, Robin. 1983. *The Ethics of Environmental Concern.* Oxford: Basil Blackwell.

Baird, Robert, and Rosenbaum, Stuart E., eds. 1991. *Animal Experimentation: The Moral Issues.* Buffalo, NY: Prometheus.

Balls, Michael. 1992. "Time to Reform Toxic Tests." *New Scientist* (May 2): 31–33.

Barnes, Donald. 1985. "A Matter of Change" In *In Defence of Animals,* ed. Peter Singer. New York: Blackwell.

Bentham, Jeremy. 1948 [1789]. *An Introduction to the Principles of Morals and Legislation.* New York: Hafner.

Capitanio, J. P., and Mason, W. A. 2000. "Cognitive Style: Problem Solving by Rhesus Macaques (Macaca mulatta) Reared with Living or Inanimate Substitute Mothers." *Journal of Comparative Psychology* 114(2): 115–125.

Carruthers, Peter. 1992. *The Animals Issue: Moral Theory in Practice.* Cambridge, Eng.: Cambridge University Press.

Cohen, Carl. 1986. "The Case for the Use of Animals in Biomedical Research." *New England Journal of Medicine* 315: 865–870.

Dawkins, Marian Stamp. 1980. *Animal Suffering: The Science of Animal Welfare.* London: Chapman and Hall.

Dawkins, Marian Stamp. 1993. *Through Our Eyes Only: The Search for Animal Consciousness.* Oxford: Freeman.

DeGrazia, David. 1996. *Taking Animals Seriously: Mental Life and Moral Status.* Cambridge, Eng.: Cambridge University Press.

DeGrazia, David. 2002. *Animal Rights: A Very Short Introduction.* Oxford: Oxford University Press.

Dresser, Rebecca. 1988. "Standards for Animal Research: Looking at the Middle." *Journal of Medicine and Philosophy* 13: 123–143.

Frey, Ray G. 1983. "Vivisection, Morals and Medicine." *Journal of Medical Ethics* 9(2): 94–97.

Gauthier, David. 1986. *Morals by Agreement.* Oxford: Oxford University Press.

Gavaghan, Helen. 1992. "Animal Experiments the American Way." *New Scientist* (May 16): 32–36.

Gray, Jeffrey. 1991a. "On the Morality of Speciesism." *Psychologist* 4(5): 196–198.

Gray, Jeffrey. 1991b. "On Speciesism and Racism: Reply to Singer and Ryder." *Psychologist* 4(5): 202–203.

Griffin, Donald. 1992. *Animal Minds.* Chicago: University of Chicago Press.

Hare, Richard M. 1981. *Moral Thinking: Its Levels, Method, and Point.* Oxford: Clarendon Press.

LaFollette, Hugh, and Shanks, Niall. 1996. *Brute Science: Dilemmas of Animal Experimentation.* London: Routledge.

Leahy, Michael P. T. 1991. *Against Liberation: Putting Animals in Perspective.* London: Routledge.

Linzey, Andrew. 1987. *Christianity and the Rights of Animals.* London: Society for the Propagation of Christian Knowledge.

McGinn, Colin. 1991. "Eating Animals Is Wrong." *London Review of Books* (January 24): 14–15.

McKeown, Thomas. 1979. *The Role of Medicine: Dream, Mirage or Nemesis?* Oxford: Basil Blackwell.

McKinlay, John B.; McKinlay, Sonia M.; and Beaglehole, Robert. 1989. "Trends in Death and Disease and the Contribution of Medical Measures." In *Handbook of Medical Sociology,* 4th edition, ed. Howard E. Freeman and Sol Levine. Englewood Cliffs, NJ: Prentice-Hall.

Midgley, Mary. 1984. *Animals and Why They Matter.* Athens: University of Georgia Press.

Mill, John Stuart. 1963–1991. *Collected Works,* ed. John M. Robinson and Jack Stillinger. Toronto: University of Toronto Press.

Orlans, F. Barbara. 1993. *In the Name of Science: Issues in Responsible Animal Experimentation.* New York: Oxford University Press.

Paton, William. 1984. *Man and Mouse: Animals in Medical Research.* Oxford: Oxford University Press.

Rachels, James. 1990. *Created from Animals: The Moral Implications of Darwinism.* Oxford: Oxford University Press.

Regan, Tom. 1983. *The Case for Animal Rights.* Berkeley: University of California Press.

Regan, Tom, and Singer, Peter, eds. 1989 (1976). *Animal Rights and Human Obligations,* 2nd edition. Englewood Cliffs, NJ: Prentice-Hall.

Rollin, Bernard. 1989. *The Unheeded Cry: Animal Consciousness, Animal Pain, and Science.* Oxford: Oxford University Press.

Rowan, Andrew. 1984. *Of Mice, Models and Men: A Critical Explanation of Animal Research.* Albany: State University of New York Press.

Ryder, Richard D. 1983 (1975). *Victims of Science: The Use of Animals in Research.* London: National Anti-Vivisection Society.

Sharpe, Robert. 1988. *The Cruel Deception: The Use of Animals in Medical Research.* Wellingborough, Eng.: Thorsons.

Sidgwick, Henry. 1963 (1907). *The Methods of Ethics,* 7th edition. London: Macmillan. First published 1874.

Singer, Peter. 1990 (1975). *Animal Liberation,* 2nd edition. New York: New York Review of Books/Random House.

Singer, Peter. 1991. "Speciesism, Morality and Biology: A Response to Jeffrey Gray." *Psychologist* 4(5): 199–200.

Singer, Peter. 1993 (1979). *Practical Ethics,* 2nd edition. Cambridge, Eng.: Cambridge University Press.

Smith, Jane A., and Boyd, Kenneth M. 1991. *Lives in the Balance: The Ethics of Using Animals in Bio-Medical Research: The Report of a Working Party of the Institute of Medical Ethics.* Oxford: Oxford University Press.

Turner, Ernest S. 1992 (1964). *All Heaven in a Rage.* Fontwell, Eng.: Centaur Press.

U. S. Congress, Office of Technology Assessment. 1986. *Alternatives to Animal Use in Research, Testing and Education.* Washington, D.C.: U.S. Government Printing Office.

White, Robert J. 1971. "Anti-Vivisection: The Reluctant Hydra." *American Scholar* 40(3): 503–512.

INTERNET RESOURCES

Center for Laboratory Animal Welfare. 2003. Available from <http://www.labanimalwelfare.org/glossary.html#LD50>.

Council for International Organizations of Medical Sciences. 1985. *International Guiding Principles for Biomedical Research Involving Animals.* Geneva. Available from <www.cioms.ch/frame_1985_texts_of_guidelines.htm>.

European Science Foundation. 2000. *Policy Briefing: The Use of Animals in Research.* Strasbourg. Available from <www.esf.org/medias/ESPB9.pdf>.

National Health and Medical Research Council. 1997. *Australian Code of Practice for the Care and Use of Animals for Scientific Purposes,* 6th edition. Canberra. Available from <www.health.gov.au/nhmrc/research/awc/code.htm>.

National Institutes of Health. 2003. Grant no: 5R37MH050479–07. Available from <http://crisp.cit.nih.gov/>.

United States Department of Defense. 2003. DoD Biomedical Research. Available from <http://www.scitechweb.com/acau/brd/>.

Tufts University School of Veterinary Medicine. 2003. "Animal Use for DVM Training." Available from <http://www.tufts.edu/vet/academic/dvmtraining.html>.

## III. LAW AND POLICY

This entry describes the laws and policies of the United States governing the care and use of animals in research, education, and testing; the history of these policies and laws since 1966; the issues addressed by these laws; and the lawsuits that have followed publication of regulations implementing these laws. Two federal laws govern the use of animals: the Health Research Extension Act of 1985 and the Animal Welfare Act, as amended. While all states have laws governing the care of animals, research usage is often exempted. Twenty states have simple facility licensure, and a few have only very general regulations governing research usage of animals. In reality, nearly all states defer to federal law in this area. A National Institutes of Health (NIH) document, *Public Health Service Policy on Humane Care and Use of Laboratory Animals,* which was revised in 2002, implements the Health Research Extension Act for all activities involving animals conducted or supported by the Public Health Service (PHS),while regulations implementing the Animal Welfare Act are in the *Code of Federal Regulations,* Title 9, Chapter 1, Subchapter A, Parts 1, 2, and 3 (known as animal welfare regulations). The PHS includes twelve health agencies within the U.S. Department of Health and Human Services (DHHS).

### History of Public Health Service Policy

Regulations have been promulgated by the PHS since 1935, originally through one of its constituents, the National Institutes of Health (Whitney). NIH guidelines have provided direction and recommendations for caring for and using laboratory animals at NIH. Subsequently, a committee of laboratory scientists assembled by the Institute of Laboratory Animal Resources of the National Research Council (NRC) wrote the *Guide for the Care and Use of Laboratory Animals* (NRC guide). First published in 1963 and updated many times since, this work has become the standard guide in the field. The first policy based upon the 1963 NRC guide came from NIH in 1971. The PHS published its first policy on animal care in 1973, with revisions in 1973, 1979, 1986, 1996, and 2002. Each successive revision increased the specificity and level of responsibility of animal-care committees in the supervision of animal use.

At the outset of NIH policymaking in animal care and use in 1971, all institutions and organizations using warm-blooded animals for the purpose of research or other projects supported by NIH were required to give assurances that facilities for animals met "acceptable standards for the care, use, and treatment of such animals." This assurance could be met either by gaining accreditation through a professional laboratory-accrediting body (such as the Association for Assessment and Accreditation of Laboratory Animal Care International [AAALAC]) or by establishing a committee to evaluate the care and housing of animals used for NIH-sponsored activities. Institutions were also obligated to follow pertinent sections of the animal welfare regulations. In 1973, the NIH policy was replaced by the first of the PHS policies. Like the NIH policy preceding it, the first PHS policy required institutions either to be fully accredited or to have a standing institutional committee with a minimum of three members, including a veterinarian for those institutions using a "significant" number of animals. These committees were required to conduct periodic facility inspections, with the review of applications and proposals involving the use of animals considered optional.

The 1979 revision to the PHS policy required all institutions using animals, regardless of numbers used and accreditation status, to have a standing committee whose responsibility was oversight of the institution's animal-care program. In addition to the establishment of a committee of at least five members, including one veterinarian, the institution was obligated to establish a mechanism to review its facilities for warm-blooded animals for adherence to the principles contained in the NRC guide. The PHS policy recommended that AAALAC accreditation was the best means of satisfying this obligation, although periodic committee review of facilities and animals' care would suffice. Absent from the 1979 PHS policy was the requirement for review of individual proposals or projects, although review was encouraged. In 1986, however, the PHS policy was revised again, this time requiring the animal-care committees of institutions to take responsibility for specific organizational and supervisory duties in an effort to strengthen the system of institutional assurance.

## History of Animal Welfare Regulations

A 1966 *Life* magazine feature titled "Concentration Camps for Dogs," along with other works published around this time, dramatized poor care and treatment of animals by some dealers who sold animals for biomedical research. This disclosure and the ensuing public outcry resulted in the introduction of twenty-nine bills in the U.S. Congress relating to the regulation of animal research. The bill that eventually became law was the Laboratory Animal Welfare Act of 1966 (LAWA; in 1970, after passage of the first amendments, the name was shortened to the Animal Welfare Act, or AWA). This act was limited to regulation of the sale and transportation of animals by dealers and the holding of animals by certain research facilities. Although the bill was passed, it was a compromise between far-reaching legislation and none at all; it did not apply to actual research usage of animals. The regulations implementing the LAWA specified that the housing facility provide shelter and protection from temperature extremes, that food and water be provided at least daily, and that cages be of a certain size and cleaned daily. These regulations also specified cage sizes and frequency of feeding and watering during transportation. Passage of amendments in 1970, 1976, 1985, and 1990 and of a law calling for the PHS policy extended federal regulations into areas covering the appropriate use and humane treatment of laboratory animals. The 1966 law regulated dogs, cats, hamsters, guinea pigs, rabbits and nonhuman primates. The 1970 amendment broadened it to include all warm-blooded animals, but regulations excluded birds, rats, and mice.

The 1970 amendments broadened the U.S. Department of Agriculture's (USDA) administrative responsibility to cover animal care throughout an animal's stay in research facilities, including the period during which research was being conducted. The 1976 amendments brought transportation carriers under the purview of the act, leading to more stringent standards for shipment of animals. The 1985 version of the AWA invested the USDA with responsibility for issuing and enforcing regulations regarding humane care, handling, and treatment of animals. Animals covered under the AWA include warm-blooded animals—such as dogs, cats, monkeys, guinea pigs, hamsters, rabbits, marine mammals, and normally wild animals—being used for research, testing, experimentation, exhibition purposes, or as a pet. Excluded from coverage are birds, rats, mice, and horses and other farm animals intended for use as food or fiber, or for use in improving animal nutrition, breeding, or management. The 1990 changes to the act added college-student work with animals to the list of areas over which a research institution has oversight responsibility.

## Public Health Service Policy

PHS policy requires that each awardee institution provide a written assurance setting forth how that institution will comply with regulations. This assurance then forms the basis for the care and use of animals in research, education, and testing at that institution and is the basis for judging the adequacy of the institution's compliance with the policy. PHS policy calls for the establishment of a program for animal care and use, using the NRC guide as a basis for developing the program. Also required is the creation of an institutional animal care and use committee (IACUC), appointed by the chief executive officer of the institution. This committee must have at least five members, including at least one veterinarian experienced in laboratory animal science, one scientist, one layperson, and one person unaffiliated with the institution. PHS policy then charges this committee with oversight responsibility for: semiannual review of the program of animal care and use; semiannual inspection of facilities; review of research protocols, or proposals for the use of animals; investigation of all concerns raised by anyone regarding the humane use of animals at the institution; recommendations for personnel training; and suspension of activities deemed improper.

An institution's program for the care and use of laboratory animals encompasses institutional policies, laboratory-animal husbandry procedures, and veterinary care practices. Institutional policies address such personnel provisions as veterinary qualifications, procedures for safely handling hazardous agents, occupational health and personal hygiene including appropriate clothing and practices, and the prohibition of smoking and eating in animal rooms; special considerations are also addressed through policies, such as those concerning prolonged physical restraint of animals and multiple surgeries on a single animal. Laboratory-animal husbandry procedures include housing systems (size of cages and provision for social interaction among animals where appropriate); temperature, humidity, ventilation, lighting control, and cage and room sanitation schedules; and methods of animal identification and of clinical record keeping. Veterinary care practices include preventive-medicine strategies; methods for detecting and treating diseases; giving investigators advice about appropriate anesthesia, analgesia, and surgical and postoperative care; and methods of euthanasia.

Facility inspection covers not only visiting the physical plant but also assessing the health of the animals and reviewing portions of the institutional program for animal care. The physical plant should be properly constructed to house the species being used and to permit sterile surgery to be performed, if necessary.

PHS policy sets forth several criteria to be followed by the IACUC in reviewing protocols. These criteria go beyond mere care and housing guidelines. The care and use of animals in proposed research must be consistent with the NRC guide, unless acceptable scientific justification is provided for any deviation. The investigator must explain the rationale for using animals at all in the proposed research as well as the appropriateness of the species to be used, the number of animals, and their proposed use. PHS policy stipulates requirements for the use of sedatives, analgesics, and anesthetics if the proposed procedure might cause more than slight pain or distress; it also requires prompt euthanasia at the end of (or, when appropriate, during) a procedure for "animals that would otherwise suffer severe or chronic pain or distress that cannot be relieved" and imposes methods of euthanasia consistent with American Veterinary Medical Association (AVMA) guidelines. All personnel involved in the use of animals in research must be appropriately trained and qualified in the procedures to be employed in the experiment.

Each IACUC must have procedures for investigating concerns raised about the care and use of animals at the institution. In addition, the IACUC must ensure that the institution has a training program for both animal-care staff (people actually caring for the animals) and research staff; videotapes and training handbooks may be used to satisfy this requirement. The final charge—the power to suspend

an improperly conducted activity—must come from an official of the institution such as the chief executive officer or the vice president. Without this official support, the IACUC cannot fulfill its duty to ensure compliance with PHS policy.

Several features of PHS policy are of special importance. While its legal force is restricted to awardee institutions, its scope includes all live vertebrates. It was the first U.S. law to call for a consideration of animal welfare during a procedure and to call for the establishment of a committee to review protocols for the appropriateness of design, the importance of knowledge sought (as set forth in the "U.S. Government Principles for the Utilization and Care of Vertebrate Animals Used in Testing, Research, and Training," published in both the PHS policy and the NRC guide), and the competency of personnel. Thus, through PHS policy, committees have been created to review the use of animals in research, much like the committees that review the participation of humans in research.

## Animal Welfare Regulations

Animal welfare regulations (AWRs) pertaining to the care and use of laboratory animals were extensively modified and rewritten following the 1985 amendments of the Animal Welfare Act to include provisions for an IACUC, for protocol review, and for more social interaction among the same species and between animals and their caretakers. These regulations are similar to PHS policy provisions because the secretary of the USDA was directed to consult with the secretary of the DHHS concerning the writing of regulations. In the AWRs, an IACUC committee with only slight differences from PHS policy is required (e.g., three members instead of five as a minimum, including an unaffiliated member and a veterinarian). The duties of the committee are very similar to the duties specified by PHS policy; instructions for reviewing protocols, however, are more detailed than those included in PHS policy. The AWRs require the investigator to search for alternatives to any procedure that may cause more than slight pain or distress and to assure that the proposed activity does not unnecessarily duplicate previous work. Several aspects of a personnel-training program are specified. In contrast to PHS policy, which requires institutions to develop an animal care and use program based upon the NRC guide, the AWRs have an extensive set of standards specifying the humane handling, care, treatment, and transport of various species of animals. The standards section of the regulations detail facility and operating standards, animal health and husbandry standards, and transportation standards for each regulated species. In addition, detailed specifications are given for marking dogs, cats, and other animals for the purpose of identification. In most, but not all, cases, the standards of the AWRs are the same as those of the PHS policy and, thus, are similar to the guidelines given in the NRC guide.

The AWA calls for the USDA to issue regulations in several areas. These regulations, which have engendered considerable public debate as well as the filing of a lawsuit, require exercise of dogs and the provision of a physical environment adequate to promote the psychological well-being of nonhuman primates. After considerable debate, the final regulations combined performance-based standards (standards that specify the desired outcome and leave the details of achieving that outcome to the regulated party) with design or engineering standards (standards that specify in measurable and objective terms how a particular outcome is to be achieved). It is the choice of performance-based standards that is especially controversial because plaintiffs in a lawsuit (see "Lawsuits" section below) alleged that they allow too much latitude for compliance by the regulated parties. It is generally true, however, that humane care and use of animals can be achieved under a variety of circumstances, making it difficult to use detailed engineering standards or specifications. For example, the regulations call for dry floors for most mammals. This can be accomplished by mopping the floor until dry, by wet-vacuuming the floor, by sloping the floor and letting water run off before placing an animal on the surface, and so on. Thus, there are a number of ways of achieving the desired goal, and it is the outcome itself that is specified rather than the steps needed to reach it. Critics of performance standards state that the goal often is not well described, leaving too much discretion to the regulated parties.

Another controversial aspect of the AWRs is that the regulatory definition of animal excludes birds, rats, and mice that have been bred for use in research; hence, these animals are not protected under the AWRs. The exclusion is a major one because more than 85 percent of animals used in research, education, and testing are rats, mice, and birds. The reason for the exclusion is to limit the scope and cost of annual USDA inspections; there are barely enough inspectors to review facilities and procedures involving larger vertebrate animals, whose use is thought to require more sensitivity and therefore more intense scrutiny. Adding rats, mice, and birds to the mandatory inspection list would exceed the capacity of the USDA, both because of the increased numbers of animals to be inspected and because there would be an increase in the number of registered research facilities requiring inspection. (A number of institutions use only rats and/or mice and therefore are not subject

to inspection.) Because PHS policy defines *animal* as any vertebrate (with no exclusions), rats, mice, and birds are covered by PHS policy. In institutions not covered by PHS policy (e.g., industry and colleges not receiving PHS funds), the use of rats and mice remains largely unregulated, a glaring oversight unique to the United States (Orlans, 2000).

## Protocol Review: Consideration of Pain and Distress and Numbers of Animals Used

Because both PHS policy and the AWRs explicitly require minimization of pain and distress of animals during research, there have been examinations of the implications and possible effectiveness of the IACUC consideration of these issues during protocol review (Dresser; Brody). Both regulations attempt to incorporate cost–benefit considerations, utilitarian theory, and some elements of a modified rights-based philosophy (Dresser). The success of PHS policy and the AWRs depends fundamentally upon the recognition that animals can experience pain and distress that can be alleviated (NRC, 1992). The USDA requires an annual report from all registered institutions that lists the numbers of animals used in research and testing, classified by the degree of pain and distress: (1) minimal, transient, or no pain or distress; (2) pain and distress relieved by anesthetics, analgesics, or tranquilizers; and (3) pain and distress not treated. A detailed statement on category 3 procedures is required, including scientific justification for withholding drugs. Another classification scheme, developed by the Scientists Center for Animal Welfare, lists six categories instead of three (Orlans, 1987). Many IACUCs use some classification scheme for pain and distress, reducing the number of animals used in research that fall into the higher categories of pain and distress by applying the "three Rs" (replacement, reduction, and refinement) of William M. S. Russell and Rex L. Burch, authors of a book first published in 1959 called *The Principles of Humane Experimental Technique*.

Some observers feel that IACUC review does not adequately reduce the number of animals used in research or the pain and distress of these animals. In a 1989 article, Mimi Brody suggested new legislation that would implement two oversight levels—first, a local committee; second, a national committee—to review uses of animals with "high ethical cost." Gary L. Francione argued in a 1990 article that open IACUC meetings, publicly announced and attended by interested members of the community, would improve the quality of protocol review. The two-committee approach has the disadvantage of delaying approval of certain types of research and has the potential for becoming excessively bureaucratic. The open-meetings approach presumes that the general public could comprehend the scientific details of the described procedures and would be able to judge the ethical and social justifications for the proposed procedure.

## Lawsuits Concerning the Animal Welfare Regulations

As mentioned earlier, the definition of animals in the AWRs excludes birds, rats, and mice specifically bred for use in research. After parts 1 and 2 of the AWRs became final in 1989, the Animal Legal Defense Fund (ALDF) and the Humane Society of the United States (HSUS) filed a rule-making petition with the USDA to amend the regulations to include rats, mice, and birds in the definition of animals. After the USDA denied the petition in 1990, the ALDF and the HSUS brought suit in federal court, seeking a declaratory judgment and an injunction preventing the USDA from excluding coverage of rats, mice, and birds. In 1992 the ALDF and the HSUS were granted summary judgment, and the USDA was ordered to reconsider its denial of plaintiffs' petition in light of the court's opinion holding the exclusion of rats, mice, and birds to be arbitrary and capricious (*Animal Legal Defense Fund v. Madigan,* 1992). The USDA appealed, and on May 20, 1994, the court of appeals vacated the district court's decision and directed the lower court to dismiss, holding that none of the petitioners had demonstrated both constitutional standing to sue and a statutory right to judicial review under the Administrative Procedure Act—leaving regulations, and presumably practice, to stand unchanged (*Animal Legal Defense Fund v. Espy,* 1994). In 1998, however, the Alternatives Research and Development Foundation filed a new suit to force the inclusion of rats, mice, and birds under AWA. The USDA settled the case (*Alternatives Research and Development Foundation v. Glickman*) in 2000, agreeing to inclusions. But the Farm Security and Rural Investment Act of 2002 blocked the settlement. This amendment permanently denied rats, mice, and birds legal protection under AWA.

The USDA regulations concerning requirements for exercise of dogs and for a physical environment adequate to promote the psychological well-being of nonhuman primates were published in February 1991. The ALDF and others sued, alleging that these regulations did not comply with the 1985 amendments of the AWA because they did not provide minimum standards for exercise of dogs and for adequate cage size and environmental enrichment for nonhuman primates as required by Congress. The district court granted plaintiffs' motion for summary judgment in February 1993 (*Animal Legal Defense Fund v. Secretary of Agriculture,* 1993). It was unclear at the time of this decision whether the federal government would appeal the decision, so the National Association for Biomedical Research (NABR) moved to intervene in the case to ensure an appeal. Although the NABR motion was originally denied, the denial was reversed by the court of appeals. The federal government subsequently decided to pursue an appeal, and the consolidated appeal was argued in May 1994. Two months later, the court of appeals vacated the district court's decision and directed the lower court to dismiss, concluding that the ALDF and the other appellees lacked standing to challenge USDA regulations (for the same reasons cited in the ALDF/HSUS case), again leaving policy unchanged.

## Conclusion

Federal laws and policies regarding the use of animals in research, education, and testing have progressed rapidly from the first enunciation of principles for the care of laboratory animals in the early days of NIH and the first animal welfare laws passed in 1966. Early policy had limited effects on the use of animals because of the generally careful practice standards already in place as well as the lack of enforcement of the new policy. Several U.S. programs and institutions had their funding suspended in the early 1980s, with increased USDA inspections and subsequent violations at numerous institutions in the years that followed, all of which serve as a warning that all animal-care policies must be followed (Rozmiarek). The evolution of policies for animal care and use shows a trend toward increased responsibility for and supervision by IACUCs, with greater emphasis on the level of assurances institutions must give, on IACUC membership, on the process of protocol review, and on the committee's power in matters involving activities using animals. This has resulted in more scrutiny of the care and use of animals in scientific research. The regulations in effect are comprehensive and, if followed, result in excellent care for animals. The penalties for not adhering to the regulations are great enough to encourage compliance and will assure that the privilege of using animals in research is carried out in a humane and careful manner.

JEFFREY KAHN
RALPH DELL (1995)
REVISED BY JEFFREY KAHN
SUSAN PARRY

**SEE ALSO:** *Animal Welfare and Rights; Law and Morality; Research Policy: Historical Aspects; Xenotransplantation;* and other *Animal Research* subentries

## BIBLIOGRAPHY

*Alternatives Research and Development Foundation v. Glickman.* 101 F.Supp.2d 7 (D.C.C. 2000).

American Veterinary Medical Association (AVMA). Panel on Euthanasia. 2001. "2000 Report of the AVMA Panel on Euthanasia." *Journal of the American Veterinary Medical Association* 218(5): 669–696.

*Animal Legal Defense Fund v. Espy.* 23 F.3d 496 (D.C. Cir. 1994).

*Animal Legal Defense Fund v. Madigan.* 781 F.Supp. 797 (D.D.C. 1992).

*Animal Legal Defense Fund v. Secretary of Agriculture.* 813 F.Supp. 882 (D.D.C. 1993).

*Animal Welfare Act, as Amended. U.S. Code.* Title 7, secs. 2131–2156.

Brody, Mimi. 1989. "Animal Research: A Call for Legislative Reform Requiring Ethical Merit Review." *Harvard Environmental Law Review* 13(2): 423–484.

"Concentration Camps for Dogs." 1966. *Life,* 4 February, 22–29.

Dresser, Rebecca. 1988. "Assessing Harm and Justification in Animal Research: Federal Policy Opens the Laboratory Door." *Rutgers Law Review* 40(3): 723–795.

Francione, Gary L. 1990. "Access to Animal Care Committees." *Rutgers Law Review* 43(1): 1–14.

*Health Research Extension Act of 1985.* U.S. Public Law 99–158.

*Laboratory Animal Welfare Act of 1966.* U.S. Public Law 89–544.

National Institutes of Health. Office of Laboratory Animal Welfare. 2002. *Public Health Service Policy on Humane Use of Laboratory Animals,* rev. edition. Washington, D.C.: Author.

National Research Council (NRC). Commission on Life Sciences. Institute of Laboratory Animal Resources. 1996. *Guide for the Care and Use of Laboratory Animals,* revised edition. Washington, D.C.: National Academy Press.

National Research Council (NRC). Commission on Life Sciences. Institute of Laboratory Animal Resources. Committee on Educational Programs in Laboratory Animal Science. 1991. *Education and Training in the Care and Use of Laboratory Animals: A Guide for Developing Institutional Programs.* Washington, D.C.: National Academy Press.

National Research Council (NRC). Commission on Life Sciences. Institute of Laboratory Animal Resources. Committee on Pain and Distress in Laboratory Animals. 1992. *Recognition and Alleviation of Pain and Distress in Laboratory Animals.* Washington, D.C.: National Academy Press.

Orlans, F. Barbara. 1987. "Research Protocol Review for Animal Welfare." *Investigative Radiology* 22(3): 253–258.

Orlans, F. Barbara. 1993. *In the Name of Science: Issues in Responsible Animal Experimentation.* New York: Oxford University Press.

Orlans, F. Barbara. 2000. "The Injustice of Excluding Laboratory Rats, Mice, and Birds from the Animal Welfare Act." *Kennedy Inst of Ethics Journal* 10(3): 229–238.

Rozmiarek, Harry. 1987. "Current and Future Policies regarding Laboratory Animal Welfare." *Investigative Radiology* 22(2): 175–179.

Russell, William M. S., and Burch, Rex L. 1959; reprint 1992. *The Principles of Humane Experimental Technique.* Potters Bar, Eng.: Universities Federation for Animal Welfare.

Southwick, Ron. "Researchers Face More Federal Scrutiny on Animal Experimentation." *Chronicle of Higher Education,* June 28, 2002, p. 23.

Whitney, Robert A., Jr. 1987. "Animal Care and Use Committees: History and Current National Policies in the United States." *Laboratory Animal Science* 37(suppl.): 18–21.

# ANIMAL WELFARE AND RIGHTS

• • •

I. Ethical Perspectives on the Treatment and Status of Animals

II. Vegetarianism

III. Wildlife Conservation and Management

IV. Pet and Companion Animals

V. Zoos and Zoological Parks

VI. Animals in Agriculture and Factory Farming

## I. ETHICAL PERSPECTIVES ON THE TREATMENT AND STATUS OF ANIMALS

Normative ethical theory may be conceived as the systematic inquiry into the moral limits on human freedom. Philosophers and theologians throughout history and across cultures have offered different, often contradictory, answers to the central question of ethics thus conceived. Some have argued, for example, that the only justified limits on human freedom are those grounded in the rational self-interest of the agent, while others have maintained that the foundations of morality, and thus the basis of morally justified limitations on human freedom, are logically distinct from self-interest, though not from the dictates of reason. Still others have alleged that the foundations of morality have nothing to do with either reason or self-interest.

In view of the variety and conflicting nature of answers to the central question of normative ethics, it is hardly surprising that ethical theories sometimes offer strikingly different accounts of the moral status of those nonhuman animals we humans raise or hunt for food and clothing, use as beasts of burden, train to entertain us, and utilize as models for purposes of biomedical research. No philosopher or theologian has gone so far as to say that, from the moral point of view, there are no justified limits on what we may do to these animals. Even René Descartes, much celebrated for his theory that nonhuman animals are automata and thus incapable of feeling either pain or pleasure (Descartes, "Animals Are Machines," in Regan and Singer, 1976; 1989), is said to have treated his dog humanely. At a certain minimal level, then, all normative ethical theories speak with one voice. But at other levels, the differences are both real and deep.

## Direct and Indirect Duties

These differences emerge clearly when we consider how competing theories answer two distinct but related questions. The first asks, What are the grounds for morally limiting human freedom when it comes to human interactions with nonhuman animals? The second asks, How extensive are these moral limits on human freedom? The former inquires as to why human freedom should be limited at all when our actions affect other animals; the latter challenges us to investigate how much our freedom should be limited. Of the two questions, the first is the more basic, for the reasons given in support of views about how much our freedom should be limited ultimately are based on views about why our freedom should be limited in the first place.

Two opposed possibilities present themselves as answers to the first, more basic question. One possibility holds that it is because of how animals themselves are affected or treated by human agents that we should limit our freedom. Viewed from this perspective, nonhuman animals are entitled to a certain kind of consideration or treatment. Because such views stress the idea that something is owed or is due directly to these animals, it is common to refer to them as "direct duty" views.

The second possibility, by contrast, locates the ground of moral constraint in some basis other than the animals. Viewed from this perspective, humans owe nothing to other animals, nor do these animals deserve any sort of treatment or consideration. Rather, human freedom should be limited because, for example, human cruelty to other animals will cause humans to treat one another cruelly. Because such views deny that we have duties directly to other animals, while recognizing that other factors should limit our freedom in our dealings with them, they are commonly referred to as "indirect duty" views.

All normative ethical theories, as they address the moral status of nonhuman animals, fall into one or the other of these two classes. That is, either they affirm that we have direct duties to nonhuman animals, or they deny that we have direct duties. Some of the major theoretical options within each class, as these have been developed by ethicists within the history of Western thought, will be considered in what follows.

## Abolition, Reform, and Status Quo

As noted earlier, a second important question asks how much our freedom should be limited in our dealings with other animals. Three sorts of options may be distinguished: abolitionist, reformist, and status quo. An abolitionist position argues on behalf of ending human practices that routinely utilize nonhuman animals (for example, as a source of food or as models in scientific research). A reformist position accepts these institutions in principle but seeks in various ways to improve them in practice (for example, by enlarging the cages for animals used in research). A status quo position, unlike the abolitionist position, accepts these institutions in principle and, unlike the reformist position, does not recognize the need to improve them. Representative examples of each outlook and their logical relationship to competing normative ethical theories will be explained below.

While the heated, sometimes acrimonious, debate among partisans of abolition, reform, and the status quo captures the attention of the media, far less attention has been devoted to the critical assessment of the competing ethical philosophies, whether of the direct or indirect duty variety. This by itself suggests the degree to which the public debate over "animal rights," broadly conceived, has assumed the greater part of what is most in need of informed, critical reflection. For clearly, whether we should favor the goals of supporters of abolition, reform, or the status quo in practice depends on determining the most adequate account of how we should treat nonhuman animals in theory. It is to a consideration of some of the major options in ethical theory that this entry now turns.

## Perfectionism

Aristotle (384–322 B.C.E.) presents the broad outlines of a moral theory that goes by the name "perfectionism." The cornerstone of this theory has a high degree of initial plausibility. Justice, it is claimed, consists in giving to individuals what they are due, and those individuals whose character is morally better (more "perfect") than the character of others prima facie deserve more of what is good in life than do other, less good people. Aristotle's accounts of what makes people morally better and of "the good of man" have helped shape much of Western moral theory. Concerning the latter first, Aristotle accepts the commonplace notion that the good we humans seek is happiness, but he argues that the true happiness we seek is not wealth, fame, or even pleasure in abundance but, rather, the possession and exercise of those virtues (those "excellences") that are uniquely human. Thus happiness, in his view, is characterized as "an activity of the soul in accordance with virtue." Those are happiest who optimally express their humanity in how they live and, in doing so, take pleasure in being the human beings they are.

As for the moral virtues (prudence, justice, courage, and temperance), Aristotle characterizes each as a mean between the extremes of excess and deficiency. A courageous person, for example, is neither foolhardy (an excess) nor cowardly (a deficiency); a courageous person has the right mix of the willingness to take risks and the fear of doing so. Among the intellectual virtues, a detached, contemplative wisdom, wherein one knows eternal truths and in this way shares in that knowledge possessed by the gods, is the highest. In the case of both the moral and the intellectual virtues, finally, the human capacity to reason plays a decisive role. For man is, in Aristotle's view, unique in being "a rational animal," and "the good of man" consists in actualizing, to the fullest extent possible, those unique potentialities that define what it is to be human. Thus, since those are happiest who optimally express their humanity in how they live, those are happiest who exercise their reason optimally.

Because it prescribes the distribution of what is good in life on the basis of one's possessing the favored virtues and, thus, on the basis of degrees of human perfection, perfectionism can—and in Aristotle's hands, does—sanction or require radically inegalitarian treatment of different individuals. In the case of nonhuman animals in particular, perfectionism provides no direct protection. Despite his teaching, in sharp contrast to Descartes's, that these animals share many of the same psychological capacities possessed by humans—including, for example, sensation and desire—Aristotle confidently denies that they share the capacity to reason. Moreover, because in his view the "lesser" exists to serve the interests or purposes of the "greater," Aristotle maintains that nonhuman animals exist for the purpose of advancing the good of human beings. He writes: "Other animals exist for the sake of man, the tame for use and food, the wild, if not all, at least the greater part of them, for food, and for the provision of clothing and various instruments" (Aristotle, "Animals and Slavery," in Regan and Singer, 1976, p. 110; 1989, p. 5). There is no implication here that Aristotle's teachings permit the wanton infliction of pain on nonhuman animals for no good reason. What is clear is that because he recognizes no greater purpose for nonhuman animals than to serve the interests of human beings, Aristotle can recognize only indirect duties in their case. Finally, while many of today's more controversial practices involving human utilization of nonhuman animals, such as factory farming and animal-to-human organ transplants, were unknown in his day, all the available evidence seems to indicate that Aristotle was well disposed to the status quo with respect to the relevant practices current while he was alive.

It is not only nonhuman animals, however, that exist for the sake of those who are more perfect. In general, women do not measure up to Aristotle's standards of "the good of man." "The male is by nature superior, and the female inferior," he writes, "and the one rules, and the other is ruled; this principle, of necessity, extends to all mankind" (ibid.). Moreover, some humans, whether male or female, lack the ability to grasp through reason those truths understood by the more virtuous among us; of such individuals Aristotle writes that they are "slave[s] by nature" (ibid.). And so it is that Aristotle affirms the obvious parallel, given the form perfectionism takes in his hands, between the moral status of human slaves and nonhuman animals: "The use made of slaves and of tame animals is not very different; for both with their bodies minister to the needs of life" (ibid.). Those humans who, because of their superior rationality, are morally more perfect are entitled to make use of those, whether human or not, who lack the virtues defining human perfection.

Few today will publicly embrace Aristotle's perfectionism. Not only does his view of women offend the emancipated gender egalitarianism of our time, but the comfortable elitism and classism that enable him to pronounce some humans "slaves by nature" will find no home among the most basic precepts of contemporary moral, political, and legal thought. The practical implications for humans of the fundamental principle of Aristotelian perfectionism—that those who are lacking in reason exist to serve the interests of those who are most virtuous—is morally offensive. It is one thing to affirm that those people who are more perfect than others prima facie deserve more of what is good in life; it is quite another to maintain that those who are less perfected exist for the sole purpose of ministering to the more virtuous. Moreover, since we cannot rationally defend the exploitation of some humans on the grounds that "by nature" they lack the potential to acquire the virtues possessed by those who exploit them, we cannot rationally defend human exploitation of nonhuman animals by offering an analogous defense—cannot, that is, rationally defend such exploitation by claiming that nonhuman animals "by nature" lack the potential to acquire uniquely human virtues.

## Despotism and Stewardship

An alternative to Aristotle's philosophy is rooted in the biblical teaching that the God of Judaism and Christianity gives human beings dominion over nature in general and other animals in particular. As so often happens, however, there is more than one way to interpret the biblical message. Two ways in which human dominion can be understood—despotism and stewardship—will be sketched here.

Despotism teaches that nature in general and the other animals in particular are created by God for the sake of humans, and thus are ordained by the divine creator to serve such myriad human purposes as a source of food and clothing. Nothing within the natural order, save humans, has value in and of itself; what value the natural world possesses is entirely dependent on the extent to which it serves human interests. In this sense, human interests *are* the measure of all things, at least all things of value. Various biblical passages are cited to confirm the despotic reading, for example, "Then God said, 'Let us make man in our image, after our likeness; and let them have dominion over the fish of the sea, and over the birds of the air, and over the cattle … and over all the earth'" (Gen. 1:26).

Seen in this light, despotism's appeal to what God has ordained provides a reason for human supremacy over nonhuman animals that Aristotle's appeal to what is guaranteed "by nature" seems to lack, and it is a small step from acceptance of the despotic interpretation of human dominion to the conclusion that we owe nothing to nonhuman animals. Thus we find Saint Thomas Aquinas (ca. 1225–1274), for example, urging in words barely distinguishable from those of Aristotle except for their reference to God that it is by "Divine ordinance that the life of animals and plants is preserved not for themselves but for man" (Thomas Aquinas, "On Killing Living Things and the Duty to Love Irrational Creatures," in Regan and Singer, 1976, p. 119; 1989, p. 11). Mindful, moreover, that some biblical passages prohibit cruelty to nonhuman animals, Aquinas firmly places himself within the indirect duty tradition when he maintains that the import of such prohibitions is, for example, "to remove man's thoughts from being cruel to other men, and lest through being cruel to animals one become cruel to human beings" (Thomas Aquinas, "Differences between Rational and Other Creatures," in Regan and Singer, 1976, p. 59; 1989, p. 9).

To the extent that Saint Thomas's philosophy is rooted in the Scripture of the Christian tradition, those who stand outside this tradition are unlikely to be persuaded that God established in nature what nature was incapable of establishing by itself. Even granting biblical underpinnings to one's ethic, moreover, questions arise concerning the accuracy of the despotic interpretation of human dominion. While the Hebrew concept of *rada*, translated as "having dominion," often is interpreted to mean human despotism over the nonhuman world—an idea that, according to some early critics (White; McHarg), is the root cause of today's environmental crisis—a significantly different interpretation has been proposed by more recent thinkers (Barr; Linzey, 1987; McDaniel; Callicott, 1993).

For *rada* can be understood as the idea of human responsibility toward and care for a created order that is good independent of the human presence. According to this latter interpretation, commonly referred to as stewardship, humans are given the task of being as loving within the natural order as God was in creating the natural order in the first place. Humans, that is, are to be the loving caretakers of an independently good creation. Because, viewed from the stewardship perspective, the natural world in general, and those nonhuman animals with whom we share it in particular, are good apart from human interests, our duties with regard to these animals emerge as direct duties owed to them rather than indirect duties owed either to other humans or to their creator.

Although when thus interpreted all of creation is seen as having a kind of value that is independent of human interests, the value of nonhuman animals arguably is especially noteworthy. One might note, first, that these animals were created on the same day—the sixth—as were humans (Gen. 1:24–27); that in the original state of perfection, in Eden, humans did not eat other animals (Gen. 1:29); and that, in God's covenant with Noah after the flood (Gen. 9:8–12), animals (but not plants) are included. Using these images, one can argue that the choice we face today is *either* to continue to move further from the sort of relationship with the animals God hoped would prevail when the world was created *or* to make daily efforts to recapture that relationship—to journey back to Eden, as it were. Given this latter reading, the practical consequences of a stewardship interpretation of dominion would depart significantly from those favored by the status quo position, just as the goals one would hope to achieve would differ from those advanced by reformists. For if our righteous relationship with the other animals, in our capacities as their caretakers and protectors, is one of nonutilization (they are not to be eaten, not to be worn, etc.), then the stewardship interpretation of human dominion would seem to support an abolitionist ideal.

However these matters are to be settled, the biblical grounding of morality characteristic of both despotism and stewardship places these moral perspectives outside the mainstream of normative ethical theory, at least from the Enlightenment forward, where rigorous, imaginative attempts have been made to ground ethics independently of belief in God and the moral authority of the Bible. One such attempt is contractarianism.

## Contractarianism

Among the most influential nontheological political and moral theories, contractarianism has a legacy that reaches at least as far back as Thomas Hobbes (1588–1679) and, among our contemporaries, includes such notable philosophers as John Rawls (1971) and Jan Narveson (1988). Like other theorists united by a common outlook, contractarians often disagree on many of the most fundamental points. It will not be possible to do justice to the rich fabric of disagreement that characterizes proponents of the theories under review.

As its name suggests, contractarianism conceives of morality as a kind of contract into which people (the "contractors") enter voluntarily. For contractarians, morality emerges as a set of mutually agreed upon and enforceable constraints on human freedom, constraints that each party to the contract rationally believes to be in his or her own self-interest. There is, then, according to contractarian theory, nothing that by its nature is morally right or wrong, just or unjust; rather, acts or institutions become right or wrong, just or unjust, as a result of the agreements reached by rational, self-interested contractors. In this sense, all of morality is conventional, and none is natural. Morality is created, not discovered, by human beings.

Both the self-interest that motivates and the rationality that guides the contractors are significant. We are not to imagine that people, as they deliberate about what limits on their freedom they will accept, are motivated by a natural sympathy for the misfortune of others or that they are willing altruistically to accept personal loss so that others might gain. Each contractor is motivated exclusively by his or her self-interest. The conception of individual self-interest each contractor has, moreover, is neither whimsical nor uninformed. Each person asks the same basic question: From the point of view of what is best for me, rationally considered, what limitations on my freedom would I be willing to accept? Morality, understood as rational, enforceable constraints on human freedom, arises when all the contractors jointly agree on the same constraints, not out of sympathy for others or because of altruistic motivations, but because each judges the outcome to be in his or her personal self-interest.

Two fundamentally opposed forms of contractarianism may be distinguished. The first permits the contractors to enter into their contractual deliberations equipped with the knowledge of who they are and what they want out of life, given their individual interests, talents, and hopes. This is the form of contractarianism favored by Hobbes and Narveson, for example. The second, favored by Rawls, requires that the contractors imagine that they lack such detailed knowledge of their individual psychology and circumstances, and instead deliberate about the terms of the contract from behind what Rawls calls "a veil of ignorance." Why Rawls would have recourse to this imaginative point of view will be explained momentarily. First, however, the implications of Hobbesian contractarianism for the treatment of nonhuman animals deserve attention.

Judged on the basis of the interests of these animals, the implications are not particularly salutary. In view of their inability to express these interests and to negotiate with others, nonhuman animals obviously are not to be counted among the potential contractors. Moreover, even while it is true that some things are in the interests of pigs and wolves, for example, the idea that these animals can have an informed understanding of what is in their rational self-interest has no clear meaning. Not surprisingly, therefore, what protection these animals are provided by Hobbesian contractarianism necessarily depends on what interests the human contractarians happen to have in them.

Narveson, for one, cheerfully indicates that this need not be very much (Narveson, "A Defense of Meat Eating," in Regan and Singer, 1989). Because many contractors have a special place in their hearts for companion animals ("pets"), these animals will be treated reasonably well, not because they are entitled to such treatment but because we owe it to their human friends not to upset them (these humans) gratuitously. In the case of most other nonhuman animals, however, including those slaughtered for food or used in research, Narveson finds no good reason to cease and desist. Clearly, then, given Hobbesian contractarianism, all our duties with respect to other animals are indirect duties owed to those human beings who help forge the contract. And just as clearly, considered from a political perspective, one finds little within this version of contractarianism that could mount an abolitionist or a far-reaching reformist approach to how other animals are treated; what one finds instead is a theory well disposed to the status quo while remaining open to modest reforms.

Critics of Hobbesian contractarianism have raised various objections (Regan, 1983). One concerns the possibility of arbitrary discrimination between people—for example, discrimination based on race. If we imagine that a large majority of potential contractors (say, 95%) are white, and the remainder black, then it is not obviously irrational for those who comprise the majority to exclude members of the minority from negotiating the contract; perhaps the majority might even agree to keep the minority in bondage, as chattel slaves, the better to advance the rational self-interests of those individuals comprising the majority. That such an arrangement would be unjust seems too obvious to need a supporting argument. And (for Hobbesian contractarianism) there's the rub. For since what is just and unjust is created by the agreements reached by the contractors, there is, within this form of contractarianism, no theoretical grounding for the evident injustice involved in excluding the minority from participating. The theory, that is, not only fails to illuminate why such discrimination is unjust, but it also seems to deprive us of the means even to raise this objection. If a moral theory is so fundamentally flawed when it comes to how human beings, given their differences in skin pigmentation, should be treated, it is unclear how it can be any nearer the truth when it comes to how nonhuman beings, given their species differences, should be treated.

Rawls's introduction of the veil of ignorance, mentioned earlier, can be interpreted as his attempt to preserve the spirit of Hobbesian contractarianism while departing importantly from the letter. Rawls invites would-be contractors to imagine themselves in what he calls the "original position," in which, because they deliberate from behind the veil of ignorance, they do not know when they will be born or where, whether they will be rich or poor, of exceptional intelligence or below average, male or female, Caucasian or non-Caucasian. The question now to be asked, by each of the contractors, is what limits on human freedom each would accept, in the face of such profound ignorance concerning such details.

The full scope of Rawls's answer need not concern us. Only two points are of particular importance here. The first concerns how Rawlsian contractarianism improves on Hobbesian contractarianism when it addresses the issue of discrimination based on race. Hobbesian contractors, as noted above, can have a self-interested reason for accepting such discrimination, given that they know they belong to a racial majority. Rawlsian contractors, in contrast, lack such a reason since, for all they know, they might be one of the minority. In this respect, Rawlsian contractarianism seems to represent a notable improvement over Hobbesian contractarianism.

Despite its apparent strengths in response to issues involving arbitrary discrimination, Rawls's account of the moral status of nonhuman animals seems to fail to live up to its own standards (VanDeVeer). While the imaginary contractors behind the veil of ignorance are denied detailed knowledge about their individual interests and circumstances, and thus do not know whether, say, they will be male or female, black or white, Rawls does permit them to know that they will be born as human beings. To allow knowledge of this detail, however, seems to prejudice the case against nonhuman animals from the start. Granted, rational, self-interested contractors, making choices from behind the veil of ignorance, will negotiate direct duties to human beings and indirect ones to nonhumans, if they know they will be born human. But this only shows that these contractors will discriminate against these animals if they are provided with an arbitrary reason for doing so. In short, neither Hobbesian nor Rawlsian contractarianism seems to offer a reasonable basis on which to ground the only duties each recognizes in the case of nonhuman animals: indirect duties.

## Kantianism

A final example of an indirect duty view is provided by the great Prussian philosopher Immanuel Kant (1724–1804). In some respects Kant's moral philosophy regarding the treatment of nonhuman animals is an amalgam of Aristotle's and, stripped of its appeals to God, Aquinas's. In concert with both, Kant emphasizes rationality as the defining characteristic of being human and, echoing Saint Thomas, objects to cruelty to animals because of the deleterious effect this has on how humans are treated. "He who is cruel to animals," Kant writes, "becomes hard also in his dealings with men," whereas "tender feelings towards dumb animals develop humane feelings towards mankind" (Kant, "Duties in Regard to Animals," in Regan and Singer, 1976, p. 123; 1989, p. 24).

Despite these historical echoes, Kant's moral philosophy is in many ways highly original. Of particular note is his thesis that humanity exists as an "end in itself." Kant does not attempt to prove this thesis by appeal to some more basic principle; rather, it is set forth as a postulate in his system. In this capacity it places humans and other rational, autonomous beings in a unique moral category that distinguishes them, as "persons," from everything else that exists. Like Aristotle and Aquinas before him, Kant views the rest of the natural order as existing to serve human interests. In particular, animals, in his words, exist "merely as a means to an end. That end is man" (ibid.). Thus, whereas in Kant's view we are morally free to use other animals as we wish, subject only to the injunction to avoid cruelty, we are not morally free to treat human beings in a comparable fashion. Because humans exist as ends in themselves, we are never to treat them merely as means, Kant argues, which is what we would be doing if we treated them as we treat other animals (for example, if we raised humans as a food source). An abolitionist, a radical reformist, Kant is not. Provided only that we are not cruel in our treatment of nonhuman animals, we do nothing wrong when we treat them as we do.

A common objection against Kant's position is the argument from marginal cases (Regan, 1983; for criticism of this argument, see Narveson, 1977). All humans, Kant implies, exist as ends in themselves. To restrict this supreme moral value to humans among terrestrial creatures is not arbitrary, Kant believes, because humans, unlike the other animals, are unique in being rational and autonomous. However, not all humans are rational and autonomous. Those who are mentally enfeebled or deranged, for example, lack these capacities. Are these humans nevertheless ends in themselves? If Kant's answer is affirmative, then it is not the presence of rationality and autonomy that ground this supreme moral value; if, on the other hand, Kant's answer is negative, then it follows that these "marginal" human beings do not exist as ends in themselves, in which case it would seem that they, no less than other animals, may be treated as mere means. Because one assumes that this latter consequence would be seen by Kant to be morally grotesque, it seems fair to assume that he would want to avoid it; but he can do so, it seems, only by accepting the view that individuals who are neither rational nor autonomous nevertheless exist as ends in themselves, a view that undermines his confident assertion that nonhuman animals, deficient in reason and autonomy, exist "merely as means to an end," the end being "man."

## Utilitarianism

The pioneering work of the nineteenth-century utilitarians Jeremy Bentham (1748–1832) and John Stuart Mill (1806–1873) represents a significant departure from the Aristotelian legacy we find in Kant's moral theory. Bentham, referring to nonhuman animals, writes, "The question is not, Can they *reason?* nor, Can they *talk?* but, Can they *suffer?*" (Bentham, "A Utilitarian View," in Regan and Singer, 1976, p. 130; 1989, p. 26). The possession of sentience (the capacity to experience pleasure and pain), not the possession of rationality, nor autonomy, nor linguistic competence, entitles any individual to direct moral consideration; and it is the possession of this particular capacity, in Bentham's and Mill's view, that creates in humans the direct duty not to cause nonhuman animals to suffer needlessly. We owe it to these animals themselves, not to those humans who might be affected by what we do, to take their (the nonhuman animals') pleasures and pains into account and, having done so, to ensure that we never make them suffer without good reason.

Both Bentham and Mill give a utilitarian interpretation of what such a good reason might be. Utilitarianism, roughly speaking, is the view that our duty is to perform that act that will bring about the best consequences for all those affected by the outcome. For value hedonists like Bentham and Mill, who recognize only one intrinsic good, pleasure, and only

one intrinsic evil, pain, the best consequences will be those that include the greatest possible balance of pleasure over pain. A good reason for permitting animal suffering, then, is that such suffering is a necessary price to pay in bringing about the best consequences, all considered. How much of the spirit of reform, abolition, or the status quo happens to characterize individual utilitarians depends on how much animal suffering is judged to be necessary. Bentham opposes hunting, fishing, and the baiting of animals for sport, for example, while Mill's name is to be found among the earliest contributors to England's Royal Society for the Prevention of Cruelty to Animals. But neither Bentham nor Mill aligns himself with the cause of antivivisection, and both are lifelong meat eaters. So reformers they are, but abolitionists they are not. Even so, in their time, and given the broader social context in which they lived, they were seen by many of their contemporaries as radicals, if not extremists.

The degree to which utilitarians can differ over important practical matters is illustrated in our time by Peter Singer and R. G. Frey. Singer is justly famous for his seminal 1975 book, *Animal Liberation,* while Frey has written two books (1980, 1983) and many essays devoted to the issues under review. The two philosophers, while agreeing on some of the most fundamental points in ethical theory, disagree on many of the most important consequences each believes follow from the application of utilitarianism, including how nonhuman animals should be treated. For example, in *Animal Liberation* Singer advocates vegetarianism, on moral grounds; Frey disagrees, appealing to the same grounds in his *Rights, Killing, and Suffering: Moral Vegetarianism and Applied Ethics* (1983). It will be useful to explain how such profound disagreements can arise between partisans of the same moral philosophy.

By its very nature, utilitarianism is a forward-looking moral theory. The consequences of our actions, and the consequences alone, determine the morality of what we do. As such, utilitarians will reach opposing judgments about what is right and wrong if they have opposing views of what the consequences of a given act will be. In the case of vegetarianism in particular, utilitarians like Singer believe that, taking everyone's interests into account, and counting equal interests equally, the consequences that flow from abstaining from animal flesh will be better than if people continue to include animal flesh in their diets; Frey, however, believes that the consequences of a vegetarian diet are not sufficiently better so as to impose an obligation on us to become vegetarians. It is, then, factual disagreements over what the future might hold that underlie the type of moral disagreement separating Singer and Frey on the issue of vegetarianism.

Some critics of utilitarianism (e.g., Clark) argue that the apparently unresolvable impasse created by Singer's and Frey's application of utilitarian theory to the particular case of vegetarianism illustrates a major weakness in utilitarian theory in general. Because so much—indeed, because everything—depends on our ability to know what will happen in the future, and in view of the limitations of human knowledge in this regard, utilitarianism, these critics maintain, reduces moral judgment to guesswork about what might or might not occur.

Despite this problem, utilitarianism may seem to be a congenial theory for those who utilize nonhuman animals in animal model research. The most common justification of such research consists in appealing to the improvements in human health and longevity to which this research allegedly has led; and while researchers may recognize the need to look for alternatives to the animal model, lest these animals be used unnecessarily, it seems clear that the moral justification they offer is utilitarian. (For dissenting voices regarding the human benefits of such research, from the perspective of the history of medicine, see McKinlay and McKinlay; for epistemological concerns, see LaFollette and Shanks). Part of the enduring greatness of *Animal Liberation* lies in Singer's relentless documentation of how much of this research prima facie fails to meet the utilitarian standard favored by researchers themselves. No less important is the way Singer exposes a prejudice that he, following Richard Ryder (1975), denominates "speciesism," and that he characterizes as "an attitude of bias in favor of the interests of members of one's own species and against those of other species" (Singer, 1990, p. 6). Research scientists, Singer believes, frequently offer at best half a utilitarian justification of their work: Human interests are considered; those of nonhuman animals are not. To be consistent, the interests of both must be counted, and counted equitably. It is Singer's considered judgment that few researchers are consistent in this regard.

Frey, too, examines the lack of moral consistency among researchers ("Vivisection, Morals, and Medicine," in Regan and Singer, 1989). Given any reasonable view about the richness and variety of psychological life, it is unquestionably true, Frey believes, that the psychological life of nonhuman primates, or even that of a cat or a dog, is richer and more varied than the psychological life of some human beings (a child born with only the stem of the brain, for example). Thus, if the moral defense of animal model research is supposed to lie in the good results allegedly produced by using these animals, then a similar defense for utilizing marginal humans is at hand. To be consistent in their utilitarianism, therefore, Frey believes that researchers should be willing to conduct their studies on marginal humans—a finding researchers are unlikely to welcome. Frey is unperturbed, insisting that researchers cannot have it both ways, using utilitarian modes of thinking when they believe it justifies their practice of using other than human animals in their studies, only to discard utilitarianism when its implications for the selection of marginal humans as research subjects are made manifest.

Whatever form utilitarianism takes, one of the principal objections its advocates face centers on questions of justice (Lyons). What limits, if any, can utilitarianism recognize on how future good is to be obtained? The theory seems to imply that good ends justify whatever means are necessary to achieve them, including means that are flagrantly unjust. Classic examples include situations in which the judicial execution of the innocent is sanctioned on the grounds that others will be deterred from committing similar offenses. Here, critics concede, good consequences are brought into being, but the means used to secure them are reprehensible because they are unjust.

Utilitarians have replies to this and similar lines of criticism that go beyond the scope of the present entry (Brandt). Suffice it to say that among those philosophers who are not utilitarians, many dissociate themselves from utilitarianism because they believe that respect for the rights of the individual is a principle that should not be compromised in the name of achieving some greater good for others. Not surprisingly, perhaps, a position of this kind, one that prohibits the use of nonhuman animals in the name of advancing the general human welfare, has been advanced (Regan, 1983). Though not the only possible theory of animal rights (see, e.g., Rollin, 1981, 1989), this particular theory (the "rights view") can be seen as an attempt to blend certain features of utilitarianism and Kant's theory.

## The Rights View

Kant, it will be recalled, recognizes only indirect duties to nonhuman animals; we humans are not to be cruel to animals, for example, not because we treat them wrongly by our cruel treatment but because cruelty to animals can lead people to be cruel to one another. By contrast, utilitarians from Bentham to Singer recognize direct duties to nonhuman animals; they believe that there are certain things we owe to these animals, apart from how humans will be effected. On this divisive issue the rights view sides with utilitarians against Kantians: Nonhuman animals are of direct moral significance; we have direct duties in their case.

In a second respect, however, the rights view sides with Kantians against utilitarians. Utilitarians believe that duty is determined by the comparative value of consequences; the right thing to do is what causes the best results. Kant and his followers take a decidedly different view: What is right does not depend on the value of consequences, it depends on the appropriate, respectful treatment of the individual—in particular, whether humans are treated as ends, not merely as means. In this regard, the rights view is cut from Kantian, not utilitarian, cloth. What is right depends not on the value of consequences but on the appropriate, respectful treatment of the individual, including individual nonhuman animals. Thus, the fundamental principle of the rights view (the respect principle) is Kantian in spirit: We are always to treat individuals who exist as ends in themselves (those who have "inherent value") with respect, which means, in part, that we are never to treat them merely as means.

One problem the rights view faces concerns which nonhuman animals possess value of this kind. Like other line-drawing issues ("Exactly how tall do you have to be to be tall?" "Exactly how old do you have to be to be old?"), this one has no precise resolution, in part because the criterion for drawing the line is imprecise. The criterion the rights view proposes is that of being the subject of a life, a criterion that specifies a set of psychological capacities (the capacities to desire, remember, act intentionally, and feel emotions, for example) as jointly sufficient. At least some nonhuman animals (e.g., mammals and birds) arguably possess these capacities, thus are subjects of a life, and thus, given the rights view, are to be treated as ends in themselves. (For criticism, see Frey, 1980).

Such a view, for obvious reasons, has massive political, social, and moral implications concerning how these animals ought to be treated. From an animal rights perspective of this kind, the abolition of human exploitation of these animals, whether on the farm, at the lab, or in the wild—not merely the reform of these practices, and certainly not approval of the status quo—is what duty requires.

Line-drawing issues aside, the rights view faces daunting challenges from other quarters. One concerns the idea of inherent value. Some critics (e.g., Sapontzis) allege that the idea is "mystifying," meaning that it lacks any clear meaning. Advocates of animal rights reply that the notion of inherent value is no less "mystifying" than Kant's idea of end in itself. As applied to human beings, Kant's idea of end in itself attempts to articulate the cherished belief that the value or worth of a human being is not reducible to instrumental value—not reducible, that is, to how useful a human being happens to be in forwarding the interests or purposes of other human beings. Neither John Doe nor Jane Doe, in Kant's view, exists as a mere resource relative to what other people want for themselves, and to treat the Does as if their value—their worth or dignity—consists merely in their

resource or instrumental value for others is morally wrong. All that the rights view alleges, then, is that to be consistent, the same moral judgment must be made in those cases where nonhuman animals that are subjects of a life are treated in a similar fashion.

Another set of challenges alleges that the philosophy of animal rights, if acted upon, would lead to catastrophic consequences, either to human interests in particular or to the community of life in general. Concerning the former challenge, some critics argue that human health and longevity would be seriously harmed if, as the philosophy of animal rights requires, nonhuman animals ceased to be used as models of human disease (see C. R. Gallistel, "The Case for Unrestricted Research Using Animals," in Regan and Singer, 1989; and Cohen). Several responses seem apposite.

First, given the massive allocation of public monies that fund such research, it needs to be asked whether abandoning reliance on the whole-animal model really is contrary to what is in the collective best interests of human beings. Some (e.g., Sharpe) argue that customary reliance on this well-entrenched scientific methodology retards the development of alternative methodologies that would be more useful in understanding and curing major human diseases; in addition, these critics insist that humans would benefit more if the dominant focus of biomedical research were shifted away from curing disease to preventing it, a goal that is more efficiently advanced, these critics allege, by methodologies other than the use of the whole-animal model.

Second, recall one of the fundamental objections raised against utilitarianism: Just as one does not justify the violation of a human being's rights because doing so will benefit others, so one does not justify the violation of the rights of nonhuman animals on similar grounds. More generally, some gains others might obtain may be ill-gotten, and they are ill-gotten if the price of obtaining them involves the violation of another's rights. Thus, even if it is true that humans stand to lose some benefits if animal model research is abandoned, this by itself does not constitute a telling moral objection to the abolitionist implications of the philosophy of animal rights, assuming that these animals, like humans, have the right to be treated as ends in themselves.

Concerning the second line of criticism—the one alleging that acting on the philosophy of animal rights would have catastrophic implications for the community of life in general—the principal objection may be summarized as follows. Predatory animals obviously live off the death and flesh of their prey. Because prey animals have the right to be treated with respect, according to the rights view, critics (e.g., Callicott, 1980; Sagoff) allege that it follows that we should intervene to stop predatory animals in their natural depredations. However, if we were to do this, there would be no check on the balance that exists in nature between predators and preys; instead, the population of prey animals would explode, and this would have the effect of irreparably damaging the balance and sustainability of life forms within the larger life community.

Advocates of the philosophy of animal rights have a number of possible replies to the predation problem, the principal one of which is the following. Situations can and do arise where the right thing to do is to come to the assistance of another, whether the potential victim is a human or a nonhuman animal. However, in these situations the potential victim not only is at risk of serious injury but also is less than capable of mounting a defense. Thus, an elderly woman who is attacked by a psychotic killer, or a puppy who is being tormented by children, merits our intervention. But the predator–prey relationship seems to bear little resemblance to such cases. Most prey animals, most of the time, are perfectly capable of eluding their predators without anyone's assistance. Thus it would seem to be human arrogance, not informed responsibility, that would lead humans to believe that because animals in the wild have rights, we are duty bound to "police" nature. From an animal rights perspective, we have no general duty to intervene in predator–prey relations; that being so, the catastrophic environmental costs alleged to be implied by acting on the rights view seem to be more in the nature of fiction than of fact. (For a different response to the predation problem, see Sapontzis.)

## Deep Ecology

Despite the significant differences separating the philosophy of animal rights and other, more traditional moral theories, such as Kant's, there are important similarities. For example, like Kant's theory, the philosophy of animal rights recognizes the noninstrumental value of the individual; and animal rights philosophy, as is true not only of Kant's theory but of utilitarianism as well, articulates an abstract, universal, and impartial fundamental moral principle—abstract because the respect principle enjoins us to treat others with respect, without regard to time, or place, or circumstance; universal because the respect principle applies to everyone capable of making moral decisions; and impartial because this principle does not favor some individuals (e.g., family members or companion animals) over others. Some contemporary moral philosophers find this approach to ethics archaic; among these critics, some of those who classify themselves as deep ecologists (see, in particular, Devall and

Sessions) command a growing audience. (For a more systematic and in some ways different version of deep ecology, see Naess. For importantly different approaches to environmental ethics, see Taylor; Rolston; Callicott, 1980.)

Both traditional moral theories and the philosophy of animal rights are doubly to be faulted, according to Devall and Sessions—first, because these moral outlooks offer an overly intellectualized account of the moral life, and second, because they perpetuate the myth of the moral preeminence of the individual. Considering this latter charge first, Devall and Sessions argue that the concept of the isolated, atomistic individual, which arises out of the anthropocentric traditions of Western philosophy, is false to the facts of all life's embeddedness in the larger life community. People are not independent bits of mind existing by themselves; they are enmeshed in networks of relationships that bind them both to their evolutionary past and to their ecological present. Expressed another way, humans do not stand "above" or "apart from" nature; they stand "within" nature. And the natural world does not exist "for us," as a storehouse of renewable human resources (a view that is symptomatic of a "shallow" view of humanity's relationship to nature); we are inseparable from the natural environment (a view that indicates a "deeper" understanding of what it means to be human).

Thus, acceptance of the illusory concept of the isolated individual, existing outside the natural order, has done, and continues to do, incalculable damage to those who seek self-understanding. So long as we carry out this quest with a fundamentally flawed preconception of our place in the larger scheme of things, the longer we search, the less we will understand. As for the charge that traditional moral theories overintellectualize the moral life, Devall and Sessions argue that the moral life should be viewed as primarily experiential, not inferential, a life that is characterized by our coming to experience certain values in the concrete particularities of day-to-day life, rather than by apprehending abstract, universal, impartial moral principles by means of our rational powers.

Among those values to be found in the concrete particularities of day-to-day life, some involve other animals; and although deep ecologists have not written extensively on some of the most pressing practical issues, the general disdain these thinkers display toward reductionist science and industrial societies' technological domination of the natural world suggests that they would be strong reformists, at a minimum, in response to such practices as factory farming and animal model research. In the case of sport and recreational hunting, however, Devall and Sessions not only find nothing wrong, they applaud the practice. In pursuit of their prey, hunters tap into natural means whereby, through the act of killing, they can obtain greater self-understanding. Viewed in this light, Devall and Sessions seem to understand our duties with respect to animals as indirect duties limited by the overarching quest for self-knowledge. While, therefore, deep ecologists like Sessions and Devall can be counted upon to add their voices to those of reformists and abolitionists in some cases, they emerge as defenders of the status quo in others.

## Ecofeminism

Ecofeminists, not just advocates of the rights view, are among those contemporary moral philosophers who differ significantly with deep ecologists. Like other isms, ecofeminism is not a monolithic position (see Adams; Diamond and Orenstein; Warren; Gaard); instead, it represents a number of defining tendencies, including in particular a principled stance that puts its advocates on the side of those who historically have been victims of oppression. For obvious reasons, women are pictured as among the oppressed, but the scope of ecofeminism's concern is not limited to women. The same ideology that sanctions oppression based on gender, ecofeminists maintain, also sanctions oppression based on race, class, and physical abilities, for example; moreover, beyond the boundaries of our species, this same ideology, ecofeminists believe, sanctions the oppression of nature in general and of nonhuman animals in particular.

In a number of fundamental ways, ecofeminism's diagnosis of the ideology of oppression resembles deep ecology's diagnosis of the deficiencies of traditional moral theory. As is true of the latter, ecofeminism challenges the myth of the isolated individual, existing apart from the world, and instead affirms the interconnectedness of all life. Moreover, no less than deep ecologists, ecofeminists abjure the overintellecutalization of the moral life characteristic of traditional moral theories, with their abstract, universal, and impartial fundamental principles. But whereas deep ecologists locate the fundamental cause of moral theory gone awry in anthropocentrism (human-centeredness), ecofeminists argue that it is androcentrism (male-centeredness) that is the real cause.

Nowhere is this difference clearer than in the case of sport or recreational hunting. Devall and Sessions celebrate the value of this practice as a means of bonding ever more closely with the natural world, of discovering "self in Self"; ecofeminists, by contrast, detect in the hunt the vestiges of patriarchy—the male's need to dominate and subdue (Kheel). More fundamentally, there is the lingering suspicion that

deep ecologists continue to view the value of the natural world instrumentally, as a means to greater self-awareness and self-knowledge. In this respect, and despite appearances to the contrary, deep ecology does not represent a "paradigm shift" away from the anthropocentric worldview it aspires to replace.

Ecofeminists believe they offer a deeper account of the moral life than do deep ecologists, one that goes to the very foundations of Western moral theorizing. The idea of "the rights of the individual" is diagnosed as a symptom of patriarchal thought, rooted in the (male) myth of the isolated individual. Morally, a "paradigm shift" occurs when, in place of assertions of rights, we freely, lovingly choose to take care of and assume responsibility for those who are victims of oppression, both within and beyond the extended human family, other animals included. Writing for the growing number of ecofeminists, Josephine Donovan states:

> Natural rights and utilitarianism present impressive and useful arguments for the ethical treatment of animals. Yet, it is also possible—indeed, necessary—to ground that ethic in an emotional and spiritual conversation with nonhuman life forms. Out of a woman's relational culture of caring and attentive love [there] emerges the basis for a feminist ethic for the treatment of animals. We should not kill, eat, torture, and exploit animals because they do not want to be so treated, and we know that. If we listen, we can hear them. ("Animal Rights and Feminist Theory," in Gaard, p. 185)

Thus, whereas the grounds for practical action offered by ecofeminists differ fundamentally from those favored by the rights view, and despite the foundational gulf that separates these two theories, both philosophies arguably have the same abolitionist practical implications.

## Conclusion

The "animal rights debate," broadly conceived, is more than a contest of wills representing professional, economic, and ethical concerns; it is also a divisive, enduring topic in normative ethical theory (Vance). Until comparatively recently, discussions of the moral status of nonhuman animals had all but disappeared from the work of moral philosophers. (For a historical overview, see Ryder, 1989.) Beginning in the 1970s (Godlovitch et al.; Singer, 1975; Linzey, 1976; Clark), however, we have witnessed a historically unprecedented outpouring of philosophical and theological interest in exploring the moral ties that bind humans to other animals, and there is every indication that this interest will intensify in the coming decades. The moral theories of philosophers are not the stuff of politics; still, the contributions philosophers make can help shape the political debate by clarifying the major theoretical options available to an informed public.

Principal among these options are those that have been canvassed here: perfectionism, despotism and stewardship, contractarianism, Kantianism, utilitarianism, the rights view, deep ecology, and ecofeminism. Doubtless other options will evolve as the discussion continues (Garner). Among these options, two in particular—utilitarianism and the rights view—have offered the most systematic accounts of those duties owed directly to nonhuman animals. It will be instructive, before concluding, to highlight some of the important practical differences, particularly as these pertain to animal model research, that flow from these competing philosophies.

Because utilitarianism is committed to reducing the total amount of suffering in the world, its proponents must be prepared to recognize the moral legitimacy of some research on nonhuman animals. Even Peter Singer, contemporary utilitarianism's most forceful critic of such research, has conceded this possibility (Singer, 1993). Moreover, utilitarians must be similarly well disposed to the activities of animal care and use committees (Singer has served as a member of such a committee), provided that these committees conscientiously work to eliminate unnecessary animal suffering. Legislative attempts to improve the well-being of animals, whether in laboratories or on the farm, find support among utilitarians. Viewed in these respects, utilitarianism offers a philosophical basis for those who would reform the ways in which nonhuman animals are utilized by humans; what it does not offer is a categorical condemnation of this utilization. For this reason utilitarianism is congenial to those individuals and groups working to advance animal welfare—who accept, that is, the morality of human utilization of nonhuman animals in principle but who seek to improve it, by making it more humane, in practice.

The rights view has a different perspective on such matters (Francione and Regan). This philosophy is opposed to human utilization of nonhuman animals in principle and seeks to end it in practice. Its practical implications are abolitionist, not reformist. Because those nonhuman animals who exist as ends in themselves are never to be treated merely as means, it is wrong to experiment on them in the name of advancing the well-being of others. Moreover, to the extent that animal care and use committees and reformist legislation help to perpetuate social acceptance of human exploitation of these animals, whether on the farm or in the laboratory, advocates of the rights view will—or, to be consistent, should—withhold their support. What animal

rights advocates *can* consistently support are incremental steps that put an end to certain practices within the larger context of animal exploitation—for example, legislation that would prohibit the use of nonhuman animals in cosmetic testing and in drug addiction experiments, and the creation of policies that end compulsory vivisection and dissection in the classroom (Francione and Charlton). When, as can often happen, utilitarians deem such practices unjustified because they cause gratuitous animal suffering, these two conflicting normative ethical philosophies—utilitarianism and the rights view—can speak with one voice. And when this happens, their potential political power is greater than the sum of its parts.

No one can predict which of the tendencies examined above—reform, abolition, or the status quo—will prevail in the coming years. Some positions (e.g., the rights view and ecofeminism) call for fundamental social change; others (e.g., Aristotelian perfectionism and Kant's view) call for much less. To the extent that people act because of their beliefs, the future of how humans treat other animals depends on what we humans believe the latter to be and how we think they should be treated. Because what we should do in practice depends on understanding what we ought to do in principle, our ability to give an appropriate response to the practical issues constituting the animal rights debate, broadly conceived—from whether we ought to be vegetarians to whether we should continue to use nonhuman animals in biomedical research—depends on our ability to make an informed, rational choice among normative ethical theories. In this respect, while a fair consideration of such theories may not be the end-all, it can make some claim to being at least part of the begin-all of a commitment to seek understanding and truth in these troubled waters.

THOMAS REGAN (1995)
BIBLIOGRAPHY REVISED

**SEE ALSO:** *Animal Research and Rights; Endangered Species and Biodiversity; Environmental Ethics; Pain and Suffering; Veterinary Ethics;* and other *Animal Welfare and Rights* subentries

### BIBLIOGRAPHY

Adams, Carol J. 1990. *The Sexual Politics of Meat: A Feminist-Vegetarian Critical Theory.* New York: Continuum.

Barr, James. 1974. "Man and Nature: The Ecological Controversy over the Old Testament." In *Ecology and Religion in History,* pp. 58–72, ed. D. Spring and E. Spring. New York: Harper & Row.

Beauchamp, Tom L. 1997. "Opposing Views on Animal Experimentation: Do Animals Have Rights?" *Ethics and Behavior* 7(2): 113–121.

Brandt, R. B. 1979. *A Theory of the Good and the Right.* Oxford: Clarendon Press.

Callicott, J. Baird. 1980. "Animal Liberation: A Triangular Affair." *Environmental Ethics* 2(4): 311–328. Reprinted in *In Defense of the Land Ethic: Essays in Environmental Philosophy,* pp. 15–38. Albany: State University of New York Press, 1989.

Callicott, J. Baird. 1993. "The Search for an Environmental Ethic." In *Matters of Life and Death: New Introductory Essays in Moral Philosophy,* pp. 322–382, 3rd edition, ed. Tom L. Beauchamp and Tom Regan. New York: McGraw-Hill.

Cavalieri, Paola. 2001. *The Animal Question: Why Non-Human Animals Deserve Human Rights,* tr. Catherine Woollard. New York: Oxford University Press.

Clark, Stephen R. L. 1977. *The Moral Status of Animals.* Oxford: Clarendon Press.

Cohen, Carl. 1986. "The Case for the Use of Animals in Biomedical Research." *New England Journal of Medicine* 315(14): 865–870.

DeGrazia, David. 1996. *Taking Animals Seriously: Mental Life and Moral Status* Cambridge, Eng.: Cambridge University Press.

Devall, Bill, and Sessions, George. 1985. *Deep Ecology: Living as if Nature Mattered.* Salt Lake City: Gibbs Smith.

Diamond, Irene, and Orenstein, Gloria Fenman, eds. 1990. *Reweaving the World: The Emergence of Ecofeminism.* San Francisco: Sierra Club.

Francione, Gary L., and Charlton, Anna E. 1992. *Vivisection and Dissection in the Classroom: A Guide to Conscientious Objection.* Jenkintown, PA: American Anti-Vivisection Society.

Francione, Gary, and Regan, Tom. 1992. "A Movement's Means Create Its Ends." *Animals' Agenda* 12(1): 40–43.

Frey, R. G. 1980. *Interests and Rights: The Case against Animals.* Oxford: Clarendon Press.

Frey, R. G. 1983. *Rights, Killing, and Suffering: Moral Vegetarianism and Applied Ethics.* Oxford: Basil Blackwell.

Frey, R. G. 1997. "Moral Community and Animal Research in Medicine." *Ethics and Behavior* 7(2): 123–136.

Gaard, Greta C., ed. 1993. *Ecofeminism: Women, Animals, Nature.* Philadelphia: Temple University Press.

Garner, Richard. 1994. *Beyond Morality.* Philadelphia: Temple University Press.

Godlovitch, Stanley; Godlovitch, Roslind; and Harris, John. 1972. *Animals, Men, and Morals: An Enquiry into the Maltreatment of Non-Humans.* New York: Taplinger.

Kheel, Marti. 1991. "Ecofeminism and Deep Ecology: Reflections on Identity and Difference." *Trumpeter* 8: 62–72.

LaFollette, Hugh, and Shanks, Niall. 1993. "Animal Models in Biomedical Research: Some Epistemological Worries." *Public Affairs Quarterly* 7(2): 113–130.

Linzey, Andrew. 1976. *Animal Rights: A Christian Assessment of Man's Treatment of Animals.* Oxford: S.M.C.

Linzey, Andrew. 1987. *Christianity and the Rights of Animals.* New York: Crossroad.

Linzey, Andrew, and Regan, Tom, eds. 1988. *Animals and Christianity: A Book of Readings.* New York: Crossroad.

Lyons, David. 1965. *Forms and Limits of Utilitarianism.* Oxford: Clarendon Press.

Magel, Charles R. 1981. *A Bibliography on Animal Rights and Related Matters.* Washington, D.C.: University Press of America.

Magel, Charles R. 1989. *Keyguide to Information Sources in Animal Rights.* Jefferson, NC: McFarland.

McDaniel, Jay B. 1989. *Of God and Pelicans: A Theology of Reverence for Life.* Louisville, KY: John Knox.

McHarg, Ian L. 1969. *Design with Nature.* Garden City, NY: Natural History Press.

McKinlay, John B., and McKinlay, S. 1977. *Health and Society.* London: Milbank.

Midgley, Mary. 1983. *Animals and Why They Matter.* Harmondsworth, Eng.: Penguin.

Naess, Arne. 1989. *Ecology, Community, and Lifestyle: Outline of an Ecosophy,* ed. and tr. David Rothenberg. Cambridge, Eng.: Cambridge University Press.

Narveson, Jan. 1977. "Animal Rights." *Canadian Journal of Philosophy* 7(1): 161–178.

Narveson, Jan. 1988. *The Libertarian Idea.* Philadelphia: Temple University Press.

Orlans, Barbara F.; Beauchamp, Tom L.; Dresser, Rebecca; et al. 1998. *The Human Use of Animals: Case Studies in Ethical Choice.* New York: Oxford University Press.

Rachels, James. 1990. *Created from Animals: The Moral Implications of Darwinism.* Oxford: Oxford University Press.

Rawls, John. 1971. *A Theory of Justice.* Cambridge, MA: Harvard University Press.

Regan, Tom. 1983. *The Case for Animal Rights.* Berkeley: University of California Press.

Regan, Tom. 1997. "The Rights of Humans and Other Animals." *Ethics and Behavior* 7(2): 103–111.

Regan, Tom. 2001. *Defending Animal Rights.* Chicago: University of Illinois Press.

Regan, Tom, ed. 1986. *Animal Sacrifices: Religious Perspectives on the Use of Animals in Science.* Philadelphia: Temple University Press.

Regan, Tom, and Singer, Peter, eds. 1976. *Animal Rights and Human Obligations.* Englewood Cliffs, NJ: Prentice-Hall.

Regan, Tom, and Singer, Peter, eds. 1989. *Animal Rights and Human Obligations,* 2nd edition. Englewood Cliffs, NJ: Prentice-Hall.

Rollin, Bernard E. 1981. *Animal Rights and Human Morality.* Buffalo, NY: Prometheus.

Rollin, Bernard E. 1989. *The Unheeded Cry: Animal Consciousness, Animal Pain, and Science.* New York: Oxford University Press.

Rolston, Holmes, III. 1988. *Environmental Ethics: Duties to and Values in the National World.* Philadelphia: Temple University Press.

Rowlands, Mark. 2002. *Animals Like Us.* New York: Verso Books.

Ryder, Richard D. 1975. *Victims of Science: The Use of Animals in Science.* London: Davis-Poynter.

Ryder, Richard D. 1989. *Animal Revolution: Changing Attitudes Towards Speciesism.* Oxford: Basil Blackwell.

Sagoff, Mark. 1984. "Animal Liberation and Environmental Ethics: Bad Marriage, Quick Divorce." *Osgoode Hall Law Journal* 22(2): 297–307.

Sapontzis, Steve F. 1987. *Morals, Reason, and Animals.* Philadelphia: Temple University Press.

Sharpe, Robert. 1988. *The Cruel Deception: The Use of Animals in Medical Research.* Wellingborough, Eng.: Thorsons.

Singer, Peter. 1975. *Animal Liberation: A New Ethics for Our Treatment of Animals.* New York: New York Review.

Singer, Peter. 1990. *Animal Liberation,* 2nd edition. New York: New York Review of Books.

Singer, Peter. 1993. "Animals and the Value of Life." In *Matters of Life and Death: New Introductory Essays in Moral Philosophy,* pp. 280–321, 3rd edition, ed. Tom Regan. New York: Random House.

Singer, Peter. 2001. *Animal Liberation,* 3rd edition. Chicago: Ecco Press.

Taylor, Paul W. 1986. *Respect for Nature: A Theory of Environmental Ethics.* Princeton, NJ: Princeton University Press.

Vance, Richard P. 1992. "An Introduction to the Philosophical Presuppositions of the Animal Liberation/Rights Movement." *Journal of the American Medical Association* 288(13): 1715–1719.

VanDeVeer, Donald. 1979. "Of Beasts, Persons, and the Original Position." *Monist* 62(3): 368–377.

Warren, Karen J. 1990. "The Power and the Promise of Ecological Feminism." *Environmental Ethics* 12(2): 125–146.

Warren, Mary Anne. 1998. *Moral Status: Obligations to Persons and Other Living Things (Issues in Biomedical Ethics).* New York: Oxford University Press.

White, Lynn, Jr. 1967. "The Historical Roots of Our Ecological Crisis." *Science* 155(3767): 1203–1207.

## II. VEGETARIANISM

Vegetarianism is traditionally defined as the practice of abstaining from eating animal flesh. Modern vegetarian societies, such as the Vegetarian Society of the United Kingdom, define the practice as abstaining from flesh, fish, and fowl, with or without the addition of dairy produce and eggs. Those who wholly or occasionally abstain from "red meat" but eat fish and/or poultry are described as "demi-" or "semi-" vegetarians. Veganism, or "pure" vegetarianism, is the practice of abstaining as completely as possible from all products and by-products of the slaughterhouse, including products derived from treatment deemed exploitative to animals. Vegans do not consume dairy produce or eggs and also exclude products such as honey on the grounds that animals are used and/or killed in producing such types of human nourishment. Most vegetarians do not wear slaughterhouse by-products such as leather, and vegans avoid wearing leather completely.

### Health Vegetarians

As late as the 1950s, the unwritten consensus among health specialists and dieticians was that animal protein in some form is essential to maintain adequate human health. While this position has not been completely reversed, medical advice from official studies increasingly recommends low-animal-fat diets, some of which eschew animal protein completely. Studies suggest that vegetarians have lower rates of diet-related cancer (Chang-Claude et al.), especially colon and rectal cancer (Phillips; Willett et al.) and prostate cancer (Giovannucci et al.). Vegetarians experience lower mortality from coronary heart disease than nonvegetarians, possibly due to their lower serum cholesterol levels (Burr and Butland). One study has shown that mortality from cardiovascular disease among vegetarians was less than half that of the general population (Chang-Claude et al.; see also Snowdon et al., 1984). Vegetarians suffer less from hypertension (Armstrong et al.; Rouse et al.), obesity (Thorogood et al.), and diabetes (Snowdon and Phillips).

Interpretation of these and other studies has become a source of controversy, with advocates for each side citing evidence in their favor (Frey, 1983; Robbins). Increasingly, however, health specialists seem to favor vegetarian diets on medical grounds alone. According to present knowledge, a balanced vegetarian diet poses no health problems and offers some indisputable advantages.

### "Green" Vegetarians

Green political parties in Europe (i.e., those parties committed to programs that give priority to ecological sustainability) increasingly advocate a vegetarian diet or, at least, reduced meat consumption for environmental reasons. For example, the policy of the Green Party of the United Kingdom "encourage[s] a reduction in consumption of animal produce and promote[s] the development and use of foods which are more healthy and humane" (Green Party, p. 15). They offer two arguments. The first is that if enough Westerners become vegetarians, worldwide food distribution will become more equitable. It is calculated that "if we all had a vegetarian diet and shared our food equally, the biosphere could support around six billion people; if 15 percent of our calories came from animal products (and again food were shared equally), the figure would come down to four billion people; if 25 percent of our calories came from animal products, then it would fall to three billion; and if 35 percent of our calories came from animal products, as in North America today, then it would fall to 2.5 billion" (Myers, discussed in Ticknell, p. 67). The second argument is that the present system of intensive farming, while cost-efficient, will prove inefficient in the long run in terms of energy and environmental costs (Porritt). Hence, Greens argue that the "expanding livestock industry contributes to … the destruction and pollution of the planet" by being "energy intensive rather than labour intensive" and contributes to "world starvation" (Green Party, p. 15).

Assessing these arguments is problematic. While intensive farming is energy inefficient and environmentally damaging—apart from concerns it raises about animal welfare—any measurement of food resources must take into account not only the quantity of food available but also the way in which complex systems of supply and demand militate against egalitarian food distribution. Again, while animal farming is not always an efficient use of food resources, it is not clear that the political will exists to adopt alternative economic policies. Those who are sympathetic to vegetarianism on environmental grounds believe that widespread and increasing vegetarianism can and will affect worldwide trade. Despite the evident increase in the number of vegetarians in the West, it is as yet unclear how far, if at all, such minorities will have lasting economic impact.

In response to the "Green" argument against vegetarianism, some environmental ethicists, while sympathetic to the view that modern industrial agriculture is environmentally damaging, hold that since nature is a predatory system, it is natural for humans as well as animals to consume sentient life forms. Frederick Ferré argues, "From the broadest biotic perspective, life is cannibalistic upon itself; an ecological ethic must begin with the affirmation of the nutrient cycle" (p. 392; see also Birch and Cobb). This view is reinforced by Holmes Rolston III, who states that "humans in their eating habits follow nature; they can and ought to do so." Rolston's argument is dependent upon a distinction between nature and culture: "Humans, then, can model their dietary habits on their ecosystems, but they cannot and should not model their interpersonal justice or charity on ecosystems" (p. 81).

Both arguments presuppose to some degree that what should be must be modeled on what is. Only faintly, if at all, do ethical considerations fundamentally apply to the human act of killing sentient animals even when it is unnecessary. Ferré and Rolston do not sufficiently consider that what is "given in nature" is as much a social construct as what may be presupposed in "human nature." No perception of nature is value-free. What we judge to be "given in nature" often turns out to be what we ourselves judge on other criteria should be the case. In sum, there is no ecological shortcut to avoiding the question of whether the human killing of sentient animals is a moral issue. Since not all ethicists, especially theological ethicists, are convinced that the natural order exists as God intended, arguments based on what is "natural" beg metaphysical questions about the justice of what is (see Linzey, 1987, 1994; Clark, 1994).

## Ethical Vegetarians

Of three main arguments for vegetarianism on ethical grounds, the first is based on the value of animal life. Even if we grant animal life secondary or even minimal value, it is difficult to see how human taste preference alone can justify killing. In general, killing for food when it is not required for human health or survival fails the test of moral necessity. Consuming flesh when we could do otherwise is "empty gluttony" (Clark, 1977, p. 183). Some philosophers have argued that it is not justifiable to kill animals even painlessly, asserting that it is logically inconsistent to care whether animals suffer without also valuing animal life itself (Godlovitch).

Other philosophers perceive gradations of value. Ferré, for example, argues against the assertion that all beings with inherent value possess that value equally. "There is no reason to suppose that the quality and intensity of the mental life—and with it its value for itself—of an oyster is on a par with that of a pheasant; but there is likewise no reason to suppose that the quality and intensity of the mental life of the pheasant is on a par with that of a human child" (p. 396). Ferré argues that "there is no 'line.' … All living beings have some degree of inherent value … but different organisms call for different forms of respect" (pp. 397–398). But even if such gradations are admitted, the case of mammals, as distinct from plants, calls for greater ethical justification. We still need to know how the killing of animals—which are sentient beings with inherent value superior to that of plants—without strict necessity is compatible with appropriate "respect" for their lives. The logic of Ferré's position is inclusive. Even the killing of plants requires strong ethical justification.

The second argument derives from considerations of animal welfare. If animals should be spared unnecessary suffering, then eating meat should be avoided, since the rearing, transport, and slaughter of farm animals invariably—and in some cases, necessarily—involves suffering, sometimes of a severe and prolonged kind (see Singer; and Frey, 1983, in response). This argument gains credibility in light of modern farming methods and the recognized fallibility of slaughtering techniques (Harrison; Mason and Singer; Johnson).

Ferré accepts that many modern farming practices are cruel but argues that "moderate" meat eating is justifiable if "nearly painless methods" of slaughter are adhered to (p. 400). If such a goal were to be achieved, fundamental changes would be required at all levels of livestock management. Minimally, slaughtering techniques would have to be indisputably humane (i.e., render the animal instantaneously unconscious), slaughterhouses would have to be regularly inspected, and regulations would need to be enforced by law. Animals would need to be killed as close as possible to their point of origin to avoid suffering in transit. Handling of animals on farms would have to be subject to a new range of welfare criteria. Conscientious meat eaters could justify eating meat only in specific circumstances when all such conditions have been met. The current failure to secure humane farm management and slaughter renders "moderate" meat eating ethically problematic. While in theory this second argument justifies only provisional vegetarianism in most, perhaps all, circumstances as a protest against animal abuse, it is difficult to envisage a time when conditions will universally prevail so as to preclude animal suffering in agriculture.

The third argument appeals to notions of animal rights. Sentient beings, or beings that can be classed as "subjects of a life," have a right to live that is equal to, or analogous with, human beings' right to live. Vegetarianism, according to the rights view, is obligatory in principle, and entails the end of commercial animal agriculture in practice. However, even this animal right not to be harmed is viewed as "a prima facie, not an absolute right" (Regan, p. 330).

The precise implications of this argument are not always clear. Do animals have in each and every case an equal right with humans to life? To what extent may individual rights be overridden in particular crisis situations? Commercial nonanimal agriculture also depends to some degree upon the control of competing species. Some animal rightists defend a stricter definition of avoidability or necessity than

others. For example, some would concede that meat eating may be justified in those limited situations were alternative resources are inadequate (Linzey, 1987).

Discussion has sometimes centered on the cultural survival of the Inuit peoples, for example, and the question of whether their cultural rights should override the rights of the animals they hunt for food and clothing. Some animal rightists would accept the legitimacy of a limited human-preference approach in such circumstances. George Woodcock maintains that there is not "a single responsible person in the animal rights movement who would object to the Indian or Inuit, where he can, following a partly subsistence life of hunting for food" (p. 5). Other animal rightists, however, would question whether cultural considerations should be paramount when considering the exploitation of animals. Both "moderate" and "strong" animal-rights positions would, however, concur with Woodcock's judgment that both indigenous peoples, as well as fur-bearing animals, "have always been the victims of the fur trade" (p. 5). The rights position may be described as the strong welfare position, more uncompromising in its insistence upon the correctness of not harming animals as a prima facie duty. The rights view may not always require absolute (as distinct from obligatory) vegetarianism, but it would contend that vegetarianism should be the ethical and social norm.

## Religious Vegetarians

Two primary motifs, ascetic and mystical, have informed an ethico-religious awareness. Vegetarianism has an established place in some Indian religious traditions, especially Jainism and, to some degree, Buddhism and Hinduism. The ascetic motif, particularly within Jainism, is based on the doctrines of nonviolence and nonpossessiveness. The goals of the spiritual life are, among other things, the renunciation of aggressive and possessive urges and following the path of purification (Jaini).

While Christianity has not formally endorsed vegetarianism, some strands of its tradition have affirmed that abstaining from meat can have value as a spiritual discipline. Some religious orders—for example, the Benedictines—eschewed meat as part of their ascetic regime (Sorrell). Self-denial as part of striving toward moral perfection has sometimes formed the basis for vegetarian lifestyles (Tolstoy). Ascetic practices may involve a vegetarian diet as a conscientious ecological response to wasteful consumerism and affluence (Lappé).

Allied to asceticism has been a mystical appreciation of other creatures as valuable beyond human calculations of utility because of their divine creation. The origins of this outlook are clear in the early and medieval periods (Sorrell). Only in modern times has this viewpoint received systematic expression in notions of reverence for life or in life-centered ethics (Schweitzer; McDaniel; Linzey, 1994). Historical Christianity has not fostered these insights, mainly because of its continuing anthropocentric theology. However, theological affirmations that animals are humans' fellow creatures, whose life or spirit belongs to God—and that they are therefore worthy of respect—undergird an ethical impulse to minimize injury and harm to them. Because of the rights of their Creator, animals can be said to bear "theos-rights," or God-rights (Linzey, 1987, p. 68).

The "modern vegetarian movement"—in the sense of organized societies specifically founded to advance ethical or religious vegetarianism—can be traced to the emergence of humanitarian sensibility from the nineteenth century onward. The Bible Christian Church, founded in 1809 by an Anglican priest, William Cowherd, made vegetarianism compulsory among its members and heralded the later growth of specifically vegetarian societies in the United Kingdom and the United States. The Bible Christian Church found its inspiration in the biblical command, recorded in Genesis 1:29, to be herbivores. Later commands to eat flesh (for example, in Gen. 9:3) were understood as permission given to humankind only after the fall and the flood (for a discussion of Judaism and vegetarianism, see Schwartz).

The Bible is, however, ambivalent about meat eating. While carnivorousness may be construed as a divine concession to human sinfulness (Baker), almost all biblical writers accepted the practice as ethically justifiable. Moreover, Jesus Christ was not a "pure" vegetarian; the gospel accounts record that he ate fish. There were various sects advocating vegetarianism in early Jewish and Christian circles, but none of their practices became normative within Judaism or Christianity (Beckwith). Carnivorousness has seldom been theologically challenged within mainstream religious traditions and only comparatively recently has ethical vegetarianism emerged as a serious option. Some modern Jewish vegetarians (see, e.g., Kook) argue that abstaining from meat is one step toward realizing the biblical vision of universal peace as described by prophets such as Isaiah (11:6f). Some Christian theologians hold that contemporary vegetarianism constitutes a more Christlike response to the evil of animal exploitation (Linzey, 1994).

The best defense of meat eating is based not only on a denial that animals have rights (Frey, 1980, 1983; Leahy; Carruthers) but also a denial that they have any moral status. According to this view, the gastronomic pleasures humans experience by consuming flesh far outweigh the value of animal life and suffering. "By comparison with animals, our lives are of an incomparably greater texture and richness, and when we say of a dying man that he has led a rich, full life we allude to something incomparably beyond to what we would allude, were we to say the same of a dying chicken, cat or chimpanzee" (Frey, 1983, p. 110).

It is difficult to see how such a position can be sustained without putting at risk the moral status of some classes of humans, for example, the mentally handicapped, the comatose, or newborns. Furthermore, it follows from the denial of animal status that a species superior to humans—as some humans now regard themselves in relation to animals—would not be morally obligated to respect human lives and suffering. The hope that "our aliens' nobility will match the quality of their imagined mentality" (Ferré, p. 406) and that therefore they will spare us unnecessary suffering and death, sadly cannot be deduced from humans' own moral record in relation to sentient nonhumans.

What has given contemporary secular and theological arguments for vegetarianism their strength and cogency is the realization that meat is not generally essential for human health and well-being. Consuming meat may have been necessary at certain times in the past; it may sometimes be necessary in the present. But eating a balanced vegetarian diet carries with it no medical or nutritional handicap. And, more important, it respects the ethical injunction to avoid killing sentient beings whenever possible.

ANDREW LINZEY (1995)

SEE ALSO: *Harm; Hinduism, Bioethics in; Jainism, Bioethics in; Moral Status; Utilitarianism and Bioethics;* and other *Animal Welfare and Rights* subentries

### BIBLIOGRAPHY

Adams, Carol J. 1990. *The Sexual Politics of Meat: A Feminist-Vegetarian Critical Theory.* New York: Continuum.

Armstrong, Bruce K.; Van Merwyck, Anthony J.; and Coates, Harvey. 1977. "Blood Pressure in Seventh-Day Adventist Vegetarians." *American Journal of Epidemiology* 105(5): 444–449.

Baker, John Austin. 1975. "Biblical Attitudes to Nature." In *Man and Nature,* pp. 87–109, ed. Hugh Montefiore. London: Collins.

Beckwith, Roger T. 1988. "The Vegetarianism of the Therapeutae, and the Motives for Vegetarianism in Early Jewish and Christian Circles." *Revue de Qumran* 13(49–52): 407–410.

Birch, Charles, and Cobb, John B., Jr. 1981. *The Liberation of Life: From Cell to Community.* Cambridge: Cambridge University Press.

Burr, Michael L., and Butland, Barbara K. 1988. "Heart Disease in British Vegetarians." *American Journal of Clinical Nutrition,* suppl. 48(3): 830–832.

Carruthers, Peter. 1992. *The Animals Issue: Moral Theory in Practice.* Cambridge: Cambridge University Press.

Chang-Claude, Jenny; Frentzel-Beyme, Rainer; and Eilber, Ursula. 1992. "Mortality Pattern of Germa Vegetarians After 11 Years of Follow-up." *Epidemiology* 3(5): 395–401.

Clark, Stephen R. L. 1977. *The Moral Status of Animals.* Oxford: Clarendon Press.

Clark, Stephen R. L. 1994. *How to Think about the Earth: The Philosophical and Theological Models for Ecology.* London: Mowbray.

Ferré, Frederick. 1986. "Moderation, Morals and Meat." *Inquiry* 29: 391–406.

Fiddes, Nick. 1991. *Meat: A Natural Symbol.* London: Routledge.

Fox, Michael W., and Wiswall, Nancy E. 1989. *The Hidden Costs of Beef.* Washington, D.C.: Humane Society of the United States.

Frey, Raymond G. 1980. *Interests and Rights: The Case against Animals.* Oxford: Clarendon Press.

Frey, Raymond G. 1983. *Rights, Killing and Suffering: Moral Vegetarianism and Applied Ethics.* Oxford: Basil Blackwell.

Giovannucci, Edward; Rimm, Eric B.; Colditz, Graham A.; Stampfer, Meir J.; Ascherio, Alberto; Chute, Chris C.; and Willett, Walter C. 1993. "A Prospective Study of Dietary Fat and Risk of Prostate Cancer." *Journal of the National Cancer Institute* 85(19): 1571–1579.

Godlovitch, Roslind. 1971. "Animals and Morals." In *Animals, Men and Morals: An Inquiry into the Maltreatment of the Non-Human,* pp. 156—172, by Stanley Godlovitch, Roslind Godlovitch, and John Harris. London: Victor Gollancz.

Green Party. 1993. "Animal Rights." In *Green Party MfSS,* 15–16. London: Author.

Harrison, Ruth. 1964. *Animal Machines: The New Factory Farming Industry.* London: Vincent Stuart.

Jaini, Padmanabh S. 1979. *The Jaina Path of Purification.* Berkeley: University of California Press.

Johnson, Andrew. 1991. *Factory Farming.* Oxford: Basil Blackwell.

Kook, Abraham Isaac. 1979. "Fragments of Light: A View as to the Reasons for the Commandments." In *The Lights of Penitence; The Moral Principles; Lights of Holiness: Essays, Letters, and Poems,* pp. 303–323; tr. Ben Zion Bokser. London: SPCK.

Lappé, Frances M. 1982. *Diet for a Small Planet,* 2nd revised edition. New York: Ballantine.

Leahy, Michael. 1991. *Against Liberation: Putting Animals in Perspective.* London: Routledge.

Linzey, Andrew. 1976. *Animal Rights: A Christian Assessment of Man's Treatment of Animals.* London: SCM.

Linzey, Andrew. 1987. *Christianity and the Rights of Animals.* London.

Linzey, Andrew. 1994. *Animal Theology.* London: SCM.

Mason, Jim, and Singer, Peter, eds. 1980. *Animal Factories.* New York: Crown.

McDaniel, Jay B. 1989. *Of God and Pelicans: A Theology of Reverence for Life.* Louisville, KY: Westminster/John Knox.

Myers, Norman. 1990. *Mass Extinctions: Palaeogeography, Palaeoclimatology, Palaeoecology.* Amsterdam: Elsevier Science Publishers.

Phillips, Roland L. 1975. "Role of Life-Style and Dietary Habits in Risk of Cancer among Seventh-Day Adventists." *Cancer Research* 35(11): 3513–3522.

Porritt, Jonathon. 1984. *Seeing Green: The Politics of Ecology Explained.* Oxford: Basil Blackwell.

Regan, Tom. 1983. *The Case for Animal Rights.* London: Routledge and Kegan Paul.

Robbins, John. 1987. *Diet for a New America: How Your Food Choices Affect Your Health,* 2nd revised edition. Walpole, NH: Stillpoint.

Rolston, Holmes, III. 1988. *Environmental Ethics: Duties to and Values in the Natural World.* Philadelphia: Temple University Press.

Rouse, Ian L.; Armstrong, Bruce K.; and Beilin, Lawrence J. 1983. "The Relationship of Blood Pressure to Diet and Lifestyle in Two Religious Populations." *Journal of Hypertension* 1(1): 65–71.

Schwartz, Richard H. 1988. *Judaism and Vegetarianism.* Marblehead, MA.: Micah.

Schweitzer, Albert. 1967. *Civilization and Ethics,* 2nd edition.; tr. C. T. Campion. London: Unwin.

Singer, Peter. 1976. *Animal Liberation: A New Ethics for Our Treatment of Animals.* London: Jonathan Cape.

Snowdon, David A., and Phillips, Roland L. 1985. "Does a Vegetarian Diet Reduce the Occurrence of Diabetes?" *American Journal of Public Health* 75(5): 507–512.

Snowdon, David A.; Phillips, Roland L.; and Fraser, Gary E. 1984. "Meat Consumption and Fatal Ischemic Heart Disease." *Preventive Medicine* 13(5): 490–500.

Sorrell, Roger D. 1988. *St. Francis of Assisi and Nature: Tradition and Innovation in Western Christian Attitudes toward the Environment.* New York: Oxford University Press.

Thorogood, Margaret; McPherson, Klim; and Mann, Jim. 1989. "Relationship of Body Mass Index, Weight and Height to Plasma Lipid Levels in People with Different Diets in Britain." *Community Medicine* 11(3): 230–233.

Tickell, Crispin. 1992. "The Quality of Life: What Quality? Whose Life?" *Interdisciplinary Science Reviews* 17(1): 19–25.

Tolstoy, Leo. 1961. "The First Step." In *Recollections and Essays,* 4th edition, pp. 123–134; tr. Aylmer Maude. London: Oxford University Press.

Willett, Walter C.; Stampfer, Meir J.; Colditz, Graham A.; Rosner, Bernard A.; and Speizer, Frank E. 1990. "Relation of Meat, Fat and Fiber Intake to the Risk of Colon Cancer in a Prospective Study Among Women." *New England Journal of Medicine* 323(24): 1664–1672.

Woodcock, George. 1989. "A Briefing on the Fur Trade and Aboriginal Cultures." In *Skinned,* pp. 1–5. Nottingham, Eng.: Lynx.

# III. WILDLIFE CONSERVATION AND MANAGEMENT

Wildlife management may be thought a contradiction in terms. The logic of "wild" precludes "managed." Wildlife lived for millions of years, unmanaged by humans. Part of what humans value in wildlife is animals that can look out for themselves. Wildlife that is managed is not wild; it is managed life. So there is logical difficulty in the idea. There is also ethical difficulty. Perhaps humans are not responsible for wildlife; wild lives are on their own. But then again, human activities affect wildlife quite adversely. Have we no duty to care for it, either because of what humans have at stake or because of what wildlife is in itself?

This entry outlines some main issues: the contemporary crisis of conserving historically evolved wildlife populations on rapidly developing human landscapes; ownership, control, management, and stewardship responsibilities for wildlife; conservation of endangered wildlife species; fishes and fisheries as managed wildlife populations; wildlife as game for hunting and trapping, including hunting as a conservation strategy; "hands-on" versus "hands-off" management; and feral animals. These are issues of management, but there are ethical questions at every point.

## Wildlife and Human Populations: An Emerging Crisis

There are more species on Earth today than there have ever been in the 2.5-billion-year history of life. Estimates run from five to thirty million species; ten million is a typical figure. Most of the vertebrate wildlife and birds are known; most unknowns are in the invertebrate animal, insect, and plant species. During evolutionary history, there was no wildlife management; wildlife conservation takes care of itself if no humans intervene. On statistical average, more species have been produced than have become extinct; diversity has gradually increased.

Some five catastrophic extinctions have been followed by rather swift regeneration of the lost species. On landscapes that have grown colder or drier, species may become fewer. Some groups of species were more numerous in the past, such as dinosaurs in the Cretaceous period, or birds in the Pleistocene. Nevertheless, diversity is at an all-time high. In one sense, all biology is conservation biology (biology that conserves life), whether or not humans are involved.

There are many more humans on Earth today than ever, and the expansion of human habitat, coupled with pollution, hunting, and trade in wildlife, threatens populations of wild animals and their habitats. Humans now threaten the biological processes that have been creating and conserving life for billions of years. Hardly an American landscape has not been impoverished of its native fauna. The larger once-dominant animals—such as eagles, wolves, cougars, grizzly bears, wolverines, bison, otters, crocodiles—are especially depleted. The New World depletion in both hemispheres is a result of Europeans entering a relatively empty continent and engaging in explosive development over recent centuries. The Amerindians had coexisted with wildlife for ten to fifteen thousand years.

Long-settled continents do not escape the problem either. Humans have inhabited Africa since evolving there over a hundred thousand years ago. Only in the twentieth century, as contemporary nations grew rapidly, was African megafauna or avifauna seriously threatened. Wildlife in China, India, and Tibet, among the oldest settled areas in the world, was greatly depleted. The crisis is as serious in the Old World as in the New.

The crisis is now potentially more urgent than at any previous time in the history of the planet. This generates unprecedented responsibilities because humans previously did not have much effect on wildlife, which took care of itself; unprecedented demands for trade-offs between human values and the welfare of wildlife; and unprecedented implications because of its global and irreversible scale.

Wildlife conservation is now challenged to mix human values with wildlife values. Fortunately, wildlife is valuable to humans and, so far, can be included among the human values. Humans wish to hunt and fish; they enjoy watchable wildlife; wildlife art is the most popular American art form. If backyard bird feeding is included, almost one in four Americans spends some time bird-watching. Animals are chosen as state animals; sports teams and automobiles are named for animals. Many animals serve useful roles in ecosystems; hawks catch mice, birds control insect populations. Wildlife can indicate the health of an ecosystem. Unfortunately, many human values conflict with wildlife on landscapes, as shown by the massive depletion of wildlife. Here human interests seem contrary to wildlife's flourishing. And what if wildlife is not valuable to humans? Have we some responsibilities for the values of wild things for what they are in themselves?

The Wildlife Society, the principal professional organization of management and conservation, affirms that "Wildlife, in its myriad forms, is basic to the maintenance of a human culture that provides quality living." The society seeks "to develop and promote sound stewardship of wildlife resources and of the environments upon which wildlife and humans depend; to undertake an active role in preventing human-induced environmental degradation; to increase awareness and appreciation of wildlife values." It also urges "ethical restraints in the use of living natural resources."

## Ownership, Control, Management, and Stewardship Responsibilities for Wildlife

According to long legal tradition in the United Kingdom, Canada, the United States, and many other nations, individual persons do not own vertebrate wildlife. Animals and birds do not belong to the landowner on whose property they are found. They move around, with dens and nests in particular places, but the larger animals and the birds can range over hundreds or thousands of square miles. They sometimes live on public land, sometimes on different tracts of private land. Continental European nations, by contrast, sometimes hold that property owners own wildlife resident on their lands.

In the Anglo-American tradition, landowners have the right to control access to their property; they control who, for instance, may hunt there. But the state determines whether and how much game may be taken. Permitted by the state, individuals can "take" wildlife—capture or kill it—at which point the animal enters their possession. State control of wildlife was long understood as state ownership, but wildlife paid no more attention to state lines than to local property boundaries; indeed, migratory birds resided in various nations. The U.S. federal government has often regulated wildlife, since much wildlife crosses state lines and much inhabits federal lands. In recent court decisions, the state ownership doctrine has been rejected as based on a flawed characterization of wildlife, which should be regulated like other natural resources considered commons, not so much owned as held in trust. State ownership of wildlife has been subsumed under the state and federal power to regulate all natural resources, an expanding public trust doctrine. Wildlife is a public good held in trust by the state for the benefit of the people (Bean).

The general idea is that there is a corporate responsibility for wildlife, a duty to persons concerning wildlife in which they have an interest, and a duty of individual persons to relate to wildlife, caring for it, tolerating it, perhaps hunting it, all within the context of a larger public interest and stewardship. Animal welfare was long subsumed under this rubric, since maintaining this public good required healthy wildlife populations. But animal welfare has increasingly become a concern in its own right, independent of human benefits. This is called the intrinsic value of wildlife, a value also held in trust. This concern becomes evident in

concern for endangered species as well as in shifting attitudes toward hunting.

## Conservation of Endangered Wildlife Species

The legal tradition arose with regard to individual animals, but protecting endangered species has increasingly figured in regulations covering both game and nongame species. State departments, once of "Game and Fish," have largely been renamed departments of "Wildlife"; though hunting and fishing remain a large part of their assignments, their interest in threatened wildlife has dramatically increased. If the government can regulate individual animals, by the same logic it can regulate species. In the fall of 1981, when black-footed ferrets were discovered on private ranches near Meeteetse, Wyoming, the ranchers were legally obligated to protect them. Furthermore, the federal government can designate critical habitat on private land.

Landowners ought not to shoot the bald eagles that fly over their property or cut the trees in which they nest. In compliance with the Endangered Species Act, in order to protect eighty bald eagle nesting sites, the Weyerhaeuser Company in the early 1980s set aside more than nine hundred acres in Washington and Oregon, representing over nine million dollars in unharvested timber. Lest it be supposed that the bald eagle, the national symbol, is a unique public good, Weyerhaeuser also, complying with the act, set aside 155 acres in southern states to protect 22 colonies of the endangered red-cockaded woodpecker. These woodpeckers prefer to nest in prime timber, eighty-year-old pine forests; loggers would rather cut these lands more often than that. Though these landowners cannot use the land as they once intended, costing them that opportunity, it does so lest they destroy, at the species level, eagles and woodpeckers that, though on their land, do not belong to them but are a common good.

The Endangered Species Act of 1973 is the most far-reaching wildlife statute adopted by any nation. The U.S. Fish and Wildlife Service is charged by the act to list both domestic and foreign wildlife species threatened with extinction. No government agency may undertake projects likely to jeopardize listed species, at home or abroad, except under authority of a high-level committee that has granted few exemptions. Jeopardizing species includes disrupting their habitat. Neither can persons take listed wildlife species on private lands. In evaluating whether to list a species, economic considerations may not be considered, a point of repeated contention but one that the U.S. Congress has reaffirmed several times. Importing species on the worldwide list into the United States is illegal except under specific conditions.

Generally this concern, enacted into legislation, reveals an increasing sense of human duty toward wildlife that comes to special focus when a species becomes endangered. Game managers who may once have thought of their responsibility as the production of an annual crop of game to shoot now see themselves as wildlife managers whose responsibility is to provide for a diverse native fauna on the landscape, both for the benefits such wildlife brings to humans and out of respect for what all species of wildlife, not just the game species, are in themselves.

## Fish and Fisheries as Managed Wildlife Populations

Analogous changes have taken place with regard to fishes. Once, what one wanted was fish to catch; and fishing remains a popular recreation. But there is an increasing concern with native fish populations, including all species.

The native fish fauna of North America has been tampered with possibly as extensively as, and certainly more rapidly than, the fish on any other continent. Managers have introduced "game" and eliminated "trash" fish; humans have made dams and water developments for domestic, industrial, and agricultural uses; polluted; caused erosional sedimentation; and accidentally introduced parasites and diseases. Of the endangered fishes of the world, about 70 percent are in North America; 56 percent are receiving some degree of protection. The fishes in the United States have been as disturbed as any other wildlife, more so in the West than in the East, most of all in the Southwest. The Endangered Species Committee of the Desert Fishes Council identifies 164 fishes in North American deserts as endangered, vulnerable, rare, or warranting various degrees of concern.

Concern for these fishes has modified or stopped water development projects. On the Virgin River and its tributaries in Utah in 1980, for example, water authorities abandoned the Warner Valley project lest it jeopardize the woundfin, and built the Quail Creek project instead. Water release from dams may be adjusted in time and volume for the benefit of endangered fish and bird species (Minckley and Deacon).

Coming to focus again in endangered species legislation, what humans think they ought to manage for is shifting from game species to native fishery populations. There is an increasing sense of duty, represented in wildlife managers, to ensure the presence of fishes as an integral part of the wildlife community, not just for the human benefits involved but out of respect for what these fishes are in themselves, as well as for their roles in the riparian ecosystems.

## Hunting and Trapping: Hunting as a Conservation Strategy

Wildlife management has traditionally meant game management. Hunting both for meat and for sport is an ancient practice. Humans evolved as omnivores; meat has been important in human nutrition, although it is quite possible for humans to be well nourished as vegetarians. The character of hunting has accentuated sport hunting in modern times; few hunters of the early twenty-first century are primarily meat hunters, although in most cases the carcass will be eaten. Most hunters have a code of ethics. They think it unethical to waste the meat. Hunters also seek a fair chase, a clean kill, minimal suffering, and respect for the animal; and hunters have long been among the most effective conservationists. Predators, especially wolves, were often eliminated as competitive hunters.

Since the mid-1960s, a strong antihunting movement has emerged, on the ground that shooting animals for sport is unethical, even if the hunter's ethic is observed. Such persons regard wildlife management for the purposes of maintaining hunting as morally wrong. A further problem is that much funding for wildlife conservation comes from hunting and fishing licenses, and if these activities are curtailed, alternative funding sources will have to be found. Hunters also argue that properly managed hunting can ensure conservation, since this activity makes wildlife valuable both to the hunter and to others who profit from the hunter's presence.

Such an argument is especially used for African wildlife. In Africa, although much hunting is legal, poaching has also been rampant, resulting in an international ban on skins, hides, horns, tusks, and other parts of various species. Wildlife managers may argue that whereas such bans may discourage poachers, they also prevent legal hunting, which can be quite profitable; this makes wildlife worthless to native peoples, who can neither hunt for food nor sell wildlife products. Even the products from culled animals (shot to reduce excess populations) cannot be sold. Ivory has been a case in point. Most world ivory trade has been made illegal, but some authorities argue that the sale of legal ivory could greatly benefit elephant conservation.

Trapping has been a traditional use of wildlife, largely for the pelts and hides made into mink coats, beaver hats, alligator-skin purses and shoes, and so on. Given available substitutes, many people object to such use of animals, on grounds that this trapping involves needless cruelty. Furs on fashion models simply flatter female vanities, somewhat as trophy animals mounted in sportsmen's dens flatter male vanities. The leghold trap is especially objectionable to opponents of trapping. A counterargument is that a high value on animal skins, with effective management, can ensure conservation. Most of the world's crocodile species are endangered; crocodiles are dangerous and often frequent rivers where humans are present. Only if the crocodiles are of considerable value to local peoples are they likely to be tolerated and saved.

## "Hands-On" versus "Hands-Off" Management

Although there is a growing consensus that humans have an urgent responsibility actively to conserve wildlife, many argue that the less wildlife is managed, the better. So far as wild animals are managed, their wildness is compromised-the paradox of wildlife management. The animals become artifacts, more like pets. This leads to a debate between "hands-on management," which favors active intervention, habitat enhancement, supplemental feeding, breeding, radio-collared monitoring, and so on, versus "hands-off management," which favors as little management as possible consistent with animal welfare.

From a medical point of view, there is contention whether veterinarians ought to treat wildlife diseases. Like all physicians, veterinarians seek good health. Colorado veterinarians treated a lungworm disease in bighorn sheep successfully. By contrast, when an epidemic of pinkeye ravaged the bighorn sheep of Yellowstone Park, authorities refused to let Wyoming veterinarians treat the disease. The welfare of the sheep, they said, required letting the disease take its course; disease-resistant sheep would survive and the genetic fitness of the herd would improve. Whether the disease is introduced by humans is a factor. The *Chlamydia* parasite producing pinkeye was not thought to be introduced; some said that the lungworm was introduced from domestic sheep, or at least that the sheep were weakened due to human disruptions, especially of their winter range. Although over half the Yellowstone herd perished by starvation and injury following partial blindness, the herd has recovered, although not yet to its former numbers.

Many argue that although hands-off management is an ideal for animals that inhabit extensive ranges, owing to development and human needs there remains insufficient habitat for hands-off management. With elephants in Africa, they say, only hands-on management is possible. Given the elephant's destructiveness and its tendencies to migrate, herds must be fenced, water holes provided, herds culled, and so on. This strikes a balance between responsibilities for elephants and for humans. A controversial case in the United States involved supplemental feeding for grizzly bears in Yellowstone Park, where, after such feeding went on for decades, park officials, preferring a wild bear over a managed bear, elected to risk letting the endangered species survive on its own.

## Feral Animals

Feral animals are those introduced by humans, not native to landscapes, that have managed to survive on their own. Management of such animals is disputed, especially of mustangs and burros in the western United States. Although not now living in their native ecosystems, such animals may have been living wild for centuries. Management policy is typically to eliminate them, on grounds that they are not authentic wildlife, although the U.S. Congress has mandated preserving mustangs in some localities. Animal-welfare advocates have protested eliminating the mustangs and burros. Other cases involve feral hogs and goats. On San Clemente Island, off the coast of California, nearly thirty thousand goats were eliminated, about half of them shot, the other half captured and relocated with poor survival rates, in order to protect endangered species of plants, as well as to prevent further degradation of the island ecosystem. The goats had been left there by the Spanish in earlier centuries. The argument here is that we have a greater responsibility to native wildlife and plants than to feral species.

HOLMES ROLSTON III (1995)

SEE ALSO: *Environmental Ethics* and other *Animal Welfare and Rights* subentries

### BIBLIOGRAPHY

Bailey, James A. 1984. *Principles of Wildlife Management.* New York: John Wiley.

Bean, Michael J. 1983. *The Evolution of National Wildlife Law,* revised edition. New York: Praeger.

*Endangered Species Act of 1973.* 1973. Publ. L. no. 93–205, 87 Stat. 884.

Hargrove, Eugene C., ed. 1992. *The Animal Rights, Environmental Ethics Debate: The Environmental Perspective.* Albany: State University of New York Press.

Minckley, Wendell L., and Deacon, James E., eds. 1991. *Battle against Extinction: Native Fish Management in the American West.* Tucson: University of Arizona Press.

Wildlife Society. 1990. *Conservation Policies of the Wildlife Society.* Bethesda, MD: Author.

## IV. PET AND COMPANION ANIMALS

The term *companion animals* refers to those animals human beings keep for purposes of control, companionship, and comfort. The word *pet,* which suggests the indulgent use of animals (Shell), is being increasingly replaced by the term "companion animals." However, the term *pet animal* seems indispensable in conveying the relationship of intimacy between some humans and selected domesticated species.

### The Emergence of Pet Keeping

The precise origins of pet keeping are obscure. There appear always to have been symbiotic relationships both between species and within species (see, for example, Kropotkin), although some argue that "almost alone among animals, humans domesticate and dwell with other animals" (Clark, 1982, p. 110). Keeping animals as companions may have been a by-product of both killing and domesticating them. Stephen Clark argues that "[p]eople who cared for their animals [kept for food] left more descendants than those who used them carelessly" and that "it 'paid' our ancestors to love what wasn't human" (1982, p. 111).

Some animals were undoubtedly kept for their own value as sources of fascination or as mediators of unusual benefits. For example, cats, although domesticated for a much briefer time than other species, have frequently been associated with the supernatural, as agents either of benign or malign forces (Clutton-Brock).

English society in the eighteenth and nineteenth centuries saw the emergence of widespread pet keeping, especially among the upper classes. Keith Thomas writes of how, as early as 1700, "symptoms of obsessive pet-keeping were in evidence," especially in the keeping of horses, cats, dogs, and pet birds (Thomas, 1983, p. 117). These species were clearly "privileged" in comparison with food animals, which were still reared and killed with hideous cruelty. Although the "idea of a pedigree did not originate in the nineteenth century," Harriet Ritvo shows how the notion of purity of species through selective breeding became widespread among the middle and upper classes, for whom particular companion animals were themselves indicators of social class and good breeding (Ritvo, 1986).

Since the nineteenth century, the phenomenon of pet keeping has increased not only among all English classes but also within European and U.S. societies. Although reliable estimates of animal populations are very difficult to obtain (partly because of nonexistent or unenforced licensing laws), one conservative estimate is that the total annual U.S. turnover in owned dogs in 1991 was 7.71 million, 4 million of which were handled by animal shelters and 2.1 million of which were euthanized (Patronek and Glickman). The current situation in the Western world of millions of animals being kept for purposes of companionship extends far beyond any reasonable interpretation of symbiosis and is historically without parallel.

Quite apart from the personal and psychological factors involved, one obvious reason accounts for this development. Pet owning has become an established part of consumer-oriented cultures in which animals are bought and sold like any other commodity. The pet industry itself, not to mention the allied supply (including veterinary) services, benefit directly or indirectly from the trade, management, and treatment of companion animals. In 1991, in the state of Washington alone, it is estimated that the number of dogs available from pet stores amounted to 11,442, and through breeders, 37,523 (Patronek and Glickman).

### The Benefits of Pet Keeping

These may be classed under three broad headings:

**PSYCHOLOGICAL BENEFITS TO HUMANS.** It seems impossible to doubt that some human–animal bonds can contribute significantly to human flourishing. Relationships with pets seem to help prevent two sources of emotional disorder: deprivation and frustration. They enable nongenital physical contact, provide tactile comfort, improve self-esteem, enhance emotional security, boost personal prowess (as when a beautiful or socially appealing animal is owned), and engender loving relationships that are sometimes seemingly impossible with other humans (Ryder; Levinson; Fogle; see also Serpell).

Potential or actual benefits for pet owners specifically include lower blood pressure (Baun et al.), lower heart rates (DeShriver and Riddick; Wilson and Nettling), reduced anxiety (Wilson, 1991), and reduced depression (Bolin). However, Cindy Wilson argues that although "much has been made over the potential benefits of a pet," it is also true that a large amount of such research "remains anecdotal, nongeneralizable, and scientifically flawed" and that a new methodology should be based on assessable "quality of life measurements" (1994, pp. 4–8).

In the absence of large amounts of data based on objective evidence, interpretation of the psychological effects of pet keeping turns on whether interspecies relations are natural and commendable. Richard Ryder warns against the view that such interspecies relationships are "unnatural or cranky" (p. 5); but that accepted, it is still questionable to what extent legitimate psychological needs are met through pet keeping and whether these needs can or should be met through relationships with members of our own species.

**BENEFITS TO HUMAN SOCIETY.** It has long been thought that pet keeping can help sensitize children, even train them in attitudes of care and respect (Rothschild). One study goes so far as to claim that "companion animals are a vital part of the healthy emotional development of children" (Robin and Bensel, p. 174). Studies have also suggested that relationships with pets can contribute to the psychological and social well-being of adult humans, especially elderly people who live alone (Connell and Lago). Animal-assisted therapy is sometimes utilized for patients in psychiatric hospitals and for individuals with special needs, such as people with the human immunodeficiency virus (HIV) or aquired immuno-deficiency syndrome (AIDS) (Gorczyca) and those suffering from chronic schizophrenia (Bauman et al.).

**BENEFITS TO PET ANIMALS.** The benefits of pet keeping to the animals themselves are difficult to quantify. Leaving aside the wider ethical question of whether animals should be domesticated at all, the impact on the individual pet depends on how well it is kept and to what degree its owners understand and meet its emotional and environmental needs. For example, although pet keeping can provide a stimulus to sensitize children, it can also conversely provide an opportunity for cruelty by abused or disturbed children or by children who lack parental supervision. Some commentators see something psychologically, even politically, perverse about indulging pet animals (see, for example, Shell), and, as discussed below, it is not clear that such indulgence is always beneficial to the animals' welfare.

## The Disadvantages of Pet Keeping

Formidable ethical and welfare problems are associated with pet keeping (Carpenter et al.). These may be classified under three headings:

**ABUSE.** Recorded acts of cruelty against pets appear to be increasing in both the United States and the United Kingdom. Living in close proximity to animals, whatever the benefits to both parties, substantially increases the risk of abuse. Apart from deliberate acts of cruelty, even sadism, unsuitable environmental conditions can cause unacceptably high levels of stress for animals. Few owners fully understand the complex psychological and physiological needs of the animals they keep. Cruelty sometimes arises through ignorance and misunderstanding rather than deliberate neglect, especially when the subjects are exotic animals. Abuse or neglect does occur despite the many and various pet-care programs available.

**OVERPOPULATION.** Present high levels of pet populations inevitably mean death, and sometimes suffering, for other animals. In order to sustain high populations of species such as cats and dogs, for example, other species such as whales, kangaroos, and horses must be killed in order to feed them. Few pet animals of any size can be sustained without meat, though it appears that dogs can live well on an appropriately balanced vegetarian diet. The commercial production of pet food has also been criticized as a waste of resources. The average cost of feeding an eighty-pound dog has been estimated at $8,353 for its lifetime (Shell).

High pet populations also raise other problems for humans. These include possible health hazards, nuisance, and social control. Dogs can communicate diseases such as *Toxicara canis,* which can cause blindness in children. Fortunately, such cases are rare, but an awareness of this hazard in the United Kingdom has recently led to local councils outlawing dogs from public parks, particularly children's parks. Animal organizations, such as the United Kingdom's Royal Society for the Prevention of Cruelty to Animals (RSPCA), have argued the case for compulsory registration of dogs as a means of ensuring responsible ownership; so far, such schemes have operated only on a voluntary or local basis. In 1992, the Dangerous Dogs Act was introduced in the United Kingdom to deal with the threat posed by aggressive dogs after some distressing incidents in which children were attacked by uncontrolled dogs.

**COMMERCIAL USAGE.** Since domestic animals have almost everywhere only the legal status of property (Sandys-Winsch; Sweeney), the breeding and sale of pets is subject to few legal constraints, save principally that direct and "unnecessary" cruelty must be avoided. The view that pets are merely human property has inevitably led, as with other consumer items, to the refashioning of pets. Nonveterinary mutilation of pets (e.g., tail docking, ear cropping, declawing, and removal of a dog's larynx to prevent barking) is not uncommon, though in the United Kingdom the British Veterinary Association refuses to authorize all nonveterinary procedures; performance of such procedures can lead to revocation of a veterinarian's license. The RSPCA opposes all "selective breeding of animals which produces changes in bodily form and/or function," in addition to the commercial sale of puppies and kittens in pet shops (Royal Society for the Prevention of Cruelty to Animals, pp. 7–8).

Animal protectionists argue that the commercial trade in animals leads inevitably to overbreeding and the consequent abandonment and disposal of millions of unwanted animals. In the United Kingdom, the RSPCA estimates that it destroys on average about 1,000 unwanted dogs every week. In the United States, estimates vary from 2.1 million to 9.1 million per year for dogs alone (Patronek and Glickman). Such a wide discrepancy in the figures indicates, among other things, the difficulty in collecting uniform data from the estimated 1,800 to 3,000 animal shelters in the United States. Current widespread euthanasia suggests a prima facie disregard for the worth of pet animals (for a discussion of the ethical problems surrounding large-scale euthanasia, see Kay et al.).

## Is Pet Keeping Immoral?

Despite the emergence of a strong animal-rights movement since the mid–1970s, the ethics of pet keeping is seldom questioned. The major works in animal ethics (Singer; Clark, 1977; Regan; Rodd) largely or entirely bypass this question, and only lone voices are raised in critical opposition (Linzey, 1976; Bryant). Animal-rights philosophy has evolved without offering any critical analysis of the pet trade, though some argue that abuse of pet animals is a "human breach of contract" (Rollin, p. 219). Since so many animal-rights thinkers oppose a purely utilitarian justification for animal exploitation, this omission is surely anomalous.

Part of the reason may be that, historically speaking, sensibility to animal suffering seems to have arisen as a necessary corollary to the practice of keeping pets (Thomas, 1983; Tester). The physical inclusion of animals into the human community seems to have signified a moral inclusiveness also. It may be no accident that the first country to found a society for the prevention of cruelty to animals—England—was also the country renowned for its love of pet animals. Moreover, one cannot but be struck by the way in which anecdotes about animal behavior, especially that of pet animals, have formed the basis for a whole string of pioneering humanitarian books appealing for greater kindness to animals and a fundamental recognition of their rights (see, for example, Youatt; Wood; Nicholson; Thomas, 1993; Lessing).

Yet questions must be asked about the ethical appropriateness of the psychological needs that pet animals apparently meet. Ryder accepts that some of these are "selfish" (p. 8). One early critique argued that "we need to distinguish between a kind of love which respects animals for what they are and allows them to pursue their own lives according to their own natural instincts, and another selfish form of love which seeks to condition animal lives in accordance with our own human desires." Pet keeping, it is argued, represents a "false anthropomorphism" in which we seek to "humanise" animals and "regard them as extensions of our own egos" (Linzey, 1976, p. 68). This view was subsequently modified on the grounds that "all loving is in practice a subtle blend of altruism and self-seeking," although "where the interests of animals are entirely subordinated to human emotional needs,

we need to beware that we are not involved in a self-deceiving tyranny" (Linzey, 1987, p. 137). According to this perspective, at least some forms of pet keeping are wrong because they are insufficiently symbiotic and fail to recognize the right of animals to their own natural life.

ANDREW LINZEY (1995)
BIBLIOGRAPHY REVISED

**SEE ALSO:** *Care; Compassionate Love; Environmental Ethics; Grief and Bereavement; Healing; Moral Status;* and other *Animal Welfare and Rights* subentries

### BIBLIOGRAPHY

Anderson, Robert S., ed. 1975. *Pets, Animals and Society.* London: Bailliere Tindall.

Bauman, Lawrence; Posner, Monte; Sachs, Karl; and Szita, Robert. 1991. "Effects of Animal-Assisted Therapy on Communications Patterns with Chronic Schizophrenics." In *Universal Kinship: The Bond Between All Living Things,* pp. 21–48, ed. the Latham Foundation Staff. Saratoga, CA: R & E.

Baun, Mara M.; Bergstrom, Nancy; Langston, Nancy F.; and Thoma, Linda. 1984. "Physiological Effects of Human/Companion Animal Bonding." *Nursing Research* 33(3): 126–129.

Bolin, S. E. 1987. "The Effects of Companion Animals during Conjugal Bereavement." *Anthrozoos* 1: 26–35.

Bryant, John. 1982 (1978, privately published). *Fettered Kingdoms: An Examination of a Changing Ethic,* rev. edition. Winchester, Eng.: Fox.

Carpenter, Edward; Bates, Angela; Beeson, Trevor; Brambell, Michael; Carpenter, Kenneth; Carpenter, Lillian; Coffey, David; Harrison, Ruth; Jennings, Sydney; Linzey, Andrew; Montefiore, Hugh; and Thorpe, William H. 1980. *Animals and Ethics.* London: Watkins.

Clark, Stephen R. L. 1977. *The Moral Status of Animals.* Oxford: Clarendon Press.

Clark, Stephen R. L. 1982. *The Nature of the Beast: Are Animals Moral?* Oxford: Oxford University Press.

Clutton-Brock, Juliet. 1993. *Cats, Ancient and Modern.* Cambridge, MA: Harvard University Press.

Connell, Cathleen M., and Lago, Daniel J. 1991. "Effects of Pets on the Well-Being of the Elderly." In *Universal Kinship: The Bond Between All Living Things,* pp. 51–62, ed. the Latham Foundation Staff. Saratoga, CA: R & E.

Davis, S. L., Cheeke, P. R. 1998. "Do Domestic Animals Have Minds and the Ability to Think? A Provisional Sample of Opinions on the Question." *Journal of Animal Science* 76(8): 2072–2079.

Dawkins, Marian Stamp. 1993. "Through Our Eyes Only?" *The Search for Animal Consciousness.* Oxford: W. H. Freeman.

Deshriver, M. M., and Riddick, C. C. 1990. "Effects of Watching Aquariums on Elders' Stress." *Anthrozoos* 4: 44–48.

Fogle, Bruce, ed. 1981. *Interrelations Between People and Pets.* Springfield, IL: Charles C. Thomas.

Francione, Gary L., and Kunstler, William M. 1995. *Animals, Property, and the Law (Ethics and Action).* New Orleans, LA: Temple University Press.

Francione, Gary L., and Watson, Alan. 2000. *Introduction to Animal Rights: Your Child or the Dog?* New Orleans, LA: Temple University Press.

Gorczyca, Ken. 1991. "Special Needs for the Pet Owner with AIDS/HIV." In *Universal Kinship: The Bond Between All Living Things,* pp. 13–20, ed. the Latham Foundation Staff. Saratoga, CA: R & E.

Kay, William J.; Cohen, Susan P.; Nieburg, Herbert A.; Fudin, Carole E.; Grey, Ross E.; Kutscher, Austin H.; and Osman, Mohamed M., eds. 1988. *Euthanasia of the Companion Animal: The Impact on Pet Owners, Veterinarians and Society.* Philadelphia: Charles.

Kropotkin, Petr Alekseevich. 1939. *Mutual Aid: A Factor in Evolution.* Harmondsworth, UK: Penguin.

Lessing, Doris. 1991. *Particularly Cats—and Rufus,* rev. edition. New York: Alfred A. Knopf.

Levinson, Boris M. 1978. "Pets and Personality Development." *Psychological Reports* 42(3) pt. 2: 1031–1038.

Linzey, Andrew. 1976. *Animal Rights: A Christian Assessment of Man's Treatment of Animals.* London: SCM.

Linzey, Andrew. 1987. *Christianity and the Rights of Animals.* London: SPCK.

Linzey, Andrew. 1994. *Animal Theology.* London: SCM.

Nicholson, Edward W. B. 1879. *The Rights of an Animal: A New Essay in Ethics.* London: C. Kegan Paul.

Patronek, G. J., and Lacroix, C. A. 2001. "Developing an Ethic for the Handling, Restraint, and Discipline of Companion Animals in Veterinary Practice." *Journal of the American Veterinary Medicine Association* 218(4): 514–517.

Patronek, Gary J., and Glickman, Lawrence T. 1994. "Development of a Model for Estimating the Size and Dynamics of the Pet Dog Population." *Anthrozoos* 7(1): 25–41.

Regan, Tom. 1983. *The Case for Animal Rights.* Berkeley: University of California Press.

Ritvo, Harriet. 1986. "Pride and Pedigree: The Evolution of the Victorian Dog Fancy." *Victorian Studies* 29(2): 227–253.

Ritvo, Harriet. 1994. "A Dog's Life." *New York Review of Books,* January 13, pp. 3–6.

Robin, Michael, and Bensel, Robert ten. 1991. "Pets and the Socialization of Children." In *Universal Kinship: The Bond Between All Living Things,* pp. 173–196, ed. the Latham Foundation Staff. Saratoga, CA: R & E.

Rodd, Rosemary. 1990. *Biology, Ethics, and Animals.* Oxford: Clarendon Press.

Rollin, Bernard E. 1992. *Animal Rights and Human Morality,* rev. edition. Buffalo, NY: Prometheus.

Rothschild, Miriam. 1986. *Animals and Man.* Oxford: Oxford University Press.

Royal Society for the Prevention of Cruelty to Animals (RSPCA). 1984. *Policies on Animal Welfare,* rev. edition. Horsham, Sussex: Author.

Ryder, Richard D. 1973. *Pets Are Good for People.* London: Pet Manufacturers' Association.

Sandys-Winsch, Godfrey. 1984. *Animal Law,* 2nd edition. London: Shaw.

Serpell, James. 1986. *In the Company of Animals: A Study of Human-Animal Relationships.* Oxford: Basil Blackwell.

Shell, Marc. 1986. "The Family Pet." *Representations* 15: 121–153.

Singer, Peter. 1976. *Animal Liberation: A New Ethics for Our Treatment of Animals.* London: Jonathan Cape.

Stallones, Lorann. 1994. "Pet Loss and Mental Health." *Anthrozoos* 7(1): 43–54.

Sweeney, Noel. 1990. *Animals and Cruelty and Law.* Bristol, U. K.: Alibi Books.

Tester, Keith. 1991. *Animals and Society: The Humanity of Animal Rights.* London: Routledge.

Thomas, Elizabeth Marshall. 1993. *The Hidden Life of Dogs.* Boston: Houghton Mifflin.

Thomas, Keith. 1983. *Man and the Natural World: A History of the Modern Sensibility.* New York: Pantheon.

Wilson, Cindy C. 1991. "The Pet as an Anxiolytic Intervention." *Journal of Nervous and Mental Disease* 179(8): 482–489.

Wilson, Cindy C. 1994. "Commentary: A Conceptual Framework for Human-Animal Interaction Research: The Challenge Revisited." *Anthrozoos* 7(1): 4–12.

Wilson, Cindy C., and Nettling, F. E. 1987. "New Directions: Challenges for Human-Animal Bond Research and the Elderly." *Journal of Applied Gerontology* 7(2): 51–57.

Wood, John George. 1874. *Man and Beast: Here and Hereafter. Illustrated by More Than Three Hundred Original Anecdotes.* London: Daldy, Isbister.

Youatt, William. 1839. *The Obligation and Extent of Humanity to Brutes, Principally Considered with Reference to Domesticated Animals.* London: Longman.

## V. ZOOS AND ZOOLOGICAL PARKS

Wild animals have been displayed in captivity for millennia (Luoma). The first known large collections were assembled in Egypt around 2500 B.C.E. Early rulers displayed their exotic menageries, captured during campaigns or expeditions, for personal amusement and as symbols of wealth and political power. Romans later maintained menageries for bloody public spectacles, sending elephants, lions, bears, and other wildlife into battle in arenas throughout Europe. Urban zoos appeared in sixteenth-century Europe and North Africa; visitors ogled strange creatures captured on colonial adventures. In 1828, the first zoo dedicated to the scientific study of captive wildlife opened in London, and in 1889, the U.S. Congress established the National Zoo for the purpose of breeding native wildlife. As zoos continued to evolve in the twentieth century, they developed a broad mission that included research, conservation, education, and entertainment.

Zoos, aquariums, safari parks, and wildlife theme parks are popular worldwide. Approximately 400 professionally managed zoos exist in the world, in addition to thousands of roadside menageries and petting zoos (Chiszar et al.). Annual zoo attendance in the United States alone exceeds one hundred million (Nelson). According to studies conducted in the United States and Canada, one-third of the public has visited a zoo within the last twelve months, and 98 percent of adults have visited a zoo in their lifetimes (Nelson).

Despite their broad popularity, zoos are increasingly criticized on ethical grounds. As the public has grown more sensitive to animal-welfare and conservation issues, animal advocates have begun to question whether or not the benefits of zoos justify the incarceration of live, and often rare, wild animals. (Although the term *zoo* may refer to a broad range of animal facilities, for the purposes of this entry it will refer only to zoos and aquariums that meet at least minimum professional standards. These minimum standards are defined by the American Association for Zoological Parks and Aquariums [AAZPA] in the United States.)

## The Ethics of Captivity

Many zoo opponents hold that wild animals should not be kept in captivity for human benefit. Dale Jamieson (1985) argues that animals taken from the wild are deprived of the opportunity to behave naturally. They are removed from their natural habitats, separated from family and social groups, and prevented from performing natural behaviors such as gathering food. Most important, the animals lose the freedom to pursue their own lives. Therefore, even under the best zoo conditions, Jamieson believes there exists a moral presumption against keeping animals in captivity.

Critics also focus on the possibility of physical or psychological suffering caused by captive conditions. Despite improvements in exhibit design, many animals remain confined in dirty, cramped, and isolated cages. Indoor facilities often lack fresh air and natural light, while outdoor enclosures may expose animals to extreme weather conditions to which they are not adapted. Without social or environmental stimulation, captive wildlife may become listless, self-abusive, or develop stereotypical behaviors such as the pacing often observed in big cats (Fox). When elephants or other potentially dangerous animals display aggression, zookeepers may respond with harsh discipline or physical restraints. The capture of animals in the wild, their transportation to zoos, and the handling required for veterinary care are other sources of stress.

Perhaps the most controversial source of potential suffering is the disposition of "surplus" animals. The zoo surplus includes aged adults and excess offspring of breeding programs. Animal activists assert that many surplus animals suffer inhumane treatment when zoos sell them to animal dealers who, in turn, sell them to research laboratories, private collectors, roadside menageries, and hunting parks (Clifton). An equally controversial disposal method is "culling," or mercy killing for management purposes. Critics decry this killing of healthy animals, especially when the surplus results from careless management. Animal advocates stress that zoos have a moral obligation to care for all zoo animals, regardless of their utility for breeding and other zoo goals.

Zoo advocates agree that culling is ethically problematic. However, they contend that responsible zoo directors manage breeding programs to avoid surpluses through contraception and segregation of sexes (Bostock). When contraception fails or a zoo's needs change, the director is expected to follow the AAZPA's code of ethics for distributing surplus animals to other qualified zoos or dealers. Euthanasia is seen as a last, though sometimes unavoidable, resort. To sustain viable captive populations of endangered species, zoo scientists must carefully balance age and sex ratios to maintain genetic diversity. Animals that are old, infertile, or genetically undesirable become surplus because zoos have limited space and financial resources. Zoo proponents defend culling these individuals as a necessary evil. Euthanasia and other disposal methods, proponents claim, allow zoos to conserve populations and species, although some individual animals must be sacrificed.

Animal welfare, according to zoo advocates, remains a high priority (Hutchins and Fascione). While recognizing that inferior enclosures still exist, they applaud the revolution in naturalistic exhibit design. At many zoos, for example, primates have been moved from isolated, tiled cells to family groupings in outdoor facsimiles of their native habitat. Tropical birds have flown from their cages into reproductions of rain forests. In addition, animal behaviorists are studying ways to stimulate animals' physical and mental activity, and veterinarians are investigating how to improve their nutrition and health. Through advances in captive breeding, zoos have also been able to reduce their demand for animals captured in the wild. Zoo advocates point proudly to these improvements, arguing that mortality and morbidity rates at zoos do not support claims that the animals are miserable (Chiszar et al.).

Furthermore, zoo proponents object to claims, such as Jamieson's, that captive animals suffer as humans would from the loss of liberty. Animals, they believe, may be happier in an enclosure free from predation and hunger than they are in the wild. Expecting animals to have the same needs and desires as humans do—an attitude called *anthropomorphism*—is viewed as a reflection of animal activists' sentimentality and biological ignorance (Robinson).

## Justifications of Zoos

Another approach to the zoo debate is to examine the reasons for keeping animals in captivity. If the benefits of zoos are negligible, animal advocates contend, then keeping wildlife captive cannot be justified. However, if significant benefits can be shown, captivity for at least some animals might be defensible.

ENTERTAINMENT. Historically, the predominant function of zoos has been entertainment. Studies of zoo visitors show that most people continue to see these facilities as parklike settings for casual family socializing (Kellert). To zoo opponents, public amusement is a trivial reason for holding animals in confinement (Jamieson). Opponents especially attack circuslike events, such as sea lion shows, that use trained animals to draw large crowds. Similarly, zoos that import animals such as giant pandas to boost attendance and revenues have been condemned. Such events are seen as denigrating the animals by exploiting them as public spectacles.

Although zoo directors vaunt high attendance rates, many de-emphasize entertainment as a zoo goal (Luoma). Baby elephant rides and similar amusements are gradually disappearing as zoos try to develop a more serious image. However, zoo educators claim that entertainment is necessary to keep visitors interested in learning. Also, zoo administrators assert that animal shows, special events, and traveling exhibits are sometimes essential to raise the funds needed to pay for research and other zoo missions (Cohn).

RESEARCH. Few visitors are familiar with the scientific efforts of zoos. Although a handful of zoos sponsor field research, most studies are conducted on site by zoo staff or affiliated researchers. Common topics include animal behavior, nutrition, reproductive biology, genetics, and pathology (Hutchins and Fascione). Animal activists challenge both the quality and usefulness of this research (Jamieson). According to critics, the experimental design of most zoo research lacks scientific rigor, rarely qualifying for publication in peer-reviewed journals. In a nutrition study, for example, a small sample size or the absence of a control group may obscure study results. Some critics also say that much of the research is aimed at improving captive husbandry and exhibit design—unnecessary benefits if wildlife were not confined in the first place. Regardless of any benefits, some animal-rights advocates oppose all animal

research. Tom Regan (1983) argues that the utility of research, whether to gain practical information of basic knowledge, is no justification for violating an individual animal's basic rights.

Zoo scientists reject the position that animal research is intrinsically wrong. They emphasize that most zoo research is noninvasive, nonterminal, and aimed at benefiting captive and wild populations (Hutchins). While acknowledging weaknesses in past studies, zoo proponents see a growing commitment to quality research at many institutions. Zoos are hiring research staff, cooperating with university faculties, and investing in major research facilities such as the U.S. National Zoo's 3,000-acre Conservation and Research Center. Much current research employs sophisticated, controversial techniques, such as embryo transfers, in efforts to improve captive breeding success. Although the experimental techniques may harm individual animals, zoo scientists contend that the long-term benefits for species conservation outweigh the costs to individual animals.

CONSERVATION. Animal advocates doubt that zoos can make a significant contribution to conservation (Fox). Although many recognize the biodiversity crisis, critics hold that zoos can do little to resolve the primary cause of extinction: habitat destruction. Nor can zoos protect more than an insignificant portion of the estimated five to thirty million species on the planet. Further, zoo conservation efforts are biased toward the charismatic large mammals preferred by zoo visitors, nearly ignoring disliked organisms such as bats and invertebrates (Kellert). When zoos do have success in maintaining a captive population, critics worry that the animals suffer from inbreeding and loss of natural behavioral characteristics. Are zoo animals and their wild relatives equivalent organisms? Could animals bred in zoos for generations be successfully reintroduced into the wild? If reintroduction is never possible, how long should the species be perpetuated in zoos? Extinction, to some zoo opponents, is more respectful of individual animals than endless confinement.

Yet conservation is viewed by many as the preeminent function of modern zoos. Zoo advocates liken the zoo to a crowded ark, struggling to accommodate as many threatened species as possible. Advocates remind critics that several organisms have already been saved from extinction by zoos, including the European bison and Mongolian wild horses (Tudge). Increasing resources are devoted to captive breeding through programs such as the AAZPA's Species Survival Plans (SSP) (Wiese and Hutchins). SSPs manage rare animal populations at zoos throughout the country, asking zoos to cooperate in breeding plans that promote genetic variability and demographic stability. SSP organizers hope that as such programs grow, world zoos will eventually be able to protect 500 to 900 endangered species (Luoma).

Zoos are also expanding efforts to reintroduce animals born in captivity to the wild, using some reintroduction projects to study techniques for managing small, isolated populations in the wild and to encourage habitat protection in developing countries. While they agree that zoos cannot directly save the majority of endangered species, zoo advocates proclaim that saving any species keeps options open for the future.

EDUCATION. The educational benefits of zoos are also viewed skeptically by animal advocates. Visitor studies indicate that relatively few people are interested in learning about animals or conservation, and there is little evidence that the zoo experience improves knowledge of biological facts or conservation issues (Kellert; Kellert and Dunlap). Given zoos' poor record of educational effectiveness, critics suggest that films, lectures, books, and nature centers may offer superior learning benefits without the ethical costs of confining wildlife. Most important, critics charge that zoos may be presenting harmful information and values (Sommer). Seeing rare animals in captivity, for example, may give visitors an inaccurate impression of human abilities to combat extinction. In addition, witnessing listless creatures in sterile cages may diminish respect for animals or concern for conservation.

Zoo advocates respond by describing the diversity of education programs and a growing commitment to educational progress (Chiszar et al.). Zoos attempt to teach casual visitors through signs, demonstrations, learning laboratories, and interactive computer technologies. Part of the revolution in exhibit design aims at enhancing learning by immersing visitors in natural environments. To extend their educational impact, zoos are developing curricula for primary and secondary students, holding workshops for teachers, visiting community centers, and organizing public lecture series. Michael Robinson (1989) promotes such changes as part of an educational revolution committed to teaching visitors about the interactions between wild animals, plants, and humans. Zoo proponents believe that, in our urbanized society, the zoo may be the only institution capable of demonstrating these vital links to the public.

Education, in fact, may offer zoos their best hope of effecting long-term, large-scale benefits (Kellert and Dunlap). If zoo educators could demonstrate positive program impacts, they could defuse criticisms and justify program expansion. Zoos should embark on a coordinated program of systematic educational evaluation and implement their findings through innovative programs dedicated to further progress. Given the wide popularity of zoos, it is doubtful

that the ethical debate will result in their abolition. If zoos can learn how to teach the public scientific information and humane and conservation values, animal advocates, zoo proponents, and wildlife will all benefit.

JULIE DUNLAP
STEPHEN R. KELLERT (1995)
BIBLIOGRAPHY REVISED

SEE ALSO: *Animal Research; Endangered Species and Biodiversity; Environmental Ethics; Veterinary Ethics;* and other *Animal Welfare and Rights* subentries

### BIBLIOGRAPHY

Bostok, Stephen. 1993. *Zoos and Animal Rights: The Ethics of Keeping Animals.* New York: Routledge.

Chiszar, David; Murphy, James B.; and Iliff, Warren. 1990. "For Zoos." *Psychological Record* 40(1): 3–13.

Clifton, Merritt. 1988. "Chucking Zoo Animals Overboard: How and Why Noah Culls the Ark." *Animals Agenda* 8(2): 14–22, 53–54.

Cohen, Carl, and Regan, Tom. 2001. *The Animal Rights Debate.* Lanham, MD: Rowman & Littlefield Publishing.

Cohn, Jeffrey P. 1992. "Decisions at the Zoo." *BioScience* 42(9): 654–659.

Fox, Michael W. 1990. "The Zoo: A Cruel and Outmoded Institution?" In *Inhumane Society: The American Way of Exploiting Animals,* pp. 145–155. New York: St. Martin's Press.

Hutchins, Michael. 1988. "On the Design of Zoo Research Programmes." *International Zoo Yearbook* 27: 9–19.

Hutchins, Michael, and Fascione, Nina. 1991. "Ethical Issues Facing Modern Zoos," In *Proceedings—American Association of Zoo Veterinarians,* ed. Randall Junge. Wheeling, W. VA: American Association for Zoological Parks and Aquariums.

Jamieson, Dale. 1985. "Against Zoos," In *In Defence of Animals,* pp. 108–117, ed. Peter Singer. Oxford: Basil Blackwell.

Kellert, Stephen R. 1987. "The Educational Potential of the Zoo and Its Visitor." *Philadelphia Zoo Review* 3(1): 7–13.

Kellert, Stephen R., and Dunlap, Julie. 1989. *Informal Learning at the Zoo: A Study of Attitude and Knowledge Impacts.* A report to the Zoological Society of Philadelphia.

Kohn, B., and Monfort S. L. 1997. "Research at Zoos and Aquariums: Regulations and Reality." *Journal of Zoo and Wildlife Medicine* 28(3): 241–250.

Luoma, Jon R. 1987. *A Crowded Ark: The Role of Zoos in Wildlife Conservation.* Boston: Houghton Mifflin.

Nelson, Andrew J. 1990. "Going Wild." *American Demographics* 12(2): 34–37, 50.

Norton, Bryan G.; Hutchins, Michael; Stevens, Elizabeth F. eds. 1996. *Ethics on the Ark: Zoos, Animal Welfare and Wildlife Conservation.* Washington, D.C.: Smithsonian Institution Press.

Regan, Tom. 1983. *The Case for Animal Rights.* Berkeley: University of California Press.

Robinson, Michael. 1989. "Zoos Today and Tomorrow." *Anthrozoos* 2: 10–14.

Sommer, Robert. 1972. "What Do We Learn at the Zoo?" *Natural History* 81(7): 26–29, 84–85.

Tudge, Colin. 1991. *Last Animals at the Zoo.* London: Hutchinson Radius.

Wiese, Robert, and Hutchins, Michael. 1993. "The Role of Captive Breeding and Reintroduction in Wildlife Conservation." In *Proceedings of the AAZPA Regional Conferences.* Wheeling, WV: American Association for Zoological Parks and Aquariums.

## VI. ANIMALS IN AGRICULTURE AND FACTORY FARMING

For almost all of human history, animal agriculture has involved human management of animals under living conditions for which the animals were biologically and evolutionarily adapted. Human intervention has consisted largely in ensuring the animals' health, nutrition, and reproduction by providing supplementary rations when forage was scarce, medical assistance, shelter from harsh elements, and so on. The symbiotic relationship between human and animal has been strongly reinforced by the cultural values of animal agricultural societies. To this day, for example, among ranchers in the American West, who are primarily traditional agriculturists and raise animals on open ranges, one finds a doctrine passed from generation to generation: "We take care of the animals, and the animals take care of us."

### Factory Farming

Intensive agriculture, also known as confinement agriculture or factory farming, differs dramatically from traditional animal agriculture. The key notion behind confinement agriculture is the application of industrial methods to producing animals or animal products. This way of thinking about agriculture emerged in the middle of the twentieth century; before that, neither the technology nor the social conditions existed to make confinement agriculture possible. After World War II, various technological developments and changing social conditions combined to alter radically the face of animal agriculture, and to model farms on factories. At about the same time, departments of "animal husbandry" in agricultural universities began to change their names to departments of "animal science." Increasingly, agriculture became a business, not merely a way of life combined with a way of making a living.

The conditions that generated confinement or intensive agriculture are relatively clear. After World War II, increasing numbers of workers moved from rural, agricultural regions into urban localities, where wages were higher and economic opportunities were perceived to be greater. At the same time, urban centers grew, encroaching onto traditional farmland, so that rising land prices and higher taxes militated against keeping that land for agricultural use. Inevitably the land was developed. Thus fewer and fewer people were directly involved in production agriculture.

With less land and fewer workers (as of 1993, 1.7 percent of Americans were engaged in production agriculture), it was difficult to keep animals under far-ranging, open, extensive conditions. With fewer people caring for them, animals were brought into closer and closer confinement, both outdoor and indoor, so that effects of temperature, rain, snow, and so on could be minimized. Instead of depending on human labor, farmers began to rely on machinery to feed, clean, water, milk, collect eggs, and so forth. Animal agricultural operations became capital-intensive rather than labor-intensive.

Animals began to be crowded together in an attempt to get as many as possible into the expensive production unit. Laying hens, for example, are typically placed 5 to 6 birds in a 12-inch-by-18-inch cage, and up to 100,000 birds may be kept in one building. Broiler chickens are raised in huge open sheds at a density of approximately two birds per square foot. Beef cattle, traditionally raised on range grass, are moved for the latter portion of their lives into feedlots, where they are fed grain diets, thus producing both increased weight gain and an outlet for U.S. grain surplus. Hogs are increasingly raised in confinement buildings where they never see the light of day—buildings holding 500 to 1000 sows are not uncommon. Most notoriously, veal calves are raised in small crates in order to restrict movement and keep their flesh tender, and are also kept anemic or near-anemic to keep the meat "white."

Thus animals are forced into environments for which they are not biologically suited. Because the operations are so expensive, producers are motivated to crowd as many animals as possible into the systems, since profit per animal is small. Thus, even though it is well known that chickens will lay more eggs if given more space, it is more profitable to crowd as many birds as possible into cages, yielding fewer eggs per bird but more eggs for the operation as a whole. Such methods would be impossible without recent technology. In the absence of antibiotics and vaccines, the spread of disease would decimate the animals in weeks. Without growth promoters< the animals could not be processed quickly enough to be profitable—broiler chickens for instance, reach full growth in eight weeks. The rise of confinement agriculture has, according to its proponents, provided cheap and plentiful food. For example, the price of chicken has remained virtually the same for more than twenty years, even in the face of inflation. Advocates of intensive agriculture also argue that confinement provides animals with shelter from extremes of weather, protection from predators, and a consistent nutritional regimen.

## Harms of Confinement

But there are hidden costs offsetting these benefits, the most important of which is the cost to the animals. The animals being produced in confinement are still essentially the animals that were genetically adapted to extensive conditions. Their fundamental biological interests are systematically violated in confinement. Thus animals that are built to move about are unable to do so. Social animals may be deprived of companionship. Air laden with dust and ammonia in confinement chicken, egg, and swine barns is execrable; in some swine operations, workers must wear respirators. Diets designed to maximize growth may lead to metabolic disease for some of the animals, even though this loss is balanced by economic gain in the other animals. In chicken and swine barns, unnatural floor surfaces such as wire and concrete slats may lead to leg, foot, and joint problems. With the advent of confinement agriculture, there has arisen a class of diseases, known as "production diseases," that result from the systems of production. Since intensive systems have a low profit margin, they are often understaffed, and care of sick or injured animals is impossible for workers whose other duties stretch them to their limit.

As a result of such systematic violation of their physical and psychological (animal scientists prefer the word "behavioral") needs, animals suffer psychologically as well as physically. Many animals in confinement show chronic signs of long- and short-term stress, which can lead to both disease and behavioral problems. Cannibalism among chickens increases in the absence of either space to flee or small enough numbers to establish a pecking order; to prevent cannibalism, producers "debeak" chickens with a hot blade and without anesthesia, sometimes producing chronic pain. Similarly, pigs are tail-docked to prevent tail-biting, a stress-induced result of confinement. Confined animals also show many bizarre, stereotypical behaviors that seem to result from the thwarting of natural inclinations and from boring, austere environments.

Confinement agriculture also exacts other social costs. In an industry requiring large amounts of capital, small operators cannot compete effectively, and large, well-capitalized corporations inevitably drive out small "family farmers." Young people cannot afford to enter agriculture.

Efficiency and productivity eclipse other values traditionally maintained in small farm communities, such as independence, self-sufficiency, and husbandry. Environmental problems such as waste disposal and water and energy consumption also arise from intensive agriculture. Lack of pasturing of animals contributes to soil erosion when land no longer used for pasture is tilled for grain. Drug residues in animal products may pose human health problems, and widespread use of antibiotics essentially breeds for resistant pathogens by eliminating microbes susceptible to the drugs. *Salmonella* and *Campylobacter* bacterial contamination are significant problems in chickens, turkeys, and eggs, since they can cause severe enteric disease in humans who consume these products.

## Toward Reform

Agriculturists have recognized that the welfare of animals in confinement represents one of the three major challenges to agriculture in the next century, the other two being food safety and environmental concerns. When the British public became aware of factory farms in the 1960s as a result of Ruth Harrison's pioneering book *Animal Machines,* the outcry generated a royal commission, the Brambell Commission, that was highly critical of confinement agriculture as violating the animals' natures. In the face of confinement agriculture, European society is moving toward legal protection for farm animals. Laws in Britain, Denmark, Germany, and Switzerland have restricted certain aspects of confinement agriculture, and Sweden has essentially abolished such agriculture and guaranteed certain rights for farm animals, in a law that has been called a "bill of rights" for farm animals because it aims at protecting their fundamental interests. In the United States, public attention was first directed toward animals in research, and certain basic protections for such animals have been legally encoded in two federal laws passed in 1985. Public attention is beginning to focus on the treatment of farm animals as well as on the environmental consequences of confinement agriculture, and articles in agricultural journals show that agriculture is starting to pay more attention to these concerns.

Until very recently, U.S. confinement agriculturists (in contrast to their counterparts in Europe and Canada) tended to deny that there were any problems of animal welfare intrinsically related to confinement agriculture, and acknowledged only occasional "bad management." This was further exacerbated by widespread skepticism in the scientific community about the existence and knowability of animal consciousness, pain, and suffering. Since the early 1990s, however, there have been indications that at least some parts of the industry and government are engaging such issues as animal deprivation, boredom, and inability to move in confinement, primarily by inaugurating research into improving animal welfare.

While it is unlikely that industrialized agriculture will ever revert to being fully or even largely extensive, it is possible to make intensive agriculture much more "animal-welfare friendly," and perhaps to change certain systems from full to partial confinement. For example, it is possible to raise swine profitably without keeping sows confined in small gestation crates for their entire lives. In addition, concern about sustainable agriculture may well result in a concerted social effort to return to less industrialized systems guided by husbandry. On the other hand, confinement agricultural systems are being introduced into Third World countries as a shortcut to rapid economic growth and as a way of adding animal products to the diets of these countries. This has generated a variety of ethical concerns, including fear of environmental despoliation, concern that successful indigenous agriculture will be lost, worries about importing Western health problems to these countries, and concern about proliferating animal suffering.

## Growing Social Concern

Animal agriculture raises other animal welfare issues beyond confinement. Although cattle ranching is highly extensive and in fact presupposes a good fit between animal and environment, management techniques such as castration without anesthesia, hot-iron branding, and dehorning without anesthesia produce pain and suffering in these animals. Transportation of agricultural animals over long distances, for example to slaughter, is very stressful, and can cause disease and injury. Handling of farm animals by people ignorant of their behavior is an extremely widespread problem that creates high levels of stress and significant injury. Slaughter of food animals raises the issue of whether these animals can be provided with a death free of pain, suffering, and fear. This problem is particularly acute in the area of Jewish and Muslim religious slaughter, where preslaughter stunning has been considered incompatible with religious demands. Genetic engineering of farm animals for traits that are desirable to producers for reasons of efficiency and productivity may well exact costs in welfare from the animals' perspective. For example, swine and chickens engineered for greater size have suffered from a variety of diseases, including foot and leg problems. A cow engineered for double muscling was unable to stand on its own and required euthanasia. On the other hand, genetic engineering can also work to the benefit of farm animals, for example, by engineering for disease resistance.

Other branches of animal agriculture rear animals for uses other than food. Raising traditionally "wild" animals for various purposes has generated concerns about the well-being of these animals—pheasants for hunting, mink for fur, and deer for antler velvet (which is considered an aphrodisiac in the Orient) provide salient examples. Numerous welfare concerns have also been raised by the production of horses for human purposes—breakdown and injury in racehorses; injury in endurance horses (those used in long, grueling, competitive rides over difficult terrain); heat, water deprivation, and poor air for urban carriage horses. Indeed, no branch of animal agriculture is being ignored by growing social concern about animal welfare.

BERNARD E. ROLLIN (1995)
BIBLIOGRAPHY REVISED

SEE ALSO: *Agriculture and Biotechnology; Animal Research; Endangered Species and Biodiversity; Enhancement Uses of Medical Technology; Veterinary Ethics;* and other *Animal Welfare and Rights* subentries

## BIBLIOGRAPHY

Dawkins, Marian S. 1980. *Animal Suffering: The Science of Animal Welfare.* London: Chapman and Hall.

Fox, Michael W. 1984. *Farm Animals: Husbandry, Behavior, and Veterinary Practice: Viewpoints of a Critic.* Baltimore: University Park Press.

Goodwin, J. L. 2001. "The Ethics of Livestock Shows—Past, Present, and Future." *Journal of the American Veterinary Medicine Association* 219(10): 1391–1393.

Harrison, Ruth. 1964. *Animal Machines: The New Factory Farming Industry.* London: Vincent Stuart.

Hodges, John, and Han, K., eds. 2000. *Livestock, Ethics and Quality of Life.* New York: Oxford University Press.

Martin, Jerome, ed. 1991. *High Technology and Animal Welfare: Proceedings of the 1991 High Technology and Animal Welfare Symposium.* Edmonton: University of Alberta Press.

Mason, Jim, and Singer, Peter. 1990. *Animal Factories,* rev. edition. New York: Harmony.

Nolen, R. S. 2001. "Welfare on the Farm: Treating Pain and Distress in Food Animals." *Journal of the American Veterinary Medicine Association* 219(12): 1657.

Rollin, Bernard E. 1981. *Animal Rights and Human Morality.* Buffalo, NY: Prometheus.

Rollin, Bernard E. 1989. *The Unheeded Cry: Animal Consciousness, Animal Pain, and Science.* Oxford: Oxford University Press.

Rollin, Bernard E. 1990. "Animal Welfare, Animal Rights and Agriculture." *Journal of Animal Science* 68: 3456–3462.

Rollin, Bernard E. 1993. *Social, Bioethical, and Researchable Issues Pertaining to Farm Animal Welfare* (USDA-CSRS Contract Research). Washington, D.C.: Government Printing Office.

Sandoe P., Nielsen B. L., Christensen L. G., et al. 1999. "Staying Good While Playing God—the Ethics of Breeding Farm Animals." *Animal Welfare* 8(4): 313–328.

Theil, D. E. 2002. "A Resource for Veterinarians on Recognizing and Reporting Animal Abuse." *Canadian Veterinary Journal* 43(2): 97–98.

Thompson, Paul B. 1998. *Agricultural Ethics: Research, Teaching, and Public Policy.* Ames: Iowa State University Press.

# ANTHROPOLOGY AND BIOETHICS

• • •

In recent years a growing number of anthropologists have turned their attention to the discipline of biomedical ethics. Bioethics traces its origins as a distinct field to the styles of reasoning and reflection found within analytic philosophy and legal scholarship. In its early decades, work in bioethics relied heavily on principle-based analysis, an approach that often led to critiques of the moral dimensions of healthcare practice divorced from underlying social, cultural and political context. Often called the "empirical turn" in bioethics, social scientists utilizing diverse theoretical and methodological programs have questioned approaches to healthcare ethics that fail to account for context (Weisz; Hoffmaster, 2001; DeVries and Subedi; Brodwin, 2000).

Researchers in medical anthropology represent one arm of a strong, and growing, internal critique of bioethics. In addition to social science voices, this critique includes diverse perspectives within philosophy, such as feminist readings of core bioethics dilemmas and a resurgence of interest in the traditions of American pragmatism and casuistry. Even philosophers working within the Kantian tradition have called attention to bioethics' need to balance attention to "institutional and professional realities and diversities" with philosophical rigor (O'Neill, p. x). O'Neill questions the primacy of autonomy, to the exclusion of a focus on relationships of trust and trustworthiness, in contemporary bioethics discourse.

This entry explores how anthropologists working in the field of bioethics bridge the gap between conceptions of medical morality grounded in local worlds and the universal understandings espoused within the western philosophical tradition. Ongoing debates about relativism from the perspectives of anthropology and philosophy also are addressed with special attention paid to the implications of a "culturally informed" practice of bioethics. Culturally diverse understandings of the meaning and expression of personhood are highlighted in order to illustrate difficulties that emerge when one tries to judge certain practices as good or bad, appropriate or inappropriate. An anthropologically informed bioethics produces a fuller account of healthcare practices, an account that grounds ethical universals such as respect for persons in local moral worlds.

The body of empirical work reviewed below reveals the thinness of bioethics accounts that disregard social context and that celebrate a particular (often American) version of individual autonomy. Ethical analyses centered exclusively on individual actors create strong barriers to understanding the troubling conflicts that emerge in multicultural worlds, especially in the arena of social justice and human rights. A simplistic application of ethical universals to particular cases discounts the complexity of lived experience and real world dilemmas. In the same way, a naïve and unqualified acceptance of ethical relativism diminishes the potential of negotiating moral consensus across cultural boundaries. An anthropologically grounded framework for bioethics requires a solid recognition of the cultural assumptions that underlie our definition of the "good" in biomedicine. An anthropologically informed bioethics calls attention to the social, political and structural factors that affect the production of scientific and clinical knowledge and its application in the practice of global biomedicine.

## Anthropological Approaches to Bioethics

Today the field of bioethics is uniquely multidisciplinary, indeed it is perhaps best understood as a cultural space in which scholars from many fields interact, joined together by topical interests. However, anthropologists and other social scientists did not play a significant role in the initial development of the field (Fox).

In his analysis of medical ethics, Lieban (pp. 221–222) suggests two key reasons why anthropologists have been absent. First, given the strong history of cultural relativism in anthropology, studies of health and illness conducted by anthropologists have generally avoided what might be construed as ethnocentric value judgments about other systems. Anthropological focus on documentation and description—as opposed to normative analysis—excludes questions about what is morally "right" or "wrong" about particular health practices.

Second, medical anthropologists have often worked in non-Western settings where the technological challenges provided by contemporary biomedicine are less salient. In addition, Marshall (1992) suggests that bioethicists—unlike anthropologists—have concentrated their attention on the individual rational actor as the primary unit of analysis. Although in recent years bioethics scholars have begun to acknowledge the importance of social milieu—for example the role of family—in constructing individual choice and shaping decision options, anthropologists, in part because of their traditional subjects, have generally theorized a more complex self, viewing the individual as firmly embedded within a broader social and cultural context. The notion of autonomy, or respect for persons, which many acknowledge has been over-celebrated in bioethics clinical discourse, presumes an individuated self, set apart from the collective experience of family or community, and triumphant over other critical values. These explanations, however, represent fairly superficial explanations for the lack of anthropological representation within or interest in bioethics. In fact, the unwillingness of anthropologists to engage with ethics (and for philosophers to reach out to social scientists generally) reflects deep seated disciplinary boundaries and conflicting epistemologies (Edel and Edel).

The concept of culture is rarely a starting point in ethics; by contrast, pioneering discussions of comparative medical ethics by anthropologists emphasized the importance of a cultural foundation for framing ethical issues in healthcare. For example, Kundstadter addressed ethical challenges associated with development projects in Third World communities, noting the relevance and importance of cultural context for understanding moral dilemmas surrounding health and illness beliefs and healing roles. Practices such as treatment of less than perfect newborns cannot be adequately understood, much less judged, without detailed local knowledge. Approximately a decade later, Fabrega and Lieban examined the potential of "ethnoethics" for cross-cultural studies of the moral dimensions of health practices. A key starting point is the recognition of variation in the issues that different societies define as morally relevant or problematic. The role of healer is also critical, including the nature of interactions between healers and their patients, interactions among healers themselves, and finally, interactions between practitioners and the larger society.

As engagement with scholars working in healthcare ethics increased, anthropologists have questioned the fundamental schema underlying bioethics, urging greater attention to the lived experience of human suffering and to the social dynamics of local context (Muller; Koenig, 1996; Kleinman, 1995, 1999; Marshall and Koenig, 1996, 2000).

Cultural interpretation situates the moral dimensions of healthcare in local ethical practices and *local* notions of the good. This traditional anthropological orientation to ethics and morality is antithetical to the universalizing discourses of both basic science—which assumes that scientific principles and rules apply to human bodies in all times and places, and to the discourse of the philosophical traditions dominant in bioethics—which define a good ethical theory as one that can produce "objective" results that yield rational standards by which to judge actions, irrespective of their history or locality (Marshall and Koenig, 1996, 2000).

Medical anthropologist Arthur Kleinman (1995), in his critical analysis of the assumptions and theoretical foundations of bioethics, suggests that the new field is fundamentally ethnocentric, psychocentric, and medicocentric, and thus shares, rather than moves beyond, biomedicine's fundamental limitations. Kleinman argues that bioethics has failed to engage with the major non-Western moral traditions or to question the "orthodox sources of the self within the western philosophical tradition" (p. 1669). The medicocentrism inherent in bioethics constrains practitioner's ability to elicit a complex illness narrative despite the fact that bioethicists are charged with listening to patients and taking account of their perspective and preferences. Although Kleinman maintains optimism that bioethics may open up space in clinical practice for genuine moral reflection and debate, he remains concerned about the limitations of a bioethics devoid of attention to cultural locality: "In the end, then, ethics, once framed as models of moral reasoning championing the reflection and rational choice of autonomous individuals in quest of objective standards, risk irrelevance to the almost always uncertain circumstances and highly contextualized conditions of human experience" (1999, p. 72).

Anthropologists have the greatest potential to make significant contributions to the field of biomedical ethics in two domains: through studies of the cultural production of scientific and clinical knowledge and its translation into medical technology and healing practices, and, secondly, through analysis of the cultural construction of canons of medical morality, including the clinical practices of bioethics itself. Note that this contribution is not linked to the traditional role of anthropology in elucidating the cultural practices of exotic peoples. Ethnographic approaches to ethical questions help clarify the contextual features that are intrinsic to problematic moral issues that arise in medical and research settings throughout the world (Koenig, 1988, 1997; Hunt; Hogle; Rapp; Marshall and Koenig, 1996, 2001; Kleinman, Fox, and Brandt; Kaufman, 2000; Brodwin, 2000; Finkler; Farmer, 2003).

## Anthropology and the Study of Biomedical Technology

A broad range of clinical issues and public health concerns have been addressed by anthropologists, including: end-of-life decision making, definitions of death, human organ and tissue transplantation therapies, disclosure of medical information, informed consent for medical treatment, reproductive technologies, genetic testing and screening, human rights, and treatment of human subjects in biomedical research. Scholars working at the boundary of anthropology and the field of science and technology studies have been central to evolving scholarship. A systematic review of the contributions of anthropologists to bioethics, and to our understanding of the moral dimensions of human suffering more generally, is beyond the scope of this review (see Marshall and Koenig 1996). Instead, several areas in which anthropologists have focused a cultural lens on moral problems in medicine are highlighted.

The development of new medical technologies has raised myriad questions at the intersection of culture, morality, and the production and application of scientific discovery (Lock, Young, and Cambrosio). New technologies in biomedicine challenge established meanings of personhood and provide fertile ground for a socially reimagined human body. Does social personhood begin with a fertilized egg, an embryo, at birth, or once the likely survival of an infant is established? How is life's end understood? Anthropological studies can reveal the ambiguous and contested boundaries between nature and culture, boundaries constantly challenged by scientific developments. Anthropological investigations of new reproductive technologies and genetics, in particular, illustrate how understandings of family are necessarily evolving, radically changing traditional notions of kinship and the cultural and biological creation and "production" of children (Ginsburg and Rapp; Lock; Becker; Finkler).

Rapp's intensive, multiyear ethnographic exploration of the use of amniocentesis for pre-natal diagnosis reveals the moral complexity of a seemingly straightforward technology. Ideally, pregnant women should make fully informed, voluntary decisions about undergoing the procedure and continuing a pregnancy if fetal anomalies are discovered. In the city of New York, where Rapp worked, the experience of testing, and the eventual decisions made, were fundamentally different for women of varying social class and ethnic background. The exercise of choice can only be understood in light of the social meanings attached to pre-natal testing. Rapp warns that a "new eugenics" is unlikely to be imposed by direct state power, but rather will be disguised under a rubric of individual choice.

Similarly, Press and Browner's 1998 study of the use of pre-natal maternal alpha fetoprotein blood testing (used to predict Down syndrome and other anomalies) illustrates the complex and culturally embedded issues surrounding women's refusal or acceptance of the procedure. Many women accepted the test believing it to be a positive way to assure the health of their baby, much like taking vitamins or other elements of routine prenatal care. In actual practice the only way to avoid the birth of an affected fetus is termination of the pregnancy, but U.S. abortion politics preclude a full and open discussion of the issues, leading to severely truncated communication in the clinic and misapprehension of the usefulness of the prenatal blood test.

Press, Fishman, and Koenig demonstrate how cultural context shapes our understanding of the meaning and practice of genetic testing for breast cancer risk, one of the first examples of a genetic test for a common adult-onset disease. Enhancing the decision-making capabilities of individual women is the most commonly suggested bioethical "solution" to the difficult dilemma of disclosing risk for cancer. Cultural analysis suggests two primary reasons for the limitations of this approach: the cultural construction of fear of breast cancer, which has been fueled in part by the predominance of a "risk" paradigm in contemporary biomedicine. The increasing elaboration and delineation of risk factors and risk numbers are in part intended to help women contend with their fear of breast cancer—fears that are inflamed by constant media attention in the form of health education campaigns. However, because there is no known cure nor foolproof prevention for breast cancer, risk designation brings with it recommendations for vigilant surveillance strategies and screening guidelines. Thus education about risks exacerbates women's fears of breast cancer, confounding decision making about genetic testing. The volatile combination of discourses of fear, risk, and surveillance has significant ethical and social consequences for women and their families.

The conceptual categories underlying our understanding of human identity and difference have been of particular concern to anthropology (Gaines; Lee, Mountain, and Koenig; Brodwin, 2002; Sankar and Cho). Is the species *homo sapiens* divided into biologically distinct races? With the advent of new knowledge about human genetic variation, as well as individualized therapies targeted to unique genetic signatures, this issue is of growing moral significance. Given profound health disparities across populations, how are we to tease out the interactions among culture, ethnicity, and most importantly, of race, in health research and clinical care? Ethnographic studies of the conduct of genetic research reveal how social categories of race inform all domains of biomedical practice. Locating disease etiology in an ethnic group's shared genetic ancestry—potentially excluding consideration of the relevant social determinants of health—may lead to group stigma as well as poor clinical outcomes.

New technologies—whether used for life-extending therapy, such as the mechanical ventilator, or diagnosis of death, such as functional brain imaging—may challenge settled understandings of the boundary between life and death (Lock). Liminal states, such as patients existing in persistent coma, are not "natural" entities, but are in fact created by new social arrangements, in this case long-term care centers dedicated to the management of those in persistent vegetative state (Kaufman, 2000). Bioethical debates about appropriate treatment for those suspended in such liminal states must take account of social forces. Anthropologists have been actively engaged in exploring the moral dimensions of changing definitions of death itself, calling attention to the powerful role that culture plays in shaping beliefs and practices for managing death and dying (Lock and Honde). Perhaps because of its potent emotional valence and symbolic salience, human organ and tissue transplantation has been studied extensively in many parts of the world. The moral questions fundamental to transplantation—whose organs should be replaced, whose may be "harvested," when is a donor "dead enough"—are deeply contingent, varying by beliefs about the location of the soul, the integrity of the physical body and the existence of an afterlife, beliefs which are negotiated within local economies and political arrangements (Lock; Ohnuki-Tierney; Sharp, 1995; Joralemon; Ikels; Hogle; Das; Gordon, E.).

A particular concern of social scientists has been the analysis of organs and their circulation, characterized initially as an elaborate system of nonmonetary gift exchange, glossed as giving the "gift of life." Sociologist Renee Fox, whose work shares many theoretical and methodological assumptions with that of anthropology, pioneered ethnographic work on transplantation. Later analysts have critiqued the status of human organs as a source of working capital for poor laborers in developing countries (Cohen), and have documented how a heart can create links of symbolic kinship between donor families and organ recipients (Sharp, 2001). Ethical quandaries stem from the commoditization of bodies that accompanies the marketing of human organs (Marshall and Daar). Most problematic is the exploitation of vulnerable individuals, especially when flows of organs go from poor nations to wealthy ones (Scheper-Hughes). Of interest is that fact that allowing individuals the right to sell their organs is justified using a neoliberal market language of rights, a discourse in many ways compatible with bioethics arguments that privilege individual choice and control of one's body. Joralemon documents the change in discourse about financial incentives for donation (from both living

and cadaveric donors) since the origins of U.S. transplantation, showing the impact of a public relations campaign formulated to minimize public resistance to donation. Bioethics debates, in response to intense pressure to increase organ supply, have tipped from vehement opposition to any financial compensation for organs to a guarded approval (Joralemon).

## Anthropological Analyses of Clinical Ethics and Research Ethics Practice

In the arena of end-of-life medical care, anthropological studies illustrate how decisions to forego technological interventions, such as intensive care, are socially negotiated (Slomka; Kaufman, 1998). Ethnographic findings allow a useful comparison with decision-making ideals based on abstract principles, providing a critique of models of care that evaluate the success of outcomes using a metric based solely on the exercise of patient choice. A review of the empirical literature suggests that the bioethics practices governing end-of-life care (a focus on self-determination, advance care planning, and explicit decisions to forgo life-sustaining treatment) are based on problematic and erroneous assumptions (Drought and Koenig). Studies of bioethics practices applied in culturally diverse clinical settings further illustrate the failure of efforts to enforce universal solutions on complex clinical problems. To fully engage with and respect a patient as a person, what is required is a nuanced understanding of each social environment (Frank et al.; Crawley et al.; Long, 2000; Koenig and Gates-Williams; Koenig and Davies). Anthropologists have also explored the ethical domain of truth-telling, demonstrating the significant impact of cultural difference on beliefs about disclosure of medical information, especially information relevant to diagnosis and prognosis of cancer and other life-threatening illness (Muller and Desmond; Gordon and Paci; Gordon and Daugherty; Orona, Koenig, Davis; Carrese and Rhodes; Kaufert; Long, 1999). Who decides which facts are truthful, whether that truth harms or helps, and who controls disclosure, are all culturally patterned.

Ethics consultation is a common and highly visible clinical application of bioethics. These services, common in U.S. hospitals, are carried out either by an expert consultant, an interdisciplinary ethics committee, or some combination of the two approaches; the goal is assistance with the identification of ethical quandaries and their resolution through bioethical analysis. Anthropological study of the actual practice of ethics consultation reveals the difficulty of simply "applying" bioethics theories in the clinic. A range of issues has been studied, including the nature of clinical disputes that are considered "ethical." In fact, consult requests often stem from non-ethical concerns, such as communication failure resulting from the social dynamics of complex hospital environments like intensive care units. Research has also examined actual decision-making processes by institutional ethics committees, power structures within organizational settings and their influence on consultation outcomes, and the potential for conflicts of interests when ethics consultants are institutional employees (Crigger; Orr et al.; Kelly et al.; Marshall, 2001a).

Voluntary informed consent is considered a universal ethical requirement for good clinical practice and for research with human subjects. However, anthropological studies reveal the ways in which the ideals of informed consent may be constrained in actual practice. The objectives of consent may be undermined by too great a reliance on a narrow conception of the exercise of personal autonomy—one excluding social relationships, by focus on consent as the articulation of a "legal" contract, rather than an ongoing process of communication, and by lack of attention to disparities in knowledge and power between professionals and lay people (Kaufert and O'Neill; Barnes et al.). Sankar demonstrates the critical value of classic observational methods by examining the actual practice of informed consent to research participation. Her analysis reveals how the informed consent process shares many characteristics with ritual; actual reflection and active decision making are not part of the dynamic. Rather, research participants offered informed consent had already made up their minds to participate in the study Sankar observed; going through the process of "consenting" the subject served primarily to inaugurate their participation in the research.

## Cross-Cultural and International Concerns

Medical interactions, including discussions of consent, are mediated by language—and the use of interpreters—and cultural beliefs about health practices, decisional authority, and professional roles (Kaufert and Putsch; Marshall et al., 1998). These interactions are complex in any environment; cross-national research projects present particular challenges. Marshall (2001b) describes the profound influence of cultural context on informed consent to genetic epidemiological studies conducted in urban and rural settings in Nigeria. Her ethnographic work highlights the challenges of translating difficult scientific concepts in cross-cultural settings; the very idea of consent may be unknown in rural settings where participants are not literate and have little experience of research. Ideal notions of individual consent, as practiced in the United States or other resource rich countries, do not easily incorporate the significance of family and community

relationships for the process of obtaining consent in diverse social environments across the world. In their work on community involvement in genetic research, Sharp and Foster outline potential strategies for representing the views of the larger community, suggesting that this may be an important component of the overall process of seeking and obtaining consent. Community consultation does not override an individual subject's right to decline or accept participation, and may serve to make individual consent more authentic. When working with international research teams, the role of the anthropologist is not simply to facilitate a particular study through in-depth knowledge of the local community, but rather to tailor the broad objectives of informed consent to fit local needs.

Issues of social justice in healthcare across the world—until recently neglected in traditional bioethics debates focused on individual choice and the dilemmas created by new technologies in resource-rich countries—are being addressed by anthropologists, particularly those working in the arena of public health (Levin and Fleischman). Anthropologists working in bioethics are deeply concerned about global health disparities, including class-based inequities in the United States (Levin and Schiller). Farmer (2003) levels a harsh critique against the narrow focus of bioethics, arguing strongly for greater attention to structural inequities that maintain health disparities in many areas of the world. The need for broadening the boundaries of bioethics beyond the confines of Western medicine and its limited attention to the political economy of social suffering is increasingly recognized by anthropologists engaged in discussions of global medical morality (Kleinman, Das, and Lock; Farmer, 1997; Kleinman, Fox, and Brandt; Das). Ethnography, which unifies the work of anthropologists, is more than a methodological orientation allowing fine-grained attention to local social and cultural processes. Rather, its theoretical foundation requires that the ethnographer draw connections between local suffering and global social and political processes.

## Culture, Morality, and the Problem of Relativism

The landscape of bioethics—in particular the "bedside" practices of clinical ethics and research procedures—is informed by the intellectual and ideological orientations of the analytic philosophers who were key figures in shaping the development of the field. Much work in bioethics reinforces and sustains an Enlightenment preoccupation with the primacy of the individual, "rational" man. Although theoretically it need not, the field's emphasis on rational decision making and individual autonomy often diminishes the importance of the social realm in ethical analysis. Culture, like emotion, may be viewed as something tangential to the core human, something that might be stripped away to reveal a rational "universal" being underneath. And many bioethics procedures seem designed with that rational man in mind. Once practices such as advance care planning or informed consent are enshrined in law and regulation, it becomes increasingly difficult to tailor those procedures to fit local conditions, even though exactly that sort of tailoring may be required to fully observe an ethical principle such as respect for persons. This silencing of culture is confusing to most anthropologists, while the anthropologists' "failure" to appreciate the preeminence of universal ethical norms may lead philosophers to the false conclusion that all anthropologists are naïve relativists.

Identifying, defining, and evaluating the nature of morality has been difficult to achieve as a common area of inquiry for bioethicists and anthropologists. While there is general agreement among the disciplines that the forms and practices of morality are inherently social, the consensus ends there. As Hoffmaster observes, "According to the prevailing positivist approach in Anglo-American philosophy, morality consists of rules and principles, which because they are *normative,* can be articulated and defended only on the basis of rational arguments directed at what *ought* to be the case" (1990, p. 242). The potential for a meaningful dialogue with anthropologists and other empirical social scientists—who, according to the tenants of moral philosophy, work only at the level of "descriptive" ethics—is thwarted given the normative and metaethical focus of moral philosophy.

Anthropologists and philosophers have approached morality and cultural pluralism from two very distinct perspectives. The unique morality expressed in diverse cultural traditions is emphasized in the "cultural relativism" of anthropology. Thus, for anthropologists, morality is viewed as an entity, like other dimensions of culture, that can be empirically described (Geertz, 1989; Hatch). It is found in social space, not argued in textbooks. Anthropologists have engaged in prolonged debates about the theoretical and methodological utility of relativism as it relates to cultural context (Herskovits; Hatch; Fabrega; Spiro; Renteln; Shweder).

Indeed, relativism has been foundational in the development of anthropology. The claims of a "moderate" descriptive relativism might be stated as follows: "Because all standards are culturally constituted, there are no available transcultural standards by which different cultures might be judged on a scale of merit or worth" (Spiro, p. 260). Thus, the only normative judgment that might be possible is one that recognizes the equal worth of moral standards (and this holds for total cultures, single cultural systems such as

religion, and specific cultural propositions). A normative claim based on this view is that because universally acceptable evaluative standards do not exist, judgments about cognition, behavior patterns, and emotions of different social groups must be relative to the variable standards of the cultures that produce them (e.g., all logic is ethno-logic or socio-logic). Epistemological relativism, the strongest form of descriptive relativism, is distinguished by its emphasis on the *particularist* theory of cultural determinism, which holds that because cultures are radically different from each other, each culture produces a unique and culturally particular set of human characteristics (Rosaldo). Epistemological relativism implies the basic incommensurability of moral standards across cultures since panhuman generalizations concerning culture are likely to be untrue; generalizations can only be true if confined to a specific group (Geertz, 1973).

The suggestion that it may be impossible to evaluate a moral system because it will always be relative to specific social traditions and historical contingencies is very problematic for many philosophers and bioethicists (Po-Wah, 2002). From the philosopher's vantage point, the sacredness and primacy of the moral sphere may be threatened by empirical descriptions of cultural variation regarding moral practices. At the heart of this debate is the presumed dichotomy of *fact* and *value.* As philosophers have asked: How can an empirical description of what "is" influence the formulation of statements about what "ought" to be? In *Against Relativism,* Macklin expresses the dominant position within Anglo-American philosophy:

> There is no denying that different cultures and historical eras exhibit a variety of moral beliefs and practices. The empirical facts revealed by anthropological research yield the descriptive thesis known as *cultural relativity.* But even if we grant that cultural relativity is an accurate description of the world's diversity, whether anything follows for normative ethics is an entirely different question. Do the facts of cultural relativity compel the conclusion that what is right or wrong can be determined only by the beliefs and practices within a particular culture or subculture? (1999, p. 4)

Macklin's (1998; 1999) argument for a strong version of anti-relativism is based upon her adherence to the idea that certain ethical principles are applicable cross-culturally. Macklin does allow that some bioethical practices might need to be compromised in culturally diverse settings. In traditional Navajo society words have enormous symbolic power; thus speaking openly about a poor prognosis is thought to actually bring on death, causing enormous difficulty for clinicians taught to disclose the truth while engaging in advance care planning or explaining the risks of clinical research (Carrese and Rhodes). In her consideration of a clinical compromise about how much information to disclose, a compromise designed to respect Navajo beliefs about the avoidance of discussing negative topics, Macklin (1999, p. 264) concedes that, "A degree of ethical relativism is undeniably present in the less-than-ideal version of informed consent, and it does admittedly constitute a 'lower' standard than that which is usually appropriate in today's medical practice." Although she acknowledges that in some cases it is appropriate to consider cultural difference in the application of ethical standards, Macklin justifies this not by recognizing that morality is culturally embedded, but instead, by noting that "flexibility" (in applying ethical rules) is "consistent with adherence to more fundamental ethical principles" (1999, p. 264).

A fear of unbridled relativism may underlie the deep seated ambivalence some bioethicists express when weighing the impact of cultural difference on beliefs about the moral. Rorty speaks directly to this concern, "Critics of moral relativism think that unless there is something absolute, something which shares God's implacable refusal to yield to human weakness, we have no reason to go on resisting evil" (p. xxxi).

The cultural relativism practiced by most anthropologists, however, is first and foremost a *methodological* position, a claim that each culture must be approached and judged initially on its own terms. The anthropologist makes every effort not to prejudge practices that are unfamiliar. Note that this methodological stance does not preclude eventual evaluation and judgment.

## Relativism, Social Justice, and Human Rights

There is an inherent tension between the universalizing discourse of bioethics and the historical celebration of cultural relativism among anthropologists. These two approaches to understanding moral practices in relation to social justice and human rights appear to be antithetical, at least in their most extreme formulations. However, in recent years, scholars in anthropology and bioethics have begun to explore, once again, the possibility of identifying transcultural or universal dimensions of the social behaviors of human groups. For example, in his attempt to develop a qualified version of ethical relativism, Shweder identifies aspects of moral behavior that are universal and culturally prescribed. Profound differences may exist between the moral codes of different people, but according to Shweder, there is more than one moral code that can be rationally defended. Universal dimensions of morality—justice and fairness, for example—are *relatively* expressed through discretionary variables such as who is designated as the moral agent, or what behavior and beliefs are judged to be morally relevant.

Renteln characterizes relativism as a metaethical theory about the nature of moral perceptions. Renteln suggests that relativism is compatible with cross-cultural universals, which could indicate support for particular human rights. It is precisely in the arena of human rights that anthropologists and bioethicists share a common concern for fundamental abuses inflicted upon individuals and communities. What is especially troubling for proponents of human rights agendas is the reliance on relativism to justify social and political practices that condone and perpetuate the systematic oppression of individuals and groups based on their gender, ethnicity, religion or political affiliation. Macklin's (1999) treatise *Against Relativism* provides a good example of the philosophical arguments against a strong form of ethical relativism. Macklin repeatedly calls attention to the dangers of moving from empirical claims about cultural variability to moral justifications in the normative sphere. Baker offers a model for negotiating value differences relevant to science and health in a multicultural world. In his discussion of bioethics and notions of the "common good" as a foundation for international human rights, Thomasma brings us closer to a conception of human rights that acknowledges fundamental human values and, simultaneously, the importance of local context and cultural difference.

Anthropologists studying human rights abuses and structural inequalities clearly differentiate between the documentation of cultural patterns and normative judgments about them. Scheper-Hughes's recent work on the global trade in human organs, for example, strongly condemns the organ trade and the dehumanizing practices surrounding it. A culturally informed bioethics must take into account the impact of globalization on social justice, human rights, and public health disparities internationally (Kleinman, Das, and Lock; Das). Anthropologist and physician Paul Farmer, who has addressed a broad range of human rights issues in international health, is especially critical when the "culture argument" is employed to rationalize, excuse or vindicate suffering and structural violence:

> Concepts of cultural relativism, and even arguments to reinstate the dignity of different cultures and 'races,' have been easily assimilated by some of the very agencies that perpetuate extreme suffering. Abuses of cultural concepts are particularly insidious in discussions of suffering in general and of human rights more specifically: cultural difference is one of several forms of essentialism used to explain away assaults on dignity and suffering. (1997, p. 278)

In his work combating the HIV epidemic, Farmer has criticized the widely held notion that only AIDS *prevention* strategies—but not *treatment*—should be used in resource-poor countries. His successful use of anti-AIDS drugs in Haiti destroyed the rationalization that therapy would not be cost effective in certain cultural groups.

## Conclusion: The Role of Anthropology

What, ultimately, will anthropology contribute to the field of bioethics, an increasingly important domain of inquiry in national and international discourses about culture, morality, and health? Whether the question is appropriate care for the dying, the donation and transplantation of human organs, the evaluation of new medical technologies, informed consent in scientific research, or national and international health disparities, the anthropological contribution will be to create carefully researched accounts of how the moral good is located in particular local worlds. Ethnographic methodologies make possible such accounts. Ethnography provides the tools for a robust description of the social dynamics of ordinary moral experience. The application of ethnography in bioethics promises to counter the prevailing policy discourse controlled by economics, decision analysis, and legal procedures, a discourse that often silences social suffering while at the same time providing the illusion of control to individuals (Kleinman, 1999, p. 89).

The paradox of relativism cannot be resolved. Instead, the work of medical anthropologists will enhance our understanding of the moral rendering and interpretation of health practices, scientific discovery, and the various uses and abuses of power in global biomedicine. A single set of universal principles or procedures will be inadequate. Bioethical approaches dominated by a simplistic application of respect for individual autonomy will fail not only in societies with a more nuanced view of the socially embedded nature of personhood, but in the West as well. In healthcare practice and in scientific research, procedures based on respectful negotiation among competing claims—measures informed by moral pragmatism—are most likely to avoid harm and contribute to the common good. Medical anthropologists have a vital role to play in furthering our understanding of the cultural construction of bioethics practices and their applications throughout the world.

BARBARA KOENIG
PATRICIA MARSHALL

SEE ALSO: *Autonomy; Beneficence; Body; Circumcision; Confidentiality; Death: Anthropological Perspectives; Death, Definition and Determination of; Eugenics and Religious Law; Health and Disease; Human Nature; Informed Consent; Medical Ethics, History of; Mental Health; Mental Illness; Population Ethics*

### BIBLIOGRAPHY

Baker, Robert. 1998. "A Theory of International Bioethics: The Negotiable and the Non-negotiable." *Kennedy Institute of Ethics Journal* 8(3): 233–274.

Barnes, Donelle; Davis, Anne J.; Moran, Tracy; et al. 1998. "Informed Consent in a Multicultural Cancer Patient Population: Implications for Nursing Practice." *Nursing Ethics* 5(5): 412–423.

Becker, Gay. 2000. *The Elusive Embryo: How Men and Women Approach New Reproductive Technologies.* Berkeley, CA: University of California Press.

Brodwin, Paul. 2002. "Genetics, Identity, and the Anthropology of Essentialism." *Anthropological Quarterly* 75: 323–330.

Brodwin, Paul, ed. 2000. *Biotechnology and Culture: Bodies, Anxieties, Ethics.* Bloomington: Indiana University Press.

Carrese, Joseph A., and Rhodes, Lorna A. 1995. "Western Bioethics on the Navajo Reservation." *Journal of the American Medical Association* 274: 826–829.

Cohen, Lawrence. 1999. "Where it Hurts: Indian Material for an Ethics of Organ Transplantation." *Daedalus* 128(4): 135–165.

Crawley, LaVera M.; Marshall, Patricia A.; Lo, Bernard; et al. 2002. "Strategies for Culturally Effective End-of-Life Care." *Annals of Internal Medicine* 136: 673–679.

Crigger, Bette. 1995. "Negotiating the Moral Order: Paradoxes of Ethics Consultation." *Kennedy Institute of Ethics Journal* 5: 89–112.

Das, Veena. 1999. "Public Good, Ethics, and Everyday Life: Beyond the Boundaries of Bioethics." *Daedalus* 128: 99–133.

DeVries, Robert, and Subedi, Janardan, eds. 1998. *Bioethics and Society: Constructing the Ethical Enterprise.* Upper Saddle River, NJ: Prentice Hall.

Drought, Theresa S., and Koenig, Barbara A. 2002. "'Choice' in End-of-Life Decision Making: Researching a Fact or a Fiction?" *The Gerontologist* 42(Suppl III): 114–128.

Edel, May, and Edel, Abraham. 1968. *Anthropology and Ethics: The Quest for Moral Understanding.* Cleveland, OH: Press of Case Western Reserve University.

Fabrega, Horatio. 1990. "An Ethnomedical Perspective of Medical Ethics." *The Journal of Medicine and Philosophy* 15: 593–625.

Farmer, Paul. 1997. "On Suffering and Social Violence: A View from Below." In *Social Suffering*, ed. Arthur Kleinman, Veena Das, and Margaret Lock. Berkeley: University of California Press.

Farmer, Paul. 2003. *Pathologies of Power: Health, Human Rights, and the New War on the Poor.* Berkeley: University of California Press.

Finkler, Kaja. 2000. *Experiencing the New Genetics: Family and Kinship on the Medical Frontier.* Philadelphia: University of Pennsylvania Press.

Fox, Renée C. 1990. "The Evolution of American Bioethics: A Sociological Perspective." In *Social Science Perspectives on Medical Ethics,* ed. George Weisz. Philadelphia: University of Pennsylvania Press.

Frank, Geyla; Blackhall, Leslie J.; Michel, Vicki, et al. 1998. "A Discourse of Relationships in Bioethics: Patient Autonomy and End-of-Life Decision Making among Elderly Korean Americans." *Medical Anthropology Quarterly* 12: 403–423.

Gaines, Atwood D. 1998. "Culture and Values at the Intersection of Science and Suffering: Encountering Ethics, Genetics, and Alzheimer Disease." In *Genetic Testing for Alzheimer Disease,* ed. S. Post and P. Whitehouse. Baltimore: Johns Hopkins University Press.

Geertz, Clifford. 1973. *The Interpretation of Cultures.* New York: Basic Books.

Geertz, Clifford. 1989. "Anti Anti-Relativism." In *Relativism: Interpretation and Confrontation,* ed. Michael Krausz. Notre Dame, IN: Notre Dame University Press.

Ginsburg, Faye D., and Rapp, Rayna, eds. 1995. *Conceiving the New World Order.* Berkeley: University of California Press.

Gordon, Deborah R., and Paci, Eugenio. 1997. "Disclosure Practices and Cultural Narratives: Understanding Concealment and Silence Around Cancer in Tuscany, Italy." *Social Science and Medicine* 4: 1433–1452.

Gordon, Elisa J. 2001. "They Don't Have to Suffer for Me: Why Dialysis Patients Refuse Offers of Living Donor Kidneys." *Medical Anthropology Quarterly* 5: 1–22.

Gordon, Elisa J., and Daugherty, Chris. 2003. "'Hitting You Over the Head': Oncologists' Disclosure of Prognosis to Advanced Cancer Patients." *Bioethics* 17(2): 142–168.

Hatch, Elvin. 1983. *Culture and Morality: The Relativity of Values in Anthropology.* New York: Columbia University Press.

Herskovits, Melville. 1972. *Cultural Relativism: Perspectives in Cultural Pluralism.* New York: Random House.

Hoffmaster, Barry. 1990. "Morality and the Social Sciences." In *Social Science Perspectives on Medical Ethics,* ed. George Weisz. Philadelphia: University of Pennsylvania Press.

Hoffmaster, Barry, ed. 2001. *Bioethics in Social Context.* Philadelphia: Temple University Press.

Hogle, Linda. 1999. *Recovering the Nation's Body: Culture Memory, Medicine, and the Politics of Redemption.* New Brunswick, NJ: Rutgers University Press.

Hunt, Linda. 1998. "Moral Reasoning and the Meaning of Cancer: Causal Explanations of Oncologists and Patients in Southern Mexico." *Medical Anthropology Quarterly* 12(3): 298–318.

Ikels, Charlotte. 1997. "Kidney Failure and Transplantation in China." *Social Science and Medicine* 44: 1271–1283.

Joralemon, Donald. 2001. "Shifting Ethics: Debating the Incentive Question in Organ Transplantation." *Journal of Medical Ethics* 27: 30–35.

Kaufert, Joseph. 1999. "Cultural Mediation in Cancer Diagnosis and End of Life Decision-Making: The Experience of Aboriginal Patients in Canada." *Anthropology and Medicine* 6: 405–421.

Kaufert, Joseph M., and O'Neil, John D. 1990. "Biomedical Rituals and Informed Consent: Native Canadians and the Negotiation of Clinical Trust." In *Social Science Perspectives on Medical Ethics,* ed. George Weisz. Philadelphia, PA: University of Pennsylvania Press.

Kaufert, Joseph M., and Putsch, Robert W. 1997. "Communication through Interpreters in Healthcare: Ethical Dilemmas Arising from Differences in Class, Culture, Language, and Power." *Journal of Clinical Ethics* 8(1): 71–87.

Kaufman, Sharon R. 1998. "Intensive Care, Old Age, and the Problem of Death in America." *The Gerontologist* 38(6): 715–725.

Kaufman, Sharon R. 2000. "In the Shadow of 'Death with Dignity': Medicine and Cultural Quandaries of the Vegetative State." *American Anthropologist* 102(1): 69–83.

Kelly, Susan E.; Marshall, Patricia A.; Sanders, Lee M.; et al. 1997. "Understanding the Practice of Ethics Consultation: Results of an Ethnographic Multi-Site Study." *Journal of Clinical Ethics* 8:136–149.

Kleinman, Arthur. 1999. "Moral Experience and Ethical Reflection: Can Ethnography Reconcile Them? A Quandary for 'The New Bioethics.'" *Daedalus* 128(4): 69–97.

Kleinman, Arthur; Das, Veena; and Lock, Margaret. 1997. *Social Suffering.* Berkeley: University of California Press.

Kleinman, Arthur; Fox, Renee C.; and Brandt, Allan M., guest eds. 1999. *Daedalus: Bioethics and Beyond: Volume 128, Number 4.* Cambridge, MA: American Academy of Arts and Sciences.

Koenig, Barbara A. 1988. "The Technological Imperative in Medical Practice: The Social Creation of a Routine Treatment." In *Biomedicine Examined,* ed. Margaret Lock and Deborah R. Gordon. Boston: Kluwer.

Koenig, Barbara A. 1996. "The Power (and Limits) of Proximity." *Hastings Center Report* 26(6): 30–32.

Koenig, Barbara A. 1997. "Cultural Diversity in Decision-Making about Care at the End-of-Life." In *Approaching Death: Improving Care at the End of Life,* ed. Marilyn J. Field and Christine K. Cassel. Washington, D.C.: National Academy of Sciences.

Koenig, Barbara A., and Davies, Betty. 2003. "Cultural Dimensions of Care at Life's End for Children and Their Families." In *When Children Die: Improving Palliative and End-of-Life Care for Children and their Families,* ed. Marilyn J. Field, and Richard E. Behrman. Washington, D.C.: National Academy of Sciences.

Koenig, Barbara, and Gates-Williams, Jan. 1995. "Understanding Cultural Differences in Caring for Dying Patients." *Western Journal of Medicine* 163: 244–249.

Kundstadter, Peter. 1980. "Medical Ethics in Cross-Cultural and Multi-Cultural Perspective." *Social Science and Medicine* 14B: 289–296.

Lee, Sandra S. J.; Mountain, Joanna; and Koenig, Barbara A. 2001. "The Meanings of 'Race' in the New Genomics: Implications for Health Disparities Research." *Yale Journal of Health Policy, Law, and Ethics* 1(1): 33–75.

Levin, Betty W., and Fleischman, Alan R. 2002. "Public Health and Bioethics: The Benefits of Collaboration." *American Journal of Public Health.* 92: 165–167.

Levin, Betty W., and Schiller, Nina G. 1998. "Social Class and Medical Decision Making: A Neglected Topic in Bioethics." *Cambridge Quarterly of Healthcare Ethics* 7: 41–56.

Lieban, Richard W. 1990. "Medical Anthropology and the Comparative Study of Medical Ethics." In *Social Science Perspectives on Medical Ethics,* ed. George Weisz. Philadelphia: University of Pennsylvania Press.

Lock, Margaret. 2002. *Twice Dead: Organ Transplants and the Reinvention of Death.* Berkeley: University of California Press.

Lock, Margaret, and Honde, Christina. 1990. "Reaching Consensus about Death: Heart Transplants and Cultural Identity in Japan." In *Social Science Perspectives on Medical Ethics,* ed. George Weisz. Philadelphia: University of Pennsylvania Press.

Lock, Margaret; Young, Alan; and Cambrosio, Alberto, eds. 2000. *Living and Working with the New Medical Technologies: Intersections of Inquiry.* New York: Cambridge University Press.

Long, Susan O. 1999. "Family Surrogacy and Cancer Disclosure: Physician-Family Negotiation of an Ethical Dilemma in Japan." *Journal of Palliative Care* 15: 31–42.

Long, Susan O. 2000. "Living Poorly or Dying Well: Decisions About Life Support and Treatment Termination for American and Japanese Patients." *Journal of Clinical Ethics* 11: 236–250.

Macklin, Ruth. 1998. "Ethical Relativism in a Multicultural Society." *Kennedy Institute of Ethics Journal* 8:1–22.

Macklin, Ruth. 1999. *Against Relativism: Cultural Diversity and the Search for Ethical Universals in Medicine.* New York: Oxford University Press.

Marshall, Patricia A. 1992. "Anthropology and Bioethics." *Medical Anthropology Quarterly* 6: 49–73.

Marshall, Patricia A. 2001a. "A Contextual Approach to Clinical Ethics Consultation." In *Bioethics in Social Context,* ed. Barry Hoffmaster. Philadelphia: Temple University Press.

Marshall, Patricia A. 2001b. "Informed Consent in International Health Research." In *Biomedical Research Ethics: Updating International Guidelines: A Consultation,* ed. Robert Levine, Samuel Gorovitz, and John Gallagher. Geneva: Council for International Organization of Medical Sciences, World Health Organization.

Marshall, Patricia A., and Daar, Abdallah. 2000. "Ethical Issues in Human Organ Replacement: A Case Study from India." In *Global Health Policy, Local Realities: The Fallacy of the Level Playing Field,* ed. Linda M. Whiteford, and Lenore Manderson. Boulder, CO: Lynne Publishers, Inc.

Marshall, Patricia A., and Koenig, Barbara A. 1996. "Anthropology and Bioethics: Perspectives on Culture, Medicine and Morality." In *Medical Anthropology: Contemporary Theory and Method,* 2nd edition, ed. Carolyn Sargent and Thomas Johnson. Westport, CT: Praeger Publishing Co.

Marshall, Patricia, and Koenig, Barbara A. 2000. "Bioethiques et Anthropologie: Situer le 'Bien' dans la Pratique Medicale [Intersection of Bioethics and Anthropology: Locating the "Good" in Medical Practices]." *Anthropologie et Sociétés* 24(2): 35–55.

Marshall, Patricia A., and Koenig, Barbara A. 2001. "Ethnographic Methods." In *Method in Medical Ethics,* ed. Jeremy Sugarman and Daniel Sulmasy. Washington, D.C.: Georgetown University Press.

Marshall, Patricia A.; Koenig, Barbara A.; Grifhorst, Paul; et al. 1998. "Ethical Issues in Immigrant Health Care and Clinical Research." In *Handbook of Immigrant Health,* ed. Sana Loue. New York: Plenum Press.

Muller, Jessica H. 1994. "Anthropology, Bioethics, and Medicine: A Provocative Trilogy." *Medical Anthropology Quarterly* 8: 448–467.

Muller, Jessica H., and Desmond, Brian. 1992. "Ethical Dilemmas in a Cross-Cultural Context: A Chinese Example." *Western Journal of Medicine* 157: 323–327.

O'Neill, Onora. 2002. *Autonomy and Trust in Bioethics.* Cambridge, Eng.: Cambridge University Press.

Ohnuki-Tierney, Eniko. 1994. "Brain Death and Organ Transplantation." *Current Anthropology* 35: 233–254.

Orona, Cecelia J.; Koenig, Barbara A.; and Davis, Anne J. 1994. "Cultural Aspects of Nondisclosure." *Cambridge Quarterly of Healthcare Ethics* 3: 338–346.

Orr, Robert; Marshall, Patricia A.; and Osborn, Jamie. 1995. "Cross-Cultural Considerations in Clinical Ethics Consultations." *Archives of Family Medicine* 4: 159–164.

Po-Wah, Julia Tao Lai, ed. 2002. *Cross-Cultural Perspectives on the (Im)Possibility of Global Bioethics.* Dordrecht: Kluwer Academic Publishers.

Press, Nancy, and Browner, Carol H. 1998. "Characteristics of Women Who Refuse an Offer of Prenatal Diagnosis: Data from the California Maternal Serum Alpha Fetoprotein Blood Test Experience." *American Journal of Medical Genetics* 78(5): 433–445.

Press, Nancy; Fishman, Jennifer R.; and Koenig, Barbara A. 2000. "Collective Fear, Individualized Risk: The Social and Cultural Context of Genetic Screening for Breast Cancer." *Nursing Ethics* 7(3): 237–249.

Rapp, Rayna. 2000. *Testing Women, Testing the Fetus: The Social Impact of Amniocentesis in America.* New York: Routledge.

Renteln, Alison D. 1988. "Relativism and the Search for Human Rights." *American Anthropologist* 90: 56–72.

Rorty, Richard. 1999. "Introduction: Relativism: Finding and Making." In *Philosophy and Social Hope,* ed. Richard Rorty. New York: Penguin.

Rosaldo, Renato. 1989. *Culture and Truth: The Remaking of Social Analysis.* Boston: Beacon Press.

Sankar, Pamela. 1996. "Informed Consent: (W)rituals of Medical Research." Paper presented at the American Anthropological Association Annual Meeting, San Francisco, CA.

Sankar, Pamela, and Cho, Mildred K. 2002. "Toward a New Vocabulary of Human Genetic Variation." *Science* 298: 1337–1338.

Scheper-Hughes, Nancy. 2000. "The Global Traffic in Human Organs." *Current Anthropology* 41: 191–224.

Sharp, Lesley. 1995. "Organ Transplantation as a Transformative Experience: Anthropological Insights into the Restructuring of the Self." *Medical Anthropological Quarterly* 9: 357–389.

Sharp, Lesley. 2001. "Commodified Kin: Death, Mourning, and Competing Claims on the Bodies of Organ Donors in the United States." *American Anthropologist* 103: 112–133.

Sharp, Richard, and Foster, Morris. 2000. "Study Populations in the Review of Genetic Research." *Journal of Law, Medicine and Ethics* 28: 41–51.

Shweder, Richard A. 1990. "Ethical Relativism: Is There a Defensible Version?" *Ethos* 18(2): 205–218.

Slomka, Jacqueline. 1992. "The Negotiation of Death: Clinical Decision Making at the End of Life." *Social Science and Medicine* 35(3): 251–259.

Spiro, Melford E. 1986. "Cultural Relativism and the Future of Anthropology." *Cultural Anthropology* 1: 259–286.

Thomasma, David C. 1997. "Bioethics and International Human Rights." *Journal of Law, Medicine and Ethics* 25: 295–306.

Weisz, George. 1990. *Social Science Perspectives on Medical Ethics.* Philadelphia: University of Pennsylvania Press.

INTERNET RESOURCE

Koenig, Barbara A., and Davies, Betty. 2003. "Cultural Dimensions of Care at Life's End for Children and Their Families." In *When Children Die: Improving Palliative and End-of-Life Care for Children and their Families,* ed. Marilyn J. Field, and Richard E. Behrman. Washington, D.C.: National Academy of Sciences. Available from <http://books.nap.edu/html/children_die/AppD.pdf>.

# ARTIFICIAL HEARTS AND CARDIAC ASSIST DEVICES

• • •

In 1964 the U.S. Congress budgeted $581,000 to establish an artificial heart program at the National Institutes of Health (NIH). This was the first large-scale effort by any nation to support systematic research into the development of an artificial heart. The effort to build a reliable, totally implantable artificial heart has yielded marginal results. But even though an effective device does not exist, the artificial heart has, since the 1960s, been at the center of a heated ethical, economic, and policy debate. The debate over the wisdom of building and testing an artificial heart has also served as a paradigm for debating the future of expensive technologies in the U.S. healthcare system.

Scientists and physicians in many countries have dreamed for centuries of curing fatal heart diseases by creating a mechanical substitute. Technological advances during the 1960s in engineering fields such as metallurgy, fluid dynamics, electronics, and computer modeling made some scientists think that it might be possible to actually construct such a device. The emergence of the kidney dialysis machine, which could mimic the functions of a human kidney, created a fundamental change in attitude in medicine about the feasibility of building an artificial heart. In the late twentieth century, the quest for the Totally Implantable Artificial Heart (TAH) was once again the catalyst for other technological advances; except for the TAH, the success of the artificial heart program to date is still up for debate.

## The Total Artificial Heart

Constructing an artificial heart requires materials such as metals, ceramics, plastics, and polymers that are lightweight and durable. At the same time, these materials must be biologically inert. They must work synergistically with other body systems and not trigger attacks by the body's natural system of immune defenses that would lead to the disruption of the circulatory system and, ultimately, death. An artificial heart also requires sufficiently smooth surfaces so as not to disrupt blood flow through the heart or damage fragile blood cells. A TAH needs a power source that can maintain an efficient and steady stream of energy for long periods of time while being small enough to fit completely inside the body. Both the pump and the power source must be capable of responding to changes in position, temperature, and pressure associated with the needs of the person using the machine.

The decision to launch a program to build a totally implantable heart had its roots in a series of exploratory meetings held during the 1950s at the NIH (Shaw). Enthusiasm for undertaking the research accelerated in the 1960s as physicians and engineers began to build and successfully use the first heart-lung machines, external pumps that could be used to support blood circulation in the body. After a few hours, these machines damaged the blood cells (Zareba). Still, the heart-lung machine was a crude, partial artificial heart that inspired physicians to think that perhaps a permanent device was not beyond reach.

Moreover, as the U.S. space program began to enjoy success, optimism grew in both scientific and government circles about the feasibility of taking on large-scale technological challenges. Many in government were impressed with the productive results being secured in the space program and the military from centrally funded, programmatic research. U.S. physicians and biomedical scientists saw themselves as being able to overcome the many technical obstacles through hard work, directed budgets, and targeted programs. The space program had as its goal putting a man on the moon before the end of the 1960s. The artificial heart program launched at the NIH in 1964 set as its goal the testing of a total artificial heart in a human being by Valentine's Day, February 14, 1970 (Bernstein).

The goal of implanting an artificial heart by the end of the 1960s was not attained. A major hurdle was the development of an energy source capable of providing long-term power to an artificial heart—while fitting inside the body. Not only was progress slow but, during the time artificial heart researchers were trying to overcome the large number of technical challenges that confronted them, an alternative to the mechanical heart appeared: cardiac transplantation. Ironically, the rationale for recent clinical trials of artificial hearts is to find a replacement for the now common cadaveric heart transplant. The increased need for organs and a stable donation rate are the main reasons why there has been renewed interest in total artificial hearts.

While Denton Cooley did implant a crude mechanical heart in a human recipient at Baylor University College of Medicine in 1969, most of the device, including the power source, remained outside the body. He explicitly stated that his sole motive for using this primitive, untested device was the desperate hope that it might help an imminently dying patient live long enough for a donor heart to become available for transplant. According to Michael DeBakey, Cooley did not believe the device he implanted was a permanent replacement for his patient's heart.

This attempt to use an artificial heart as a *bridge* to keep a patient alive in the hope that a transplant could be done took place without the approval of Cooley's superiors or any government agency. The recipient, Haskell Karp, died shortly after the implant. Cooley's decision set off a storm of controversy within his medical center. Karp's wife later filed suit against Cooley for failure to obtain proper informed consent to the experiment. Texas courts held that since the

procedure was experimental, there was no agreed-upon informed-consent standards that governed artificial heart implant surgery and dismissed the suit.

The power source for the TAH has been a persistent problem. Some researchers in the late 1960s believed that the problem of how to power a TAH could be solved by using a small, implantable capsule of plutonium. In 1972 a specially convened NIH panel, the Artificial Heart Assessment Panel, conducted the first governmental review of such technology. It concluded in 1973 that while the "advent of the totally implantable artificial heart" would be "an earth-shaking event," the use of atomic power to drive a mechanical heart posed unacceptable radiation-exposure risks to the public health (Artificial Heart Assessment Panel, 1973, p. 187). Current devices rely on access to external power and small batteries. More than thirty years after Cooley's first implant, battery technology still has proven to be a limit on how long a patient can safely remain on an artificial heart.

## The Artificial Heart Goes Private

In 1976, Willem Kolff (a physician and the inventor of kidney dialysis and one of the first artificial hearts) and some of his Utah colleagues formed a private company, Kolff Medical Associates, to attract venture capital to support their research. In order to interest private investors, they had to create a marketing program for their mechanical heart. The decision to proceed with a private company constituted a first step into the emerging and often ethically controversial world of public-private partnerships intended to advance medical research.

After further testing and redesign of models previously tested in calves, Clifford Kwan-Gett, Willem Kolff, and later Robert Jarvik managed to use a Jarvik-7 to keep some animals alive for as long as eight months. In 1980, Kolff Medical Associates applied for permission from the institutional review board (IRB) of the University of Utah Medical Center to try the device on a human being. They also sought permission from the U.S. Food and Drug Administration (FDA), which, since 1976, had authority to regulate the testing and marketing of medical devices. While awaiting approval, members of the Utah artificial heart group traveled to Philadelphia and conducted a series of three practice implants of a Jarvik-7 heart on brain-dead patients at Temple University Medical Center. Permission from family members to use the cadavers was obtained by Jack Kolff, Willem Kolff's son, then a surgeon at Temple.

After many weeks of resubmissions and revisions, the IRB at Utah and the FDA granted approval to undertake a series of seven implants of a Jarvik-7 heart in human beings at the University of Utah. The subjects were to be patients with very severe, life-threatening congestive heart failure resulting from cardiomyopathy, a poorly understood condition that causes irreversible fatal damage to the muscle of the heart (Scherr et. al.). Kolff and Jarvik, who had renamed their company Symbion, selected a young surgeon, William DeVries, to perform the first implant in a human recipient.

## The Experiment on Barney Clark

Barney B. Clark, a retired dentist who had been admitted to the University of Utah Medical Center on November 29, 1982, with cardiomyopathy, was deemed to be an ideal candidate for the first implant of the Jarvik heart (Fox and Swazey) as he was educated, enthusiastic, and had a very supportive family. He signed the eighteen-page consent form the night he was admitted to the hospital. When his heart began to fail on December 1, he was taken to the operating room, and after a nine-hour operation he became the first human being to receive an artificial heart intended as a permanent replacement for his own.

Jarvik and DeVries spent many hours speaking with the media about the operation, the device, and their patient's health status. In the days after the implant, the healthcare team made many optimistic pronouncements to the media about Clark's chances for survival. But Clark followed a very rocky course during the 112 days he lived with the Jarvik-7 device. He suffered a wide range of complications that required three additional surgical procedures. After a few weeks on the machine, his emotional and cognitive state deteriorated severely, and on more than one occasion, he asked that the artificial heart be turned off. This was not done. After his death, more than 1,300 people, including political figures, members of the governing council of the Latter-Day Saints (Mormon) Church, of which Clark was a member, many of his doctors, and media representatives from around the world attended his funeral in Seattle, Washington.

DeVries and the Utah group pronounced the Clark experiment a success. They had kept a man alive in the final stages of heart failure for well over three months. But the IRB at Utah, troubled by the many complications that had arisen during the experiment, asked for many changes and clarifications in the research protocol before giving DeVries permission to try another implant. Among other things, the Clark experiment raised questions about the adequacy of informed consent of potential recipients. Could those facing certain death really be said to choose? And were those

conducting the research so enthusiastic and hopeful about its prospects that they could not provide a realistic picture of the risks and dangers inherent in the experiment (Fox and Swazey)?

Between 1984 and 1987, four more implants were done using artificial hearts as permanent replacements for the human heart. William J. Schroeder received his implant of a Jarvik heart on November 29, 1984, less than two months after the IRB at Humana-Audubon gave its approval. Schroeder initially did well on the heart, but within nineteen days he suffered a stroke. During the course of the next 620 days he spent on the device, he had three more strokes; the last brought about his death. The other recipients of total artificial hearts, two at Louisville, one in Sweden, and one in Arizona—all experienced similar difficulties and ultimately died. It became clear from these experiments that the Jarvik-7 was not suitable for use as a permanent replacement device.

In January of 1988 the new director of the National Heart, Lung, and Blood Institute, Claude Lenfant, decided to cancel the NIH program to build a total artificial heart. The recent experience with artificial hearts, he believed, clearly indicated that such devices could be best used to assist failing hearts or for temporary use until a transplant could be found. Lenfant argued that a totally implantable artificial heart was still at least ten years away and might well wind up benefiting a relatively small number of patients at great cost. The threat of shutting down research on the TAH created a whirlwind of political protest in Congress. Legislators from states such as Utah and Massachusetts, where heart research was being conducted, fought to block Lenfant's plan. By the end of 1988, $20 million had been awarded to four centers to continue this research.

In July of 1991, the National Academy of Sciences' Institute of Medicine issued a study in which they recommended continued federal funding for both Left-Ventricular Assist Devices (LVADs) and TAHs. They predicted that a reliable LVAD should become available in the late 1990s and a TAH by around 2005 (Institute of Medicine). Federal funding for research on both permanent and temporary artificial hearts continued.

In July of 2001 the first Totally Implantable Artificial Heart replaced Robert Tools's own heart. Abiomed, Inc., started the controversial clinical trial of the Abiomed artificial heart. The FDA has approved fifteen patient implants.

## The Left-Ventricular Assist Device

The left chamber, or ventricle, of the human heart does the greatest share of the work of circulating blood throughout the body. Heart attacks and other forms of heart disease frequently damage this portion of the heart. An LVAD is a pump capable of supplementing the function of the left ventricle, thus allowing a weakened or damaged heart to support life. It does not require an implantable power source and its design can be simpler since it does not have to duplicate all the functions of a heart for prolonged periods of time.

In the United States the ventricular assist device is used primarily for three groups of patients: those who cannot be weaned from cardiopulmonary bypass after a cardiac procedure; those who have an acute heart attack that results in cardiogenic shock; and the largest group, those who have end-stage heart disease and need some support while waiting for a heart transplant. In several European countries the LVAD is used as destination therapy. This is prohibited in the United States because the FDA has only approved the device as a bridge to transplant.

Starting in 1973, the NIH spent approximately $10 million per year over the next decade and a half on research on LVADs for damaged hearts. The first implant of an LVAD in a patient who could not be weaned from bypass was done in August of 1966 (Goldstein et al.). In the ten days after surgery the patient's continued improvement allowed her to be successfully weaned from the pump (DeBakey). It was not, however, until the early 1990s that a number of universities and private companies in a wide variety of countries undertook formal clinical trials of LVADs. Currently LVADs are a relatively common treatment for patients who are candidates for heart transplantation.

## Ethics and Mechanical Hearts and Cardiac Assist Devices

The history of artificial heart research and use raises many ethical issues. Among these there are several issues that are especially important. These issues are both specific to the artificial heart and also apply more generally to all forms of new and expensive high-technology healthcare.

The use of human subjects in a clinical trial is one of the most important dilemmas of artificial heart research. The existing protections for persons who participate in medical research are informed consent and review by local committees of scientists (IRBs) of research proposals. The history of artificial heart research has called into question the adequacy of both protections.

Patients asked to serve as subjects in the use of artificial hearts and during the development of LVADs are extremely

vulnerable. They face certain death if the device is not implanted. In many cases their heart failure came about suddenly and unexpectedly, and in others the opportunity to receive a device is not introduced until the patient is facing imminent death. For many of the subjects, the complexities of the research and the rigorous post-implant monitoring of the device in the past have been extremely intimidating and continue to be. Moreover, subjects may hear the risks and benefits of participation only from researchers who themselves have a powerful interest in wanting their work to proceed. Those who sought subjects to receive artificial hearts in past trials did so as both clinician and researcher to the recipients of the device, generating a strong conflict of interest.

The threat of imminent death tends to coerce subjects to make particular choices; furthermore, those charged with reviewing requests to use artificial hearts have faced serious moral challenges. There has been a great deal of pressure associated with the race to be the first medical center to use a mechanical heart or to be the first to use one successfully. Considerable financial and publicity stakes are involved for the researcher, the institution, and any companies in which the institution or researcher might have an interest. Local IRBs usually do not have the requisite expertise or independence to evaluate exactly what sorts of criteria to use to govern subject selection, consent forms, or the methods for accumulating data on subjects over long periods of time. Because of limited time and resources, local IRBs often do not adequately monitor clinical trials over time, which provides little protection for research subjects.

Once it became clear in the 1980s that the devices then available could not safely support long-term heart function in human beings, enthusiasm for artificial hearts turned to their temporary use. Here, too, tough ethical questions must be confronted. If artificial hearts are to be used on a temporary basis, is it permissible to implant them without the explicit consent of a person who has undergone a sudden, unexpected heart failure? Which patients would constitute the best patient population for testing devices intended for temporary use only: those nearest death and thought to have the lowest risk for the greatest potential benefit, or those not quite as sick, who are most likely to recover if given a *respite* by an LVAD or temporary use of an artificial heart? It is not clear that those who are given artificial hearts or LVADs on a temporary basis understand what their rights are to turn off these devices. Nor is it clear, according to George Annas, that the use of these devices will contribute to an overall increase in the number of lives saved. When cadaver hearts are scarce, the use of artificial hearts or bridge devices as a prelude to transplant means only that the identity of those getting a chance at a transplant may change while the overall number of transplants done remains the same (Caplan). Many believe that assist devices will not save more lives since there are only a small number of cadaver hearts available for transplant. One must find the balance between simply extending life versus improving its quality and happiness.

## The Societal Impact of the Artificial Heart

One of the obvious moral questions raised by research to develop an artificial heart is whether developing this device is the best way to spend limited research dollars in meeting the healthcare needs of Americans or of the world's population as a whole. Artificial heart research is expensive. The costs of doing the first TAH implants ran into the hundreds of thousands of dollars, and current research promises to be much more costly. Approximately 40,000 people die annually from heart disease so the life saving potential of the artificial heart appears significant, yet the development of expensive new medical technology raises ethical questions about where money should be allocated and what diseases should be the priority for research.

Many experts note that to develop, test, and manufacture a fully perfected artificial heart would probably cost billions of dollars. Those most likely to benefit from access to such a device would likely be those who could afford insurance to pay for mechanical hearts. The quest for a totally implantable artificial heart, as with many other new procedures, devices, and pharmaceuticals, brings to mind questions of equity and justice in asking all to bear the cost of research for a device that would only be available to some. Questions of fairness also exist in the decision to build a machine that may add years of life to those at the end of their life span, when tens of millions of persons around the globe die before reaching adolescence from diseases and injuries that can be prevented. Explicit debates about fairness have not been very much in evidence regarding how best to allocate resources to perfect new therapies in American healthcare policy. If the pursuit of a TAH is to continue, it would seem prudent to make considerations of fairness a more central part of the policy debate.

Finally, the development of the total artificial heart and the use of ventricular assist devices have gained popularity and are believed to be one solution to the problem of a limited number of donor hearts and an ever-increasing transplant waiting list. It is imperative as we seek new technology to replace organs that cease to function effectively that we continually ask, what are the acceptable limits of our drive for prolonging life through radical replacement technologies?

ARTHUR L. CAPLAN (1995)
REVISED BY ARTHUR L. CAPLAN
SHELDON ZINK

**SEE ALSO:** *Biomedical Engineering; Cybernetics; Healthcare Resources, Allocation of; Informed Consent; Justice; Research, Human: Historical Aspects; Transhumanism and Posthumanism*

### BIBLIOGRAPHY

Annas, George J. 1994. *Standard of Care: The Law of American Bioethics.* New York: Oxford University Press.

Artificial Heart Assessment Panel, National Heart, Lung, and Blood Institute. 1973. *The Totally Implantable Artificial Heart: Economic, Ethical, Legal, Medical, Psychiatric, and Social Implications: A Report.* Bethesda, MD: National Institutes of Health.

Artificial Heart Assessment Panel, Working Group on Mechanical Circulatory Support, National Heart, Lung, and Blood Institute. 1985. *Artificial Heart and Assist Devices: Directions, Needs, Costs, Societal and Ethical Issues.* Bethesda, MD: Author.

Bernstein, Barton. 1984. "The Misguided Quest for the Artificial Heart." *Technology Review* 87(6): 12–17.

Blakeslee, Sandra, ed. 1986. *Human Heart Replacement: A New Challenge for Physicians and Reporters.* Los Angeles: Foundation for American Communications.

Caplan, Arthur L. 1992. *If I Were a Rich Man Could I Buy a Pancreas? and Other Essays on the Ethics of Health Care.* Bloomington: Indiana University Press.

DeBakey, Michael E. 2000 "The Odyssey of the Artificial Heart." *Artificial Organs* 24(6): 405–411.

DeVries, William C.; Anderson, Jeffrey L.; Joyce, Lyle D.; et al. 1984. "Clinical Use of the Total Artificial Heart." *New England Journal of Medicine* 310(5): 273–278.

Fox, Renée C., and Swazey, Judith P. 1992. *Spare Parts: Organ Replacement in America.* New York: Oxford University Press.

Gil, Gideon. 1989. "The Artificial Heart Juggernaut." *Hastings Center Report* 19(2): 24–31.

Goldstein, D. J.; Oz, M. C.; and Rose, E. A. 1998. "Implantable Left Ventricular Assist Devices." *New England Journal of Medicine* 339(21): 1522–1533

Institute of Medicine Committee to Evaluate the Artificial Heart Program of the National Heart, Lung, and Blood Institute. 1991. *The Artificial Heart: Prototypes, Policies and Patients,* ed. John R. Hogness and Malin Van Antwerp. Washington, D.C.: National Academy Press.

Jonsen, Albert R. 1973. "The Totally Implantable Artificial Heart." *Hastings Center Report* 3: 1–4.

Jonsen, Albert R. 1986. "The Artificial Heart's Threat to Others." *Hastings Center Report* 16(1): 9–11.

Miles, Stephen; Siegler, Mark; Schiedermayer, David L.; et al. 1988. "The Total Artificial Heart: An Ethics Perspective on Current Clinical Research and Deployment." *Chest* 94(2): 409–413.

Scherr, Kimberly; Jensen, Louise; and Koshal, Arvind. 1999. "Mechanical Circulatory Support as a Bridge to Cardiac Transplantation: Toward the 21st Century." *American Journal of Critical Care.* 8(5): 324–337.

Shaw, Margery W., ed. 1984. *After Barney Clark: Reflections on the Utah Artificial Heart Program.* Austin: University of Texas Press.

Zareba, Karolina M. 2002. "The Artificial Heart-Past, Present and Future." *Medical Science Monitor* (8)3: RA72–77.

# ARTIFICIAL NUTRITION AND HYDRATION

• • •

The ability to deliver nutrition and hydration artificially is a powerful tool; in many clinical settings patient weight, nitrogen balance, visceral protein markers, and other parameters are favorably affected. While it has been difficult to document impact on survival in many clinical settings, artificial nutrition and hydration have become an essential component of multidisciplinary care in acutely ill or injured patients.

The means for providing nutrition and fluids under these circumstances are twofold. One is parenteral nutrition, called total parenteral nutrition (TPN). Fluid and nutrients are administered intravenously, most often via a large central vein accessed by a catheter placed using a minor surgical or radiological procedure. The other is enteral nutrition, in which nutrients are artificially pumped into the stomach or small intestine through a transnasal tube or ostomy (gastrostomy, jejunostomy). While nutritional goals can often be met with either method, TPN is costly and subject to complications, particularly infection. Unless precluded by medical conditions, enteral feeding is most often chosen when non-oral feeding is to be initiated.

The benefits of generally short-term nutritional support can be significant. Not surprisingly, as a result of these experiences, chronic, indefinite use of enteral feeding has been proposed for patients who have permanently lost the ability to take in adequate calories. However, the benefits of long-term enteral feeding in many settings have, for the most part, not been defined in controlled clinical trials. While observational studies with case-control or cohort design have provided insight into this area, ultimately, a decision to live with enteral tube feedings when oral intake ability has been lost or impaired becomes an individual one and personal values can be a critical variable. Advanced dementia, terminal cancer, and catastrophic neurological injury are clinical circumstances in which this option is often considered.

In the past, when long-term artificial feeding was considered, surgical gastrostomy provided enteral access. This has been largely replaced by endoscopic gastrostomy that can be performed, if necessary, at the bedside. This technique does not require general anesthesia, has less associated morbidity, and can be performed for a fraction of the cost of that for surgical techniques. Endoscopic placement, or percutaneous endoscopic gastrostomy (PEG), was first reported by Michael Gauderer in pediatric patients. It has since been adapted to many clinical situations, involving patients of all ages who are unable to eat and are thought to need nutritional support. In the Medicare population alone, PEG procedures more than doubled from 1991 to 1999, numbering more than 160,000 annually.

## Opposing Viewpoints

There are disagreements about the use of artificial nutrition and hydration (Lipman). One viewpoint favors enteral feeding in most situations in which the ability to eat and drink has been lost. After all, it is a relatively simple and straightforward process, and while there is some risk involved in providing access, it is relatively small. Many would argue that doing so is, in fact, an obligation, that food and water are basic human needs under all circumstances. They do not view feeding tubes as medical or life-sustaining therapy. Moreover, there is the concern that because food and water are often viewed as a good, withholding or withdrawing them will cause suffering, akin to the traditionally held concepts of starvation.

On the other hand, an alternative and competing concept is based on the view that this traditional position just described, while at first glance justified by the clinical circumstances, is one for which factual support is lacking. Further, there is evidence that in some clinical settings, particularly terminal conditions, artificial nutrition and hydration may actually be harmful and may add to the burden of suffering that medical providers are trying to minimize. This viewpoint also holds that in the setting of illness, forced administration of nutrition and hydration, provided artificially via alternative access to the digestive system using specially designed equipment, represents medical treatment. As such, it contrasts with oral ingestion of food and water, which provide nurture and comfort.

In view of these contrasting perspectives, it becomes necessary to consider the variables that impact on a decision about the use of artificial nutrition and hydration.

## Experience in Specific Disorders

ADVANCED DEMENTIA. An extensive literature has evolved over the past several years addressing the long term use of artificial enteral feeding in patients with advanced dementia, including advanced Alzheimer's dementia, a terminal disorder. Survival is the variable most often measured. Thomas Finucane reviewed fifteen studies quantifying mortality after feeding tube placement in patients with neurogenic (including dementia) and mixed disorders. Nearly all of these studies failed to identify a survival benefit afforded by feeding tube placement. Moreover, up to 50 percent of advanced dementia patients may die within a month of PEG placement.

Finucane also reviewed available evidence about other outcome parameters: prevention of aspiration pneumonia, prevention of the consequences of malnutrition, prevention or improvement of decubitus ulcers, prevention of other infections, improvement of functional status, and improvement of patient comfort. In this review of the literature from 1966 through March 1999, there were no reports documenting improvement in any of these outcomes with tube feeding.

TERMINAL CANCER. The role of nutritional support as an adjunct to managing cancer patients, not just those with incurable disease, has long been a subject of discussion and opinion. Ten years ago, a review of the status of nutritional support in cancer patients concluded that with the possible exception of bone marrow transplantation, no benefit had been documented for any outcome parameter, including survival. In 1997 Samuel Klein summarized a conference sponsored by the National Institutes of Health (NIH) and two nutrition societies, which concluded that at least short-term enteral or parenteral support does not decrease mortality or complications in cancer patients receiving cancer therapy; no good trials of long-term support were available to analyze. The conference further noted that while one might expect nutritional support to improve quality of life, no data existed that demonstrated this. Although no trials have specifically addressed terminal cancer patients there is consensus that artificial nutrition would not be beneficial.

CATASTROPHIC NEUROLOGICAL INJURY. Supplemental nutrition is commonly provided in patients in the neurological intensive care unit, be it patients with stroke or head trauma with brain injury. Most such patients have altered consciousness and are unable to eat. Some stroke patients will have dysphagia as a manifestation of neurological injury, although many will eventually recover swallowing function. In the initial assessment of these patients, outcome cannot always be defined. Moreover, in young patients with head trauma, for example, families cannot easily accept the prospect of death or at best, permanent loss of cognitive function requiring indefinite custodial care. It is thus reasonable to implement artificial nutritional support during the acute care of patients with severe neurological injury. With failure of recovery, however, the decisions regarding long-term support, including enteral tube feedings, must at some point be confronted. At the very least, any benefits and adverse effects of continued support become items of discussion.

Devastating neurological injury from trauma or nontraumatic etiology (e.g., hypoxic encephalopathy, extensive cerebral hemorrhage or infarction) are a common cause of permanent vegetative state (PVS) in which patients may exhibit wakefulness but otherwise have no detectable awareness. These patients have been particularly visible in the public eye because of the Karen Ann Quinlan and Nancy Cruzan cases in which the courts have also played a role.

There are no trials of enteral tube feedings in patients with PVS. This disorder is different from advanced dementia, and terminal cancer in which supplemental nutrition is considered as an adjunct to management in dying patients but does not affect outcome. In PVS, it is clearly life sustaining treatment: Brain injury, this devastating, is lethal and it is only with artificial provision of nutrition and fluids, and in some cases other supportive interventions, that these patients continue to live. The mechanics of providing nutrition differ little, however, and because feeding may be indefinite, PEG is the route most often chosen.

## Adverse Effects of Non-Oral Enteral Feeding

While placement of enteral feeding tubes is often taken for granted on a clinical hospital unit, complications are possible. These complications can be associated with placement itself, the mechanical effects of the tube once it has been placed, and the effects of the nutritional supplements themselves. Placement and mechanical complications, while unusual, include head and neck trauma (e.g., bleeding, infection, sinus perforation), inadvertent intubation of the tracheobronchial tree, esophagitis and esophageal stricture, and several issues related to dysfunction of these generally small caliber tubes. Many of these problems are not seen with gastrostomy or jejunostomy. However, the surgical or endoscopic procedures needed to place these tubes, while safe, have a small but measurable risk, primarily infection and, rarely, even death.

Regardless of delivery route, diarrhea and aspiration are the two most common problems that can occur when tube feeding is begun. In hospital patients, diarrhea and often incontinence occur in 25 percent of patients on general units and as many as 65 percent of patients in critical care units. The feeding solutions themselves are responsible for many of these cases. The problem is likely less in nursing homes and patients cared for at home. In most cases, instilling feeding solutions into the stomach, duodenum, or jejunum probably has little impact on the likelihood of aspiration, although reports are conflicting. Upper airway secretions are a more important variable in the risk for aspiration.

Sometimes adding to the suffering burden in dementia patients is the common need for restraints in patients with enteral feeding tubes. Restraining patients is often viewed as humiliating and demeaning, their dementia notwithstanding. In PVS patients, while pain and suffering are not experienced, indirect adverse effects such as incontinence and the requirement for diapers may jeopardize individual dignity.

## Withholding Food and Water: The Patient Experience

Not surprisingly, there is little information that precisely defines the patient experience when food and water are withheld. Two aspects of this issue are worth noting, however. First, while a decision might be made to forego supplemental nutrition, oral intake will often continue. Examples are advanced dementia and terminal cancer. Either the patient will choose to eat or drink as desired, or family or providers will assist oral feeding; in this situation, a patient need is being met. The second aspect is the circumstance in which the dying patient makes a conscious decision not to eat or drink, or tube feedings are withdrawn in a patient with PVS. Are pain and suffering aggravated when food and water are withheld?

Independent of the healthcare setting, fasting does not cause physical suffering, although such individuals are presumably healthy and, in most cases, water is not withheld. Nonetheless, the prospect of going without food or water may be untenable for a healthy individual. However, in dying patients, anecdotal reports in the medical literature consistently note that they appear comfortable without food and water and even euphoria has been described. Further, urine volumes fall and respiratory and gastrointestinal secretions decrease, lessening cough, congestion, vomiting, and

diarrhea. Robert McCann reported an experience with thirty-two dying cancer patients in a hospice-like setting. These patients were sufficiently aware to judge hunger and thirst, and were offered food and water as desired. Nearly two-thirds experienced neither hunger nor thirst; one-third had hunger only initially. Oral feeding as desired and/or mouth lubrication effectively met needs when they occurred and caregivers could focus on patient comfort.

The physiological basis for these effects is incompletely understood, but at least a few suggestions have been offered, based largely on both human and animal studies in which food and water are withheld. For example, accumulation of ketones, which accompanies fasting, may cause anorexia. Increased levels of salutary endogenous opioids have been found in the plasma and hypothalamus of laboratory rodents deprived of food and water. Metabolic changes that occur with dehydration can cause decreased awareness, obtundation, and coma; death follows naturally and without suffering.

There are no reports in PVS patients, but given the loss of awareness in this condition, pain and suffering are not likely to occur.

## Perceptions about Artificial Feeding

Perceptions about enteral tube feedings vary, but in general, surveys of elderly patients show that the majority would not want artificial feeding were they to develop advanced dementia; these opinions were common in groups educated about the procedures involved and the adverse effects, in particular the possible need for restraint. Surveys of physicians generally support not placing feeding tubes when elderly patients, or those at end of life, are no longer eating; yet in reality feeding tubes appear to be used more often than such surveys would predict. Surrogates opt for feeding tubes more often than the patients would, but these decisions rely on an incomplete knowledge base of benefits and adverse effects.

A number of variables are likely at play in the outcome of tube feeding decisions. Historically the roots of artificial feeding are deep. For centuries, it was a foregone conclusion that food must be provided when patients were not eating. Supplemental nutrition has also been intrinsic to sound surgical management for over 100 years. Another major variable, as just noted, is poor understanding of benefits and risks. This deficit seems to be most evident in families and non-physician providers. Physician surveys suggest that these providers are knowledgeable but because tubes are placed anyway, other factors are likely at work. One is found in federal regulations for nursing homes, which require adequate nutrition for residents. However, this is not the only variable. Mildred Solomon surveyed physicians who reported acting "against their conscience" (Solomon, p. 16) in providing certain life-sustaining treatment. Others have cited a fear of litigation were a tube not to be placed. Christopher Callahan has suggested that practice patterns tend to dictate PEG placement when patients stop eating. Moreover, the underlying illness may serve as a distraction by occupying center stage such that the placement of a feeding tube is relegated to a lower priority. To completely educate patients and/or families is time consuming and it is simply easier for tube placement to be the default position when the question of supplemental nutrition arises. Often this proceeds without disclosure and hence without informed consent.

## Legal Issues in Non-Oral Enteral Feeding

The controversy and concerns surrounding withholding nutrition and fluids in the clinical circumstances discussed herein have also extended to the courts. To the extent that death is predictable in a period of hours, days, or even weeks, these intellectual and emotional struggles are less intense. This is less likely to be the case in patients with terminal disorders in whom the timing of death is less certain or in PVS patients who might live for years with artificial feeding. As a result, disagreement has spilled over into the legal system. Subsequent judgments have provided legal support for the following concepts:

1. Artificial feeding is medical treatment, and can be viewed on a level with other life-sustaining interventions (mechanical ventilation, dialysis, antibiotics, etc.).

2. Competent patients may refuse life-sustaining treatment and this is a right also afforded to incompetent patients, particularly when there has been prior indication of this desire. State interests do not trump these rights.

3. Withholding and withdrawing life-sustaining treatment, including artificial feeding, are equal under the law. There is no requirement to continue a treatment once started if the proportionality of benefits and burdens is unfavorable.

4. Withholding or withdrawing life-sustaining treatment in a patient with terminal disease is neither killing nor euthanasia.

## Obligations and Options in Artificial Nutrition and Hydration

A wealth of experience and a burgeoning literature, supported by sound ethical and legal principles, are questioning the appropriateness of artificial nutrition and hydration in clinical settings like the ones discussed here. (Among these

are Finucane; Cillick; Lynn; Post; Slomka; Steinbrook; and Winter.) Yet many providers and laypersons are unaware, or because of personal views rooted in their own moral background, do not accept these concepts. It is important, therefore, to first educate patients and families to insure that knowledge and understanding are on an even par so that decision making may be shared. A second step is to define goals as one might with any treatment modality. Considerations include the patient's prognosis, and how feeding is expected to either positively or negatively affect the medical condition (benefits and burdens), taking into account expected life span, patient comfort, and, as applicable, any previously expressed wishes about use of life sustaining treatment. The availability of technology is coercive and constitutes a challenge to the physician; yet a recommendation to withhold or withdraw a useless, burdensome treatment can be a more caring act than any other. Nonetheless, in the event of uncertainty about prognosis, or with failure to reach a consensus, initiation of artificial feeding as a trial, for an agreed-upon time frame with defined goals, may be an appropriate option, which does not jeopardize the relationship between physician and the patient or surrogate. Decisions about continuation or withdrawal can then be made with more confidence.

Providing food for dying patients is much more likely rooted in the act of eating than in the provision of nutrition and fluid by an alternate route. While both options offer physiological benefits, oral feeding provides comfort and pleasure to the extent one wants to eat. It also respects autonomy in that one is left in control of oral intake. Assisting in this process is a nurturing act. Even thought artificial feeding may be rejected, assisted oral feeding should be considered an obligation rather than an option, as permitted by the clinical situation.

With disagreements about management that involves ethical issues for some, the institutional ethics committee can be helpful by shedding light on the pertinent issues and improving communication among the involved parties. This is a valuable resource when conflicts are looming, but also in providing support for providers and family in emotionally charged situations.

## Summary and Conclusion

The symbolism associated with eating a meal, and wanting to provide nutrition when this is not possible, involves concepts that have been deeply ingrained in society for centuries. They traverse cultural boundaries. Technology affords society a relatively easy means of artificially providing food and fluids when oral intake diminishes or ceases. Thus, placing a feeding tube relieves the provider of liability concerns for not treating, and family or surrogates are relived of guilt for not feeding. Yet a tension exists. The idea of a seemingly simple way to provide food when a patient is not eating conflicts with the more ominous themes in the clinical settings considered herein of failing to benefit, adding to suffering, and using technology that may be dehumanizing and disrespectful.

Howard Brody has suggested that artificial nutrition and hydration in terminal illness may be "...a textbook case of disproportionate care, which patients may choose to forgo" (p. 740). A principlist analysis would likewise argue that both beneficence and autonomy might be in jeopardy if artificial nutrition and hydration are initiated in patients with terminal illness. Lastly, while the definition of medical futility is debatable, a physician is not obligated to provide treatment so judged; while sometimes considered an affront to autonomy, an element of paternalism may contribute to effective medical decision making, although physicians may hesitate to exercise it.

In many patients with advanced dementia, terminal cancer, and neurological devastation, artificial feeding is inappropriate. The ethical and legal basis for withholding this treatment discussed earlier is sound. While a morally pluralistic society will always generate different views because of competing value systems, the differences may not be as great as they might seem. While respecting these views, the goal of ethically sound decision making can realistically be achieved in most cases in a manner satisfactory to all.

LARRY D. SCOTT

SEE ALSO: *Aging and the Aged; Autonomy; Chronic Illness and Chronic Care; Clinical Ethics; Dementia; DNR; Harm; Informed Consent; Judaism, Bioethics in; Long-Term Care; Technology; Surrogate Decision-Making*

### BIBLIOGRAPHY

Brett, Allan, S., and Rosenberg, Jason C. 2001. "The Adequacy of Informed Consent for Placement of Gastrostomy Tubes." *Archives of Internal Medicine* 161(5): 745–748.

Brody, Howard. 2000. "Evidence-Based Medicine, Nutritional Support, and Terminal Suffering." *The American Journal of Medicine* 109: 740–741.

Callahan, Christopher M.; Haag, Kathy M.; Buchanan, Nancy Nienaber; et al. 1999. "Decision-Making for Percutaneous Endoscopic Gastrostomy among Older Adults in a Community Setting." *Journal of American Geriatric Society* 47(9): 1105–1109.

Curran, William J. 1985. "Defining Appropriate Medical Care: Providing Nutrients and Hydration for the Dying." *The New England Journal of Medicine* 313(15): 940–942.

Finucane, Thomas E.; Christmas, Colleen; and Travis, Kathy. 1999. "Tube Feeding in Patients with Advanced Dementia: A Review of the Evidence." *Journal of the American Medical Association* 282(14): 1365–1370.

Gauderer, Michael W.; Ponsky, Jeffrey L.; and Izant, Robert J., Jr. 1980. "Gastrostomy without Laparotomy: A Percutaneous Endoscopic Technique." *Journal of Pediatric Surgery* 15(6): 872–875.

Gillick, Muriel R. 2000. "Rethinking the Role of Tube Feeding in Patients with Advanced Dementia." *The New England Journal of Medicine* 342(3): 206–210.

Gjerdingen, Dwenda K.; Neff, Jennifer A.; Wang, Marie; et al. 1999. "Older Persons' Opinions about Life-sustaining Procedures in the Face of Dementia." *Archives of Family Medicine* 8(5): 421–425.

Klein, Samuel; Kinney, John; Jeejeebhoy, Khursheed; et al. 1997. "Nutrition Support in Clinical Practice: Review of Published Data and Recommendation for Future Research Directions. Summary of a Conference Sponsored by the National Institutes of Health, American Society for Parenteral and Enteral Nutrition, and American Society for Clinical Nutrition." *American Journal of Clinical Nutrition* 66(3): 683–706.

Larson, David E.; Burton, Duane D.; Schroeder, Kenneth W.; et al. 1987. "Percutaneous Endoscopic Gastrostomy. Indications, Success, Complications, and Mortality in 314 Consecutive Patients." *Gastroenterology* 93(1): 48–52.

Lipman, Timothy O. 1997. "Enteral Nutrition and Dying: Ethical Issues in the Termination of Enteral Nutrition in Adults." In *Clinical Nutrition: Enteral and Tube Feeding,* ed. John L. Rombeau and Rolando H. Rolandelli. Philadelphia: W. B. Saunders Company.

Lynn, Joanne, ed. 1989. *By No Extraordinary Means: The Choice to Forgo Life-Sustaining Food and Water.* Bloomington: Indiana University Press.

Mackie, Sarah Breier. 2001. "PEGS and Ethics." *Gastroenterology Nursing Journal* 24(3): 138–142.

McCann, Robert M.; Hall, William J.; and Groth-Juncker, Annmarie. 1994. "Comfort Care for Terminally Ill Patients: The Appropriate Use of Nutrition and Hydration." *Journal of the American Medical Association* 272(16): 1263–1266.

Meier, Diane E.; Ahronheim, Judith C.; Morris, Jane; et al. 2001. "High Short-Term Mortality in Hospitalized Patients with Advanced Dementia." *Archives of Internal Medicine* 161: 594–599.

Meyers, Roberta M., and Grodin, Michael A. 1991. "Decisionmaking Regarding the Initiation of Tube Feedings in the Severely Demented Elderly: A Review." *Journal by the American Geriatrics Society* 39(5): 526–531.

Mitchell, Susan L.; Berkowitz, Randi E; Lawson, Fiona M.E.; et al. 2000. "A Cross-National Survey of Tube-Feeding Decisions in Cognitively Impaired Older Persons." *The American Geriatrics Society* 48(4): 391–397.

Post, Stephen G. 2001. "Tube Feeding and Advanced Progressive Dementia." *Hastings Center Report* Jan.–Feb. 31(1): 36–42.

Rabeneck, Linda; Wray, Nelda P.; and Petersen, Nancy J. 1996. "Long-Term Outcomes of Patients Receiving Percutaneous Endoscopic Gastrostomy Tubes." *Journal of General Internal Medicine* 11: 287–293.

Rabaneck, Linda; McCullough, Laurence B.; and Wray, Nelda P. 1997. "Ethically Justified, Clinically Comprehensive Guidelines for Percutaneous Endoscopic Gastrostomy Tube Placement." *The Lancet* 349(9050): 496–498.

Slomka, Jacquelyn. 1995. "What Do Apple Pie and Motherhood Have to Do with Feeding Tubes and Caring for the Patient?" *Archives of Internal Medicine* 155: 1258–1263.

Solomon, Mildred Z.; O'Donnell, Lydia; Jennings, Bruce; et al. 1993. "Decisions Near the End of Life: Professional Views on Life-Sustaining Treatments." *American Journal of Public Health* 83(1): 14–23.

Steinbrook, Robert, and Lo, Bernard. 1988. "Artificial Feeding-Solid Ground, Not A Slippery Slope." *The New England Journal of Medicine* 318(5): 286–290.

Sullivan, Robert J., Jr. 1993. "Accepting Death without Artifical Nutrition or Hydration." *Journal of General Internal Medicine* 8: 220–224.

Winter, Stephen M. 2000. "Terminal Nutrition: Framing the Debate for the Withdrawal of Nutritional Support in Terminally Ill Patients." *The American Journal of Medicine* 109: 723–726.

# AUTHORITY IN RELIGIOUS TRADITIONS

• • •

Religious authority is a complex and ever-contested issue. Historical studies of religion demonstrate that religions are always changing; nevertheless, most religions anchor themselves in the concept that there is an unchanging truth to which they are always loyal. Between this ideal of unchanging truth and the reality of historical contingency, issues of religious authority are played out. Some factions of a religious community push for change; others pull against the tide of new ideas, social practices, or technology. Balance or synthesis among these competing factions may be temporarily achieved, but changing circumstances will again challenge that consensus. Just as often, no consensus is possible and religious communities split, giving rise to new denominations and even to new religions. Thus, the existence of religious diversity is closely linked to conflicts about appropriate and reliable religious authority and the inability of religious communities to agree upon the same sources of authority.

## Overview: Types of Religious Authority

Four major types of religious authority, usually combined in some way, are found in the world's religions. In most cases, tradition itself is regarded as authoritative. Religions tend to appeal to a more remote past, the true tradition, especially when current authorities are being challenged. In only a few religions, however, is tradition regarded as the major source of authority. A second source of authority is the world of nature, used as a model for human behavior and often thought to set limits for humans. While some appeal to nature is common, again only a few religions regard it as the major religious authority.

Against that background of appeal to tradition or nature, texts, both oral and written, and often regarded as revealed, vie with people for the status of highest or final authority. The authority accorded to texts varies greatly, but they are always important, regarded as repositories of wisdom from ancient times, trustworthy because they represent sacred wisdom from long ago. According to many religions, the sacred text should always be more authoritative than any reader of that text; that is to say, the readers should submit to the authority of the text, not the other way around. However, the problem with texts is that they cannot function in an unmediated fashion, directly transmitting their contents. They have to be understood and made relevant for contemporary people by contemporary readers, which means that people interpreting the texts can have equal, or even greater, authority than the texts on which a religion bases itself, no matter what that religion may assert about the superior authority of texts. Other religions do not trust a text, by itself, to give clear guidance and rely more on learned or realized human beings who have experienced the text's meaning for reliable authority. Thus, at least to scholars of religion, it is clear that the people who receive and interpret texts, are, in fact, the most important sources of religious authority, though few religions openly declare that to be the case.

## Types of Religious Leaders

The types of people in whom religious authority is vested vary greatly and struggles among different claimants to religious authority often occur. Frequently, an educated, elite group claims authority by virtue of its training and credentials. In some cases, entry into that group depends on heredity and almost universally in traditional settings, women are barred from that group. Among the various types of religious leaders, these people often function as priests who perform rituals on behalf of the whole community and often they are conservative, rather than innovative or radical in religious matters.

Another elite group found in many religious traditions consists of charismatic leaders who often claim to have been chosen by the spirits for their vocation. Such leaders can have great authority among rank and file members of a religious community, and, because they owe their authority to unseen spiritual forces rather than to routine processes of education and licensing, they are difficult to control. But many religions expect leaders directly inspired by the spirits to be part of the mix of religious authorities and have an honored place for them. Such leaders can be avenues by which innovation comes into a tradition, or they may argue that a more traditional practice would be more pleasing to the spirits. They also may cause the development of new denominations or religions.

Especially in some Asian traditions, a sage or *guru* (teacher) who has personally experienced the truths taught by that religion is the highest religious authority. These leaders also are often innovators in their tradition because they have been thoroughly trained, authorized to lead by their own teachers, and are trusted to advise people on matters of spiritual disciplines such as meditation.

Finally, religious authority is always vested to some extent in the whole community. Those with authority may wish to lead the community in a certain direction, but find that their followers simply are not willing to be led in that direction. Who is more innovative and who is more conservative in these struggles also varies. Sometimes, religious leaders want to push their followers to accept new elements into the tradition, such as the ordination of women to clerical roles in twentieth-century Judaism and Christianity. In other cases, such as the frequent use of birth control by North American Roman Catholics, the ordinary members of the tradition defy the more conservative stances of religious authorities. But, in any case, however uneasy the consensus may be, religious communities and those who claim religious authority have to come to some common understandings. If that does not happen, the religious tradition would fall apart and become something else—either a purely secular community or a new religion.

## When Authorities Clash

Clashes between religious authorities are common. One type of clash is that between completely different religions, for example, the contemporary hostility between Islam and Hinduism on the Indian subcontinent. In such cases, differences in worldview are so great that the only resolution is some accord permitting coexistence. A more common clash of religious authorities occurs within traditions, when some individuals argue very strongly for one way of practicing or interpreting the religion and another group argues just as

strongly for a different method. Denominations within one religion or the formation of a new, closely related religion often are the result of disagreements between religious leaders, all of whom claim authority. In these cases, both leaders claim to revere that tradition's ultimate religious authority, but also claim that responsibility to care for and interpret that religion has fallen into the wrong hands. At least three major kinds of protest have arisen repeatedly.

First, individuals or groups protest that the wrong people have been put in authority or that they have too much power. The major division between the Sunni and Shi'ite branches within Islam arose from controversy over who was the legitimate successor to the Prophet Mohammed, meant to rule over a unified Islam. While the Protestant movement is complex, one major initial cause certainly was German Reformation leader Martin Luther's (1483–1546) defiance of papal authority. According to Luther, the pope had usurped the authority that should reside directly in the Bible and believers should form their faith directly on the Bible rather than relying on the decisions of a human intermediary. Luther's protests were only the first of many movements claiming to abandon various human institutions to return to the sacred text as ultimate and final authority. Today, numerous individuals and movements within Christianity claim to have found that unmediated text, but each claim is contested by another contender.

Second, individuals or groups often claim that those with formal authority have lost contact with the spiritual sources of the tradition and no longer can speak for the deity or interpret texts accurately. Claims of corruption on the part of established authorities are also common, found in every religion. Protestors often claim direct contact with the spiritual sources of the tradition, which they say is more authoritative than the mere rote learning or heredity power of those with formal authority. Usually they do not wish to form a separate group but long for a more vibrant, ecstatic spiritual experience within their tradition. Sometimes these movements can be incorporated into the larger tradition, as happened with many monastic movements in European Christianity and with many of the great Christian mystics. The Sufi movement within Islam also sought and provides more direct religious experience. The medieval mystical branch of Judaism, the Kabbalah, became quite popular, though it is not well-known or frequently practiced today. Some groups break away from their parent body, as did the English Quakers who believe that clergy are not necessary because deity can speak to anyone who waits in silence, only to become established groups themselves. Variations on this theme are infinite, as spirit-filled individuals and groups, dissatisfied with what they experience as dead and rigid ways of those with formal authority, refuse to remain silent.

Third, countless movements of social protest and reform have arisen when groups of believers claim that, while the religion dictates charity and concern for the poor and underprivileged, the religious authorities have sided with the rich and powerful. Many of the great reform movements of the nineteenth and twentieth centuries—abolition, the civil rights movement, feminism, war protest, environmental activism and anti-colonial movements—have been fueled in part by the inspiration that their religion authorizes social protestors to act against religious authorities who have lost their mandate because they ignored an important part of the sacred heritage.

## The Predominance of Texts: Monotheistic Religions

Texts believed to be revealed are more definitive sources of authority in the three monotheistic religions than in other religions. Furthermore, the most serious disagreement among the monotheistic religions concerns which of them possesses the truly revealed, authoritative scripture. Judaism, Christianity, and Islam all claim to believe in a monotheistic deity and all three claim that the deity has spoken to humankind in trustworthy, definitive revealed scriptures. But each claims its scripture as the one reliable scripture, and predictably, as each of the three religions emerged into history, it claimed that its scriptures fulfilled and replaced previously recognized texts. Also predictably, those who did not follow the new revelation claimed it to be the work of misguided usurpers. Thus, Jews regard the Hebrew Bible, the oldest monotheistic scripture, as the valid revelation and do not recognize either the Christian New Testament or the Muslim Qur'an as revelations. Christians recognize the Hebrew Bible, virtually identical with what they call the Old Testament, as genuine revelation, but claim that their New Testament is the culmination and fulfillment of that scripture. However, they pay little attention to the Qur'an, which emerged later. Muslims, on the other hand, claim that both the Hebrew Bible and the New Testament were genuine messages from the deity, valid in their own time, but now made obsolete by their own final and definitive revelation.

Fundamental to claims of authority for these scriptures is the claim that revelation has now ceased; each of the three monotheistic religions in turn makes the claim that the deity said all it intends to say now that its scripture has been revealed and that humans can expect no further revealed messages. Thus each religion in turn has declared the canon to be closed.

Within each of the three monotheistic traditions, similar problems have developed in the process of living with a definitive, final revealed text that cannot be amended or changed. First, who determines that the canon is, indeed, closed? In the Muslim tradition, this issue was solved relatively easily. The entire Qur'an was revealed during the lifetime of the prophet Mohammed (570–632 C.E.) and Muslims of his own day and later times never questioned whether any other texts could be part of the Qur'an. But the issue was not so easily solved with the New Testament or the Hebrew Bible, in part because the idea of a definitive revealed scripture as the charter of the religious community was not yet well established.

By the beginning of the common era, the contents of the Hebrew Bible had been roughly agreed upon, though one class of literature, the Apocrypha, usually included in Roman Catholic Bibles but not in Protestant or Jewish Bibles, had an ambiguous status. Many new texts about Jesus and the meaning of his life were being circulated in the Roman Empire as Christianity began to form and to split from Judaism. Were they revealed scriptures? Many texts about Jesus did not make it into the New Testament canon as Christianity gradually defined its orthodoxy and rejected the texts of the defeated Christian groups. Bishops began to circulate lists of texts that they regarded as appropriate reading material for their congregations; they had a list in common sometime between the second and the fourth centuries C.E. that closed the New Testament canon. Christians also accepted the texts that had already become sacred to Jews, but they read them in Greek (or later in Latin), not in Hebrew. The Apocrypha circulated as part of the already established Greek translation, which is why Christians continued to regard it as scripture until the Reformation.

Jews experienced very chaotic times after the destruction of the Second Temple in 70 C.E., when they were dispersed to all parts of the Roman empire, and Christianity became dominant. In these conditions a group of rabbis regarded as religious authorities met to come to a firm decision about which texts were authoritative for Jews. They came to the conclusion that the Apocrypha should be set aside, leaving the Torah, the Prophets, and the Writings as the three parts of the Hebrew Bible.

One way or another, the authority of a specific text is established. All three monotheistic religions agree that life should be based on that text, that the text is the final arbiter of the deity's wishes and commands for human beings. But how is what the text really says determined, and who gets to make those determinations? These are the fundamental issues about religious authority in the monotheistic religions. Deeming the text authoritative does not solve the problem of which persons or institutions should determine the text's meaning or the text's solution to various unforeseen circumstances that inevitably arise.

This problem is solved by authorizing a specific group of people to determine the text's meaning. In all three monotheistic religions, these people must be well educated in the text and commentaries upon it because they should derive their interpretations from the text, not impose them upon the text. In time, commentaries become as important, if not more important than the root text, as each generation adds its layer of commentary, which becomes part of the whole authoritative tradition.

In Judaism and Islam, the revealed text is regarded above all as the guideline for daily life. Religious authority involves not only questions of belief or ethical behavior but also of diet, inheritance, marriage and divorce, testimony in court, and all the other myriad details that make up a whole society. The most respected scholars in the tradition are those who know the all-encompassing religious legal code and how to bring it to bear on any new situation that develops. The revealed text has often been compared to a constitution and the process of interpreting it to the development of constitutional law. This fact helps explain why the separation of religion and government is so difficult for many Muslim societies; there can be no real separation between religion and the affairs of daily life that governments oversee if the revealed sacred text is, in fact, a constitution setting forth a daily routine and way of life. Muslims and Jews usually regard this code for daily living as a great blessing rather than a burden. They say that having such matters as diet or family law predetermined by religious authority makes life simpler and less stressful.

Valid "constitutional law" that develops in this process is regarded as having equal authority with the original text. In Judaism, the *oral Torah* of the Mishnah and the Talmud, compiled in the early centuries of the common era, is regarded as having been contained, in a hidden way, in the written Torah, the first five books of the Hebrew Bible (which Christians call the Old Testament). It was the job of skilled, well educated rabbis to draw out those meanings, for often Jewish law as practiced in contemporary Orthodox Judaism goes well beyond the literal text of the written Torah. In a similar fashion, Muslims rely on the Hadith, the sayings of the prophet Mohammed that are not part of the Qur'an, to answer questions seemingly left unanswered by it. If more resources are needed, reasoning from the text is considered a valid source of authority in Islam. The fourth source of authority in Islam is the consensus of the whole community, a source of authority much less explicitly recognized in most other religions.

Christianity did not develop the same kind of overarching blueprint for daily living and so the same kind of detailed attention to the development of religious law did not occur. However, matters of theological doctrine drew the same intense scrutiny, the same creative reasoning to prove that doctrines most historians would regard as later developments really are present in the Biblical text itself. Early Christianity was very diverse and many different forms of Christianity competed for dominance, especially before the legalization of Christianity under the Emperor Constantine in 313 C.E. and the formation of the Nicene Creed in 325 C.E. With those events, a dominant form of Christianity, under the authority of the bishop of Rome (the popes) emerged.

## Living Lineages of Oral Transmission: Asian and Indigenous Traditions

It is more common for accomplished religious practitioners to advise individuals and communities about what practices need to be followed and how to do that rather than to rely primarily on texts. Thus, religious authority is invested first in persons, who often use traditional texts extensively, but whose main basis for authority comes from their own realization of the meanings encoded in the texts. Another person, equally well versed in study of the texts, but lacking personal realization of their meaning, would not command the same prestige or be approached by others seeking religious guidance. In such religions, there is a well-established body of traditions, both textual and oral, but the canon of tradition and text is not closed; it is quite possible for contemporary teachers and their writings eventually to come to be as highly regarded as those of past leaders. Most important of all, the meaning of the text or tradition is regarded as locked and inaccessible to most ordinary people without the guidance of a teacher who has fathomed the meaning of the text.

In such traditions, the guarantor of authenticity rather than wholesale freelance creativity is the lineage of oral transmission. Locating reliable religious authority in a lineage of oral transmission depends upon two major premises. The first is that, because of the brittle, unreliable character of the written word, it can be rather dangerous and misleading for untutored individuals to try to rely directly on texts, particularly those that discuss advanced exercises in meditation and mystical experience. Such danger exists because the written word cannot fully capture or express the truths it tries to communicate. Instead, communication of the deeper meanings of a text or tradition depends on the oral instruction from someone who has already understood the text fully and can transmit it in an appropriate manner. A very different evaluation of the reliability and potency of written or memorized texts from that found in monotheistic religions drives this idea about reliable religious authority. However, protection from dangerous or misleading innovations is also needed so that the oral transmission does not become completely idiosyncratic. Such protection comes through insistence on lineage, the second major premise basic to a lineage of oral transmission as religious authority. Only those teachers who have been authorized to do so by their teachers can transmit the oral teachings, and it is believed that this lineage of transmission is unbroken from the current teacher back to the founder of the specific religious movement. Within that protective restriction of who can teach, it is believed that appropriate innovations will be introduced safely and as needed. In fact, in religions that rely upon a lineage of oral transmission for religious authority, innovations and new lineages occur frequently, often without opposition or divisiveness.

The clearest examples of investing religious authority in the authorized teacher are found in Vajrayana and Zen Buddhism, some lineages of Hinduism, and some indigenous religions. These religions value direct religious experience highly and mistrust anything else to satisfy the longings that drive people to religions in the first place.

Buddhism depends on the ineffable enlightenment experience of one man, Siddartha Gautama (563–483 B.C.E.), and his ability to teach his students to experience for themselves the peace and freedom he had found. What he experienced has never been put into words and most Buddhists would regard the attempt to do so as futile and unnecessary. However, he did teach methods to lead people toward their own enlightenment and others can teach these as well. The voluminous texts of the many denominations within Buddhism are primarily attempts to provide instruction on how to cross over from the confusion that Buddhists regard as the inevitable normal human condition to the freedom and peace that is the birthright of each human being.

Throughout Buddhist history, many types of Buddhism have evolved and some of these developments have included serious disagreement over the most reliable sources of authority. The major division in Buddhism is between the Theravadin Buddhists who prevail in Southeast Asia and the many forms of Mahayana Buddhism, which prevails in Tibet, China, Japan, and Korea. The name *Theravada* means *the way of the elders,* and this name indicates precisely what these Buddhists believe about themselves; they rely on the texts and traditions taught by the earliest generations of the Buddha's disciples and claim that Mahayana Buddhism is based on later, fraudulent ideas and practices that crept into Buddhism when some ignored the genuine oral transmissions. By contrast, Mahayanists claim that they possess oral transmissions going back to the historical Buddha,

which were taught to only a few students during the Buddha's lifetime, but gradually were made more public (and written down) when conditions were appropriate. Among the many forms of Mahayana Buddhism, Vajrayana Buddhism of Tibet and Zen Buddhism (the Japanese name) of China, Japan, Korea, and Vietnam rely most heavily on a lineage of authorized teachers to communicate the core teachings and practices. In these forms of Buddhism, texts are sometimes ignored almost completely, so great is the mistrust of the written word and the emphasis on the student's direct personal experience as opposed to their competence in intellectual knowledge of philosophical traditions.

Hinduism is a much more complex and diverse religion than is Buddhism, and by no means do all forms of Hinduism rely on lineages of living teachers for authority. For some forms of Hinduism, tradition, as passed down in communal memory and in texts, to a lesser extent, is the final authority. However, forms of Hinduism more concerned with philosophy and meditation do rely on such living teachers and the transmission of their authority from generation to generation. Each teacher or group has its own history and dynamic and they are endlessly diverse. Summarizing them is impossible.

Indigenous traditions worldwide are also impossible to discuss in general. Among them, one important authority is a figure often referred to as a *shaman* in Western sources. It is believed that shamans gain their authority through direct encounter with the spirits. Who might become a shaman cannot be predicted and it is also widely believed that an individual who has been chosen to be a shaman cannot resist that call. Shamans do not usually learn much of their craft from other human teachers, but because of their ability to communicate between the human world and the spirit world, they are trusted authority figures in their communities. Usually, they function as advisors and healers, not lawgivers. Though shaman-like individuals can be found in many indigenous settings, some of the most famous and best known are found among groups of indigenous North and South Americans. One can also study shaman-like individuals in the religions of aboriginal Australia, but they are not characteristic of indigenous African religions. Formerly, they were common in the northernmost parts of Asia.

## The Force of Tradition: Collective Memory as Religious Authority

Many religious communities are not especially oriented either to a sacred text or an authorized teacher. Instead, for them, what counts is what has always been done, what they believe their forbears always did, and what tradition dictates.

Tradition as the ultimate religious authority can be found in segments of the religions already discussed because convention has always had great appeal and force. However, in at least two major religions, large segments of Hinduism and the Confucian perspective, tradition and custom have been explicitly elevated to the highest rank of religious authority.

*Hinduism* is a modern European term for the religious behavior Europeans encountered in India, which is one reason why Hinduism as an overarching tradition is so difficult to summarize. For the vast majority of Hindus, tradition is the foundation of religious life, upon which other elements may be cast, but often tradition is the entire content of religious life. This is especially true for those segments of Hinduism not oriented to enlightenment and ultimate release but to doing one's duty well in this world—and this type of Hinduism is, at least theoretically, the bottom line for all Hindus, no matter what else they might add on to this foundation. For traditional Hindus, life is a vast complex of duties and relationships, all of them laid out in the *eternal dharma,* the law code that no one quite understands fully, that is contained in no single source, and that differs from person to person depending on one's caste and stage of life. Nevertheless, duty is absolute and cannot be avoided.

The mystery and complexity of understanding one's duty is discussed in many Hindu texts, including the national epic, the *Mahabharata* (The Great War). For starters, there is the complexity of the duty of caste and stage of life. India's controversial caste system was considered to be of ultimate authority in classical Hinduism, of cosmic or divine origins and not subject to human moral qualms about its effects on individuals and society. Part of one's required duty is to conform to the requirements of one's caste status, as determined by birth. Individual abilities and desires were meaningless against this bank of tradition. Furthermore, one should conform to the duties required by one's stage in life. It is not appropriate for young people to seek individual religious fulfillment; they must first fulfill their family and professional roles, as laid out by sex and caste. Countless authorities, from the Buddha to Mahatma Gandhi, have tried to modify or eliminate the caste system, but the force of tradition has always prevailed over them. Today, the caste system is illegal in India, and *affirmative action* that tries to elevate the status of the less privileged castes is deeply resented by many in the more privileged castes.

Rather than being the timeless traditions of ordinary believers, the Confucian system was the ruling ideology of the Chinese elite for most of Chinese history. Though many well known human authors, including Confucius (551–479 B.C.E.) and Mencius (372–289 B.C.E.), wrote texts that are regarded as foundational to the Confucian movement, the authors always claimed that they were not inventing anything but only urging return to the trustworthy customs of the ancients. These traditions turned on maintaining the proper hierarchical relationships between, among others, rulers and subjects, elder and younger family members, and husbands and wives. If each person truly fulfilled the duties appropriate to his or her role, harmony would prevail and society would prosper. However, in this hierarchical system, those with power had an obligation to be fair and generous, rather than to take advantage of their power. If they took advantage of their power, that would disturb cosmic harmony and warfare or poverty would result. An important part of the Confucian system is *Li,* the accumulated customs of civilized people which included everything from how to greet someone to how to use one's eating utensils. According to Confucian thought, having a custom or rule to govern every possible occasion led to social harmony and contentment.

## The Ways of Nature as Religious Authority

Finally, for some religions, the natural world itself is the highest religious authority and the model upon which humans should base their lives.

A second religion indigenous to China—Daoism, whose founder is the legendary Lao Tzu (604 B.C.E., traditional birth date)—does not rely primarily on people or texts for authority, even though it is the source of the famous *Dao De Jing.* Rather, the Dao itself, the natural cosmic law that cannot be put into words but governs everything is the authority to which humans and everything else should submit and which they should imitate in every act of living. All human woe is said to derive from ignoring cosmic natural law and trying to impose human norms upon it. A wise person observes nature and trains until he or she can follow its ways in complete spontaneity, no matter where that may lead.

Finally, Shinto, the indigenous religion of Japan, is famous for not regarding texts as important. Ritual traditions and the cultivation of beauty are its primary means of expressing itself. Priests know how to perform the beautiful rituals and maintain beautiful temples, often located in places of great natural beauty, but they are not regarded as religious authorities or leaders either. Rather, the delightful natural world itself is of supreme value. It is the sacred source of all life and nothing human can compete with it for value.

This model of religion that orients itself more to the ways of the natural world than to texts or people is also common among indigenous religions around the world.

They commonly have a keen understanding of and appreciation for nature and regard the entire natural world as sacred, of ultimate value.

## Religious Authority and Modern Thought

All traditional sources of religious authority are being challenged by modern thought, especially science, empirical history, and secular movements of social reform.

Religions respond to these developments in various ways, from significant internal changes accommodating modern thought to complete resistance.

In many ways, the religions most oriented to texts have had the most difficult time dealing with modern thought; the texts often contain science, history, and social systems that do not fit well with modernity and the texts are supposed to be eternally valid and binding. Many interpreters have found ways to combine the deepest insights of religious texts with modern thought by considering some aspects of the text to stem from its social context rather than divine revelation, and by regarding many stories in the text as metaphorical rather than literal truths. Others have refused to concede any aspect of traditional religious thought where it conflicts with modern science or history, with the result that fundamentalism is a dominant religious movement in the twenty-first century, especially in monotheistic religions.

The traditional religions of China have also been deeply affected by modern thought, largely in negative ways. The triumph of Communism deeply weakened the hold of both Confucian and Daoist thought on Chinese people. It also led to the severe repression of Buddhism in both Tibet and China.

Secularism or indifference to religion is also common in many parts of the modern world, especially Japan and Europe. Religion has become a minor ceremonial affair having little real authority for many people.

In other parts of the world, especially India and the Middle East, religion has become a major source of conflict as different religions claim that their texts and traditions give them alone control over land and sacred places. Both sides in the conflict claim the authority of their religious tradition and ignore similar claims by their opponents as illegitimate.

## Conclusion

In every situation, religious authority will depend on a complex mix of tradition, views about nature, various types of religious leaders, and texts or oral traditions possessing varying levels of sanctity. Usually one or two of these sources of authority are dominant. Sometimes those sources of authority will try to push the religious community into new practices or understandings. Sometimes those sources of authority will try to conserve current practices and understandings in the face of intellectual or ethical challenges. Few generalizations regarding authority in religious traditions can be made with any reliability.

RITA M. GROSS

SEE ALSO: *Autonomy; Coercion; Conscience; Conscience, Rights of; Responsibility; Trust*

### BIBLIOGRAPHY

Berndt, Ronald M., and Berndt, Catherine H. 1964. *The World of the First Australians: An Introduction to the Traditional Life of the Australian Aborigines.* Chicago: University of Chicago Press.

Bornkamm, G. 1960. *Jesus of Nazareth.* New York: Harper.

Cole, W. Owen. 1982. *The Guru in Sikhism.* London: Dartman, Longman and Todd.

Coulson, N. G. 1964. *A History of Islamic Law.* Edinburgh: Edinburgh University Press.

Denny, Frederick M., and Taylor, Rodney. 1985. *The Holy Book in Comparative Perspective.* Columbia: University of South Carolina Press.

Earhart, H. Byron. 1982. *Japanese Religion: Unity and Diversity,* 3rd edition. Belmont, CA: Wadsworth.

Garry, Ron, tr. 1999. *The Teacher-Student Relationship: A Translation of "The Explanation of the Master and Student Relationship and How to Teach and Listen to the Dharma" by Jamgon Kongtrul Lodro Thaye.* Ithaca, NY: Snow Lion Publications.

Gill, Sam D. 1982. *Native American Religions: An Introduction.* Belmont, CA: Wadsworth.

Graham, William A. 1987. *Beyond the Written Word: Oral Aspects of Scripture in the History of Religions.* New York: Cambridge University Press.

Gross, Rita M. 1996. *Feminism and Religion: An Introduction.* Boston: Beacon Press.

Hopkins, Thomas J. 1971. *The Hindu Religious Tradition.* Belmont, CA: Wadsworth.

Jaini, Padmanabh. 1979. *The Jaina Path of Purification.* Berkeley: University of California Press.

Kimball, Charles. 2002. *When Religion Becomes Evil.* San Francisco: Harper.

Kinsley, David. 1993. *Hinduism: a Cultural Perspective,* 2nd edition. Englewood Cliffs, NJ: Prentice-Hall.

Larson, Gerald James. 1995. *India's Anguish over Religion.* Albany: State University of New York.

Ludwig, Theodore M. 1996. *The Sacred Paths: Understanding the Religions of the World,* 2nd edition. Upper Saddle River, NJ: Prentice-Hall.

Mitchell, Donald W. 2002. *Buddhism: Introducing the Buddhist Experience.* New York: Oxford University Press.

Needham, Joseph. 1969. *Science and Civilization in China,* vol. 2: *History of Scientific Thought.* Cambridge, Eng.: Cambridge University Press.

Neihardt, John. 1961. *Black Elk Speaks: Being the Life Story of a Holy Man of the Oglala Sioux.* Lincoln: University of Nebraska Press.

Nuesner, Jacob. 1987. *The Way of Torah: An Introduction to Judaism,* 4th edition. Belmont, CA: Wadsworth.

Rahman, Fazlur. 1979. *Islam.* Chicago: University of Chicago Press.

Rahula, Walpola. 1974. *What the Buddha Taught,* rev. edition. New York: Grove Press.

Ray, Benjamin C. 1976. *African Religions: Symbol, Ritual and Community.* Englewood Cliffs, NJ: Prentice-Hall.

Ray, Reginald A. 2001. *Secret of the Vajra World: The Tantric Buddhism of Tibet.* Boston: Shambhala Publications.

Robinson, Richard, and Johnson, Willard. 1997. *The Buddhist Religion: A Historical Introduction,* 4th edition. Belmont, CA: Wadsworth.

Saso, Michael. 1978. *The Teachings of Taoist Master Chuang.* New Haven, CT: Yale University Press.

Schwartz, Regina M. 1997. *The Curse of Cain: The Violent Legacy of Monotheism.* Chicago: University of Chicago Press.

Sekida, Katsuki. 1985. *Zen Training: Methods and Philosophy.* New York: Weatherhill.

Sered, Susan Starr. 1994. *Priestess, Mother, Sacred Sister: Religions Dominated by Women.* New York: Oxford University Press.

Taylor, Rodney L. 1986. *The Way of Heaven: An Introduction to Confucian Religious Life.* Leiden, Netherlands: Brill.

Thompson, Laurence C. 1996. *Chinese Religion: An Introduction,* 5th edition. Belmont, CA: Wadsworth.

Van Voorst, Robert E. 1997. *Anthology of World Scriptures.* Belmont, CA: Wadsworth.

Weaver, Mary Jo. 1998. *Introduction to Christianity,* 3rd edition. Belmont: CA: Wadsworth.

# AUTOEXPERIMENTATION

• • •

Autoexperimentation, which refers to the practice of intentionally utilizing oneself as an experimental subject, is not a rare event. Over the past four centuries, more than 135 examples have been documented, and the true incidence is undoubtedly much higher (Altman; Franklin and Sutherland). Although the preponderance of recorded autoexperimentation has been conducted in the name of biomedical research, investigators in the physical and social sciences have also engaged in this practice.

Autoexperimentation has long enjoyed a measure of romantic appeal in the scientific and popular tradition. "The experimenter," wrote Sir George Pickering, "has one golden rule to guide him as to whether the experiment is justifiable. Is he prepared to submit himself to the procedure? If he is, and if the experiment is actually carried out on himself, then it is probably justifiable. If he is not, then the experiment should not be done" (p. 229). Henry K. Beecher suggested that any scientist wishing to engage in human experimentation ought to experiment on himself "as evidence of good faith."

Despite a reputation for nobility of purpose, the practice of autoexperimentation has been the focus of substantial scientific and ethical debate. The scientific controversy concerns the methodological limitations of autoexperimentation and its capacity to yield useful data. The ethical debate is more complicated. Superficially, it concerns the extent to which autoexperimentation ought to be regulated. At its heart, however, lies a fundamental conflict between two opposing views of scientific research. The libertarian view advocates a relatively laissez-faire policy toward all forms of scientific inquiry, including autoexperimentation. The paternalistic view, in contrast, emphasizes the importance of protecting experimental subjects from risk, whether self-imposed or imposed by others. While this entry presents various perspectives on the issue, the author is opposed to autoexperimentation in most cases and will make clear why this view is plausible as the entry unfolds.

Neither the methodological nor the ethical aspects of this debate can be fully understood without examining the historical and cultural context in which autoexperimentation developed.

## Historical Perspectives

One important factor in the history of autoexperimentation, upon which many investigators have remarked, is the existence of an extremely powerful and deeply rooted obligation to pursue scientific knowledge regardless of personal risk. A good example is John Hunter's unfortunate experiment with venereal disease. Throughout the eighteenth century, physicians debated whether gonorrhea and syphilis were two separate entities or different manifestations of the same disease. Hunter, a prominent surgeon, anatomist, and fellow of the Royal Society, believed they were the same. In 1770, to prove the point, he inoculated his own penis with the fresh urethral discharge of a man with gonorrhea. When syphilitic chancres developed at the site of inoculation, Hunter erroneously concluded that his theory was correct. Even though he thought he had contracted gonorrhea, Hunter eventually died of syphilis (Franklin and Sutherland). It is clear, in retrospect, that the discharge most probably transmitted both diseases.

Closely related is the idea that the true scientist must always be prepared to engage in resolute acts of personal daring (including, though not necessarily limited to, autoexperimentation) to overcome impediments to research. There are two famous cases in point. In 1929, despite the direct prohibition of his department chief, Werner Forssmann surreptitiously passed an intravenous catheter into his own heart to prove the feasibility of cardiac catheterization in humans. He later shared the Nobel Prize for these experiments (Altman). The second case pertains to the thymidine experiments of Beppino Giovanella during the late 1970s. Thymidine had been shown to be a promising cancer drug in animals, but the U.S. Food and Drug administration (FDA) refused to authorize clinical trials on the grounds that its safety had not been established. Giovanella proceeded to ingest huge doses of thymidine, thereby proving its safety and overcoming the objections of the FDA (Franklin and Sutherland).

A third factor has to do with the problem of justifying human research before the safety of an experiment has been established. Experimenting on oneself or one's colleagues signals the conviction that the experiment is at least worthwhile, if not necessarily safe (see Beecher; Pickering; Bok). In 1997, the International Association of Physicians in AIDS Care (IAPAC) announced that many of its members had agreed to be subjects in trials of a live attenuated HIV-1 vaccine. Some AIDS researchers said the vaccine was too dangerous to be tested in people, but the head of the IAPAC initiative argued that 8,500 new HIV infections every day made further delay in testing vaccines unethical (McCarthy). As of March 1998, more than 270 physicians, healthcare professionals, and healthcare advocates had volunteered for the trials, which had not yet commenced in early 2003 (IAPAC).

A fourth factor derives from the observation that autoexperimentation is usually the best, and sometimes the only, way to ensure absolute adherence to an exacting research protocol. In 1962, for example, Victor Herbert undertook an investigation to explore a possible link between nutritional folic acid deficiency and megaloblastic anemia. To deplete the body of folic acid reserves, he subsisted for eighteen weeks upon an extraordinarily insipid and unpalatable diet (Altman). Herbert commented that the experiment would probably have failed had he not experimented upon himself.

Finally, autoexperimentation has often been fostered when it appeared that certain researchers, by virtue of special training and experience, might extract significantly more from an experiment by participating than by observing. Data obtained uniquely through autoexperimentation proved critical, for example, in the development of protective clothing for ultrahigh-altitude airplane ejection, in studies of extreme acceleration and deceleration, in investigations of decompression sickness, and in studies of human physiology in space (Gibson and Harrison; Dille; Franklin and Sutherland).

## Criticisms of Autoexperimentation

Critics of autoexperimentation object to the practice on both methodological and ethical grounds.

**METHODOLOGICAL ISSUES.** The worth of an experiment depends upon its scientific merit, upon its permissibility from ethical and legal perspectives, and upon its advisability on other grounds. Before any experiment is carried out, each of these elements must be assessed. Autoexperimentation suffers from three major methodological problems. First, there is an inherent difficulty in observing oneself dispassionately. This difficulty often leads to the confusion of objective and subjective data. Second, it is virtually impossible to establish adequate controls, particularly because autoexperiments tend to involve serial observations of one individual. Third, it is very difficult to extract statistically valid information because of the typically very small numbers of subjects and experiments. As a general rule, the likelihood that useful data will result from experiments on very small groups is determined by the likelihood that the data would not be materially affected by iterations (repetitions of the experiment) on larger groups.

Because of these weaknesses, autoexperimentation rarely proves to be a wholly satisfactory experimental method. There may be two important exceptions, however: pilot studies to establish the feasibility of a procedure or the safety of a pharmacological agent in normal subjects; and studies in which the scientist consents to be treated as an ordinary research subject and to remain under the supervision of other investigators for the duration of the experiment. It is worth noting that the second exception complies with the provisions of the Declaration of Helsinki stipulating that "the responsibility for the human subject must always rest with a medically qualified person and never rest on the subject of the research" (World Medical Association, p. 3).

**ETHICAL ISSUES.** Autoexperimentation is clearly often heroic, but the basis for the alleged obligation to engage in this practice is less clear, for it is not clear that there are good moral reasons to encourage—let alone require—autoexperimentation. As discussed above, autoexperimentation is not always good science, for it may lack adequate controls and sufficient subjects to generate meaningful results. Therefore, autoexperimentation makes sense more as a potential condition to involving noninvestigator subjects in further testing than as a substitute for using such subjects. However, autoexperimentation may not be sufficient to establish that lay persons may appropriately participate in an experiment, for the investigator may be more risk-accepting than other subjects, or may not be medically representative of all potential subjects, or may not meet the physiological qualifications for subjects in that experiment. It is also unclear that autoexperimentation is necessary to establish that noninvestigators should participate in an experiment, for the processes of institutional ethics review and informed consent are probably better ways to determine whether that is appropriate. Of course, these points may not apply when the risks are exceptionally high and the need for the research exceptionally urgent.

To the extent there is an obligation for researchers to engage in autoexperimentation, that obligation does not always outweigh the problems with autoexperimentation. The fundamental issue is whether any of the precautions required to protect the subject in other forms of human experimentation may be legitimately suspended in the case of voluntary autoexperimentation.

The three basic arguments that have been brought to bear on this question are not easily reconciled: (1) Individuals are entitled to assume voluntarily risks they may never impose on others; (2) under proper circumstances, both self-sacrifice (martyrdom) or assumption of high risk for good reason (heroism) are universally lauded; and (3) societies have a vested interest in protecting the welfare of their members, and some degree of regulation in recognition of this interest is required or, at the very least, ought to be permissible.

Libertarians argue that the principle of autonomy grants scientists the right to engage voluntarily in risky behavior. On this basis, they refute the applicability of regulations for the protection of human subjects in autoexperimentation. Champions of a more paternalistic approach, in contrast, oppose unlimited risk taking in any experimental context because of the following concerns:

1. Many risks have been undertaken for unimportant goals;

2. Habitual risk takers might turn to autoexperimentation even when other, more desirable forms of investigation exist;

3. Investigator–subjects may be at greater risk than other potential subjects because curiosity, enthusiasm, and other intangible factors may induce them to ignore risks that would otherwise deter a prudent individual from participation (Bok);

4. Certain levels of risk are, or ought to be, beyond consent (Bok);

5. Investigators reckless with respect to their own safety are wont to become reckless in other aspects of their investigations;

6. The autonomy of investigator–subjects might be tainted by various levels of institutional or peer coercion, or even by self-imposed psychological pressures (Dagi and Dagi); and

7. Large-scale, unregulated autoexperimentation might subvert accepted guidelines for the protection of human subjects under other experimental conditions.

The apparent contradiction between concerns (3) and (4), on the one hand, and the respect and admiration traditionally accorded to martyrs and heroes in Western society on the other, is not easily reconciled.

Finally, because most scientific research is now done in teams, the simple model from earlier days of a lone researcher experimenting upon himself does not fit all current autoexperimentation. "Group autoexperimentation" can involve vulnerable subjects when junior investigators, students, or laboratory technicians participate as subjects. Some recent research ethics policies addressing autoexperimentation reflect concern for such investigator–subjects.

## Policies and Regulations

While it is generally agreed that institutions are ultimately responsible for the regulation of all forms of experimentation carried out within their jurisdiction, there is no consensus regarding how—or even whether—autoexperimentation should be regulated. The Nuremberg Code tacitly encourages autoexperimentation through the provisions of Article 5: Perilous human experimentation is prohibited "except, perhaps, in those experiments where the experimental physicians also serve as subjects" (Germany [Territory Under Allied Occupation]). The World Medical Association's Declaration of Helsinki does not address autoexperimentation directly, but does say that responsibility for the subject always rests with a "medically qualified person," never on the subject (p. 15–16), and that, when the subject is in a dependent relationship with the researcher, informed consent should be obtained by a physician who is not engaged in the investigation and is "completely independent" of the relationship (p. 16). The U.S. National Institutes of Health promulgated a code for self-experimentation "to provide the same safeguards for physician–subjects as for the normal volunteer" (Altman). The Office for Protection of Research Risks of the U.S. Department of Health and Human Services has ruled that autoexperimentation is subject to the same regulations as other human research, including review by institutional review boards (IRB).

Some institutional ethics codes and policies now advise against or even prohibit autoexperimentation, even when it takes the form of "group" autoexperimentation, and involves residents, students, or employees. The *IRB Guidebook* issued by the Office for Human Research Protections of the U.S. Department of Health and Human Services suggests advertising for subjects, rather than recruiting students directly, and notes that some universities prohibit or severely restrict student participation. The research ethics policy of Massachusetts General Hospital is more stern: "Studies of volunteers in the investigator's own department or who are the investigator's students should be avoided and will usually be disapproved by the Human Research Committee because of the subtle coercive factors that could be present in even the most harmonious situations." The University of Maryland Baltimore County requires IRB approval to enroll students and employees.

## Conclusion

No act of autoexperimentation, no matter how worthy or well intentioned, should be sanctioned until three conditions are fulfilled: (1) The proposed experiment has been fully described; (2) potential sources of coercion influencing the experimenter have been investigated and excluded; and (3) the institutional and social consequences of the experiment have been thoroughly explored, particularly with respect to risks such as the appearance of condoning inconsistent standards for the protection of human subjects. In most cases, fulfillment of these conditions will result in autoexperimentation being held to the same standard of review as any other forms of human investigation. These conditions are expressly designed to protect both the experimenter–subject *and* the institution, in equal measure.

The decision-making process associated with autoexperimentation should, therefore, involve peer review, and it should accord with established criteria for determining the acceptability of experimental protocols. At the very least, judgments about the permissibility of autoexperimentation

must weigh questions of risk, benefit, voluntariness, and scientific significance, as well as the more elusive issues comprehended by the term *institutional interests*. While the requirement for institutional review may induce some scientists to experiment on themselves outside the scientific mainstream, this effect is unlikely to prevail and, as a practical matter, is virtually impossible to repress.

TEODORO FORCHT DAGI (1995)
REVISED BY JOHN K. DAVIS

**SEE ALSO:** *Autonomy; Harm; Paternalism; Research, Human: Historical Aspects; Research, Unethical*

### BIBLIOGRAPHY

Altman, Lawrence K. 1987. *Who Goes First? The Story of Self-Experimentation in Medicine.* New York: Random House.

Beecher, Henry K. 1959. "The Experimentation in Man." *Journal of the American Medical Association* 169(5): 461–478.

Bok, Sissela. 1978. "Freedom and Risk." *Daedalus* 107(2): 115–127.

Dagi, T. Forcht, and Dagi, Linda Rabinowitz. 1988. "Physicians Experimenting on Themselves: Some Ethical and Philosophical Considerations." In *The Use of Human Beings in Research with Special Reference to Clinical Trials,* ed. Stuart F. Spicker, Ilai Alon, André de Vries, and H. Tristram Engelhardt, Jr. Dordrecht, Netherlands: Kluwer.

Dille, J. Robert. 1984. "Introduction to the First of Two Aerial Voyages of Dr. Jeffires and Mons. Blanchard." *Aviation, Space, and Environmental Medicine* 55(11): 993–999.

Forssmann, Werner. 1964. "The Role of Heart Catheterization and Angiocardiography in the Development of Modern Medicine." In *Physiology or Medicine, 1942–1962,* vol. 3 of *Nobel Lectures.* Amsterdam: Elsevier.

Franklin, Jon, and Sutherland, John. 1984. *Guinea Pig Doctors: The Drama of Medical Research Through Self-Experimentation.* New York: Morrow.

Germany (Territory under Allied Occupation, 1945–1955: U.S. Zone) Military Tribunals. 1947. "Permissible Medical Experiments." In "The Nuremberg Code," excerpted from vol. 2 of *Trials of War Criminals before the Nuremberg Tribunals under Control Council Law No. 10.* Washington, D.C.: U.S. Government Printing Office. Reprinted in Sugarman, Jeremy, Mastroianni, Anna C., and Kahn, Jeffrey P., eds. 1998. *Ethics of Research with Human Subjects: Selected Policies and Resources.* Frederick, MD: University Publishing Group.

Gibson, T. Mike, and Harrison, Mike H. 1984. *Into Thin Air: A History of Aviation Medicine in the RAF.* London: Robert Hale.

Herbert, Victor. 1962. "Experimental Nutritional Folate Deficiency in Man." *Transactions of the Association of American Physicians* 75: 307–320.

McCarthy, Michael. 1997. "AIDS Doctors Push for Live-Virus Vaccine Trials." *The Lancet* 350(9084): 1082.

Pickering, George W. 1949. "The Place of Experimental Method in Medicine." *Proceedings of the Royal Society of Medicine* 42(1): 229–234.

World Medical Association. 1998. "Declaration of Helsinki." In *Ethics of Research with Human Subjects: Selected Policies and Resources,* eds. Jeremy Sugarman, Anna C. Mastroianni, and Jeffrey P. Kahn. Frederick, MD: University Publishing Group.

INTERNET RESOURCES

Institutional Review Board, University of Maryland Baltimore County. 2003. "Enrollment of Participants and Use of Data." Available from <http://www.umbc.edu/irb/Enrollme.html>.

International Association of Physicians in AIDS Care (IAPAC). "IAPAC's HIV Vaccine Initiative." Available from <http://www.iapac.org>.

Massachusetts General Hospital. 2003. "Selection of Human Subjects." In "Responsible Conduct of Human Studies," internal publication. Available from <http://healthcare.partners.org/phsirb>.

Office for Human Research Protections. 2003. *IRB Guidebook.* Available from <http://ohrp.osophs.dhhs.gov>.

# AUTONOMY

• • •

The concept of autonomy in moral philosophy and bioethics recognizes the human capacity for self-determination, and puts forward a principle that the autonomy of persons ought to be respected. At this level of generality, there is not much with which to take issue; a full account of autonomy must further define self-determination and state how and to what extent autonomy should be respected. Autonomy as a capacity of persons must be distinguished from autonomy as a property of actions and decisions, for a person with the capacity for autonomy may act nonautonomously on particular occasions, for example, a person who is coerced to do something. Autonomy as a fundamental value and a basic right is part of the moral and political theory of liberal individualism. According to this view, autonomous individuals are the ultimate source of value: The basis for an action, social practice, or government policy to be right or good is in the values, preferences, or choices of autonomous individuals. In social philosophy, individual autonomy as a basic value and a fundamental right is in tension with community values, such as caring for others, promoting the good of society, and preserving and enhancing the moral practices of society. In clinical bioethics, the right to autonomy of individual patients is in tension with healthcare professionals' obligations to benefit patients. These conflicts will be examined in what follows.

## Autonomy as Capacity

There are three elements to the psychological capacity of autonomy: agency, independence, and rationality. Agency is awareness of oneself as having desires and intentions and of acting on them. (Desire includes inclinations, aversions, wants, and similar terms.) When people have a desire for some state of affairs, they form an intention to do what they believe will bring about the desired state of affairs; further, they want their desire to determine their action (Benn; Haworth).

The capacity for agency distinguishes persons from inanimate objects and from nonhuman animals. Inanimate objects can be affected by objects and conditions external to them, as can persons, but unlike persons, inanimate objects cannot be said to act on desires. Nonhuman animals have desires, but there is no (noncontroversial) reason to believe that they have the capacity for self-consciousness that is manifest in having an awareness of desires and wanting them to be effective in action. Agency does not imply that persons are never influenced by external forces or that persons never act impulsively. It is an account of how persons are able to act and not how they always act.

Independence is the absence of influences that so control what a person does that it cannot be said that he or she wants to do it. This may seem a feature of an autonomous action rather than an element of psychological capacity. However, there are cases in which a person's course of life is under constant threat of violence from others, and the person acts always to avoid harm: war, poverty, abusive relationships, police states. When the whole of a person's beliefs, plans, self-image, and ways of relating to others are the result of unrelenting coercion and manipulation, then that person has little or no capacity for autonomy.

Autonomy also requires that persons have an adequate range of options. Coercion and manipulation limit options, but options are also limited by social and physical environments. If a person's options are numerous and noncoerced but are trivial in relation to what is valued by the person, then there is no capacity for autonomy in a significant sense (Raz). This would be the case in a totalitarian, caste, or slave society where a combination of coercion and ideology suppress the aspirations and real options of a segment of the members of the society. A full account of the conception of autonomy must distinguish external influences that defeat autonomy from external influences that are consistent with being autonomous. The former includes coercion and manipulation, and the latter includes persuasion and the normal limitations of physical and social environments.

The third element of the capacity for autonomy is *means-end rationality,* or *rational decision making.* In addition to the self-consciousness of agency, the capacity for rational decision making requires a person: (1) whose beliefs are subject to standards of truth and evidence; (2) with ability to recognize commitments and to act on them; (3) who can construct and evaluate alternative decisions; (4) whose changes in beliefs and values can change decisions and actions; and (5) whose beliefs and values yield rankings of action commitments. Another way to understand rationality as an element of the capacity for autonomy is as the capacity for reflection on desires. A rational person can have a desire for or fear of something, such as a desire for food or a fear of surgery, and also have the wish that he or she not have that desire or not be moved by that fear (Dworkin, 1976, 1988; Childress). Persons who lack the psychological capacity for rational decision making are those who are severely mentally ill—paranoiacs, compulsive neurotics, schizophrenics, and psychopaths. Such persons have the capacity for agency, that is, they are aware of acting on their desires, but they fail to meet one or more of the above conditions. For example, a paranoid patient who persists in a delusion that the healthcare professionals are Martians attempting to capture him is unable to adjust beliefs and actions to a reality confirmed by evidence (Benn).

## Principle of Respect for Autonomy

Principles that support autonomy can be directed at the everyday relationships and encounters between persons; at the constitution, laws, and regulations of a nation-state; and at the policies of institutions such as hospitals, insurance companies, schools, and corporations. What ought to be done to respect autonomy will not be the same at all these levels and will be a function of a broad social ideology.

The minimal content for a principle of respect for autonomy is that persons ought to have independence, that is, be free from coercion and other similar interferences. John Stuart Mill made this the main principle in *On Liberty* (1947): No one should interfere with the liberty of action of another except to prevent harm to others. This obligation not to coerce others is defensible as an obligation binding on individuals, private organizations, and governments. Mill defended his principle of liberty, not because he believed that there is a fundamental right to autonomy nor that autonomy is valuable in itself, but because the recognition of

liberty is supported by the principle of utility. This principle is that an action or policy is right to the extent that it promotes the greater happiness for the greater number. However, securing negative liberty does not establish autonomy as fundamental in moral theory. Other philosophers have gone further than Mill in their defense of autonomy.

The most widely quoted principle of respect for autonomy is one of Immanuel Kant's versions of the categorical imperative: "Treat others and oneself, never merely as a means, but always at the same time as an end in himself" (p. 101). This is frequently expressed as treating others as persons, and its distinctive Kantian claim is that others should be treated as rational beings who have their own ends. A further explanation of this principle is that persons should be seen as having interests in two senses. First, interests in those things that are a benefit to nearly everyone, for example, being free of pain, not being killed, being saved from dying. A physician can treat a patient without that person's consent and still protect these interests. Second, autonomous persons "take an interest" in things, that is, have preferences, projects, and plans. Acting only with concern to serve interests in the first sense, as is sometimes alleged against uses of the principle of utility, is not sufficient for respecting another's autonomy; we must also discover and take into account the individual's values and objectives (Benn). For example, a physician may believe that a surgical procedure is an effective treatment to relieve the pain of a patient's ulcer, but the patient may have a greater aversion to the risks of surgery than the physician does, and would prefer a restricted diet and medication. To not solicit, or to ignore, the patient's preferences in this matter would not respect his or her autonomy.

## Autonomy, Rights, and Liberty

The concept of rights presupposes that right-holders are beings who have the capacity for autonomy, who make choices and can use discretion to exercise a right or not. Basic liberties in a liberal democracy are protected by constitutional and other legal rights. The idea of a right has three elements: the right-holder (the person who has the right); the object of the right (the activity or thing that the right-holder has a right to); and the duty-bearer (the person or institution who must do what the right requires). Negative rights are rights not to be interfered with; for example, everyone has the right not to be given medical treatment without consent, and all healthcare providers must respect this right. Positive rights are rights that a person be provided with something—for example, the right of all senior citizens in the United States to Medicare payment for healthcare, a right that is binding on government agencies and healthcare providers.

Recognizing the negative right to autonomy imposes on everyone the obligation not to coerce or otherwise interfere with the action of another. This protection of autonomy is not as costly to social institutions as recognizing positive rights to autonomy. If there is a positive right to $X$, this means that someone is under an obligation to provide $X$ to the right-holder(s). For example, if every citizen has a fundamental positive right to the best-quality medical care, then the state must provide full access to medical care to all citizens. While there cannot be a positive right to autonomy per se—for autonomy as capacity is not something that can simply be given to persons who do not have it—there can be rights to other things that are required for, or supportive of, autonomy. Among them are rights to a decent minimum of healthcare, education, a decent standard of living, political participation, freedom of inquiry and expression, and equal opportunity to compete for positions in society. These goods contribute to autonomy in two ways: First, they make possible the development of the capacity for autonomy; second, they make autonomy meaningful by establishing the personal and social powers and range of options for autonomously chosen projects and plans. Discrimination against minorities and women decreases their autonomy by explicitly excluding them from desirable positions in society and by implicitly agreeing to the limited range of options offered to minorities and women.

## Autonomy as an Ideal

There is no sharp line separating accounts of autonomy as an ideal from autonomy as an actual capacity of persons. Autonomy can be described as a high level of self-determination that few persons will actually achieve, and yet it can still be regarded as a capacity for all persons, if it is believed that all persons under suitable conditions could acquire it and use it to direct their lives. Views that describe autonomy at a level that nearly all normal adult persons can and do exercise are views of autonomy as capacity, and views that describe it at a higher level are accounts of autonomy as an ideal.

Autonomy as an ideal will center on a person's use of the capacity for deliberation and reflection. The person who realizes the ideal of autonomy is, first, one who is consciously aware of having the capacity, someone who believes that he or she can use it to shape his or her life. Second, the autonomous person will make particular decisions with a sense of control—creating and evaluating options. That person will also reflect on how values, preferences, attitudes, and beliefs received in the socialization process function in

his or her own decision making, examine the kind of person this makes him or her, consider alternatives, and make a commitment to accept or try to alter who he or she is. This is of course a matter of degree; like every virtue, it can be realized well and thoroughly or in some small measure. The ideal of autonomy does not require individuals to make conscious, deliberated decisions before every action. A person who has accepted a set of preferences, beliefs, and attitudes can respond without much thinking to common situations that fall into recognized patterns.

## Autonomy of Actions

In a clinical setting, it is often important to determine whether a patient's decision regarding treatment, or the decision of a proxy in the case of an incompetent patient, is autonomous. A person who has the capacity for autonomy may, for a variety of reasons, not act autonomously on a particular occasion. Determining whether a particular action or decision is autonomous is a matter of how the three elements of the capacity for autonomy (agency, independence, and rationality) are involved in the process of deciding. The autonomy of actions is a matter of degree because independence and rationality are matters of degree, though agency is not.

Ruth Faden and her colleagues describe the three elements of autonomy as intentionality, freedom from controlling influence, and understanding. They point out that controlling influences and understanding can be seen on two independent continua. An action can be performed within the range of full understanding to full ignorance, and within the range of completely uncontrolled to completely controlled.

Bruce Miller views the autonomy of actions and decisions on four levels: (1) as free action (agency and independence); (2) as authenticity (the decision is consistent with what is known about the person's values, preferences, and plans); (3) as effective deliberation (rationality); and (4) as moral reflection (deliberation about one's values, preferences, and plans). The decision of a patient may be autonomous at one or more, but not all levels. For example, a patient who accepts a recommended treatment without reflecting much about the decision, acted autonomously at the level of free action, and perhaps authenticity, but not at the levels of rationality and moral reflection.

The legal concept of competence is closely related to the concept of autonomy. A competent person is one who has the capacity for autonomy, and a competent decision is one that is autonomously made.

David Jackson and Stuart Youngner present six cases of decision making in an intensive-care unit that "illustrate specific situations in which superficial preoccupation with the issues of patient autonomy and death with dignity could have led to inappropriate clinical and ethical decisions …" (p. 407). In one of the cases, a patient with multiple sclerosis appeared to autonomously refuse further lifesaving treatment following a suicide attempt. However, psychiatric evaluation showed that the patient had become depressed and withdrawn at the time his wife and sons began spending time with his mother-in-law who had been diagnosed with inoperable cancer.

Jay Katz has said that insufficient attention has been given to the unconscious and irrational motivations of behavior. It is not only patients' motivations that should be examined, but physicians' as well, for example, their denial of uncertainty. Whether a patient's decision to consent to or refuse treatment is autonomous depends on more than the patient's statement of decision and reasons. Physicians and patients must engage in conversations; physicians are obligated to facilitate patients' opportunities for reflection to prevent ill-considered decisions, and patients are obligated to participate in the process of thinking about their choices. The U.S. President's Commission (1982) echoes this view in its discussion of the importance of communication between patient and health professional to attain shared decision making based on mutual trust.

## Privacy, Informed Consent, and Paternalism

Autonomy as a fundamental right is used to justify rights to privacy, confidentiality, refusal of treatment, informed consent, and a decent minimum of healthcare. The legal right to privacy has two components. The right to control information about oneself is protected in medicine as the patient's right to confidentiality of information gained by health professionals. The right not to be interfered with and to make one's own decisions is protected in medicine as a competent patient's right to refuse recommended treatment and as the obligation of health professionals to obtain a patient's informed consent to treatment. Informed consent requires that a patient be informed of a recommended treatment and of the options for treatment and their likely consequences, and that the patient give express permission for a treatment (often in writing). The right to autonomy also requires that patients be told the truth about their medical status and prognosis, that their questions be answered, and that they receive assistance from healthcare providers in making rational decisions. Meaningful exercise of the right to autonomy in living requires that individuals possess physical and psychological capacities within the normal, human range. So the positive right to autonomy supports a right to a level of healthcare that will return and

maintain a person to the normal range of functioning. This includes acute care, for example, repair of a broken bone; chronic care, for example, treatment of diabetes or heart disease; and supportive care for permanent disability, for example, wheelchairs for paraplegics.

Paternalism in healthcare is treating a patient against his or her wishes on the grounds that the healthcare provider is professionally obligated to provide care that will benefit patients, and that the healthcare provider knows better than the patient what is good for the patient. When paternalism is justified, it overrides patient autonomy, at least partially. An example of justified paternalism could be when a physician does not accede to a patient's refusal of emergency treatment because the patient believes he or she will surely die.

## Criticisms of Autonomy

Some authors (Clements and Sider; Callahan; Thomasma) have criticized the centrality of autonomy in medical decision making. Their argument states that the primary obligation of healthcare providers is to maintain and restore health. There are two aspects to this claim. First, if patient autonomy is given primacy over the obligations of health professionals, physicians and other providers may violate their obligation to maintain and restore the health of patients; for example, a patient may refuse a treatment that will save his or her life or prevent a serious illness. These conflicts between autonomy and patient benefit have often been decided by courts, usually in the form of a request by a terminally ill patient's family member, or other agent, that life-preserving treatments such as respirators be withdrawn, a request denied by physicians who cite their obligation to preserve life.

A second aspect of the criticism of autonomy recognizes the centrality of patients' values and wishes in cases of deciding whether to forgo life-preserving treatment for a terminally ill patient, but other sorts of medical-care decisions depend less on respecting patients' rights to autonomy and more on the value of restoring and maintaining the capacity for living a meaningful life. In this sort of case, autonomy is secondary to principles of beneficence, compassion, and caring.

Defenders of autonomy can make several replies to this critique. (1) Some of the attacks on autonomy wrongly assume that it is simply a principle of negative freedom, that is, the right not to be interfered with. (2) The claim of the centrality of patient autonomy in medicine does not imply that it is the only value. The principles of beneficence or nonmaleficence may, in some circumstances, justify paternalism. (3) Autonomy cannot be ignored in medical decision making. Knowing what will be most beneficial for a patient often requires input from the patient on values, objectives, and preferences. This is true not only in morally difficult situations that call for a decision about preserving the life of a terminally ill patient, but in less dramatic cases as well, for example, whether a patient should have surgery for a condition that causes minor discomfort and dysfunction but will not develop into something more threatening to health, or whether the patient should simply "live with" the condition. In cases of acute and severe injury or illness where there is clearly a best treatment that will almost certainly restore the patient to health, it can usually be safely assumed that whatever else the patient values, he or she will value the restoration of health, and hence, discussion of the relative value of options and their consequences is not required to respect the autonomy of the patient.

Criticisms of autonomy have also been launched from a broader, communitarian perspective (MacIntyre; Sandel; Callahan). Communitarians charge that the political theory of liberal individualism states that individuals are fully self-determining and that rights to autonomy are the primary or sole standard for individual behavior, institutional practices, and government policy. Communitarians object to liberal individualism on several grounds. First, the socialization process determines, or shapes, the values and preferences of individuals, hence, the idea of autonomously chosen values is factually incorrect. Second, an individual's actions, desires, and objectives are comprehensible only within the context of social conventions and institutions. For example, a person cannot report that he or she is thinking about depositing a check without the conventions of language and the institution of banking. Third, the view that an autonomous individual chooses his or her own values, preferences, and desires presupposes a self that does the choosing. This self will have to have a core of values with which to choose, in which case either there are values not autonomously chosen, or it is inexplicable how individuals come to have a set of values. Communitarians also claim that liberal individualism regards persons as separate from others in the sense that individuals have no obligations to others or society that are not voluntarily assumed, other than the obligation to respect the individual rights of others. A society that respects only the autonomy rights of all its members is not morally complete. A good society must recognize obligations to help others; its members must have virtues such as compassion, caring, and love, and they should recognize a commitment to society to maintain social practices and institutions that establish and promote these obligations and virtues (Callahan).

There may be theories of autonomy that are susceptible to these criticisms, but the fundamental value of autonomy can be defended without embracing such versions of liberal individualism (Sher; Taylor, 1985). The conceptions of autonomy presented above recognize that persons are social beings whose values and preferences are shaped by society and that the capacity for autonomy is itself socially determined. Being autonomous requires language and reason, and these abilities are not possible without socially given practices and standards. Reflecting on socially given values and preferences and either accepting them as one's own or changing them in some measure, which is a feature of autonomous persons, cannot be done unless there is a social environment that encourages autonomy. A free society makes autonomy possible.

However, a society in which no one does more or less than respect everyone else's liberal rights, in which there is no caring, love, or friendship and no neighborhood associations, political parties, or civic groups, is not one we would want, though it may be a liberal society (Gutmann). On the other hand, a society organized to promote civic virtues and obligations such as beneficence, caring, and compassion, but which does not recognize a right of individuals to be different, to make their own decisions about matters of importance to them or to find a style of life that makes them happy, is also not one we would want. Love and care can be stifling if they do not recognize an individual's own view of what his or her good is. Finally, a defensible theory of the nature and value of individual autonomy will fall between radical individualism and extreme collectivism. It must explain the obligations to create and maintain social and political institutions that support the exercise and flourishing of autonomy. It must explain how the exercise of autonomy depends upon the opportunity range and values given in the traditions and structure of society. It will also recognize other fundamental values and explain their place in decision making.

In the early period of contemporary medical ethics, much attention was on medical paternalism in cases of life-and-death decision making for terminally ill patients and on what can be called "medical opportunism" in research on human subjects. Critics of these practices brought the rights of patients and subjects to the forefront of medical ethics. In a climate of concern for allocation of healthcare resources and other issues of social policy, autonomy appears less frequently in medical ethics literature than do moral concepts such as justice, fairness, equality, economic efficiency, and cost-containment. This shift in issues should not lead to the view that autonomy has lost its importance in moral and social theory and in bioethics.

BRUCE L. MILLER (1995)
BIBLIOGRAPHY REVISED

SEE ALSO: *Beneficence; Coercion; Conscience; Ethics: Social and Political Theories; Freedom and Free Will; Human Dignity; Human Rights; Informed Consent; Justice; Professional-Patient Relationship; Research Policy: Subjects; Sexism*

### BIBLIOGRAPHY

Benn, Stanley I. 1988. *A Theory of Freedom.* Cambridge, Eng.: Cambridge University Press.

Berg, Jessica; Appelbaum, Paul S.; Lidz, Charles W.; and Parker, Lisa S., eds. 2001. *Informed Consent: Legal Theory and Clinical Practice,* 2nd edition. New York: Oxford University Press.

Callahan, Daniel. 1984. "Autonomy: A Moral Good, Not a Moral Obsession." *Hastings Center Report* 14(5): 40–42.

Childress, James F. 1990. "The Place of Autonomy in Bioethics." *Hastings Center Report* 20(1): 12–17.

Clements, Colleen D., and Sider, Roger C. 1983. "Medical Ethics' Assault on Medical Values." *Journal of the American Medical Association* 250(15): 2011–2015.

Davis J. K. 2000. "The Concept of Precedent Autonomy." *Bioethics* 16(2): 114–133.

Donchin, A. 2001. "Understanding Autonomy Relationally: Toward a Reconfiguration of Bioethical Principles." *Journal of Medicine and Philosophy* 26(4): 365–386.

Dworkin, Gerald. 1976. "Autonomy and Behavior Control." *Hastings Center Report* 6(1): 23–28.

Dworkin, Gerald. 1988. *The Theory and Practice of Autonomy.* Cambridge, Eng.: Cambridge University Press.

Ells, C. 2001. "Shifting the Autonomy Debate to Theory as Ideology." *Journal of Medicine and Philosophy* 26(4): 417–430.

Faden, Ruth R.; Beauchamp, Tom L.; and King, Nancy M. P. 1986. *A History and Theory of Informed Consent.* New York: Oxford University Press.

Gaylin W. 1996. "Worshiping Autonomy." *Hastings Center Report* 26(6): 43–45

Gutmann, Amy. 1985. "Communitarian Critics of Liberalism." *Philosophy and Public Affairs* 14(3): 308–322.

Haworth, Lawrence. 1986. *Autonomy: An Essay in Philosophical Psychology and Ethics.* New Haven, CT: Yale University Press.

Kant, Immanuel. 1956. *Groundwork of the Metaphysics of Morals,* tr. and ed. Herbert James Paton. New York: Harper & Row.

Katz, Jay. 1984. *The Silent World of Doctor and Patient.* New York: Free Press.

Jackson, David L., and Youngner, Stuart. 1979. "Patient Autonomy and 'Death with Dignity.'" *New England Journal of Medicine* 301(8): 404–408.

MacIntyre, Alasdair C. 1981. *After Virtue: A Study in Moral Theory.* Notre Dame, IN: University of Notre Dame Press.

Mill, John Stuart. 1947. *On Liberty,* ed. Aubrey Castell. New York: Appleton-Century-Crofts.

Miller, Bruce L. 1981. "Autonomy and the Refusal of Lifesaving Treatment." *Hastings Center Report* 11(4): 22–28.

Pantilat, S. Z. 1996. "Patient-Physician Communication: Respect for Culture, Religion, and Autonomy." *Journal of the American Medical Association* 275(2): 107–110.

Raz, Joseph. 1986. *The Morality of Freedom.* Oxford: Clarendon Press.

Sandel, Michael J. 1982. *Liberalism and the Limits of Justice.* Cambridge, Eng.: Cambridge University Press.

Schneider, Carl E. 1998. *The Practice of Autonomy: Patients, Doctors, and Medical Decisions.* New York: Oxford University Press.

Sher, George. 1989. "Three Grades of Social Involvement." *Philosophy and Public Affairs* 18(2): 133–157.

Taylor, Charles. 1985. "Atomism." In *Philosophical Papers,* vol. 2 of *Philosophy and the Human Sciences.* Cambridge, Eng.: Cambridge University Press.

Taylor, Charles. 1991. *The Ethics of Authenticity.* Cambridge, MA: Harvard University Press.

Thomasma, David C. 1984. "Freedom, Dependency, and the Care of the Very Old." *Journal of the American Geriatrics Society* 32(12): 906–914.

U.S. President's Commission for the Study of Ethical Problems in Medicine and Biomedical and Behavioral Research. 1982. *Making Health Care Decisions: A Report on the Ethical and Legal Implications of Informed Consent in the Patient-Practitioner Relationship.* Washington, D.C.: Author.

Wear, Stephen; Engelhardt, H. Tristam; and Wildes, Kevin W., eds. *Informed Consent: Patient Autonomy and Clinician Beneficence within Health Care,* 2nd edition. (Clinical Medical Ethics Series). Washington, D.C.: Georgetown University Press.

# B

## BEHAVIORISM

• • •

I. History of Behavioral Psychology
II. Philosophical Issues

## I. HISTORY OF BEHAVIORAL PSYCHOLOGY

The earliest human communities undoubtedly appreciated the systematic application of rewards and punishments as an effective means to control behavior. The domestication of animals throughout prehistory, and the numerous early historical references to the proficiency of animal trainers, further establish a form of behavioral psychology as the most venerable of the folk psychologies. Thus, if the term *behavioral psychology* is taken to mean only a set of techniques useful for the prediction and control of behavior, then its history is coeval with human history.

As it is generally understood, however, behavioral psychology is not merely a collection of methods for controlling behavior. It also represents a judgment on the nature of psychology itself—a position informed by identifiable traditions within philosophy and the philosophy of science, as well as by the larger scientific context within which psychology seeks a proper place.

Understood in this light, the subject has its origins in the first great age of modern science, the seventeenth century—the century of Francis Bacon, Johannes Kepler, Galileo, Thomas Hobbes, René Descartes, and Isaac Newton, to mention only some of the more celebrated figures. Setting aside the many and fundamental conceptual and scientific disagreements of this era, a coherent theme exists; namely,

that an unprejudiced and objective inquiry into the operations of the natural world will yield lawful and useful knowledge. The older world of logical analysis, occult powers, hidden forces, revealed truths, and scriptural authority was now to be replaced by the more modest—but more solid—discoveries of direct experience. The knowable cosmos, from this perspective, is just the observable cosmos.

The two divisions of science most fully developed in the seventeenth century were mechanics and optics, and both of these served as models and metaphors for phenomena only poorly understood. The well-ordered Hobbesian state, the clockwork precision of the Newtonian heavens, and Descartes's stimulus-response psychology are all based upon the metaphor of the machine, as well as on the conviction that fuller explanations in these areas will be drawn from the science of mechanics. Descartes's (1596–1650) psychology of animal behavior, which he extended to include those aspects of human psychology not dependent upon language and abstract thought, is entirely mechanistic and behavioristic, even in the more modern senses of these terms. His explanations for all animal, and most human, behavior were grounded in what would now be called instinctual reflex mechanisms and acquired (but still reflexive) habits. The nervous system, in this view, is an elaborate input-output system organized in such a way that specific patterns of stimulation lead to organized and adaptive patterns of behavior. The tendency to focus on Descartes's famous dualistic solution to the mind–body problem, and his emphasis on the cognitive, rational, and linguistic uniqueness of human beings should not obscure the essentially behavioristic content of his overall psychology.

Criticized in Descartes's own time by Thomas Hobbes and Pierre Gassendi, among others, Cartesian psychology was stripped of its introspective features in the eighteenth century, where it survived within progressive circles as a primitive biological psychology. In British philosophy, David Hartley (1705–1757) stands out in the movement to adapt Newtonian and Cartesian mechanistic principles to the needs of an emerging mental science. His *Observations on Man* (1749) provides a richly argued and illustrated defense of a behavioristic psychology grounded in (Humean) associationistic principles operating within the sort of reflex framework advocated by Descartes. In France, Julien de La Mettrie's *L'Homme-machine* (1748) presented an uncompromisingly materialistic psychology, at once antispiritual, reductionistic, and behavioristic. The circle of French philosophes included stridently mechanistic theorists (e.g., Paul-Henri Dietrich, Baron d'Holbach), but also those with a radically environmentalistic orientation (e.g., Claude-Adrien Helvétius), who insisted that social and familial pressures were totally responsible for human psychological development.

As the philosophes and natural philosophers of the eighteenth century were assembling strong rhetorical arguments on behalf of a fully naturalistic psychology, the medical and scientific communities were broadening and deepening its empirical foundations. Robert Whytt's (1714–1766) pioneering studies of spinal reflexes are illustrative. These were accomplished while La Mettrie was offering little more than polemical defenses of psychological materialism. Whytt's research exemplified the steady, modest, and entirely experimental approach of scientists loyal to what they took to be the methods of Newton and Bacon. Early in the nineteenth century, programmatic research of this sort had unearthed the distinct sensory and motor functions of the spinal cord (the Bell-Magendie Law) and had put the mechanistic-behavioristic perspective on firm anatomical foundations. By the 1830s, Marshall Hall (1790–1857), in a tradition of Scottish medical science that includes Whytt and Charles Bell, would put the concept of "reflex function" at the very center of a nascent biological psychology that would influence the ultimate character of modern behaviorism.

It should be noted that it was during this same period (1750–1850) that the so-called animal model became accepted, and, in the early decades of the nineteenth century, a single laboratory might perform vivisection on *thousands* of animals, none of them anesthetized. Cartesianism, in still another sense, was the gray eminence here, fortifying the scientific community in the belief that nonhuman animals were merely a species of machinery. This perspective, shorn of its horrific surgical practices, would survive in the confident antimentalism of twentieth-century behaviorism.

By the middle of the eighteenth century, the medical clinic was also yielding an ever more coherent account of the causal efficacy of the nervous system in human sensory and behavioral functions. By the end of the century, and as a result of his own original and exhaustive studies (including postmortem examinations of exceptional as well as feeble and felonious persons) Franz Joseph Gall (1758–1828) would offer the "science" of phrenology as a developed and systematic psychology—a psychology grounded in the principle that all sensory, motor, affective, and cognitive functions are brought about by conditions in the brain and its numerous subsystems. Once again, the evidence all pointed to a quasi-mechanistic system, both complex and law-governed, functioning in such a manner as to adjust (or fail to adjust) behavior to the demands of the environment.

## The Evolutionary Perspective

By the time Charles Darwin published *On the Origin of Species* (1859), the "Darwinian" perspective was already dominant in scientific and progressive circles. Adam Smith's *The Wealth of Nations* (1776), Jacques Turgot and his party of "physiocrats," and the writings of any number of philosophes point to a (more or less) settled Enlightenment position: The free movement of ideas, goods, and persons—constrained by no more than "natural" forces—produces an ever more refined, successful, and robust stock.

But Darwin's monumental contribution went beyond this general perspective and reached the level of a developed and richly integrative theory. Its implications for psychology were clear: As there is no sharp line dividing places along the broad evolutionary continuum that humanity shares with the balance of the animal economy, there is no reason to confine inquiries into complex psychological functions to the study of human beings.

## Antecedents in Psychology

Darwin's evolutionary theory emphasized differences in degree, not in essence. Thus, the most complex human psychological attributes could, in principle, be examined in a more systematic fashion by studying their simpler, but kindred, manifestations in nonhuman animals. Studies of this sort, it was assumed, would establish psychology's own independent scientific status. As Herbert Spencer (1820–1903) declared:

> The claims of Psychology to rank as a distinct science … are not smaller but greater than those of any other science. If its phenomena are contemplated objectively, merely as nervo-muscular adjustments by which the higher organisms from moment to moment adapt their actions to environing coexistences and sequences, its degree of

specialty, even then, entitles it to a separate place. (*Principles of Psychology,* p. 141)

In the patrimony of Darwin, and influenced chiefly by his *Descent of Man* (1871), specialists in animal psychology appeared before the end of the nineteenth century and made their own contributions toward a behavioral science. For all his anthropomorphic tendencies, George Romanes (1848–1894), in his *Animal Intelligence* (1882) and *Mental Evolution in Animals* (1883), put the study of animal behavior on the map of the new psychology. All that was needed to prepare this Darwinian psychology for adoption by the forthcoming generations of behaviorists was to strip it of just this anthropomorphism. C. Lloyd Morgan, in his *Introduction to Comparative Psychology* (1894), delivered his famous canon:

> In no case may we interpret an action as the outcome of the exercise of a higher psychic faculty, if it can be interpreted as the outcome of the exercise of one which stands lower in the psychological scale. (p. 53)

Thus, with this insistence on explanatory parsimony, did the "ism" in behaviorism begin to take shape.

It is customary, if misleading, to date the birth of experimental psychology with Wilhelm Wundt's founding of the discipline's first university laboratory at Leipzig in 1878–1879. Wundt (1832–1920) was perhaps the discipline's most prolific writer. His texts, which were wideranging and immensely influential at the time psychology departments were being formed in Europe, England, and the United States, emphasized experimental over ethological (naturalistic) modes of inquiry. But the reading of Wundt was rather selective. In his less-consulted multivolume *Völkerpsychologie* (best rendered as "anthropological psychology") he developed and defended the nonexperimental and essentially historical anthropological mission of psychology, drawing attention to the limits of reductionistic strategies and explanations. Even with this broadened perspective, Wundt remained loyal to the scientific views of his age, acquired in his medical education and as he assisted the great Hermann von Helmholtz. In these respects he was representative of an entire generation of thinkers committed to the scientific study of psychology and the abandonment of purely philosophical modes of analysis, wherever the scientific and experimental alternative was practicable.

In the Wundtian tradition, however, the subjects of scientific inquiry were taken to be mental processes and functions—those now generally dubbed *cognitive*. Moreover, although he did much to advance comparative psychology in his textbooks, the bulk of his theoretical writings, and all of the research undertaken in the Leipzig laboratory, focused on *human* psychology and the development of a *science of mental life*. To this extent, Wundtian psychology formed a path distinct from that so heavily trod by the neurophysiologists, anatomists, and clinicians, a path more readily associated with the introspective philosophical psychologists (e.g., John Locke and David Hume). Nor was it clear that Wundtian psychology had a place within the larger naturalistic context of Darwinian science.

Labels offer useful shortcuts, but they can be misleading. It may be said, with ample qualifications, that the Wundtian perspective, at least in the hands of his most influential students (e.g., Edward B. Titchener), was structuralist. Any number of passages and entire chapters in books by Wundt are devoted to the (hypothetical) constituents or components of thought. And, if *structuralism* (according to which the task facing a scientific psychology requires an analysis of the structure of consciousness) and *functionalism* (which focuses instead on the functions served by the behavior of animals or the functions of the nervous system itself) are to be understood in essentially dialectical terms, it is also the case that Wundt's major works are not beholden to the idiom of functionalism. But his attention to the workings of the nervous system, his attempts to provide a loosely evolutionary framework for both human and animal psychology, and his problem-centered cognitive psychology are all anticipations of the functionalist psychology so explicit in the works of William James (1842–1910).

What is relevant here in the tension (real or apparent) between structuralism and functionalism in the history of modern psychology is the claim later made by John B. Watson (1878–1958) that behaviorism was to replace both. In significant respects, it may be said to have replaced both by merging the two rather than by fully rejecting either. Structuralism, which was never a central feature of Wundt's own agenda for the discipline, has this much in common with behaviorism: It is a reductionistic theory or strategy, according to which complex and psychologically significant ensembles can be analyzed into more elementary components. Further, both posit that the only valid evidence is the observable and repeatable evidence gleaned by laboratory investigations. For all their differences, then, behaviorism and structuralism, in their mechanistic and reductive commitments, were faithful to that "religion of science" launched in the seventeenth century.

Functionalism, of course, is the immediate precursor to behaviorism and even a version of it, depending on how the term is to be understood. One account of it is defended by Alexander Bain (1818–1903), the founder of the journal *Mind* and intimate friend of John Stuart Mill. In *The Senses and the Intellect* (1855) and *The Emotions and the Will* (1859), Bain argued that the discipline of psychology was to be advanced by merging its issues and findings with the science of physiology in such a way as to ground psychological processes in the functions of the nervous system. Functionalism, in this sense, is a function-based psychology whose general laws are derived from neurophysiology. From still another (but quite compatible) perspective, such as that defended by William James, the question to ask of any psychological process or phenomenon is what *function* it serves in the larger context of the organism's (person's) overall and long-term interests. The psychological event is explained when the functions it serves are delineated. These, in the most general sense, are *adaptive* functions, rendering the organism more successful in its transactions with the environment. In the writings of William James, this orientation is tied to a *pragmatism* that anticipates the central tenets of modern behaviorism.

## Modern Behavioral Psychology

The Nobel Prize–winning research of Ivan Pavlov (1849–1936) addressed gastric physiology and the chemistry of digestion. But in the process of studying the formation and secretion of digestive enzymes, Pavlov discovered that initially automatic or innate reflex mechanisms could be controlled externally by associating them with specific events in the environment. His theories of *classical conditioning* were grounded in neurophysiology and were intended to replace the mentalistic approach of traditional psychology. In this aim he was joined by the American psychologist John B. Watson, widely regarded as the father of behaviorism.

In his influential essay "Psychology as the Behaviorist Views It" (1913), and in his widely read and cited *Psychology from the Standpoint of a Behaviorist* (1919), Watson waged relentless war on introspective psychology, structuralism, "folk" psychology, and the entire tradition of philosophical speculation regarding the nature of human nature. He insisted that the only proper subject matter of any science is directly observable events, which for psychology means observable *behavior*. In tying his recommendations to a version of the Pavlovian theory, Watson failed to produce the sort of behavioral psychology compatible with the functionalistic and pragmatic bent already dominant in America. But his writing did much to put mentalistic psychologies on notice and promote a seemingly objective, scientific, and descriptive discipline, practical in its aims and stridently antimetaphysical.

This much of the Watsonian legacy was accepted by the most influential figure in the history of behavioral psychology, B. F. Skinner (1904–1991). In numerous books and articles, in scores of laboratory demonstrations, and through a veritable legion of students and coworkers, B. F. Skinner dominated psychology in the United States and, indeed, much of psychology around the world, for a quarter of a century. From 1950 until the 1970s, specialists in a wide variety of psychological employments came to regard themselves as "behavioral scientists," adopting the idiom and perspective of "Skinnerian" psychology and fashioning methods and measurements akin to those of the "Skinner box" and the cumulative recorder.

As early as 1938, in *The Behavior of Organisms,* Skinner had argued for the independence of *behavioral* science from physiology or other (even if somehow related) sciences. The facts of observed behavior, he insisted, remain what they are, no matter what the nervous system is found to be doing, no matter what the genetic composition of the organism proves to be, and no matter what theory is invented or adopted to account for these facts. Taking his lead from the research of Edward L. Thorndike (1874–1949), Skinner devoted himself to the study of *operant,* or *instrumental,* behavior—the behavior that is instrumental in securing positive reinforcers or in avoiding aversive stimulation. Unlike Pavlovian reflexes (or *respondents,* in Skinner's terminology), operant behaviors actually operate on and alter the animal's environment. Behavior that results in positive reinforcement (food, for example) becomes statistically more probable. Nonreinforced behavior—behavior that has no systematic effect on the environment—simply drops out. Thus, behavior within an environment containing reinforcing contingencies is not unlike the evolutionary arena itself. Those behaviors that result in more successful adaptations survive, while those that do not are extinguished.

As developed by Skinner, behavioral psychology is a descriptive, empirical science—more akin to engineering, perhaps, than to physics—and is able to identify the conditions under which behavior is rendered more or less probable. Useless to this enterprise are theories laden with hypothetical processes, hidden variables, or private "states." Perhaps the most concise philosophical defense of the perspective was provided by Gilbert Ryle in *The Concept of Mind* (1949), in which the Cartesian "ghost in the machine" was analytically exorcised, leaving in its wake a collection of psychological attributes uniquely specified by observable behavioral events and dispositions.

Skinner's version of behavioral psychology, though the most influential, is but one of several developed in the twentieth century. The main points of division among various schools or types are three: (1) the level of explanation to be attained by a behavioral psychology; (2) the room within such a psychology for nonobservable (mental) events and processes; (3) the proper place of such a psychology within the larger context of the natural (biological) sciences. On each of these points, major and self-proclaimed behaviorists have taken positions at variance with Skinner's.

Clark Hull (1884–1952), for example, adopted the nomological-deductive model of scientific explanation. According to the dominant version of the model, an event is explained when it is shown to be deducible from a general law, not unlike explanations in classical physics. He attempted to develop a formal theory of behavior based on a number of hypothetical constructs (e.g., "habit-strength") and intervening variables (e.g., fatigue-substances generated by muscular activity). Hullian behavioral psychology is characterized by pages of mathematical equations expressing such relationships as that between learning and practice, between strength of response and magnitude of reward, or between speed of response and hours of food-deprivation.

E. C. Tolman (1886–1959) defended a form of *cognitive-behavioral* psychology that grounded explanations of problem solving on the part of nonhuman animals in such notions as "cognitive maps." Rats, for example, who learn the various turns in a maze and are later placed on top of the maze box will run directly toward the goal rather than retracing the successful learned paths. What the rats have, in Tolman's theory, is a map or representation of the situation, and very different patterns of behavior can be arranged to achieve the same results.

Yet other behavioristic psychologists, notably Karl Lashley (1890–1958), retained their commitment to the study of observable behavior, while insisting that a science of behavior had to be fully integrated into the brain sciences, and had to make contact with the well-established cognitive dimensions of human and animal psychology. In this, the influences and criticisms of such Gestalt psychologists as Wolfgang Köhler (1887–1967) wrought changes on the behavioristic outlook—or otherwise rendered the outlook itself dubious.

## Ethical Implications

From the first, the Darwinian, reductionistic, and positivistic character of behaviorism targeted it for criticism from expected (humanistic) quarters. Yet, unlike the value-neutral orientation of much of modern science, behaviorists have tended to defend their perspective on ethical grounds. Both Watson and Skinner were explicit in this regard. Skinner's *Beyond Freedom and Dignity* (1971), though dismissive of traditional moral theories and their supporting "folk" psychologies, contended nonetheless that a behaviorally engineered society would achieve the most precious of the ends envisaged by ethical theorists. His work inspired the formation of several small communities organized around principles of operant conditioning, with desired behavior brought about without the moral tags of "praise" and "blame." His work also provided the theoretical and technical foundations for various "behavior therapies" applied to disturbances ranging from bed-wetting to catatonic withdrawal. Considered ethically, these methods would seem to be neither more nor less coercive than those arising within other theoretical contexts and employed for the benefit of consenting patients.

In viewing human nature as part of nature at large, and as impelled by the same evolutionary pressures faced by the balance of the animal kingdom, behavioral psychology is neither more nor less humanistic than, say, psychoanalytic theory or, for that matter, the contemporary neurocognitive psychologies that have all but replaced behaviorism. Skinner rejected moral theories grounded in deontological or transcendental arguments, but accepted the proposition that complex societies require the imposition of constraints, and that coercive principles and practices must be justified in ways conducive to a flourishing and productive life within such societies.

It was clear by the end of the twentieth century that the central precepts and methodology of behaviorism would be steadily overtaken and replaced by what is generally referred to as *cognitive neuroscience*. Though the term is new, the perspective is not, for it has been the guiding perspective within physiological psychology at least since early in the nineteenth century. Rejected is the claim that the chief sources of behavioral control are external to the organism. Rather, what is assumed is the evolution of the nervous system as "pre-wired" (though not necessarily "hard-wired"); that is, it is able to perceive the environment selectively, to code or represent it in quasi-computational ways, and to do so by way of distinguishable "modular" processes in the brain.

If cognitive neuroscience has overtaken behaviorism within the theoretical and experimental domains, the complexities of mental and social life have rendered it suspect in the wider realms of thought and action. Life, as depicted by Watson and Skinner and otherwise implicit in the very language of behavioral psychology, matches up poorly with the life actually lived by most human beings and many other species. In ignoring or depreciating the richly social, self-moving, and self-conscious dimensions of life—and thus the irreducibly moral terms that rational beings must invoke to live together in a principled way—the architects and defenders of radical versions of behavioral psychology have more or less resigned from the domain of ethical discourse.

DANIEL N. ROBINSON (1995)
REVISED BY AUTHOR

SEE ALSO: *Autonomy; Behavior Modification Therapies; Coercion; Freedom and Free Will; Informed Consent; Mental Health Therapies; Mental Illness; Neuroethics; Patients' Rights, Mental Patients' Rights; Psychiatry, Abuses of; Psychoanalysis and Dynamic Therapies;* and other *Behaviorism* subentries

### BIBLIOGRAPHY

Hartley, David. 1998 (1749). *Observations on Man.* Washington, D.C.: Woodstock Books.

Morgan, C. Lloyd. 1978 (1893). *Introduction to Comparative Psychology: The Limits of Animal Intelligence.* Significant Contributions to the History of Psychology, Series 2, ed. Daniel N. Robinson. Westport, CT: Greenwood Press.

Robinson, Daniel N. 1986. *An Intellectual History of Psychology.* Madison: University of Wisconsin Press.

Robinson, Daniel N. 1998. *The Mind: An Oxford Reader.* Oxford: Oxford University Press.

Ryle, Gilbert. 1949. *The Concept of Mind.* London: Hutchinson.

Skinner, B. F. 1938. *The Behavior of Organisms: An Experimental Analysis.* New York: Appleton Century.

Skinner, B. F. 1971. *Beyond Freedom and Dignity.* New York: Knopf.

Spencer, Herbert. 1896. *The Principles of Psychology,* 3rd edition. New York: Appleton.

Tolman, Edward C. 1948. "Cognitive Maps in Rats and Man." *Psychological Review* 55(4): 189–208.

Watson, John B. 1919. *Psychology from the Standpoint of a Behaviorist.* Philadelphia: Lippincott.

## II. PHILOSOPHICAL ISSUES

Behaviorism involves two basic views: (1) the proper subject matter of psychology is not consciousness but the behavior of persons and animals, and (2) the proper goal of psychology is the prediction and control of behavior through "stimulus control." There are many forms of behaviorism, and they evoke varied philosophical responses. Behaviorism arose out of frustration with older, introspective approaches to mind and consciousness that appeal to direct awareness of mental states and processes, and out also of the desire to turn psychology into a proper natural or physical science with an empirical methodology and subject matter.

### Methodological and Metaphysical Behaviorism

Methodological behaviorism does not deny the existence of mind and consciousness. Rather, it holds merely that such things are causally ineffective and irrelevant in psychology. To be scientific, psychology must adopt an empirical, scientific methodology applied to the empirical, physical subject matter of observable human behavior.

Metaphysical behaviorism of the sort espoused by John B. Watson (1878–1958) and his followers makes a much stronger claim. It denies the existence of mind and consciousness and proposes that all mentalistic concepts be properly defined (or redefined) in terms of observable behavior. Watson maintained that behavior can be explained entirely in terms of stimulus and response, without the intervention of mental or conscious events and activities. For Watson, all behavior is environmentally derived and cannot be explained by appeals to heredity, instincts, the unconscious, human nature, or internal predispositions.

Some behaviorists recognize two different kinds of observable behavior: external behavior, which is sometimes characterized as overt, external, or molar (pertaining to the whole); and internal behavior, which is alternatively called covert, implicit, deep, or central behavior. If *thinking* is defined as "talking" or "speaking," an account must be given of what transpires when people are thinking silently "to themselves." The wife of a philosopher once complained that she could never tell whether he was working or loafing. Many psychological processes and activities seem, at times, to involve no external behavior. Behaviorists may either deny the reality of private events or affirm that they involve internal behaviors or processes. Thus, thinking becomes "motion in the head," as Thomas Hobbes (1588–1679) put it, or "sub-vocal speech," as Watson suggested.

Behaviorism is usually associated with some form of metaphysical materialism, of which there are many varieties (Foss). When internal behavior is identified with neurophysiological activity, behaviorism becomes *central-state materialism,* or *neuromaterialsim,* according to which the reality of mental states and processes is identical with that of physical states and processes in the brain and central nervous system. This theory identifies mental processes with electrical and chemical processes within the central nervous system ("motion in the head"). Modern brain-scanning devices give indirect sensory access to these neurophysiological motions and processes, though not to the mental processes that are supposedly embodied in them. Brain scans can picture structures and electrochemical changes within the brain, but an enormous and highly controversial conceptual leap, or explanation gap, exists when these are designated as thoughts, feelings, volitions, or emotions.

Taking both consciousness and neuroscience seriously need not involve mind–matter dualism, which affirms that matter but not mind has spatial properties. If, contrary to the

Cartesian tradition, people's thoughts, feelings, and volitions are spatially extended, then they can be located within specific regions of the brain. Whether psychological events are identical with or merely correlated with brain events is at present unknown.

This discussion, however, concentrates on the behaviorism of John B. Watson, B. F. Skinner, and those philosophers of language who focus on observable acts, or on dispositions to behave in observable ways. It raises questions about whether behaviorism is or is not incompatible with presuppositions that are commonplace in ethical theory and bioethics.

## Logical or Linguistic Behaviorism

Many philosophers are attracted to behaviorism's original emphasis on observable external behavior, either for metaphysical or methodological reasons. Some want to escape from Cartesian mind–body dualism—from "the ghost in the machine," as Gilbert Ryle (1900–1976) put it—though this may be done without resorting to behaviorism. Members of the positivistic Vienna Circle, an influential group of scientifically oriented philosophers who flourished in Vienna from the early 1920s to the mid-1930s, wanted to avoid introspective methodology, and so do those influenced by them. They are attracted to the behavioristic methodology of theoretically redefining mentalistic language in terms of external, overt, publicly observable behavior because of its compatibility with the empiricist, or verification criterion, of meaning: that meaning consists exclusively in sensory reference.

Logical, or linguistic, positivism attempts to analyze or redefine the meanings of concepts and beliefs in terms of sensory reference and verifiability. Many recent and contemporary philosophers with a bent toward this form of positivism have tried to formulate in observable behavioral terms the meanings of psychological concepts such as thought, understanding, intelligence, doubt, imagination, and memory, as well as the classes and manifold subclasses of feelings, sensations, pleasures, pains, emotions, desires, and purposes.

Gilbert Ryle, a prominent British linguistic philosopher, was convinced that ordinary language is a behavioristic language, and that ordinary meanings of psychological terms are behavioral meanings. Without denying the existence of inner mental events, he believed that the ordinary meanings of mental concepts can be captured by reference to observable behaviors (or the dispositions to manifest them), without appeal to private or privileged access. Most philosophers and psychologists since Ryle, however, have believed that psychological concepts in ordinary language and "folk psychology" cannot be analyzed purely behaviorally without an

important loss of significance. Many see this as a reason for abandoning familiar psychological terminology for a technically or theoretically constructed psychological vocabulary. Others have found self-awareness to be too evident and significant to be abandoned, believing that a purely behavioral outlook only fosters trivialities and ignores the obvious.

Although Ludwig Wittgenstein (1889–1951), a highly influential linguistic philosopher, did not deny the existence of consciousness and its contents, features of his philosophy of mind can be interpreted to support a behavioristic outlook. He argued convincingly against private languages and purely private experience, contending that human infants originally learn to use psychological concepts by reference to behavioral criteria in a social setting, and that these criteria are themselves integral aspects of the meaning of such concepts. Few philosophers today would deny this intimate connection between mental concepts and behavior. Nevertheless, "How do we learn mentalistic concepts?" and "To what do mentalistic concepts refer?" seem to be very different questions.

Some of Wittgenstein's interpreters subsequently dropped his conviction that psychological concepts point to something internal and mental, adopting only the view that the meanings or referents of psychological concepts consist entirely in behavioral criteria. Thus, the meaning of *pain* consists solely in pain behaviors such as screaming, crying, or moaning, and internal states do not need external criteria, for there are no internal states. Psychological concepts are identical in meaning with their external criteria, just as good Watsonian behaviorists contended.

## Objections to Behaviorism

Behaviorism has been criticized from many philosophical and psychological perspectives, and developments in psychology often have a significant bearing on philosophical issues raised by behaviorism.

PSYCHOLOGICAL AND PHILOSOPHICAL DIFFICULTIES. The technical language that behaviorism aspired to generate was certainly not ordinary everyday language, for it never lost sight of consciousness, its complexity, and its manifold contents, purposes, and values. Since the middle of the twentieth century, more and more philosophers, psychologists, neuroscientists, and psychotherapists have acknowledged the centrality of consciousness for their own activities. Consciousness is now seen as being complex, ranging from minimal awareness devoid of conceptual representation, through symbolic awareness, to self-awareness, while a great deal of nonconscious data-processing occurs (Gazzaniga et al.).

Consciousness and immediate self-awareness are indispensable for people to understand their uniqueness and their personal, ethical, professional, and therapeutic relations with each another. Initially, behaviorists aspired to explain what people do on a simple Pavlovian stimulus–response model; but the terms *stimulus, response,* and *behavior* have been used quite loosely. Muscles, glands, and organs (and who knows what else) react to external (and, they confessed later, to internal) stimuli; and no conscious processing or activities intervene. This view, however, proved to be too simple, too ambiguous, and too devoid of comprehensiveness, to be true—which does not deny that valuable lessons can be learned from the study of behavior.

Gestalt psychologists recognized that empirical stimuli or data are processed internally and holistically, and that no simple stimulus–response theory could explain how humans perceive continuous motion from discontinuous and still motion-picture frames. Noam Chomsky argued effectively that psychological conditioning and associationist learning theory, according to which learning occurs solely through repeated exposures that form connecting links, are too weak to account for the genetically prestructured dispositions of human infants to learn human languages—and for the creative and rule-governed ways in which languages are employed. Abraham Maslow (1971) reported that having a child of his own made behavioristic views of conditioned associationist learning look so foolish that he could not stomach them anymore. To Maslow, the presence of conscious, creative processing of information in his own children was too obvious to be denied. Cognitive psychologists emphasized the indispensability of conscious cognitive or conceptual maps in understanding how people understand, anticipate the future, plan ahead, and act accordingly. According to evolutionary psychology, the evolutionary process has prepared and predisposed people to act, feel, think, and choose in certain ways; and conscious comprehension, insight, information processing, and problem solving have immense significance for purposive and voluntary activity, adaptation, and survival.

The teleological (consciously purposive) and the intentional (consciously focused on an object) features of much psychological discourse cannot be accounted for by a purely descriptive language that completely eliminates teleology, intentionality, and all "final causes." Purposive acts, like trying to persuade psychologists that behavior is the only proper subject matter of psychology, cannot be redescribed as nonpurposive behaviors without losing essential meaning. Denying the existence of consciousness, purpose, or intentionality is refuted by that very act, which is a conscious, purposive, and intentional event.

Behaviorists are asked why they adopt and espouse behaviorism, why they want psychology to be strictly sensory and empirical, and why they want to control the behavior of others. They repudiate conscious rationality, and with it the possibility of justifying any beliefs on rational or scientific grounds. To behavioralists, all that people are and do is a product of stimulus control, which means that behaviorists are behaviorists only because they have been conditioned to be, not because the preponderance of evidence supports the theory.

Stipulating that psychological processes and events are identical with behavioral processes and events is self-contradictory, some critics argue, for two different things cannot be metaphysically identical. Responding that the psychological and the behavioral are only one thing, not two, begs the question. Critics also suspect that the identity of the mental and the behavioral (or the mental and the neurophysiological in central-state materialism) is established by decree, not by observation or scientific method. Watsonian behaviorists solve the problem of other minds by stating that no problem exists because there are no minds at all, while for Skinner's behaviorism, minds do not matter.

First-person self-knowledge based on direct introspective experience has been a great obstacle to the acceptance of behaviorism. To be sure, introspection is not always reliable and is often confused; but direct self-awareness is often quite clear and trustworthy. Individuals are not always mistaken about what they think, how they feel, or what they select. Critics of behaviorism contend that individuals know many things about themselves before, not after, they receive overt expression. For example, authors solve many conceptual problems before they express their ideas in writing. There can be thought without speech (silent thought) and speech without thought (e.g., a parrot's speech). Most people can tell whether they are feeling well or ill before looking into the mirror in the morning or bouncing their countenances off the countenances of others. Further, one can deceive others about one's mental states and processes by playing public roles that do not match one's private self-awareness. A person might be in great pain and yet sit passively and unresponsively in a dentist's chair. Short- and long-range plans are made without a purpose being overtly expressed, and a person can change his or her mind about many things with no one ever knowing.

Nonbehaviorists are convinced that people frequently know many things about their psychological states and processes that are not identical with, and find no expression in, overt behavior. Further, attempts to establish the identity or correlation of mentalistic concepts with behaviors must rely initially upon the self-reports of individual experimental subjects, as well as upon ordinary language with its imbedded folk psychology. When the brain regions and events are examined through brain scanners, they are not labeled as "thinking," "remembering," "hearing," or "seeing a rainbow." Once the initial connections are made, an immense amount of information can be derived about the intimate associations of consciousness functions with brain regions and electrochemical activities through neuroimaging, electroencephalograms, brain stimulation, and studies of genetics, or brain disorders and injuries, as well as by experimenting on individual subjects, both animal and human (Gazzaniga et al.).

## Behaviorism, Ethical Theory, and Bioethics

Other objections to behaviorism arise from its incompatibility with concepts and beliefs that are presupposed in most ethical theories, people's common moral life, and the practice of bioethics. This suggests a choice: either to give up behaviorism or abandon much that ethics takes with utmost seriousness, such as consciousness, pleasure and pain, agency or autonomy, freedom, and human dignity, just as Skinner advocated.

CONSCIOUSNESS. Ethics asks questions about right and wrong, and about good and evil. The notions of intrinsic goodness (that which is desirable or valuable in itself or for its own sake) and intrinsic evil (that which is undesirable and to be avoided for its own sake) are of central importance to ethical theory. In teleological theories of right and wrong, right acts result in intrinsic goodness, while wrong acts fail to do so or produce intrinsic evil. Doing good and avoiding or preventing evil are momentous moral duties even in deontological theories (except for Immanuel Kant's). Doing one's duty usually, if not always, involves understanding and acting in accord with moral ideals and rules—none of which even exist, according to metaphysical behaviorism. Ethicists may disagree about answers to questions like "What acts are right or wrong?" or "What things are good or evil?" There is, however, agreement that no moral obligations and no intrinsic good or evil would exist in a world without consciousness. Moral right and wrong and intrinsic good and evil exist only in and for conscious active beings.

Almost all the philosophers who have considered the question agree that ethics would have no point in a world devoid of conscious beings. Yet Watsonian metaphysical behaviorism gives us just such a world—one in which all behavior is caused by external or environmental stimuli and no behavior is caused by inner conscious mental states and processes. Skinner's radical behaviorism may allow that some activities are spontaneous rather than environmentally caused, but these behaviors are repeated only if their consequences are positively reinforcing. (He doesn't use the terms *pleasurable* or *enjoyable*.) When Skinner admits the existence of inner mental states and processes, he denies their causal efficacy in explaining behavior and providing reasons for action, as well as their relevance to the science of psychology. They are always the effects of stimuli, never the causes of behavior; they exist only epiphenomenally, that is, as ineffective appearances. Scientific psychology can disregard them, for scientifically knowing, controlling, and predicting behavior do not require them.

Some behaviorists retain the notion of consciousness and redefine it in purely behavioral terms—as overt wakeful behavior, for example, as opposed to sleep behavior. Most ethicists, however, are convinced that ethics is concerned with wakefulness itself, as directly experienced by conscious subjects, not merely with wakeful behavior and muscle jerks as experienced by external observers.

Medical professionals are concerned primarily with wakeful consciousness itself, not solely with its public or overt expressions. They often prescribe analgesics or other pain management strategies for suffering patients. During invasive medical procedures, general anesthesia is administered, not to circumvent external pain behaviors, but to prevent conscious pain. After a lapse of consciousness, a patient's return to awareness is eagerly awaited. Lost consciousness is the tragedy of comatose patients, while death involves the irreversible loss of embodied consciousness and its necessary physiological conditions. The seriousness of these medical interests seems to be quite incompatible with a concern only for overt behavior.

PLEASURES AND PAINS. Philosophical ethicists are keenly interested in consciously experienced pleasures and pains, and medical professionals give considerable attention to conscious pains, if not also to pleasures. Most ethicists believe that pointless pains (those that are not necessary for the achievement of goals knowingly and freely accepted) are to be avoided if possible; and most recognize that happiness, conceived of as a surplus of conscious pleasures over pains for extended periods of time, is one of the great goods of life (if not the only good, as hedonists maintain). Medical professionals accept the duties of relieving pain and not inflicting unnecessary conscious pain as serious professional obligations. Patients want relief from real pains, not merely the suppression or elimination of pain behaviors. *Pleasures* usually means "conscious inner qualities of feeling that persons or other sentient beings normally wish to cultivate and sustain for their own sake," and *pains* means "conscious inner qualities of feeling that persons or other sentient beings normally wish to avoid and eliminate for their own sake" (Edwards, pp. 74, 92–96).

Although pain behaviors are indispensable for describing or communicating inner sufferings to others, most ethicists and bioethicists do not believe that overt pain behaviors, completely divorced from conscious suffering, are intrinsically bad, or that they are duty bound to relieve and not induce pain behaviors as such. Reflex responses to pain stimuli may be evoked from irreversibly comatose patients with only brain-stem, but no upper-brain, functioning, yet no one believes that these patients are thereby subjected to intrinsic evil, or that moral duties are being violated or shirked. No one, not even behaviorists, really believes that happiness consists merely of overt expressions of pleasure. Neither pain behavior nor pleasure behavior is of significance to ethics unless they indicate inner conscious pains or pleasures themselves.

Skinner maintains that only positive and negative reinforcers, not conscious pleasures and pains, are relevant to a correct theory of good and evil. Good things are nothing but external positive reinforcers, and bad things are nothing more than external negative reinforcers. Secondarily, those stimuli, responses, or consequences that promote cultural survival may be good things, and those that threaten cultural survival may be evil things. The words *good* and *bad* may also be used to reinforce other behaviors, positively or negatively. Positive reinforcers are stimuli that strengthen the behaviors that produce them, and negative reinforcers are stimuli that reduce or terminate the behaviors that produce them. Just why some stimuli reinforce positively and others negatively is obscure for behaviorists. They cannot maintain that consciously experienced pleasures or pains are the mechanisms that induce or inhibit behaviors. According to Skinner, identifying values with reinforcers results in a purely descriptive, empirical, and scientific ethics that overcomes the "is-ought" gap that plagued traditional ethical theory.

A few philosophers accept Skinner's behaviorist ethics (Hocutt), but most are unconvinced. Most hold that G. E. Moore's "open question" ("Granted that $x$ possesses some descriptive property, but is $x$ good?") is not a senseless or self-answering question, not even when the $x$ is a positive reinforcer. Skinner's position might avoid this objection, however, if construed as an answer to Moore's second question of ethics, "What things are good?" rather than to his first question, "What is the meaning of 'good'?"

Skinner's theory contains no purely empirical or descriptive method for resolving value conflicts. Suffering patients may beg stoic physicians for pain medication, who might refuse to give it because they believe that patients should be allowed, or even required, to suffer for their own good in order to strengthen their characters and powers of resolution. This value conflict is not eliminated by the behaviorist's explanation that these patients find pain-relieving behavior to be positively reinforcing, while the stoic physicians find it to be negatively reinforcing. Whether any other theory of the good can resolve value conflicts is another matter, but other theories generally do not claim to offer purely descriptive solutions to internal normative value problems. A behaviorist's recommendation to give pain medication because doing so has adaptation and survival value would be a prescriptive, not a descriptive, resolution.

Skinner often prescribes norms. He cannot resolve value disagreements about "good" and "ought" merely by describing what is positively reinforcing to individuals or to their communities of value, which are groups of individuals who find similar things to be reinforcing. The behaviorist's contention that psychology should be a strictly descriptive behavioral science does not describe the beliefs and practices of most professional psychologists and psychotherapists. It is a value prescription that, if analyzed in Skinner's own terms, means merely that he and the few psychologists who agree with him find it positively reinforcing to practice psychology behavioristically. Most psychologists and philosophers have not been so conditioned, and they cannot accept the narrow strictures that behaviorism places on psychological inquiry and practice. Skinner's program, which purports to eliminate purposes and prescriptive norms, can be advanced only purposively and as a prescriptive norm.

AGENCY, FREEDOM, AND DIGNITY. Most philosophical ethicists are rationally persuaded that moral obligation and responsibility presuppose internal, autonomous, rational agency, self-control, and choice, and that the denial of the existence or efficacy of informed conscious choice in bringing about moral action is fundamentally incompatible with morality. Ethicists may disagree about whether autonomous moral choice is compatible with rigid metaphysical determinism. Some maintain that autonomous moral choice must be creative and spontaneous, while others hold that conscious choice is sufficient for moral autonomy, even if it is strictly caused by a desire to do right (or wrong). However, ethicists seldom doubt that consciousness, agency, and self-control are essential for of morality.

Informed voluntary consent is a cardinal ethical principle in modern bioethics. This principle affirms that no diagnostic, therapeutic, or experimental medical procedures should be performed on patients unless they have consciously, knowingly, and voluntarily consented to them. The principle affirms that the rational agency or autonomy of patients—the capacity of conscious patients to make informed choices for themselves—is of paramount importance in the medical setting. When behaviorism affirms that all behaviors result from external or environmental stimuli, it denies the reality, or at least the efficacy, of inner mental processes and activities, including inner understanding and decisions.

Behaviorism affirms that people are controlled entirely by their environment, which includes other clever people trained to know how to condition them. People never control themselves or their circumstances through their conscious knowledge or efforts. Although stimulus controls can be self-administered, the "prediction and control of behavior" at which behaviorism aims is primarily meant for other people. But who controls the controllers? Where do they get, and how do they justify, the norms they impose on others by psychological manipulation?

Skinner sometimes writes as if inner conscious ideas, ideals, purposes, feelings, and choices simply do not exist (Blanshard and Skinner). At other times he makes an epiphenomenal (causally ineffective) place for inner activities like self-control, choice, agency, or autonomy. He recognizes that freedom of action is important because it allows individuals to avoid aversive or negatively reinforcing stimuli, but he can make no place for conscious moral agency.

In Skinner's view, human dignity consists of behaviors that cultivate the positive reinforcement of praise or credit from others for behaving well, or as others want them to behave. By contrast, most ethicists agree that human dignity involves conscious self-awareness, self-control, and rational persuasion. They abhor manipulative techniques that bypass these qualities, and they approve of educative and persuasive techniques that develop and appeal to them.

Escaping aversive stimuli and cultivating social credit have their proper place, but most moral philosophers would balk at Skinner's behavioral reduction of freedom and dignity to solicitous activity. Behavioral freedom means little without inner personal autonomy, and human dignity, however difficult to define, is something that persons constantly have as conscious persons; and it makes all people equals. Dignity is not just something that people possess during those rare moments when others credit them for behaving as they see fit.

Thus, behaviorism is incompatible with the ideal of informed voluntary consent as it functions in applied bioethics, as well as with many fundamental principles of ethics. In sum, it seems that one must give up either behaviorism or ethics and bioethics.

REM B. EDWARDS (1995)
REVISED BY AUTHOR

SEE ALSO: *Autonomy; Behavior Modification Therapies; Coercion; Freedom and Free Will; Human Nature; Informed Consent; Mental Health Therapies; Mental Illness; Neuroethics; Patients' Rights: Mental Patients' Rights; Psychiatry, Abuses of; Psychoanalysis and Dynamic Therapies;* and other *Behaviorism* subentries

## BIBLIOGRAPHY

Blanshard, Brand. 1955. *The Nature of Thought,* vol. 1. New York: Macmillan.

Blanshard, Brand, and Skinner, Burrhus Frederic. 1967. "The Problem of Consciousness—A Debate." *Philosophy and Phenomenological Research* 27: 317–337.

Chomsky, Noam. 1964. "A Review of B. F. Skinner's Verbal Behavior." In *The Structure of Language: Readings in the Philosophy of Language,* ed. Jerry A. Fodor and Jerrold J. Katz. Englewood Cliffs, NJ: Prentice Hall.

Dennett, Daniel Clement. 1978. *Brainstorms: Philosophical Essays on Mind and Psychology.* Montgomery, VT: Bradford Books.

Edwards, Rem Blanchard. 1979. *Pleasures and Pains: A Theory of Qualitative Hedonism.* Ithaca, NY: Cornell University Press.

Foss, Jeffrey E. 1995. "Materialism, Reduction, Replacement, and the Place of Consciousness in Science." *Journal of Philosophy* 92(8): 401–429.

Gazzaniga, Michael S., et al., eds. 2000. *The New Cognitive Neurosciences,* 2nd edition. Cambridge, MA: The MIT Press.

Hocutt, Max. 1977. "Skinner on the Word 'Good': A Naturalistic Semantics for Ethics." *Ethics* 87(4): 319–338.

Huxley, Aldous. 1960. *Brave New World.* New York: Harper & Row.

Kim, Jaegwon. 1996. *Philosophy of Mind.* Boulder, CO: Westview Press.

Malcolm, Norman. 1964. "Behaviorism as a Philosophy of Psychology." In *Behaviorism and Phenomenology: Contrasting Bases for Modern Psychology,* ed. Trenton W. Wann. Chicago: University of Chicago Press.

Maslow, Abraham. 1971. *The Farther Reaches of Human Nature.* New York: Viking Press.

Mattaini, Mark A., and Thyer, Bruce A., eds. 1996. *Finding Solutions to Social Problems: Behavioral Strategies for Change.* Washington, D.C.: American Psychological Association.

Modgil, Sohan, and Modgil, Celia, eds. 1987. *B. F. Skinner: Consensus and Controversy.* New York: Falmer Press.

Newman, Bobby. 1992. *The Reluctant Alliance: Behaviorism and Humanism.* Buffalo, NY: Prometheus Books.

O'Donohue, William, and Kitchener, Richard F., eds. 1996. *The Philosophy of Psychology.* London: Sage.

Ryle, Gilbert. 1949. *The Concept of Mind.* New York: Barnes and Noble.

Scriven, Michael. 1956. "A Study of Radical Behaviorism." In *The Foundations of Science and the Concepts of Psychology and Psychoanalysis,* ed. Herbert Feigl and Michael Scriven. Minneapolis: University of Minnesota Press.

Skinner, B. F. 1948. *Walden Two.* New York: Macmillan.

Skinner, B. F. 1953. *Science and Human Behavior.* New York: Free Press.

Skinner, B. F. 1971. *Beyond Freedom and Dignity.* New York: Knopf.

Skinner, B. F. 1974. *About Behaviorism.* New York: Knopf.

Smith, Laurence D., and Woodward, William R., eds. 1996. *B. F. Skinner and Behaviorism in American Culture.* Bethlehem, PA: Lehigh University Press.

Staddon, John. 2001. *The New Behaviorism: Mind, Mechanism, and Society.* Philadelphia, PA: Psychology Press.

Stevenson, Leslie. 2000. *The Study of Human Nature: A Reader,* 2nd edition. New York: Oxford University Press.

Strawson, Galen. 1994. *Mental Reality.* Cambridge, MA: MIT Press.

Taylor, Charles. 1964. *The Explanation of Behaviour.* London: Routledge.

Thyer, Bruce A., ed. 1999. *The Philosophical Legacy of Behaviorism.* Dordrecht: Kluwer.

Watson, John B. 1913. "Psychology as the Behaviorist Views It." *Psychological Review* 20: 158–177.

Watson, John B. 1914. *Behavior: An Introduction to Comparative Psychology.* New York: Henry Holt.

Watson, John B. 1930. *Behaviorism,* 2nd edition. New York: Norton.

Wittgenstein, Ludwig. 1953. *Philosophical Investigations.* New York: Macmillan.

Wozniak, Robert H., ed. 1993. *Theoretical Roots of Early Behaviourism: Functionalism, the Critique of Introspection, and the Nature and Evolution of Consciousness.* London: Routledge.

# BEHAVIOR MODIFICATION THERAPIES

• • •

Since the 1960s and 1970s, numerous developments have occurred in both the theory and the practice of behavior therapy. There has been a significant shift away from a reliance on models of classical and operant conditioning (derived largely from animal studies) as the theoretical basis for behavior therapy, and toward a more cognitive approach in both theory and practice. These two developments have "humanized" behavior therapy to a great extent. In addition, radical or metaphysical behaviorism has reemerged in a gradual, limited way as a basis for new therapeutic technologies and conceptual formulations. These changes imply a growing recognition by behavior therapists that human behavior is the result of a complex interaction of environmental, social, cognitive, genetic, physiological, and emotional factors (Fishman and Franks).

## Criticisms of Early Behavior Therapy

Prior to 1970, behavior therapy was strongly criticized by proponents of other therapeutic schools (typically humanistic or psychodynamic) as being mechanistic and authoritarian. It was alleged, for example, that terms such as *behavior control* carried with them the implicit, and sometimes explicit, message that irrevocable and often involuntary behavioral changes could be induced by the selective application of conditioning techniques. The protestations of behavior therapists notwithstanding, psychosurgery, electroconvulsive therapy, and the enforced ingestion of psychotropic medications were lumped together with mainstream behavior therapy as further examples of this authoritarian approach to behavior change.

The behavior therapy of this era was also accused of attempting to impose therapy goals on unwilling or unaware clients, and of utilizing punishment and other aversion procedures to bring this about. Behavior therapists, it was believed, had the power to impose their wills upon a hapless society through a sinister manipulation of environmental responses to behavior in the form of carefully chosen rewards and punishments.

Finally, early behavior therapy was viewed by its most extreme critics as a nefarious attempt to maintain an unjust status quo, as an imposition of majority demands upon a socially deviant minority (e.g., prisoners, the developmentally disabled, chronic psychiatric patients) helpless to resist the behavioral juggernaut. Behavior therapists were viewed as willing agents of a ruling class unable to tolerate any deviation from the prevailing ethos.

While a small proportion of early behavior-therapy practice did reflect these values to some extent, most behavior therapists eschewed such methods of coercive behavior change, preferring a much more egalitarian approach to therapeutic goal setting and behavior change. Then, as now, most behavior-therapy techniques lacked the potency to bring about involuntary behavior change. Most behavior therapists, then as now, considered it unethical to "enforce" behavior changes against a client's wishes, even when such changes appeared, from the therapist's perspective, to carry with them potential client benefits. Regardless of theoretical basis, the "humanization" of behavior therapy referred to above has resulted in an increasing emphasis on teaching clients "self-control."

## Cognitive Approaches in Behavior Therapy

In the early 1970s, behavior therapists began to explore the possibility of integrating cognition and self-guided behavior change (see Bandura, 1977; Beck; Lazarus; Mahoney). With the exception of those who espouse a radical perspective, most cognitive behavior therapists implicitly assume that human behavior is guided in part by an internal "self" that consists of cognitive structures called *schemas*. Schemas comprise learned patterns of information processing that guide both immediate behavior and general perceptions of the world. These perceptions, in turn, have a significant impact on affective states. Cognitively oriented behavior therapists believe that to change behavior one must change the schemas through which the environmental information is processed. By helping the client to alter maladaptive schemas, the therapist enables the client to engage in broader, more effective information processing, thereby producing changes in attributions that ultimately lead to changes in both behavior and affect.

Most cognitive approaches to behavior therapy still reflect a primarily linear, mechanistic view of behavior. For example, the rational emotive therapy (RET) of Albert Ellis (1962), one of the earliest attempts at integration of cognitive and behavioral approaches, affirms that emotional states occur as the result of an information-processing sequence in which an external event triggers a set of beliefs (a schema), which in turn triggers an emotional response. Thus, a rational emotive therapist would view the emotion of anger as being triggered by the patient's thoughts about the event to which the patient responded with anger, rather than by the event itself. In the view of RET, to paraphrase Shakespeare, nothing is good or bad but thinking makes it so.

Effective treatment enables the client to alter irrational beliefs that lead to negative emotional states or other maladaptive behaviors. This is accomplished by directly challenging irrational beliefs in a Socratic fashion and by devising behavioral exercises to assist the client in learning that irrational beliefs are, in fact, incorrect. For example, in order to combat irrational feelings of shame and self-consciousness, which are presumably based on an irrational fear of sanction or ridicule for particular types of behavior, a rational emotive therapist might assign a client to perform the behavioral exercise of boarding a commuter train and loudly announcing each stop to the other passengers. The objective is to demonstrate that such behavior, absurd and inappropriate though it may seem to the client, does not necessarily evoke public sanction or ridicule, and that, even if it does, such responses from others are not catastrophic.

In one form or another, this combination of restructured irrational beliefs and behavioral exercises is the hallmark of most cognitive approaches to behavior therapy. Albert Bandura's social learning theory (1977), for example, aims at altering specific cognitive structures called "self-efficacy expectations" through teaching clients new behavioral skills and helping these clients practice them both in the therapist's office and in the daily world. Self-efficacy is assumed to determine, in part, whether or not a given set of environmental contingencies will be responded to with a particular behavior by the client. Therapy consists, in part, of designing graded behavioral exercises leading to both new behavior and a revision of self-efficacy expectations. Accomplishing these goals is presumed to facilitate a change in client behavior in previously problematic situations.

Research has consistently demonstrated that, in spite of the heavy emphasis by many theorists on the "cognitive" component of cognitive-behavior therapy, the most effective means of promoting both cognitive and behavioral changes is through performance-based treatments; that is, by actively engaging in new behaviors that are incompatible with older, problematic ones (see Rachman and Wilson). Engaging in new behavior, under the guidance of a therapist, seems to be an effective approach to the treatment of a variety of emotional and behavioral disorders. For example, a client who suffers from a fear of cats might be encouraged, with the therapist's assistance, to engage in closer and closer contacts with cats, moving from merely approaching a cat to actually holding one, until the fear subsides.

## Radical Behaviorist Approaches to Behavior Therapy

In contrast to cognitively oriented behavior therapists, radical behaviorists reject outright the concept of "self." They view cognition as simply a form of behavior that occurs in correlation to a person's responses to environmental contingencies, but not as a cause of those responses. All behavior is presumed to be "caused" by a relationship between external events (contingencies) and behavior. According to radical behavior therapists (e.g., Hayes, 1987, 1989; Kohlenberg and Tsai), people learn sets of "rules" that guide their behavior through the experience of being rewarded or punished for particular behaviors in specific situations. Rules, considered to be verbal representations of environmental contingencies (the relationship between behavior and reward or punishment), are largely determined by an individual's cultural and linguistic milieu and prior learning history. According to radical behaviorists, rules and the linguistic milieu constitute a context that forms the causal matrix within which behavior is produced. Emotional disorders result from rigid adherence to "rules" of behavior that do not apply in a particular context, or to misattributing the causes of one's behavior to emotions rather than environmental contingencies. Thus, rules themselves are potential causes of emotional or behavioral problems.

A similar situation can arise from responding to inappropriately formed environmental contingencies, usually those derived from the structure of the individual's language. These inappropriately formed contingencies reinforce aspects of a person's subjective experience (e.g., the association of emotions with events) in a way that leads the person concerned to misattribute behavior to emotions rather than to the external contingencies that, in the radical behaviorist view, actually cause behavior.

Radical behaviorist approaches to treatment place strong emphasis on the role of an individual's linguistic community and language structure in guiding behavior. Cognition per se is irrelevant, except to the degree that thought is a part of the client's use of language. Behavior change is brought about by teaching new linguistic structures that lead to less affective upset. This is accomplished by attempting to alter the way in which clients use language to form attributions about the causes and meanings of their emotional experience. Most often, this involves teaching clients that emotions are not experiences that can or should be avoided. Rather, they are to be viewed as natural accompaniments to the process of living. Clients are taught to accept and utilize in a positive fashion affective and other inner experiences that their linguistic community has taught them should be avoided or eliminated (e.g., anxiety). Clients are also shown how to alter the contexts (contingencies) that control their behavior. Curiously, radical behaviorist approaches to behavior therapy are in some ways philosophically more similar to psychoanalysis than they are to traditional behavior or cognitive-behavior therapy, in that clients are taught that negative emotions are a natural part of life and cannot be eliminated. Eschewing mechanistic, linear views, radical behavior therapists prefer to view behavior as the product of an interaction between person and context.

Although formally rejecting any direct consideration of cognition, radical behaviorist and cognitive approaches to behavior therapy are consistent in other ways. For example, radical behavior therapists view the person as an active influencer of an environment that, in turn, influences the person. This is similar to Bandura's notion of reciprocal determinism (1982), a key concept in social learning theory. In addition, both radical and cognitive-behavior therapists adopt as a treatment goal the empowerment of the client to control aspects of behavior or experience that are presumed to be at the root of his or her problems. While the pathways to change are different, direct attempts to alter thoughts and behavior by cognitively oriented behavior therapists and the alteration of environmental or personal contingencies by radical behavior therapists are predicated upon the same goal: enabling people to exert more control over the causes of the problems that brought them to treatment in the first place.

## Therapist-Client Relationships in Behavior Therapy

From the beginning, most behavior therapists have been intensely concerned with the ethical aspects of the application of behavior therapy, the ethical implications of the relationship between therapist and client, and the role of each in treatment. In contrast to other psychotherapeutic approaches, behavior therapy is characterized by a heavy emphasis on the responsibility of the therapist for successful treatment outcome. In behavior therapy, failure to achieve treatment goals is presumed to be the result of therapist errors or environmental hazards beyond the therapist's control, rather than of client resistance. The therapist is viewed as an "expert" guide who brings to the situation a body of teachable knowledge. In collegial fashion, as a mutual collaborative process, the patient is shown how to use this knowledge to bring about desired change. In this view, therapeutic failures result from several sources of therapist error, particularly: (1) errors in selection of therapeutic goals due to inadequate assessment; (2) errors in the selection, teaching, or application of techniques; (3) failure to consider client values in the selection of therapeutic goals, or the placing of societal or therapist values above those of the client in the process of goal selection; and (4) variables beyond the therapist's control.

While early behavior therapists tended to neglect the importance of a workable therapeutic relationship with the client, as the field has evolved such issues have become increasingly important in behavior therapy (see Wilson and Evans). Most behavior therapists recognize that without a therapeutic relationship characterized by mutual respect, empathy, trust, and equality, the first three types of therapist error noted above cannot be avoided, and treatment is unlikely to be successful. An increasing emphasis on thought and feeling leads to recognition that an adequate therapeutic relationship is essential to assessment and treatment. Changes in thoughts and emotions can, in and of themselves, be appropriate outcomes of treatment, as can changes in overt behavior. These changes can be facilitated by the establishment of a good therapeutic relationship.

## Ongoing Ethical Concerns in the Practice of Behavior Therapy

Ethical practice has been a priority among behavior therapists. Nonetheless, concerns continue to arise. Particularly in cases where, at least potentially, the application of a technique can inflict pain, or where clients are relatively powerless or are involuntarily the subject of treatment, areas of ethical concern still remain.

USE OF AVERSION PROCEDURES. The use of aversion procedures (the application of subjectively unpleasant stimulation contingent upon performance of an undesirable behavior) has been, and remains, a source of criticism of behavior therapists. Particularly when procedures such as low-level electric shocks are applied to clients who lack the ability to offer informed consent to the use of such procedures, behavior therapists face a dilemma in which the desirability of treatment outcome goals has to be weighed against the rights of the client. Even when aversion therapy seems to be the best, most rapid means of suppressing other, perhaps more injurious, behavior, such as self-destructive behaviors in clients suffering from pervasive developmental disorders, behavior therapists are ethically bound to attempt to reduce the target behavior through nonaversive means before considering an aversion procedure. Only when the target behavior has been conclusively shown to be impervious to other means should aversion therapy be used.

The use of aversion techniques with clients for whom rapid, permanent behavior change is not essential, or for whom there may be some question as to the desire or willingness to change, raises significant ethical concerns. The application of aversion procedures to clients in powerless positions, or where the goals of the agent of behavior change seem directly counter to those of the client, requires careful assessment of the interests of all involved parties, with extra weight perhaps being given to the client's right to be free from external influence over his or her behavior. Practices such as those reported to have occurred in the former Soviet Union, including the use of aversion procedures or drugs for the subjugation of prisoners and psychiatric patients, are clearly not in keeping with the ethical application of behavior therapy or any other form of therapy. When aversion procedures are used, clear guidelines need to be established. Review by an institutional ethics board in order to set up extensive safeguards of client rights has to precede treatment.

TOKEN ECONOMIES IN INSTITUTIONAL SETTINGS. Token economies are based on the notion that behavior can be changed by systematically rewarding desired behaviors contingent upon performance. Token economies set up a microeconomy in which desired behaviors are "rewarded" by contingent distribution of tokens, or "points," that can later be exchanged for rewards (often food or privileges). Early proponents of token economies in institutional settings frequently sought to enhance the effects of this process by withholding basic needs, which could be regained only by compliance with token-reinforced behavioral contingencies imposed by therapist fiat. This practice is now judged to be both legally and ethically unacceptable. Clients forced to reside in facilities where token economies are in effect are entitled to have basic needs for food, shelter, clothing, and social companionship met, regardless of ability to earn token reinforcers. As with the application of aversion procedures, the legitimate parameters of reinforcers need to be clearly spelled out, and the application of contingencies monitored, through continuing and independent peer review. It is the obligation of the therapist to develop effective reinforcers that are consistent with these values.

Token economies present another ethical and theoretical dilemma: the degree to which behavior changes effected through a token economy either will or should generalize to other settings in which the client may be placed in the future. Much research suggests that the sort of reinforcement contingencies that prevail in most token-economy programs do not characterize most naturally occurring reinforcers. When a client who has learned a new behavior under conditions of monitored and controlled reinforcement in a token economy moves to a setting in which different contingencies apply, there is substantial risk that the new behavior may disappear, leaving the client bereft of adequate, meaningful reinforcers.

The consequences for both the client and society of such a failure of generalization can be significant. For example, psychiatric patients who acquire workplace social skills in a consistent and regulated token-economy program and then enter a "real world" workplace where reinforcement is inconsistent may not be able to respond adequately to the new contingencies, and will therefore be unable to cope with the new setting, even though they functioned well under the token-economy conditions. This may lead to a financial inability to live independently, and even to homelessness and the need for welfare benefits that might not have been required had attention been paid to the generalization of token-economy-acquired skills to the outside world. This possibility makes it essential for behavior therapists to address the issues of generalization and maintenance of behavior change across various settings.

COMPUTER-ASSISTED AND ADMINISTERED THERAPY AND SELF-HELP BOOKS. Since the mid-1990s there has been an increasing interest among behavior and cognitive-behavior therapists in the development of computer-assisted and administered treatments, as well as in the dissemination of self-help books that detail, for the lay person, ways to cope with one's problems without the assistance of a therapist. This movement has been driven by the ready availability of computer technology and the Internet, and by a desire to bring the benefits of behavior therapy to people who might otherwise have limited access to therapists (such as those in remote rural areas).

The promulgation of treatments that involve minimal or no professional guidance, but rely instead upon the theories and techniques of behavior and cognitive-behavior therapies, as well as the claims made by these therapies in such a context, raises important ethical issues. Specifically, to what extent is a human therapist necessary to produce effective behavior change, and is it ethically responsible to promote these approaches in this way?

Many of these programs function by attempting to mimic the interaction between therapist and patient using decision tree programming that provide standardize computer responses to a variety of specific client input statements.

Researchers have also validated a number of computer-assisted and administered treatments using "virtual reality" and computer-assisted interviewing to treat panic disorder (Newman, Kenardy, Herman, and Taylor), anger (Timmons, Oehlert, Sumerall, Timmons, et al.), acrophobia (Vincelli), and problem drinking (Hester and Delaney). To the extent that these treatments have been found to be as effective as their human-delivered counterparts, they pose no more ethical concerns than do other behavioral therapies. However, there is a danger that untested approaches and methods will be used, possibly to the detriment of patients, and it is incumbent upon all behavior therapists to insure that computer or Internet-based treatments are subjected to thorough research testing prior to full dissemination.

Similar issues adhere to the publication of self-help books. As with computer- and Internet-based applications, it is incumbent upon the authors of these books to insure that they have reasonable research evidence for their efficacy.

Authors and users of both computer-assisted and administered applications of behavior therapy and self-help books need to be attentive to possible misapplication of these techniques, particularly by persons whose problems may be more complex and difficult than such approaches can address. Clear disclaimers and cautions to potential users with respect to the limitations of these approaches are necessary to insure their ethical dissemination and use. On the positive side, these approaches are entirely consistent with the traditional emphasis in behavior therapy on active client participation in treatment.

## The Image of Behavior Therapy

As noted, the image of early behavior therapy among nonbehavioral professionals and the lay public was often extremely negative. Grossly inaccurate notions about the nature of behavior therapy were commonplace, and behavior therapy was lumped with such alien procedures as psychosurgery and Erhard Seminar Training. Such misconceptions are now infrequent. This is due largely to the incorporation of behavior therapy into the mental health mainstream, to increased sophistication and greater acceptance of behavior therapy by the general public, and, perhaps above all, to the concerted attempts of behavior therapists, both as individuals and as members of professional organizations, to correct these misconceptions and thereby improve the image of behavior therapy.

There is a continuing need to modify misconceptions through well-planned public education. Behavior therapists also need continuing educational training in the maintenance of good ethical practice. Measures of consumer satisfaction are the rule rather than the exception in both clinical research and treatment. Behavior therapists must increasingly think in terms of public relations and the necessity for keeping patients informed at all stages of the intervention process. For example, behavior therapists in private practice are beginning to make available written descriptions of the treatment procedures and policies for discussion and review before treatment begins (Franks).

## Conclusion

Contemporary behavior therapy is characterized by an emphasis on client participation in therapeutic goal setting and a balancing of client rights (particularly when the client is relatively powerless) against societal needs, values, and expectations. Even in institutional settings the application of techniques is much less mechanistic and intrusive, and behavior therapists are trained to apply their techniques with stringent safeguards of client rights.

An increasing awareness of the roles of thoughts and feelings in the production and maintenance of behavior has led to behavior therapists' becoming more client-centered and humanistic in their approaches to behavior change. This awareness has also produced an increasing emphasis on teaching clients self-control techniques rather than "applying techniques to clients" without consideration of the active role the client should play in the process of changing behavior.

By virtue of the inclusion of cognitive and contextual variables in theory and application, contemporary behavior therapy is a considerably advanced over early behavior therapy, which was based largely on animal models of learning. Behavior therapy is unique among current psychotherapeutic schools in that practitioners rely on repeated, data-based, objective assessments of client behaviors, thoughts, and feelings to aid in the establishment of therapeutic goals and the continuous assessment of therapeutic progress. Contemporary behavior therapy is a diverse field in which theoretical progress and practice are based on demonstrable advances in scientific knowledge, rather than on the pronouncements of authorities or "gurus." Although not yet fully integrated into behavior-therapy practice, developments in basic psychology, human rule-governed behavior (Hayes), cognitive sciences, and computer science all hold promise for enhancing both treatment efficacy and sensitivity to ethical constraints. As practitioners of a discipline and through organizations such as the Association for Advancement of Behavior Therapy, behavior therapists are learning how to apply these rigorous standards to themselves and to their personal interactions with clients, colleagues, students, and society at large.

FREDERICK ROTGERS
CYRIL M. FRANKS (1995)
REVISED BY AUTHORS

SEE ALSO: *Autonomy; Behaviorism; Coercion; Freedom and Free Will; Informed Consent; Mental Health Therapies; Mental Illness; Neuroethics; Patients' Rights: Mental Patients' Rights; Psychiatry, Abuses of; Psychoanalysis and Dynamic Therapies*

### BIBLIOGRAPHY

Bandura, Albert. 1977. *Social Learning Theory.* Englewood Cliffs, NJ: Prentice Hall.

Bandura, Albert. 1982. "Self-Efficacy Mechanism in Human Agency." *American Psychologist* 37(2): 122–147.

Beck, Aaron T. 1976. *Cognitive Therapy and Emotional Disorders.* New York: International Universities Press.

Ellis, Albert. 1962. *Reason and Emotion in Psychotherapy.* Secaucus, NJ: Citadel.

Fishman, Daniel B., and Franks, Cyril M. 1992. "Evolution and Differentiation Within Behavior Therapy: A Theoretical and Epistemological Review." In *History of Psychotherapy: A Century of Change,* ed. Donald K. Freedheim. Washington, D.C.: American Psychological Association.

Franks, Cyril M. 1994. "Basic Concepts and Models: Behavioral Model." In *Advanced Abnormal Psychology,* ed. Vincent B. Van Hasselt and Michel Hersen. New York: Plenum.

Hayes, Steven C. 1987. "A Contextual Approach to Therapeutic Change." In *Psychotherapists in Clinical Practice: Cognitive and Behavioral Perspectives,* ed. Neil S. Jacobson. New York: Guilford.

Hayes, Steven C., ed. 1989. *Rule-Governed Behavior: Cognition, Contingencies, and Instructional Control.* New York: Plenum.

Hester, R. K., and Delaney, H. D. 1997. "Behavioral Self-Control Program for Windows: Results of a Controlled Clinical Trial." *Journal of Consulting and Clinical Psychology* 65(4): 686–693.

Kohlenberg, Robert J., and Tsai, Mavis. 1991. *Functional Analytic Psychotherapy: Creating Intense and Curative Therapeutic Relationships.* New York: Plenum.

Lazarus, Arnold A. 1981. *The Practice of Multimodal Therapy: Systematic, Comprehensive, and Effective Psychotherapy.* New York: McGraw-Hill.

Mahoney, Michael J. 1974. *Cognition and Behavior Modification.* Cambridge, MA: Ballinger.

Newman, M. G.; Kenardy, J.; Herman, S.; and Taylor, C. B. 1997. "Comparison of Palmtop-Computer-Assisted Brief Cognitive Behavioral Treatment to Cognitive-Behavioral Treatment for Panic Disorder." *Journal of Consulting and Clinical Psychology* 65(1): 178–183.

Rachman, Stanley J., and Wilson, G. Terence. 1980. *The Effects of Psychological Therapy,* 2nd edition. Oxford: Pergamon.

Timmons, P. L.; Oehlert, M. E.; Sumeral, S. W.; Timmons, C. W.; et al. 1997. "Stress Inoculation Training for Maladaptive Anger: Comparison of Group Counseling versus Computer Guidance." *Computers in Human Behavior* 13(1): 51–64.

Vincelli, F. 1999. "From Imagination to Virtual Reality: The Future of Clinical Psychology." *Cyberpsychology and Behavior* 2(3): 241–248.

Wilson, G. Terence, and Evans, Ian M. 1977. "The Therapist-Client Relationship in Behavior Therapy." In *Effective Psychotherapy: A Handbook of Research,* ed. Alan S. Gurman and Andrew M. Razin. New York: Pergamon.

# BENEFICENCE

• • •

*Beneficence* denotes the practice of good deeds. In contemporary ethics, the principle of beneficence usually signifies an obligation to benefit others or to seek their good. It is a principle of major importance in bioethics and has been prominent in the codes of physicians since antiquity.

## Beneficence and Benevolence

Beneficence as a principle that guides decisions should be distinguished from the virtue that motivates actors. The

*Oxford English Dictionary* defines "beneficence" as "doing good, the manifestation of benevolence, or kindly feeling" (emphasis added). This definition bespeaks the etymology of both terms. *Beneficence* is derived from the Latin *bene* (well; from *bonus,* good) and *facere* (to do), whereas *benevolence* is rooted in *bene* and *volens* (a strong wish or intention) (Partridge). Philosophers who emphasize a more rationalist approach, calculated to guide principled choices, tend to endorse beneficence. Those who see ethics as primarily concerned with virtue, character, and the psychological dimensions of the moral life emphasize benevolence.

David Hume, for example, conceived of benevolence as one of the instincts originally implanted in human nature. Like Joseph Butler, Francis Hutcheson, Adam Smith, and other eighteenth-century English-speaking philosophers, Hume was not so much concerned with ethical problem solving as with describing the role and place of benevolence in the moral topography of human beings. Adam Smith used the term *beneficence,* but employed it to describe the virtue of goodwill, and saw it as a moral passion rather than a principle. Of concern to all these philosophers was a task set for them by Thomas Hobbes a century earlier.

Hobbes set the modern polemical context for discussions not only of beneficence and benevolence but also of ethics more generally. His moral philosophy was determinist, denying any capacity for choice based on values, and relativist, denying any independent reference for the terms good and evil: Liberty he saw as merely the ability to enact one's desires, not freedom to deliberate and choose. Good and evil simply denoted human appetites and aversions. "Will" was just another desire, not a distinctive moral capacity. Obviously such a philosophy was no place for beneficence as a principle of choice or benevolence as a motivation for the good of others. Ethics devolves into a deterministic egoism. Butler, Hutcheson, Hume, and Smith, in a variety of ways, took as their task a survey of the moral psyche, with special regard for the place of benevolence as something innate or natural to human life.

Unless Hobbes's egoistic portrait is correct, any well-rounded view of ethics will include ways of describing and evaluating both the motivational and character-laden aspects, and the decisional, action-oriented elements of ethics—that is, both benevolence and beneficence.

A principle of beneficence can be broadly or narrowly defined. William Frankena views beneficence as an inclusive principle involving elements of refraining from inflicting harm and preventing or removing evil, as well as an obligation actively to promote good. James Childress adopts Frankena's elements but reclassifies them according to two distinct principles: nonmaleficence, the obligation not to inflict harm; and beneficence, the obligations to prevent harm, to remove harm or evil, and positively to promote good. This refinement has the merit of following an intuitive division between refraining and active doing. It elucidates why refraining from harm is usually seen as a universal duty to others, while actively promoting good or helping others is typically seen as a less stringent obligation and often as resulting from specific role obligations (being a parent or a doctor) or contractual agreements. A broader-ranging sense of beneficence is, nevertheless, endorsed by some philosophers. For example, in *The Right and the Good,* W. D. Ross claimed that duties of beneficence are incurred because of "the mere fact that there are other human beings in the world whose condition we can make better …" (p. 21).

## Relation to Utility

Beneficence has natural affinities with a principle of utility. Tom Beauchamp and James Childress, for example, claim that promoting good always involves a calculation of what harms might also be incurred. A principle of utility is a way to assess harms and benefits. In his *Utilitarianism,* John Stuart Mill asserted in 1863 that the measure of "good" by which all actions are to be judged is whether they promote the greatest happiness for the greatest number. Mill saw his principle of utility as a systematic expression of the teaching of Jesus, for example, as embodied in the "golden rule."

When defined through Mill's utility principle, beneficence becomes vulnerable to two criticisms frequently leveled at utilitarianism. The first is the problem of adequacy. A focus on beneficence as the promotion of happiness, to the exclusion of other kinds of goods and obligations, seems too narrow. People value things other than happiness, however broadly defined. Promoting the happiness of others can conflict with treating them fairly or respecting them as persons. The second problem is idealism. For Mill at least, utilitarianism presented a stringent requirement. "As between his own happiness and that of others utilitarianism requires him to be as strictly impartial as a disinterested and benevolent spectator" (1979, p. 16). To count the good of strangers equally with our own good, or that of our families or friends, seems saintly and perhaps impossible to achieve.

These problems have led some philosophers to question utilitarianism as a system but also to see beneficence as only one principle among others, and as usually (if not always) an imperfect or supererogatory duty. While some principle of utility is necessary to enact beneficence, it need not be Mill's rendition. A utility principle that recognized a variety of goods would at least moderate the force of the criticisms above.

## Beneficence and Autonomy

How beneficence is put into practice depends on how it is modified by other principles. Especially important in this regard is respect for autonomy or self-determination. Another way to put this is to ask whose notion of *good* will be definitive. Respect for autonomy means that *good* will be defined by the recipient of the action rather than the agent. Beneficence not so defined leads to paternalism, in which the beneficent actor overrides or ignores the recipient's ideas of good and imposes his or her own. The history of medical ethics is largely (but not entirely) a history of paternalistic beneficence. In the mid-twentieth century, consistent challenges arose to beneficent paternalism through assertions of patient rights. Defenders of simple paternalism in healthcare relationships are now rare, and most ethicists would agree with Erich Loewy that paternalistic actions generally represent a "caricature" rather than a natural extension of beneficence.

Autonomy as a moral principle is historically rooted in freedom as a political principle, to which John Locke's *Second Treatise of Government* (1690) gave definitive expression. Freedom, Locke asserted, is not license "but a *liberty* to dispose, and order as he lists, his person, actions, possessions, and his whole property, within the allowance of those laws under which he is, and therein not to be subject to the arbitrary rule of another, but freely follow his own" (p. 32). The eighteenth-century monument to autonomy is the work of the German philosopher Immanuel Kant. Whereas Locke was concerned to protect individuals from the power of the state, Kant focused on freedom of the will. His "practical imperative" requires that others be treated as ends in themselves and never only as a means. For Kant this respect for the moral freedom of others was grounded in a recognition of their rational nature. In bioethics this raises the difficult issue of when and to what extent the rational capacities of patients are compromised and in which cases autonomy should give way to medical beneficence.

The grounds for limiting beneficence through respect for autonomy were most powerfully stated by John Stuart Mill. In *On Liberty* (first published in 1859) he cautioned against supposing that the principle of liberty necessitates a "selfish indifference." Indeed, he asserted, "there is need of a great increase of disinterested exertion to promote the good of others." But, he continued, "disinterested benevolence can find other instruments to persuade people to their good than whips and scourges, either of the literal or of the metaphorical sort" (p. 74).

While advocacy for autonomy as the preeminent principle of medical ethics was powerful during the 1970s and 1980s, there are still substantial voices for a beneficence-based theory. Edmund Pellegrino and David Thomasma argue that "medicine as a human activity is of necessity a form of beneficence" (p. 32). Rather than espousing the older traditions of paternalism, however, they argue for an enlarged beneficence, "beneficence-in-trust"—a non-rights-based approach that includes respect for autonomy but emphasizes a fiduciary grounding for doctor–patient encounters. This approach has an advantage over single-principle approaches that ground medical obligations in simple beneficence or simple autonomy, conceived as mono-lithic norms. Beneficence, unleavened by respect for autonomy, can lead to paternalism, while autonomy alone obviates trust and often deteriorates into indifference. Still the feasibility of trust depends upon shared values and goals, or at least stable role expectations between providers and patients. The greater the pluralism in a society, the less likely it is that the trust Pellegrino and Thomasma commend can be established.

## Health Professional Codes

While beneficence is important to many philosophical and religious systems of ethics, it is central to the health professions. The Hippocratic Oath clearly states that the physician's actions are "for the benefit of the sick" (see Appendix for this and other codes and oaths). The Declaration of Geneva begins with a pledge to "consecrate" one's life to "the service of humanity." The 1980 "Principles" of the American Medical Association (AMA) opens with the declaration that these principles are established "primarily for the benefit of the patient." The International Code for Nurses devised in 1973 begins with a broad-ranging assertion of beneficence. The "fundamental" responsibility of the nurse, it states, is to promote and restore health, alleviate suffering, and prevent illness. While duties to specific persons are recognized, the obligation to perform beneficent actions is seen as universal, because the need for nursing services is universal.

The U.S. Code for Nurses of 1976 differs from all physician codes in recognizing that services not only should promote good but also should be guided by the values of those served. The first principle in this formulation asserts the "self-determination of clients." As noted above, self-determination, or autonomy, is frequently seen as a limiting factor in gauging the extent of beneficence, yet this factor is rarely mentioned in the ethical formulations of health professionals. For example, the practice of soliciting consent from patients was evident in medical practices in the United States in the eighteenth century. Yet these solicitations were not commensurate with today's notion of informed consent.

Consent was sought in the eighteenth century primarily to enhance therapy rather than to encourage independent decision making by patients (Faden et al.). Jay Katz presses this point by asserting that consent is largely "alien" to medical thinking, which prefers "custody" over "liberty."

Still, claims for the modern uniqueness of informed consent should be viewed with caution, especially when they tend to valorize an "autonomy model" over a "beneficence model" (Faden et al.). It would be anachronistic to believe that eighteenth-century physicians worked with the mid-twentieth-century concept of consent. Yet it is too sweeping and dualistic to believe that, by default, they were under the sway of a "beneficence model." Medical practices, or moral practices more generally, do not lend themselves to easy encapsulation into models, just as beneficence as a practice is not identical with the philosophical principle of beneficence.

While all versions of professional ethics agree that the acceptance of a patient or a client creates a specific obligation of beneficence, some codes go further and talk of a general duty to seek the public good in matters of health. Here the 1847 Code of the American Medical Association is notable. Chapter III of that code enumerates "Duties of the Profession to the Public." Among those listed are vigilance for the welfare of the community, counsel to the public on health matters, and advice about epidemics, contagion, and public hygiene. Twentieth-century medical codes tend to be more parsimonious in their interpretations of what beneficence entails.

Not even the more generous beneficence in the 1847 AMA Code, however, takes it to cover what Charles Fried calls "the duty to work for and comply with just institutions" (p. 129). Fried here follows and extends the thinking of Kant, who saw beneficence in terms of a duty of mutual aid. Such aid is required because all persons (including ourselves) will at some time need the help of others, so to neglect aiding others would be self-defeating. The societal and public policy implications of beneficence in healthcare are poorly worked out at present. The issues that require attention include general programs of prevention, medical assistance to specific groups (such as AIDS patients), and healthcare for the indigent and uninsured. Most proposals for a more equitable healthcare system in the United States build on notions of justice as an independent principle rather than deriving their justifications from an extension of duties of beneficence.

## Limits

If beneficent duties are more than supererogatory, or optional, a persistent issue is how to discern their proper scope. Where do obligations to benefit others end? Are we morally required to give away all our surplus income and, beyond that, to chasten ourselves to more modest patterns of consumption? Are physicians obligated never to say "no" to patients so long as any thread of hope for improvement exists? Would beneficence require acceptance of higher taxes to fund universal health coverage, or does acting for my fellow citizens' good require me to die cheaply and forgo expensive treatments with low probability of benefit?

Beneficent duties may be limited in two ways. The first limiting force is duties to oneself. Self-respect, and an appropriate attention to one's own well-being, will of necessity restrict activities for the good of others, unless beneficence is given a preemptive place and is conflated with saintliness. Hume, for example, believed persons can be "too good," carrying "attention for others beyond the proper bounds," blunting a due sense of pride and the self-assertive virtues (p. 93). A second kind of limit involves our psychological capacity for identification of and sympathy with those who could use our help. The press of human suffering that could be alleviated by our actions is immense. To conceive of this larger and seemingly inexhaustible world of suffering as our charge would likely be debilitating. Jonathan Glover has suggested that a restricted but feasible beneficence may be the price we pay for our sanity. Limits to the duty to promote good restrict us, but also orient and direct our finite capacities. But perhaps the greater risk is that we will draw a circle around duties in a niggardly fashion, that our imagination will not be too large, risking paralysis, but too stingy and self-serving. It is this narrow and parochial tendency that concerns the advocates of a robust and extensive beneficence.

## Relational Selves

The recent challenges to ethical theory from psychological studies of moral experience have profound implications for beneficence. In 1982 Carol Gilligan published her research on the moral development of women, titled *In a Different Voice.* She claimed that females tend to see moral problems in terms of relationships. They are prone to think of their choices in problem solving as issues of care and responsibility for those relationships. By contrast, males tend to see moral problems in terms of rules and principles, and are prone to think of their choices as logical adjudications. Women's moral orientations tend toward valuing and preserving ties among persons, while men's tend toward abstract thinking by an agent largely removed from and impartial to the parties involved. Gilligan's claim is not that there are precise gender types for moral experience but that the model of the moral self as an abstract, isolated, principled, and hierarchical thinker is insufficient.

Consider the case of Jake and Amy, two eleven-year-olds, who discuss the question "When responsibility to oneself and responsibility to others conflict, how should one choose?" (Gilligan, pp. 35ff.). While Jake adjudicates these responsibilities as if it were a problem of rule application, Amy's response is pragmatic and assumes a relational self. Jake seeks fairness in the manner of a judge; Amy is concerned to see that others' needs are met and relationships are nurtured. The point is not so much that Jake and Amy offer different answers but that they see different issues, and see themselves in different ways.

The implications for a principle of beneficence in bioethics, and in the ethical codes of health professionals, are substantial. Gilligan's research directly challenges the adequacy of thinking of beneficence simply as a principle to be applied to cases, and recommends a notion of beneficence grounded in complex, relational understandings of the self. Hence, the issues of beneficence can no longer be formulated as if the agent were essentially solitary and could contemplate the scope of his or her duties from afar. The self is already, and essentially, immersed in a web of convivial responsibilities. The ethical formulations of most health professions exhibit precisely the hierarchical distancing and the assumption of optional relationships depicted in the "male" model. Attending to the second voice in moral experience would mean moving bioethics beyond an exhaustive reliance on applying beneficence, as a principle, to problem cases. It would also mean taking the ethical codes of health professionals beyond the contract model and into a recognition of a deeper and more integral bond between healers and the sick, and between health professionals and society.

LARRY R. CHURCHILL (1995)

SEE ALSO: *Autonomy; Bioethics; Compassionate Love; Confidentiality; Ethics: Normative Ethical Theories; Justice; Paternalism; Professional-Patient Relationship*

### BIBLIOGRAPHY

Beauchamp, Tom, and Childress, James. 1989. *Principles of Biomedical Ethics.* 3rd edition. New York: Oxford University Press.

Beauchamp, Tom, and McCullough, Lawrence. 1984. *Medical Ethics: The Moral Responsibilities of Physicians.* Englewood Cliffs, NJ: Prentice-Hall.

Childress, James F. 1982. *Who Should Decide?: Paternalism in Health Care.* New York: Oxford University Press.

Faden, Ruth, and Beauchamp, Tom, with Nancy King. 1986. *A History and Theory of Informed Consent.* New York: Oxford University Press.

Frankena, William. 1973. *Ethics.* 2nd edition. Englewood Cliffs, NJ: Prentice-Hall.

Fried, Charles. 1978. *Right and Wrong.* Cambridge, MA: Harvard University Press.

Gilligan, Carol. 1982. *In a Different Voice: Psychological Theory and Women's Development.* Cambridge, MA: Harvard University Press.

Glover, Jonathan. 1977. *Causing Death and Saving Lives.* London: Penguin.

Hobbes, Thomas. 1947. *Leviathan,* ed. Michael Oakeshott. New York: Oxford University Press.

Hume, David. 1966 (1777). *An Enquiry Concerning the Principles of Morals.* 2nd edition. La Salle, IL: Open Court.

Kant, Immanuel. 1959. *Foundations of the Metaphysics of Morals,* tr. Lewis White Beck. New York: Macmillan.

Katz, Jay. 1984. *The Silent World of Doctor and Patient.* New York: Free Press.

Locke, John. 1980 (1690). *Second Treatise of Government,* ed. Crawford B. MacPherson. Indianapolis: Hackett.

Loewy, Erich. 1991. *Suffering and the Beneficent Community: Beyond Libertarianism.* Albany: State University of New York Press.

Mill, John Stuart. 1978 (1859). *On Liberty.* Indianapolis: Hackett.

Mill, John Stuart. 1979 (1863). *Utilitarianism.* Indianapolis: Hackett.

Partridge, Eric. 1983. *Origins: A Short Etymological Dictionary of Modern English.* New York: Greenwich House.

Pellegrino, Edmund D., and Thomasma, David C. 1988. *For the Patient's Good: The Restoration of Beneficence in Health Care.* New York: Oxford University Press.

Ross, W. D. 1930. *The Right and the Good.* Oxford: Clarendon Press.

# BIAS, RESEARCH

• • •

In the behavioral sciences, the difficulties of studying complex, changing interactions among living beings led to investigations of possible sources of bias. For example, the gender, race, class, and even presence of a researcher during an interview have been shown to influence the responses of the interviewee (Oakley). Researchers sought to apply the scientific method to problems in the behavioral sciences, in an attempt to eliminate bias.

Like all scholars, scientists hold, either explicitly or implicitly, certain beliefs concerning their enterprise. Most scientists try to use what they assume to be the best information to collect data and draw theories to elucidate the laws and facts that will be constant, providing that experiments have been done correctly. But the individuals who make observations and create theories are people who live in a particular country at a certain time in a definable socioeconomic condition, and their situations and mentalities impinge on their discoveries. Aristotle "counted" fewer teeth in the mouths of women than in those of men—adding this dentitional inferiority to all the others he asserted characterized women (Arditti). Galen, having read the book of Genesis, "discovered" that men had one less rib on one side than women did (Webster and Webster). Neither is true, and both would be refuted easily by observation of what would appear by today's standards to be easily verifiable facts. Although they also could count, they took these to be "nonclassical cases" because what we take to be facts can vary depending upon the theory or paradigm—the specific problematics, concepts, theories, language, and methods—guiding the scientist.

Because most scientists, feminists, and philosophers of science recognize that no individual can live a life and be entirely neutral or value-free since science and values are both very important. To some, "objectivity is defined to mean independence from the value judgments of any particular individual" (Jaggar, p. 357). The paradigms themselves, however, also are far from value-free. The values of a culture, in the historical past and the present society, heavily influence the ordering of observable phenomena into a theory. The worldview of a particular society, time, and person limits the questions that can be asked, and thereby the answers that can be given. Therefore, the very acceptance of a particular paradigm that appears to cause a "scientific revolution" within a society may depend at least in part upon the congruence of that theory with the institutions and beliefs of the society (Kuhn).

Elizabeth Potter (2001) documented Boyle's choice of the mechanistic model to explain his Law of Gases both because it comported well with the data and because it supported the status quo of conservative religion and monarchy of the seventeenth century with regard to class and gender compared to the competing animistic model seen as more radical socially. Scholars suggest that Darwin's theory of natural selection was ultimately accepted by his contemporaries (whereas they did not accept similar theories as described by Alfred Russel Wallace and others) because Darwin emphasized the congruence between the values of his theory and those held by the upper classes of Victorian Britain (Rose and Rose). Social Darwinists used Darwin's theory to base the political and social rights to their wealth and power held by men and the upper classes in biological determinism. In this manner Darwin's data and theories

reinforced the natural superiority of wealthy men, making his theories acceptable to the leaders of Victorian English society. Fausto-Sterling's research (1999) revealed how different societies at particular historical periods have also used varying biological and genetic data as determinants for the social construction of gender and race.

Not only what is accepted, but what and how we study, have normative features. Helen Longino (1990) has explored the extent to which methods employed by scientists can be objective, in the sense of not being related to individual values, and lead to repeatable, verifiable results while contributing to hypotheses or theories that are congruent with nonobjective institutions and ideologies such as gender, race, and class that are socially constructed in the society: "Background assumptions are the means by which contextual values and ideology are incorporated into scientific inquiry" (p. 216). For example, scientists may calculate rocket trajectories and produce bombs that efficiently destroy living beings without raising the ethical questions of whether the money and effort for this research to support the military could be better spent on other research questions that might be solved by using similar objective methods.

## Unintended Research Bias

Given the high costs of sophisticated equipment, maintenance of laboratory animals and facilities, and salaries for qualified technicians and researchers, little behavioral or biomedical research is undertaken without governmental or foundation support. The choice of problems for study in medical research is substantially determined by a national agenda that defines what is worthy of study, that is, worth funding. As Marxist (Zimmerman et al.), African-American (Campbell, Denes, and Morrison), and feminist (Harding, 1998) critics of scientific research have pointed out, the scientific research undertaken in the United States reflects the societal bias toward the powerful, who are overwhelmingly white, middle/upper class, and male. Members of Congress and the individuals in the theoretical and decision-making positions within the medical and scientific establishments that set priorities and allocate funds for research exemplify these descriptors. The lack of diversity among Congressional and scientific leaders may allow unintentional, undetected flaws to bias the research in terms of what we study and how we study it. Some have characterized the diversion of scarce resources away from public health measures known to prevent diseases for the masses towards the multibillion dollar Human Genome Project as an example of placing the interests of the powerful above those of the general public, since gene therapy and designer genes are likely to benefit fewer, wealthier people.

Examples from research studies demonstrate that unintentional bias may be reflected in at least three stages of application of the scientific method: (1) choice and definition of problems to be studied; (2) methods and approaches used in data gathering, including whom we choose as subjects; and (3) theories and conclusions drawn from the data.

### CHOICE AND DEFINITION OF PROBLEMS TO BE STUDIED.

Many diseases that occur in both sexes have been studied in males only and/or used a male-as-norm approach. Cardiovascular diseases serve as a case in point. Research protocols for large scale studies (MRFIT; Grobbee et al.; Steering Committee of the Physicians' Health Study Group) of cardiovascular diseases failed to assess gender differences. Women were excluded from clinical trials of drugs, they said, because of the desire to protect women or fetuses (and fear of litigation) from possible teratogenic effects on fetuses. Exclusion of women from clinical drug trials was so pervasive that a meta-analysis surveying the literature from 1960 to 1991 on clinical trials of medications used to treat acute myocardial infarction found that women were included in less that 20 percent and the elderly in less than 40 percent of those studies (Gurwitz, Nananda, and Avorn).

Many of these studies, including the Physicians' Health Study, were flawed not only by the factors of gender and age but also by factors of race and class. Susceptibility to cardiovascular disease is known to be affected by lifestyle factors such as diet, exercise level, and stress, which are correlated with race and class. Since physicians in the United States are not representative of the overall male population with regard to lifestyle, the results may not be applicable to most men. The data from these studies should not have been generalized to the population as a whole. (Some argued they directed studies to the group that they care about most, namely, people like themselves.)

Designation of certain diseases as particular to one gender, race, or sexual orientation not only cultivates ignorance in the general public about transmission or frequency of the disease; it also results in research that does not adequately explore the parameters of the disease. Most of the funding for heart disease has been appropriated for research on predisposing factors for the disease (such as cholesterol level, lack of exercise, stress, smoking, and weight) using white, middle-aged middle-class males. Much less research has been directed towards elderly women, African-American women who have had several children, and other high-risk groups of women. Virtually no research has explored predisposing factors for these groups, who fall outside the disease definition established from the dominant perspective.

Recent data indicate that the initial designation of AIDS as a disease of male homosexuals, drug users, and Haitian immigrants not only has resulted in homophobic and racist stereotypes but also has particular implications for women of color. In 1981 the first official case of AIDS in a woman was reported to the Centers for Disease Control and Prevention (CDC). By 1991, $80 million had been spent since the inception of the Multicenter AIDS Cohort Study (MACS), designed to follow the natural history of HIV among gay and bisexual males (Faden, Kass, and McGraw). Although by 1988, the case reports for women were higher than the number for men in 1983, the year the MACS began (Chu, Buehler, and Berelman), it was not until the final quarter of 1994 that the first study on the natural history of HIV infection in women began. In 1998, the CDC reported that AIDS remains the leading cause of death among black females aged 25 to 44, and the second leading cause of death overall among those aged 25 to 44 (CDC, 1998). The majority of women diagnosed with AIDS are black or Hispanic.

These types of bias raise ethical issues. Healthcare practitioners treat the majority of the population, which consists of females, minorities, and the elderly, based on information gathered from clinical research in which women and minorities have not been included. Bias in research thus leads to further injustice in healthcare diagnosis and treatment. Understanding this bias led to changes in policies in the 1990s. Investigators now receiving federal money must give a compelling reason if their studies fail to include both men and women, young and old, as well as individuals of diverse races. Although this increases the cost of research, since the sample must be larger, cost alone does not stand as a compelling reason.

### APPROACHES AND METHODS USED IN DATA GATHERING.

Using the white, middle-aged, heterosexual male as the "basic experimental subject" not only ignores the fact that females may respond differently to the variable tested; it also may lead to less accurate models even for many men. For example, the standard dosage of certain medications is not only inappropriate for many women and the elderly, but also for most Asian men, because of their smaller body size and weight. Certain surgical procedures such as angioplasty and cardiac bypass result in higher death rates for women (Kelsey) and Asian men and may require modification for the same reason (Chinese Hospital Medical Staff; Manley et al.).

When women of color are used as experimental subjects, clinicians often hold stereotypical and racist views that limit accurate diagnosis. For example, numerous research studies have focused on sexually transmitted diseases in prostitutes in general (CDC, 1987; Cohen et al; Rosser, 1994) and African-American women as prostitutes in particular. Several studies have also revealed that practitioners recognize and report at higher rates crack-cocaine abuse in African-American women and alcohol abuse in American Indian women, compared to white women seeking prenatal care. An American Civil Liberties Union study revealed that in forty-seven out of fifty-three cases brought against women for drug use during pregnancy in which the race of the woman was identifiable, 80 percent were brought against women of color (Pattrow, p. 2).

Frequently it is difficult to determine whether these women are treated disrespectfully and unethically due to their gender or whether race and class are more significant variables. From the Tuskegee syphilis experiment (1932–1972), in which the effects of untreated syphilis were studied in 399 men over a period of 40 years (Jones), it is clear that men who are black and poor may not receive appropriate treatment or information about the experiment in which they are participating. Scholars (Clarke and Olesen) explore the extent to which gender, race, and class become complex, interlocking variables that may affect access to and quality of healthcare.

Using only a particular discipline's established methods may result in approaches that fail to reveal sufficient information about the problem being explored. This may be a difficulty for research surrounding medical problems particularly important to the elderly, women, men of color, and homosexual males. Pregnancy, childbirth, menstruation, menopause, lupus, sickle-cell disease, AIDS, and gerontology represent healthcare issues for which the methods of one discipline are clearly inadequate.

Methods that cross disciplinary boundaries or include combinations of methods traditionally used in separate fields may provide more appropriate approaches. For example, heart disease is caused not only by genetic and physiological factors but also by social/psychological factors such as smoking and stress. Jean Hamilton (1985) has called for interactive models that draw on both the social and the natural sciences to explain complex problems. Some of the biological solutions such as Depo-Provera or Norplant implants (Washburn) favored for addressing teen pregnancy in some African-American and American Indian populations will be less effective without accompanying strategies based upon research from the social and behavior sciences on raising self-esteem, increasing education, and dealing with underlying family dynamics. Stripped of the complex of social, economic, educational, and family dynamics issues that may contribute to teen pregnancy, Norplant implants and Depo-Provera may prevent a particular pregnancy. Without information about family planning, counseling to deal with family problems, and education and job skills, however, such approaches do not solve the basic problems causing the teen pregnancy.

**THEORIES AND CONCLUSIONS DRAWN FROM THE DATA.** Emphasis upon traditional disciplinary approaches that are quantitative and maintain the distance between observer and experimental subject supposedly removes the bias of the researcher. Ironically, to the extent that these "objective" approaches are synonymous with a particular approach to scientific phenomena, they may introduce bias. As a corrective to such bias to a science that is too narrow, Sandra Harding proposes the notion of "strong objectivity" which recognizes the cultural, social, and historical forces that shape the questions asked by scientists, their approaches, and the theories and conclusions drawn from their data (1993, 1998).

Theories may be presented in androcentric, ethnocentric, or class-biased language. An awareness of language should aid experimenters in avoiding the use of terms such as "tomboyism" (Money and Erhardt), "aggression," and "hysteria," which reflect assumptions about sex-appropriate behavior (Hamilton). Researchers should use evaluative terms such as "prostitute" with caution. Often the important fact for AIDS research is that a woman has multiple sex partners or is an IV drug user, rather than that she has received money for sex. The use of such terms as "prostitute" may induce bias by promoting the idea that women are vectors for transmission to men when, in fact, the men may have an equal or greater number of sex partners to whom they are transmitting the disease. Even more important, by emphasizing AIDS in "prostitutes," healthcare practitioners are able to distance themselves and their patients from the risk of AIDS. This may also lead to practitioners treating prostitutes as less than human and underdiagnosing AIDS in women who are not prostitutes. Focus on group characteristics such as "prostitute" or "poor, black, unmarried woman" repeats the initial mistake of identifying the disease by group rather than by behavioral risk.

Once a bias in terminology is exposed, the next step is to ask whether that terminology leads to a constraint or bias in the theory itself. Theories and conclusions drawn from medical research may be formulated to support the status quo of inequality for oppressed groups. Not surprisingly, the androcentric bias in research that has led to exclusion of women from the definitions and approaches to research problems may result in differences in management of disease and access to healthcare procedures based on gender. In a 1991 study in Massachusetts and Maryland, John Z. Ayanian and Arnold M. Epstein (1991) demonstrated that women were significantly less likely than men to undergo coronary angioplasty, angiography, or surgery when admitted to the hospital with a diagnosis of myocardial infarction, unstable or stable angina, chronic ischemic heart disease, or chest pain. This significant difference remained even when the variables of race, age, economic status, and other chronic diseases (such as diabetes and heart failure) were controlled. A similar study (Steingart et al.) revealed that women have angina before myocardial infarction as frequently and with more debilitating effects than men, yet they are referred for cardiac catheterization only half as often. Gender bias in cardiac research has therefore been translated into bias in management of disease, leading to inequitable treatment for life-threatening conditions in women. Women exhibited higher death rates from angioplasty (Kelsey et al.) and thrombolytic therapy (Wenger, Speroff, and Packard).

Recognizing the possibility of bias is the first step toward understanding the difference it makes and combating it. Perhaps white male researchers have been less likely to see flaws in and question biologically deterministic theories that provide scientific justification for their superior status in society because they gain social power and status from such theories. Researchers from outside the mainstream (women and people of color, for example) are much more likely to be critical of such theories because they lose power from those theories.

In order to eliminate bias and recognize the cultural, social, and historical forces impacting their research, the community of scientists needs to include individuals who serve as members on review panels and as leaders to review studies from backgrounds of as much variety and diversity as possible with regard to race, class, gender, and sexual orientation (Rosser, 2000). Only then is it less likely that the perspective of one group will bias research design, approaches, subjects, and interpretations. Since the scientific method itself is supposed to be "self-correcting," if results are continually tested and subject to critical review, these biases are likely to be exposed.

SUE V. ROSSER (1995)
REVISED BY AUTHOR

**SEE ALSO:** *AIDS; Feminism; Genetic Discrimination; Metaphor and Analogy; Prisoners as Research Subjects; Privacy and Confidentiality in Research; Race and Racism; Research Policy; Sexism*

### BIBLIOGRAPHY

Arditti, Rita. 1980. "Feminism and Science." In *Science and Liberation,* pp. 350–368, ed. Rita Arditti, Pat Brennan, and Steven Cavrak. Boston: South End Press.

Ayanian, John Z., and Epstein, Arnold. 1991. "Differences in the Use of Procedures between Women and Men Hospitalized for Coronary Heart Disease." *New England Journal of Medicine* 325: 221–225.

Campbell, George, Jr.; Deanes, Ronni; and Morrision, Catherine, eds. 2000. *Access Denied: Race, Ethnicity and the Scientific Enterprise.* Oxford: Oxford University Press.

Centers for Disease Control. 1987. "Antibody to Human Immunodeficiency Virus in Female Prostitutes." *Morbidity and Mortality Weekly Report* 36: 157–161.

Centers for Disease Control. 1998. "Guidelines for Evaluating Surveillance Systems." *Morbidity and Mortality Weekly Report* 37: 1–18.

Chinese Hospital Medical Staff and University of California School of Medicine. 1982. Conference on health problems related to the Chinese in America. San Francisco, May 22–23.

Chu, S.Y.; Buehler, J. W.; and Berelman, R. L. 1990. "Impact of the Human Immunodeficiency Virus Epidemic on Mortality in Women of Reproductive Age, United States." *Journal of the American Medical Association* 264: 225–229.

Clarke, Adele E., and Olesen, Virginia L., eds. 1999. *Revisioning Women, Health, and Healing: Feminist, Cultural, and Technoscience Perspectives.* New York: Routledge.

Cohen, J., et al. 1988. "Prostitutes and AIDS: Public Policy Issues." *AIDS and Public Policy Journal* 3: 16–22.

Faden, R.; Kass, N.; and McGraw, D. 1996. "Women as Vessels and Vectors: Lessons from the HIV Epidemic." In *Feminism and Bioethics: Beyond Reproducion,* pp. 252–281, ed. S. M. Wolf. New York: Oxford University Press.

Fausto-Sterling, Anne. 1999. "Gender, Race, and Nation: The Comparative Anatomy of Hottentot Women in Europe, 1815–1817." In *Deviant Bodies: Critical Perspectives on Difference in Science and Popular Culture,* pp. 19–48. NY: Routledge.

Grobbee, Diederick E.; Rimm, Eric B.; Giovannucci, Edward; et al. 1990. "Coffee, Caffeine, and Cardiovascular Disease in Men." *New England Journal of Medicine* 323(15): 1026–1032.

Gurwitz, J. H.; Nananda, F. C.; and Avorn, J. 1992. "The Exclusion of the Elderly and Women from Clinical Trials in Acute Myocardial Infarction." *Journal of the American Medical Association* 268(2): 1417–1422.

Hamilton, Jean. 1985. "Avoiding Methodological Biases and Policy-Making Biases in Gender-Related Health Research." In vol. 2 of *Women's Health: Report of the Public Health Service Task Force on Women's Health Issues,* pp. 54–64, ed. Ruth L. Kirschstein and Doris H. Merritt. Washington, D.C.: U.S. Dept. of Health and Human Services, Public Health Service.

Harding, Sandra. 1993. *The Racial Economy of Science.* Bloomington, IN: Indiana University Press.

Harding, Sandra. 1998. *Is Science Multicultural? Postcolonialisms, Feminisms, and Epistemologies.* Bloomington, IN: Indiana University Press.

Jaggar, Alison M. 1983. *Feminist Politics and Human Nature.* Totowa, NJ: Rowman & Allanheld.

Jones, James H. 1981. *Bad Blood: The Tuskegee Syphilis Experiment.* New York: Free Press.

Kelsey, Sheryl F. et al., and Investigtors from the National Heart, Lung, and Blood Institute Percutaneous Transluminal Coronary Angioplasty Registry. 1993. "Results of Percutaneous Transluminal Coronary Angioplasty in Women: 1985–1986 National Heart, Lung, and Blood Institutes Coronary Angioplasty Registry." *Circulation* 87(3): 720–727.

Kuhn, Thomas S. 1970. *The Structure of Scientific Revolutions.* 2nd edition. Chicago: University of Chicago Press.

Longino, Helen. 1990. *Science as Social Knowledge: Values and Objectivity in Scientific Inquiry.* Princeton, NJ: Princeton University Press.

Manley, Audrey; Lin-Fu, Jane S.; Miranda, Magdalena; et al. 1985. "Special Health Concerns of Ethnic Minority Women." In vol. 2 of *Women's Health: Report of the Public Health Service Task Force on Women's Health Issues,* pp. 37–47, ed. Ruth L. Kirschstein and Doris H. Merritt. Washington, D.C.: U.S. Dept. of Health and Human Services.

Money, John, and Erhardt, Anke. 1972. *Man and Woman, Boy and Girl: The Differentiation and Dimorphism of Gender and Identity from Conception to Maturity.* Baltimore: Johns Hopkins University Press.

Multiple Risk Factor Intervention Trial Research Group. 1990. "Mortality Rates after 10.5 Years for Participants in the Multiple Risk Factor Intervention Trial: Findings Related to A Priori Hypotheses of the Trial." *Journal of the American Medical Association* 263(13): 1795–1801.

Oakley, Ann. 1981. "Interviewing Women: A Contradiction in Terms." In *Doing Feminist Research,* pp. 30–61, ed. Helen Roberts. London: Routledge & Kegan Paul.

Pattrow, Lynn M. 1990. "When Becoming Pregnant Is a Crime." *Criminal Justice Ethics,* (Winter/Spring): 41–47.

Rose, Hilary, and Rose, Stephen. 1980. "The Myth of the Neutrality of Science." In *Science and Liberation,* pp. 17–32, ed. Rita Arditti, Pat Brennan, and Steve Cavrak. Boston: South End Press.

Rosser, Sue V. 1994. *Women's Health: Missing from U.S. Medicine.* Bloomington, IN: Indiana University Press.

Rosser, Sue V. 2000. *Women, Science, and Society: The Crucial Union.* New York: Teachers College Press.

Steering Committee of the Physicians' Health Study Group. 1989. "Final Report on the Aspirin Component of the Ongoing Physicians' Health Study." *New England Journal of Medicine* 321: 129–135.

Steingart, Richard M.; Packer, Milton; Hamm, Peggy; et al. 1991. "Sex Differences in the Management of Coronary Artery Disease." *New England Journal of Medicine* 325(4): 226–230.

Washburn, Jennifer. 1996. "The Misuses of Norplant: Who Gets Stuck?" *Ms.* 7(3): 232–236.

Webster, Douglas, and Webster, Molly. 1974. *Comparative Vertebrate Morphology.* New York: Academic Press.

Wenger, N. K.; Speroff, L.; and Packard, B. 1993. "Cardiovascular Health and Disease in Women." *New England Journal of Medicine* 329: 247.

Zimmerman, B., et al. 1990. "People's Science." In *Science and Liberation,* pp. 299–319, ed. Rita Arditti, Pat Brennan, and Steve Cavrak. Boston: South End Press.

# BIOETHICS

• • •

"There is," says the biblical book of Ecclesiastes, "no new thing under the sun." Those words are worth pondering in light of the emergence of the field of bioethics since the 1950s and 1960s. From one perspective it is a wholly modern field, a child of the remarkable advances in the biomedical, environmental, and social sciences. Those advances have brought a new world of expanded scientific understanding and technological innovation, seeming to alter forever what can be done about the vulnerabilities of nature and of the human body and mind, and about saving, improving, and extending human lives. Yet from another perspective, the kinds of questions raised by these advances are among the oldest that human beings have asked themselves. They turn on the meaning of life and death, the bearing of pain and suffering, the right and power to control one's life, and our common duties to each other and to nature in the face of grave threats to our health and well-being. Bioethics represents a radical transformation of the older, more traditional domain of medical ethics; yet it is also true that, since the dawn of history, healers have been forced to wrestle with the human fear of illness and death, and with the limits imposed by human finitude.

It is wholly fitting that an encyclopedia of bioethics devote some of its space to defining and understanding the field that it would examine in both breadth and depth. Yet that is not an easy task with a field that is still evolving and whose borders are hazy. The word *bioethics,* of recent vintage, has come to denote not just a particular field of human inquiry—the intersection of ethics and the life sciences but also an academic discipline; a political force in medicine, biology, and environmental studies; and a cultural perspective of some consequence. Understood narrowly, bioethics is simply one more new field that has emerged in the face of great scientific and technological changes. Understood more broadly, however, it is a field that has spread into, and in many places has changed, other far older fields. It has reached into law and public policy; into literary, cultural, and historical studies; into the popular media; into the disciplines of philosophy, religion, and literature; and into the scientific fields of medicine, biology, ecology and environment, demography, and the social sciences.

The focus here will be on the broader meaning, place, and significance of bioethics. The aim will be to determine not only what the field means for specific ethical problems in the life sciences, but also what it has to say about the interaction of ethics and human life, and of science and human values. Bioethics is a field that ranges from the anguished private and individual dilemmas faced by physicians or other healthcare workers at the bedside of a dying patient, to the terrible public and societal choices faced by citizens and legislators as they try to devise equitable health or environmental policies. Its problems can be highly individual and personal—what should I do here and now?—and highly communal and political—what should we together do as citizens and fellow human beings?

While the primary focus of this entry will be on medicine and healthcare, the scope of bioethics—as the encyclopedia as a whole makes clear—has come to encompass a number of fields and disciplines broadly grouped under the rubric *the life sciences.* They encompass all those perspectives that seek to understand human nature and behavior, characteristically the domain of the social sciences, and the natural world that provides the habitat of human and animal life, primarily the population and environmental sciences. Yet it is the medical and biological sciences in which bioethics found its initial impetus, and in which it has seen the most intense activity. It thus seems appropriate to make that activity the center of attention here.

## Historical Background

An understanding of the emergence of bioethics will help to capture the panoramic breadth and complexity of the field. The 1960s is a pertinent point of departure, even though there were portents of the new field and issues in earlier decades. That decade brought into confluence two important developments, one scientific and the other cultural. In biomedicine, the 1960s was an era of extraordinary technological progress. It saw the advent of kidney dialysis, organ transplantation, medically safe abortions, the contraceptive pill, prenatal diagnosis, the widespread use of intensive-care units and artificial respirators, a dramatic shift from death at home to death in hospitals or other institutions, and the first glimmerings of genetic engineering. Here was a truly remarkable array of technological developments, the palpable outcome of the great surge in basic biomedical research and application that followed World War II. At the same time, stimulated by Rachel Carson's book *Silent Spring,* there was a gradual awakening to the environmental hazards posed by the human appetite for economic progress and the domination of nature. Taken together, these developments posed a staggering range of difficult, and seemingly new, moral problems.

Bioethics as a field might not have emerged so strongly or insistently had it not been for parallel cultural developments. The decade was the spawning ground for a dazzling array of social and cultural reform efforts. It saw a rebirth, within the discipline of moral philosophy, of an interest in normative and applied ethics, both out of a dissatisfaction with the prevailing academic emphasis on theoretical issues and in response to cultural upheavals. It was the era of the civil-rights movement, which gave African Americans and other people of color new rights and possibilities. It was the era that saw the rebirth of feminism as a potent social movement, and the extension to women of rights often previously denied them. It was the era that saw a fresh surge of individualism—a by-product in many ways of postwar affluence and mobility—and the transformation of many traditional institutions, including the family, the churches, and the schools. It was an era that came to see the enormous possibilities the life sciences offer to combat disease, illness, and death—and no less to see science's possibilities for changing the way human beings could live their lives.

Some of these possibilities had been foreseen in the important book *Medicine and Morals,* written by Joseph Fletcher, an Episcopal theologian who eventually came to reject religious beliefs. He celebrated the power of modern medicine to liberate human beings from the iron grip of nature, putting instead in their hands the power to shape lives of their own choosing. This vision began to be lived out in the 1960s. That decade brought together the medical advances that seemed to foreshadow the eventual conquest of nature and the cultural changes that would empower newly liberated individuals to assume full control of their own destinies. There was in this development both great hope and ambition, and perhaps great hubris, the prideful belief that humans could radically transcend their natural condition.

The advances of the biomedical sciences and their technological application had three great outcomes that came clearly into full view by the 1960s. They transformed first many traditional ideas about the nature and domain of medicine, then the scope and meaning of human health, and, finally, cultural and societal views of what it means to live a human life. Medicine was transformed from a diagnostic and palliative discipline into a potent agent able to cure disease and effectively forestall death. Human "health" more and more encompassed the 1947 World Health Organization definition with its broad emphasis on health as "a state of complete physical, mental, and social well-being and not merely the absence of disease or infirmity." Traditional notions of the living of a life were changed by longer life expectancies, the control of procreation, and powerful pharmacological agents able to modify mood and thought.

The advent of bioethics can be seen as the principal social response to these great changes. If there was any single, overarching question, it might have been this: How were human beings wisely to confront the moral puzzles, perplexities, and challenges posed by the confluence of the great scientific and cultural changes? But this large question concealed an intimidating range of more specific issues. Who should have control over the newly emergent technologies? Who should have the right or privilege to make the crucial moral decisions? How could individuals be assisted in taking advantage of the new medical possibilities or, if need be, protected from being harmed by them? How could the fruits of the medical advances be most fairly distributed? What kind of character or human virtues would be most conducive to a wise use of the new technologies? What kind of institutions, or laws, or regulations would be needed to manage the coming changes in a moral fashion?

## Facts and Values

It soon became evident that such questions required more than a casual response. Two important tasks emerged. One of them, logically the first, was to distinguish the domain of science from that of ethics and values. As a consequence of the triumphalist positivism that during the late nineteenth and the first half of the twentieth century had come to dominate the general understanding of science, matters of ethics and values had been all but banished from serious intellectual discussion. A sharp line could be drawn, it was widely believed, between scientific facts and moral values (MacIntyre, 1981b). The former were solid, authoritative, impersonally true, while the latter were understood to be "soft," relativistic, and highly, even idiosyncratically, personal. Moreover, doctors should make the moral decisions no less than the medical decisions; indeed, a good medical decision was tantamount to a good moral decision. The first task of bioethics, then, was to erase the supposedly clear line that could be drawn between facts and values, and then to challenge the belief that those well trained in science and medicine were as capable of making the moral decisions as the medical decisions.

The second important task was to find or develop the methodologies necessary to come to grips with the new moral problems. If there is no sharp line between facts and values, how should their relationship be understood? If there is a significant difference between making a medical (or scientific) decision and making a moral decision, how are those decisions different and what kinds of skills are needed to make the one or the other? Who has a right to make the different kinds of decisions? If it is neither sensible nor fair to think of moral and value matters as soft and capriciously personal, hardly more than a matter of taste, then how can rigor and objectivity be brought to bear on them?

As the scope and complexity of these two large tasks became more obvious, the field of bioethics began to emerge. From the first, there was a widespread recognition that the moral problems would have to be approached in an interdisciplinary way (Callahan, 1973). Philosophy and religion, long the characteristic arenas for moral insight, analysis, and traditions, should have an important place, as should the historical moral traditions and practices of medicine and biology. Ample room would also have to be made for the law and for the social and policy sciences. Moral problems have important legal, social, political, and policy implications; and moral choices would often be expressed through court decisions, legislative mandates, and assorted regulatory devices. Hardly less important was the problem of which moral decisions should be left to private choice and which required some public standards. While there was a strong trend to remove procreational choices from public scrutiny, and thus to move toward the legal use of contraception and abortion, environmental choices were being moved from private choice to governmental regulation. Debates of this kind require the participation of many disciplines.

While the importance of an interdisciplinary approach was early recognized, three other matters were more troublesome. First, what should be the scope of the field? The term *bioethics,* as it was first used by the biologist Van Rensselaer Potter, referred to a new field devoted to human survival and an improved quality of life, not necessarily or particularly medical in character. The term soon was used differently, however, particularly to distinguish it from the much older field of medical ethics. The latter had traditionally been marked by a heavy, almost exclusive emphasis on the moral obligations of physicians and on the doctor–patient relationship. Yet that emphasis, while still important, was not capacious enough to embrace the huge range of emerging issues and perspectives. *Bioethics* came to refer to the broad terrain of the moral problems of the life sciences, ordinarily taken to encompass medicine, biology, and some important aspects of the environmental, population, and social sciences. The traditional domain of medical ethics would be included within this array, accompanied now by many other topics and problems.

Second, if the new bioethics was to be interdisciplinary, how would it relate to the long-standing disciplines of moral theology and moral philosophy? While those disciplines are able to encompass some interdisciplinary perspectives, they also have their own methodologies, developed over the years to be tight and rigorous. For the most part, moreover, their methodologies are broad, aimed at moral problems in general, not just at biomedical issues. Can they, in their broad, abstract generality, do justice to the particularities of medical or environmental issues?

Another problem becomes apparent. An interdisciplinary field is not necessarily well served by a tight, narrow methodology. Its very purpose is to be open to different perspectives and the different methodologies of different disciplines. Does this mean, then, that although parts of bioethics might be rigorous—the philosophical parts taken by themselves or the legal parts—the field as a whole may be doomed to a pervasive vagueness, never as strong as a whole as its individual parts? This is a charge sometimes leveled against the field, and it has not been easy for its practitioners to find the right balance of breadth, complexity, and analytical rigor.

## Varieties of Bioethics

As the field has developed, it has become clear that because of the range of diversity of bioethics issues, more than one methodology is needed; by the same token, no single discipline can claim a commanding role. At least four general areas of inquiry can be distinguished, even though in practice they often overlap and cannot clearly be separated.

THEORETICAL BIOETHICS. Theoretical bioethics deals with the intellectual foundations of the field. What are its moral roots and what ethical warrant can be found for the moral judgments made in the name of bioethics? Part of the debate turns on whether its foundations should be looked for within the practices and traditions of the life sciences, or whether they have philosophical or theological starting points. Philosophers and theologians have a central place in this enterprise, but draw strongly upon the history and practices of the life sciences to grasp the aims and developments of these fields.

CLINICAL ETHICS. Clinical ethics refers to the day-to-day moral decision making of those caring for patients. Because of that context, it typically focuses on the individual case, seeking to determine what is to be done here and now with a patient. Should a respirator be turned off? Is this patient competent to make a decision? Should the full truth be disclosed to a fearful cancer patient? Individual cases often give rise to great medical and moral uncertainty, and they evoke powerful emotions among those with a role in the

decisions. Decision-making procedures, as well as the melding of theory and practice—what Aristotle called "practical reason"—come sharply into play. It is the concreteness of the judgment that is central here: What is to be done for this patient at this time? The experience of practicing physicians, other healthcare workers, and patients themselves takes a prominent place, yet on occasion can require a collaborative interplay with those trained more specifically in ethics.

REGULATORY AND POLICY BIOETHICS. The aim of regulatory and policy bioethics is to fashion legal or clinical rules and procedures designed to apply to types of cases or general practices; this area of bioethics does not focus on individual cases. The effort in the early 1970s to fashion a new legal definition of clinical death (from a heart-lung to a brain-death definition), the development of guidelines for the use of human subjects in medical research, and hospital rules for do-not-resuscitate (DNR) orders are examples of regulatory ethics. It can also encompass policies designed to allocate scarce healthcare resources or to protect the environment. Regulatory ethics ordinarily seeks laws, rules, policies, and regulations that will command a wide consensus, and its aim is practical rather than theoretical. The law and the policy sciences are highly important in this kind of bioethics work; but it also requires a rich, ongoing dialogue among those concerned with theoretical bioethics, on the one hand, and clinical ethics and political realities, on the other. Regulatory bioethics seeks legal and policy solutions to pressing societal problems that are ethically defensible and clinically sensible and feasible.

CULTURAL BIOETHICS. Cultural bioethics refers to the effort systematically to relate bioethics to the historical, ideological, cultural, and social context in which it is expressed. How do the trends within bioethics reflect the larger culture of which they are a part? What ideological leanings do the moral theories undergirding bioethics openly or implicitly manifest? A heavy emphasis on the moral principle of autonomy or self-determination can, for example, be said to display the political and ideological bias of culturally individualistic societies, notably the United States. Other nations—those in central and eastern Europe, for instance—give societal rather than individual concerns a more pronounced priority (Fox). Solidarity rather than autonomy would be their highest value.

The social sciences, as well as history and the humanities, have a central place in this interpretive effort (Marshall). If done well, the insights and analysis they provide can help everyone to a better understanding of the larger cultural and social dynamic that underlies the ethical problems. Those problems will usually have a social history that reflects the influence of the culture of which they are a part. Even the definition of what constitutes an ethical "problem" will show the force of cultural differences. Countries with strong paternalistic traditions may not consider it necessary to consult with patients about some kinds of decisions; they will not see the issue of patient choice or informed consent as a moral issue at all—yet they may have a far livelier dedication to equality of access to healthcare.

## General Questions of Bioethics

While bioethics as a field may be understood in different ways and be enriched by different perspectives, at its heart lie some basic human questions. Three of them are paramount. What kind of a person ought I to be in order to live a moral life and to make good ethical decisions? What are my duties and obligations to other individuals whose life and well-being may be affected by my actions? What do I owe to the common good, or the public interest, in my life as a member of society? The first question bears on what is often called an ethic of virtue, whose focus is that of personal character and the shaping of those values and goals necessary to be a good and decent person. The second question recognizes that what we do can affect, for good or ill, the lives of others, and tries to understand how we should see our individual human relationships—what we ought to do for others and what we have a right to expect from them. The third question takes our social relationships a step further, recognizing that we are citizens of a nation and members of larger social and political communities. We are citizens and neighbors, sometimes acquaintances, and often people who will and must live together in relatively impersonal, but mutually interdependent, ways.

These are general questions of ethics that can be posed independently of the making of biomedical decisions. They can be asked of people in almost any moral situation or context. Here we encounter an important debate within bioethics. If one asks the general question "What kind of person ought I to be in order to make good moral decisions?" is this different from asking the same question with one change—that of making "good moral decisions in medicine"? One common view holds that a moral decision in medicine ought to be understood as the application of good moral thinking in general to the specific domain of medicine (Clouser). The fact that the decision has a medical component, it is argued, does not make it a different kind of moral problem altogether, but an application of more general moral values or principles. A dutiful doctor is simply a dutiful person who has refined his or her personal character to respond to and care for the sick. He or she is empathic to

suffering, steadfast in devotion to patients, and zealous in seeking their welfare.

Another, somewhat older, more traditional view within medicine is that an ethical decision in medicine is different, precisely because the domain of medicine is different from other areas of human life and because medicine has its own, historically developed, moral approaches and traditions. At the least, it is argued, making a decision within medicine requires a detailed and sensitive appreciation of the characteristic practices of medicine and of the art of medicine, and of the unique features of sick and dying persons. Even more, it requires a recognition of some moral principles, such as *primum non nocere* (first, do no harm) and beneficence, that have a special salience in the doctor–patient relationship (Pellegrino and Thomasma). The argument is not that the ethical principles and virtues of medical practice find no counterpart elsewhere, or do not draw upon more general principles; it is their combination and context that give them their special bite.

## The Foundations of Bioethics

There may not be a definitive resolution to the puzzle of whether bioethics should find its animating moral foundations within or outside medicine and biology. In any case, with time these two sources become mixed, and it seems clear that both can make valuable contributions (Brody, 1987). Perhaps more important is the problem of which moral theories or perspectives offer the most help in responding to moral issues and dilemmas.

Does an ethic of virtue or an ethic of duty offer the best point of departure? In approaching moral decisions, is it more important to have a certain kind of character, disposed to act in certain virtuous ways, or to have at hand moral principles that facilitate making wise or correct choices? The traditions of medicine, emphasizing the complexity and individuality of particular moral decisions at the bedside, have been prone to emphasize those virtues thought to be most important in physicians. They include dedication to the welfare of the patient and empathy for those in pain. Some philosophical traditions, by contrast, have placed the emphasis on *principlism*—the value of particular moral principles that help in the actual making of decisions (Childress; Beauchamp and Childress). These include the principle of respect for persons, and most notably respect for the autonomy of patients; the principle of beneficence, which emphasizes the pursuit of the good and the welfare of the patient; the principle of nonmaleficence, which looks to the avoidance of harm to the patient; and the principle of justice, which stresses treating persons fairly and equitably.

The advantage of principles of this kind is that, in varying ways and to different degrees, they can be used to protect patients against being harmed by medical practitioners and to identify the good of patients that decent medical and healthcare should serve. Yet how are such principles to be grounded, and how are we to determine which of the principles is more or less important when they conflict? Moral principles have typically been grounded in broad theories of ethics—utilitarianism, for example, which justifies acts as moral on the basis of the consequences of those acts (sometimes called consequentialism). Utilitarian approaches ask which consequences of a choice or an action or a policy would promote the best possible outcome. That outcome might be understood as maximizing the widest range of individual preferences, or promoting the greatest predominance of good over evil, or the greatest good of the greatest number. Just what one should judge as a "good" outcome is a source of debate within utilitarian theory, and a source of criticism of that theory. Such an approach to healthcare rationing, for instance, would look for the collective social benefit rather than advantages to individuals.

A competing theory, deontology, focuses on determining which choices most respect the worth and value of the individual, and particularly the fundamental rights of individuals. The question of our basic obligations to other individuals is central. From a deontological perspective, good consequences may on occasion have to be set aside to respect inalienable human rights. It would be wrong, for instance, to subject a human being to dangerous medical research without the person's consent even if the consequences of doing so might be to save the lives of many others. Our transcendent obligation is toward the potential research subject.

Not all debates about moral theory come down to struggles between utilitarianism and deontology, though that struggle has been central to much of the moral philosophy that influenced bioethics in its first decades. Other moral theories, such as that of Aristotle, stress neither principles nor consequences but see a combination of virtuous character and seasoned practical reason as the most likely source of good moral judgment. For that matter, a morality centering on principles raises the problems of the kind of theory necessary to ground those principles, and of how a determination of priorities is to be made when the principles conflict (Clouser and Gert). A respect for patient autonomy, stressing the right of competent patients to make their own choices, can conflict with the principle of beneficence if the choice to be made by the patient may actually be harmful. And autonomy can also conflict with the principle of nonmaleficence if the patient's choice would seem to require that the physician be the person who directly brings harm to the patient.

Another classical struggle turns on the dilemma that arises when respect for individual freedom of choice poses a threat to justice, particularly when an equitable distribution of resources requires limiting individual choice. Autonomy and justice are brought into direct conflict. Recent debates on healthcare rationing, or setting priorities, have made that tension prominent.

Even if principles—like autonomy and justice—are themselves helpful, their value declines sharply when they are pitted against each other. What are we supposed to do when one important moral principle conflicts with another? The approach to ethics through moral principles—often called *applied ethics*—has emphasized drawing those principles from still broader ethical theory, whose role it is to ground the principles. Moral analysis, then, works from the top down, from theory to principles to case application. An alternative way to understand the relationship between principles and their application, far more dialectical in its approach, is the method of *wide reflective equilibrium*. It espouses a constant movement back and forth between principles and human experience, letting each correct and tutor the other (Daniels).

Still another approach is that of casuistry, drawn from methods commonly used in the Middle Ages. In contrast with principlism, it works from the bottom up, focusing on the practical solving of moral problems by a careful analysis of individual cases (Jonsen and Toulmin). A casuistical strategy does not reject the use of principles but sees them as emerging over time, much like the common law that has emerged in the Anglo-American legal tradition. Moral principles derive from actual practices, refined by reflection and experience. Those principles are always open to further revision and reinterpretation in light of new cases. At the same time, a casuistical analysis makes prominent use of analogies, employing older cases to help solve newer ones. If, for instance, general agreement has been reached that it is morally acceptable to turn off the respirator of a dying patient, does this provide a good precedent for withdrawing artificially provided hydration and nutrition? Is the latter form of care morally equivalent to the former, so that the precedent of the former can serve to legitimate the latter? Those are the kinds of questions that a casuistical analysis would ask. At the same time, a casuistical analysis runs the risk of being too bound to past cases and precedents. It can seem to lack the capacity to signal the need for a change of moral direction (Arras).

Still another principle-oriented approach proposes a new social contract between medicine and society (Veatch).

Such a contract would be threefold. It comprises basic ethical principles for society as a whole, a contract between society and the medical profession about the latter's social role, and a contract between professionals and laypersons that spells out the rights and prerogatives of each. This strategy is designed both to place the ethics of medicine squarely within the ethical values of the larger society and to make sure that laypeople have sufficient choice and power to determine the kind of care they, and not paternalistic physicians, choose. Still another approach, more skeptical about finding any strong consensus on ethical foundations, stresses an ethic of secular pluralism and social peace, devising a minimal ethic for the community as a whole but allowing great play to the values and choices of different religious and value subcommunities (Engelhardt).

Contemporary feminist approaches to bioethics, like casuistry, reject the top-down rationalistic and deductivist model of an ethic of principles (Baier; Sherwin). They reject even more adamantly what is seen as the tendency of an ethic of principles to universalize and rationalize. Feminist ethics lays a far heavier emphasis on the context of moral decisions, on the human relationships of those caught in the web of moral problems, and on the importance of feeling and emotion in the making of moral decisions. Feminist approaches, rooted in ways of thinking about morality that long predate the feminist movement of recent decades, also reflect a communitarian bias, reacting against the individualism that has been associated with a principle-oriented approach. Feminist thinkers commonly argue that those who lack power and status in society are often well placed to see the biases even of those societies that pride themselves on equality. While feminism has gained considerable prominence in recent years, it is only one of a number of efforts to find fresh methods and strategies for ethical analysis and understanding. These include phenomenological analyses, narrative-based strategies, and hermeneutical, interpretive perspectives (Zaner; Brody, 1987).

## How Important is Moral Theory?

There can be little doubt that the quest for the foundations of bioethics can be difficult and frustrating, no less so than the broader quest for the foundations of ethics in general (MacIntyre, 1981a). Yet how important for bioethics are moral theory and the quest for a grounding and comprehensive theory? Even the answers to that question are disputed. At one extreme are those who believe that bioethics as a discipline cannot expect intellectual respect, much less legitimately affect moral behavior, unless it can show itself to be grounded in solid theory justifying its proposed virtues,

principles, and rules. At the other extreme are those who contend that—even if there is no consensus on theory—social, political, and legal agreement of a kind sufficient to allow reasonable moral decisions to be made and policy to be set can be achieved. The President's Commission for the Study of Ethical Problems in Medicine and Biomedical and Behavioral Research of the early 1980s, and the National Commission for the Protection of Human Subjects in the mid-1970s, were able to achieve considerable agreement and gain general public and professional respect even though individual members disagreed profoundly on the underlying principles of the consensus. There is of course nothing new in that experience. The American tradition of freedom of religion, for instance, has been justified for very different reasons, both theological and secular—reasons that in principle are in fundamental conflict with each other, yet are serviceable for making policy acceptable to believers and nonbelievers alike.

What kind of authority can a field so full of theoretical and practical disputes have? Why should anyone take it seriously? All important fields, whether scientific or humanistic, argue about their foundations and their findings. Bioethics is hardly unique in that respect. In all fields, moreover, agreement can be achieved on many important practical points and principles even without theoretical consensus. Bridges can be built well even if theoretical physicists disagree about the ultimate nature of matter. But perhaps most important, one way or another, moral decisions will have to be made, and they will have to made whether they are well grounded in theory or not. People must do the best they can with the material at hand. Even in the absence of a full theory, better and worse choices can be made, and more or less adequate justification can be offered. As the field progresses, even the debates on theory can be refined, offering greater insight and guidance even if the theories are still disputable.

Where, then, lies the expertise and authority of bioethics (Noble)? It lies, in the end, in the plausible insight and persuasive rationality of those who can reflect thoughtfully and carefully on moral problems. The first task of bioethics—whether the issues are clinical, touching on the decisions that must be made by individuals, or policy-oriented, touching on the collective decisions of citizens, legislators, or administrators—is to help clarify what should be argued about. A closely related task will be to suggest how these issues should be argued so that sensible, moral decisions can be made. Finally, there will be the more advanced, difficult business of finding and justifying the deepest theories and principles. There can, and will, be contention and argument at each of these stages, and it well may appear at first that no resolution or agreement can be found. Endless, unresolved disagreement in fact rarely occurs in practice, and that is why, if one looks at bioethics over a period of decades, achieved agreement and greater depth can be found, signs of progress in the field. The almost complete acceptance of such concepts as *patient rights, informed consent,* and *brain death,* for instance—all at one time heatedly disputed concepts—shows clearly enough how progress in bioethics is and can be made.

## Making Good Moral Decisions

Good individual decision making encompasses three elements: self-knowledge, knowledge of moral theories and traditions, and cultural perception. Self-knowledge is fundamental because feelings, motives, inclinations, and interests both enlighten and obscure moral understanding. In the end, individual selves, alone with their thoughts and private lives, must wrestle with moral problems. This sort of struggle often forces one to confront the kind of person one is, to face one's character and integrity and one's ability to transcend narrow self-interest to make good moral decisions. And once a decision is made, it must be acted upon. A decision of conscience blends moral judgment and the will to act upon that judgment (Callahan, 1991). A complementary kind of knowledge, not easy to achieve, is also needed. Even as individuals we are social creatures, reflecting the times in which we live, embodied in a particular society at a particular time. Our social embeddedness will shape the way we understand ourselves, the moral problems we encounter, and what we take to be plausible and feasible responses to them. Moral theory by itself is hardly likely to be able to give us all the ingredients needed for an informed, thoughtful moral judgment. Only if it is complemented by self-understanding and reflectiveness about the societal and cultural context of our decisions can moral theory be fleshed out sufficiently to be helpful and illuminating. Good moral judgment requires us to move back and forth among the necessary elements: the reflective self, the interpreted culture, and the contributions of moral theory. No one element is privileged; each has an indispensable part to play.

Yet something else is needed as well: a vision of the human good, both individual and collective. The biomedical, social, and environmental sciences produce apparently endless volumes of new knowledge about human nature and its social and natural setting. However, for that knowledge to be useful or meaningful, it must be seen in light of some notions of what constitutes the good of human life. What should human beings seek in their lives? What constitute good and worthy human ends? Proponents of the technological advances that emerge from the life sciences claim they can enhance human happiness and welfare. But that is likely to be possible only to the extent we have some decent idea of just what we need to bring us happiness and an enhanced welfare.

Bioethics must pay sustained attention to such issues. It cannot long and successfully attend only to questions of procedure, or legal rules and regulations, without asking as well about the ends and goals of human life and activity. Ethical principles, rules, and virtues are in part a function of different notions of what enhances human life. Implicitly or explicitly, a picture of human life provides the frame for different theories and moral strategies of bioethics. This picture should animate living a life of our own, in which we develop our own understanding of how we want to live our individual lives, given the vast array of medical and biological possibilities; living our life with other human beings, which calls up ideas of rights and obligations, bonds of interdependency, and the creation of a life in common; and living our life with the rest of nature, which has its own dynamics and ends but provides us with the nurturing and natural context of our human lives.

Is there such a thing as the human good, either individually or collectively? Is there something we can, in an environmental context, call the good of nature? There is no agreement on the answer to those questions; on the contrary, there is fundamental disagreement. Some would argue that ethics can proceed with a relatively thin notion of the human good, placing the emphasis on developing those moral perspectives that would make it most possible to live with our differences about the meaning and ends of life. Others stress the importance of the substantive issues and reflect some basic doubt about whether ethics can proceed very far, or have sufficient substance, without trying to gain some insight into, and agreement upon, those basic matters (Kass; Callahan, 1993). Those debates must continue.

The greatest power of the biomedical, social, and environmental sciences is their capacity to shape the way we as human beings understand ourselves and the world in which we live. At one level—the most apparent—they give us new choices and thus new moral dilemmas. At another level, however, they force us to confront established views of our human nature, and thus to ask what we should be seeking: What kind of people do we want to be? A choice about artificial reproduction, say surrogate motherhood, is surely a moral choice. But it is also a way into the question of how we should understand the place of procreation in our private lives and in society. To see that is to appreciate profound challenges to our understanding of sexual and familial roles and purposes. The boundaries of bioethics cannot readily be constrained. The expanding boundaries force us to take up larger and deeper problems, much as a small stone tossed into the water creates larger and larger ripples.

## Summary

In its early days, contemporary bioethics was generally seen as an activity on the fringes of research and practice in the life sciences; it had no place within environmental analysis. The dominant view was that the life sciences were a strictly scientific endeavor, with questions of morality and values arising only now and then in the interstices. That view has gradually changed. The life sciences are increasingly understood as, at their core, no less a moral endeavor than a scientific one. Ethics lies at the very heart of the enterprise, if only because facts and values can no longer be clearly separated—any more than the ends of the life sciences can be separated from the means chosen to pursue them.

No less important, questions of the moral means and ends of the life sciences cannot be long distinguished from the moral means and ends of the cultures and societies that pursue and deploy them. Here, fundamental questions must be asked. First, what kind of medicine and healthcare, what kind of stance toward nature and our environment, do we need for the kind of society we want? Such a question presupposes that we have some end in view for our society, though that may not be all that clear. What is clear, however, is that it is almost impossible to think for long about bioethics without being forced to think even more broadly about the society in which it will exist and whose ends—for better or worse—it will serve.

The second question reverses the first: What kind of a society ought we to want in order that the life sciences will be encouraged and helped to make their best contribution to human welfare? The contribution bioethics makes will in great part be a function of the goals sought by the life sciences, and those in turn will be stimulated or formed by society's goals. The life sciences shape the way we think about our lives, and thus they increasingly provide some key ingredients in society's vision of itself and in the lives of the citizens who comprise society.

Understood in terms of these two broad questions, bioethics takes its place at the heart of the enterprise of the life sciences. Only a part of its work will bear on dealing with the daily moral dilemmas and ethical puzzles that are part of contemporary healthcare and environmental protection. A no less substantial part will be to help shape the social context in which those dilemmas and puzzles play themselves out. At its best, bioethics will move back and forth between the concreteness of necessary individual and policy decisions and the broad notions and dynamic of the human situation. It is still a new field, seeking to better define itself and to refine its methods. It has made a start in shaping its direction and possible contribution, but only a start.

DANIEL CALLAHAN (1995)

SEE ALSO: *Abortion; Animal Welfare and Rights; Bioethics Education; Clinical Ethics; Death, Definition and Determination of; Environmental Ethics; Ethics; Eugenics and Religious Law; Fertility Control; Genetic Testing and Screening; Health and Disease; Healthcare Resources; Informed Consent; Life, Quality of; Life Sustaining Treatment and Euthanasia; Medical Ethics, History of; Mental Health; Population Ethics; Reproductive Technologies*

### BIBLIOGRAPHY

Arras, John D. 1991. "Getting Down to Cases: The Revival of Casuistry in Bioethics." *Journal of Medicine and Philosophy* 16(1): 29–51.

Baier, Annette C. 1992. "Alternative Offerings to Asclepius?" *Medical Humanities Review* 6(1): 9–19.

Beauchamp, Tom L., and Childress, James F. 1989. *Principles of Biomedical Ethics*. 3rd edition. New York: Oxford University Press.

Brody, Baruch A. 1988. *Life and Death Decision Making*. New York: Oxford University Press.

Brody, Howard. 1987. *Stories of Sickness*. New Haven, CT: Yale University Press.

Callahan, Daniel. 1973. "Bioethics as a Discipline." *Hastings Center Studies* 1(1): 66–73.

Callahan, Daniel. 1993. *The Troubled Dream of Life: Living with Mortality*. New York: Simon and Schuster.

Callahan, Sidney Cornelia. 1991. *In Good Conscience: Reason and Emotion in Moral Decision Making*. San Francisco: HarperSanFrancisco.

Carson, Rachel. 1962. *Silent Spring*. Boston: Houghton Mifflin.

Childress, James F. 1989. "The Normative Principles of Medical Ethics." In *Medical Ethics*, pp. 27–48, ed. Robert M. Veatch. Boston: Jones and Bartlett.

Clouser, K. Danner. 1978. "Bioethics." In vol. 1 of *Encyclopedia of Bioethics*, pp. 115–127, ed. Warren T. Reich. New York: Free Press.

Clouser, K. Danner, and Gert, Bernard. 1990. "A Critique of Principlism." *Journal of Medicine and Philosophy* 15(2): 219–236.

Daniels, Norman. 1979. "Wide Reflective Equilibrium and Theory Acceptance in Ethics." *Journal of Philosophy* 76(5): 256–282.

Engelhardt, H. Tristram, Jr. 1986. *The Foundations of Bioethics*. New York: Oxford University Press.

Fletcher, Joseph F. 1954. *Morals and Medicine: The Moral Problems of: The Patient's Right to Know the Truth, Contraception, Artificial Insemination, Sterilization, Euthanasia.* Boston: Beacon.

Fox, Renée C. 1990. "The Evolution of American Bioethics: A Sociological Perspective." In *Social Science Perspectives on Medical Ethics,* pp. 201–217, ed. George Weisz. Philadelphia: University of Pennsylvania Press.

Hoffmaster, Barry. 1991. "The Theory and Practice of Applied Ethics." *Dialogue* 30(2): 213–234.

Jonsen, Albert R., and Toulmin, Stephen E. 1988. *The Abuse of Casuistry: A History of Moral Reasoning.* Berkeley: University of California Press.

Kass, Leon R. 1985. *Toward a More Natural Science: Biology and Human Affairs.* New York: Free Press.

MacIntyre, Alasdair. 1981a. "A Crisis in Moral Philosophy: Why Is the Search for the Foundations of Ethics So Frustrating?" In *The Roots of Ethics: Science, Religion, and Values,* pp. 3–20, ed. Daniel Callahan and H. Tristram Engelhardt, Jr. New York: Plenum.

MacIntyre, Alasdair. 1981b. *After Virtue.* Notre Dame, IN: University of Notre Dame Press.

Marshall, Patricia A. 1992. "Anthropology and Bioethics." *Medical Anthropology Quarterly* 6(1): 49–73.

Noble, Cheryl N. 1982. "Ethics and Experts." *Hastings Center Report* 12(3): 7–9.

Pellegrino, Edmund D., and Thomasma, David C. 1981. *A Philosophical Basis of Medical Practice: Toward a Philosophy and Ethic of the Healing Professions.* New York: Oxford University Press.

Potter, Van Rensselaer. 1971. *Bioethics: Bridge to the Future.* Englewood Cliffs, NJ: Prentice-Hall.

Sherwin, Susan. 1992. *No Longer Patient: Feminist Ethics and Health Care.* Philadelphia: Temple University Press.

Toulmin, Stephen. 1981. "The Tyranny of Principles." *Hastings Center Report* 11(6): 31–39.

Veatch, Robert M. 1981. *A Theory of Medical Ethics.* New York: Basic Books.

Zaner, Richard M. 1988. *Ethics and the Clinical Encounter.* Englewood Cliffs, NJ: Prentice-Hall.

# BIOETHICS: AFRICAN-AMERICAN PERSPECTIVES

• • •

The type of healthcare delivery system used by a society says a great deal about what that society thinks of its most vulnerable citizens. African Americans in U.S. society have historically been treated unfairly in every dimension of group and individual life—subjected to segregated and inferior medical services, housing, employment, education, as well as racist environmental policies and practices. These are all factors that determine the collective and individual health of African Americans, which has been, and continues to be, worse than that of white people in the United States.

Until recently, mainstream bioethics paid little attention to the role of race, racism, and ethnicity in bioethical discourse. As opposed to specific issues like stem cell research, abortion, or end-of-life discussions, race plays a role in every ethical conundrum from violation of informed consent to allocation of organ donations. Notably, over the last few years, more bioethicists are devoting serious scholarship to the examination of race as a topic for debate.

An African-American perspective on bioethical issues brings to the table concerns that are important to the health and well-being of African Americans, concerns that are marginalized in mainstream bioethics. They include racial disparities in health status; racial disparities in access to healthcare and technologies; continued medical research abuses; and other factors contributing to poor health such as toxic dumping in communities of color, poor housing, dangerous jobs, and lack of adequate health insurance. African-American perspectives address a major principle: The health disparities of U.S. racial and ethnic groups are a fundamental bioethics issue.

## Bioethics Perspective I: Health Disparities

What are health disparities and why are they ethical violations? Olivia Carter-Pokras and Claudia Baquet discuss a number of definitions that have emerged since 1985, when the U.S. Department of Health and Human Services issued the *Report of the Secretary's Task Force on Black and Minority Health.* The Task Force defines health disparities as excess mortality of minorities as compared to that of whites. Healthy People 2010, whose goal is to eliminate disparities, defines them as differences that occur by gender, race or ethnicity, education or income, disability, and residence in rural localities. The National Institutes of Health (NIH) defines disparities as differences in incidence, prevalence, mortality, and burden of disease (Carter-Pokras and Baquet).

According to reports from the Centers for Disease Control (CDC), African Americans have higher death rates than whites due to cancers, diabetes, cirrhosis, homicide, AIDS, and cardiovascular diseases. Maternal death is between three and four times higher for black women than for white women. More white women have breast cancer, but the death rate is higher in black women and is increasing.

The excessive rates of illness contribute to the higher mortality rate of African Americans; the National Vital Statistics Report puts life expectancy for white women at 80.0 years; 74.9 years for black women; 74.8 years for white men; and for black men it is 68.2 years (Arias).

Beginning with slavery and continuing throughout the twentieth century, a persistent and disturbing gap has characterized the health status of African Americans and whites. At emancipation public health officials predicted that freedom would lead to the extinction of the former slaves, who did, in fact suffer numerous health problems, including tuberculosis, malaria, excessive malnutrition, pellagra, and syphilis. The disparities continued throughout the twentieth century and into the beginning of the twenty-first.

A number of reports and policies established goals and recommendations to improve the alarming state of African Americans' health. With the launching of Medicare and Medicaid in 1966, the health of blacks improved, as did that of whites, but the health gap remained. In 1985 the previously mentioned Task Force made recommendations for reducing the disparities. In 1990 the American Medical Association (AMA) Council on Ethical and Judicial Affairs published an influential and much cited article on the disparities. In 1998 President Bill Clinton established the *Initiative to Eliminate Race and Ethnic Disparities* in health by 2020.

Despite some improvement over the years, the health gaps persevere and in some instances have gotten worse as the twenty-first century began. In 1970 infant mortality in blacks was twice that of whites; at the beginning of the twenty-first century, black infant mortality is still twice that of whites. In 1970 deaths due to asthma were about three times higher in blacks; at the beginning of the twenty-first century, deaths due to asthma have increased: They are now five times higher than in whites (Centers for Disease Control, 1996). Researchers Robert Levine and his colleagues report that the disparities have not improved since the end of World War II, despite decades of funding for health-related programs.

Some observers attribute the health gap to biology, suggesting that excess infant deaths and disproportionate incidences of lung cancer and breast cancer deaths are due to genetic differences. Others attribute the high rate of sickness and death to *irresponsible lifestyles*. According to this explanation, African-American women and men refuse or neglect to get timely cancer screenings until it is too late to curb the spread of the condition, or they prefer to smoke high-nicotine content cigarettes and drink high-alcohol content liquor that increase lung and liver disease (Moore, Williams, and Qualls). Still others attribute the disparity in health status to cultural attitudes and deficits that prevent health-seeking behaviors that take advantage of available health services; patient and family beliefs at variance with those of medical professionals; and negative attitudes toward healthcare providers. This explanation, for example, asserts that African Americans prefer dialysis to a kidney transplant (Ayanian et al.). In particular, many authors single out suspicion of the healthcare system as a barrier to seeking care. Indeed, many African Americans fear that they will become guinea pigs for unethical medical research (Thomas and Quinn; Dula).

Health researchers are beginning to acknowledge that health disparities do not merely reflect class, lifestyle choices, or genetics. They are also a result of current and accumulative racism and discrimination in U.S. society (Peterson et al.). Yet the word racism is grudgingly used even though it is a statistical fact that one's race often determines the quality and quantity of services, procedures, and healthcare that one receives. Health disparities must be understood as a bioethical issue if they result in more sickness and shorter life spans for African-American populations as compared to white populations. If these disparities are a result of racial discrimination, they ought to be ethically unacceptable in a just society.

## Bioethics Perspective II: Race and Racism in Access to Healthcare

Differential treatment based on race or the group to which one belongs is an ethical problem because such treatment usually has a negative impact on life opportunities, education, and physical and mental well-being. African Americans have always been sicker and lived fewer years than whites; they have historically had—and continue to receive—different, unequal, and inferior access to healthcare. The prestigious Institute of Medicine's (IOM) March 2002 report evaluated over 100 studies focusing on health disparities published over the previous ten years. The IOM panel found that minorities who have the same income, education, medical conditions, and insurance as whites still receive poorer care than do the latter, showing that race is a significant variable in the health and healthcare of African Americans. Even though heart disease is a top killer of African Americans, whites get more aggressive treatment. Blacks with coronary heart disease are significantly less likely than whites to undergo bypass surgery, angioplasty, and a host of other services and procedures. Differential and racist treatment regarding kidney transplants, intensive care unit (ICU) treatment, and even the kind of information provided to pregnant women of different races have all been thoroughly documented.

Differential treatment is illustrated in government programs that provide health insurance for poor people on

Medicaid, elders insured by Medicare, and U.S. veterans. In these systems, no money is passed between patient and provider; thus, one assumes that patient enrollees in these three programs would be treated fairly, regardless of race. Studies of the distribution of services under all three programs show that blacks get a lower quality of care that whites. Under Medicare Managed Care, African Americans are less likely to receive breast cancer screening, diabetic eye examinations, beta-blockers for myocardial infarction, and mental health follow-up (Schneider, Zaslavsky, and Epstein). In Veterans Administration (VA) hospitals, black U.S. veterans get substantially fewer treatments for Acute Myocardial Infarction (AMI) than do white veterans and are less likely to undergo cardiac catheterization and to receive coronary bypass surgery (Peterson et al.). Medicaid too offers differential and substandard treatment to people of color. African-American children have a disproportional incidence of asthma; prevalence is twice that of whites, and death rates between 1980 and 1993 were four to six times higher (Centers for Disease Control, 1997; National Institute of Allergy and Infectious Diseases). Yet black and Latino children with worse asthma status are prescribed fewer preventive asthma medications than are white children within the same managed Medicaid plan (Lieu, Lozano, and Finkelstein).

Government programs also perpetuate disparities in health status and access to services in other ways. Due to federal medical criteria, African Americans receive proportionately fewer kidneys and they wait twice as long for them as whites. World-renowned transplant surgeon Thomas Starzl and his colleagues report that the national kidney allocation system inherently favors white patients because of the heavy emphasis placed on donor-recipient compatibility. They argue that antigen matching should not weigh so heavily in deciding who gets a kidney since differences in survival rates (the justification for current donor allocation) are negligible (Starzl, Aliasziw, and Gjertson).

Whether disproportional access to healthcare and services is intentional, it is clear that race is a factor in the delivery of healthcare in the United States. Although discussions of racism in healthcare and services have been prominent in other academic disciplines, it has been insufficiently explored in the area of bioethics. Differential treatment in access to healthcare is unassailably a bioethics issue.

## Bioethics Perspective III: Informed Consent and Racism in Research

Informed consent in research is an ethical principle that has particular relevance to African Americans and similarly vulnerable populations. Throughout the history of this country, medical research has supported racist social institutions. The Tuskegee Syphilis Experiment (TSS) is the most egregious violation of informed consent against a specific group of people, but it certainly is not an isolated example. Enslaved women were used to conduct painful research on urine leaks into the vagina and black women were used to perfect Cesarean sections (Reverby). More recently, President Clinton's Advisory Committee on Human Radiation Experiments observed that in several studies, research subjects were disproportionately chosen from minority populations. Questions have also been raised about an early 1990s measles vaccine trial that involved mostly minority children in several inner cities (Marwick). All these studies are examples of research without consent.

Although blacks have been over-represented in unethical research, generally they have been excluded from ethically conducted research studies that might benefit future populations of African Americans. In an attempt to remedy this, the NIH Revitalization Act of 1993 mandated that women and minorities be included in federally funded research. However, during the ten years since the enactment, despite attempts at aggressive recruitment, researchers still have difficulty enrolling African Americans in clinical trials. Low participation is due to mistrust of the medical/scientific community because of real and perceived medical abuse; poor access to primary care physicians who make most referrals to trials; scarcity of minority health professionals who might facilitate enrollment; potential enrollees' lack of knowledge about clinical trials; and language and cultural barriers. The most significant factor that contributes to low participation in clinical trials is African American suspicion of the healthcare system. Until researchers understand the psychic, physical, and emotional damage done by racism in medicine and in the larger society, they will continue to have trouble recruiting African Americans for research. Despite possible benefits from research, an African-American perspective reminds one that research still offers a potent possibility for continued abuse.

## Bioethics Perspective IV: Difference and Biology

One goal of the TSS was to show that the course of syphilis was different in blacks, suggesting biological differences between blacks and whites. Similarly, an underlying motive behind the enactment of the aforementioned NIH Revitalization initiative was that minorities and women sometimes respond differently from white men to the same drug, again suggesting the possibility of biological difference among races.

Belief in biological difference has long been used to justify different treatment in social arrangements. Aristotle said that from their birth, some people were set out for subjection and others to rule. Slaves were to be ruled by their masters, women by their husbands, and children by their parents. Difference has been used to establish authority and hierarchies; dominance and subordination; superiority and inferiority; the rulers and the ruled; us and them; good and evil; the beautiful and the ugly; and the civilized and the savage. Concepts of difference have been used to oppress, exploit, maintain the status quo, strip people of their rights, and prevent them from making decisions regarding their own well-being. For the most part these hierarchies in the United States have separated whites from nonwhites.

The construction of *difference* or *the other* was used as a rationale so that one group—the group in power—could do as they wished with another group. The political uses of difference led to slavery, colonialism, racism, classism, and sexism, as well as other atrocities and racist brutalities like lynching, rape, medical neglect, and research abuse. The construction of the other worked well for those in power; if people were biologically different—not quite human—they did not have to be treated as moral agents. This of course was part of the implicit justification for the TSS. The men were different (they were black), so they could be treated differently.

Scientists have long been fascinated with the possibility of genetic differences between blacks and whites and they continue to search for *black* genes that explain disproportionate susceptibility to breast and lung cancers, heart disease, violent behavior and intelligence deficits, poverty, and the relation between race and detrimental health effects of environmental pollution.

In the March 20, 2003, issue of the *New England Journal of Medicine,* two articles highlight the controversy surrounding race and disease susceptibility. On the one hand, Esteban Gonzalez Burchard and his colleagues argue that there are racial and ethnic differences in the causes and expressions of various diseases. Richard Cooper and his colleagues, on the other hand, see race as a social category, not biological, and think that doctors have been too quick to suggest genetics as the reason for the greater susceptibility of African Americans to certain diseases. As with the TSS, race is again explicitly linked to ideas of biological differences between racial and ethnic groups (Cooper, Kaufman, and Ward).

As the debate about biology and disease susceptibility continues, the TSS is a reminder of the hazards of research on race-based differences. Genetic explanations often neglect or gloss over the interactions of genes and the environment. It is important to remember that when blacks receive comparable treatment for lung cancer or breast cancer, their survival rate is comparable to that of whites (Bach, Schrag, and Brawley) and that when black VA patients receive the same treatment as whites, they also receive a survival advantage (Jha et al.).

## Bioethics Perspective V: The Colorblindness of Bioethics

Bioethicists, in efforts to be colorblind, *white* out the experience of color as a bioethical issue, as well as the harmful effects of racism on health. A colorblind bioethics has the unfortunate potential of increasing health inequalities if it recognizes only the larger ethical issue in a policy or practice, and not also how that policy might affect less dominant populations. When ethicists ignore race, they remove racism and its effects on health from ethical debate. In a sense, a colorblind bioethics is misleading because it makes judgments based on incomplete information. Regrettably, race and racism are not high priority topics in bioethics.

The TSS is the paradigm case of the intersection of race, bioethics, and the healthcare system. In Macon County, Alabama, between 1932 and 1972, the U.S. Public Health Service conducted a study involving 399 African-American men and 200 controls to determine the course of untreated syphilis in the male Negro. During the study the men were told that they were being treated for bad blood. When the case came to public attention in 1972, a great deal of the bioethical discussion and debate centered around the lack of informed consent; deception and lying; the ethical and scientific benefits of research; the ethics of withholding treatment once penicillin became available; and the ethics of active intervention to prevent treatment. At the time of public disclosure of the study, there was little analysis of racism as a bioethics issue, even though the ethical violations clearly involved only black men and their families. The early failure to address the racism underlying the experiment illustrates the misguided colorblindness of bioethics.

Certainly mainstream bioethicists have done extremely valuable work from which society as a whole has benefited. Nonetheless white bioethicists have defined and shaped the field, deciding what is important. The interests, problems, and standpoints of those in power have obscured the unique concerns—race and racism in the healthcare system and in society at large—of African American and other people of color.

Happily, this is changing. More mainstream bioethicists are stepping outside their traditional role as white bioethicists, to consider race, racism, and white privilege as a valid bioethics concern. Bioethicist Catherine Myser—in an article dedicated to the late African-American bioethicist Marian Secundy—argues in the 2003 Spring issue of the *American Journal of Bioethics* that the cultural construction of bioethics in the United States has not sufficiently questioned the dominance and normativity of whiteness. The September–October 2001 issue of the *Hastings Center Report* also presented several articles on race and bioethics, including pieces by historian Susan Reverby and bioethicist Lawrence Gostin. Editor Greg Kaebnick comments on the movement of bioethicists to consider little talked about topics like race. Reverby revisits the TSS, and Gostin discusses the rights of pregnant women drawing on the late 1980s Medical University of South Carolina policy, which tested poor black pregnant women on Medicaid—without their consent—for drugs.

This entry has focused on some issues that make up a framework for African-American bioethcs: the ethics of health disparities, unequal access to healthcare based on race, and informed consent in research. Other framing issues include religion and suspicion of the healthcare system. Religion and spirituality play dominant roles in the lives of a majority of African Americans and is connected to social change. Any worldview that ignores this will fail to represent African-American reality. Also, any worldview that purports to represent African-American perspectives must take into account the widespread suspicion of the healthcare system. Suspicion has inhibited African Americans from participating in clinical trials for fear of being used as guinea pigs; it has led to false beliefs that the U.S government purposely infected the TSS men with syphilis; and it is responsible for the belief that the U.S. government is capable of genocide of the black population. Some think suspicion keeps African Americans from seeking timely care. The source of the suspicion resides in historically abusive treatment of African Americans at the hands of the healthcare system and the larger society. Annette Dula and Sara Goering's 1994 book *"It Just Ain't Fair": The Ethics of Health Care for African Americans* outlines additional considerations for African-American perspectives on bioethics.

When examined in this framework, from this perspective, every bioethics issues has a race/ethnicity element. For example, an African-American perspective challenges mainstream assumptions around end-of-life discussions. One mainstream assumption is that at the end of life, people will get unwanted healthcare that will compromise their dignity. Many African Americans believe the opposite; they are afraid that they will not get any treatment, let alone unwanted treatment, at the end of life. As a result they want all the care they can get at the end of life, even if it makes no sense. Given the lack of fair access to healthcare, the fear makes sense. Another assumption around end-of-life care is

that people want to die with dignity. Mainstream bioethics associates dignity with quality of life. Most African Americans prefer quantity to quality of life, challenging the mainstream definition of dignity. Again this is reasonable since quantity of life for blacks has always been less than that for whites, and is often due to unfair practices of the healthcare system.

In a March 6, 2002, News Release, the Commonwealth Fund reported that African Americans are more likely than whites to experience difficulty communicating with physicians and to feel as if they were treated with disrespect when receiving healthcare. The doctor–patient relationship influences the quality of communication and health outcome. Doctor–patient communication is an important bioethics issue and has generated tomes of information. Just as African Americans have less access to healthcare, they also have fewer discussions with their physicians and their visits are less participatory. In many instances there is no meaningful communication because more blacks than whites lack a regular physician.

This discussion is meant not to vilify mainstream bioethics, but to show the need for a perspective and interpretation that focuses on bioethics issues that have a unique relevance for African-American populations.

ANNETTE DULA

**SEE ALSO:** *African Religions; Christianity, Bioethics in; Genetics and Racial Minorities; International Health; Islam, Bioethics in; Justice; Medical Ethics, History of Africa; Medicine, Anthropology of; Medicine, Sociology of; Minorities as Research Subjects; Organ Transplants, Sociocultural Aspects of; Race and Racism; Research, Multinational*

### BIBLIOGRAPHY

Advisory Committee on Human Radiation Experiments. 1996. *The Human Radiation Experiments.* New York: Oxford University Press.

Ayanian, John Z.; Cleary, Paul D.; Weissman, Joel S.; and Epstein, Arnold M. 1999. "The Effect of Patients' Preferences on Racial Differences in Access to Renal Transplantation." *New England Journal of Medicine* 341(1): 1661.

Bach, Peter; Schrag, Deborah; and Brawley, Otis. 2002. "Survival of Blacks and Whites after a Cancer Diagnosis." *Journal of the American Medical Association* 287(16): 2106–2113.

Burchard, Esteban Gonzalez; Ziv, Elad; Coyle, Natasha; et al. 2003. "The Importance of Race and Ethnic Background in Biomedical Research and Clinical Practice." *New England Journal of Medicine* 348(12): 1170–1175.

Carter-Pokras, Olivia, and Baquet, Claudia. 2002. "What Is a Health Disparity?" *Public Health Reports* 117: 426–434.

Centers for Disease Control. 1996. "Mortality Patterns—United States, 1993." *Morbidity and Mortality Weekly Report* 45(8): 161–163.

Centers for Disease Control. 1997. "Asthma Hospitalizations and Readmissions Among Children and Young Adults—Wisconsin, 1991–1995." *Morbidity and Mortality Weekly Report* 46(31): 726–728.

Cooper, Richard. S.; Kaufman, Jay. S.; and Ward, Ryk. 2003. "Race and Genomics." *New England Journal of Medicine* 348(12): 1166–1170.

Council on Ethical and Judicial Affairs. 1990. "Black-White Disparities in Health Care." *Journal of the American Medical Association* 263(17): 2344–2346.

Dula, Annette. 1994. "African American Suspicion of the Healthcare System is Justified: What Do We Do about It?" *Cambridge Quarterly of Healthcare Ethics* 3(3): 47–57.

Dula, Annette, and Goering, Sara, eds. 1994. *"It Just Ain't Fair!": The Ethics of Health Care for African Americans.* Westport, CT: Praeger.

Gostin, Lawrence O. 2001. "The Rights of Pregnant Women: The Supreme Court and Drug Testing." *Hastings Center Report* 31(5): 8–9.

Jha, Ashish K.; Shlipak, Michael G.; et al. 2001. "Racial Differences in Mortality among Men Hospitalized in the Veterans Affairs Healthcare System." *Journal of the American Medical Association* 285(3): 297–303.

Levine, Robert S.; Foster, James E.; Fullilove, Robert E.; et al. 2001. "Black-White Inequalities in Mortality and Life Expectancy, 1933–1999: Implications for Healthy People 2010." *Public Health Reports* 116(5): 474–483.

Lieu, Tracy A.; Lozano, Paula; and Finkelstein, Jonathon A. 2002. "Racial/Ethnic Variation in Asthma Status and Management Practices among Children in Managed Medicaid." *Pediatrics* 109(5): 857–865.

Marwick, Charles. 1996. "Questions Raised about Measles Vaccine Trial." *Journal of the American Medical Association* 276(16): 1288–1289.

Moore, David J.; Williams, Jerome D.; and Qualls, William J. 1996. "Target Marketing of Tobbaco and Alcohol-Related Products to Ethnic Minority Groups in the United States." *Ethnicity and Disease* 6(1,2): 83–99.

Myser, Catherine. 2003. "Differences from Somewhere: The Normativity of Whiteness in Bioethics in the United States." *American Journal of Bioethics* 3(2).

Peterson, Eric D.; Shaw, Linda K.; DeLong, Elizabeth R.; et al. 1997. "Racial Variation in the Use of Coronary-Revascularization Procedures—Are The Differences Real? Do They Matter?" *New England Journal of Medicine* 336(7): 480–486.

Reverby, Susan. 2001. "More Than Fact and Fiction." *Hastings Center Report* 31(5): 22–28.

Schneider, Eric C.; Zaslavsky, Alan M.; and Epstein, Arnold M. 2002. "Racial Disparities in the Quality of Care for Enrollees in Medicare Managed Care." *Journal of the American Medical Association* 287(10): 1288–1294.

Starzl, Thomas E.; Aliasziw, M. E.; and Gjertson, D. 1997. "HLA and Cross-Reactive Antigen Group Matching for Cadaver Kidney Allocation." *Transplantation* 64(7): 983–991.

Thomas, Stephen B., and Quinn, Sandra Crouse. 1991. "The Tuskegee Syphilis Study, 1932 to 1972: Implications for HIV Education and the AIDS Risk Programs in the Black Community." *American Journal of Public Health* 81(11): 1498–1505.

INTERNET RESOURCES

Arias, Elizabeth. 2002. "United States Life Tables." *National Vital Statistics Reports* 51(3): 1–39. Available from <http://www.cdc.gov/nchs/data/nvsr/nvsr51/nvsr51_03.pdf>.

Commonwealth Fund. "Minority Americans Lag Behind Whites on Nearly Every Measure of Health Care Quality." Available from <http://www.cmwf.org/media/releases/collins523_release03062002.asp>.

National Institute of Allergy and Infectious Diseases. 2001. Asthma: A Concern for Minority Populations. Available from <http://www.niaid.nih.gov/factsheets/asthma.htm>.

# BIOETHICS EDUCATION

• • •

I.   Medicine

II.  Nursing

III. Secondary and Postsecondary Education

IV.  Other Health Professions

## I. MEDICINE

Education in medical ethics is as old as medical education itself. The Hippocratic school of medicine of fourth-century B.C.E. Greece is best remembered for the Hippocratic oath, which has provided moral guidance to students of medicine for more than two millennia.

For most of medicine's history, efforts to inculcate ethical precepts relied on the apprenticeship model, through which medical students were guided in the simultaneous development of their knowledge, technical skill and judgment, and evolving sense of proper professional conduct (Bosk). Direct observation and emulation were the primary methods apprentices used to develop clinical judgment regarding right action.

In the second half of the twentieth century, however, the emerging field of biomedical ethics catalyzed a radical reexamination of the ways in which students learn to understand and manage ethical issues that arise in professional medical practice. Initially, this effort was led by nonphysician humanists—philosophers, theologians, and others—who developed interests in applied ethics and the medical humanities. In the early 1970s, medical schools, led by Penn State University, hired these humanists and began to offer first elective, then required, ethics courses for medical students. Rather than concentrating on the importance of mentorship and role modeling, these courses were rooted in a philosophical model, stressing ethical concepts such as autonomy and the importance of learning to apply ethical principles to discern the proper course of action. Lectures and seminars became the dominant method used to teach these cognitive skills. Unfortunately, with rare exceptions, the content of ethics training, particularly in the clinical years, has been either on the extreme ends of life or on technological innovations rather than on the day-to-day work of doctoring or justice-based concerns. Starting in the late 1990s, the difference in goals and methods between an apprenticeship model and a philosophical model of teaching medical ethics began to blur as programs focusing on professionalism arose. These programs concentrate more on physician character and offer the opportunity for medical ethics to focus more on the mundane ethical issues of doctoring.

## The Growth of Medical Ethics Education

A series of empirical studies in the 1970s and 1980s documented the rapid growth of teaching programs. In a 1974 survey, 97 of 107 responding medical schools reported teaching medical ethics (Veatch and Solitto). Only six of these schools, however, reported a required exposure to medical ethics. In 1982 a majority of physicians reported that they had never received formal education in clinical ethics, and many felt inadequately prepared for common ethical problems in medicine (Pellegrino et al.). A 1985 study found that 84 percent of U.S. medical schools had some form of human values curricula during the first two years (Bickel). By 1989, 43 of 127 U.S. medical schools reported separate required courses in medical ethics (Miles et al.). In 2000, of the 125 American medical schools, 46 reported separate, required courses in medical ethics, 104 taught medical ethics as part of a required course, and 44 had separate electives in medical ethics; the numbers for teaching in medical humanities were 8, 87, and 51, respectively. The 2002 Association of American Medical Colleges (AAMC) graduation survey found that between 70 and 80 percent of students felt they had received adequate training in medical ethics.

It was not until the latter part of the 1980s that educators began to advocate explicit teaching in medical ethics during residency training. This is a critical formative period, because it is during their residency that physicians first acquire decision-making responsibilities, and thus can fully appreciate the relevance of medical ethics to patient care. In 1984 researchers found that residents in 40 percent of internal medicine residencies had no formal exposure to clinical ethics teaching (Povar and Keith). Two reports by the American Board of Internal Medicine and American Board of Pediatrics in the 1980s provided strong impetus to the development of teaching programs during the residency years. Since then, a growing number of other boards have issued recommendations regarding the teaching of medical ethics during residency. Moreover, residency requirements in medicine, surgery, pediatrics, and obstetrics-gynecology all require education in medical ethics, and the 2003 description of general competencies promulgated by the Accreditation Council for Graduate Medical Education (ACGME) requires that all residents "demonstrate a commitment to ethical principles pertaining to provision or withholding of clinical care, confidentiality of patient information, informed consent, and business practices" (ACGME website).

There was a long tradition of teaching medical deontology (study of moral obligation) in both Europe and Latin America, particularly in Catholic medical schools. But the 1980s saw in these countries, as in North America, a steady expansion of the number and scope of medical ethics programs. In Great Britain, the General Medical Council created a committee in 1984 to study the teaching of medical ethics in British medical schools and make recommendations. The resulting 1987 "Pond Report" recommended that the teaching of medical ethics be encouraged in medical school, but no specific guidelines were advocated (Institute of Medical Ethics). While initially little progress was made, a later study found that most medical schools included ethics education (Goldie).

A 1991 study in Canada found that fifteen of the sixteen Canadian medical schools provided medical ethics education and some sort of examination, with the number of required hours ranging from 10.5 to 45 (Baylis and Downie). Almost all of the schools used physicians as instructors and focused on specific ethical issues (e.g., euthanasia), as opposed to ethical theory or professional codes of ethics. The College of Family Physicians of Canada and the Royal College of Physician and Surgeons of Canada require ethics training, and there is increasing interest in continuing education in bioethics (McKneally and Singer).

In numerous other countries, medical schools have developed curricula in medical ethics. At Lagos University in Nigeria, two-day workshops were initiated in 1982 for fourth-year students, at which lawyers, doctors, and patients all participated in lectures and discussions of issues in medical ethics (Olukoya). In Australia, medical graduates are required to understand basic medical ethics principles, and in the early 2000s educators promulgated a core curriculum (Working Group).

During this period of rapid growth in formal medical ethics education, a wide variety of activities were subsumed under the general heading of "ethics programs." There was great variability in the establishment of explicit curricular goals, the identification and support of teaching faculty, the teaching methods that were employed, and the attempts (if any) at evaluation of educational success. Although a degree of consensus evolved for some areas, important areas of controversy remain.

## Goals

Ambitious and diverse goals have been proposed for medical ethics education, including increased awareness of ethical issues; a cultivation of basic ethical commitments; more humane medical practice; tolerance of conflicting views; development of analytic skill in moral reasoning; enhanced intellectual development in ethics and the humanities; positive attitudes toward patients; less paternalism in clinical practice; higher professional conduct; and improved clinical decision making (Callahan; Miles et al.).

Despite this dauntingly heterogeneous list, a consensus has developed regarding some core objectives. First, the primary goal of clinical ethics education is to prepare physicians to deal effectively with ethical issues in clinical practice. Accomplishing this requires that students learn to: (1) recognize ethical issues as they arise in clinical care and identify hidden values and unacknowledged conflicts; (2) think clearly and critically about ethical issues in ways that lead to an ethically justifiable course of action; and (3) apply the practical skills needed to implement an ethically justifiable course of action. Each of these objectives in turn requires that the students possess specific knowledge, attitudes, and skills.

To recognize ethical issues as they appear in clinical care usually requires a positive attitude concerning the importance of the humanistic and value-laden aspects of medical care. For example, a physician's decision regarding chemotherapy for a woman with breast cancer involves the physician's awareness of the biomedical issues and of the morbidity and mortality of the disease, as well as of the patient's own views regarding continued life, her body image, and the morbidity of treatment. Recognizing the presence of an ethical issue also requires knowledge of the nature of common ethical issues and how they arise in clinical practice.

Finally, proficiency in recognizing these issues requires students to learn certain behaviors. Highly motivated students who understand the importance of autonomy and recognize the ways in which patients' values are frequently ignored or overridden will still have difficulty incorporating respect for autonomy into care unless they become skilled in eliciting their patients' personal values, concerns, and goals.

A general consensus was also developed in the 1980s regarding most of the core content areas for medical ethics education. In the 1985 report of the DeCamp Conference (Culver et al.), leading physicians and ethicists proposed "basic curricular goals in medical ethics," stressing knowledge and ability as the primary targets of medical ethics education in medical schools. Among the seven items in the "minimal basic curriculum" are the ability to obtain a valid consent to treatment or a valid refusal of treatment, knowledge of how to proceed if a patient refuses treatment, and knowledge of the moral aspects of the care of patients with a poor prognosis, including patients who are terminally ill. Notably absent from this "core list," because of a lack of consensus, were issues related to financial aspects of medical care (including distributive justice and access to healthcare), doctor's societal obligations, and questions related to abortion. Interestingly, the U.K. and Australian consensus statements on core curricula are much broader and include both issues of resource distribution and physicians' role in society in their purview. (Whether this influences what is taught is unknown.) Building on these earlier reports, subsequent teaching programs increasingly stressed the importance of ensuring that educational goals are appropriate to students' specific level of training and future career choices. Courses for first- and second-year medical students, who have limited clinical experience, generally focused on developing an awareness of the complex moral issues that arise in contemporary medicine and on developing skill in moral reasoning. In contrast, teaching programs for physicians in subspecialty residency programs tended to focus on the specific issues that those physicians were already encountering in their fields of practice and the specific knowledge, attitudes, and skills needed to address those problems.

Attempts to teach medical ethics through "professionalism" began in the late 1990s. Professional organizations, such as the American Board of Internal Medicine and the ACGME, define professionalism in terms of virtues such as altruism, respect for others, honor, integrity, accountability, competence, and duty/advocacy. These statements typically stress physicians' public role in promoting health in terms of quality and access as much as they stress individual patient care (ABIM Foundation). Interesting the 2001 AAMC graduate medical student survey assessed professionalism separately from medical ethics, reflecting some confusion between the two content areas.

## Methods

Given the diverse objectives of ethics education, it is no surprise that a variety of methods have been developed to help students develop the knowledge, attitudes, and skills needed to become proficient in dealing with ethical issues in clinical practice. Teaching methods have ranged from large group lectures providing conceptual and historical overviews of issues in medical ethics, to seminar room discussions of "paper cases," to participation in discussions of actual cases encountered during clinical rotations, to participation in ethics consultation programs, with each of these supplemented by readings and in some cases videotapes or films. During the clinical years and the years of residency training, there has been a slow but steady increase in the use of practical teaching exercises, with an emphasis on the communication skills deemed necessary for the identification and resolution of ethical problems. Achieving a thorough conceptual understanding of the doctrine of informed consent, for example, is increasingly understood to be of limited value if physicians are not able to explain information clearly to patients. More recently, end-of-life ethics education has been highlighted through the growth of palliative care education, both at the medical school level and during residency (EPERC).

By the early 1990s, there was widespread agreement that in almost all settings instruction should be primarily case-based, because using real or detailed hypothetical cases emphasizes the difference that clinical ethics can make in actual patient care. Moreover, there is some empirical literature supporting the use of case- or problem-based education in promoting students' knowledge of professional judgments regarding ethical issues. In addition, case discussions allow for integrating moral reasoning with the other tasks of patient care.

Some educators, however, have raised concerns about overreliance on the use of the case method in teaching medical ethics (Barnard; Kass). Case discussions typically emphasize problem solving and ethical dilemmas, and they may ignore essential issues of clinical ethics, such as what constitutes informed consent in routine office care. Critics point out that cases typically deal with either the beginning or end of life or an exotic use of technology. Issues of daily practice or resource allocation are typically ignored. In addition, by concentrating on what should be done in a specific case, participants often ignore the institutional or interpersonal factors that may have led to the problem.

Analyzing the institutional factors that lead to family–physician conflict or how to treat families more respectfully in the intensive care unit may be more important in improving ethical care than teaching house staff about when it is ethically justifiable to override surrogate decision makers (Goold; Levine and Zuckerman, 1999, 2000). Institutional factors play an important and frequently overlooked role in influencing ethical decisions and behavior; discussion of institutional reforms may constitute an essential part of medical ethics education. Finally, while the cases presented often raise intellectually interesting ethical dilemmas, in practice, ethical conflicts are often attributable to communication problems.

In general, mirroring debates in moral philosophy, considerable disagreement remains about the importance of theory to ethical analysis. Tom L. Beauchamp and James F. Childress, authors of one of the most widely used texts in medical schools, emphasize the important role of the principles of respect for autonomy, nonmaleficence, beneficence, and justice, both as a framework for identifying moral issues and as a structure for moral justification. Others, such as K. Danner Clouser, argue against a primary stress on principles, for both theoretical and pedagogical reasons. In addition to intellectual concerns about the nature of proper moral justification, Clouser and others stress the importance of training students to attend to the highly specific biotechnical, psychological, and social complexities of individual cases in their moral reasoning, reporting that through a series of case discussions, students often arrive inductively at general precepts that they can then apply to other cases.

For different reasons, feminist theorists, virtue theorists, and casuists also have argued for less emphasis on theoretical principles. Rather than viewing cases as ways to illustrate principles, for example, casuists argue that they are the primary locus of moral meaning (Arras). Rather than using short, theoretically driven hypothetical cases, casuists encourage the use of real cases that illustrate the complexities and uncertainties of clinical practice. John D. Arras stated that these cases "display the sort of moral complexities and untidiness that demand the (nondeductive) weighing and balancing of competing moral considerations and the casuistical virtues of discernment and practical judgment (*phronesis*)" (p. 32). Feminists have argued for greater attention to social, economic, and political factors and their effect on the nature and dynamics of healthcare (Sherwin). Finally, according to Alisa L. Carse, virtue theorists and feminist theorists suggest that bioethical discussions should address questions such as 'What kind of person ought I be?' and 'What traits and capacities ought I to develop?' In an attempt to enhance students' moral imagination and empathy, and to stress the narrative aspects of medical ethics, educators include literature and film in teaching bioethics. These resources force students to critically reflect on the larger context and meaning of their work and, according to William T. Branch, to "conceptualize and generalize their behavioral changes into their mental structure of knowledge, skills and values" (p. 505).

Technological innovations also have spawned new approaches to teaching medical ethics. Computers and the Internet allow, for instance, attempts to combine ethics education with communication skills (an example is the MedEthEx Online website). Interactive DVDs dealing with difficult issues force the learner to confront challenges to their position in a structured manner. Telemedicine allows students at distant sites to interact in real time with faculty trained in medical ethics.

Most programs have adopted eclectic approaches to teaching medical ethics. In the preclinical years, a combination of lecture and small group case-based discussions predominate. Film and short stories are often used to promote self-reflection and discussion. In the clinical years, ethics education is usually structured as case-based small group discussions. Communication skills are often integrated with ethics education, and the focus of the discussion is practice-based.

The different programs, unfortunately, have some common limitations. First, as noted above, until very recently, the day-to-day life and behavior of physicians received little attention. The curricula are designed by faculty who are often unaware of the issues that students actually confront. (Student-run programs have focused more attention on issues that students are concerned about, such as "abuse" or being asked to violate their personal conscience.) Similarly, issues that are not directly applicable to patient care are discussed less frequently. Thus, for example, the medical-pharmaceutical-industrial complex and the ethical issues that it poses to both physicians and patients gets short shrift. Second, mirroring the lack of work in philosophy of medicine, there is little discussion of what it means to be a doctor in today's society. Third, the programs are, in general, cognitively physician-focused. Thus, despite the (re)inclusion of the humanities that has been taking place, students' ability to be empathic or to think creatively about ethical options may not be challenged. Attempts to integrate ethics, the humanities, and the social sciences in medical education may help with this situation.

## Faculty and Program Development

As in other areas of medical education, the evolution of teaching in medical ethics has been heavily shaped by the availability (or, for many programs, the scarcity) of qualified faculty. Throughout the 1970s and early 1980s, a central debate involved the question of whether medical ethics teaching should be done primarily by physicians or by those trained in the humanities, such as philosophy or religious studies. Mark Siegler, for example, stressed the ways in which the knowledge and professional experience of clinicians was central to an understanding of the true complexities and realities of clinical-ethical problems and their possible solutions. He therefore urged that primary teaching responsibility should lie with the physician-ethicist. Respected clinical teachers who emphasize the importance of medical ethics can be important role models who can help shape students' ethical sensibilities. On the other hand, strong reasons for using nonphysicians to teach medical ethics have been offered. First, many important aspects of the identification, analysis, and resolution of ethical problems in medicine do not fall within a physician's own specialized training or expertise, but depend instead on the intellectual background and analytic skills of individuals trained in other disciplines. Second, involving nonphysicians in teaching medical ethics can help sensitize students to the importance of other viewpoints and improve physicians' ability to communicate with nonphysicians—two primary educational goals. This controversy regarding who should teach has largely been replaced by a consensus that a variety of disciplines have important and distinct contributions to make.

The limited number of trained faculty, more than disputes regarding the academic background of those faculty, restricted the growth of ethics education. Many programs depended on faculty who, despite an interest in medical ethics, had little formal background in the field. Over time, this problem has abated as the number of faculty with prior training in ethics has increased. Moreover, in part to address this shortcoming, both short courses and longer master's programs in medical ethics have been developed around the world. The growth of healthcare providers with graduate training in ethics reflects the degree to which medical ethics has become integrated in the culture of medical education.

In their attempts to develop ethics curricula, medical ethics faculty have encountered a number of other barriers, including financial and time constraints, students' attitudes toward medical ethics, and the lack of reinforcement by other faculty (Strong, Connelly, and Forrow). Ethics teaching programs occupy a tenuous position in most medical schools. Although the inclusion of ethics test questions in certifying exams has improved this situation a bit, ethics training is rarely viewed as central to the education of physicians in the way that the "basic sciences" and traditional biotechnical clinical training are.

Economic constraints are a limiting factor in ethics education. Ethics education, conducted in small groups, is very faculty intensive. Moreover, at the same time that ethics has become integrated into medical schools, funding for teaching programs has decreased. This has happened during a period in which physicians are under increasing pressure to generate income. Thus, trained faculties' availability for teaching may again become a rate-limiting factor in ethics education.

## Evaluation

Evaluation, both of teaching programs themselves and of individual students, is still in flux. Most formal courses have included a pass–fail grading system based on class participation and written exercises, usually either papers or in-class essay examinations. These efforts convey to students the importance of medical ethics in the medical school (as has the addition of questions to the national boards and many of the specialty boards).

Efforts to develop formal and valid evaluation techniques have remained hampered, however, by uncertainty about what specific teaching goals are most important, about how best to measure whether any of those goals have in fact been accomplished, and about what is realistic to expect from ethics courses. (Similar constraints plague efforts to teach professionalism [Arnold].) Underlying the challenge of evaluating the impact of teaching medical ethics is a deeper debate regarding what teaching ethics does. Ethics as an academic discipline can be taught; one can evaluate a student's knowledge of ethical concepts and cognitive skills. Philosophers in undergraduate ethics courses have done this for centuries. Most attempts at evaluation in medical school have tried to measure this aspect of the ethics curriculum using essay or short-answer tests.

In arguing for the importance of formal ethics education, teachers of medical ethics typically have emphasized more ambitious goals, such as improving students' ability to address ethical issues in clinical practice or promoting humanistic qualities such as integrity. Efforts at evaluation, however, have not always distinguished among residents' attitudes, knowledge, or behavior. Moreover, there are numerous methodological problems, particularly in evaluating ethical behavior or character, problems that are compounded if one tries to determine whether improvements are attributable to formal ethics teaching. Some faculty involved in ethics programs question whether stricter standards of evaluation should be required of their curricula, arguing that courses in the traditional areas of anatomy, biochemistry, and physiology have rarely, if ever, been required to prove their ultimate effectiveness.

Attempts to develop innovative methods of evaluation have included measuring students' moral reasoning, evaluating students' behavior by nonphysicians (such as nurses or patients), and using formal tools such as the Objective Standardized Clinical Examination. These exercises have attempted to move beyond merely evaluating cognitive skills to analyzing students' actual behavior. Although these efforts show a great deal of promise as formative educational tools, few schools use these tools as summative evaluation methods. Limitations in their psychometric properties and the large number of raters needed for reliable ratings have limited their general use.

## Conclusion

While formal teaching programs in medical ethics were practically nonexistent in 1970, by the early 1990s there was extraordinary diversity both in the United States and elsewhere in formal teaching activities from the undergraduate to the postgraduate level. Bioethics education in the early twenty-first century is an accepted part of education for students in almost all medical schools and for residents in many programs.

Nevertheless, despite this growth and an evolving consensus that began in the 1980s regarding some core goals and teaching methods, many questions remain only partially answered. What should the primary goals of such teaching be—analytic ability, behavioral skills, or actual practice? What is the relationship between professionalism and medical ethics? How should those goals vary according to the developmental stage of the health professional and according to the person's specific field of practice within medicine? How can (or should) the attention on ethical attention be expanded beyond conflicts at the beginning and end of life to the day-to-day activities of doctoring? Who are the most appropriate faculty members to lead teaching efforts in various settings? What teaching methods are most effective and efficient in accomplishing curricular goals in each of the various settings? Finally, what is the proper role of formal evaluation efforts, both of individual students and of overall teaching programs? What methods of evaluation are both valid and feasible?

The difficulty in finding answers to these questions ensures that designing and implementing effective medical ethics education will remain challenging well into the twenty-first century.

ROBERT M. ARNOLD
LACHLAN FORROW (1995)
REVISED BY AUTHORS

**SEE ALSO:** *Casuistry; Conscience, Rights of; Literature and Bioethics; Medical Ethics, History of; Medicine, Anthropology of; Narrative; Nursing, Profession of; Professionalism and Professional Ethics;* and other *Bioethics Education* subentries

### BIBLIOGRAPHY

ABIM Foundation, ACP–ASIM Foundation, and European Federation of Internal Medicine. 2002. "Medical Professionalism in the New Millennium: A Physician Charter." *Annals of Internal Medicine* 136(3): 243–246.

American Board of Internal Medicine. Subcommittee on Evaluation of Humanistic Qualities in the Internist. 1983. "Evaluation of Humanistic Qualities in the Internist." *Annals of Internal Medicine* 99(5): 720–724.

American Board of Pediatrics. Medical Ethics Subcommittee. 1987. "Teaching and Evaluation of Interpersonal Skills and Ethical Decision Making in Pediatrics." *Pediatrics* 79(5): 829–834.

Arnold, Louise. 2002. "Assessing Professional Behavior: Yesterday, Today, and Tomorrow." *Academic Medicine* 77(6): 502–515.

Arras, John D. 1991. "Getting Down to Cases: The Revival of Casuistry in Bioethics." *Journal of Medical Philosophy* 16(1): 29–51.

Barnard, David. 1988. "Residency Ethics Teaching: A Critique of Current Trends." *Archives of Internal Medicine* 148(8): 1836–1838.

Baylis, Françoise, and Downie, Jocelyn. 1991. "Ethics Education for Canadian Medical Students." *Academic Medicine* 66(7): 413–414.

Beauchamp, Tom L., and Childress, James F. 2001. *Principles of Biomedical Ethics,* 5th edition. New York: Oxford University Press.

Bickel, Janet W. 1986. *Integrating Human Values Teaching Programs into Medical Students' Clinical Education.* Washington, D.C.: Association of American Medical Colleges.

Bosk, Charles L. 1979. *Forgive and Remember: Managing Medical Failure.* Chicago: University of Chicago Press.

Branch, William T. 2000. "Supporting the Moral Development of Medical Students." *Journal of General Internal Medicine* 15(7): 503–508.

Burling, S. J.; Lumley, J. S. P.; McCarthy, L. S. L, et al. 1990. "Review of the Teaching of Medical Ethics in London Medical Schools." *Journal of Medical Ethics* 16(4): 206–209.

Callahan, Daniel. 1980. "Goals in the Teaching of Ethics." In *Ethics Teaching in Higher Education,* ed. Daniel Callahan and Sissela Bok. New York: Plenum.

Carse, Alisa L. 1991. "The 'Voice of Care': Implications for Bioethical Education." *Journal of Medicine and Philosophy* 16(1): 5–28.

Clouser, K. Danner. 1989. "Ethical Theory and Applied Ethics: Reflections on Connections." In *Clinical Ethics: Theory and Practice,* ed. Barry Hoffmaster, Benjamin Freedman, and Gwen Fraser. Clifton, NJ: Humana.

Culver, Charles M.; Clouser, K. Danner; Gert, Bernard; et al. 1985. "Basic Curricular Goals in Medical Ethics." *New England Journal of Medicine* 312(4): 253–256.

DeWachter, Maurice A. M. 1978. "Teaching Medical Ethics: University of Nijmegen, The Netherlands." *Journal of Medical Ethics* 4(2): 84–88.

Drane, James F. 1988. *Becoming a Good Doctor: The Place of Virtue and Character in Medical Ethics.* Kansas City, MO: Sheed and Ward.

Goldie, John. 2000. "Review of Ethics Curricula in Undergraduate Medical Education." *Medical Education* 34(2): 108–119.

Goold, S.; Williams, B.; Arnold, R.A. 2000. "Conflicts Regarding Decisions to Limit Treatment." *Journal of American Medical Association.* 283(7): 909–914.

Institute of Medical Ethics. Working Party on the Teaching of Medical Ethics. 1987. *Report of a Working Party on the Teaching of Medical Ethics,* ed. Kenneth M. Boyd. London: Author.

Kass, Leon. 1990. "Practicing Ethics: Where's the Action?" *Hastings Center Report* 20(1): 5–12.

Levine, C., and Zuckerman, C. 1999. "The Trouble with Families: Toward an Ethic of Accommodation." *Annals of Internal Medicine* 130: 148.

Levine, C., and Zuckerman, C. 2000. "Hands On / Hands Off: Why Health Care Professionals Depend on Families but Keep Them at Arm's Length." *Journal of Law and Medical Ethics* 28: 5.

McKneally, Martin F., and Singer, Peter A. 2001. "Bioethics for Clinicians: 25. Teaching Bioethics in the Clinical Setting." *Canadian Medical Association Journal* 164(8): 1163–1167.

Miles, Steven H.; Lane, Laura Weiss; Bickel, Janet; et al. 1989. "Medical Ethics Education: Coming of Age." *Academic Medicine* 64(12): 705–714.

Olukoya, A. A. 1984. "A Workshop on Medical Ethics at the College of Medicine, Lagos University." *Journal of Medical Ethics* 10(4): 199–200.

Pellegrino, Edmund D.; Hart, Jr., Richard J.; Henderson, Sharon R.; et al. 1985. "Relevance and Utility of Courses in Medical Ethics: A Survey of Physicians' Perceptions." *Journal of the American Medical Association* 253(1): 49–53.

Povar, Gail J., and Keith, Karla J. 1984. "The Teaching of Liberal Arts in Internal Medicine Residency Training." *Journal of Medical Education* 59(9): 714–721.

Sherwin, Susan. 1992. *No Longer Patient: Feminist Ethics and Health Care.* Philadelphia: Temple University Press.

Siegler, Mark. 1978. "A Legacy of Osler: Teaching Clinical Ethics at the Bedside." *Journal of the American Medical Association* 239(10): 251–256.

Strong, Carson; Connelly, Julia E.; and Forrow, Lachlan. 1992. "Teachers' Perceptions of Difficulties in Teaching Ethics in Residencies." *Academic Medicine* 67(6): 398–402.

Veatch, Robert M., and Solitto, Sharmon. 1976. "Medical Ethics Teaching: Report of a National Medical School Survey." *Journal of the American Medical Association* 235(10): 1030–1033.

A Working Group, on behalf of the Association of Teachers of Ethics and Law in Australian and New Zealand Medical Schools. 2001. "An Ethics Core Curriculum for Australasian Medical Schools." *Medical Journal of Australia* 175(4): 205–210.

INTERNET RESOURCES.

Accreditation Council for Graduate Medical Education. 2003. Available from <http://www.acgme.org>.

Association of American Medical Colleges. 2003. Available from <http://www.aamc.org>.

End of Life/Palliative Education Resource Center (EPERC). 2003. Available from <http://www.eperc.mcw.edu.2003>.

Novack, Dennis. MedEthEx Online. 2003. Available from <http://griffin.auhs.edu/medethex/index.html>.

## II. NURSING

Ethics has received increased attention in nursing education programs; however, problems remain. This entry provides an overview of nursing ethics education in the United States and in other countries addressing both the advances made and the issues remaining.

### Nursing Ethics Education in the United States

Nursing ethics has been incorporated to some degree in nursing education since the early twentieth century. In the early 1900s ethics was taught as a science necessary to the education of the competent nurse who put patient safety and welfare first (Robb). Ethics teaching, reflecting religious and military influences, focused on the character and ethics of the nurse, the virtues required of nurses (e.g., loyalty and obedience), the duties and obligations nurses owed physicians and the hospitals that employed them, and proper etiquette for nurses. Obligations that nurses have as citizens of the community to participate in public policy and political areas to achieve healthcare goals first emerged in the *Code of Ethics* proposed by the American Nurses' Association (2001) in 1926 and adopted in 1950, and in the nursing literature of the first half of the twentieth century (Goodrich; Densford and Everett; Fowler). These wider obligations of nurses as citizens continue to be a very minor theme in nursing ethics education.

Ethics as a distinct part of the nursing curriculum almost disappeared in the 1950s and 1960s, except in programs affiliated with religious traditions and institutions. The 1970s brought renewed attention to nursing ethics education, partly because of the resurgence of medical ethics and the appearance of bioethics in the professional and academic worlds. These were responses to challenges emerging from medical technologies, abuses in research, and changes in the healthcare environment, challenges for which no ready-made responses were available. Some nurse educators and philosophers recognized, however, that nurses faced ethical issues and challenges different from those faced by physicians, largely because of nurses' positions as employees rather than as independent professionals in healthcare organizations. The National Student Nurses' Association and the American Nurses' Association passed resolutions calling for more attention to ethics in nursing education programs.

A survey conducted to assess the status of ethics teaching in accredited baccalaureate and graduate nursing programs (Aroskar) disclosed that most schools offered limited opportunities for study of ethical aspects of nursing and that these opportunities were often integrated into other nursing courses. Only 7 percent of the programs required work in ethics or medical ethics. Codes of ethics such as the *Code for Nurses* (American Nurses' Association, 1976) were identified as priority content in ethics courses, followed by patients' rights and obligations. No nursing faculty had primary responsibilities for teaching ethics.

Beginning in the late 1970s and early 1980s, nursing ethics education that incorporates values clarification and a more philosophical, principled approach to ethical issues received increased attention in nursing programs. This continuing development, however, depends on administrative support, faculty priorities, interests, and expertise, and varies greatly from school to school. A few nursing programs have full-time faculty in teaching and research activities devoted to ethics in nursing. Usually these are schools with master's and doctoral programs in nursing that offer studies in ethics, bioethics, and philosophy as electives or as a minor field. Teaching resources such as textbooks and nursing journal articles on ethics have increased significantly. Since 1975, activities to enhance the teaching of ethics in nursing have been supported by the Joseph P. Kennedy, Jr., Foundation, the National Endowment for the Humanities, The Hastings Center, the Fund for the Improvement of Post Secondary Education (FIPSE), and other institutions. There are more than fifty-five academic bioethics centers in the United States offering undergraduate, graduate, or continuing education courses in bioethics. However, few have dedicated programs or joint appointments for nursing ethics education (National Reference Center for Bioethics Literature [NRCBL], 2002a).

Baccalaureate education provides the foundations for professional nursing practice that requires knowledge of ethical obligations of the profession and ethical decision-making skills for the practitioner. Not all baccalaureate nursing programs have required or elective courses in ethics. Ethics education is still not required for program accreditation. Where ethics is a required curriculum component, content may be offered through separate courses or modules (Payton); integrated throughout the curriculum in existing courses (Ryden et al.); or presented in some combination of separate courses and integrated into classroom and clinical experiences. New approaches focus on case discussion, writing portfolios, and web-based interaction to encourage application of core concepts to clinically encountered situations (Pinch and Graves; Sorrell et al). An overall goal is to develop morally accountable practitioners who have a clear conceptual framework and the skills for ethical decision making in practice (Cassells and Redman; Fry, 1989). Ethics education is required core content for master's education in nursing and for the preparation of advanced practice nurses (American Association of Colleges of Nursing, 1996; American Nurses' Association, 1996; Kenney).

Sara T. Fry identified four models of ethics teaching used in undergraduate and graduate nursing programs and clinical settings:

1. The *moral-concepts model* incorporates three general areas: historical foundations of the nursing ethic, including codes of ethics and medical versus nursing ethics; the value dimensions of nursing, such as advocacy, loyalty, and moral obligations; and the skills needed for ethical decision making.

2. The *moral-issues model* focuses on common moral problems in healthcare relationships, such as confidentiality and informed consent, and issues of moral concern in healthcare, such as abortion, termination of treatment, and allocation of healthcare resources. Course content includes historical and contemporary legal cases that illustrate the legal and ethical aspects of specific issues in patient care.

3. The *clinical-practice model,* developed by bioethicists and nurse ethicists, incorporates clinical conferences on moral issues in patient care usually specific to a clinical area, case-study presentations, and ethics rounds that focus on ethical issues pertaining to a patient's care rather than to a patient's clinical condition.

4. The *ethics-inquiry model,* found primarily at the graduate level, incorporates the forms of traditional philosophical inquiry such as descriptive, normative, and metaethics; explores diverse methods of ethical inquiry; and looks at the relationship of ethical inquiry to other forms of inquiry in science and nursing. Additional topics in ethics education include the role of the nurse as a moral agent; roles of gender and ethnicity in nursing ethics; major ethical theories and principles and their application

in nursing practice; and the ethics of nursing research.

Since the early 1990s, caring as a foundation of nursing ethics has received a great deal of attention (Bishop and Scudder; Harbison). Curriculum change based upon theories of caring has been proposed and, in many places, implemented. However, strong critiques of theories of caring and the ethics of care persist and the success of these curricular changes has yet to be established.

The ethics of end-of-life care and pain management have also received much attention since the mid-1990s. Reviews of standard nursing texts found very little content related to pain management, end-of-life care, or the ethical issues at the end of life (Ferrell et al.). Concern over these shortcomings was mobilized into national projects to develop resources for teaching nurses the clinical skills needed for pain and symptom management as well as an understanding of the myriad ethical issues that arise in the provision of end-of-life care. The End-of-Life Nursing Education Collaboration Project (ELNEC) developed a standardized curriculum on end-of-life care and provided train-the-trainer programs for nursing school faculty, continuing education providers, and state boards of nursing across the country (American Association of Colleges of Nursing, 1996). The Toolkit for Nursing Excellence at End-of-Life Transitions (TNEEL) was provided free of charge to all nursing schools (Wells et al.). TNEEL is a computerized learning tool provided on CD-ROM that contains multimedia components such as audio, video, graphics, photographs, and animation to create an interactive program. Both of these projects contain specific ethics content as a prominent component of the suggested curricula.

Examples of specific outcome objectives for nursing ethics education include:

Identification of ethical dilemmas in the delivery of nursing care;

Identification of the components of an ethical decision-making framework;

Participation in ethical decision making in client care;

Leadership participation in ethics rounds and institutional ethics committees;

Analysis of impediments to the ethical practice of nursing;

Distinguishing the ethical elements of nursing practice from medical or technical elements; and

Analysis of nursing codes as they relate to client advocacy (NRCBL 2002b).

There are underlying tensions and ongoing debates in nursing ethics education. Argument continues over the question of whether nursing ethics does or should exist as a separate field of inquiry. Differences have arisen between those who teach ethics based on cognitive-moral-development theory and those who teach ethics based on moral philosophy and ethical theory. Evaluation of the effectiveness of ethics teaching has been a continuing challenge. Although research on ethics in nursing education has been expanding, it needs to be developed more systematically if it is to contribute to effective curriculum change (Silva and Sorrell). A shortage of adequately prepared faculty and overcrowded nursing curricula impede ethics teaching in nursing programs.

## Nursing Ethics Education in Other Countries

The fact that nursing ethics education in the international arena varies so greatly reflects the state of nursing and nursing education, as well as the priority of healthcare problems and issues, in many different countries. The lack of systematic, international information about nursing ethics education creates problems in providing a general overview of the topic.

The International Council of Nursing (ICN), Geneva, in an effort to address the uneven development of nursing ethics education, has provided ethics education through publications, programs, and conferences. The ICN's code of ethics serves as the nursing code in many countries. The code was revised in 2000. Since these countries have different histories, cultures, and priorities, the question arises as to whether or not all countries have common ethical values and principles regarding nursing and nursing education. In addition, much of nursing ethics education in the United States focuses on the issues that arise from advanced medical technology, whereas the main issue in many other countries is primary healthcare. More recently, numerous countries have developed their own codes of ethics for nurses.

Since the early 1990s, ICN has scheduled a special interest group in nursing ethics at its major open international meetings. This has been very successful in identifying nurses around the world with this professional focus.

The Journal of Nursing Ethics, which began in 1994, provides an arena for information and research from an international perspective. In conjunction with the journal, the editors and editorial board members established an International Centre for Nursing Ethics at the University of Surrey, England, that provides a place for researchers and educators to visit or come for more extended work.

In the United Kingdom nursing education is well developed, and higher education has been available to nurses for many years. In some colleges or departments of nursing, ethics is either taught as a separate course or integrated into other courses. During recent decades, the Royal College of Nursing actively articulated nursing ethics. In addition, nurse educators and others have published numerous papers, research reports, and books focused on nursing ethics. A major British nursing journal includes an ethics column that deals with clinical ethical problems. The Center for Midwifery and Nursing Ethics in London publishes a newsletter, runs educational programs, and serves as a clearinghouse for ethics materials. In 1990, Swansea University, Wales, sponsored the first national conference on nursing ethics and nursing ethics education. Over the past several years, Swansea has also sponsored conferences on Nursing Philosophy and since 1999 has published a journal with this title that includes ethics articles (De Raeve).

In Canada, numerous conferences have focused on nursing ethics and ethics education. An annual conference to discuss philosophy and nursing touches on many ethical themes. Several schools of nursing have invited visiting professors to teach ethics and have prepared some Canadian nursing professors to teach this subject as well. Canada has revised its own nursing code of ethics in 2002.

The ethics committee of the Swiss Nursing Association wrote a code of ethics in the 1980s and has been instrumental in increasing nurses' awareness of the need for more systematic approaches to teaching ethics in nursing programs. The association includes in its annual conference papers on ethics in curriculum content and clinical practice. For some years, one nurse educator has taught courses in Switzerland and France on ethical issues in dying and death with a special focus on suffering.

Nurse educators in Finland have offered seminars around the country on nursing ethics. One nurse educator has published a book on the topic. Several nurse educators in Finland and other Nordic countries have conducted research on ethical questions and have participated in multinational research projects examining selected ethical issues.

The board of directors of the Center for Medical Ethics at the University of Oslo, Norway, consists of people from diverse health-related professions. It continues to work with nurse educators and nurse researchers in developing educational programs and research focused on ethical issues.

Universities in both Norway and Sweden have invited nurse educators from overseas to lecture on nursing ethics. The annual, week-long seminar held in Sweden for doctoral students in nursing, which has either a primary or secondary focus on nursing ethics, has been of special interest because of its potential impact on nursing education. Extensive research on the ethics of various clinical problems with elderly patients has been undertaken at the University of Umea, Sweden. In Stockholm, two nurse educators teach and conduct research in nursing ethics.

One nurse educator in Budapest developed an ethics course for nursing students and wrote a textbook to use in this education. Another nurse educator teaches an ethics class at the Academy of Medicine in Lublin, Poland. In the Baltic States and Eastern Europe, physicians often are the major or only faculty teaching in nursing schools. For example, Estonia has a shortage of nurses prepared to teach nursing. In this context, emphasis has been placed on the medical model and little, if any, ethics has been included because the teachers have had limited exposure to ethics content. Nursing leaders in Estonia and other countries with similar problems are developing alternatives to this situation.

Throughout Latin America, Colombia has been the most active in nursing ethics education. The National Association of Nursing Schools has an ethics committee working with schools of nursing, the Ministry of Health, and the Nursing Association to increase ethical content in nursing education. The ethics committee sponsors workshops on nursing ethics and has been involved in research projects on nursing ethics. Chile has a nurse who has dealt with ethical issues working in the national nursing association. Brazil nurse educators teach nursing ethics and conduct research on ethics topics. Increasingly, nurses, and colleagues in other professions, are developing collaborative activities in teaching and research in healthcare ethics. Some of these activities involve Spain.

Australian nursing education throughout the country has supported conferences, seminars, and consultation in nursing ethics. One nurse ethicist in Melbourne has taught in a nursing program and has published several books in the field. The Center for Human Bioethics in Melbourne, established in 1980, examined the state of nursing ethics in Australia and has continued to work with nurses seeking education in ethics. In Queensland, a professor in the university nursing department served as a member of the research ethics committee at her institution. Both Australian and New Zealand nurses contribute regularly to the nursing ethics literature.

Numerous nurse educators present papers at the ongoing World Congress on Law and Ethics which recently elected a Swedish nurse to its board. In Israel, Jewish ethics has been taught throughout the nursing curricula and several educators conduct research in healthcare ethics.

The High Institute of Nursing, University of Alexandria, Egypt, held a nursing ethics conference in 1993 on ethics in education and practice. More recently, the Aga Khan University College of Nursing, Pakistan, held a conference and invited a keynote paper on nursing ethics.

In Asia, the People's Republic of China has developed eleven bachelor of science in nursing programs. The curriculum has included an ethics course that combines Confucian and Maoist ethics. The political slogan "serve the people" translates in nursing into respect for patients as persons. One Hong Kong educator conducted extensive research focused on nursing ethics in China. Korean nursing has developed an interest in ethics that manifests the influences of Christian missionary work. At Japan's national and international nursing research conferences, nurses present papers on nursing ethics from a clinical and an educational perspective. The Japanese Association of Bioethics includes nurses as speakers and participants in its conferences. The Japanese Nursing Association has an ethics committee and increasingly, the many new colleges of nursing are developing research ethics committees.

This discussion reflects great differences and many activities in nursing ethics education on the international scene. The lack of teachers and resources to teach nursing ethics remains a serious problem in many countries. However, one of the most striking developments in nursing ethics education is the amount of international research being conducted. Collaboration among Europeans and among European, Asian, and North and South American nursing colleagues has increased and provides a rich source of data for teaching.

## Conclusion

The last two decades of the twentieth century have seen a significant, worldwide resurgence and expansion of nursing ethics education activities and programs. These efforts have varied greatly. Many serious challenges remain for the twenty-first century, including a lack of formal ethics teaching in many programs, inadequate resources such as prepared nursing faculty to teach ethics, and the need for evaluation of the impact of existing nursing ethics education courses and programs on nursing practice.

MILA A. AROSKAR
ANNE J. DAVIS (1995)
REVISED BY THERESA DROUGHT
ANNE J. DAVIS

SEE ALSO: *Bioethics; Literature and Bioethics; Narrative; Nursing Ethics; Nursing, Profession of; Nursing, Theories and Philosophy of; Sexism; Teams, Healthcare; Women as Health Professionals;* and other *Bioethics Education* subentries

### BIBLIOGRAPHY

American Association of Colleges of Nursing. 1986. *Essentials of College and University Education for Professional Nursing: Final Report.* Washington, D.C.: Author.

American Association of Colleges of Nursing. 1996. *The Essentials of Master's Education for Advanced Practice Nursing.* Washington, D.C.: Author.

American Nurses' Association. 1976. *Code for Nurses with Interpretive Statements.* Kansas City, MO: Author.

American Nurses' Association. 1996. *Scope and Standards of Advanced Practice Registered Nursing.* Washington, D.C.: Author.

American Nurses' Association. 2001. *Code of Ethics for Nurses with Interpretive Statements.* Washington, D.C.: Author.

Aroskar, Mila A. 1977. "Ethics in the Nursing Curriculum." *Nursing Outlook* 25(4): 260–264.

Bishop, Ann H., and Scudder, John R., Jr. 1991. *Nursing: The Practice of Caring.* New York: National League for Nursing.

Blasszauer, Robert, and Rozsos, Elizabeth. 1991. "Ethics Teaching for Hungarian Nurses." *Bulletin of Medical Ethics* 69: 22–23.

Cassells, Judith M., and Redman, Barbara K. 1989. "Preparing Students to Be Moral Agents in Clinical Nursing Practice: Report of a National Study." *Nursing Clinics of North America* 24(2): 463–473.

Davis, Anne J.; Davidson, Bonnie; Hirschfeld, Miriam; et al. 1993. "An International Perspective of Active Euthanasia: Attitudes of Nurses in Seven Countries." *International Journal of Nursing Studies* 30(4): 301–310.

Densford, Katharine J., and Everett, Millard S. 1946. *Ethics for Modern Nurses.* Philadelphia: W. B. Saunders.

De Raeve, Louise. 2002. "Trust and Trustworthiness in Nurse-Patient Relationships." *Nursing Philosophy* 3(2): 152–162.

Ferrell, Betty R.; Grant, Marcia; and Virani, Rose. 1999. "Strengthening Nursing Education to Improve End-of-Life Care." *Nursing Outlook* 47(6): 252–256.

Fowler, Marsha D. M. 1997. "Nursing's Ethics." In *Ethical Dilemmas and Nursing Practice,* 4th edition. Stamford, CT: Appleton and Lange.

Fry, Sara T. 1989. "Teaching Ethics in Nursing Curricula: Traditional and Contemporary Models." *Nursing Clinics of North America* 24(2): 485–497.

Goodrich, Annie W. 1932. *The Social and Ethical Significance of Nursing: A Series of Addresses.* New York: Macmillan.

Harbison, Jean. 1992. "Gilligan: A Voice for Nursing?" *Journal of Medical Ethics* 18(4): 202–205.

Kenney, Janet W. 1996. *Philosophical and Theoretical Perspectives for Advanced Nursing Practice.* Boston: Jones and Bartlett.

Payton, Rita J. 1980. "A Bioethical Program for Baccalaureate Nursing Students." In *Ethics in Nursing Practice and Education.* Kansas City, MO: American Nurses' Association.

Pinch, Winifred J., and Graves, Janet K. 2000. "Using Web-Based Discussion as a Teaching Strategy: Bioethics as an Exemplar." *Journal of Advanced Nursing* 32(3): 704–712.

Robb, Isabel H. 1909. *Nursing Ethics: For Hospital and Private Use.* Cleveland, OH: E. C. Koeckert.

Ryden, Muriel B.; Duckett, Laura; Crisham, Patricia; et al. 1989. "Multi-Course Sequential Learning as a Model for Content Integration: Ethics as a Prototype." *Journal of Nursing Education* 28(3): 102–106.

Silva, Mary C., and Sorrell, Jeanne Merkle. 1991. *Research on Ethics in Nursing Education: An Integrative Review and Critique.* New York: National League for Nursing.

Sorrell, Jeanne M.; Brown, Hazel N.; Silva Mary C.; et al. 1997. "Use of Writing Portfolios for Interdisciplinary Assessment of Critical Thinking Outcomes of Nursing Students." *Nursing Forum* 32(4): 12–24.

Wells, Marjorie J.; Wilkie, Diana J.; Brown, Marie-Annette; et al. 2002. "Technology Available in Nursing Programs: Implications for Developing Virtual End-of-Life Educational Tools." *Journal of Cancer Education* 17(2): 92–96.

### INTERNET RESOURCES

American Nurses' Association. 2001. *Code of Ethics for Nurses with Interpretive Statements.* Available from <http://www.nursingworld.org/ethics/ecode.htm>.

International Centre for Nursing Ethics. 2002. Available from <http://www.freedomtocare.org/iane.htm>.

International Council of Nursing. 2000. Code of Ethics for Nurses. Available from <http://www.icn.ch/icncode.pdf>.

National Reference Center for Bioethics Literature. 2002a. "Educational Opportunities in Bioethics, Spring 2002." Available from <http://www.georgetown.edu/research/nrcbl/edopps.html#usa>.

National Reference Center for Bioethics Literature. 2002b. "Syllabus Exchange Catalogue, 2002." Available from <http://www.georgetown.edu/research/nrcbl/syllabus/sylbcat.htm>.

## III. SECONDARY AND POSTSECONDARY EDUCATION

Since the early 1970s, there has been a marked increase in bioethical reflection within the secondary and postsecondary curricula. On the high school level there is a growing movement to incorporate questions concerning public policy and values into science teaching and to raise bioethical issues in social science classes. Many colleges and universities offer courses in bioethics that are popular with students bound for the health professions and with others simply interested in the topical issues raised in such courses. There has also been a proliferation of postgraduate programs offering advanced degrees or certificates in bioethics, which has become an autonomous and accredited discipline.

## High School Level

It is a rare high school that offers its students a specialized course in bioethics. Bioethical reflection, however, may be embedded within the standard science offerings. To some degree this is an outcome of what has been called the "STS" movement—the acronym standing for "science, technology, and society." This movement reflects an attempt by U.S. secondary schools to include within the science curriculum the profound ethical and policy issues raised by developments in science and technology. This movement is not without its obstacles. For example, the training of science teachers, shaped by the traditional division of science from the humanities, has often placed little emphasis on developing teaching skills for ethical reflection. Nevertheless, the integrative movement has made inroads.

For example, bioethics issues may be raised in high school biology courses, during discussions of genetics, human and animal research, or environmental science. The treatment of such topics may be limited to brief case presentations or to discussions designed to help students with values clarification. There is a growing body of opinion, however, that such strategies can be insufficient; not all opinions are of equal value, and students need to develop the critical reasoning skills to evaluate their stances in the light of scientific evidence, material implications, and logical consistency. This approach, emphasizing the evaluation of ethical positions, may eventually prove most appealing to science educators for it dovetails well with aspects of the scientific method they are trying to transmit.

Bioethics teaching on the secondary level need not be restricted to the science curriculum. The High School Bioethics Curriculum Project of the Kennedy Institute of Ethics seeks to train and support teachers in using bioethical case studies in a wide range of courses, including those in social studies, civics, history, philosophy, and religion. The project has prepared curriculum units covering topics such as neonatal ethics, organ transplantation, human subjects research, and eugenics. High school teachers are introduced to these units through workshops and are assisted with ongoing curriculum development, networking, and resource identification.

## College Level

On the college level, offerings in bioethics are a well-established feature. Certain institutions offer, or allow students to construct, an interdisciplinary major in bioethics.

More common is a minor or concentration in bioethics, interdisciplinary in nature or offered through a philosophy, religion, or social-science-based department.

Though most colleges have neither major or minor, they are likely to offer one or more courses in bioethics. A typical course might use one of the standard textbooks of bioethics, either written from a unitary perspective or offering an edited collection of canonical "pro" and "con" articles on bioethical issues. The instructor may choose to supplement this with a collection of cases or to replace it with an assembled course packet of the instructor's choosing.

A number of didactic approaches may be used to help students become experientially involved with the topics. Most popular is the case analysis mode where students grapple with the dilemmas raised by actual or constructed cases. Class debates can provoke spirited dialogue, and a growing library of films and videotapes vividly portrays for students the human impact of these issues. Some professors may bring in, or team-teach with, healthcare professionals, or ask students to visit a healthcare setting as part of the course. Bioethics can lend itself well to a "service-learning" approach, where student service in healthcare-related fields can be used by the instructor as a way to make bioethical issues come alive.

Most bioethics textbooks and many instructors begin from a framework of ethical theories and principles that are then applied to specific issues, such as informed consent, abortion, and euthanasia. However, this "standard approach"—and indeed the "standard issues" of bioethics—have been criticized by professionals associated with fields such as phenomenology, pragmatism, hermeneutics, feminism, casuistry, virtue ethics, and narrative theory. Critics argue, for example, that to base ethical analysis on high-level theory may obscure the richness of particular cases and the complex modes of interpretation that real-life decision makers employ. Moreover, simply to stick to recognized "ethical quandaries" is to risk overlooking the sociopolitical biases and the metaphysics of self and body that have shaped contemporary Western medical systems in ethically significant ways.

Instructors may therefore choose to supplement the medical ethics textbook with other kinds of resources. For example, a brief selection from the seventeenth-century French mathematician and philosopher René Descartes might be used to reflect on the model of body-as-machine that has powerfully influenced the doctor–patient relationship. A literary work such as "The Death of Ivan Ilyich" (1886), by the Russian novelist and philosopher Leo Tolstoy, can render vivid and lucid the experience of illness, the significance of truth telling, and the dilemmas surrounding death and dying. A work of social critique, such as a feminist history of women and medicine, can raise issues concerning the power relations embodied in medical practice and disease categories. The growing diversity of methodologies used within professional bioethics can thus "filter down" to diversify the methods and materials used in college-level teaching.

## Postgraduate Level

On the postgraduate level, a number of centers and universities around the country offer advanced degree programs specializing in bioethics. One popular model is the master's or Ph.D. program, often in philosophy, less frequently in religion, with a bioethics concentration. The program may include a series of courses focused on bioethical issues, some exposure to a clinical setting, and a thesis written on a topic relevant to bioethics. Such programs may attract individuals looking to pursue this field as a primary academic career. Alternatively, healthcare professionals may enter such programs, usually for the master's degree, in preparation for teaching and/or service on ethics committees, or out of personal interest. Then, too, certain programs are designed to offer joint degrees through collaborative arrangements, allowing students to complete a medical or a legal degree along with an M.A., M.P.H. (master of public health), or Ph.D. degree. While most degree programs focus on bioethics or medical ethics as such, others define themselves more broadly as teaching the medical humanities and thus may incorporate diverse disciplines such as history, sociology, anthropology, and literature.

In addition to degree programs, there are many options for those seeking more limited preparation in bioethics. A number of centers, for example, offer intensive courses in bioethics lasting from one to four weeks or involving sessions spread out over a longer period. There are continuing education courses and certificate programs in bioethics. Special bioethics fellowships are also available, often directed toward those already engaged in clinical practice.

## Conclusion

Much of what this entry details concerning bioethics teaching on the high school, college, and postgraduate level has become available since 1978, when the first edition of the *Encyclopedia of Bioethics* appeared. Academic interest in bioethics has been growing apace. With the continued expansion of the healthcare industry, the constant development of new and troubling biomedical technologies, and the daily bioethics headlines in the popular press, it is likely that this interest will continue unabated.

DREW LEDER (1995)
REVISED BY AUTHOR

**SEE ALSO:** *Bioethics; Care; Casuistry; Ethics; Law and Bioethics; Literature and Bioethics; Narrative;* and other *Bioethics Education* subentries

### BIBLIOGRAPHY

Jennings, Bruce; Nolan, Kathleen; Campbell, Courtney; et al. 1991. *New Choices, New Responsibilities: Ethical Issues in the Life Sciences: A Teaching Resource on Bioethics for High School Biology Courses.* Briarcliff Manor, NY: Hastings Center.

Levine, Carol, ed. 2000. *Taking Sides: Clashing Views on Controversial Bioethical Issues,* 9th edition. Guilford, CT: Dushkin/McGraw-Hill.

Thornton, Barbara C., and Callahan, Daniel. 1993. *Bioethics Education: Expanding the Circle of Participants.* Briarcliff Manor, NY: Hastings Center.

#### INTERNET RESOURCES

"Bibliographic Resources." Georgetown University, Kennedy Institute of Ethics, National Reference Center for Bioethics Literature. Available from <http://www.georgetown.edu/research/nrcbl/home.htm>.

"Educational/Teaching Resources." Georgetown University, Kennedy Institute of Ethics, National Reference Center for Bioethics Literature. Available from <http://www.georgetown.edu/research/nrcbl/home.htm>.

"Study Opportunities in Practical and Professional Ethics." Indiana University, Association for Practical and Professional Ethics. Available from <http://php.indiana.edu/~appe/>.

## IV. OTHER HEALTH PROFESSIONS

Bioethics education in health professions other than medicine and nursing takes place both in professional schools and in continuing-education settings. The group to which *other health professions* refers is so diverse that no generalizations embrace all of the professions equally. Some major groups include therapists (e.g., occupational, recreational, respiratory, physical), technologists (e.g., radiologic, medical laboratory), physician assistants, pharmacists, dietitians, dentists, and medical social workers. This entry emphasizes major common themes that have emerged in the content and pedagogy of their educational offerings; it also describes common factors that have led to the introduction of bioethics teaching in these fields.

## Common Themes in Content and Pedagogy

A set of guidelines for professional conduct has been one of the first types of documents produced when a new health field emerges. Up until the 1960s the documents often were called codes of ethics, but focused on dress codes and the importance of good manners and a cheerful disposition. They also emphasized the importance of keeping one's proper place in the bureaucracy, so that all documents except those for dentistry stressed deference to the physician's authority. Dedication to one's profession was considered essential. This list served as a foundation for teaching "ethics" to students in that field. The predictable result was that early ethics education was a presentation of a list of "dos and don'ts" that detailed a professional etiquette and morality punctuated by loyalty to one's group.

The educational emphasis has changed, as a result of changes in the focus of ethics documents and developments in the field of bioethics. There is also a growing consensus about the pedagogical methods that should be employed for bioethics education.

Late twentieth century codes of ethics reflect basic ethical principles and virtues relevant to professional practice. For instance, the Code of Ethics of the National Association of Social Workers is designed around the central notion of ethical responsibility. The American Academy of Physician Assistants followed the model of several others by delineating its major types of interactions and specifying principles for each. Many groups provide accompanying guides for professional conduct that attempt to elaborate behaviors consistent with those principles and virtues. For example, the American Dental Association includes "advisory opinions" for most of its principles, and the American Physical Therapy Association issues a separate guide detailing each of its eight principles. Faculty have adopted these documents as a basis for education, with the predictable result that there is less focus on simply indoctrinating students into behaviors and attitudes and more on urging them to think about the ethical principles and virtues that underpin professional roles and responsibilities.

The development of bioethics as a field also has influenced education in these fields. Teachers focus on basic bioethics theory and methods of ethical analysis. Students are taught to think critically, recognize ethical issues, and reflect on them. Character traits or virtues are not simply declared essential; rather, students are encouraged to understand the significance of behaviors and attitudes that express compassion, honesty, and integrity (to name some). Materials introduced from the social sciences highlight how ethnic, religious, age, sex, class, and other differences among individuals and groups influence situations in which bioethical problems arise. In short, the teaching of ethics has evolved to foster analysis of and reflection on practical issues.

There is a growing consensus about pedagogical methods that should be utilized to teach bioethics. Educational programs actively promote the integration of theoretical content with case examples. The case method is especially effective in allowing students readily to recognize key ethical issues as they arise in everyday practice and to grasp the relevance of bioethics to their chosen professions. A larger proportion of bioethics instruction is taking place in small group discussions during the clinical period of professional preparation, so that challenging cases can be highlighted in discussion. Some programs utilize real or simulated patients with the goal of integrating ethical aspects of a patient's situation into the diagnostic, treatment, and social aspects.

There is less consensus about who should teach bioethics. Some schools of thought favor a stronger emphasis on theory, so that persons formally trained in philosophical ethics or moral theology are thought to be ideal. Others argue that an understanding of the clinical peculiarities and "facts" is most important, so clinicians are favored, especially if they have taken advanced work (or even a short course) in bioethics. Another alternative is a teaching team composed of a bioethicist and clinician working together. Preferences for one or another of these approaches seem less profession-specific than idiosyncratic of particular regions or institutions. In spite of the differences of opinion, the debates revolve around the common goal of effectively integrating theoretical and practical dimensions of bioethics.

## Common Factors Leading to the Necessity of Bioethics Education

At least three major factors have led to the need for bioethics teaching, with its focus on thoughtful deliberation about complex ethical issues.

The issue of professional autonomy in relation to physicians is the crucial distinguishing feature of bioethics education in the groups being discussed. Their predicament is shared with nurses, and nursing ethics has provided valuable insights into the dilemma that is created. Such groups must gain understanding of their peculiar situation: having moral authority without ultimate decision-making authority. In some states, groups such as physician assistants, physical therapists, and social workers have legal license to evaluate or practice independently. But this does not resolve the thorny questions of how to coordinate care for patients in a system largely centered on physician autonomy. The different levels of progress toward full professional status among the groups compound the issue.

A second factor distinguishing bioethics education for the groups under discussion is that many claim, as the rationale for their very existence, the mastery of a particular technology. Reliance on technology may drastically alter the complexion of the traditional health professional–patient relationship. First, technology may create a detrimental distance between health professionals and patients. Patients and health professionals alike may place unrealistic expectations on technologies to bring about "miracles," creating dissent and distrust when they fail to do so. And the high cost of many technologies may add undue burdens on patients and families.

Since the professional–patient relationship is at the heart of professional ethics, germane bioethics education is crucial so that health professionals can respond well to the larger human dilemmas created by technology. The types of technology the various professions employ will differ, but the generic challenges are similar for all. A list of "dos and don'ts" will not suffice. The concepts and methods of ethics are needed for thinking through and acting on technology-related challenges.

A third factor is the presence of inequities in healthcare. The tools of bioethics enable students to understand why inequities are morally unacceptable in the healthcare system. They also provide an opportunity to encourage reflection on how professionals can contribute to the advancement of just and fair policies.

Since bioethics education in the professions under discussion in this entry encourages critical thinking, considered action, and the exercise of ethically appropriate character traits, it will continue to be a powerful resource as new developments in healthcare and society give rise to ethical issues.

RUTH B. PURTILO (1995)
BIBLIOGRAPHY REVISED

SEE ALSO: *Bioethics; Dentistry; Literature and Bioethics; Narrative; Nursing Ethics; Nursing, Profession of; Nursing, Theories and Philosophy of; Pastoral Care and Healthcare Chaplaincy; Sexism; Teams, Healthcare; Women as Health Professionals;* and other *Bioethics Education* subentries

### BIBLIOGRAPHY

Golden, David G. 1991. "Medical Ethics Courses for Student Technologists." *Radiologic Technology* 62(6): 452–457.

Haddad, Amy M. 1988. "Teaching Ethical Analysis in Occupational Therapy." *American Journal of Occupational Therapy* 42(5): 300–304.

Haddad, Amy M., and Becker, Evelyn S., eds. 1992. *Teaching and Learning Strategies in Pharmacy Ethics.* Omaha, NE: Creighton University Biomedical Communications.

Hope, Tony. 2000. *Oxford Practice Skills Course Ethics, Law, and Communication Skills in Health Care Education.* New York: Oxford University Press.

McMillan, J. 2002. "Ethics and Clinical Ethics Committee Education." *Healthcare Ethics Comittee Forum* 14(1): 45–52.

Nilstun, T.; Cuttini, M.; and Saracci, R. 2001. "Teaching Medical Ethics to Experienced Staff: Participants, Teachers and Method." *Journal of Medical Ethics* 27(6): 409–412.

Ozar, David T. 1985. "Formal Instruction in Dental Professional Ethics." *Journal of Dental Education* 49(10): 696–701.

Parker, Michael, and Dickenson, Donna. 2001. *The Cambridge Medical Ethics Workbook: Case Studies, Commentaries and Activities.* New York: Cambridge University Press.

Purtilo, Ruth B. 1990. *Health Professional and Patient Interaction,* 4th edition. Philadelphia: W. B. Saunders.

Purtilo, Ruth B., and Cassel, Christine K. 1993. *Ethical Dimensions in the Health Professions,* 2nd edition. Philadelphia: W. B. Saunders.

Rogers, Joan C. 1983. "Clinical Reasoning: The Ethics, Science and Art." *American Journal of Occupational Therapy* 37(9): 601–616.

Seebauer, Edmund G., and Barry, Robert L. 2000. *Fundamentals of Ethics for Scientists and Engineers.* New York: Oxford University Press.

# BIOLOGY, PHILOSOPHY OF

• • •

While it may seem that the philosophy of biology, a field known for its focus on metaphysical, epistemological, and conceptual issues in biology, is far removed from the concerns of bioethics, there is a trend in philosophy of biology towards descriptivism that paradoxically allows for significant bridges with the predominantly normative concerns of bioethics.

About the same time that bioethics was born (the 1960s), the field of philosophy of biology took its first steps. Initially, it looked a lot like the rest of philosophy of science, which often meant focusing on the kinds of concerns that had their roots in physics. David Hull, Michael Ruse (1973) and others created a field that was dominated by formal concerns in evolutionary biology, including the nature and structure of its theories. Questions for the field included the nature of any reductions from the theories of Mendelian and transmission genetics to molecular genetics, whether it was possible to axiomatize evolutionary theory, how to account for the apparent teleology of evolutionary explanations, whether species are classes or individuals, and what the units of selection are. Many of these topics have remained active sub-fields to the present day.

Over time, philosophy of biology came to include much richer and detailed involvement with both current biology and the history of biology. Many philosophers came to ground their philosophical insights in rich historical accounts of various periods in the history of biology or in contemporary debates of active concern to practicing biologists. This *naturalistic* turn occurred in many parts of philosophy of science, but seems to have been most acute in philosophy of biology, at least partly for institutional reasons, including the creation of the International Society for the History, Philosophy, and Social Studies of Biology (Callebaut).

Through these developments, the field still largely avoided normative issues and focused on evolutionary biology. Recently several attempts have been made to move the field to other parts of biology. There are a number of philosophers working on developmental biology and using it as an alternative for framing traditional issues (Oyama, Griffiths, and Gray). Kenneth Schaffner has made a notable and unusual attempt to discuss the more medical parts of biology. Paul Thagard has similarly attempted to use work in the biomedical sciences (attempts at explaining the causes of ulcers) to address general philosophical issues in the nature of explanation.

There are a number of topics within philosophy of biology that especially bear on issues within bioethics.

## Biological Function

One of the central concepts in the more medical parts of biology, particularly physiology, is the concept of function. It is impossible to understand the way we classify organ systems without this concept. The function of the heart is to pump blood. Hence any blood pump is a heart—even if there are some structural differences between the hearts of different species or (as mechanical hearts demonstrate) differences in the material makeup of the heart. So, what makes something a heart is fundamentally its function or purpose. This poses a philosophical problem, because the concept of function is a teleological notion. The function of the heart is to pump blood is simply another way of saying that the heart is designed to pump blood. But, who is the designer? Prior to Darwin the answer would have been an appeal to God.

Philosophers have attempted to account for the apparent goal-directed nature of biological science in two different ways. One solution is to accept that functions are goal directed, but to appeal to natural selection. Rather than a conscious designer, natural selection *designed* the heart to pump blood. The etiological view of functions (sometimes called Wright functions) gives an explanation of why a function is there in historical terms. More precisely, "The function of X is Z means (a) X is there because it does Z and (b) Z is a consequence (or result) of X's being there" (Wright, p. 139–168). To Larry Wright, "a heart beats *because* its beating pumps blood" (p. 40).

In contrast, in 1975 Robert Cummins rejected the goal-directed, historical approach to functions. What matters in thinking of functions is the contribution it makes to a whole system, the role that it plays in bringing about the performance of that system.

Early-twenty-first-century commentators have concluded that each approach captures a different notion of function. Where Larry Wright attempts to account for why a function is there (a function as opposed to an accident), Cummins explains what a function does, what it is good for (whether it is an accident or not). Continued debate over whether an etiological account can be developed in the Wright mode and how to overcome various problems continues (Cummins and Perlman).

The concept of function plays an especially important role in medicine since health and disease are often understood as normal (species typical) functioning or dysfunction respectively.

## Concepts of Disease and Health

This is perhaps the most important area of research in philosophy of biology for bioethics. Arthur Caplan explains it as follows:

> It may strain credulity to believe that the analysis of concepts such as *health, disease,* or *normality* can shed light on the ethical and policy issues associated with the vast amounts of new knowledge being generated by the human genome project and related inquiries in biomedicine. However credulity must be strained. The focus of attention *qua* philosophy tends to be on who owns the genome or whether an insurance company can boot you off the rolls if you are at risk of succumbing to a costly disease. But this is not really where the ethical and philosophical action is with respect to the ongoing revolution in genetics. (p. 128)

There are two important distinctions that must be understood in the debates over concepts of disease. First, there is a distinction between ontological and nominalist concepts of disease. On the ontological (realist) view of disease, diseases are real entities that exist in the world. Nosologies represent a true classification of the world—they carve nature at the joints. The paradigm diseases on this view would be either discrete disease causing agents that are at the same time identified as the diseases themselves or as discrete lesions. Thus, poliovirus is not the cause of poliomyelitis, it *is* poliomyelitis.

In contrast, the nominalist about disease would appeal to the old saying, "there are no diseases, only sick people." On this view, nosologies are merely conventional systems of classification. They may have a great deal of practical value, but they are not in any meaningful sense true descriptions of reality. In some cases we classify diseases based on the pathogen that causes the disease. In other cases we classify based on the signs and symptoms. In others we focus on the organ system that is damaged, regardless of the causes or the symptoms. Thus, the nominalist would use the current lack of unity in the organization of our taxonomy of diseases as support for the view that it is merely a conventional (and somewhat arbitrary) system. Realists would respond by appealing to the role of disease in medical science and point to similar problems with other taxonomic systems in science that are nonetheless regarded as capturing reality.

One of the arenas where this debate has been most heated has been over the issue of the status of the Diagnostic and Statistical Manual of Mental Disorders (DSM) in all of its versions. The fact that there are so many changes in the different versions of the DSM can be interpreted either as an indication that the classification scheme is merely a convention, or that the science of psychiatry is progressing (as any science does).

The second related distinction in debates over the concept of disease is over the role of values in the development of the nosologies. For the non-normativist, the starting point for understanding disease is to understand species typical functioning. Disease is malfunction of the organism, a failure to function as organisms are *designed* to do. To understand disease, one needs only to understand physiology. The concepts are the same in humans as in understanding disease in nonhuman organisms. Therefore, (non-scientific or epistemological) values play no role in the development of the classification and understanding of disease (Boorse).

In contrast, normativists believe that identifying a condition as a disease is a value-laden exercise. To say that a condition is a disease is to say something about what we value. Labeling something as a disease is a way of signaling the undesirability of the state. Normativists appeal to many

examples that illustrate the way social values seem to permeate nosology. The early versions of the DSM identified homosexuality as a disease. The tendency of some slaves to attempt to escape was identified as a disease in the United States in the nineteenth century. Foot binding in Japan produces a condition that would be recognized as a disease in many parts of the world, but is seen as normal in Japan. Normativists deny that an account of disease solely in terms of species typical functioning can work. It is *normal* in some sense for humans to develop osteoarthritis in old age, normal for teeth to decay, normal to develop many ailments at advanced age. Yet medicine is committed to these things as disease. In fact age itself may be conceived of as both normal and a disease (Caplan et al.).

Finally, there is a dispute over the meaning of health. Non-normativists tend to think of health as the absence of disease. In that case, an organism is functioning within the normal parameters of its species at its age. In contrast there are those who adopt a much broader concept of health. On this view health is not the mere absence of disease, but is the full flourishing of a person in multiple dimensions, including psychological, economic, physical, and social well being. These different conceptions of health and disease lead to very different views about the obligations of medicine towards society, the scope of the medical field, and the nature of medical care.

## What Counts as a Genetic Trait?

What does it mean to call something a *genetic* trait or disease? Clearly, at least part of that judgment rests on some kind of causal assessment. If a disease is genetic, then it is caused by one or more of an organism's genes. Indeed, this seems to fit a more general concept of disease, in which the causal basis of disease is incorporated into our nosologies. As Richard Hull has explained:

> In its efforts to understand, control, and avoid disease, modern medicine has incorporated into the very identification of a disease the notion of the cause of the syndrome. This permits the individuation of similar syndromes with distinct causes into different diseases. (p. 61)

There is a fairly obvious problem with this as a way of distinguishing between genetic and epigenetic diseases. That is because there are genetic and nongenetic factors which are causally relevant to every trait, a fact recognized by virtually all commentators on the concept of genetic disease (see Gifford; Hull, 1979). So the real issue in deciding that something is a genetic disease, is whether the causal factors which are genetic are the most important causes. How do we decide whether genetic factors or environmental factors are more important in the production of various diseases? In response to the selection problem, a number of solutions have been proposed. These can be grouped into a few major categories.

One approach is to try to tease out a notion of genes as *direct* causes of disease. In 1990 Fred Gifford tried to capture this notion in one of his two definitions:

> …the trait must be the specific effect of some genetic cause, that the trait must be described or individuated in such a way that it is properly matched to what the gene causes specifically. (p. 329)

However, this approach seems hopeless in the face of the actual complexity of development. Quite simply, this definition probably does not identify any diseases or traits as genetic. As Kelly Smith argued in 1990, "genes do not directly cause anything of immediate phenotypic significance" (p. 338).

Perhaps the most obvious and promising approach to the selection problems is to try a statistical approach. A number of variants on this have been attempted.

> The first and central sense of *genetic* is this: a trait is genetic if genetic *differences* in a given population account for the phenotypic *differences* in the trait-variable amongst members of that population. (Gifford, p. 334)

This seems to exactly capture at least something important about society's concept of genetic disease. It can be put perhaps more precisely in terms of covariance. When some trait is identified as genetic, it can be argued that (in that population) the covariance of the trait with some genetic factor(s) is greater than the covariance of the trait with other (nongenetic) factors. This solves the selection problem neatly by allowing us to pick out which causal factors are irrelevant (the ones which are fixed) and highlight the important ones (the ones that *make the difference*). In one of the canonical examples of causality, one is inclined to say that the lighting of a match (under normal circumstances) was the cause of the fire, while the presence of oxygen (while a contributing causal factor) was not. In contrast, in an environment where fire was normally present and oxygen was not, one might well pick out the (unusual) presence of oxygen as the cause of a fire.

There are several advantages to this approach to the selection problem. First, it corresponds to the use of analysis of variance that is used by biologists to measure the causal contribution of hereditary and environmental factors in a population. Second, it is capable of clear explication. Third, it has at least some intuitive support. However, this account seems to conflict with common usage in cases where pathogens typically identified as *the* cause of disease are nearly ubiquitous (so that, for example, genetic factors may make the difference between which people exposed to the pathogen become ill).

In spite of its advantages, the statistical approach fails to capture all of the myriad uses of the concept of genetic disease. Another approach has been developed from the way the most important causal factor in an explanation is picked out.

Philosophers have claimed on quite general grounds that the most important cause is chosen in terms of the manipulability of the various factors. Whatever the general virtues of this approach, it is promising when it comes to medicine. In the natural sciences, it could be argued that there is a strong interest in prediction and explanation. In contrast it has been argued that the medical realm is more concerned with the prevention and treatment of disease than with explanation (Wulff; Engelhardt). Instrumentalist interests play a much more central role in medical practice than in science. Hence, the appropriate solution to the selection problem can be formulated in terms of manipulability. The most important cause is the one that is identified as the most easily manipulated to prevent or treat disease. A disease is genetic if it is genes that play this role and epigenetic if it is non-genetic factors that are most easily manipulated.

Like the statistical definition, the manipulability definition captures something important about our usage of the term. In addition it is often an implicit aspect of the justification for the extension of the concept of genetic disease to new cases. However there are some problems with this approach as well. The obvious problem seems to be that on this analysis, no disease could be classified as genetic. Many of the paradigm genetic diseases (phenylketonuria [PKU], cystic fibrosis [CF]) involve treatments that are not molecular. Indeed, in the case of PKU, the standard treatment involves a change in diet. At the same time the tests for PKU were developed before the actual mutation responsible for the disease had been identified. It is impossible to adhere to the manipulability definition and accept that PKU is a genetic disease. This seems to be a fatal flaw in the manipulability definition. In addition, it is not true that biomedical science is always instrumentally oriented. A great deal of effort is aimed not just at treating and preventing disease, but at understanding it. This may lead to a conflict over which causal factor is most important (the factor most easily manipulated for treating or preventing a disease may not be the most revealing for the purposes of understanding a disease).

It is worth noting that both the statistical approaches and the manipulability approaches seem to imply a relativity in the concept of genetic disease. In the case of the statistical notion, something will count as a genetic disease or not, depending on the population it is a part of. The manipulability definition implies that technological advances will affect what counts as a genetic disease as the *reach* of our technology is extended. Yet, this result seems to be incompatible with an ontological conception of disease. If diseases are real entities (and independent of values) then the solution to the selection problem should not depend on factors outside of the organism (Boorse). Thus the normativist or constructivist position on disease seems to be supported by these analyses (however inadequate they are as a general account).

## Evolutionary Ethics

As philosophy has become more *naturalized*, it is unsurprising that philosophers (and especially philosophers of biology) would attempt to find a way to ground ethics in a biological account of human nature. Perhaps even more significantly, the development of sociobiology and its subsequent incarnation, evolutionary psychology, meant that biologists were looking to explain the origins of morality in an evolutionary account (Wilson; Farber; Wright, 1995). Michael Ruse has been perhaps the most influential voice on evolutionary ethics (1991, 1993).

Ruse argues that evolutionary theory offers *the* explanation of the origin of altruism and other moral sentiments. He follows the explanatory strategy of the sociobiologists (and evolutionary psychologists) by appealing to the apparent universality of cooperative behaviors and moral sentiments, combined with the obvious adaptive value that cooperative strategies represent. Indeed there are a number of game theoretic accounts to demonstrate the adaptive value of altruistic behavior in at least some circumstances (Smith, 1982).

Ruse then claims that the fact that evolution explains morality undermines moral realism. He offers two arguments. First, although human moral sentiments evolved, it is quite possible that an alternative set of sentiments could have produced the same effects. The contingency of evolution means that morality itself is contingent. Second, Ruse takes great care in dispelling any teleological interpretation of evolution. Evolution is a directionless process with no end or goal. Since morality is founded on a directionless process, it follows that realism towards ethics is undermined. Evolution is meaningless, and without value. Organisms that survived and adapted are not *better* in a normative sense. Hence there is no normative foundation for ethics.

Critics have attempted a number of strategies, including questioning the extent to which evolution can really account for morality (Lewontin), or denying the relevance of the facts of evolution to normative issues (Nagel). Other critics have argued that a fully naturalized ethics that accepts evolution as the foundation of morality is fully compatible with ethical realism (Maienschein and Ruse).

## What Is Life?

A recently emerging research area at the intersection of philosophy of biology and bioethics is over the definition of life. This question has multiple dimensions. National Aeronautics and Space Administration (NASA) scientists wonder about the definition as they pursue research into the question of life on other planets. How will researchers know whether what they find is a living organism or a (nonliving) chemical reaction? Biologists interested in the origins of life similarly strive to understand the demarcation between the living and nonliving as they construct their models. Genomic scientists attempt to better understand gene function by trying to determine the minimal number of genes necessary for life—life's genetic essence. Public policy makers and scientists debate the moral significance of ex vivo fertilized egg cells and the stem cells that can be derived from them. Are the embryos living? Are they alive when they are frozen? Are the stem cells that can be derived from them living beings deserving of respect or are they research tools to be used to help people suffering from disease?

The process of development, from an early embryo to a fully differentiated and functioning organism is a long, complex process. Determining the moral status of that embryo at different stages of the process is a difficult task (Green). Prior to implantation, an embryo's undifferentiated blastomeres are each capable of creating separate and unique individuals (through twining). Other traits emerge later as the nervous system develops. At what point is there a (human) life? And is life (as opposed to, for instance, personhood) the right concept to be considering? And what is the status of the derived stem cells themselves? As Arthur Caplan and Glen McGee have argued, the problem of "What's in the dish?" remains one of the key concepts in this policy debate. At heart though, the issue turns on precisely the kinds of metaphysical and biological issues that philosophy of biology has been exploring for decades. Surprisingly few have weighed in (Maienschein) but more can be expected to do so in the future.

Debates about the origins of life have produced very different approaches to the meaning of life (Rizzotti). More reductionist accounts place a heavy emphasis on genetic features—the ability to replicate is key and the genes are seen as what make cells alive. In contrast, metabolists have long focused on the interactive elements of living things. Recent attempts to define the minimal genome represent the latest in the reductionist approach to defining life (Cho et al.).

## Reductionism and Genetic Determinism

One of the themes that runs through much of the intersection of philosophy of biology and bioethics is the question of reductionism and its most criticized form, genetic determinism. To what extent is behavior and character dictated by genes? Popular images in magazines hype genes as the new Rosetta stone, the key to unlocking who and what people are (Nelkin and Lindee). Many biologists have defended the view that genes are the primary determinants of key traits (Hamer; Koshland).

Philosophically there are multiple meanings of reductionism that can be distinguished. There is theory reductionism in which theories at one level are explained by other theories that are seen as more *fundamental*. Recent philosophy of science has moved away from traditional views about theories, requiring alternative accounts of formal reductionism that looks at models and mechanisms (Sarkar). Reductionism can be epistemological in character—it can be about what provides the epistemological force to claims at different levels. So, for example, the force of rules in psychology could be dependent on the force of genetic rules that would explain the rules in psychology. Ontological reductionism would claim in one way or another that the only real entities are those at lower levels. Ultimately, the ideal reductionist picture would show the unity of science—behavioral accounts can be reduced to population genetics, population genetics can be reduced to molecular genetics, molecular genetics reduced to chemistry, and chemistry to physics. The only real entities are the entities posited by physics.

There have been many criticisms of reductionism (Sarkar; Moss; Kaplan; Lewontin; Keller; Kitcher). These have ranged from technical difficulties with reducing theories from biology to other levels (the only plausible laws in Mendelian genetics are not only false, transmission genetics is a measure of the degree of falsity of the law of independent assortment) to criticisms of specific *popular* reductions which purport to demonstrate the fundamental importance of genes as the determinants of human characteristics. Reductionism (especially the popular version) is largely a promissory note, one that the critics show is virtually impossible to pay off.

## Conclusion

Philosophy of biology continues to grapple with conceptual issues that concern bioethicists. The meaning of disease, health, genetics, and even life are all issues that are full of import for normative concerns with how research should proceed, what sorts of science and medicine should be funded, and the moral status of different entities. The turn towards thick descriptions of biology and a growing interest in parts of biomedical science beyond evolution should fuel continued overlap between philosophy of biology and bioethics.

DAVID MAGNUS

**SEE ALSO:** *Body: Cultural and Religious Perspectives; Healing; Life; Medicine, Philosophy of; Natural Law; Science, Philosophy of*

### BIBLIOGRAPHY

Boorse, Christopher. 1981. "On the Distinction between Disease and Illness." *Philosophy and Public Affairs* 5: 49–68.

Callebaut, Werner. 1993. *Taking the Naturalistic Turn.* Chicago: University of Chicago Press.

Caplan, Arthur. 1992. "If Gene Therapy is the Cure, What is the Disease?" In *Gene Mapping,* ed. G. Annas and S. Elias. Oxford: Oxford University Press.

Caplan, Arthur; Englehardt, Tristram H.; et al., eds. 1981. *Concepts of Health and Disease: Interdisciplinary Perspectives.* Reading, MA: Addison-Wesley Publishing Co.

Caplan, Arthur, and McGee, Glenn. 1999. "What's in the Dish?" *Hastings Center Report* 29(2): 36–38.

Cho, Mildred; Magnus, David; Caplan, Arthur; et al. 1999. "Ethical Implications of Synthesizing a Minimal Genome." *Science* 286: 2087–2090.

Cummins Robert. 1975. "Functional Analysis." *Journal of Philosophy* 72: 741–765.

Cummins, Robert, and Perlman, Mark, eds. 2002. *Functions: New Essays in the Philosophy of Psychology and Biology.* Oxford: Oxford University Press.

Engelhardt, T. 1981. "The Concepts of Health and Disease." In *Concepts of Health and Disease: Interdisciplinary Perspectives,* ed. Arthur Caplan, H. Tristram Engelhardt, and James J. McCartney. Reading, MA: Addison-Wesley Publishing Co.

Farber, Paul. 1998. *The Temptations of Evolutionary Ethics.* Berkeley: University of California Press.

Gifford, Fred. 1990. "Genetic Traits." *Biology and Philosophy* 5(3): 327–347.

Green, Ronald M. 2001. *The Human Embryo Research Debates: Bioethics in the Vortex of Controversy.* Oxford: Oxford University Press.

Hamer, Dean. 1998. *Living with Our Genes.* New York: Doubleday.

Hull, David. 1974. *Philosophy of Biological Science* Engelwood Cliffs, NJ: Prentice-Hall.

Hull, Richard. 1979. "Why *Genetic Disease?*" In *Genetic Counseling: Facts, Values and Norms,* ed. Alexander Capron, Marc Lappé, Robert Murray, Jr., et al. New York: National Foundation March of Dimes Birth Defects Original Article Series.

Kaplan, Jonathan. 2000. *The Limits and Lies of Human Genetic Research.* New York: Routledge Press.

Keller, E. F. 1995. *Refiguring Life: Metaphors of Twentieth Century Biology.* New York: Columbia University Press.

Kitcher, Philip. 1984. "A Tale of Two Sciences." *Philosophical Review* 93: 335–373.

Koshland, Daniel. 1990. "The Rational Approach to the Irrational." *Science* 250: 189.

Lewontin, Richard. 1992. *Biology as Ideology: The Doctrine of DNA.* New York: Harper-Perennial.

Maienschein, Jane. 2003. *Defining Life.* Cambridge, MA: Harvard University Press.

Maienschein, Jane and Michael Ruse, eds. 1999. *Biology and the Foundations of Ethics.* Cambridge, Eng.: Cambridge University Press.

Moss, Lenny. 2001. *What Genes Can't Do.* Cambridge, MA: MIT Press.

Nagel, Thomas. 1997. *The Last Word.* Oxford: Oxford University Press.

Nelkin, Dorothy, and Lindee, Susan. 1995. *The DNA Mystique.* New York: W.H. Freeman Press.

Oyama, Susan; Griffiths, Paul; and Gray, Russell, eds. 2001. *Cycles of Contingency: Developmental Systems and Evolution.* Cambridge, MA: MIT Press.

Rizzotti, M, ed. 1996. *Defining Life, the Central Problem in Theoretical Biology.* Padova, Italy: University of Padova.

Ruse, Michael. 1973. *The Philospohy of Biology.* London: Hutchinson.

Ruse, Michael. 1991. "The Significance of Evolution." In *A Companion to Ethics,* ed. Peter Singer. Cambridge, Eng.: Blackwell.

Ruse, Michael. 1993. "The New Evolutionary Ethics." In *Evolutionary Ethics,* eds. Matthew Nitecki, and Doris Nitecki. Albany: State University of New York Press.

Sarkar, Sahotra. 1998. *Genetics and Reductionism.* Cambridge, Eng.: Cambridge University Press.

Schaffner, Kenneth. 1993. *Discovery and Explanation in Biology and Medicine.* Chicago: University of Chicago Press.

Smith, John Maynard. 1982. *Evolution and the Theory of Games.* Cambridge, Eng.: Cambridge University Press.

Smith, Kelly. 1990. "Genetic Disease, Genetic Testing, and the Clinician." *Medical Student Journal of the American Medical Association* 285: 327–347.

Thagard, Paul. 1999. *How Scientists Explain Disease.* Princeton, NJ: Princeton University Press.

Wilson, E. O. 1988. *On Human Nature.* Cambridge, MA: Harvard University Press.

Wright, Larry. 1973. "Functions." *Philosophical Review* 82: 139–168.

Wright, Robert. 1995. *The Moral Animal.* New York: Vintage Books.

Wulff, Henrik. 1984. "The Casual Basis of the Current Disease Classification." In *Health, Disease, and Casual Explanation in Medicine,* eds. Lennart Nordenfeld and Ingemar B. Lindahl. Dordrecht, The Netherlands: Reidel.

# BIOMEDICAL ENGINEERING

• • •

Since the early 1960s biomedical engineering has transformed healthcare in industrialized countries, confronting healthcare professionals and the lay public with new problems, decisions, and possibilities. The need to understand those problems, decisions, and possibilities has contributed to the importance of bioethics in healthcare.

## Biomedical Engineers and Biomedical Engineering

Biomedical engineers develop sophisticated quantitative methods of measurement and analysis for the diagnosis and treatment of health problems. Those methods typically draw on an understanding of various biomedical sciences, including normal and pathological physiology. For example, biomedical engineers use engineering methods to study the stresses and pressures in human joints so that they can develop replacements and study the mechanisms of cellular excitation and electrical propagation in tissue so that they can improve cardiac pacemakers. Their work includes the design, development, testing, and refinement of medical devices and procedures to prevent, diagnose, and treat trauma and disease. For example, biomedical engineers developed magnetic resonance imaging (MRI) not only as a new technique for noninvasive diagnosis but also to guide the treatment of tumors. Other biomedical engineers develop and oversee the manufacture, marketing, and maintenance of high-technology medical products.

In doing this work biomedical engineers collaborate with medical research investigators, healthcare providers, and other mechanical, electrical, chemical, aero/astro, and nuclear engineers. The collaborators often lack a biomedical background but may address special technical problems that arise in the design and development of medical products.

The devices that biomedical engineering makes possible vary from "smart" thermometers for home use to multi-million-dollar MRI equipment. Some biomedical devices come into direct contact with patients, becoming "the machine at the bedside" (Reiser and Anbar); other machines become part of the patient's body, such as cardiac defibrillators; these are new elements in the public's experience of healthcare.

## Current Practices and Approaches

There are more than 3 million engineers in the United States, but engineering work is not well understood by the public, which often confuses the engineer who designs or develops a device with the technician who operates it or the skilled worker who assembles it. The most common, and mistaken, view of engineering in general and biomedical engineering in particular is that it entails only the application of science. This "applied science" model disregards the central place of design and synthetic or creative thinking.

Engineers invent, design, develop, and adapt devices, constructions, materials, and processes in response to human needs and wants. Their concern is the actual behavior of the objects and systems they study; that behavior results from many simultaneous influences, only some of which are the object of study in the natural sciences. Biomedical engineers, like other engineers, often enhance and extend the distinct body of knowledge known as engineering science.

In the early twenty-first century the dominant fields of engineering—mechanical, civil, electrical, computer, chemical, and materials—are based on the physical and mathematical-computer sciences. Biomedical engineering may draw on engineering knowledge from any of those fields to help solve health problems by using state-of-art technology. In being defined by an area of human concern—medicine—biomedical engineering is similar to another new field or area of engineering: environmental engineering.

Biomedical engineering has a somewhat different character within each of the established engineering fields. Electrical engineering informs the biomedical investigation of the bioelectric phenomena involved in nerve and muscle function and the designs of devices, such as pain-blocking stimulators and implanted electrodes, to aid hearing. Mechanical engineering illuminates problems in biomechanics, the large-scale and small-scale solid and fluid mechanics of the living body. Biomechanics leads to the production of devices such as artificial joints and has many of its applications in orthopedic surgery, physical therapy, rehabilitative medicine, and other empirical areas of healthcare. Advances in biomechanics include the investigation of cartilage at the cellular and subcellular levels and even at the molecular level.

Since the 1990s bioengineering as practiced by chemical engineers has been transformed by advances in molecular biology that have provided the theoretical and experimental basis for predicting how the human body will interact with nonhuman materials. It has produced major new tools, such as monoclonal antibodies. Therefore, molecular biology informs the design of devices in which there is dynamic exchange between human and nonhuman systems, for example, dialysis machines, heart-lung machines, artificial organs, and implants for the sustained delivery of medications. It also informs nondevice research areas such as therapeutic protein research and lends important techniques to tissue engineering: the use of engineering theory and methods to develop cell-based artificial organs. New skin for burn patients is the first of many therapies expected from tissue engineering.

Most biomedical engineers are employed outside healthcare facilities. However, a small percentage of biomedical engineers are "clinical engineers" who work in healthcare facilities and oversee the use, adaptation, integration, maintenance, and repair of an increasingly sophisticated array of devices. In rehabilitation technology, for example, "rehabilitation engineers" often collaborate in prescribing appropriate devices and designing unique devices for individuals.

Because cutting-edge technology often finds ready application in the development of military and medical devices, engineers who are attracted to such work may choose biomedical engineering as an alternative to military work. The desire to avoid military work may explain in part why the proportion of biomedical engineers in the United States who are women is high in comparison to the proportion in other engineering fields. The high proportion of women also may be due to women's interest in the helping professions, the relative openness of new fields to women, and the high rate of representation of women in the life sciences.

Collaborations between engineers and physicians in the United States highlight the cultural differences between those professions in this country. Although corporate management or "the market" may constrain engineering work, engineers thoroughly discuss and "brainstorm" how best to deal with all existing constraints. In contrast, physicians, especially surgeons and others who must make critical decisions quickly, are accustomed to unilateral decision making. Engineers often find the hierarchical organization and authoritarian practices of medicine perplexing and even counterproductive.

The naming of devices illustrates the dominance of medicine over engineering in collaborations on medical devices. Medical devices that are named for individuals (e.g., in orthopedic surgery the Harris hip and the Galante hip) bear the names of the physicians who collaborated on them or brought them into clinical use even when the design is largely the work of a single biomedical engineer. The influence of physicians on biomedical engineering in the United States is demonstrated further by the fact that the U.S. market for medical technologies, especially technologies used in healthcare facilities, is driven by physicians and the administrators of healthcare facilities. Even when U.S. physicians do not collaborate in design and development, their demands as major customers have a much greater effect on the design of biomedical engineering devices than do those of other health professionals. In contrast, in Sweden, where the healthcare system is government-sponsored, all the healthcare workers who are expected to use a device are involved in setting the requirements for the device to be designed or purchased.

## Biomedical Engineering, Medical Technology, and Issues in Bioethics

One reason for the growing public interest in bioethics is the rapid change in healthcare practice that has resulted from biomedical innovation. The resulting technology has both desirable and undesirable effects as well as many effects that, although not clearly negative or positive, alter the responsibilities of professionals and laypersons in regard to birth and death, illness, and injury. As people confront new information and new possibilities, they are faced with difficult decisions that were unknown to previous generations. New biomedical technology forces people to become "moral pioneers" (Rapp).

There are several major categories of medical technology that have important implications for the definition of decisions and responsibilities. Medical information systems are computer-based systems that store patient information and assist in clinical problem solving. Rehabilitation devices are designed to give patients greater independence, comfort, and dignity. Drug delivery systems often alter patient participation in administering medications as well as affecting the safety, reliability, and efficacy with which medications

are administered. Teaching devices enable students to learn and practice clinical skills, often reducing patient suffering and lessening guilt and stress among student-practitioners during clinical training. Finally, some technologies improve the use of healthcare technology. For example, assessment systems help clinicians match rehabilitation technology to an individual patient's needs and abilities.

New technologies also change responsibilities by altering the healthcare labor force. Devices that require special skills to operate or for the interpretation of their output have created new healthcare occupations with new responsibilities. Other devices have reduced or eliminated the need for other kinds of work. Some devices, such as imaging technologies and therapeutic X rays, have tended to centralize care in large university or urban centers because of the expense or massiveness of the equipment or the requirements for its installation and maintenance (Reiser). For example, the powerful magnets used in magnetic resonance imaging require extensive shielding so that they do not affect metal objects in the vicinity. Other kinds of technology, such as information technology, have fostered decentralization by giving practitioners in less populated areas ready access to both specialized medical knowledge and patient information (Reiser).

New medical technology often makes healthcare more effective. However, some devices have become deeply entrenched in practice before their clinical value or lack of diagnostic clinical value has been established. This is illustrated by the electronic fetal heart monitor used during childbirth. After its introduction, this monitor was adopted quickly in hospital obstetrics units, but it was shown later not to improve birth outcome even for high-risk births (see Luthy et al.).

Medical technology has had a variety of profound effects on family-care as well as healthcare practice. For example, some people have criticized the intrusiveness of intensive-care technology in light of the relatively high frequency with which people die in intensive-care units. The unit isolates a critically ill patient from family members, making it impossible for them to care for and comfort the patient in his or her final hours and disrupting the grieving process.

Engineering innovations often change "standards of care" when the use of a particular device becomes required for care to qualify as competent. For example, a physician who does not order a diagnostic X ray in certain cases may be liable to charges of negligence.

Lasers, fiber-optic and endoscopic technology, and ultrasound irradiation have made some surgeries less invasive.

Other areas of surgery, especially invasive neonatal surgery, have grown dramatically as new devices for surgery and new intensive-care technology for postsurgical recovery have been introduced. The outcome of these surgeries is sometimes problematic. The U.S. Congress, Office of Technology Assessment, reported that largely as a result of such heroic interventions, there were 17,000 "technologically dependent" children chronically dependent on respirators, intravenous nutrition, and other medical devices for life support.

Bioethics has devoted much attention to effective but sometimes harrowing new therapies and means of life support. Diagnostic and monitoring devices have received less discussion. Diagnostic and monitoring technology often changes the character of medical decisions, along with their basis and the parties to them. For example, when a pregnancy can be terminated if prenatal testing shows an abnormality, a test, such as amniocentesis, which is done halfway through pregnancy, transforms the pregnancy into a "tentative pregnancy" even if the test results are normal (Rothman).

Some of the effects of technological devices and improvements are at least in part the responsibility of the engineers who design them. The engineering profession recognizes that engineers are responsible for both the safety and the performance of their products. The issue of safety in diagnostic, monitoring, and life-critical devices is especially prominent because a failure is often life-threatening. The scope of the biomedical engineer's responsibility for how devices are used has begun to be discussed widely among biomedical engineers only recently. That discussion has considered whether engineers bear some guilt for the suffering caused by the use of respirators in patients who have no hope of recovery (Lewis). This suggestion proposes a particularly stringent standard of professional responsibility for engineers because respirators perform their intended function very well and often enable people to resume active lives. However, when they are used on terminally ill patients, respirators may only prolong suffering for patients and families and use precious healthcare resources. This kind of misuse must be distinguished from, for example, the use of a device in a wet environment. Devices in the home or in a hospital frequently are used in areas that become wet, thus presenting the risk of electrocution. That risk is eliminated through the installation of groundfault-interrupt circuit breakers. There are no similar engineering measures to ensure that respirators are used only in patients who have some hope of recovery.

Because the basis of professional responsibility is the special knowledge that a professional possesses, professional responsibility must originate in the knowledge that enables a professional to recognize or remedy a particular class of ill effects and promote good ones. In recent years state and national legislation has strengthened the legal standing of patients' advance directives, such as living wills and healthcare proxy statements, about their care. Those measures have had some success in addressing problematic use of life-support technology. The engineers who design and develop medical technology have some responsibility to ensure that it furthers human welfare, but in a democracy all citizens bear some responsibility for government policies governing its use.

CAROLINE WHITBECK (1995)
REVISED BY AUTHOR

SEE ALSO: *Artificial Hearts and Cardiac Assist Devises; Artificial Nutrition and Hydration; Cybernetics; Dialysis, Kidney; Human Dignity; Nanotechnology; Organ Transplants, Medical Overview of; Pharmaceutical Industry; Research Policy; Technology; Transhumanism and Posthumanism*

## BIBLIOGRAPHY

Cravalho, Ernest G., and McNeil, Barbara J., eds. 1982. *Critical Issues in Medical Technology.* Boston: Auburn House.

Lewis, Steven M. 1988. "A Sense of Sin." *Biomedical Engineering Society Bulletin* 12(1): 1–2.

Luthy, David A.; Syn, Kirkwood K.; van Belle, Gerald; et al. 1987. "A Randomized Trial of Electronic Fetal Monitoring in Preterm Labor." *Obstetrics and Gynecology* 69(5): 687–695.

Mann, Robert W. 1985. "Biomedical Engineering: A Cornucopia of Challenging Engineering Tasks—All of Direct Human Significance." *IEEE Engineering in Medicine and Biology Magazine* 4(3): 43–45.

Rapp, Rayna. 1987. "Moral Pioneers: Women, Men, and Fetuses on a Frontier of Reproductive Technology." *Women and Health* 13(1 and 2): 101–117.

Reiser, Stanley. 1978. *Medicine and the Reign of Technology.* Cambridge, Eng.: Cambridge University Press.

Reiser, Stanley J., and Anbar, Michael, eds. 1984. *Machine at the Bedside: Strategies for Using Technology in Patient Care.* Cambridge, Eng.: Cambridge University Press.

Rothman, Barbara Katz. 1986. *The Tentative Pregnancy: Prenatal Diagnosis and the Future of Motherhood.* New York: Viking.

Saha, Subrata, and Bronzino, Joseph D., eds. 2000. "Ethical Issues Associated with the Use of Medical Technology." In *The Biomedical Engineering Handbook,* 2nd edition., Vol. II, ed. Joseph D. Bronzino. Boca Raton, FL: CRC Press.

Shaffer, Michael J., and Shaffer, Michael D. 1989. "The Professionalization of Clinical Engineering." *Biomedical Instrumentation and Technology* 23(5): 370–374.

U. S. Congress, Office of Technology Assessment. 1987. *New Developments in Biotechnology,* 5 vols. Washington, D.C.: U.S. Congress, Office of Technology Assessment.

Whitbeck, Caroline. 1991. "Ethical Issues Raised by New Medical Technologies." In *The New Reproductive Technologies: Medical, Psychosocial, Legal, and Ethical Dilemmas,* ed. Judith Rodin and Aila Collins. Hillsdale, NJ: Lawrence Erlbaum.

Whitbeck, Caroline. 1998. *Ethics in Engineering Practice and Research.* Cambridge, Eng.: Cambridge University Press.

# BIOTERRORISM

• • •

The issues associated with bioterrorism are as broad in their scope and as challenging in their complexity as any in bioethics. These issues engage the resources of basic sciences, history, political philosophy, sociology, healthcare administration, and public health, as well as clinical medicine. In some instances they present unique concerns, in others they are variations on more familiar bioethical problems. In providing a sound bioethical account of these problems this entry will presuppose that the terrorist threat in question is morally unjustifiable either because the cause it represents or the means used to advance this cause cannot be rationally defended.

## Public Health and Civil Liberties

There is broad agreement that individual liberties of speech, movement, and personal privacy may be abrogated when they present an imminent risk of serious harm to other persons and when no other means of ameliorating this risk is available. This doctrine is familiar within the traditional domain of public health. An additional element presents itself when there is an intentional threat to public safety from persons or states that seek to advance a political agenda.

Whether the political element is in itself sufficient justification for permitting the state to have greater latitude in the abrogation of civil liberties than it would in a naturally occurring public health emergency is an issue that may be raised. One might argue that the intentionality of a terrorist act, expressed through a biological attack, is liable to sow panic in a fashion that differs from the psychological effects of a naturally occurring epidemic. Whether that is the case or not is an empirical matter, and whether it is sufficient justification for a more aggressive response is a matter of political philosophy.

It is clear that the tactics required to minimize the harms of a disease outbreak are not substantially altered by the cause of the contagion. In the case of highly contagious and dangerous diseases like smallpox, public health theory calls for the identification and isolation of primary cases and the creation of a ring around plausible secondary cases. This surveillance and containment strategy requires that all those exposed, and their immediate contacts, be vaccinated, isolated, and quarantined if they become ill. Treatment of all cases within that ring should be sufficient to control the epidemic.

Conceivably a disease might be more likely to appear simultaneously in several distant places as part of a terrorist conspiracy than it would as part of a natural event. There is disagreement among public health experts concerning the point at which a certain number of far-flung individual cases would constitute a dire emergency that would render the ring strategy inadequate.

Although bioethics has emphasized self-determination, the public health context presents demands that are incompatible with strict adherence to individual rights. Some have argued that, especially in an emergency, effective public health interventions may entail justifiable limitations on civil liberties that would at other times be unacceptable. Limitations on such rights as speech, privacy, and travel should not be excessive or arbitrary, and they must be rationally linked to protection of the public. They may be imposed no longer than required by the circumstances.

Not all agree that more stringent restrictions on civil liberties may be required by a bioterrorism event. Some oppose abrogating the right to refuse treatment and any requirement that doctors treat patients against their will. These critics also question the practicality and effectiveness of large-scale quarantine. All these actions tend to undermine the most important defense against panic, which is trust in government authority. Adequate and equitable healthcare for all would, under this view, go farther than draconian measures to build public trust and elicit cooperation in an emergency.

## Resource Allocation in a Response to Bioterrorism

Standard accounts of a formal principle of justice require that similar cases be treated similarly. In an extreme event healthcare institutions may not have the capacity to absorb large numbers of patients that suddenly present themselves. An important problem is whether differential treatment is always morally wrong, or whether it can be justified in some instances.

The classic approach to sorting battlefield injuries is triage, a nineteenth-century French policy based on the strictly utilitarian principle of the greatest good for the greatest number. Depending on the particular model, triage utilizes three or five categories that range from *urgent* to *non-urgent* to *care not needed.* Although triage has become a familiar term in the civilian medical world, especially in busy emergency rooms, in its original military context the idea included a criterion of social merit, that the argument for care in any particular case turned on the potential for the individual to return to duty.

Under ordinary circumstances clinical triage differs from battlefield triage. In the former case the most seriously ill are not simply set aside. Rather, resources are made available through such ad hoc means as the temporary diversion of ambulances to other emergency rooms (Kipnis). Under extreme conditions these routine bypass procedures may not be feasible. A social worth criterion could be transferred to civilians if the circumstances were sufficiently dire that, for example, the very survival of the community was threatened. According to theologian Paul Ramsey, the comparative social worth of individuals can justifiably be measured in these highly defined circumstances.

First priority must be given to victims who can quickly be restored to functioning. They are needed to bury the dead to prevent epidemic. They can serve as amateur medics or nurses with a little instruction—as the triage officer directs the community's remaining medical resources to a middle group of the seriously but not-so-seriously injured majority. Among these, one could argue, a physician should first be treated (Ramsey).

A social worth criterion applied to extreme conditions appears to be incompatible with respect for each individual person, for the inevitably unsuccessful act of treating some is sacrificed in exchange for the potential survival of a valuable individual whose survival would in turn benefit the larger number. However, an argument can be made that the unequal treatment is justifiable precisely because one respects all of the others whose survival is made more likely because of the treatment of this one. Respect for all the others that might survive is respect for each of them as individuals, hence egalitarianism is preserved (Childress, 2003).

But not all who are possessed of critical skills may be required for the benefit of the community. Rather, only a few may be needed, therefore it would be unfair to guarantee all of these individuals a place at the head of the queue. Instead, to ensure that at least some of them survive without providing inappropriate advantages to all of them, essential workers may be entered into a weighted lottery in such a way that their selection is more likely, on average, than that of others (Childress, 2003).

As has been observed, the successful management of a bioterrorism event requires a high degree of public trust. Therefore, criteria for triage and resource allocation should be formulated as part of a public consensus process. Transparency in the development and application of resource allocation principles under extreme conditions should include their defense and readjustment in light of public reaction. Precedent can be found in the case of the allocation of organs (Childress, 1997). The articulation and adjustment of allocation principles must take place well in advance of the event itself.

## The Obligations of Emergency Health Workers

Healthcare workers are often expected to undergo a degree of discomfort and inconvenience in executing their duties. This expectation is justified by the vulnerability of those under their care, a vulnerability grounded in illness and in the knowledge differential between doctor and patient. Similar role-related obligations apply to other professionals, such as attorneys or securities analysts, whose clientele is inherently vulnerable by virtue of social status or lack of relevant information. Perhaps because of the concreteness and intimacy of their work, no other professional group is held to as high a standard in this regard as are those in healthcare.

The degree to which healthcare workers must compromise their own well being for the sake of others is often unclear. The role-related duties of healthcare professionals imply at least a modest degree of self-sacrifice for the sake of others who are in need of their services. Ordinarily these sacrifices are limited to brief periods of discomfort or inconvenience, particularly embodied in the rigors of the medical residency. At the extreme, martyrdom and other supererogatory acts spell out the limits of these duties, but detailed guidance is lacking. Although emergency health workers have been designated as a special group with more extensive duties under circumstances that demand urgent attention, this designation is not informative about the boundaries of their obligations (World Medical Association, Pan American Health Organization).

One set of considerations has to do with the support emergency healthcare workers are given in executing their tasks. Professionals cannot be expected to perform their responsibilities in the absence of adequate materials, much less expose themselves to conditions that put them at risk. Governments must provide "an effective and centralized authority to coordinate public and private efforts." (World

Medical Association). In the context of terrorism the society under threat should also provide the material support required for emergency healthcare workers to do their job, particularly as there is an expectation that their personal welfare is at somewhat greater risk than that of other health professionals (Eckenwiler). The failure to provide suitable support is not an excuse for the healthcare worker to abandon his or her post. Rather it reflects the reciprocity that skilled professionals may fairly expect considering the physical and psychological stresses to which they are exposed.

Another consideration relevant to the question of the limits of emergency healthcare workers' duties is that of moral responsibilities to distant others, as compared to appropriate concerns for one's own welfare or that of significant persons in one's life. As the victims of catastrophe are less familiar to us, as they become more distant in space or culture, it may become more psychologically challenging to relate to their circumstances, especially if their plight competes with that of someone in greater geographic or social proximity.

A feature of the healthcare workers' morality that should, in principle, set them apart from the rest of society is that their circle of concern knows no distance. Yet it is worth asking if this presumption of universal concern, of impartiality, is always sound when it competes with more local concerns about one's own family, friends, and colleagues. Further, partiality is not a vice if it is conceived as one way in which human beings express their individuality through the uniqueness of their relationships (Eckenwiler). Healthcare professionals functioning in emergencies may not be expected and should not be required to subvert justifiable tendencies to place primary value on personal relationships when forced to allocate their caregiving under extreme conditions.

## The Role of Private Sector Institutions

Many of the human and material resources that may be required in catastrophic circumstances are in the private sector, especially pharmaceutical manufacturers and managed care organizations. Nonpublic entities are generally agreed to have some responsibilities to the society that provides a stable framework for their business activities, responsibilities that must only increase in the event of social emergency. The contours of these corporate social responsibilities assume a special character in the context of bioterrorism.

Yet private industry cannot be expected or required to resolve all societal problems that are more appropriately considered the province of public entities, such as providing access to medication or healthcare for all. Rather, these private interests have a duty to participate in the public discourse that seeks the resolution of policy problems and to engage in business practices, such as fair pricing policies, that make solutions practicable. The rationale for this duty can be expressed in terms of the primary moral purpose of any business, to produce goods or services that contribute to the pursuit of the good life (DeRenzo).

Within this scheme drug companies can be said to have certain obligations with regard to the bioterror threat. For example, they are obligated to provide security to guard against any potential vulnerabilities in their production activities or storage arrangements. They should make positive efforts to help ensure that medications are available for the treatment of bioweapons injuries with a wide therapeutic range and based on different mechanisms, rather than simply produce medications similar to those already available. For cases wherein there is only one patented drug for a certain indication that is related to a bioterror threat, government may consider a *stop the clock* mechanism that permits at least temporarily lifting the patent so that production and distribution can be accelerated. (DeRenzo)

Managed care organizations (MCOs) have concentrated a large portion of the highly skilled healthcare work force in the private sector. Not limited to bioterrorism, this arrangement raises questions about the relationship between corporate responsibilities and threats to the public health. Controlling of costs while also providing excellent healthcare has proven to be a significant challenge to the industry, and quality improvement efforts have proven disappointing in resolving the cost-quality tension. Because public health agencies have limited resources, any severe public health problem would further tax the private healthcare system as MCOs would be obligated to provide care for victims even if they are not enrolled in some defined health or insurer plan (Mills and Werhane).

In one sense, as the burden of providing care for a potentially large patient population at risk from bioterrorism falls on MCOs—in the form of vaccination, treatment of victims and planning for attacks—the tension between cost and quality will become still more pronounced. In another sense, however, the requirements of physical survival in extreme circumstances render the cost issue moot, as the best possible care will simply have to be provided. From an economic standpoint the goods and services involved are *decommodified* or removed from the marketplace because market mechanisms are unable to deal with such conditions. Instead, MCOs should think of themselves as part of a wider system of healthcare, along with government agencies, the pharmaceutical industry and academia. Paradoxically, the threat of bioterrorism introduces a community perspective into privatized healthcare in a way that normal economic and political conditions do not (Mills and Werhane).

## Research Ethics and National Security

The development of human research ethics, and of biomedical ethics itself, has been decisively influenced by experience with the involvement of human subjects in national security experiments. The signal event in this often dispiriting history was the exploitation of concentration camp prisoners in experiments under the cover of World War II, many sponsored by the Nazi German military apparatus. The culmination of the Nazi doctors' trial in 1947 was the creation of the Nuremberg Code, which set down rules for human subjects' research and is generally considered a landmark document in biomedical ethics (Moreno).

Subsequent policies regulating human experiments on biological, chemical and atomic warfare in the U.S. military during the cold war specifically referenced the Nuremberg Code. However, these policies were not always followed, in some instances because the activity in question was not considered to be a medical experiment but a training exercise. Secrecy has itself proven to be among the greatest single obstacles to developing consistently applied ethical standards in this area.

The populations that have been involved in national security research represent a wide range, from military personnel, conscientious objectors, and institutionalized persons including prisoners, mental patients and medical patients. Military personnel in particular occupy a complex role because they are expected to subject themselves to risks that would not be required of others, and must accept medical interventions that will preserve or reestablish their fitness for duty (Moreno). Certain basic ethical standards have been recommended, such as appropriate security clearance for all parties, including subjects, prior review by an institutional review board, an appeals process, informed consent, and record keeping (Advisory Committee on Human Radiation Experiments).

Like the other bioethical issues associated with bioterrorism, the development of ethical standards for the involvement of human beings in national security experiments requires the resources of several disciplines. Still more challenging, is the application of these standards, which requires a level of engagement with the political system that clearly identifies bioethics as a practical moral activity.

JONATHAN D. MORENO

SEE ALSO: *Coercion; Epidemics; Freedom and Free Will; Harm; Hazardous Wastes and Toxic Substances; Holocaust;* *Homicide; Immigration, Ethical and Health Issues of; Race and Racism; Warfare: Chemical and Biological Weapons*

### BIBLIOGRAPHY

Advisory Committee on Human Radiation Experiments. 1996. *Final Report of the Advisory Committee on Human Radiation Experiments.* New York: Oxford University Press.

Childress, James F. 1997. *Practical Reasoning in Bioethics.* Bloomington, IA: Indiana University Press.

Childress, James F. 2003. "Triage in Response to a Bioterrorist Attack." In *Bioethics after the Terror,* ed. Jonathan D. Moreno. Cambridge, MA: MIT Press.

DeRenzo, Evan G. 2003. "The Rightful Goals of a Corporation and the Obligations of the Pharmaceutical Industry in a World with Bioterrorism." In *Bioethics after the Terror,* ed. Jonathan D. Moreno. Cambridge, MA: MIT Press.

Eckenwiler, Lisa A. 2003. "Emergency Health Professionals and the Ethics of Crisis." In *Bioethics after the Terror,* ed. Jonathan D. Moreno. Cambridge, MA: MIT Press.

Kipnis, Kenneth. 2003. "Overwhelming Casualties: Medical Ethics in a Time of Terror." In *Bioethics after the Terror,* ed. Jonathan D. Moreno. Cambridge, MA: MIT Press.

Mills, Anne E., and Werhane, Patricia H. 2003. "After the Terror: Healthcare Organizations, the Healthcare System, and the Future of Organization Ethics." In *Bioethics after the Terror,* ed. Jonathan D. Moreno. Cambridge, MA: MIT Press.

Moreno, Jonathan D. 2001. *Undue Risk: Secret State Experiments on Humans.* New York: Routledge.

Ramsey, Paul. 1970. *Patient as Person.* New Haven, CT: Yale University Press.

*U.S. v. Karl Brandt et al., Trials of War Criminals before the Nuremberg Military Tribunals under Control Council Law No. 10* (October 1946–April 1949).

# BODY

• • •

I. Embodiment in the Phenomenological Tradition

II. Cultural and Religious Perspectives

## I. EMBODIMENT IN THE PHENOMENOLOGICAL TRADITION

Philosophical and ethical issues are closely connected with medical and health professional self-understanding, knowledge, research, and practice. The human body occupies a central place in those contexts, but especially within medicine—certainly one of the sources for understanding the human body. In this entry, after a brief review of ideas about the body in the history of medicine, its place in philosophical thought since René Descartes is addressed. This history plays an important role in more recent philosophical reflections on human life, especially in writings directed to the experience of embodiment. After reviewing that history and the understanding of embodiment, some suggestions are made about the relationship between embodiment and the variety of ethical issues presented by medicine, biomedical research, and clinical practice. This discussion is unavoidably difficult, because both that history and the issues raised by efforts to explicate and understand embodiment are complex. Addressing those complexities, however briefly, will be helpful in delineating the specific concepts, terms, and methods used in the phenomenological tradition regarding embodiment.

From the earliest stirrings of human fetal life through old age, individuals are embodied. Whether their bodies are more or less healthy, or are sick, injured, compromised by congenital or genetic defects, or are such that they arouse social prejudice, individuals experience the surrounding world by means of a particular body. Being embodied, furthermore, means having a certain sexuality and thus experiencing the milieu in ways that both structure and are socially structured by that sexuality. Even slight reflection also shows that the human body has aesthetic, economic, political, and other dimensions specific to every cultural time: the body figures prominently in clothing styles, pornography, labor, torture, and the like. The experience of the body by oneself and others plays other important roles in broader terms: in the "body politic," for instance, or in the manufacture of automobiles, or in contexts such as physical examinations in the military.

Underlying all of these, however, is a striking phenomenon: regardless of the state of health, skin coloration, sexuality, or sociopolitical usages, one body is uniquely singled out for a person's experience as "mine," as that sole body through which anything else is experienced. While any full explication of embodiment must address each of these fascinating dimensions, the first question concerns that core sense of "mineness": How are we to understand that? It is to this that the present entry is devoted. First, however, an equally brief word is needed about the place of the body in medicine.

## The Body in Medicine

Historically, physicians have sought to understand the body's structures (anatomy), functions (physiology), cellular makeup (biology, biochemistry), activating and regulatory mechanisms (neurology, immunology), the several organ systems and their connections (cardiac, pulmonary, renal, hepatic, etc.), and the variety of diseases, injuries, noxious environmental influences, and genetic and congenital conditions that govern the body's development and underlie personal life.

Even with this focus, however, historical medical views of the body have varied over time (Edelstein). For example, the "dogmatic" or "rational" view understood the human body as fundamentally causal in nature—events inside the body were thought to cause outer symptoms (a pathological understanding of the body and disease). By contrast, according to the "empiricist" and "skeptical" traditions, the body and the embodied person form an experiential, temporally developing "whole" in continuous and multiple interactions with the surrounding world (a holistic view). Physicians in later historical times who were convinced of the dogmatic, rational view literally looked inside the body—by dissection and vivisection—and understood its structures and functions. Those who held the empiricist view turned instead to history (the patient's history and the collective histories of other physicians) in treating diseases. These two basic, conflicting models have continued to have an important place in medical understanding (Leder; Zaner, 1988).

Although these views continue to be present in medicine, the rationalist tradition (emphasizing the body as a material, causally determined organic system) has been clearly dominant in more recent times. The first major steps in the historical development of a rationalist view of the human body were taken in the early fourteenth century by Mondino de' Luzzi and his student Guido da Vigevano (Singer). By far the most significant steps are found in the seminal work on anatomy by Andreas Vesalius (1514–1564) and later in the important discoveries in physiology by William Harvey (1578–1657), strongly endorsed by René Descartes and continued in the work of seventeenth- and eighteenth-century post-Cartesian physicians, such as Robert Boyle (1627–1691) and Friedrich Hoffmann (1660–1742) (King) and Jerome Gaub (1705–1780) (Rather).

In modern times, the body was first proposed as a fundamentally causally determined organic system by Giovanni Battista Morgagni (1682–1771) and Xavier Bichat (1771–1802). Before this time, even though abundant autopsy reports had been published, such recorded data had not offered any correlation between clinical and anatomical findings (King). With Morgagni and Bichat, however, this changed profoundly. The introduction of the "clinicopathological correlation" radically altered medical understanding. For the first time, what was found at autopsy was taken as "explaining" clinical symptoms observed while the patient was alive. Now disease took on a highly specific form—the "organic lesion" found inside the body—and was no longer associated with a more or less loosely collected set of clinically observed symptoms or patient reports (King; Zaner, 1988). Because this "correlation" fundamentally changed the way physicians understood disease, it has been called a "revolution" (Laín Entralgo) comparable to what Copernicus effected in astronomy when he proposed that instead of thinking that the sun moves around the earth, we should perceive it to be the other way around.

The marriage of clinical medicine to biological science, definitively begun in the nineteenth century, was consummated through the work of neurologists such as John Hughlings Jackson (1834–1911) and clinicians such as William Osler (1849–1919), and the educational reforms recommended by Abraham Flexner (1866–1959) in the early twentieth century. Medical thinking then incorporated the idea that the body is a complex system of physiologically interacting structures and mechanisms governed by multiply interrelated controls seated in the neurological system. Some physicians, appreciating that this complex organism (or set of organ systems) serves as the embodied person's means of expression and action, advocated a type of "medical dualism" or "epiphenomenalism"—there must be a place for the "person," whether thought of as a distinct entity or as a causal consequence of the body complex's functional stability across time.

## The Body in Philosophy

While the history of philosophical and moral deliberations about human life is quite as sophisticated and colorful as medical history, the bulk of reflections have focused on *mind* (*person, self, subjectivity,* and related notions) (Zaner, 1980). With some notable exceptions, however, there has not been nearly as much reflection about *body* per se. In large part, a basically traditional view of these matters was assumed: that body and soul are distinct (or even separate) realities, and that what is essential in human life is to be found in the soul, not the body. The soul (mind, reason) is the pure and unchanging essence of the human; the body, on the other hand, is a baser sort of affair, belonging to the changeable, the temporal, and the corrupt. The soul, imprisoned within the corporeal, is subject to the body's peculiar "nature," its appetites and inclinations, but has its true destiny and nature elsewhere—a destiny it must pursue by becoming freed from its worldly, bodily prison.

There have been exceptions to this view of the human body. René Descartes (1596–1650), for example, argued that mind (*res cogitans*) and body (*res extensa*) are to be understood as "substances": mutually exclusive, self-subsistent, and ontologically distinct entities, neither of which requires the other to be or to be known. This familiar bifurcation of reality (dualism), often said to be at the basis of modern medicine and modern thought more generally (Cassell, 1991; Eccles), led Descartes to the view that mind and body "interact" in some manner, although specifying that the form of this interaction proved to be inordinately difficult and highly problematic (Leder).

Hardly satisfied with that, and challenged by Princess Elizabeth (daughter of the exiled king of Bohemia, living at the time in Holland), Descartes's reflections on the body show a surprising turn—one that has not been well appreciated. The mind, he thought, is not "in" the body in the way a boatman is "in" a boat—contingently or accidentally. Rather, the mind is "intimately" connected to the body, an "intimate union" that led him to the view that the human body is intrinsically complex and not at all the simple "extended substance" posited in his metaphysics (Zaner, 1988). As Descartes remarked to Princess Elizabeth, neither mathematics nor metaphysics is capable of apprehending this union. It can be known only in "daily conversation" and in clinical encounters—one might say that the union is essentially a matter of concrete experience (Descartes, 1967; Descartes, 1973; Lindeboom).

To be sure, from his early work in anatomy, Descartes had learned that the cadaver does indeed seem to be little more than such "extension." But from his earnest attempts to provide medical diagnosis, he knew full well that while it is alive, the body is far more than merely a material entity extended in space. For example, writing of the "dropsical patient" in his *Meditations* (Descartes, 1955), he took pains to point out that there are in fact *two* "natures": the one subject to the laws of nature, the other with its own specific characteristics that must be understood in quite different ways than the other (Kennington). Indeed, Neils Stenos (1638–1686), a younger physician contemporary of Descartes who specialized in the brain, contended that nature in the first sense was merely heuristic, a "manner of speaking" (*une pure dénomination* is Descartes's phrase), and should not be taken literally (Lindeboom). This intrinsic complexity of the body—as cadaver and as embodying the mind— did not attract the attention of many philosophers (or, for that matter, physicians) (Zaner, 1988).

Addressing the Cartesian idea of the "intimate union" of soul and body, Blaise Pascal (1623–1662) argued that one must be able to account for this intimacy. He noted with marked irony that if, like Descartes, one "composes all things of mind and body," surely that mixture would be intelligible—especially to one who so composes all things. Yet not only do we not understand the body, and even less the mind; least of all do we know "how a body could be united to a mind. This is the consummation of [our] difficulties, and yet it is [our] very being" (Pascal, pp. 27–28).

Benedict de Spinoza (1632–1677) thought that Descartes's bifurcation created insuperable difficulties for understanding how the mind could possibly be connected to the body, much less "intimately" connected. Like others at the time, Spinoza's argument is couched in metaphysical terms: he argued that what Descartes termed "substance" (mind and body) could only be "attributes" of the one and only substance, reality itself. Mind and body are essential to one another; the way in which they are "united," he concluded, then becomes comprehensible. The body is a mirror of the soul; mind, the idea of the body (Spinoza).

Understanding the body continued to preoccupy physicians but did not become a focal issue for philosophers until the early writings of Henri Bergson (1859–1941). Although he did not fully probe the matter, Bergson argued that the human body should be seen as the person's placement or locus in the world. What makes the body, a sui generis phenomenon, unlike any other worldly object is, he believed, that it is experienced as "mine," as "my center" of action and experience. While it is physical, it is not simply that; it is the "center" of experience, and thus the field of physical objects is spatially organized around it. In addition, the human body and its perceptual capacities are in the service of action. The body is fundamentally an actional center. It is that by means of which the embodied person is able to engage in actions in and on the field of objects. Spatial location and the familiar sensory qualities are thus always experienced within specific contexts of action: for the perceiver, "things" are "menacing," "helpful," "handy," "obstacles," and so on (Bergson). Correlated to the body as the center of action, physical things are organized as "poles of action" appearing only within specific activities directed toward them, as Jean Piaget (1896–1980) later emphasized. Because of these characteristics, the human body is a critical factor in the development of language and culture.

In the early days of the twentieth century, Max Scheler (1874–1928) devoted serious reflection to the "lived body" (Leib), in particular as regards the performance of "deeds" in moral conduct. Scheler's analysis suggests that both "ego" and the ego's "acts" are distinct from what he terms "lived bodiliness" (Leiblichkeit). At the same, lived bodiliness must be sharply distinguished from the "thing body" (Körper). Although Scheler does not mention it, this idea is a clear echo of the earlier Cartesian insight. The body that embodies the person ("my body") is uniquely singled out for, and experienced by, the person as "mine" (and in this sense is "intimately connected"). As the person's experiential "center," it is that by means of which the person is, as it were,

worlded: in the midst of objects, people, language, culture, and so on. These points, which had also impressed Bergson, came to be regarded as fundamental to embodiment, and are crucial for understanding subsequent discussions.

Edmund Husserl (1859–1938) grappled with this phenomenon throughout his career. Its primary feature, he contended, is the experiential relationship of consciousness to its own embodying organism (Husserl, 1952). Granted that this organism (Leibkörper) is uniquely singled out (Husserl, 1956–1959), the problem of embodiment is to determine in what sense and in what ways it is actually experienced by the person as his or hers, since it is solely by means of that experience that it is at all possible for the person to experience worldly things (physical, biological, cultural).

What had so impressed and troubled Descartes—the "intimate union"—Husserl calls the experiential relationship to the "body-as-mine"; however, he did not appreciate Descartes's insight any more than had Bergson or Scheler. Descartes seems clearly to have recognized that while a person is alive, there is an "intimate union" between body and soul; yet how are we to understand this "union"—a connection that is all the more peculiar when death occurs and this "alive" body becomes a cadaver that seems no different in kind from any other material thing? Although apparently appreciating this puzzle, Descartes nevertheless obscured matters (as did many others after him) by trying to resolve the very different metaphysical question of the "mind–body" relation.

It is to the embodiment phenomenon that Gabriel Marcel's analysis of the fundamental opacity (the elemental "feeling" or, as he termed it, Urgefühl) at the heart of personal life—my body qua mine—is addressed (Marcel, 1940). It is here, too, that Maurice Merleau-Ponty locates the essential ambiguity intrinsic to the body itself (Merleau-Ponty). So "intimate" is this "union," both Marcel and Merleau-Ponty point out, that one is tempted to say, with Jean-Paul Sartre, "I am my body." "My body qua mine" is thus the paradigm of "belonging" or "having": the sense in which things belong to a person is ultimately derived from the ways in which the "own" body is experienced as belonging to the person. The latter is the condition for the former (Marcel, 1935). This existential source of "belonging" becomes apparent especially in instances where mental disturbances occur and the sense of "mineness" becomes severely compromised or remains seriously undeveloped (Bosch). A central issue then emerges: By virtue of what is this one animate organism uniquely singled out to exist in my experience as that whereby everything else in the world is experienced? Which specific processes are there without which this organism would cease to be experienced by me as mine, or which give it its sense as mine (Straus, 1958)?

The problem is exceedingly complex and subtle, and is by no means settled (Zaner, 1971, 1980). It is one of those regions where philosophy and medicine can productively learn from one another. Within philosophy, however, there seems at least some agreement that the animate organism becomes and remains an embodying organism solely to the extent that (1) it is not just a physical body but a genuinely animate organism, the sole "object" within which the person's own fields of sensation (that whereon sensations occur) belong; (2) it is the only object "in" which the person immediately "rules and governs," within and from each of its "organs" and the total organism itself; (3) it is that whereby the person's "I can" (walk, perceive, move, grasp, and the like) is most immediately realized and enacted; (4) it is that "by means of which" the person perceives and otherwise experiences the field of worldly objects (things, people, language, etc.) and thus is the person's access to the world and the focus of the world's (objects, people) actions on the person; and (5) it is not only that whereby the person experiences other things, but it is itself experienced by the person (in health and sickness, and these in specific individual ways)—that is, the person's embodying organism is reflexively related to itself (Husserl, 1956, 1959).

## The Body in Medicine and Philosophy

It should of course be recognized that, given the uniqueness of each embodiment, individuals experience their bodies (and, correlatively, the surrounding world) in different ways, depending on initial biological endowments, native and cultivated abilities, activities that are available and/or encouraged, and others. Thus, a boy who from birth has been unable to walk experiences "I can" in quite different ways from a boy who has that ability. If the latter has an accident that renders him unable to walk, moreover, his inability is experienced quite differently from that of the former—indeed, while the one undergoes a "loss," the other may not, except perhaps in the indirect way of realizing that while others can walk, he has never been able to. One who is born blind experiences the surrounding world quite differently from one who goes blind due to an accident—while neither experiences a "visual world," the one has "to get used" to the absence of visual space while the other has never experienced anything else. Even in cases where an individual may from birth lack several bodily capabilities (such as Helen Keller), or loses them through illness or injury, the features suggested above still hold: the embodying organism is that whereby one experiences sensations, which most immediately embody wishes and movements, by means of

which one perceives (in whatever ways), and through which other things are experienced. Moreover, there are many other meanings the human body acquires—social, political, economic, and others—that a more complete explication of embodiment must address—bodily abilities, stances, comportments, and movements (Buytendijk) that have their sense and place within the spheres of nature, culture, and history.

Embodiment is thus fundamentally connected with various levels and modalities of bodily actions, attitudes, stances, and movements (Buytendijk), personal striving or willing, and perceptual awareness of things (including the body itself). Wishing, desiring, noticing, attending, and the like are or can be actualized (embodied, enacted) by means of corporeal movements (kinesthetic flow patterns correlated with muscle activations) that are functionally correlated with the several perceptual fields and what appears in them (turning one's head and looking at …). Only to that extent can one sensibly say that this organism is "uniquely singled out" from the field of worldly objects as "mine." Involved in embodiment are processes of sensory "feeling"—coenesthetic (of inner body, e.g., of hunger), kinesthetic (of body motion), proprioceptive (of body stance or posture)—and elementary strivings (reaching, squinting, locomotion, etc.). Together, these contribute not only to the sensing of "this" organism as "belonging to me" but also to the forming of the surrounding field of objects as correlated to bodily feelings and movements, positions, and actions.

But it needs to be emphasized that there is quite another dimension to embodiment. Although surprisingly little attention has been devoted to it, it turns out to be quite essential. However tempting it is to say "I am my body" (when, for example, someone strikes me in the face, I say "Don't hit me!"), many cases in psychopathology literature (Binswanger), and situations in daily life, suggest that matters are more complicated. The relation between self and its embodying organism seems as much a matter of "otherness" as of "mineness." However intimate and profound the relation between the person and the person's body, it is equally true that a person experiences his or her body as strange and alien, in ways that can be understood (Leder).

I am my body; but in another sense I am not my body, or not simply that. This otherness is so profound that we inevitably feel forced to qualify the "am": it is not identity, equality, or inclusion. It is "mine," but this means that the person is in a way distanced from it, for otherwise there would be no sense to "belonging"; it would not be characterizable in any sense as "mine." So close is the union that a person's experience of his or her "own" body can be psychologically unnerving (its happy obedience that the person notices for the first time, or its hateful refusal to obey his or her wish to do something) (Binswanger). So intimate is it that the person has moments of genuinely feeling "at home" with it. Yet so other is it that there are times when the person treats the body as a mere thing that is other, obsessively stuffing it with food or otherwise mistreating it; or when it is encountered as "having a life of its own" to which the person must willy-nilly attend: like it or not, "my" hair grows and must be trimmed for certain purposes, "my" hands cleaned, "my" bowels moved, "my" cold cured, and so on (Zaner, 1980; Leder).

The person finds himself or herself embodied by an animate organism whose peculiar connections to the person (and the person to it) give embodiment its uniquely uncanny character. Nothing is so much "me-myself," yet nothing seems so strange; so deeply familiar (Who else could "I" be?) yet so oddly alien (Who, indeed, am "I"?). This experience is not indicative of an inability to make up one's mind but, rather, suggests the peculiarity of embodiment. What seems distinctive is this "mineness/otherness" (the most familiar yet the most alien) dialectic that is the core of human body-as-experienced (Engelhardt; Zaner, 1980).

In these terms, to speak of embodiment is to speak of something that "I" am and not something that can be placed over against me (ob-jectum) as an object. As embodied, "I" am in a clear sense a fundamental puzzle to myself—precisely what Pascal had appreciated with remarkable insight. What is expressed by "the problem of the body" is precisely the person's "being as embodied," that is, the fundamental sense of being human in the first place. The "self-body" (or "mind-body") problem is, therefore, a matter of experience: It is enacted at every moment in the ongoing life of the person. These considerations make it easier to appreciate that the human body is essentially expressive. It is that by means of which the person enacts and expresses feelings, desires, strivings, and so on (albeit in culturally and historically different manners) (Merleau-Ponty, 1945). This expressiveness signifies that embodiment is valorized, that is, deeply textured with a sense of worth (whether positive or negative, as the case may be). After all, what happens to it happens to me: the person, as that which "rules and governs," is at the same time subject to its conditions. What happens to the person's body, in still different terms, matters to the person whose body it is: The embodying organism lies at the root of the moral sense of inviolability of personhood—of the "privacy," "integrity," "consent," "respect," and "confidentiality" that play such profound roles in research ethics, bioethics, and clinical ethics. Nor does the fact that people can and do dissemble and deceive themselves and others—as in cases of factitious illness when a person is thought to "fake" symptoms (Ford)—belie the body's expressivity.

Indeed, these are themselves expressive phenomena, however difficult it may be to discover and to interpret them (Hauerwas and Burrell).

This value character of the embodying organism also helps elucidate more fully why the continuing discussions of many bioethical issues—pregnancy, prenatal diagnosis, abortion, psychosurgery, withdrawal of life support, euthanasia—are so highly charged and deeply personal. On the other hand, the profound moral feelings evoked by certain medical practices (surgery, chemotherapy) and much biomedical experimentation (in particular the Human Genome Project) are understandable, as they are in effect ways of intervening or intruding into that most intimate and integral of spheres: the embodied person. The person is embodied, enacts himself or herself through that specific animate organism that is his or her own, and is thus expressive of that very person. Bodily schemata, attitudes, movements, actions, and perceptual abilities are all value modalities by which one enacts and expresses one's character, personality, habits, goals, moral beliefs—in short, by which the person is alive as such.

To view medical practice and biomedical research from the perspective of embodiment is to appreciate them as planned or potential interventions into the sphere of personal intimacy, whether this sphere be initial (as in infancy) or more developed. Whether or not such interventions are mainly directed to the body (medicine, surgery) or to the person's mental life or status (psychiatry, psychotherapy), they all unavoidably affect the individual. The person's life as a whole is necessarily affected by surgery no less than by psychotropic medication. Psyche and soma are inextricably bound together as constituents of an integral, contextual whole (Zaner, 1980). The expressive and valuative character of this whole, the embodied person, helps to explain why every medical intervention falls within the moral order. Recognizing this, of course, does not of itself settle any of the ethical issues present in research or clinical situations: when it is morally permissible to withdraw life support, for instance, or whether it is right to restrict a retarded person's ability to procreate. However any such issues may eventually be settled, the point here is that medicine is an inherently moral enterprise, in no small way due to the nature of embodiment and the interventional character of medicine (Cassell, 1973, 1991).

Clearly, the effort to settle the specific ethical issues associated with medical practice and biomedical research requires that the fundamentally ethical nature of any intervention be explicitly recognized and appreciated (Zaner, 1988). It can also be appreciated that the ethical issues associated with the medical profession (medical ethics) can be distinguished from those that arise in research (biomedical ethics) as well as from those that occur in clinical settings (clinical ethics). Each set of issues poses important and distinctive problems.

While embodiment has a place in each of these disciplines, perhaps it is more important in clinical ethics deliberations. Because embodiment is essentially individual, the tasks of identifying, discussing, and (one hopes) settling moral issues that arise in clinical situations require that the specific circumstances of each individual situation be determined. Personal integrity and respect for the unique person are not concerns somehow imported into clinical situations from the outside; they are, on the contrary, intrinsic to the very nature of biomedical research and clinical practice. It might be added that in problematic cases (interventions for an unconscious or incompetent patient, for instance), the decision to intervene in ways that do not or cannot include the patient's own perspective nevertheless requires other ethical grounds, and thus must be subject to critical ethical assessment. Other problematic situations—involving mental retardation, disabled infants, and so on—do not escape the necessity to respect the patient, though they do require special ways of taking it into account (e.g., consulting family or surrogate) along with the ethical issues involved in decision making (identifying and respecting the moral frameworks of each decision maker).

Medical and other health issues are not only inherently within the moral order but also context-specific. No bioethical or clinical ethics issue can be settled in the abstract. Every medical practice, no matter how apparently trivial, is value-laden to begin with, which means that it either explicitly or (most often) implicitly expresses some vision of what is, or is thought to be, morally good. The primary issue for ethics in clinical situations is to help primary decision makers make explicit what each believes to be most worthwhile, of greatest value, as this is found in ongoing clinical or research situations. Only subsequently does it become possible to make informed judgments about the particular context-specific practices and issues facing people in clinical or research contexts (Zaner, 1988).

How one can come to such truly informed judgments is an obvious problem, but it is not within the scope of this entry. It is, one hopes, enough to have delineated the philosophical and ethical dimensions of the human body—in particular, the phenomenon of embodiment, its expressive and value character, and consequently the ethical nature of medicine and biomedical research. What remains to be done is also clear: not only to find appropriate ways to incorporate these philosophical and ethical considerations into the teaching and practices of the health professions and the research community, but also to study the important aesthetic, political, sexual, and other dimensions of the body in social life more broadly.

RICHARD M. ZANER (1995)

SEE ALSO: *Biology, Philosophy of; Feminism; Gender Identity; Human Dignity; Human Nature; Life; Women, Historical and Cross-Cultural Perspectives;* and other *Body* subentries

### BIBLIOGRAPHY

Bergson, Henri. 1953. *Matière et mémoire.* 54th edition. Paris: Presses Universitaires de France. Tr. Nancy Margaret Paul and W. Scott Palmer under the title *Matter and Memory.* London: Allen & Unwin, 1970.

Binswanger, Ludwig. 1958. "The Case of Ellen West," tr. Werner M. Mendel and Joseph Lyons. In *Existence: A New Dimension in Psychiatry and Psychology,* pp. 237–364, ed. Rollo May, Ernest Angel, and Henri F. Ellenberger. New York: Basic Books.

Bosch, Gerhard. 1970. *Infantile Autism: A Clinical and Phenomenological-Anthropological Investigation Taking Language as the Guide,* tr. Derek Jordan and Inge Jordan. New York: Springer Verlag.

Buytendijk, Frederik J. J. 1957. *Attitudes et mouvements: Étude fonctionelle du mouvement humain.* Paris: Desclée de Brouwer.

Cassell, Eric. 1973. "Making and Escaping Moral Decisions." *Hastings Center Studies,* 2: 53–62.

Cassell, Eric. 1991. *The Nature of Suffering and the Goals of Medicine.* New York: Oxford University Press.

Descartes, René. 1955. *Philosophical Writings,* tr. Elizabeth S. Haldane and George R. T. Ross. 2 vols. New York: Dover.

Descartes, René. 1963–1973. *Oeuvres philosophiques,* ed. Ferdinand Alquié. 3 vols. Paris: Garner Frères.

Eccles, Sir John. 1979. *The Human Mystery.* New York: Springer International.

Edelstein, Ludwig. 1967. *Ancient Medicine: Selected Papers of Ludwig Edelstein,* ed. Owsei Temkin and C. Lillian Temkin. Baltimore: Johns Hopkins University Press.

Engelhardt, H. Tristram, Jr. 1973. *Mind-Body: A Categorial Relation.* The Hague: Martinus Nijhoff.

Ford, Charles V. 1983. *The Somatizing Disorders: Illness as a Way of Life.* New York: Elsevier Biomedical.

Gurwitsch, Aron. 1964. *Field of Consciousness.* Pittsburgh: Duquesne University Press.

Hauerwas, Stanley, and Burrell, David. 1974. "Self-Deception and Autobiography: Theological and Ethical Reflections on Speer's Inside the Third Reich." *Journal of Religious Ethics* 2: 99–118.

Husserl, Edmund. 1952a. *Allgemeine Einführung in die reine Phänomenologie*, vol. 1 of *Ideen zu einer reinen Phänomenologie und phänomenologischen Philosophie*, vol. 3 of *Husserliana: Gesammelte Werke*. The Hague: Martinus Nijhoff, tr. Fred Kersten under the title *Ideas Pertaining to a Pure Phenomenology and to a Phenomenological Philosophy: First Book: General Introduction to a Pure Phenomenology*. The Hague: Martinus Nijhoff, 1982.

Husserl, Edmund. 1952b. *Phänomenologische Untersuchen zur Konstitution*, vol 2 of *Ideen zu einer reinen Phänomenologie und phänomenologischen Philosophie*, vol. 4 of *Husserliana: Gesammelte Werke*. The Hague. Martinus Nijhoff.

Husserl, Edmund. 1956–1959. *Erste Philosophie (1923–1924)*, vols. 7 and 8 of *Husserliana: Gesammelte Werke*. The Hague: Martinus Nijhoff.

Kennington, Richard. 1978. "Descartes and Mastery of Nature." In *Organism, Medicine, and Metaphysics: Essays in Honor of Hans Jonas on his 75th Birthday, May 10, 1978*, pp. 201–223, ed. Stuart F. Spicker. Dordrecht, Netherlands: D. Reidel.

King, Lester. 1978. *The Philosophy of Medicine: The Early Eighteenth Century*. Cambridge, MA: Harvard University Press.

Laín Entralgo, Pedro. 1969. *Doctor and Patient*. New York: McGraw-Hill.

Leder, Drew. 1990. *The Absent Body*. Chicago: University of Chicago Press.

Lindeboom, Gerrit A. 1978. *Descartes and Medicine*. Amsterdam: Rodopi.

Marcel, Gabriel. 1935. *Être et avoir*. Paris: F. Aubier.

Marcel, Gabriel. 1940. *Du refus à l'invocation*. Paris: Gallimard.

Merleau-Ponty, Maurice. 1945. *Phénoménologie de la perception*. Paris: Gallimard, tr. Colin Smith under the title *Phenomenology of Perception*. London: Routledge and Kegan Paul, 1962.

Pascal, Blaise. 1941. *Pensées: The Provincial Letters*, tr. William F. Trotter and Thomas McCrie. New York: Modern Library.

Piaget, Jean. 1952. *The Origins of Intelligence in Children*, tr. Margaret Cook. New York: International Universities Press.

Rather, L. J. 1965. *Mind and Body in Eighteenth Century Medicine: A Study Based on Jerome Gaub's De regimine mentis*. Berkeley: University of California Press.

Sartre, Jean-Paul. 1943. *L'être et le néant*. Paris: Gallimard, tr. Hazel E. Barnes under the title *Being and Nothingness*. New York: Washington Square Press, 1953.

Scheler, Max. 1973. *Formalism in Ethics and Non-Formal Ethics of Values: A New Attempt toward the Foundation of an Ethical Personalism*, 5th rev. edition, tr. Manfred S. Frings and Roger L. Funk. Evanston, IL.: Northwestern University Press.

Singer, Charles J. 1925. *Evolution of Anatomy: A Short History of Anatomical and Physiological Discovery to Harvey*. New York: Alfred Knopf.

Spinoza, Benedict de. 1951. "Ethics." In vol. 2 of *Chief Works*, tr. Robert Harvey Monro Elwes. New York: Dover.

Straus, Erwin W. 1958. "Aesthesiology and Hallucinations," tr. Erwin W. Straus and Biyard Morgan. In *Existence: A New Dimension in Psychiatry and Psychology*, pp. 139–169, ed. Rollo May, Ernest Angel, and Henri F. Ellenberger. New York: Basic Books.

Straus, Erwin W. 1966. *Phenomenological Psychology: The Selected Papers of Erwin Straus*. New York: Basic Books.

Zaner, Richard. 1971. *The Problem of Embodiment*, 2nd edition. Phaenomenologica, no. 17. The Hague: Martinus Nijhoff.

Zaner, Richard. 1980. *The Context of Self: A Phenomenological Inquiry Using Medicine as a Clue*. Athens: Ohio University Press.

Zaner, Richard. 1988. *Ethics and the Clinical Encounter*. Englewood Cliffs, NJ: Prentice-Hall.

## II. CULTURAL AND RELIGIOUS PERSPECTIVES

Scholarly and popular thought alike have typically assumed that the human body is a fixed, material entity subject to the empirical rules of biological science. Such a body exists prior to the mutability and flux of cultural change and diversity, and is characterized by unchangeable inner necessities. Beginning with the historical work of Michel Foucault and Norbert Elias, the anthropology of Pierre Bourdieu, and phenomenological philosophers such as Maurice Merleau-Ponty, Hans Jonas, Max Scheler, and Gabriel Marcel, however, scholarship in the social sciences and humanities has begun to challenge this notion. Late twentieth-century commentators argue that the body can no longer be considered as a fact of nature, but is instead "an entirely problematic notion" (Vernant, p. 20); that "the body has a history" insofar as it behaves in new ways at particular historical moments (Bynum, 1989, p. 171); that the body should be understood not as a constant amidst flux but as an epitome of that flux (Frank); and that "the universalized natural body is the gold standard of hegemonic social discourse" (Haraway, 1990, p. 146).

This scholarly perspective—that the body has a history, and is not only a biological entity but also a cultural phenomenon—goes hand in hand with the increasing number and complexity of bioethical issues in contemporary society, many of which have strong religious overtones. Some decades ago the only such issue arose in cases where religious and biomedical priorities conflicted in the treatment of illness. Within the majority population, various groups such as Christian Scientists, some Pentecostal Christians, and members of small fundamentalist sects occasionally have created controversy by refusing medical treatment on the grounds that faith in medicine undermined faith in God, in other words, that since healing should occur only at the will and discretion of the deity, human medicine was presumptuous upon divine prerogative. This was especially problematic when young children suffered and were kept from medical treatment by their parents. In Native American communities it has been, and occasionally remains, the practice for ill people to seek biomedical treatment only after having exhausted the resources of their spiritually based traditional medical systems. This occasionally results in the discovery of serious illness such as cancer or tuberculosis at a very advanced stage, and creates a dilemma for healthcare personnel who are supportive of indigenous traditions yet concerned that their patients also receive timely biomedical treatment.

More recently, the number of bioethical issues with religious overtones has multiplied. The legality of and right of access by women to abortion have been defined not only as issues of civil rights and feminist politics, but also as religious and moral issues. Surrogate motherhood and donorship of sperm and eggs raise ethical dilemmas regarding the biological, legal, and spiritual connections between parent and child. There is also concern about the apparently godlike ability of biotechnology to determine the genetic makeup of the human species; some see this approaching with the increasing sophistication of genetic engineering and the massive Human Genome Project, which will catalogue all possible human genetic characteristics. At the other end of the life course, the problems of euthanasia, technological prolongation of vital functions by means of life-support machines, and physician-assisted death raise moral and spiritual questions about the prerogative to end the life of oneself or of another. Legal and ethical acceptance of the definition of death as "brain death" has particular significance in that the brain dead individual's other organs are still viable for transplantation to other persons. In the United States the bioethical dilemma is whether the brain-dead person can morally be considered dead until all other vital functions have ceased, or whether removing those organs constitutes killing the patient. In Japan an added dilemma is that a person's spiritual destiny as a deceased ancestor depends in part on maintaining an intact physical body.

Each of these issues has to do with religion, not only because religions often define them as within their moral purview, but also because at a more profound level, each taps a concern that is at the very core of religious thought and practice: the problem of what it means to be human. More precisely, the problem is the nature of human persons, of what it means to have and be a body, of life and death, and of the spiritual destiny of humankind. In the succeeding sections of this entry these issues are placed in the context of recent thought about the cultural and historical nature of the human body, about religious conceptualizations of the body, and about religious practices that focus on the body.

## The Body as a Cultural Phenomenon

It has been suggested that in contemporary civilization the human body can no longer be considered a bounded entity, in part because of the destabilizing impact of "consumer culture" and its accompanying barrage of images. These images stimulate needs and desires, as well as the corresponding changes in the way the social space we inhabit is arranged with respect to physical objects and other people (Featherstone et al.). In this process, fixed "life-cycle" categories have become blurred into a more fluid "life course" in which one's look and feel may conflict with one's biological and chronological age; some people may even experience conflict between age-appropriate behavior and subjective experience. In addition, the goals of bodily self-care have changed from spiritual salvation, to enhanced health, and finally to a marketable self (Featherstone et al.; cf. Foucault; and Bordo). As Susan Bordo has observed, techniques of body care are not directed primarily toward weight loss, but toward formation of body boundaries to protect against the eruption of the "bulge," and serve the purposes of social mobility more than the affirmation of social position. Bodily discipline is no longer incompatible with hedonism but has become a means toward it, so that one not only exercises to look good, but also wants to look good while exercising. This stands in sharp contrast not only to early historical periods but to other societies such as that of Fiji where the cultivation of bodies is not regarded as an enhancement of a performing self but as a responsibility toward the community (Becker).

This transformation in the body as a cultural phenomenon has been related by Emily Martin (1992) to a global change in social organization. In her view the "Fordist body" structured by principles of centralized control and factory-based production is on the decline. It is being replaced by a body characteristic of late capitalism, a socioeconomic regime characterized by technological innovation, specificity, and rapid, flexible change. She sees these changes particularly vividly in the domains of reproductive biology, immunology, and sexuality, all of which are increasingly intense loci of bioethical debate.

With respect to immunology in particular, Donna Haraway (1991) understands the concept of the "immune system" as an icon of symbolic and material systematic "difference" in late capitalism. The concept of the immune system was developed in its present form as recently as the 1970s, and was made possible by a profound theoretical shift from focus on individual organisms to focus on cybernetic systems. The result has been the transformation of the body into a cybernetic body, one that for Haraway requires a "cyborg ethics and politics" that recognizes radical pluralism, the inevitability of multiple meanings and imperfect communication, and physical groundedness in a particular location.

This groundedness thus extends to biology itself. In addition to immunology, this is evident in recent feminist theory that eliminates "passivity" as an intrinsic characteristic of the female body and reworks the distinctions between sex and gender, female sexual pleasure, and the act of conception (Jacobus et al.; Bordo; Haraway, 1990). With biology no longer a monolithic objectivity, the body is transformed from object to agent (Haraway, 1991). The bioethical implications of the body as experiencing agent are evident in recent social science work on the experience of illness (Kleinman; Murphy), pain (Good et al.), and religious healing (Csordas, 1990, 1994). New disciplinary syntheses grounded in a paradigm of embodiment are emerging in disciplines such as anthropology (Csordas, 1990, 1994), sociology (Turner), and history (Berman).

Many of these new syntheses are predicated on a critique of tenacious conceptual dualities such as those between mind and body, subject and object, and sex and gender (Haraway, 1991; Frank; Ots; Csordas, 1990; Leder). Drew Leder, for example, begins his critique of Cartesian mind–body dualism with the observation that in everyday life our experience is characterized by the disappearance of our body from awareness. He contrasts this with a description of *dysappearance*, the vivid but unwanted consciousness of one's body in disease, distress, or dysfunction. He then argues that it is the very sense of disappearance, itself an essential characteristic of our bodily existence, that leads to the body's self-concealment, and thus to a mistaken notion of the immateriality of mind and thought. That such a notion is cultural is evident in the technological domain if one compares Western navigational techniques, which are based on intellectualist mathematical instruments and calculations, with traditional Polynesian navigation, which in contrast relied on concrete sensory information regarding clouds and light, wave patterns, star movement, and the behavior of birds (Leder). Leder further suggests that the Western tradition compounds the error by construing the body as a source of epistemological error, moral error, and mortality. In contrast, based on a phenomenological appreciation of unitary embodiment, he suggests the possibility of a new ethics of compassion, absorption, and communion.

The contemporary cultural transformation of the body can be conceived not only in terms of revising biological essentialism and collapsing conceptual dualities, but also in discerning an ambiguity in the boundaries of corporeality itself. Haraway points to the boundaries between animal and human, between animal/human and machine, and between the physical and nonphysical (Haraway, 1991). Michel

Feher construes the boundary between human and animal or automaton (machine) at one end of a continuum whose opposite pole is defined by the boundary between human and deity. Cultural definitions of the boundary between human and divine can be significant given the circumstances of corporeal flux and bodily transformation sketched above. This is especially the case when the question goes beyond the distinction between natural and supernatural bodies, or between natural corporeality and divine incorporeality, to the question posed by Feher of the kind of body with which members of a culture endow themselves in order to come into relation with the kind of deity they posit to themselves (Feher). Thus, if the body is a cultural phenomenon in a way that makes its understanding essential to questions of bioethics, religion is an important domain of culture to address in understanding the body.

## Religious Conceptualizations of the Body

Perhaps the most vivid example from the domain of religion that the body is a cultural phenomenon subject to cultural transformations is given in the classic work on New Caledonia by Maurice Leenhardt, the anthropologist and missionary. Leenhardt recounts his discovery of the impact of Christianity on the cosmocentric world of the New Caledonian Canaques via a conversation with an aged indigenous philosopher. Leenhardt suggested that the Europeans had introduced the notion of "spirit" to the indigenous way of thinking. His interlocutor contradicted him, pointed out that his people had "always acted in accord with the spirit. What you've brought us is the body" (Leenhardt, p. 164). In brief, the indigenous worldview held that the person was not individuated but was diffused with other persons and things in a unitary sociomythic domain:

> [The body] had no existence of its own, nor specific name to distinguish it. It was only a support. But henceforth the circumscription of the physical being is completed, making possible its objectification. The idea of a human body becomes explicit. This discovery leads forthwith to a discrimination between the body and the mythic world. (Leenhardt, p. 164)

There could be no more powerful evidence that the body is a cultural and historical phenomenon. Insofar as the objectification of the body has the consequences of individuation of the psychological self and the instantiation of dualism in the conceptualization of human being, it has implications for defining a very different regime of ethical relationships and responsibilities. This is not only a relative difference, but—as is clear in the missionary example of

Leenhardt—one that has consequences for relations between different cultures.

**ANCIENT GREEK CONCEPTUALIZATIONS.** There is much more to the cultural and historical variability of the human body, however. For the ancient Greeks, as described by Jean-Pierre Vernant, the distinction between the bodies of humans and the bodies of deities was not predicated on that between corporeality and incorporeality, but on the notion that the divine bodies were complete and human bodies incomplete. Furthermore, this distinction emphasized not bodily features or morphology, but the being's place on a continuum of value and foulness. Bodies were understood as mutable along these dimensions without losing their identity, and thus deities could be simultaneously very heavy and very light, moving over the earth without quite touching it while leaving exceedingly deep footprints (Vernant). The deities thus had bodies that were not bodies, but they had characteristics that never ruptured their continuity with human bodies, and which therefore defined human bodies by their very otherness. The existence of the deities guaranteed that in Greek culture qualities such as royalty and beauty were not abstract concepts or categories, since they were concretely embodied in beings like Zeus and Aphrodite (Vernant).

**HINDU CONCEPTUALIZATIONS.** In the Hindu worldview *atman,* "self," is understood not as soul in distinction to body, but as the center in relation to an existential periphery, or as whole in relation to parts (Malamud). The ritual act of sacrifice is personified and has a body, or in other words the body is both the model for and origin of sacrifice (Malamud). The individual bodies are inherently sexual and are portrayed as couples, or *mithuna.* The masculine is invariably singular and the feminine plural, as in the sun of day in relation to the multiple stars of night, or the singularity of act/mind/silence in relation to the multiplicity of speech. In contrast to the mutable but distinctly individual body of the Greek deities, Hindu ritual portrays a rich "combinatory of the sexes" that constitutes a way of mythically thinking with the body. The mithunas achieve cosmic engenderment (begetting) through diverse body operations including dismemberment, multiplication of body parts, replication of bodies, birth, coupling/copulation, merging/incorporation, transformation and transgendering, and the emission of body products/fluids (Malamud).

**JEWISH AND CHRISTIAN CONCEPTUALIZATIONS.** If, in Hinduism, engenderment is timeless and instantiated in the cosmos by the sacrificial act, in Judaism it is linear and instantiated in history by the act of procreation. Creation and engenderment are two moments of the same process, a "hiero-history" in which human generation does not imitate a divine process, but is that process (Mopsik). Whereas in the Christian perspective the biblical injunction for man and woman to "become one flesh" is understood to refer to the indissolubility of marriage, in the Jewish perspective it is understood as the production of a child, and the birth of Christ outside the historical chain of engenderments is the basis for the Pauline splitting of the spiritual and carnal individual (Mopsik). This view is elaborated further in the Jewish kabbalistic tradition's notion of the *sefirot,* the ten-gendered emanations of the Infinite that are represented as combining to form a body (Mopsik).

In sharp contrast to the Jewish kabbalistic elaboration of engenderment as life, the Christian gnostic tradition elaborates it as death (Mopsik). Gnosticism sees the corporeal form as the creation of monstrous demiurges or archons, foremost among whom is Ialdabaoth, the equivalent of Jehovah. The human condition is symbolized in the gnostic tale of the archons' rape of Eve, who escapes with her psychic body while her "shadow" or material body is defiled (Williams). The latter is a prison or garment, beastly because humans are created by beasts. Sexuality is an aspect of this beastliness, and hence cannot be part of an embodied sacred process, while the upright posture that distinguishes us from animals is attributed to a separate spark from the authentically spiritual Human (Williams).

From a more mainstream Christian perspective, the profound cultural implications of Feher's question of the kind of body people endow themselves with in order to come into relation with the sacred (Feher) can be seen by considering the Eucharist. That the consumption of bread and wine transubstantiated into the body and blood of Christ is essentially a form of ritual cannibalism is emphasized by the story of a miracle in which a priest who doubted the divine reality of the Eucharist was forced to experience the bloody flesh, so that he could come to appreciate God's graciousness in presenting it in the tamer appearance of bread and wine (Camporesi; see also Bynum, 1989). In earlier periods of Christianity the spiritual power of the Eucharist extended to the nourishment of the body, and this, not through ingestion but by means of its aroma (Camporesi). Unlike ordinary food, however, it does not become us, but we become it through its sanctifying power (Camporesi). Great anxiety was created among priests with regard to the immense responsibility of transforming something dead into something alive by the utterance of a few words, and among communicants because of the inclusion of such a sacred substance in such a profane terrain as the digestive tract—hence the importance of a fast before communion (Camporesi). Yet because the Eucharist was thought to release its grace only in the stomach, sick people who could not eat were excluded (Camporesi). When later the substantial bread was replaced by thin wafers, it became common to let the wafer melt in one's mouth. Well into the twentieth century, Catholics were taught that biting or chewing the Eucharist was an insult and injury to the deity that could result in divine retribution.

MEDIEVAL CONCEPTUALIZATIONS. Recent work on medieval Christian spirituality relates to the notion of the body as a cultural phenomenon. Caroline Walker Bynum (1989) has documented the prominence during the years 1200–1500 of a "somatic spirituality" that stands in contrast to gnostic rejection of the body, and that reflects a less dualist mentality than has heretofore been attributed to the thought of this period. In general, a great deal of concern with embodiment was evidenced in speculation about whether the final "resurrection of the body" might be a natural consequence of human nature rather than a discrete divine act to occur at the Last Judgment, and whether we will taste and smell heaven as well as see it.

The medieval body was defined less by its sexuality than by notions of fertility and decay, but the contrast between male and female was as important as that between body and soul. Somatic spirituality was especially evident among female mystics, who—in contrast to their more cerebral male counterparts' experience of stillness and silence—tended to blur the boundaries among the spiritual, psychological, bodily, and sexual by cultivating a sensualized relationship of human body with divine body. Bynum draws on the cultural-historical context to understand why the male-dominated ecclesiastical hierarchy allowed this female spirituality to flourish: evidence was needed against the contemporary dualist heresy of the Cathars; because they were denied education in Latin, they wrote in the less linear and more oral style of the vernacular; they were encouraged to act out maternal roles vis-à-vis Christ (1989).

In this context the relation between the genders took on remarkable properties. Although ideally a woman would die to defend her holy chastity, it was as likely for a holy man to be resurrected in order to complete a virtuous task. In other ways the genders were blurred, since it was thought that all had both genders within, and that men and women had identical organs with only their internal and external arrangements being different. Because of the powerful symbolic association of the female and the fleshly, while holy women sometimes experienced being the mother or lover of Christ, their nature often allowed them to mystically *become* the flesh of Christ. By the same reasoning, since body is

equivalent to female, the incarnate Christ had a female nature, and the image of Christ as mother became a feature of medieval iconography (Bynum, 1989).

## Religious Practices and the Body

FASTING. The cultural-historical transformation of the body is highlighted by comparison of fasting as a technique of the body in the medieval somatic spirituality with the phenomenon of anorexia nervosa in the late twentieth century. In a study of 261 holy women in Italy since the year 1200, Rudolf Bell distinguishes between contemporary anorexia nervosa and what he calls "holy anorexia." While the former is regarded as a syndrome of clinical pathology, in the latter, "the suppression of physical urges and basic feelings—fatigue, sexual drive, hunger, pain—frees the body to achieve heroic feats and the soul to commune with God" (p. 13). There are parallels between the two conditions and historical epochs. Bell suggests that the observation that the internal locus of evil as a corrupting force for women in the Middle Ages, in distinction to the external locus of sin as a response to external stimulus for men, corresponds to the Freudian model of anorexia nervosa as a food/sex oral fixation. In addition, in both, "the main theme is a struggle for control, for a sense of identity, competence, and effectiveness" (Hilde Bruch, quoted in Bell, p. 17). However, there is a critical difference, and "whether anorexia is holy or nervous depends on the culture in which a young woman strives to gain control of her life" (Bell, p. 20).

Bynum (1987) warns against the assumption that these are precisely the same phenomenon, given theological meaning in one epoch and psychiatric meaning in another. She points out that even medieval writers had more than one paradigm for explaining fasting—that it could be supernaturally caused, naturally caused, or feigned—and that there was a clear distinction between choosing to renounce food and the inability to eat. In both historical cases, the behavior "is learned from a culture that has complex and long-standing traditions about women, about bodies, and about food," including what kind of behaviors are in need of cure (p. 198). It is a profoundly cultural fact that in the patristic era miraculous fasting was attributed largely to men, while in the medieval period it was characteristic of women; likewise it is cultural that in the medieval period the illnesses of men were more likely thought of as needing to be cured, while those of women were to be endured. Furthermore, in the later Middle Ages fasting was associated with a wider array of miracles and practices of somatic spirituality, including subsistence on the Eucharist, stigmata, espousal rings, sweet-smelling bodies, bodily elongation, and incorruptibility. Some of the behavior of these women fits the pattern of nineteenth-century "hysteria," some is clearly the result of other illnesses, and some follows the thematic of control, altered body concept/perceptions, and euphoria. Yet one cannot be sure whether symptoms are associated with an inability to eat or are the result of freely chosen ascetic fasting. Finally, insofar as psychodynamic explanation can explain only individual cases, Bynum concludes that it is less helpful to know that contemporary labels can in some cases be applied to the medieval phenomenon than to account for cultural symbols that give meaning to the phenomenon, such as body, food, blood, suffering, generativity, or hunger (1987).

FAITH HEALING. Other contemporary religious practices equally require an appreciation of the body as a cultural phenomenon. How, for example, can we understand the imputed efficacy of "faith healing" among contemporary Christians? An understanding of the body as a cultural phenomenon suggests that ritual healing operates on a margin of disability that is present in many conditions. It is well known, for example, that some people who become "legally blind" are able to engage in a wide range of activities, while others retreat to a posture of near total disability and inactivity. Likewise, persons with chronic pain in a limb may be physically able to move that limb, but refrain from doing so for lack of sufficient motivation to make the risk of pain worthwhile. Disability is thus constituted as a habitual mode of engaging the world. The process of healing is an existential process of exploring this margin of disability, motivated by the conviction of divine power and the committed participant's desire to demonstrate it in himself or herself, as well as by the support of the other assembled devotees and their acclamation for a supplicant's testimony of healing. To be convinced of this interpretation one need only consider the hesitant, faltering steps of the supplicant who, at the healer's request, rises from a wheelchair and shuffles slowly up and down a church aisle; or the slowly unclenching fist of the sufferer of chronic arthritis whose hand is curled by affliction into a permanent fist. Ritual healing allows this by challenging the sensory commitment to a habitual posture, by removing inhibitions on the motor tendency toward static postural tone, and by modulating the somatic mode of attention, that is, a person's attention to his or her own bodily processes in relation to others.

Consider also the practice of "resting in the Spirit" or being "slain in the Spirit" among Charismatic and Pentecostal Christians as evidence for the kind of body with which people endow themselves in order to come into relation with the sacred. In this practice, which occurs primarily in healing services, a person is overcome with divine power, and falls into a semi-swoon characterized by tranquility and motor dissociation. Despite its popularity, or perhaps because of it, resting in the Spirit is a controversial phenomenon for Charismatics, and the heart of the issue is its authenticity. More specifically, critics challenge its authenticity while apologists argue for its beneficial effects in terms of healing and spiritual development. Both sides invoke the same biblical scenarios, such as Saul on the road to Damascus and the apostles confronted by the transfiguration of Jesus, and the same religious writers, including the ecstatic mystics Theresa of Avila and John of the Cross, and both sides draw opposing conclusions about whether these constitute examples of resting in the Spirit. They likewise draw opposing conclusions about the historical prototypes of healers known for similar practices, extending backward in time from Kathryn Kuhlman to Charles Finney, George Jeffreys, George Fox, John Wesley, and the fourteenth-century Dominican preacher John Tauler. To be sure, such analogies and precedents suggest that it would be possible to examine the varying meanings of religious falling or swooning across historical and cultural contexts. In the contemporary context, however, the ideological/theological/pastoral debate about authenticity is predicated on the recurrent, constitutive North American psychocultural themes of spontaneity and control, and on the Charismatic cultural definition of the tripartite person as a composite of body, mind, and spirit.

SPIRIT POSSESSION. The sacred swoon leads also to the complex issue of dissociation, common to discussions of "spirit possession." Spirits who inhabit people may be regarded either as malevolent, in which case they must be expelled or exorcised, or as benevolent, in which case becoming possessed is an act of worship and devotion. Possession of both types is widely reported in ethnological literature (Bourguignon), and is increasingly common in contemporary Western society. Not only is the negative, or demonic, variant reported among some varieties of Christian religions, but the positive variant of possession by deities is characteristic of rapidly growing African religions. These include religions based on the Yoruba tradition of Nigeria, such as *santeria, candomble,* and the related *vodun.* The Yoruba religion, in which the possessing deities are called *orixas,* is rapidly aspiring to membership in that select group of "world religions" that once included only so-called "civilized" faiths such as Christianity, Judaism, Islam, Hinduism, Buddhism, Taoism, and Confucianism. This cultural development requires a more sophisticated understanding of the possession phenomenon not as mental or cognitive dissociation but as physical and existential incarnation; not as a pathological hysterical amnesia to which the devotee becomes abandoned, but as a form of habitual body memory in which the deity's characteristics are enacted in a contemporary form of somatic spirituality.

**ABORTION HEALING RITUALS.** A final example of the interplay of religion and bioethics with respect to bodily practices pertains to the contemporary cultural debate over abortion. Among participants in the North American Christian religious movement known as the Charismatic Renewal, and in Japan as a facet of what are called the New Religions, healing rituals are conducted both for the removal of guilt presumed to be experienced by the woman, and for the fetus in order to establish its spiritual status. The American practice is largely a private one that takes place within the membership of a discrete religious movement within Christianity, and is a specific instance of the healing system elaborated within that movement. The Japanese practice has a relatively public profile not limited to a particular social group, and is an instance of a type of ritual common to a variety of forms of Buddhism.

In both societies the affective issue addressed by the ritual is guilt, but whereas in American culture this is guilt occurring as a function of sin, in Japan it is guilt as a function of necessity. For the Americans abortion is an un-Christian act, and both perpetrator and victim must be brought back ritually into the Christian moral and emotional universe; for the Japanese both the acceptance of abortion as necessary and the acknowledgment of guilt are circumscribed within the Buddhist moral and emotional universe. Both rites are intended to heal the distress experienced by the woman, but the etiology of the illness is somewhat differently construed in the two cases. For Charismatics any symptoms displayed by the woman are the result of the abortion as psychological trauma compounded by guilt, along with the more or less indirect effects of the restive fetal spirit "crying out" for love and comfort. In Japan such symptoms are attributed to vengeance and resentment on the part of the aborted fetal spirit that is the pained victim of an unnatural, albeit necessary, act. Finally, not only the etiology but the emotional work accomplished by the two rituals is construed differently. For the Charismatics, this is a work of forgiveness and of emotional "letting go." For the Japanese, in whose cultural context gratitude and guilt are not sharply differentiated, it is a work of thanks and apology to the fetus. Thus, "[t]here is no great need to determine precisely whether one is addressing a guilt-pre-supposing 'apology' to a fetus or merely expressing 'thanks' to it for having vacated its place in the body of a woman and having moved on, leaving her—and her family—relatively free of its physical presence" (LaFleur, p. 147).

## Conclusion

The contemporary transformation of the human body and scholarly formulations of it, placed alongside the transformative power of religion in its task of defining what it means to be human, offers an important perspective on issues relevant to bioethics. These range from abortion to brain death, from fasting to resting in the Spirit, from consumer culture to dissociation, and bear on the relation between genders, between cultures, and between the poles of dualities such as mind and body. Such phenomena, and new ways of understanding them, will increasingly come to light with continuing elaboration of the body/culture/religion nexus.

THOMAS J. CSORDAS (1995)

**SEE ALSO:** *Anthropology and Bioethics; Buddhism, Bioethics in; Christianity, Bioethics in; Death; Embryo and Fetus; Healing; Judaism, Bioethics in; Medical Ethics, History of; Medicine, Art of; Native American Religions, Bioethics in; Sexual Ethics;* and other *Body* subentries

### BIBLIOGRAPHY

Becker, Anne. 1994. "Nurturing and Negligence: Working on Others' Bodies in Fiji." In *Embodiment and Experience: The Existential Ground of Culture and Self,* ed. Thomas J. Csordas. Cambridge, Eng.: Cambridge University Press.

Bell, Rudolph M. 1985. *Holy Anorexia.* Chicago: University of Chicago Press.

Berman, Morris. 1989. *Coming to Our Senses: Body and Spirit in the Hidden History of the West.* New York: Simon and Schuster.

Bordo, Susan. 1990. "Reading the Slender Body." In *Body/Politics: Women and the Discourses of Science,* pp. 83–112, ed. Mary Jacobus, Evelyn Fox Keller, and Sally Shuttleworth. New York: Routledge.

Bourguignon, Erika. 1976. *Possession.* San Francisco: Chandler and Sharp.

Bynum, Caroline Walker. 1987. *Holy Feast and Holy Fast: The Religious Significance of Food to Medieval Women.* Berkeley: University of California Press.

Bynum, Caroline Walker. 1989. "The Female Body and Religious Practice in the Later Middle Ages." In pt. 1 of *Fragments for a History of the Human Body,* pp. 160–219, ed. Michel Feher. New York: Zone.

Camporesi, Piero. 1989. "The Consecrated Host: A Wondrous Excess." In pt. 1 of *Fragments for a History of the Human Body,* pp. 220–269, ed. Michel Feher. New York: Zone.

Csordas, Thomas J. 1990. "Embodiment as a Paradigm for Anthropology." *Ethos* 18(1): 5–47.

Csordas, Thomas J., ed. 1994. *Embodiment and Experience: The Existential Ground of Culture and Self.* Cambridge, Eng.: Cambridge University Press.

Featherstone, Mike; Hepworth, Mike; and Turner, Bryan S., eds. 1991. *The Body: Social Process and Cultural Theory.* London: Sage.

Feher, Michel. 1989. Introduction. In pt. 1 of *Fragments for a History of the Human Body,* pp. 10–17, ed. Michel Feher. New York: Zone.

Foucault, Michel. 1986. *The Care of the Self,* vol. 3 of *The History of Sexuality,* tr. Robert Hurley. New York: Pantheon.

Good, Mary-Jo Delvecchio; Brodwin, Paul E.; Good, Byron J.; and Kleinman, Arthur, eds. 1992. *Pain as Human Experience: An Anthropological Perspective.* Berkeley: University of California Press.

Haraway, Donna J. 1990. "Investment Strategies for the Evolving Portfolio of Primate Females." In *Body/Politics: Women and the Discourses of Science,* pp. 139–162, ed. Mary Jacobus, Evelyn Fox Keller, and Sally Shuttleworth. New York: Routledge.

Haraway, Donna J. 1991. *Simians, Cyborgs, and Women: The Reinvention of Nature.* New York: Routledge.

Jacobus, Mary; Keller, Evelyn Fox; and Shuttleworth, Sally, eds. 1990. *Body/Politics: Women and the Discourses of Science.* New York: Routledge.

Kleinman, Arthur. 1988. *The Illness Narratives: Suffering, Healing, and the Human Condition.* New York: Basic Books.

Leder, Drew. 1990. *The Absent Body.* Chicago: University of Chicago Press.

Leenhardt, Maurice. 1979. *Do Kamo: Person and Myth in the Melanesian World.* Chicago: University of Chicago Press.

Malamud, Charles. 1989. "Indian Speculations about the Sex of the Sacrifice." In pt. 1 of *Fragments for a History of the Human Body,* pp. 48–73, ed. Michel Feher. New York: Zone.

Martin, Emily. 1992. "The End of the Body?" *American Ethnologist* 19(1):121–140.

Mopsik, Charles. 1989. "The Body of Engenderment in the Hebrew Bible, the Rabbinic Tradition, and the Kabbalah." In pt. 1 of *Fragments for a History of the Human Body,* pp. 48–73, ed. Michel Feher. New York: Zone.

Murphy, Robert F. 1987. *The Body Silent.* New York: Henry Holt.

Ots, Thomas. 1991. "Phenomenology of the Body: The Subject-Object Problem in Psychosomatic Medicine and Role of Traditional Medical Systems Herein." In *Anthropologies of Medicine: A Colloquium on West European and North American Perspectives,* pp. 43–58, ed. Beatrix Pfleiderer and Gilles Bibeau. Brunswick, Germany: Vieweg.

Turner, Bryan. 1986. *The Body and Society: Explorations in Social Theory.* New York: Basil Blackwell.

Vernant, Jean-Pierre. 1989. "Dim Body, Dazzling Body." In pt. 1 of *Fragments for a History of the Human Body,* pp. 18–47, ed. Michel Feher. New York: Zone.

Williams, Michael A. 1989. "Divine Image—Prison of Flesh: Perceptions of the Body in Ancient Gnosticism." In pt. 1 of *Fragments for a History of the Human Body,* pp. 128–147, ed. Michel Feher. New York: Zone.

# BUDDHISM, BIOETHICS IN

• • •

Buddhism originated in India around 500 B.C.E. In the early twenty-first century Buddhist traditions exist in South, Southeast, and East Asia, as well as Australia, Western and Eastern Europe, and North and South America. The diversity found in these traditions makes it impossible to speak of Buddhism in the singular or to assert an "official" Buddhist perspective. For the purpose of formulating an overview of Buddhist bioethics, however, Buddhist traditions can be categorized into two primary trajectories: Theravada and Mahayana. Theravada traditions are closely identified with the teachings of the historical Buddha, and include both early South Asian Buddhist traditions as well as contemporary South Asian traditions in Sri Lanka, Thailand, and Myanmar (formerly Burma). Mahayana traditions include some later forms of Indian Buddhism, Tibetan and other Himalayan-region Buddhisms (also referred to as Tibetan, Vajrayana, Tantric, and Esoteric Buddhism), and Central and East Asian Buddhist traditions. Both Theravada and Mahayana Buddhism are practiced in such places as Australia, Europe, and North and South America.

Historically, bioethics has been a field of inquiry primarily in Western cultures and thus centers on Western cultural assumptions and moral perspectives. Genetic engineering, cloning, and stem cell research—and the ethical dilemmas they engender—pivot on recent advances in biomedical technology and Western emphases on the value of medical progress. However, moral issues raised by biomedical technology are no longer confined to Western cultural contexts. Predominately Buddhist countries have begun to confront the ethical implications of biomedicine. Not surprisingly, Buddhist ethical perspectives stem from assumptions that are sometimes very different from Western views, and these concerns affect how Buddhists engage with bioethical issues.

Individuals from North American and European cultural backgrounds may be troubled at the specter of "playing God" in making ethical decisions. From a Buddhist perspective, however, emphasis is placed, for instance, on investigating how the Buddha's exemplary life and compassion might reveal satisfying solutions to problems never envisioned by past Buddhists. After outlining some fundamental Theravada and Mahayana Buddhist ideas, this entry considers ways that Buddhists might respond to bioethical dilemmas and which

Buddhist religious ideas could be invoked to make sense of diverse bioethical issues.

## Theravada Buddhist Thought and Practice

Western interpretations of the Buddhist Dharma—Buddha's law or teaching—often treat it as a philosophy. Although it is possible to view the Dharma this way, Buddha emphasized the centrality of religious practice over philosophy and doctrines. Intellectual understandings merely point at what must ultimately be realized through experience. Buddha posited a religious path attainable through a rigorous tripartite practice of wisdom, morality, and meditation. These three were the foundations of the Noble Eightfold Path, Buddha's outline for how to live the religious life.

Theravada Buddhism focuses particular attention on the life of the historical Buddha (c. 563–483 B.C.E.). Buddha ("The Enlightened One") was a human being who, through assiduous spiritual practices, was able to comprehend the true nature of the universe. The realization of this transcendent wisdom is the achievement of *nirvana,* or enlightenment. Buddha, therefore, is a model for humanity, an example of what is possible by diligent practice of the Dharma.

The biography of the historical Buddha recounts the story of an entitled prince, Siddhartha Gautama of the Sakya clan, who is provided with material comforts and sensual pleasures by the king, his father. Wishing that his son will become a great leader, the king arranges for the prince to be sequestered in the palace, shielded from the pain and suffering that afflicts human beings. Over time, the prince—now grown and married with a young son—becomes curious about the world beyond the confines of the palace. Against his father's wishes, he ventures outside the palace walls on four separate occasions. Each time he encounters an aspect of human experience hitherto unknown to him. The four encounters—a sick person, an elderly person, a corpse, and a religious ascetic—result in the prince's realization of the fundamental suffering of human existence. The encounter with the ascetic prompts Prince Siddhartha's quest to attain an understanding of the world that would end suffering.

Prince Siddhartha subsequently decides to leave the palace and pursue the spiritual life of an ascetic renunciant. Single-minded in his resolve to attain spiritual liberation from the bonds of human existence by denying material needs, he nearly starves to death. As a result, he recognizes that liberation must lie somewhere between extreme hedonism and severe asceticism. He embarks on what becomes known as the Middle Path, a practice that allows sufficient bodily nourishment to carry out meditation and other spiritual practices. Through deep and persistent meditation he attains nirvana, thereby becoming Buddha. A reluctant teacher, he eventually accedes to the desire of others that he expound upon what he has learned. Thus begins Buddha's lifelong teaching of the Dharma.

Buddha's teaching centers on wisdom attained through enlightenment, a transcendent awareness of both the problem in the human condition and a means to its solution. This problem finds expression in the Three Marks of Existence, a description of the nature of life within the unenlightened world of *samsara* (the cycle of birth-death-rebirth). Individual status in the samsaric cycle is determined by actions (*karma*) and their moral consequences. Moral behavior leads to a higher spiritual rebirth, while immoral actions result in movement away from enlightenment. Buddha recognized that the samsaric world is fundamentally unsatisfactory and human beings eventually seek escape from it. According to the Three Marks, all existence is characterized by: (1) impermanence (*anitya*); (2) suffering (*duhkha*); and (3) absence of a permanent ground or essence (*anatman*).

Impermanence refers to the idea that all aspects of the samsaric world are in constant flux. While the world might appear to have stability and solidity, deeper scrutiny reveals that samsara is characterized by perpetual instability. Human beings mistake the temporary coming together of constituent elements (*dharma*s) for permanence. Thus, the world is best characterized not in terms of the atomistic existence of discrete enduring objects, but rather as a state of dependent origination, or interdependence—*pratitya-samutpada.* Samsaric entities—including human beings—exist as a result of cause and effect. Nothing has an intrinsic foundation or essence that gives rise to its own existence. *Samsara* itself is understood as constituted by conditioned reality, that is, arising from a series of causes and effects.

The second mark of existence is suffering. The Buddhist term *duhkha* refers to both physical and mental suffering—especially the latter. *Duhkha* signifies the anxiety and insecurity prompted by the impermanent, transitory nature of the human condition. Markers of impermanence include the cycle of birth, disease, old age, and death, as well as anticipation of the inevitable loss of happiness and other temporarily pleasant emotions. Buddha did not deny the reality of happiness, but simply noted that it too is fleeting and impermanent. Suffering results from ignorance of the true nature of the samsaric world as transitory, momentary, and subject to constant flux.

The third mark of existence, *anatman* (no-self), refers to the absence of a permanent self or eternal soul that persists after physical death. Human ignorance engenders a misperception of current identity or sense of self as an enduring, independent essence. This idea is illustrated in an

Indian Buddhist text that relates a dialogue between King Milinda and the monk Nagasena. In the *Simile of the Chariot,* Nagasena asserts that the self, like a chariot, has no essence. The King protests, so Nagasena describes the process of disassembling a chariot. Once the chariot has been reduced to a pile of parts, the King concedes that there is no essence of the chariot that persists. Like the chariot, human beings consist of constituent elements. These elements coalesce to form both animate and inanimate objects. Upon death, the *dharma*s disperse and re-form due to cause and effect, but no aspect of self, soul, or personality persists. Thus, *anatman* asserts that all existence is causally conditioned. The five aggregates of *dharma*s that constitute human beings are constantly arising and ceasing, but they do not produce a discrete, identifiable self or soul.

In accord with the worldview expressed by the Three Marks of Existence, Buddha taught that liberation from suffering may be attained though the Four Noble Truths:

1. All existence is suffering.
2. Suffering is caused by desire.
3. Cessation of desire results in the cessation of suffering.
4. The Eightfold Path leads to liberation (nirvana).

Like a medical analysis of the human condition, the Four Noble Truths mirror the steps of diagnosing a disease (suffering), understanding its cause (desire), identifying the cure for the disease (cessation of desire), and prescribing medicine that effects the cure (Eightfold Path). An outline of attitudes and actions necessary for spiritual advancement and enlightenment, the Eightfold Path offers a foundation for understanding Buddhist ethics in general and Theravada Buddhist bioethics in particular.

Buddha expounded the Eightfold Path as the mental and physical practices necessary to reach liberation from the samsaric world. The Eightfold Path consists of three components: wisdom (*prajna*): (1) right views and (2) right intention; morality (*sila*): (3) right speech, (4) right conduct, and (5) right livelihood; and concentration (*samadhi*): (6) right effort, (7) right mindfulness, and (8) right concentration.

Wisdom refers to the fundamental mental states necessary to practice Buddha's Dharma. Right views include knowledge and acceptance of the Four Noble Truths and other aspects of the Dharma. Right intention refers to cultivating qualities such as compassion, benevolence, and detachment from the fruits of actions, and a commitment to harm no living creatures.

Morality is conceptualized in terms of speech, conduct, and occupation. Right speech requires that Buddhists abstain from verbal abuses such as slander, lying, and gossip.

Right conduct refers to the avoidance of actions that harm others, such as killing, stealing, and sexual impropriety. Right livelihood extends the ideal of moral actions and prohibits specific occupations. Thus, one must refrain from work that leads—either directly or indirectly—to harming other living beings.

Concentration entails mental practices aimed at purifying the mind of evil and other distracting thoughts, and gaining mastery of mental processes and feelings in order to engage in advanced meditation.

The practice of the Eightfold Path is neither linear nor sequential. Rather, all eight aspects must be cultivated simultaneously. Through self-effort these practices eventually effect a spiritual transformation from ignorance to a state of transcendent wisdom—*nirvana*. One who has cultivated of the Eightfold Path and achieved liberation is known as an *arhat* (holy one)—the model of Theravada Buddhist religiosity that all endeavor to follow.

## Mahayana Buddhist Thought and Practice

Even a brief survey of Mahayana Buddhism, which arose less than 500 years after the historical Buddha's lifetime, strongly suggests that "Buddhist bioethics" cannot be approached in singular terms. Mahayana refashions Theravada perspectives through the concept of *sunyata* (emptiness), while adding a new soteriological possibility based on faith: birth in a Buddhist paradise as the goal of religious praxis. Thus, Mahayana Buddhism incorporates the ideal of enlightenment achieved through individual self-effort—Zen Buddhism is the most well-known exemplar of this—as well as potential for salvation through birth in a Buddhist paradise. Particularly noteworthy is the Western Paradise, or Pure Land, of Amitabha Buddha who vows to save all sentient beings that call on him for assistance. Further, anyone—monastic or layperson—could practice devotion to the "other power of Amitabha," emphasizing for the first time nonmonastic practice leading to salvation.

In contrast to Theravada emphasis on the arhat, Mahayana focuses on the figure of the *bodhisattva,* a concept that has two primary significances. First, meditation-based Mahayana centers on the bodhisattva vow, a pledge to follow the Buddha's Dharma in order to achieve enlightenment and to compassionately assist others in the same quest. Through meditation, the *bodhisattva* aims to perceive the reality of the universe—that all *dharma*s are empty of self-nature. The concept of emptiness (*sunyata*) asserts that all dualistic perceptions are misperceptions, and that *nirvana* and *samsara* are the same thing. Otherwise, a duality or opposition between the enlightened and the unenlightened is being expressed. The Mahayana goal is not to transcend *samsara,* but rather to understand—experientially—that dualities result from a mistaken view of nirvana as permanent and eternal, existing outside of *samsara.*

Second, in faith-based Mahayana, the term *bodhisattva* describes compassionate figures, like Avalokitesvara (Known in China as Guanyin and in Japan as Kannon), who have advanced along the path to enlightenment and gained great spiritual powers. They are called upon for assistance with both spiritual and material difficulties. Faith-based Mahayana recognizes that, for most lay Buddhists, following the Dharma is too difficult. In a degenerate age far removed from the teachings of the historical Buddha, the only hope for release from *samsara* is by calling—single-mindedly and with devotion—on those whose spiritual progress far exceeds our own. Devotions may be made to Amitabha Buddha for spiritual and material assistance in addition to the intervention of *bodhisattva*s.

Mahayana conceptions of the *bodhisattva* critique the Theravada *arhat* ideal, arguing that in an interdependent world individuals must assume responsibility not only for personal enlightenment, but also for assisting others in the quest. Thus, spiritual compassion becomes significant in Mahayana ethics in general, and in bioethics in particular.

## Approaches to Buddhist Bioethics

Buddhist ethical perspectives, unlike some Western views, seldom characterize morality in absolute terms. For Buddhists, ethical behavior is a necessary component of successful adherence to the Dharma rather than an end in itself. Once enlightenment is attained, dualities expressed in ethical problems cease to exist. Action is judged not against an absolute moral standard (such as the Ten Commandments), but rather on the basis of its relative merit in leading toward or away from enlightenment. From an enlightened perspective, actions can no longer be characterized as moral or immoral. Rather, action (*karma*) has a neutral value, transcending moral distinctions. As such, ethics are important to the spiritual practice of human beings, but they have no larger significance.

Historically, Buddhist monastics and lay people have expressed ethical concern for the poor, the sick, and the elderly. Yet Buddhists differ in their approaches to bioethical dilemmas. In part, competing bioethical interpretations arise from Theravada and Mahayana distinctions. Further, as Buddhism has traveled across Asia and other parts of the world, diverse indigenous cultural traditions have informed Buddhist notions of morality. The divergent views of Buddhist practitioners and scholars of Buddhism add another

dimension to understanding Buddhist bioethics. Finally, interpretive concerns arise when contemporary bioethical problems are evaluated using Buddhist texts composed centuries before the advent of current biomedical technologies. Despite these complexities, concepts such as nonharm (*ahimsa*) in Theravada and compassion (*karuna*) in Mahayana—though they do not posit an explicit bioethics—offer a way to measure the morality of bioethical issues.

## Theravada Buddhist Bioethics

Precepts for both monastics and laypersons provide a starting point for investigating Theravada bioethics. Although the number of precepts and issues addressed differs depending on individual religious status, there is nevertheless a core set of values applied to all Theravada practitioners. Buddha's moral conduct serves as a behavioral model for those who wish to pursue *nirvana.*

The *sangha,* or monastic community, is bound by a code of moral conduct inscribed in monastic rules (*vinaya*) that were established to promote the rigorous mental and physical discipline required to achieve the Theravada religious goal. These detailed rules regulate monastic life and spiritual practice. The first five of the ten Theravada precepts, which apply to both monastics and laity, are:

1. abstention from causing injury to all living beings;
2. abstention from theft and cheating;
3. abstention from sexual misconduct;
4. abstention from lying and other forms of injurious speech; and
5. abstention from intoxication.

Of these five, injunctions against killing, lying, and sexual misconduct have specific relevance to Theravada bioethics. These precepts carry additional significance when coupled with other Theravada Buddhist concepts. For example, respect for life and non-injury to living beings (*ahimsa*) is linked to the idea of *pratitya-samutpada,* the interdependence of existence and consequentially the moral responsibility of all beings.

As noted above, Theravada Buddhist traditions assert that the universe is fundamentally impermanent. Given this assumption, Theravada ethics strongly advocate comforting the terminally ill rather than trying to extend life through any means available. The value of life is not commensurate with lifespan, and death is understood as an inevitable consequence of unenlightened existence in an ephemeral world. Attempts to postpone death are unnatural acts that suggest a morbid (and ignorant) fear of death and an ego-motivated attachment to life.

Theravada principles both inform and complicate responses to contemporary bioethical dilemmas. For example, in Thailand, Theravada Buddhism is intimately connected to all aspects of life. Abortion in Thailand is prohibited by legislation that makes exception only in circumstances such as danger to the mother's life, rape, or incest. Theravada precepts against killing and doing harm to others are used to justify this legislation. Thai Buddhists apply the precepts to the unborn because a fetus is considered a human being from conception, and often cite traditional Theravada texts that oppose abortion.

However, orthodox Buddhist views sometimes clash with the realities of contemporary life in Thailand. In fact, abortions are performed in Thailand (although illegally), and Thais advocate different interpretations of Theravada ethical principles to justify or deny the morality of abortion. While some Buddhists invoke the nonharm precept, others maintain that abortion—in cases such as pregnancy due to rape or incest—can contribute to positive karmic consequence if performed with selfless intention.

On the other hand, in situations where abortions might be morally justified—at least in the United States—this is not necessarily the case in Thailand. Malee Lerdmaleewong and Caroline Francis list reasons that Thais cite for seeking illegal abortions, including economic difficulties and the lack of adequate or effective contraception. Yet, when a Thai woman learns that her fetus is developing abnormally due to Down's syndrome or some other serious disease, abortions are rarely sought (Ratanakul, 1998). In such cases, women are reluctant to seek an abortion because they believe that the fetus's disease is the result of negative karmic consequence produced by both the mother and the fetus (in a prior existence). To abort the fetus would only increase the negative effect. (Ratanakul, 1998). Fear of detrimental karmic consequence, then, is a deterrent to having an abortion.

## Mahayana Buddhist Bioethics

Mahayana Buddhist bioethics often center on the ideal of the bodhisattva. In devotional Mahayana, bodhisattvas such as Avalokitesvara embody compassion and the power to save those in material or spiritual distress—thus serving as ethical exemplars. In meditation-based Mahayana, emphasis is often placed on the ethical implications of a *bodhisattva*'s wisdom and experience of emptiness (*sunyata*). Despite positing different ethical ideals, the moral import of compassion and wisdom are interrelated in faith- and meditation-based Mahayana. Wisdom without compassion is no wisdom at all, and compassion without wisdom is potentially dangerous because action might originate in desire and attachment. Realization of compassion and wisdom results from actualizing attitudes and mental conditions—such as generosity, patience, and diligence—that are among the six perfections that bodhisattvas strive to achieve.

In part, the Mahayana bodhisattva ideal resulted in an increased emphasis on both monastic and lay concern for the spiritual and material well-being of others. Bodhisattvas enact the virtues of compassion and wisdom by striving to alleviate suffering and attending to the sick and elderly, among other selfless activities. When bodhisattvas declare the "thought of enlightenment" (*bodhicitta*), they vow not only to attain enlightenment, but also pledge to overcome defilements and to utilize compassion and wisdom to save all sentient beings.

For some Mahayana Buddhists, the imperative of compassionate action can override injunctions against harming others, lying, and other apparent violations of Buddhist morality. In essence, precepts may be broken in order to help others. This is possible because of the related notion of *upaya*—an expedient device. According to this important Mahayana concept, the historical Buddha used expedient means to expound the Dharma. That is, he presented his teachings in accord with variations in individual ability to comprehend his religious message. However, these alternate versions of the Dharma ultimately lead to the same truth. Similarly, *bodhisattva*s employ efficacious devices according to the needs of those who seek their aid. Japanese stories, for example, recount instances in which *bodhisattva*s assume the guise of a thief in order to be thrown in jail and thereby gain access to incarcerated individuals in need of spiritual solace. While this expedient device seems to transgress the precepts, the act is justified by virtue of compassion. In this and similar situations, the motivation for a behavior becomes central—a *bodhisattva* can only perform such actions if detached from any idea of self-benefit. As a being liberated from dualistic distinctions such as good and evil, the *bodhisattva* demonstrates action informed by the realization of *sunyata*, and the moral efficacy of integrating compassion and wisdom.

Bodhisattva virtues of compassion and wisdom impact Mahayana perspectives on bioethical issues such as abortion. For instance, in Japan, Buddhists do not officially condone abortion. Nevertheless, Japanese Buddhism generally tolerates abortion and sometimes plays a significant role in assuaging the negative karmic consequence that accrues from abortion.

In Japan, abortion is considered a *necessary sorrow* (LaFleur, 1990). That is, while never a moral good, sometimes abortion can be justified over carrying a child to term.

From a Japanese perspective, it is morally problematic and socially irresponsible to bring more children into the world than a family can support and nurture. In addition, Buddhist beliefs about rebirth characterize abortion as postponing the fetus's entry into the samsaric world. However, there are moral consequences to aborting the fetus. In order to try to rectify the negative karmic consequence that accrues from an abortion, Japanese Buddhist rituals, known as *mizuko kuyo,* are performed in order to speed the soul of the aborted fetus (*mizuko*) to a more positive rebirth. In addition, *mizuko kuyo* are intended to comfort aborted fetuses. Such rites also serve as a way for parents to repent sexual misconduct that results in unwanted pregnancy. Repentance helps alleviate the effects of immoral behavior, especially when admitted to a Buddha or *bodhisattva.*

Abortions are a common form of birth control in Japan and temples devoted to *mizuko kuyo* flourish to meet the spiritual needs of both mother and aborted fetus. The *bodhisattva jizo* (in sanskrit, *Ksitigarbha;* literally *Earth Womb*) is usually a focus of worship at these temples. Jizo is believed to aid sentient beings in their movement through the samsaric cycle and to protect deceased children as well as miscarried and aborted fetuses. Small statues of *jizo,* representing the fetus, are often dressed in children's clothing and presented with offerings of toys. Making offerings to *jizo* is a way to rectify negative karmic consequence of killing the fetus.

## Buddhist Bioethics: Prospects

This entry has offered an overview of the relationship between Buddhist ideas and bioethical issues. The fundamental logic introduced concerning abortion, for example, also pertains to Buddhist discussions of other bioethical dilemmas. Most likely, ongoing Theravada and Mahayana debates over the morality of euthanasia or human cloning will also pivot on concepts of nonharm and compassion.

At least three areas remain for further study that will undoubtedly raise new and important questions about Buddhist bioethics. First, the Buddhist textual record that currently exists represents mostly the views of Buddhist males. What are the ethical perspectives, both past and present, of Buddhist women? Do Buddhist women have different views of bioethical issues than men? Second, as medical technology continues to impact traditionally Buddhist cultures, what new conflicts and challenges will emerge? Finally, in what ways will Western Buddhist (for instance, American Buddhist) syntheses of bioethical issues impact traditional Buddhist bioethics?

WILLIAM E. DEAL

**SEE ALSO:** *Authority in Religious Traditions; Compassionate Love; Death: Eastern Thought; Environmental Ethics: Overview; Ethics: Religion and Morality; Eugenics and Religious Law; Hinduism, Bioethics in; Medical Ethics, History of South and East Asia; Population Ethics: Religious Traditions, Buddhist Perspectives*

### BIBLIOGRAPHY

Barnhart, Michael G. 1998. "Buddhism and the Morality of Abortion." *Journal of Buddhist Ethics* 5: 276–297.

Barnhart, Michael G. 2000. "Nature, Nurture, and No-Self: Bioengineering and Buddhist Values." *Journal of Buddhist Ethics* 7: 126–144.

Becker, Carl B. 1990. "Buddhist Views of Suicide and Euthanasia." *Philosophy East and West* 40: 543–556.

Becker, Carl B. 1993. *Breaking the Circle: Death and Afterlife in Buddhism.* Carbondale: Southern Illinois University Press.

Feldman, Eric A. 2000. *The Ritual of Rights in Japan: Law, Society, and Health Policy.* Cambridge, Eng.: Cambridge University Press.

Florida, Robert E. 1993. "Buddhist Approaches to Euthanasia." *Studies in Religion Sciences Religieuses* 22(1): 35–47.

Florida, Robert E. 1994. "Buddhism and the Four Principles." In *Principles of Health Care Ethics,* ed. Raanan Gillon and Ann Lloyd. New York: John Wiley & Sons.

Florida, Robert E. 1998. "The Lotus Sūtra and Health Care Ethics." *Journal of Buddhist Ethics* 5: 170–189.

Hardacre, Helen. 1994. "Response of Buddhism and Shinto to the Issue of Brain Death and Organ Transplant." *Cambridge Quarterly of Healthcare Ethics* 3: 585–601.

Hardacre, Helen. 1997. *Marketing the Menacing Fetus in Japan.* Berkeley: University of California Press.

Harvey, Peter. 2000. *An Introduction to Buddhist Ethics: Foundations, Values and Issues.* Cambridge, Eng.: Cambridge University Press.

Hughes, James J., and Keown, Damien. 1995. "Buddhism and Medical Ethics: A Bibliographic Introduction." *Journal of Buddhist Ethics* 2: 105–124.

Keown, Damien. 1992 (reprint 2001). *The Nature of Buddhist Ethics.* Basingstoke, Eng.: Palgrave.

Keown, Damien. 1995 (reprint 2001). *Buddhism and Bioethics.* Basingstoke, Eng.: Palgrave.

Keown, Damien. 1999. "Attitudes to Euthanasia in the Vinaya and Commentary." *Journal of Buddhist Ethics* 6: 260–270.

Keown, Damien, ed. 1998. *Buddhism and Abortion.* London: MacMillan.

Keown, Damien, ed. 2000. *Contemporary Buddhist Ethics.* Richmond, Surrey, Eng.: Curzon Press.

LaFleur, William R. 1990. "Contestation and Confrontation: The Morality of Abortion in Japan." *Philosophy East and West* 40(4): 529–542.

LaFleur, William R. 1992. *Liquid Life: Abortion and Buddhism in Japan.* Princeton, NJ: Princeton University Press.

Lerdmaleewong, Malee, and Francis, Caroline. 1998. "Abortion in Thailand: a Feminist Perspective." *Journal of Buddhist Ethics* 5: 22–48.

Lock, Margaret. 2002. *Twice Dead: Organ Transplants and the Reinvention of Death.* Berkeley: University of California Press.

Lopez, Donald S., Jr. 2001. *The Story of Buddhism: A Concise Guide to Its History and Teachings.* San Francisco: HarperCollins.

Mettanando, Bhikkhu. 1991. "Buddhist Ethics in the Practice of Medicine." In *Buddhist Ethics and Modern Society: An International Symposium,* ed. Charles Wei-hsun Fu and Sandra A. Wawrytko, Westport, CT: Greenwood Press.

Perrett, Roy W. 1996. "Buddhism, Euthanasia and the Sanctity of Life." *Journal of Medical Ethics* 22(5): 309–313.

Ratanakul, Pinit. 1986. *Bioethics: An Introduction to the Ethics of Medicine and Life Sciences.* Bangkok: Mahidol University.

Ratanakul, Pinit. 1988. "Bioethics in Thailand: The Struggle for Buddhist Solutions." *Journal of Medicine and Philosophy* 13: 301–312.

Ratanakul, Pinit. 1998. "Socio-Medical Aspects of Abortion in Thailand." In *Buddhism and Abortion,* ed. Damien Keown. London: MacMillan.

INTERNET RESOURCES

Barnhart, Michael G. 1998. "Buddhism and the Morality of Abortion." *Journal of Buddhist Ethics* Available from <http://jbe.gold.ac.uk/5/barnh981.pdf>.

Barnhart, Michael G. 2000. "Nature, Nurture, and No-Self: Bioengineering and Buddhist Values." *Journal of Buddhist Ethics* Available from <http://jbe.gold.ac.uk/7/barnhart001.pdf>.

Florida, Robert E. 1998. "The Lotus Sūtra and Health Care Ethics." *Journal of Buddhist Ethics* Available from <http://jbe.gold.ac.uk/5/flori981.pdf>.

Hughes, James J., and Keown, Damien. 1995. "Buddhism and Medical Ethics: A Bibliographic Introduction." *Journal of Buddhist Ethics* Available from <http://jbe.gold.ac.uk/2/hughes.pdf>.

Keown, Damien. 1999. "Attitudes to Euthanasia in the Vinaya and Commentary." *Journal of Buddhist Ethics.* Available from <http://jbe.gold.ac.uk/6/keown993.pdf>.

Lerdmaleewong, Malee, and Francis, Caroline. 1998. "Abortion in Thailand: a Feminist Perspective." *Journal of Buddhist Ethics* Available from <http://jbe.gold.ac.uk/5/aborti1.pdf>.

Tsomo, Karma Lekshe. 1998. "Prolife, Prochoice: Buddhism and Reproductive Ethics." Feminism and Nonviolence Studies Association. Available from <http://www.fnsa.org/fall98/tsomo.html>.

# C

## CANCER, ETHICAL ISSUES RELATED TO DIAGNOSIS AND TREATMENT

• • •

Significant advances in cancer control and prevention have emerged from the front lines of medicine since the 1970s. Sophisticated diagnostic modalities aid in the timely detection of the disease. The benefits of established treatments such as chemotherapy and radiation therapy have been maximized gradually but steadily, and the risks have been minimized. Major changes in other aspects of cancer care have followed. For example, oncology personnel today pay far more attention than did their predecessors to issues such as the frank disclosure of diagnoses and treatment options, long-term quality of life for cancer patients and their families, and ethically complex scenarios that range from gaining consent from incompetent adults to the participation of children in discussions and decision making about cancer clinical trials.

These and other developments also have created new problems and concerns for clinicians, ethicists, and other stakeholders in the struggle against cancer. These issues include complicated questions about the nature, quality, and outcomes of oncologist-patient communication and decision making. Is there a preferred way for an oncologist to disclose a diagnosis of cancer to patients and their families that is frank *and* compassionate, truthful *and* hopeful? Should children diagnosed with cancer participate in discussions and critical decisions about their disease and its treatment? Can one envisage a continued role for paternalism in contemporary cancer care, and how effective or

realistic are the models proposed as alternatives? Are oncologists responding to the growing ethnic diversity of their patients? What sorts of opportunities and obstacles will confront oncologists as people with cancer organize and inform themselves through online advocacy groups, websites that promote "alternative" treatments, and other high-technology resources?

### Cancer and the Oncologist's Ethical Duties: Some General Considerations

An oncologist's ethical responsibilities typically begin with a positive diagnosis of cancer, an event that triggers shock and anxiety in patients and their families. Cancer is associated by many people with disfigurement, dying, and death; therefore, the first ethical duty of an oncologist and his or her team is to convey the diagnosis in a way that balances the reality of the disease and its implications with the overall need to maintain optimism and hope. Whereas the obligation to be honest about the reality of cancer derives from the ethics of truth telling in cancer care and in medicine generally (see below), the duty to foster hope taps several sources (Kodish et al., p. 2974):

1. The poorly understood relationship between the mind and the body and the ability of the body to respond positively to a positive frame of mind.
2. The physician's responsibility to attend to the patient's psychological as well as physical welfare.
3. A need for humility on the physician's part in light of the limitations of her or his ability to predict the future for any individual patient.

How much hope should an oncologist foster in patients and their families? Researchers point out that the language of hope is a critical part of the culture of oncology in the United

States. It "articulates fundamental American notions about personhood, individual autonomy, and the power of thought (good and bad) to shape life course and bodily functioning" (Good et al., p. 61). Several factors have to be assessed in promoting hope in a specific case, including the type and stage of cancer, the patient's age, and the point of evolution in the disease and treatment at which the discussion occurs (Kodish et al., p. 2974). Cultural factors also may have to be considered. Cancer carries different connotations in different cultures and may require a discussion tailored to the degree of fatalism, fear, or "social death" that the disease inspires in different ethnic groups (Taylor; Good et al.; Gordon; Good).

From the reinforcement of hope flow other responsibilities: to time the disclosure of survival chances sensitively; to discuss the available treatment options and their respective risks and benefits fully; to discuss, among other rights, the patient's right to withdraw from a clinical trial if one is offered; to encourage patients and their families to ask questions; and to give honest answers to all the questions patients ask. Special attention has to be paid to clarifying key concepts in oncology such as the distinction between remission and cure. *Remission* means that there is no clinical or radiographic evidence of active tumor and often is accompanied by the hope of a cure. Unfortunately, relapse often occurs and brings a much more grave prognosis. Many oncologists and patients are reluctant to use the term *cure* because of the implied guarantee that there will be no relapse.

Care must be taken so that patients are neither overburdened with information nor underinformed. To strike this balance an oncologist initially should meet several times with a patient rather than only once and space the meetings to give the patient time to absorb sensitive or complicated information. Institutional review board–approved consent scripts and other written materials on cancer or cancer clinical trials may help literate patients understand their options and rights (Meade; Flores et al., p. 847).

These are some of the key ethical responsibilities that face oncologists in their daily encounters with patients. Many more exist and depend largely for their successful outcome on oncologists' ability to take into account the physical, emotional, and social needs of their patients. Some of those needs may be dictated by the ways in which cancer is conceptualized.

## The Concept of Cancer: An Overview

Although the biological, epidemiological, and genetic origins and indicators of cancer are vitally important—they are the frontiers on which the disease is being battled—cancer is more than the sum of its physical parts. It is also a socially imagined disease that is collectively thought about, embellished, and reacted to in ways that mesh with a people's established social and cultural norms. In some African countries, for example, perceptions of cancer as a stealthy, insidious disease mesh with notions of malice and witchcraft (Bezwoda et al., p. 123; El-Ghazali, p. 101). In parts of Italy cancer poses the threat of social as well as physical disruption and death, a viewpoint that meshes with the importance Italians place on defining themselves and their worth in relationship to others (Gordon). In the United States, by contrast, "having" cancer sometimes is considered a personal failing and responsibility, a notion that clearly draws on deeply ingrained concepts of individuality and the individual's role in determining his or her destiny (Good et al.).

Ideas and perceptions about cancer are not, however, unchanging or static. Cancer was widely viewed in pre-nineteenth-century art and literature as a distinctly romantic disease. Susan Sontag has linked this view to evidence that for a long time cancer was confused with tuberculosis, a disease historically infused with a romantic mythology (Sontag). Gradually, however, after tuberculosis was identified in 1882 as being bacterial in origin, cancer developed a separate and far less romantic identity, characterized in Sontag's view by a highly deleterious and stigmatizing image that persists to this day.

In the United States the situation can be made worse by the punitive and often militaristic paradigm of the disease (Sontag, pp. 65–67; Payer). People with cancer are treated aggressively, sometimes without much concern for their quality of life, perhaps partly as a result of the way in which cancer treatment is framed as a "war" that should be "waged" with "weapons" such as chemotherapy and radiation therapy. Such language is widespread and public: Cancer research institutions have worked it into their mission statements, and high-profile cancer "survivors" such as Lance Armstrong use it to encourage others.

So detrimental do some scholars consider this metaphoric expression of cancer that they recommend a shift away from the use of metaphor to understand and define cancer and other diseases (such as AIDS). Writes Sontag: "The most truthful way of regarding illness—and the healthiest way of being ill—is one most purified of, most resistant to, metaphoric thinking" (p. 3). Metaphors can hurt, Sontag suggests; they are a rhetorical means by which diseases can acquire meanings that inflict additional pain and suffering on people with diseases such as cancer and AIDS.

Sontag's argument has to be considered in light of two other observations. First, cancer patients are rarely passive victims of the collective lore or mythology surrounding their disease. One cancer patient, in an advice column published online by the American Cancer Society, rejected the notion of cancer as a purely individual, unshakable disease: "I find myself more comfortable telling people, 'I was diagnosed with cancer' instead of saying, 'I have cancer.' On some deep level, I don't want to 'own' this illness." The writer goes on to offer the following advice to other cancer patients: "Choose language that suits you when you share your news. And keep in mind that there is no one 'right' way of doing this" (Murray).

Individually or as members of self-help organizations, cancer patients can and do actively oppose the aspects of their disease and its conception or management that they consider negative and unfair.

Second, metaphors do not only hurt or damage; they also may help patients cope with cancer. Studies show, for example, that cancer patients frequently draw on religion, nature, art, the military, and many other sources of imagery to help them visualize their diseases, treatments, and recoveries (Skelton; Tompkins and Lawley). Psychologists have reported considerable success working with the many different kinds of metaphors that cancer patients can adopt throughout the course of their disease (Tompkins and Lawley). Ethnographic evidence indicates that even oncologists and other specialists use metaphors to help them understand and confront cancer and "routinize" new technologies and treatments (Koenig; Simon; Skelton et al.).

"In the healing process the most important part of communication takes place at the metaphoric level," states the medical anthropologist Margaret Lock in Capra's *Uncommon Wisdom* (1989, p. 289). "Therefore, you have to have shared metaphors" (chapter 19). This may be especially true in the case of cancer because of the seriousness of the disease and the onus on patients and their caregivers to utilize the full range of resources—medical, social, and metaphoric—available to them in their joint effort against cancer.

## The Doctor–Patient Relationship in Cancer Care: Four Models

The doctor–patient relationship has particular relevance in the context of cancer. Frequently life-threatening, clinically complex, and requiring sustained, repeated face-to-face interactions, cancer and its treatment raise the fundamental question of what exactly is involved when patients and clinicians enter into a "relationship." For months and perhaps years a cancer sufferer and his or her clinician or clinicians must meet, talk, listen to, and learn from one another in an atmosphere built on mutual trust, good communication and understanding, competency and compassion, and openness. Without these interpersonal characteristics the doctor–patient relationship is likely to be a rocky one, leading to possible patient and clinician dissatisfaction, mistrust, and a compromised quality of care.

The respective roles that patients and clinicians ideally should adopt, however, are not widely agreed on or easily implemented. Different models ranging from strict paternalism to complete patient autonomy have been suggested. Below, four of these models and their relevance to the cancer care setting are reviewed. Although paradigmatic in several important ways, these are not the only models that are relevant to cancer care. Variations on these models and other alternatives have been proposed (Ong et al.; Gattellari et al.).

THE PATERNALISTIC MODEL. Definable as the overriding or restricting of the rights or freedom of individuals for their own good, paternalism entails clinicians ensuring that patients receive the interventions that best promote their health and well-being regardless of the patients' preferences (Goldman). Although many scholars oppose strict paternalism, arguing that it is too coercive, some concede that paternalism has moral validity and limited practical relevance. Paternalism may be useful and necessary in emergency situations in which the time taken to discuss treatment options or obtain informed consent may harm the patient irreversibly (Emanuel and Emanuel, p. 73). Otherwise, strict paternalism rarely is advocated or considered tenable in the treatment of diseases such as cancer.

Nevertheless, patients and/or their families may at times express a desire for a paternalistic approach. In a large behavioral cancer study, for example, the authors audiotaped the parent of a young boy with leukemia in a discussion with an oncologist who was trying to explain the option of enrolling the child in a Phase III clinical trial. The parent interrupted the clinician and said, "Anything you gotta do to fix him! I don't care." The clinician persisted, saying she felt obligated to inform him about the clinical trial. She again was interrupted by the parent, who insisted: "You don't have to tell me all the lingo. Just fix him [the patient]!"

Clearly, a paternalistic approach in which the clinician calls all the shots may be preferred by some healthcare consumers. Other studies have highlighted similar preferences, finding that some cancer patients prefer to relinquish decision-making control in favor of a more passive or deferential role, a phenomenon that may be rooted in the inordinate trust some people place in their doctors or in prevalent cultural norms and values that discourage shared decision making and patient autonomy (Flores).

**THE INFORMATIVE OR CONSUMER MODEL.** Like all patients, cancer patients can be viewed as consumers, and their clinicians as providers of information and treatment. This model supports a view of the doctor–patient relationship as a neutral and transactional one in which the clinician furnishes, without trying to influence the patient, the facts relevant to the patient's diagnosis, prognosis, treatment options and their risks and benefits, and aspects of care. The goal of this approach is to empower the patient with as much information as possible so that the patient can make a fully informed, autonomous decision about treatment. Although this approach may prove beneficial to patient understanding and informed decision making, it also may lead to information overload and patient dissatisfaction. The burden of choice and decision making falls squarely on patients in this model, an outcome that not all cancer patients find desirable or helpful (Gattellari et al., p. 1867).

**THE INTERPRETIVE MODEL.** Also based on a view of the clinician as an information provider, the interpretive model suggests that clinicians furnish the facts and go several steps further to help the patient understand them and make a decision about treatment. The clinician may have to act as a counselor of sorts, supplying relevant information, elucidating the patient's values and preferences, and suggesting which treatment options best match the patient's values. An oncologist adopting this role, for example, might listen to a breast cancer patient, articulate the patient's values and then inform the patient that it is important for him or her to fight the cancer but that the treatment must leave the patient with a healthy self-image and quality time outside the hospital. Without recommending a particular course of action, the oncologist might suggest that the patient's values seem compatible with radiation therapy but not with chemotherapy because the former would do better at maximizing the patient's chance of survival while preserving the patient's breast.

Patient autonomy is conceived as self-understanding in this model; the patient "comes to know more clearly who he or she is and how the various medical options bear on his or her identity" (Emanuel and Emanuel, p. 69). Objections to this model include the possibility that clinicians may misinterpret the patient's values or impose their own values under the guise of articulating those of the patient.

**THE DELIBERATIVE MODEL.** From the standpoint of this model the clinician acts as the patient's teacher or friend, helping the patient *deliberate* on various aspects of the disease, prognosis, and treatment options. The clinician aims at most for moral persuasion, not coercion, and tries to engage the patient in a dialogue about what treatment is best in light of the patient's condition and health-related values. An oncologist adopting this role might begin by pointing out the facts, articulating the patient's values, and then balancing the options with the patient in a discussion of their risks and benefits and potential impact on the patient's life. This model supports an oncologist who goes on to recommend a particular course of action, suggesting, for example, that radiation therapy may be the best option because it offers maximal survival with minimal risk, disfigurement, and disruption of the patient's life (Emanuel and Emanuel, p. 71).

In contrast to the interpretive model and its emphasis on self-understanding, the deliberative model conceives of patient autonomy as "moral self-development" (Emanuel and Emanuel, p. 69). A major criticism of the deliberative model is that clinicians should not be entitled to act as moral teachers or guardians; their role is to heal without regard to a patient's personal values or morals. However, this criticism is subject to the counterargument that many people may not want or expect their clinicians to be simply mechanistic healers and may desire help—especially when faced with the prospect of cancer treatment—in developing a personal moral foundation for their long-term health and well-being.

In their classic work on the subject Thomas Szasz and M. H. Hollender make the point that the doctor–patient relationship is a relatively novel concept in modern medicine. Instead of fostering its relationship with patients as people, they argue, medicine has cared primarily about its relationship to such "things" as anatomic structures, cells, lesions, bacteria, and viruses (p. 278). Certainly this characterization rings true for oncology during the early and intermittent phases of the "war on cancer" (Proctor). Patients' rights, truth telling, and other ethical components of cancer care that are taken for granted today were not always high on the agenda in much of the twentieth century, when efforts were directed primarily toward developing a basic understanding of cancer and options for treating it. Before 1970 the paternalistic model was widely accepted, entitling oncologists to decide unilaterally what sorts of information and treatment their patients should get.

As different models of patient autonomy in cancer care are developed and debated by experts ranging from medical sociologists and anthropologists to oncologists and research nurses in oncology, the doctor–patient relationship in cancer care increasingly is undergoing scrutiny and refinement. Few experts still advocate the paternalistic model. The debate centers more on whether the model for cancer care should be informative, interpretive, or deliberative or should involve some combination of these models and their respective strengths. At the same time researchers across a spectrum of disciplines increasingly are consulting cancer patients and their communities for input on the merits or drawbacks of particular ways of gaining information, making decisions, adhering to drug regimens, and developing effective coping mechanisms for cancer. Such informant-based, empirical research will continue to play a vital role in understanding and developing the oncologist–patient relationship in ways that promote quality of care and quality of life for people with cancer.

## Telling the Truth about Cancer and Its Treatment

In the United States attitudes toward truth telling in cancer care have changed markedly in the last few decades. In 1946 Charles Lund wrote that a patient diagnosed with cancer should not be told the "whole truth." He advised physicians to use a "loosely descriptive word" such as *cyst* or *lesion* in place of the word *cancer* and to give patients only "some rough idea" of the extent of treatment. That was sufficient information, Lund felt, on which to base a diagnostic discussion and consent to treatment. In the same vein, a 1961 survey reported that 90 percent of 219 Chicago doctors did not tell patients the truth about a diagnosis of cancer (Oken). Maintenance of hope, in contrast, was considered the single most important factor for physicians to take into account when discussing cancer with a patient. By contrast, 97 percent of physicians surveyed at the same Chicago institution in 1979 reported a preference for telling cancer patients the truth about their diagnoses, a dramatic reversal of earlier findings (Kodish et al., p. 2974). Since that time it has become widely accepted that patients should be told the truth about their diagnoses and prospects, although not all studies find that this happens in practice. Omission or concealment of the truth remains an issue in cancer care because of the traditional and cultural resonances of dread associated with the disease (Freedman, p. 572).

Studies reveal a number of benefits associated with an open, truthful approach to a patient's diagnosis of cancer, chances of survival, treatment options, and progress over time. Honest disclosures build trust and ameliorate conflict between clinicians and patients and their families. They satisfy legal and ethical norms of patient autonomy. Truthfulness also ultimately may help patients understand and cope with cancer. Nevertheless, a clinician should take into account several factors before initiating a frank discussion with a cancer patient.

Foremost among these factors is whether the patient has been diagnosed with cancer for the first time. Such patients may require a more sensitive approach than do relapsed patients or patients with long-standing symptoms, who generally will be less surprised and more prepared for a diagnosis of cancer. Also "the truth" must be balanced against the fact that a clinician can share openly with a patient only what is clinically knowable. The natural history of a particular cancer and the way a patient will respond cannot always be predicted at the time of diagnosis. This may add to a discussion an element of uncertainty that can make the truth appear murky and confusing as well as uncomfortable for patients. Finally, a frank approach to a cancer diagnosis may not be welcomed by all patients and their families. Comparative studies illustrate, for example, that the culture of oncology may vary from country to country. Cancer patients in parts of Italy, for example, fear that disclosure of the true nature and implications of their disease may lead to "social death" (Gordon). Similarly fearful, some Latino and Japanese immigrants in the United States consider American styles of disclosure and prognosis cruel and unnecessary (Good et al.).

In light of these and other contrasting cultural norms, oncologists practicing in diverse ethnic environments may need to approach their commitment to truth telling with special sensitivity and "cultural competence" (Flores). They may have to enlist the support of social workers, interpreters, and other appropriate support personnel to counteract the fear of social isolation and loss of hope that may strike some cancer patients harder than others.

## Childhood Cancer and Its Ethical Challenges

Cancer kills more children than does any other disease. Recent data show that after unintentional injury, childhood cancer continues to be the most common cause of death for children ages one to nineteen years in the United States (Hoyert et al., p. 257). Beyond the impact on mortality, the disease burden of childhood cancer is very significant. The quality of life of an afflicted child and his or her family are affected profoundly. The time of a new diagnosis is a particularly difficult period, with parents reporting tremendous stress and emotional turmoil (Dahlquist et al., p. 111; Levi et al., p. 244).

Unlike most areas of clinical medicine, randomized clinical trials are the norm for pediatric oncology (Hirschfield et al., p. 256). Most often the "standard" therapy for a particular disease is determined by a previous study and then embedded in the randomized design of clinical trial along with one or more alternative regimens. Children in typical pediatric oncology randomized clinical trials may be assigned to the "standard" arm or to an "experimental" arm that is generally either more intensive (with hopes of improving the cure rate with tolerable toxicity) or less intensive (with hopes of maintaining the cure rate with less toxicity than the "standard" arm). If a parent or an older child declines study participation, the treating oncologist generally will elect to provide the "standard" therapy without collecting data for the research study.

Ethical issues in childhood cancer are complex and potentially difficult to resolve. Until recently children were compared to incompetent adults, for whom treatment-related decisions are made by a close family member. Ethicists now point out that this comparison fails to acknowledge a key distinction between children and incompetent adults: The former are different because in most cases their competency is still in a state of growth or evolution. In most prominent legal cases, by contrast, incompetent adults were never expected to regain competency (Truog et al., p. 1411). This places most children in a category different from that of incompetent adults, one that challenges doctors to preserve their future autonomy as opposed to the former autonomy that doctors strive to respect when offering multiple treatment options to incompetent adults. In light of this critical difference, how involved should children be in discussions and decision making about the treatment they will receive?

Answers to this question typically make use of the concept of "assent" for treatment, which first was proposed for pediatric patients in the 1970s by the National Commission for the Protection of Human Subjects of Biomedical and Behavioral Research (Truog et al., p. 1412). The commission proposed that children between ages seven and fourteen be asked for their assent to medical treatment, whereas older children would be presumed to have full decision-making capacity. The American Academy of Pediatrics sanctioned this approach in 1995, with its Committee on Bioethics adding that physicians should take the following steps to assure assent:

- Help the patient achieve a developmentally appropriate awareness of the nature of his or her condition.
- Tell the patient what he or she can expect with tests and treatments.
- Make a clinical assessment of the patient's understanding of the situation and the factors influencing how he or she is responding (including whether there is inappropriate pressure to accept testing or therapy).
- Solicit an expression of the patient's willingness to accept the proposed care.

The last of these four requirements is perhaps the most controversial in the context of childhood cancer, in which the unwillingness of a child to accept treatment most likely would be considered insufficient grounds to forgo that treatment. For this reason the American Academy of Pediatrics is careful to account for situations in which children will receive a particular treatment despite their objection, noting that they should be told that and not be deceived (Truog et al., p. 1412). Although this approach helps ensure that children do not naively forgo treatments that could save their lives, it also raises questions about the sincerity of "assent" as a concept that is intended to foster patient autonomy. Also, achieving assent in practice may have unintended effects. Although more research is needed on the topic, at least one study of children with leukemia suggests that the consent process may be compromised when children and parents participate in the same discussions. With the oncologist typically focusing her or his comments and attention on the patient, the parents may ask fewer questions and display lower levels of understanding than do parents whose children are approached separately and who receive the undivided attention of their oncologists. These findings suggest an urgent need for further research on the practical compatibility of assent and parental permission.

## Other Ethical Dilemmas in Pediatric Oncology

Parents sometimes express the wish that their children not know the diagnosis or severity of their disease. At one time this sentiment would have received support in most segments of the pediatric oncology community, in which the culture of nondisclosure widely included the notion that children had to be protected from the psychological trauma of finding out about cancer and their chances of survival (Truog et al.). However, evidence indicates that children cope remarkably well with the shock of a diagnosis such as cancer and may adjust better psychologically to their disease and its treatment if they are informed early (Slavin et al.; Truog et al., p. 1412). Oncologists may legitimately use such findings to convince reluctant or fearful parents of the importance of disclosing to their children the nature of their disease.

The refusal by some parents to consent to any kind of medical intervention for their child poses another dilemma for oncologists. Cancer is typically a life-threatening illness, and oncologists subsequently display a relatively low level of tolerance for parents who deny them permission to treat a child diagnosed with the disease. Court orders usually are obtained to override such parental decisions. The situation can become more complicated, however, when a parent's decision not to treat a child biomedically is backed by a community whose values and life views differ dramatically from the mainstream, such as the ultraconservative segments of the Amish community in the Midwest. Careful negotiation aimed at building mutual trust and confidence may be required in such instances so that the best interest of the child and the community can be served.

## Cancer and End-of-Life Care

In the past oncologists typically greeted with foreboding and mistrust the prospect of relinquishing treatment in favor of palliative, end-of-life support such as hospice care. That open opposition has been replaced in most cases with careful circumspection. Many oncologists recognize a threshold beyond which continued treatment does more harm than good even though they may struggle to unite that recognition with the Hippocratic imperative to heal. This threshold, however, may not always coincide with patient or family preferences.

An oncologist may be asked to taper off or stop treatment at a juncture where the oncologist foresees, with statistical and collegial support, that continued treatment is still likely to benefit the patient. In equally problematic situations the reverse may occur. Crawley and her colleagues cite as an example an African-American man with metastatic colon cancer who angrily rejected his physician's suggestion that they had reached a point where the interventions would be costly and would serve only to prolong the man's suffering (Crawley et al., pp. 673–675). The patient demanded that he receive every medical test and procedure available regardless of the cost. This insistence, the physician felt, was based on the man's inability to grasp the limitations of the technological options still available to him.

The provision of good end-of-life care for cancer patients frequently is complicated by disagreements, poor communication, and cultural differences. However, there are strategies that oncologists can adopt to alleviate end-of-life pain and suffering among their patients. Foremost is a willingness by a physician to probe beneath the surface for explanations of why patients and/or families may or may not desire an option such as hospice care. Investigating the case mentioned above further, Crawley et al. discovered that the physician, a European-American, consulted an African-American colleague for advice. As an ethnic "insider," the colleague was able to point out that African-Americans who have suffered discrimination may fear neglect if they do not insist on maximal care. The colleague also stated that many patients seek aggressive treatment because they value the sanctity of life, not because they misunderstand the limits of the technology available to them, as the patient's doctor had suspected (Crawley et al., p. 675). Enlightened by this and other information, the doctor met again with his patient and reopened the discussion with greater understanding about the patient, his cultural background, and his preferences.

A unique problem in end-of-life care arises when the physician's best-intentioned efforts appear to resemble physician-assisted suicide or euthanasia. The classic case involves the terminally ill patient whose death may be hastened by high doses of morphine. Discerning clinicians and ethicists usually can recognize whether a physician's goal in such cases is to relieve pain or respiratory distress—a fundamental clinical obligation in the eyes of many—or whether the objective is to hasten the patient's death, a goal that remains ethically controversial (Kodish et al., p. 2979).

The growing worldwide hospice movement provides an important avenue for improving end-of-life care for cancer patients. Hospice philosophy calls for providing patients and their families with medical, psychological, and spiritual support as they encounter terminal illness. The primary goal is palliation of symptoms and improvement of the quality of life. Antineoplastic therapy may be a part of hospice care, but cure of cancer is no longer attainable and the focus is on comfort. Although tension between the goals of cancer treatment and the goals of hospice care may arise, they need not be incompatible. Patients who develop a trusting relationship with an oncologist may feel abandoned if their care is transferred abruptly to a hospice team. For this reason oncologists should remain active in the care of patients with terminal cancer, using hospice services as an adjunct rather than a replacement for providing excellent care.

## Cancer Care and the Future

Future developments in cancer care will be affected by advances in the clinical control and prevention of the disease. Ongoing genetic and molecular research promises not just more effective treatments for cancer but also less invasive procedures for patients, greater patient autonomy, and improved quality of life. Potential problems may include a compounding of concerns about informed consent for cancer clinical trials and genetic susceptibility testing, as well as more "macro" issues such as the inequitable distribution of cancer care resources in the United States and globally. Also, current trends suggest continued growth in "informal" cancer care resources ranging from online information networks to holistic alternatives to conventional cancer care. Many of these resources have the potential for linking together and empowering cancer patients but also of misinforming them or undermining the oncologist's authority and purpose through the exposure of patients to multiple, conflicting messages. Surveys and other kinds of behavioral research may be needed so that providers of cancer care may better grasp the pluralistic knowledge- and treatment-seeking tendencies of their patients and the way in which they affect physician-authority, treatment adherence, and other key clinical issues.

Finally, demographic trends at the beginning of the twenty-first century strongly suggest that cancer care will be provided amid growing ethnic and cultural diversity in the United States and elsewhere. Already many providers of cancer care feel the impact of this diversity through their daily struggles with language barriers, conflicting expectations, lack of treatment adherence, and other problems. Learning more about patients and their backgrounds provides an important way to address these and other problems. Clearly, however, it is unrealistic to expect caregivers to identify the countless cultural norms and behaviors that may affect their patients' preferences and decisions. An approach tailored to a particular institution's patient demographic is needed, and for this there are handbooks and other tools that may assist a cancer caregiver practicing in any region of the United States. Leading cancer care institutions also increasingly hire professional, culturally astute interpreters who can help oncologists and patients bridge the cultural and linguistic differences that may hinder effective communication and understanding. Conferences and workshops on "cultural competence" and "cultural sensitivity" increasingly are organized for researchers, ethicists, and caregivers to use in response to growing patient heterogeneity.

CHRISTIAN M. SIMON
ERIC D. KODISH

**SEE ALSO:** *Alternative Therapies; Autonomy; Beneficence; Clinical Ethics; Double Effect, Principle or Doctrine of; Grief and Bereavement; Healing; Informed Consent; Life, Quality of: Quality of Life in Clinical Decisions; Life Sustaining Treatment and Euthanasia; Palliative Care and Hospice; Surrogate Decision-Making*

### BIBLIOGRAPHY

American Academy of Pediatrics Committee on Bioethics. 1995. "Informed Consent, Parental Permission, and Assent in Pediatric Practice." *Pediatrics* 95: 314–317.

Bezwoda, W. R.; Colvin, H.; and Lehoka, J. 1997. "Transcultural and Language Problems in Communicating with Cancer Patients in Southern Africa." In *Communication with the Cancer Patient: Information and Truth,* ed. M. Zwitter. New York: New York Academy of Sciences.

Capra, Fritjof. 1989. *Uncommon Wisdom: Conversations with Remarkable People.* NY: Bantam Books.

Crawley, L. M.; Marshall, P. A.; Lo, B.; et al. 2002. "Strategies for Culturally Effective End-of-Life Care." *Annals of Internal Medicine* 136(9): 673–679.

Dahlquist, L. M.; Czyzewski, D. I.; Copeland, K.G.; et al. 1993. "Parents of Children Newly Diagnosed with Cancer: Anxiety, Coping, and Marital Distress." *Journal of Pediatric Psychology* 18(3): 365–376.

El-Ghazali, Sawsan. 1997. "Is It Wise to Tell the Truth, the Whole Truth, and Nothing but the Truth to a Cancer Patient?" In *Communication with the Cancer Patient: Information and Truth,* ed. M. Zwitter. New York: New York Academy of Sciences.

Emanuel, E., and Emanuel, L. 1992. "Four Models of the Physician-Patient Relationship." *Journal of the American Medical Association* 267: 2221–2226.

Flores, Glenn. 2000. "Culture and the Patient-Physician Relationship: Achieving Cultural Competency in Health Care." *Journal of Pediatrics* 136(1): 14–23.

Flores, Glenn; Milagros, Abrue; Schwartz, I.; et al. 2000. "The Importance of Language and Culture in Pediatric Care: Case Studies from the Latino Community." *Journal of Pediatrics* 137(6): 842–848.

Freedman, Benjamin. 1993. "Offering Truth: One Ethical Approach to the Uninformed Cancer Patient." *Archives of Internal Medicine* 153: 572–576.

Gattellari, M.; Butow, P. N.; Tattersall, M.H.; et al. 2001. "Sharing Decisions in Cancer Care." *Social Science and Medicine* 52(12): 1865–1878.

Goldman, Alan. 1999 (1980). "The Refutation of Medical Paternalism." In *Ethical Issues in Modern Medicine,* ed. J. D. Arras and B. Steinbock. Mountain View, CA: Mayfield.

Good, Byron J. 1994. *Medicine, Rationality, and Experience: An Anthropological Perspective.* Cambridge, Eng.: Cambridge University Press.

Good, M. J. Delvecchio; Good, B. J.; Schaffer, C.; et al. 1990. "American Oncology and the Discourse on Hope." *Culture, Medicine and Psychiatry* 14: 59–79.

Gordon, Deborah R. 1990. "Embodying Illness, Embodying Cancer." *Culture, Medicine and Psychiatry* 14: 275–297.

Hirschfield, S.; Shapiro, A.; Dagher, R.; et al. 2000. "Pediatric Oncology: Regulatory Initiatives." *The Oncologist* 5(6): 441–444.

Hoyert, D. L.; Freedman, M. A.; Strobino, D.M.; et al. 2001. "Annual Summary of Vital Statistics: 2000." *Pediatrics* 108(6): 1241–1255.

Kodish, E.; Singer, P. A.; et al. 1997. "Ethical Issues." In *Cancer: Principles and Practices of Oncology,* ed. S. A. Rosenberg. Philadelphia and New York: Lippincott-Raven.

Koenig, Barbara. 1988. "The Technological Imperative in Medical Practice: The Social Creation of a Routine Treatment." In *Biomedicine Examined,* ed. D. Gordon. Boston: Kluwer.

Levi, Rachel B.; Marsick, Rebecca; Drotar, Dennis; and Kodish, E. D. 2000. "Diagnosis, Disclosure, and Informed Consent:

Learning from Parents of Children with Cancer." *Journal of Pediatric Hematology/Oncology* 22(1): 3–12.

Lund, Charles C. 1999 (1946). "The Doctor, the Patient, and the Truth." In *Ethical Issues in Modern Medicine,* ed. J. D. Arras and B. Steinbock. Mountain View, CA: Mayfield.

Meade, Cathy D. 1999. "Improving Understanding of the Informed Consent Process and Document." *Seminars in Oncology Nursing* 15(2): 124–137.

Oken, D. 1961. "What to Tell Cancer Patients: A Study of Medical Attitudes." *Journal of the American Medical Association* 175: 1120–1128.

Ong, L. M.; de Haes, J. C.; Hoos, A.M.; et al. 1995. "Doctor-Patient Communication: A Review of the Literature." *Social Science and Medicine* 40(7): 903–918.

Payer, Lynn. 1996. *Medicine and Culture.* New York: Henry Holt.

Proctor, Robert. 1995. *Cancer Wars: How Politics Shapes What We Know and Don't Know about Cancer.* New York: Basic Books.

Simon, C. 1999. "Images and Image: Technology and the Social Politics of Revealing Disorder in a North American Hospital." *Medical Anthropology Quarterly* 13(2): 141–162.

Skelton, J. R.; Wearn, A. M.; Hobbs, F. D.; et al. 2002. "A Concordance-Based Study of Metaphoric Expressions Used by General Practitioners and Patients in Consultation." *British Journal of General Practice* 52(475): 114–118.

Slavin, L. A.; O'Malley, J. E.; Koocher, J. P.; et al. 1982. "Communication of the Cancer Diagnosis to Pediatric Patients: Impact on Long-Term Adjustment." *American Journal of Psychiatry* 139: 179–183.

Sontag, Susan. 1989 (1977). *Illness as Metaphor and AIDS and Its Metaphors.* New York: Farrar, Straus and Giroux.

Szasz, Thomas, and Hollender, M. H. 1997. "The Basic Models of the Doctor-Patient Relationship." In *The Social Medicine Reader,* ed. Gail E. Henderson, Nancy M. P. King, Ronald P. Strauss, Sue E. Estroff, and Larry E. Churchill. Durham, NC: Duke University Press.

Taylor, Kathryn M. 1988. "Physicians and the Disclosure of Undesirable Information." In *Biomedicine Examined,* ed. D. Gordon. Dordrecht, Netherlands: Kluwer Academic.

Tompkins, Penny, and Lawley, James. 2002. "The Mind, Metaphor, and Health." *Positive Health* vol. 78.

Truog, R. D.; Burns, J.; et al. 2002. "Ethical Considerations in Pediatric Oncology." In *Principles and Practices of Pediatric Oncology,* ed. D. G. Poplack. Philadelphia: Lippincott Williams and Wilkins.

INTERNET RESOURCE

Murray, Lorraine V. 2002. "Breaking the News about Your Diagnosis: Tips from a Breast Cancer Survivor." American Cancer Society. Available from <www.cancer.org/>.

# CARE

• • •

## I. HISTORY OF THE NOTION OF CARE

Prior to 1982 scarcely anyone spoke of an "ethic of care." The word "care" had never emerged as a major concept in the history of mainstream Western ethics—as compared, say, with the concepts of freedom, justice, and love. Yet, starting with the 1982 publication of a book by Carol Gilligan that spoke of a care perspective in women's moral development and throughout the 1980s and into the 1990s, an ethic of care emerged very rapidly, questioning earlier assumptions and setting new directions for bioethics. (These contemporary publications and discussions will be reviewed in the third subentry in this entry.) One characteristic of the literature on an ethic of care is that it has paid virtually no attention to the history of the notion of care prior to 1982. Yet one finds in this history a broad range of meanings and models that both illuminate and challenge the emerging ethic of care.

### The "Cura" Tradition of Care: Ancient Rome

Ancient literary, mythological, and philosophical sources form the roots of the "Cura" tradition of care, named after a mythological figure. The background for this tradition is found in the ambiguity of the term *cura* (care) in the Latin literature of ancient Rome. The term had two fundamental but conflicting meanings. On the one hand, it meant worries, troubles, or anxieties, as when one says that a person is "burdened with cares." On the other hand, care meant providing for the welfare of another; aligned with this latter meaning was the positive connotation of care as attentive conscientiousness or devotion (Burdach).

A literary instance of the first meaning of care—the care that is so burdensome that it drags humans down—is found in the work of the Roman poet Virgil (70–19 B.C.E.), who placed the personified "vengeful Cares" (*ultrices Curae*) before the entrance to the underworld. The philosopher Seneca (4 B.C.E.—65 C.E.), by contrast, saw care not so much as a burdensome force that drags humans down as the power in humans that lifts them up and places them on a level with God. For Seneca, both humans and God have reasoning powers for achieving the good; in God, the good is perfected simply by his nature, but in humans, "the good is perfected by care (*cura*)"(pp. 443–444). In this Stoic view, care was the key to the process of becoming truly human. For Seneca, the word *care* meant *solicitude*; it also had connotations of attentiveness, conscientiousness, and devotion (Burdach; Seneca).

The struggle between the opposing meanings of care—care as burden and care as solicitude—as well as the radical importance of care to being human, were elements in an influential Greco-Roman myth called "Care," found in a second-century Latin collection of myths edited by Hyginus (Hyginus; Grant). More than any other single source, this little-known myth, narrated below, has given shape to the idea of care in literature, philosophy, psychology, and ethics through the intervening centuries.

As Care (Cura) was crossing a river, she thoughtfully picked up some mud and began to fashion a human being. While she was pondering what she had done, Jupiter came along. (Jupiter was the founder of Olympian society, a society of the major gods and goddesses who inhabited Mount Olympus after most of the gods had already appeared.) Care asked him to give the spirit of life to the human being, and Jupiter readily granted this. Care wanted to name the human after herself, but Jupiter insisted that his name should be given to the human instead. While Care and Jupiter were arguing, Terra arose and said that the human being should be named after her, since she had given her own body. (Terra, or Earth, the original life force of the earth, guided Jupiter's rise to power.) Finally, all three disputants accepted Saturn as judge. (Known for his devotion to fairness and equality, Saturn was the son of Terra and the father of Jupiter.) Saturn decided that Jupiter, who gave spirit to the human, would take back its soul after death; and since Terra had offered her body to the human, she should receive it back after death. But, said Saturn, "Since Care first fashioned the human being, let her have and hold it as long as it lives." Finally, Jupiter said, "Let it be called *homo* (Latin for human being), since it seems to be made from *humus* (Latin for earth)" (see Grant; Shklar).

The meaning of the word *care* in this myth reflects the Stoic sense of an uplifting, attentive solicitude; it is in light of this positive side of care that we can understand the deeper meaning of the Myth of Care. Yet the word *care* is not without tension: The lifelong care of the human that would be undertaken by Cura entails both an earthly, bodily element that is pulled down to the ground (worry) and a spirit-element that strives upward to the divine (Burdach;

Grant). The positive side of care dominates in this story, for the primordial role of Care is to hold the human together in wholeness while cherishing it.

It is significant that a myth communicates the meaning of care, for one of the major functions of myths is to offer ancient narratives that make it possible for people to understand the meaning of their experiences regarding the basic characteristics of human life (Doty; Frye). The Myth of Care conveys an understanding of how care is central to what it means to be human and to live out a human life. It also provides a genealogy of care in light of which to rethink the value of care in human life.

Myths of origins have often been used to question the established order, both divine and human, and to establish radical moral claims, including claims about power and the social order (Shklar). Although several prominent political philosophies that have shaped much of modern bioethics are based on myths of origin that emphasize adversarial struggles as the starting point for human societies, the Myth of Care offers a subversively different image of human society, with very different implications for ethics in general and bioethics in particular (Reich). Indeed, the Myth of Care presents an allegorical image of humankind in which the most notable characteristic of the origins, life, and destiny of humans is that they are cared for (cf. Grant). At the same time, this gentle myth also speaks about the roots of power. Modern psychology teaches us that those who are cared for from birth (which is the image conveyed in this myth) develop the nurturing power to care for self and others. Furthermore, the fact that the myth's first human being is not named for the most powerful of the gods and goddesses, which would have been a symbol of being dominated by them, suggests that truly solicitous care protects humans from oppressive and manipulative power. The myth also suggests that humankind as a social totality is brought into the world and sustained by care. Since it binds humans together, care is the glue of society.

## The Care of Souls Tradition

The moral meaning of care is not only shaped by narratives, it is also historically embedded in practices such as the care of souls (*cura animarum*). The care of souls refers to the care of troubled persons whose difficulties—whether spiritual, mental, or physical—are approached in the context of the pursuit of the religious goals of life or, in nonreligious contexts, the search for ultimate meanings (cf. Clebsch and Jaekle; Browning). The care of souls tradition—the explanations offered in its literature and the interpretation of its practices—sheds light on the origins and content of contemporary ideas about care.

The word *care* in the care of souls refers both to the tasks involved in the care of a person or group and to the inner experience of solicitude or carefulness concerning the object of one's care. In the framework of the first meaning of the word, the care of souls consists of helping acts that are directed principally toward "healing" and the means by which healing is brought about, for example, reconciliation (including penitential reconciliation for those who have sinned), sustaining (including compassionate consolation), and guiding (spiritual and moral guidance).

The selection of the term *care of souls* to designate these activities (the word *cura* in the term *care of souls* is frequently translated as "cure" of souls) reflects the historical emphasis on a comprehensive idea of healing in the care of souls tradition (McNeill; Clebsch and Jaekle). Socrates regarded himself as the physician or healer of the soul, as did other philosophers (McNeill); and Gregory of Nazianzus (362 C.E.) said all pastors are physicians of souls, "who must prescribe medicines, or cautery, or the knife"(McNeill, p. 108).

The word *soul* in the care of souls can have a variety of meanings, depending on the philosophical explanation chosen or the religious tradition in which the term is used. John McNeill calls the soul "the essence of human personality" (p. vii). It is spirit intertwined with the body without being a mere expression of bodily life. The soul is regarded as being susceptible to disorder and anguish, while being endowed with possibilities for well-being and blessedness. The care of souls, then, is the healing treatment of persons in those matters that reach beyond the requirements of physical life, in pursuit of the "health of personality" (p. vii). But the welfare of the soul was not isolated: Caring for the healing of the soul, mind, and body have often been integrated (May, 1982). Thus, when we speak of "the care of the whole person," we are speaking of something comparable to the ancient idea of the care of souls.

The care of souls conveys the primary message that there is invariably a hierarchy of values in what it is that humans choose to care about, and that among those values, care for the spiritual should be preeminent. Socrates exhorted his hearers in Plato's *Apology* "not to care for your bodies or for money above and beyond your souls and their welfare"; and in the *Phaedo* he argued that "the cultivation of the soul is the first concern"(McNeill, p. 20). Some scholars believe his exhortation greatly influenced the emergence of the idea of the care of the soul in ancient Greece and in Christianity (McNeill).

Another prominent feature of the care of souls has been the way in which it calls attention to the subjective experience of those who are suffering and their need for relief in the form of personal attention. In the Hebrew scriptures, the Psalmist speaks out of bitter anguish: "I looked … and beheld, but … no man cared for my soul" (Ps. 142:4–5; McNeill). The sufferer then appealed to the Lord to be his refuge in the land of the living. In the care of souls tradition, God, self, and other humans care for the troubled soul. The one who gives care must be very attentive to the needs of the individual sufferer. For example, Gregory the Great, renowned for his pastoral leadership in the Western church (590–604), taught that the guide of souls must be a compassionate neighbor to all, a shrewd observer, and watchful and discerning like the physician of the body (McNeill). But one problem remains constant: whether the sufferer will seek and/or accept care (McNeill).

The contrast between negative and positive care that one finds in Seneca and the Myth of Care was also presented by Jesus, who contrasted the heavy burdens (the "yoke") that many people bear—the worrisome cares of life—with relief or solicitous care (Matt. 11:28–30). He exhorted his followers not to be anxious about the necessities of life, but instead to trust that they would be cared for by the heavenly Father who knows their needs (Matt. 6:25–34; Davies).

The care of souls tradition produced three major bodies of literature that are of special historical interest to contemporary bioethics. First, casuistry arose within the context of the *cura animarum*. In contrast to the rigid ethics of the medieval penitential documents, in which priest-confessors were instructed on how to deal with various categories of sinners, casuistry had the objective of bringing the lives of ordinary people under the influence of religious and moral standards by emphasizing practical, case-based moral reasoning that avoided excessive abstractions and complications (McNeill).

Second, those who cared for souls cared for the sorrows and anxieties of individuals, partly by writing a body of so-called Consolation literature. For example, Seneca and Plutarch in the classical age and Cyprian and Ambrose in the third and fourth centuries C.E. composed Consolation literature, offering sympathy for the ills of life, suffering, and persecution (McNeill).

Third, in the fourteenth and fifteenth centuries, when the idea of death was so vivid, the care of souls tradition produced a vast *Ars moriendi* literature, commending the art of dying well (willingly and joyfully, rather than in despair) and how to help the dying person (Clebsch and Jaekle; McNeill).

Finally, care had the constantly changing function of sustaining souls through the pitfalls of the earthly pilgrimage of each period of history. For example, during the seventeenth and eighteenth centuries, sustaining the troubled soul became the dominant function of the care of souls. Because of the Enlightenment, hopes and human aspirations for this life ran very high, and pastoral sustenance attempted principally to keep believers mindful of their individual destinies beyond this life (Clebsch and Jaekle). This was precisely the environment in which care (*Sorge*) appeared in Goethe's *Faust*.

## Goethe: A Romanticist Portrayal

The mythic idea of care made a major appearance in German literature in the eighteenth and early nineteenth centuries—a time when the meaning and relevance of myth were being rediscovered as never before—in the work of Johann Wolfgang von Goethe (1749–1832). Taking the Myth of Care from his teacher Johann Gottfried Herder (1744–1803)—specifically from Herder's poem titled "The Child of Care"—Goethe wove the major themes of that myth into his masterpiece, the dramatic poem *Faust* (Grant; Burdach).

Dr. Faust, passionately committed to the pursuit of reason and science, also wants to be care-free, that is, free of the disturbing anxieties of care that the pursuit of his goals would entail in working with ordinary human resources. He enters into a pact with Mephistopheles (the devil). In exchange for the knowledge and magical assistance of Mephistopheles, Faust agrees to be his slave; it is agreed at the outset that Faust may lose his soul to the devil in the process (Goethe, 1985).

In the final act of the drama, Faust has become powerful and wealthy, the ruler of a flourishing land that he has reclaimed from the sea. He discovers that the deceitful Mephistopheles, working under orders from Faust, has horribly destroyed by fire the last cottage destined for demolition in the reclamation project; consumed by the flames was a peaceful old couple to whom Faust had promised relocation. Appalled by the horrific consequences of his thoughtless order, Faust breaks with Mephistopheles and his magic. He wants to stand before Nature as the "mere" human being he had been before his pact with the devil. This internal change sets the stage for the struggle over Faust's character, and for the appearance of Care (Goethe, 1959; Burdach).

Care (*Sorge*), a gray hag calling herself the "eternally anxious companion" (*Ewig ängstlicher Geselle*), chides Faust for never having known her: "Have you never known Care?" (*Hast du die Sorge nie gekannt?*). She denounces the darkness and ambiguity of Faust's soul—and blinds him because he refuses to acknowledge her fully. The terrible power of the burdens of Sorge's care almost overwhelms Faust but fails to conquer his soul. Linked with Faust's profound horror over

his own crime, Sorge's denunciation has the effect of bringing about Faust's turn from burdensome care to the uplifting solicitude of positive care. His "striving," which led him to ruthless acquisition, the oppressive manipulation of masses of people, and the destruction of the old couple, is transformed during his blindness into a genuine solicitude for his people (Jaeger, pp. 41–43). Faust's experience of a new and very satisfying solicitude (the greatest moment of his life) is represented by his vision of millions of free people living in comfort and freedom on an earth that has been reconciled with itself through human effort.

Goethe's Faustian narrative demonstrates that striving for one's own life goals while shutting out a sometimes worrisome and painful concern for people and institutions results in terrible external and internal harm. In the pursuit of one's destiny, a human cannot avoid care. One must first deal with the heavy side of care, rejecting its power to engulf and destroy, and then convert this care, which is the root of all human striving, into a positive, solicitous concern for people and institutions. For Goethe, care becomes conscientiousness and devotedness (Burdach). At the same time, care relates in a fundamental way to the human condition, for it may be the key to one's moral "salvation," as it was for Faust. In contrast to today's tendency to associate care exclusively with interpersonal devotion, Goethe works out the meaning of care in a political setting; the problem for Faust is whether he will show solicitous care as a ruler. As a result, Goethe's portrayal of care has important implications for political philosophy.

## Kierkegaard and Heidegger: Existentialist and Phenomenological Approaches

**KIERKEGAARD.** Søren Kierkegaard (1813–1855), the Danish philosopher and religious thinker, was the first major philosopher to make significant use of the notion of care or concern, albeit in embryonic fashion. Intimately familiar with the *Sorge* of Goethe's *Faust* (Collins), Kierkegaard offered creative philosophical explanations of themes that had appeared both in the Myth of Care and in Goethe: that care is central to understanding human life and is the key to human authenticity. The extensive influence of Kierkegaard's idea of care or concern on subsequent thought can be seen in the context of his role as father of existentialism: It was Kierkegaard's idea of the "concerned thinker," pivotal for his own philosophy, that became the central theme of existentialist philosophy and theology (Bochenski).

***Concern and care in Kierkegaard's philosophy.*** Kierkegaard introduced notions of concern, interest, and care to counteract what he considered the excessive objectivity of philosophy and theology as they were formulated in the early nineteenth century. To recover the sense and significance of individual human existence that he believed modern philosophy's abstract and universal categories had obliterated, Kierkegaard called attention to what he saw as the missing element of concern or care in the kind of philosophical reflection that those systems utilized (Copleston).

Kierkegaard distinguished between disinterested reflection, on the one hand, and consciousness, which entails interest or concern, on the other. Reflection, he argued, focuses on the objective or hypothetical; it is a merely disinterested process of classifying things in opposition to each other (e.g., the ideal and the real, soul and body); it has "no concern with, or interest in, the knower" (1958, p. 150), or with what happens to the individual person as a result of this kind of knowing.

Consciousness is inherently concerned both with the knower and with the collision of opposites that come to be known through reflection. Indeed, consciousness brings the merely objective elements of reflection into a real relationship with the knowing subject through care or concern (Kierkegaard, 1958). A personal (i.e., a concerned) relationship to truth is the basis of Kierkegaard's whole theory of knowledge (Croxall). For Kierkegaard the issue of concerned knowledge is a moral issue. To adopt the stance of the impersonally knowing subject rather than that of the concerned human being "as a refuge from the chaos and pain of life," he believes, "is cowardice and escapism" (Rudd, p. 28).

Kierkegaard also uses the notion of concern to express the nature of the human being and its moral choices. Humans are beings whose greatest interest or concern is in existing; concern or care is subjectively chosen as an intimate part of the individual's being (Kierkegaard, 1958; Stack). The individual gives form and direction to his or her life, and expresses his or her true self, not by being caught up in a large social system, but by exercising free choice and commitment (Kierkegaard, 1940; Copleston).

The fundamental question of ethics is: How shall I live? Objective reasoning plays a part in answering this question; but an ethical argument is valid only insofar as it articulates a concerned individual's search for meaning (Rudd). Thus, ethics starts with the individual. "As soon as I have to act, interest or concern is laid upon me, because I take responsibility on myself ..." (Kierkegaard, 1958, pp. 116–117, 152–153). Without care or concern, action would not be possible: Concern is the impetus for the resolute moral action of the self-reflecting individual who acts with purpose

(Stack). Always in the process of becoming, lacking the security of knowledge and facing contradiction, the human is constrained to mold his or her integrity through decision and action. One cannot do this without an "unrelieved and unceasing concern" for the passion and possibility of becoming oneself (Mackey, p. 71; Hannay).

***Being burdened with cares; being cared for.*** Kierkegaard offers profound insights into the experience of being laden with cares and being cared for in writings that fall into the category of care of souls literature. He takes the traditional struggle between negative and positive care, previously discussed in the Myth of Care and in Goethe, in a new direction, by turning the subjective experience of worrisome care into reasons for caring for one's self and seeking the care of others.

In his writings on a biblical exhortation regarding human solicitude for material versus spiritual things (Matt. 6:19–34), Kierkegaard remarks that by contemplating the lilies of the field and the birds of heaven, who are not neglected, humans realize that even when they themselves are "outside all human care," neither are they neglected: They are still cared for by a caring God (1940, p. 16). Humans must work to fill their needs; but the human capacity to be weighted down by material care is a mark of perfection, for it also signals the human capacity to cast one's care from oneself, find consolers, accept their sympathy, and choose a caring God. On the other hand, humans can trap themselves into a care-ridden state of mind by worrying about future needs, being convinced they need total security against their anxieties, feeling an exaggerated sense of self-sufficiency, and comparing themselves unfavorably to others.

For Kierkegaard, a special kind of anxious care is created when, in the course of an illness, the question arises whether the sick person is confronting life renewing itself or the looming decay of death. The pathos of this question, which is more moving than the prospect of a terrifying death, can move the sick person to reduce his or her resistance to accepting consolation from others (1940). Finally, Kierkegaard remarks that caring for someone is not always a gentle art. When, for example, there is much that the sick person can do to improve his or her health, stern demands made by the authoritative doctor—sometimes even at the request of the patient—are the expression of concern for the anxious sick person.

**HEIDEGGER.** For Martin Heidegger (1889–1976), one of the most original and influential philosophers of the twentieth century, care was not just one concept among many; it was at the very center of his philosophical system of thought. Conceptually, Heidegger was strongly influenced by Kierkegaard's teachings on concern and care; yet there is a notable difference. Whereas Kierkegaard saw care or concern always in an individualized, subjective, and psychological fashion, Heidegger used the word at an abstract, ontological level to describe the basic structure of the human self. Although Heidegger insisted that he was not speaking of concrete and practical aspects of care, such as worry or nurturing, it can also be argued that his writings on care do have existential moral significance. He certainly developed some ideas that provide useful insights for a practical ethic of care (Stack).

Heidegger's starting point and lifelong interest was the philosophical question of being—in particular, the question of the meaning of being. He used the term *Dasein,* or "being-there," to represent the human experience of being in the world through participation and involvement (1973, 1985). Heidegger's interest was to show how care is the central idea for understanding the meaning of the *human self,* which is another word for *Dasein.* His philosophy explains how, at a deeper level than the psychological experience of care, care is what accounts for the unity, authenticity, and totality of the self, that is, of *Dasein.* Briefly, Heidegger claims that we are care, and care is what we call the human being (Gelven).

Heidegger explains the radical role of care by pointing to the tendency of the human self to turn away from its own authentic being to seek security in the crowd. It accommodates itself to what "they" think and forms its conduct in accordance with the expectations of public opinion. Care (*Sorge*) summons the self (*Dasein*) back from the feeling of insignificance and anxiety found in this flight from the self, and instead enables one to be one's own self, that is, to be authentic (Flynn; Martinez).

Heidegger also explains care in the context of openness to future possibilities. We are not simply "spectators for whom in principle, nothing would 'matter'" (Olafson, p. 104). To say that the self (*Dasein*) is care means that we understand and care about ourselves-in-the-world in terms of being connected with what we can and cannot do. Because of the connectedness brought about by care, it matters that we can act, and we must act to choose among our own possibilities (Olafson). In so doing, *Dasein* chooses itself; and the meaning of its existence unfolds in every resolute act. This is all implicit in care (Martinez).

For Heidegger, care has the double meaning of anxiety and solicitude—the same duality we found among the Romans—and these two meanings of care represent two conflicting, fundamental possibilities (1973). Anxious, worrisome care (*Sorge*) represents our struggle for survival and for favorable standing among our fellow human beings. It continually drives us to avoid the significance of our finitude,

by immersing ourselves in conventionality and triviality, so as to "conceal from ourselves the question of the meaning of being, and in the process truncate our humanity as well" (Ogletree, p. 23). Yet care also bears the meaning of solicitude or "caring for" (*Fürsorge*): tending to, nurturing, caring for the Earth and for our fellow human beings as opposed to merely "taking care of" them. However, anxious care never totally dissolves: In the everyday world we cannot avoid the dual sense of care-as-anxiety and care-as-solicitude. Accepting the kinds of beings we are entails embracing a deep ambiguity in which we know that worrisome cares may drive us to escape and that solicitous care can open up all our possibilities for us (Ogletree).

Heidegger also contrasts *Besorgen* (taking care of, in the sense of supplying the needs of others) with *Fürsorge* (solicitous care). The human self (*Dasein*), which is essentially related to others, enters the world of others by way of care in two ways. On the one hand, we can take care of the "what" that needs to be done for the other, in a rather functional way. This sort of minimal taking care (*Besorgen*) requires few qualities—principally circumspection, so that the service is done correctly. Yet other humans are never merely things like equipment that need to be taken care of in this way; for they, too, are selves oriented to others. Hence they are not simply objects of service but of solicitude (*Fürsorge*). Solicitous care is guided by the subsidiary qualities of considerateness and forbearance. But Heidegger insists that when someone nurses the sick body as a mere social arrangement, that is, without considerateness, the nursing care should still be regarded as solicitude, albeit a deficient solicitude, and never as (mere) service-care (1973).

Heidegger also speaks of two extreme forms of solicitous care. Intending to show solicitous care, one can "jump in" and take over for the other, who then is dominated and dependent in the caring relationship. Doing what the other can do for himself or herself, the "solicitous" person is actually taking "care" away from the other. In contrast, Heidegger continues, there is a solicitous care that "jumps ahead" of the other, anticipating his or her potentiality—not in order to take away his or her "care" but to give it back. This kind of solicitude is authentic care, for it helps the other to know himself or herself in care, and to become free for care (Heidegger, 1973; Bishop and Scudder).

Heidegger's substantive development of the notion of care drew from and contributed to the "Cura" tradition of care. At the "high point" of his inquiry (Heidegger, 1973), Heidegger directly cited the Myth of Care as a primordial justification of his central claim that the human self (*Dasein*) has the stamp of care (Klonoski, p. 65). In spite of Heidegger's complexities, some writers are attempting to develop elements of an ethic of care from his insights; and some scholars, such as Anne Bishop and John Scudder, are utilizing Heidegger's ideas in their arguments regarding the moral practice of healthcare.

## Rollo May and Erik Erikson: Psychological Developments

**ROLLO MAY.** Rollo May (1909–1994), a pioneer of the humanistic school of psychology, introduced to U.S. psychology the views of European existentialists. He made Heidegger's views on care more accessible to the average reader by pointing to their psychological and moral implications.

May's 1969 book *Love and Will* was written in a historical period in which, he argued, humans were experiencing a general malaise and depersonalization resulting in cynicism and apathy, which he regarded as "the psychological illnesses of our day" (p. 306). What the youth of the 1960s were fighting in their protests, May claimed, was the "creeping conviction that nothing matters …, that one can't do anything." The threat was apathy. Care "is a necessary antidote" to apathy, for care "is a state in which something does matter; care is the opposite of apathy." It is "the refusal to accept emptiness …, the stubborn assertion of the self to give content to our activities, routine as these activities may be" (p. 292). Care, regarded as the capacity to feel that something matters, is born in the same act as the infant: If the child is not cared for by its mother, it withers away both biologically and psychologically.

May was concerned that the idea of care would not be taken seriously if it were regarded as mere subjective sentiment. To counteract this attitude, he argued that care is objective. With care, "we are caught up in our experience of the objective thing or event we care about" and about which we must do something (1969, p. 291). Following Heidegger and citing the text of the Myth of Care, May holds that care constitutes the human as human: Care is "the basic constitutive phenomenon of human existence" (1969, p. 290). Drawing from these sources the idea that the human being is constituted in its human attitudes by care, May claimed: "When we do not care, we lose our being; and care is the way back to being." This has moral implications: "If I care about being, I will shepherd it with some attention paid to its welfare …" (May, 1969, p. 290).

We could not will or wish if we did not care to begin with; and if we do authentically care, we cannot help wishing or willing. Care makes possible the exercise of will and love; and it is also the source of conscience: "Conscience is the call of Care" (May, 1969, p. 290, quoting Heidegger). Care is a state composed of the recognition of a fellow human being, of the identification of one's self with the pain or joy of the other … and of "the awareness that we all stand on the base of a common humanity from which we all stem." Care of self psychologically precedes care of the other, for care gains its power from the sense of pain; but pain begins with one's own experience of it. "If we do not care for ourselves, we are hurt, burned, injured." And this is the source of identification with the pain of the other (May, 1969, p. 289).

According to May, care must be at the root of ethics, for the good life comes from what we care about. Ethics has its psychological base "in the capacities of the human being to transcend the concrete situation of the immediate self-oriented desire," and to live and make decisions "in terms of the welfare of the persons and groups upon whom his own fulfillment intimately depends" (1969, p. 268).

**ERIK ERIKSON.** Partly under the influence of Heidegger's philosophy, Erik Erikson (1902–1994) constructed a richly humanistic theory of psychosocial development in which care played a major role. Like May, Erikson made the idea of care more accessible to the average person; but he went far beyond all his predecessors by developing a fairly comprehensive psychological account of care that is relevant to many of the interests of contemporary ethics.

Based on his study of case histories and of life histories, Erikson developed a theory of psychosocial development in which the human life cycle has eight stages, each of them characterized by a developmental crisis or turning point. From the resolution of that crisis a "specific psychosocial strength" or a "basic virtue" emerges.

In the seventh stage, "adulthood," the developmental crisis is generativity versus self-absorption and stagnation. Generativity—"the concern with establishing and guiding the next generation" (Erikson, 1987, p. 607)—encompasses procreativity, productivity, and creativity. It entails the generation not only of new human beings but also of new products and new ideas, as well as a self-generation concerned with further personal development. Generativity struggles with a sense of self-absorption or stagnation, "the potential core pathology of this stage" that might manifest itself through regression to an obsessive need for pseudo-intimacy (Erikson, 1982, pp. 67–68; 1963, pp. 266–268). The virtue or "basic strength" that emerges from this crisis is care.

Adult caring is "the generational task of cultivating strength in the next generation" (Erikson, 1982, pp. 55, 67–68; 1963, p. 274; 1978, p. 22); that task may be parental, didactic, productive, or curative (1982). For Erikson, care is "the concrete concern for what has been generated by love, necessity, or accident"; it is "a widening commitment to take care of the persons, the products, and the ideas one has learned *to care for*" (1978, pp. 27–28).

The impetus to care has instinctual roots in the "impulse to 'cherish' and to 'caress' that which in its helplessness emits signals of despair" (Erikson, 1982, pp. 59–60). The infant's demeanor awakens in adults a strength that they need to have confirmed in the experience of care; conversely, maternal care enables the infant to trust rather than mistrust and to develop hope rather than a sense of abandonment (1987, p. 600).

The tasks of taking care of new generations must be given continuity by institutions such as extended households and divided labor (Erikson, 1987). "[A] man and a woman must [define] for themselves what and whom they have come to care for, what they care to do well, and how they plan to take care of what they have started and created" (1969, p. 395). Even if individuals choose not to have children, they have a relationship to "care for the creatures of this world" through participation in those institutions that safeguard and reinforce generative succession (1963, pp. 267–268). Some, like Gandhi, choose, as an expression of their care, to become "father and mother, brother and sister, son and daughter, to all creation ..." (1969, 399). The task of taking care of the new generation also falls to organized human communities (1987); social and political leadership often entails giving direction to people's capacity to care (1969).

The framework for Erikson's ethic of care is one of dialectic dynamics, that is, it depends on a process of development and change through the conflict of two opposing forces; the moral task is to see to it that a new strength emerges. The negative aspect of adulthood (self-absorption) continues to interact dynamically with the positive aspects (generativity) throughout life (1963). Personal growth and the strength of care emerge from this conflict through an active adaptation that requires that one change the environment, including social mores and institutions, while making selective use of its opportunities (1978).

For Erikson, part of the ethics of care involves the struggle between the willingness to embrace persons or groups in one's generative concerns (a *sympathic* strength, which is the virtue of care) and the unwillingness to include specified persons or groups in one's generative concern (an *antipathic* inclination, which Erikson calls rejectivity). With rejectivity, "one does not care to care for" certain individuals or groups, or may even express hostility toward them (1982, p. 68). Because care must be selective, some rejectivity is unavoidable. "Ethics, law, and insight" must define the allowable extent of rejectivity in any given group. With the

purpose of reducing rejectivity among humans, "religious and ideological belief systems must continue to advocate a more universal principle of care for specified wider units of communities" (1982, p. 69). Consequently, for Erikson, the ethics of care expresses itself in both "small but significant gestures" (1978, p. 15) and in global struggles against uncaring attitudes that contribute to the destruction of public and private morals.

## Milton Mayeroff: A Personalist Vision

The 1971 book *On Caring* by American philosopher Milton Mayeroff (1925–1979) provides a detailed description and explanation of the experiences of caring and being cared for. Although he drew on several major themes from the history of the notion of care, he took the idea of care in new, personalist directions. Mayeroff's book is a philosophical essay that at the same time shares some of the characteristics of the care of souls tradition, inasmuch as Mayeroff's purpose was to show how care could help us understand and integrate our lives more effectively.

To care for another, according to Mayeroff, is to help the other grow, whether the other is a person, an idea, an ideal, a work of art, or a community; for example, the basic caring stance of a parent is to respect the child as striving to grow in his or her own right. Helping other persons to grow also entails encouraging and assisting them to care for something or someone other than themselves, as well as for themselves (1971).

The caring relationship is mutual: The parent feels needed by the child and helps him or her grow by responding to the child's need to grow; at the same time, the parent feels the child's growth as bound up with his or her own sense of well-being. Caring, Mayeroff says, is primarily a process, not a series of goal-oriented services. For example, if the psychotherapist regards treatment as a mere means to a future product (the cure), and the present process of therapeutic interaction is not taken seriously for its own sake, caring becomes impossible (1971).

According to Mayeroff, caring entails devotion, trust, patience, humility, honesty, knowing the other, respecting the primacy of the process, hope, and courage. Knowledge, for example, means being able to sense "from inside" what the other person or the self experiences and requires to grow. Devotion, which gives substance and a particular character to caring for a particular person, involves being "there" for the other courageously and with consistency. But caring does not entail "being with" the other constantly: That is a phase within the rhythm of caring, followed by a phase of relative detachment (1971).

Caring involves trusting the other to grow in his or her own time and way. There is a lack of trust when guarantees are required regarding the outcome of our caring, or when one cares "too much." One who "cares" too much is not showing excessive care for the other so much as deficient trust in the other's process of growing (Mayeroff, 1971).

In Mayeroff's vision, moral values are inherent in the process of caring and growth. When cared for, one grows by becoming more self-determining and by choosing one's own values and ideals grounded in one's own experience, instead of simply conforming to prevailing values. Mayeroff's moral approach to care is that of an ethic of response: He emphasizes the values and goods that are discovered in caring, and the fitting sort of human responsiveness to self and other that these engender. Care-related responsibilities and obligations—such as those that derive from devotion to one's children—arise more from internal sources related to character and relational commitments than from external rules (1971). When caring engages one's powers sufficiently, it has a way of ordering the other values and activities of life around itself, resulting in an integration of the self with the surrounding world.

The conviction that life has meaning corresponds with the feeling of being uniquely needed by something or someone and of being understood and cared for. Mayeroff concludes that the more deeply we understand the central role of caring in our own life, the more we realize it is central to the human condition (1971). Mayeroff's idea that care is central to the human condition reaches back through several philosophers to the Myth of Care, while his rich descriptions of the nature and effects of care set the stage for an ethic of care in the contemporary healthcare setting.

## Parallel Concepts

SYMPATHY. The history of the ethics of sympathy provides useful insights for the developing notion and ethics of care. A number of philosophers writing between the end of the seventeenth century and the beginning of the twentieth—principally Joseph Butler (1692–1752), David Hume (1711–1776), Adam Smith (1723–1790), Arthur Schopenhauer (1788–1860), and Max Scheler (1874–1928)—developed an ethic of sympathy. Taken from the Greek word *sympatheia,* meaning "feeling with," sympathy referred to a "felt concern for other people's welfare" (Solomon, p. 552).

There are several reasons for considering some highlights of an ethic of sympathy in the context of this entry. First, there are some links between care and sympathy: Some of the authors who have developed the notion of care include sympathy, empathy, or compassion as elements of care, for example, Rollo May and Milton Mayeroff; yet sympathy differs from care, for care has a deeper role in human life, is broader than sympathy in its tasks, and entails a more committed role with other people and projects. Second, the ethics of sympathy offers sustained philosophical examination of issues that are of interest to the ethics of care, which has been subjected to relatively little systematic philosophical inquiry. In particular, an ethics of care has much to learn from an ethics of sympathy regarding its most distinctive formal feature: It is based on a fundamental human emotion that is viewed as the central feature of the moral life and the basis of an ethic—a fundamental characteristic that it shares with the ethics of sympathy.

Accordingly, there are questions significant for an ethic of care that could be examined in the context of the ethics of sympathy. For example, there is the question regarding justification for the use of a passion or emotion such as care as the starting point or central point in ethics. Joseph Butler, writing in the sympathy tradition, argued against the view of psychological egoism, which asserted that we cannot be motivated simply by a concern for others, for human psychology is such that we cannot help but act in our own interests when we act on emotion. Against this, Butler argued that passions and affections, which are "instances of our Maker's care and love," contribute to public as well as private good and naturally lead us to regulate our behavior. Benevolence for others and the self-love that prompts care of the self are distinct; they are not in conflict; and they are both governed by moral reflection or conscience. David Hume went much further: Passions, or moral emotions, are primary, for they alone move humans to action; reason must serve the passions by providing the means for achieving the ends that sentiment selects. Consequently, moral judgments, which are the motives moving us to action, must be based primarily on moral sentiments or feelings, not on reason (Hume, 1983; Raphael).

Another question is whether an altruistic virtue traditionally regarded as soft could have much effect on the ethics of the practice of medicine, which emphasizes principles and objectivity. A comparable issue arose particularly in the writings of John Gregory (1724–1773), a prominent Scottish physician-philosopher, who applied the ethics of "sympathy" and "humanity" (the paired terms were taken from David Hume) to the medical care of the sick. Gregory held that the chief moral quality "peculiarly required in the character of a physician" is humanity, namely "that sensibility of heart which makes us feel for the distresses of our fellow creatures, and which, of consequence, incites us in the most powerful manner to relieve them" (1817, p. 22). The moral quality paired with humanity is sympathy, which "produces an anxious attention to a thousand little circumstances that may tend to relieve the patient" and "naturally engages the affection and confidence of a patient, which, in many cases, is of the utmost consequence to his recovery" (1817, p. 22).

Gregory speaks of the development of a balanced skill of medical compassion in the clinician: Physicians who are truly compassionate, "by being daily conversant with scenes of distress, acquire in process of time that composure and firmness of mind so necessary in the practice of physic. They can feel whatever is amiable in pity, without suffering it to enervate or unman them" (1817, p. 23). In this way, Gregory closely tied the virtue of sympathy to the art of medicine and to medical benefit, while answering the objection that sympathy causes an emotional imbalance in the practitioner.

Not only does Gregory defend the role of the "soft" altruistic virtue in medicine; he pointedly identifies the core of the objection against them. Rejecting as "malignant and false" the view that compassion is associated with weakness, Gregory argues that rough manners are "frequently affected by men void of magnanimity and personal courage" in order to conceal their defects (1817, pp. 22–24). Men can gain from women both "humanity" and "sentiment," qualities that are at the very core of the moral life (1765).

**ATTENTION**. Attention (or heed or regard) has, for centuries, been one of the meanings of care; it remains an element of care today. To care for someone is to pay solicitous attention to him or her and to have a disposition of attentiveness. To take good (conscientious) care of a patient means to be attentive both to the needs of the patient and to the duties of proper care. The "attending physician" is one who has primary responsibility for the care of, and is ready for service to, the patient. Thus, the notion of attention is not only a concept parallel to care; it is an ingredient in care. The philosopher Gilbert Ryle says, "To care is to pay attention to something …" (p. 135).

The most significant and stimulating thinker on the topic of attention was Simone Weil (1909–1943), a French philosopher and mystic who makes attention the central image for ethics. Attention, she explains, is a negative effort consisting of suspending one's thought, leaving it detached, empty, and ready to receive the being one is looking at, "just as he is, in all his truth" (1977, p. 51).

Weil says that solving a philosophical problem (including one dealing with morality) requires a kind of caring contemplation: "clearly conceiving the insoluble problems in all their insolubility, … simply contemplating them,

fixedly and tirelessly, … patiently waiting" (1970, p. 335). Being attentive is being open to illumination (Weil, 1978, p. 92); we should look at these problems "until the light suddenly dawns" (1952, p. 174). What we sometimes fail to see is what Weil perceives: that solving moral problems sometimes entails facing mystery. Thus, to discover what is causing a person's suffering and how to respond to it, the caring nurse may need to employ Weil's contemplative attention to all details; and even that exercise of attention is itself a caring act.

Attention offers a powerful approach to ethics. For example, Simone Weil thinks of equality and justice not as abstract concepts or principles that serve the well-ordered society; she conceives of them as virtues that can only be illuminated and developed through attentive knowledge. Thus, for Weil, equality is a certain kind of attention, "a way of looking at ourselves and others" (Teuber, p. 223). Respect for another person is not respect insofar as the other has a rational nature or is a person: Weil states bluntly that she could put out a man's eyes without touching his person or personality. Rather, we show respect for individuals in their concrete specificity: "There is something sacred in every man, but it is not his person [nor] the human personality. It is this man.… The whole of him. The arms, the eyes, the thoughts, everything …" (1981, p. 13). Respect for others is based more in compassion than in awe for personhood, and compassion does not depend on familiarity: We can and should foster compassion for individuals who are very different from ourselves (Teuber, p. 225).

Attention is also a key part of the practice of compassion. Weil explained that those who are suffering "have no need for anything in this world but people capable of giving them their attention." She contended that the capacity to give one's attention to a sufferer is a very rare and difficult thing; "it is almost a miracle; it is a miracle …" (Weil, 1977, p. 51).

Attention and the equality it discovers do not suffice for all problems in ethics: They do not in themselves define any principles for adjudicating conflicts; but they can and do convey certain attitudes and forms of conduct without which we would lose sight of the meaning and substance of our obligations and rights (Teuber, p. 228). In addition, Weil's sort of attention can show us duties we did not see before (Nelson, p. 13) and can instruct us in the skills required for caring.

## Conclusion

In a variety of settings—mythological, religious, philosophical, psychological, theological, moral, and practical—the notion of care has developed throughout history, influencing moral orientations and behaviors. The tasks for the future will be to more fully understand the richness and complexity of the history of the idea of care, do justice to the texts that have imaginatively portrayed it and the thinkers who have made this idea central to their work, and enter into dialogue with them.

This history reveals, not a unified idea of care, but a family of notions of care. Yet it is a fairly closely related family, for the ideas of care are united by a few basic sentiments, some formative narratives whose influence stretches over time, and several recurring themes. Furthermore, in the history of the English word *care,* this single word serves a range of meanings but with a subtle coherence.

The meanings of the word *care* fall into four clusters. The basic meaning is associated with the origins of the word, which are found in the Middle High German word *kar* and more remotely in the Common Teutonic word *caru,* meaning "trouble" or "grief" (Simpson and Weiner, pp. 893–894). Correspondingly, the primary meaning of the word *care* is anxiety, anguish, or mental suffering. A second meaning of *care* is a basic concern for people, ideas, institutions, and the like—the idea that something matters to the one who is concerned. Two other meanings of care, sometimes in conflict, are found at a more practical level. One is a solicitous, responsible attention to tasks—taking care of the needs of people and one's own responsibilities; and the other is caring about, having a regard for, or showing attentive care for a person, for his or her growth, and so forth. In a sense, all the meanings of *care* share to some extent a basic element: One can scarcely be said to care about someone or something if one is not at least prepared to worry about him, her, or it. The truly caring health professional is one who worries about—is concerned about—his or her patients, especially the patients who cannot take care of themselves.

Several distinctive features stand out in this history of care. The metaphysical and religious dimensions of care appear forcefully and repeatedly in history, emphasizing that care is essential to understanding humans and the human condition. The history of care shows that, at one level, care is a precondition for the whole moral life. It also manifests various frameworks for an ethic of care, including evolutionary ethics, virtue ethics, an ethic of growth, an ethic of response, and duty ethics, yet one does not find a formal and systematic ethics of care in the sources examined.

Repeatedly in this history one encounters a dialectical element in which pairs of ideas of care struggle against each other: care as worry or anxiety versus care as solicitude; the care that enables growth versus the effort to care that robs a person of self-care; or taking technical care of the other versus caring about the other. There is much to learn from history about the dark side of care and how humans might deal with it.

A key historical puzzle is why the notion of care has not become better known and has not exerted more influence in ethics, in view of its highly significant, if somewhat limited, history. The answer lies, in part, in the fact that care has always been a minority tradition of thought and practice. As this survey exemplifies, care is a deeply engaging emotion/idea that has confronted and challenged rationalist, abstract, and impersonal systems of thought, with far-reaching social, political, ethical, and religious implications. In this sense, care has had a countercultural role.

More recently, care may be acquiring a "mainstream" importance, especially in the area of the ethics of healthcare. The following two entries will show how some elements in the history of the idea of care have become ingredients in an emerging ethic of care in the context of healthcare, while other historical elements have been overlooked.

All ethics assumes a vision of the human condition. The ethics of care rests on a vision of the capacity to care or be concerned about things, persons, a whole life-course, a society, one's self. The history certainly is not compatible with reducing care to caregiving. The Myth of Care suggestively offers a care-based genealogy of morals that is deeply ingrained in human psychology, anthropology, religion, and altruistic service. The philosophical and psychological developments in the idea of care have built on this basic vision of being well cared for. That the history of the idea of care also suggests many practical ideas—for example, the call and the limits of taking care of others; dealing with the negative side of care; and the intergenerational function of care—makes it all the more useful for a contemporary ethic of care.

WARREN THOMAS REICH (1995)

SEE ALSO: *Alternative Therapies; Beneficence; Chronic Illness and Chronic Care; Compassionate Love; Feminism; Human Dignity; Long-Term Care; Nursing Ethics; Obligation and Supererogation; Paternalism; Professional-Patient Relationship; Women, Historical and Cross-Cultural Perspectives;* and other *Care* subentries

### BIBLIOGRAPHY

Baier, Annette C. 1980. "Master Passions." In *Explaining Emotions,* pp. 403–423, ed. Amélie Oksenberg Rorty. Berkeley: University of California Press.

Baier, Annette C. 1987. "Hume, the Women's Moral Theorist?"In *Women and Moral Theory,* pp. 35–55, ed. Eva Feder Kittay and Diana T. Meyers. Totowa, NJ: Rowman and Littlefield.

Bishop, Anne H., and Scudder, John R., Jr. 1991. "Nursing as Caring." In *Nursing: The Practice of Caring,* pp. 53–76. New York: National League for Nursing Press.

Blum, Larry; Homiak, Marcia; Housman, Judy; and Scheman, Naomi. 1973. "Altruism and Women's Oppression."*Philosophical Forum* 5: 222–247.

Bochenski, Joseph M. 1968. *The Methods of Contemporary Thought.* New York: Harper and Row.

Browning, Don S. 1983. *Religious Ethics and Pastoral Care.* Philadelphia: Fortress.

Bryant, S. 1961. "Sympathy." In *Encyclopaedia of Religion and Ethics,* vol. 12, pp. 152–155, ed. James Hastings. New York: Charles Scribner's Sons.

Burdach, Konrad. 1923. "Faust und die Sorge." *Deutsche Vierteljahrsschrift für Literaturwissenschaft und Geistesgeschichte* 1: 1–60.

Butler, Bishop Joseph. 1950 (1726). *Five Sermons Preached at the Rolls Chapel; and, A Dissertation upon the Nature of Virtue.* New York: Bobbs-Merrill.

Clebsch, William A., and Jaekle, Charles R. 1964. *Pastoral Care in Historical Perspective: An Essay with Exhibits.* New York: Harper and Row.

Collins, James D. 1953. *The Mind of Kierkegaard.* Chicago: Henry Regnery.

Copleston, Frederick. 1966. *Contemporary Philosophy: Studies of Logical Positivism and Existentialism.* Westminster, MD: Newman.

Croxall, Thomas Henry. 1958. "Assessment." In *Johannes Climacus; or, De Omnibus Dubitandum Est; and A Sermon.* By Søren Kierkegaard, tr. Thomas Henry Croxall. Stanford, CA: Stanford University Press.

Davies, Paul E. 1962. "Care, Carefulness."In vol. 1 of *The Interpreter's Dictionary of the Bible,* p. 537, ed. George Arthur Buttrick. New York: Abingdon.

Doty, William G. 1991. "Myth, the Archetype of All Other Fable: A Review of Recent Literature." In *Soundings: An Interdisciplinary Journal* 71(1–2): 243–274.

Erikson, Erik H. 1963. *Childhood and Society,* 2nd edition, rev. New York: W. W. Norton.

Erikson, Erik H. 1964. *Insight and Responsibility: Lectures on the Ethical Implications of Psychoanalytic Insight.* New York: W. W. Norton.

Erikson, Erik H. 1969. *Ghandi's Truth: On the Origins of Militant Nonviolence.* New York: W. W. Norton.

Erikson, Erik H. 1974. *Dimensions of a New Identity.* New York: W. W. Norton.

Erikson, Erik H. 1978. "Reflections on Dr. Borg's Life Cycle." In *Adulthood: Essays,* pp. 1–31, ed. Erik H. Erikson. New York: W. W. Norton.

Erikson, Erik H. 1980a. *Identity and the Life Cycle: Selected Papers.* New York: W. W. Norton.

Erikson, Erik H. 1980b. "On the Generation Cycle: An Address." *International Journal of Psycho-Analysis* 61, pt. 2: 213–223.

Erikson, Erik H. 1982. *The Life Cycle Completed: A Review.* New York: W. W. Norton.

Erikson, Erik H. 1987. *A Way of Looking at Things: Selected Papers from 1930 to 1980,* ed. Stephen Schlein. New York: W. W. Norton.

Flynn, Thomas R. 1980. "Angst and Care in the Early Heidegger: The Ontic/Ontologic Aporia." *International Studies in Philosophy* 12 (Spring): 61–76.

Frye, Northrop. 1971. *The Critical Path: An Essay on the Social Context of Literary Criticism.* Bloomington and London: Indiana University Press.

Gelven, Michael. 1989. *A Commentary on Heidegger's Being and Time,* rev. edition. De Kalb: Northern Illinois University Press.

Gilligan, Carol. 1982. *In a Different Voice: Psychological Theory and Women's Development.* Cambridge, MA: Harvard University Press.

Goethe, Johann Wolfgang von. 1959. *Faust.* Part 2, tr. Philip Wayne. London: Penguin.

Goethe, Johann Wolfgang von. 1985. *Faust,* Part 1. German/English rev. edition, tr. Peter Salm. New York: Bantam.

Goethe, Johann Wolfgang von. 1989. *Faust: Der Tragödie erster und zweiter Teil; Urfaust,* ed. Erich Trunz. Munich: C. H. Beck.

Grant, Mary A., tr. and ed. 1960. *The Myths of Hyginus.* Lawrence: University of Kansas.

Gregory, John. 1765. *A Comparative View of the State and Faculties of Man with Those of the Animal World.* London: J. Dodsley.

Gregory, John. 1817. *Lectures and Duties on the Qualifications of a Physician.* Philadelphia: M. Carey and Son.

Hannay, Alastair. 1982. *Kierkegaard.* London: Routledge and Kegan Paul.

Heidegger, Martin. 1973. *Being and Time,* tr. John Macquarrie and Edward Robinson. New edition. Oxford: Basil Blackwell.

Heidegger, Martin. 1985. *History of the Concept of Time: Prolegomena,* tr. Theodore Kisiel. Bloomington: Indiana University Press.

Herder, Johann Gottfried. 1990. "Das Kind der Sorge."In *Volkslieder, Übertragungen, Dichtungen,* pp. 743–744, ed. Ulrich Gaier, vol. 3 of *Herder's Werke,* ed. Martin Bollacher, Jürgen Brummack, Ulrich Garer, Gunter E. Grimm, Hans Dietrich Irmscher, Rudolf Smend, and Johannes Wallmann. Frankfurt am Main: Deutscher Klassiker Verlag.

Hume, David. 1983. *An Enquiry Concerning the Principles of Morals.* Indianapolis, IN: Hackett.

Hume, David. 1992. *A Treatise of Human Nature.* Buffalo, NY: Prometheus.

Hyginus. 1976 (1535). *Fabularum Liber.* New York: Garland.

Jaeger, Hans. 1968. "The Problem of Faust's Salvation." In his *Essays on German Literature, 1935–1962,* pp. 41–98. Bloomington: Department of Germanic Languages, Indiana University.

Kaelin, Eugene Francis. 1988. *Heidegger's "Being and Time": A Reading for Readers.* Tallahassee: Florida State University Press.

Kierkegaard, Søren. 1940. *Consider the Lilies: Being the Second Part of "Edifying Discourses in a Different Vein,"* tr. Amelia Stewart Ferrie Aldworth and William Stewart Ferrie. London: C. W. Daniel.

Kierkegaard, Søren. 1958. *Johannes Climacus; or, De Omnibus Dubitandum Est; and A Sermon,* tr. Thomas Henry Croxall. Stanford, CA: Stanford University Press.

Kierkegaard, Søren. 1960. *Kierkegaard's Concluding Unscientific Postscript,* tr. David F. Swenson and Walter Lowrie. Princeton, NJ: Princeton University Press.

Kierkegaard, Søren. 1967. *Stages on Life's Way,* tr. Walter Lowrie. New York: Schocken.

Kierkegaard, Søren. 1971. *Christian Discourses; and The Lilies of the Field and the Birds of the Air; and Three Discourses at the Communion on Fridays,* tr. Walter Lowrie. Princeton, NJ: Princeton University Press.

Klonoski, Richard J. 1984. "Being and Time Said All at Once: An Analysis of Section 42." *Tulane Studies in Philosophy* 32: 62–68.

Knowles, Richard T. 1986. *Human Development and Human Possibility: Erikson in the Light of Heidegger.* Lanham, MD: University Press of America.

Mackey, Louis. 1972. "The Poetry of Inwardness." In *Kierkegaard: A Collection of Critical Essays,* pp. 1–102, ed. Josiah Thompson. New York: Anchor.

Martinez, Roy. 1989. "An 'Authentic' Problem in Heidegger's Being and Time." *Auslegung* 15(1): 1–20.

May, Gerald G. 1982. *Care of Mind, Care of Spirit: Psychiatric Dimensions of Spiritual Direction.* San Francisco: Harper and Row.

May, Rollo. 1969. *Love and Will.* New York: W. W. Norton.

Mayeroff, Milton. 1965. "On Caring." *International Philosophical Quarterly* 5(3): 462–474.

Mayeroff, Milton. 1971. *On Caring.* New York: Harper and Row.

McNeill, John T. 1951. *A History of the Cure of Souls.* New York: Harper and Brothers.

Mercer, Philip. 1972. *Sympathy and Ethics: A Study of the Relationship Between Sympathy and Morality with Special Reference to Hume's Treatise.* Oxford: Oxford University Press.

Mooney, Edward F. 1992. "Sympathy." In vol. 2 of *Encyclopedia of Ethics,* pp. 1222–1225, ed. Lawrence C. Becker and Charlotte B. Becker. New York: Garland.

Nelson, Hilde. 1992. "Against Caring." *Journal of Clinical Ethics* 3(1): 11–15.

Ogletree, Thomas W. 1985. *Hospitality to the Stranger: Dimensions of Moral Understanding.* Philadelphia: Fortress.

Olafson, Frederick A. 1987. *Heidegger and the Philosophy of Mind.* New Haven, CT: Yale University Press.

Raphael, David D. 1973. "Moral Sense." In vol. 3 of *Dictionary of the History of Ideas,* ed. Philip P. Wiener. New York: Charles Scribner's Sons.

Reich, Warren Thomas. 1993. "Alle origini dell'etica medica: Mito del contratto o mito di Cura?" In *Modelli di Medicina: Crisi e Attualità dell'Idea di Professione,* ed. Paolo Cattorini and Roberto Mordacci. Milan: Europa Scienze Umane Editrice.

Rudd, Anthony. 1993. *Kierkegaard and the Limits of the Ethical.* Oxford: Clarendon Press.

Ryle, Gilbert. 1949. *The Concept of Mind.* London: Hutchinson.

Scheler, Max. 1954. *The Nature of Sympathy,* tr. Peter L. Heath. London: Routledge and Kegan Paul.

Schopenhauer, Arthur. 1965. *On the Basis of Morality.* Indianapolis, IN: Bobbs-Merrill.

Seneca. 1953. *Seneca ad Lucilium Epistulae.* vol. 3 of *Epistulae Morales,* tr. Richard M. Gummere. Cambridge, MA: Harvard University Press.

Shklar, Judith N. 1972. "Subversive Genealogies." *Daedalus* 101(1): 129–154.

Simpson, J. A., and Weiner, S. C., eds. 1989. *The Oxford English Dictionary,* 2nd edition, vol. 2. Oxford: Oxford University Press.

Solomon, Robert C. 1985. *Introducing Philosophy: A Text with Readings,* 3rd edition. San Diego, CA: Harcourt Brace Jovanovich.

Stack, George J. 1969. "Concern in Kierkegaard and Heidegger." *Philosophy Today* 13(Spring): 26–35.

Teuber, Andreas. 1982. "Simone Weil: Equality as Compassion." *Philosophy and Phenomenological Research* 43(2): 221–237.

Weil, Simone. 1952. *Gravity and Grace.* New York: G. P. Putnam's Sons.

Weil, Simone. 1970. *First and Last Notebooks.* London: Oxford University Press.

Weil, Simone. 1977. *The Simone Weil Reader,* ed. George A. Panichas. New York: David McKay.

Weil, Simone. 1978. *Lectures on Philosophy.* Cambridge, Eng.: Cambridge University Press.

Weil, Simone. 1981. *Draft for a Statement for Human Obligations.* Lebanon, PA: Sowers.

## II. HISTORICAL DIMENSIONS OF AN ETHIC OF CARE IN HEALTHCARE

In the context of healthcare, the idea of care has two principal meanings: (1) taking care of the sick person, which emphasizes the delivery of technical care; and (2) caring for or caring about the sick person, which suggests a virtue of devotion or concern for the other as a person. At times these two aspects of care have been united; at other times they are in conflict.

## Taking Care of: Competent, Technical Care

When speaking of the medical aspects of "taking care of" the patient, one often uses the language of taking good care, or receiving appropriate care. This practical vision of care can be viewed historically from the perspectives of medical competence and technical excellence. The Greek demigod Asklepios, because of his reputation for competence, became the "patron of human healers" (Jonsen). The virtue that motivated the physician of classical Greece was *philotechnia,* or love of the art (May, 1983; Laín Entralgo). In the Greek tradition, "the love of technical skill included not only an appreciation of the good which the application of that skill might achieve but also a kind of natural piety that recognized the limits of the art" (May, 1983, pp. 92–93). The ethic of competent care can also be called a Hippocratic ethic, after Hippocrates (c. 460–378 B.C.E.), the "father of medicine." One phrase in the Hippocratic oath—"I will act for the benefit of my patient according to my ability and judgment"—implies the imperative of the competent practice of the art of medicine (Jonsen). Under these historical influences, competence, "in the sense of a disciplined understanding of the science and skilled manipulation of the art [of medicine]," was regarded as the first virtue of medical care at least through the seventeenth century (Jonsen, p. 22).

In modern times, competence has become the essential and comprehensive virtue of medicine; medical practice and education came to emphasize ever-more-complete scientific knowledge and ever-more-competent clinical performance. This demanding standard of competence in turn fueled a drive toward biomedical excellence and deepened the sense of meaning and pleasure gained from practicing the art of medicine (May, 1983; Jonsen).

At the turn of the twentieth century, as medical competence focused more and more intently on the principles of pathophysiology and factual diagnostics, medical "care" came to be defined by objective data. Clinical and laboratory efforts to comprehend, apply, and evaluate medical data led physicians increasingly to divorce the disease from the patient, thus marginalizing personal care. The desire for liberation from the sometimes oppressive consequences of emotional involvement in "caring for" the person who is in critical condition may have contributed to this trend. As increased technical expertise raised expectations of what "taking care" should mean, legal and ethical requirements of "due care" spelled out the criteria for medical care, prompting clinicians to focus even more on the technical ideal of competence in "taking care of the sick" (Annas).

By the 1920s, competent care was becoming the moral meaning of "taking care of" the patient. Richard C. Cabot (1868–1939), a renowned professor at Harvard Medical School, articulated and championed this new ethic of competence. The humanistic virtue of "caring for" the patient was quickly pushed to the periphery of medicine, for that sort of care was viewed as bearing no apparent relation to the highly esteemed "hard data." This narrowing of the notion of care placed medical ethics in crisis (Jonsen).

## Caring for the Sick Person

While "taking care of the patient" in competence had been pushing "caring for" the patient to the periphery of medical concerns, "caring for" the patient received a major impetus at Harvard during the 1920s. This section will consider what altruistic terms and virtues "caring for" replaced, why they had lost their meaning, an account of the onset of the term *caring for,* and its meaning in healthcare prior to 1982.

The moral term *caring for* was turned to at a time when the altruistic virtues that had shaped the care of the sick for centuries had lost much of their luster, particularly terms like hospitality, philanthropy, charity, love, and sympathy.

For example, hospitality, which meant the friendly and cordial taking in of strangers or travelers, had enormous influence as an altruistic virtue for healthcare; it was a model in rabbinic Judaism, early Christianity, and Islam (Exod. 23:9). Christianity had transformed hospitality from a private into a public virtue of mercy and beneficence that was often directed to the sick stranger (Bonet-Maury). Hospitality prompted establishment of travelers' inns, which evolved into hospices where healthcare was sometimes provided, and eventually to hospitals, especially in the Byzantine East but also eventually in the Latin West (Miller). But by the 1920s, this religious term had lost its force; even Christians no longer spoke of hospitality as a major public virtue motivating healthcare.

Philanthropy had, for centuries, been a dominant altruistic motive for "caring for" the sick in most religious traditions, but it has virtually disappeared from the moral sphere of healthcare. The ideal of philanthropy (from the Greek *philanthropos,* meaning humane or benevolent) encouraged a love of humankind that expressed itself in concrete deeds of service to others. Philanthropy, associated with the Christian ideal of charity, made it possible for the sick person to assume a preferential position in society (Sigerist) and motivated the establishment of hospitals starting in the fourth century in the East, until modern times in the West. The ideal of philanthropy also appeared strongly in the first code of medical ethics, adopted by the American

Medical Association in 1847. But by the 1920s, professional philanthropy, from which modern professionals had derived much of their authority and prestige, had lost much of its respect, and the significance of the word *philanthropy* had been reduced to its meaning of private (and to some extent, public) support of the arts, education, and research (May, 1983, 1986).

Sympathy and compassion have exerted a strong public influence on caring for the sick in times past, in particular by motivating the sensitivities of individual medical practitioners. Codes and oaths have exhorted health practitioners throughout the ages to care for the sick out of motives of compassion and sympathy. John Gregory (1724–1773) spoke of the sensibility of heart that makes us feel for the sick and arouses in us the desire to relieve their distresses. Use of the word *sympathy* to motivate personalized medical care appeared commonly right up to the 1920s and beyond. But the word *sympathy* lost its effectiveness as it often came to be regarded as the condescending manifestation of pity; the word *compassion* was looked on with some disfavor as it came to suggest too much identification with the suffering person.

In addition, there is an overarching reason why the previous caring virtues were discounted, leaving room for the new, secular term of care. In criticizing ecclesiastical institutions in the eighteenth century, Enlightenment thinkers denounced charity for the sick and philanthropic hospitals because these activities were tainted by the essentially self-centered gifts and legacies of pious people who sought to atone for their sins by acts of charity in support of the hospitals. Eighteenth-century rationalists emphasized that the poorly organized philanthropic hospitals of Christian Europe did little to help the sick get well; and some Enlightenment thinkers blamed the very concept of Christian charity for these abuses. Furthermore, Christian charity was regarded as too closely linked to dead traditions and blind superstitions to have a close relationship with science (Locke). The attempt by some philosophers in the eighteenth, nineteenth, and twentieth centuries to base an altruistic care of the sick on a secular notion of sympathy was, in part, a result of these developments.

By the 1920s, the secular term *care* had begun to replace the earlier altruistic terminology. By this time, the history of the idea of care had progressed to the point that the term was coming to be known for its moral implications. In addition, *care* had special appeal as a virtue for healthcare because the same word had—for centuries and in a variety of languages—been the descriptive term for "taking care of" sick people. It should be no surprise, then, that for a number of decades prior to 1982—when the idea of care began capturing widespread contemporary attention—there appeared a small body of literature in the clinical ethics of physicians and nurses as well as in religious medical ethics that focused attention on the moral meaning and practice of care, as well as on an ethic of care.

## "Caring for" in Clinical Medical Ethics, 1920–1982

In championing the fast-developing technical art of medicine, Richard C. Cabot acknowledged and seemed to acquiesce in the fact that doctors and nurses were not caring for the whole patient: Their attention was "too strongly concentrated" on the difficult tasks of diagnosis and treatment, and "there is not enough attention left to go round" (Cabot, p. 16). He was certainly in favor of manifesting courtesy and patience with sick people; but under some conditions, he said, it is not advisable for the physician to care for anything but the patient's body; and when care for the whole person is desirable, others—medical students, social workers, and even ministerial students—can suitably offer that kind of care (Cabot). To carry out his purpose of designating surrogates who would "care for" the patient, Cabot was instrumental in establishing the professions of medical social work and clinical pastoral care.

The following year, Francis Peabody, a physician-professor colleague of Cabot at Harvard, offered the opposite point of view. "Caring for" the patient is essential to the practice of medicine, he argued; physicians must engage in this sort of care in order to achieve the goals inherent in medicine. His 1927 essay "The Care of the Patient" is one of the foundation stones of an ethic of care in twentieth-century medicine in the United States (Peabody).

Peabody acknowledged that the "enormous mass of scientific material" to which a young doctor must be exposed, the depersonalized aspects of modern hospital practice, and physicians' bias toward organic disease could jeopardize the personal aspects of the art of medicine. To remedy these problems, he urged the physician to form and be attentive to a personal relationship with the patient and with the patient's "environmental background." The treatment of a disease, which may be impersonal, "takes its proper place in the larger problem of the care of the patient" (p. 396), which "must be completely personal" (p. 389). His oft-quoted principle was: "One of the essential qualities of the clinician is interest in humanity, for the secret of the care of the patient is in caring for the patient" (p. 401).

The physician must be attentive to particular circumstances of the patient, "not from the abstract point of view of the treatment of the disease, but from the concrete point of view of the care of the individual" (p. 398). Peabody was clearly attempting to exonerate the usefulness—indeed, the necessity—of care in the practice of good clinical medicine when he argued that neglect of careful attention to the true situation of the whole patient, including functional disorder, jeopardizes diagnosis, treatment, and effectiveness of care. Furthermore, the mere caring effort in the relationship with the patient, aside from drugs or other treatments, can help patients get well. This sort of care requires attentiveness and alertness to what kind of a person the patient is; sympathy for the patient's total situation; friendliness that elicits trust; and a consideration expressed in "little incidental" actions that assure the patient's comfort—which may require that the physician learn much from the nurse regarding practical care and comfort of the patient.

Following Peabody's clarion call for care in 1927, several physicians, writing in the 1960s and 1970s, advocated a caring perspective in professional attitudes, practices, and moral analysis in medicine. The starting point that convinced these writers of the need for "caring for" was the depersonalization of medical care in hospitals. Clinical care oriented to the disease in the body leads caretakers to allow technical considerations to dominate, avoid death at any cost, and ignore patients' preferences; this produces indignities for patients and suffering for caregivers (Benfield).

The concept of caring is defined in the literature of the 1960s and 1970s as implying a broader concern for the whole patient, or for the quality of the patient's life, rather than just for the patient's disease (Menninger; Benfield). Caring involves sympathy with the patient, which entails entering into or sharing the feelings of the patient. To prevent loss of objectivity and perspective, "compassionate detachment" (Blumgart, p. 451) is recommended, which is "to sense the patient's experience empathically without becoming so involved sympathetically that the physician's rational and effective clinical judgment is impaired by emotional involvement" (Menninger, p. 837).

Caring for the patient embraces both the science and art of medicine; both are oriented to the patient, and both should meet in the individual physician (Blumgart). A caring solicitude for the individual patient is integral and essential in the practice of clinical medicine (Tisdale); failure to practice caring medicine leads to incomplete or inaccurate diagnosis and ineffective treatment (Blumgart). On the other hand, patients manifest care-seeking behavior (Tisdale). Receiving the sought-for care can be crucial for the patient's "adaptation to various maladjustments, including illness" (Menninger, p. 836). The role of the physician and other healthcare providers in our society is one of a surrogate caregiver, who has the power to give attention to the ill and excuse them from the performance of everyday duties (Menninger).

There are several obstacles to caring in medicine. The demands of the scientific and technological aspects of medicine, combined with physicians' fascination with disease, achieve great progress for humankind but tend to block out compassionate attention to suffering and the particular needs of the ill individual who has the disease. In addition, patients and families are reluctant to communicate their feelings with health professionals, who are too busy monitoring the patient's physical condition to listen. Other factors that obstruct person-oriented caring are (1) lack of teamwork among healthcare providers, coupled with overemphasis on the physician's hierarchical authority; (2) caregivers' feelings of inadequacy due to lack of training in caring for critically ill or dying patients and their families; and (3) time pressures on health professionals (Blumgart; Benfield).

Acts of caring, some of which counteract the obstacles to caring, include: listening to patients with personal attentiveness, particularly as a history-taking technique that enables patients to relate their experiences in terms of their own values and concerns (Tisdale; Blumgart); being attentive to both the physical and the emotional components of illness (even though medical education and practice tend to focus on the physical—in fact, all medicine is psychosomatic, since the emotional and bodily factors always interact in every disease) (Blumgart; Menninger); and offering maximum understanding, freedom, and support to the individual patient (Tisdale).

Caring is also expressed through acting as companion to a bereaved family; solicitous communication regarding the nature of the illness and its expected course; sharing the patient's and family's responsibility and agony of deciding whether to continue care; relieving the patient of suffering from pointless dehumanizing treatment; and caring for caretakers who suffer the stress of the combined roles of technical caregiver and concerned caregiver (Benfield).

William Tisdale, writing in 1979, contended that modern medical ethics, with its concern for "the neon problems" of high controversy, is ill-adapted to account for an ethic of care. Because clinical caring pertains to the usual and the commonplace in medicine, it is more difficult to isolate and analyze. William Tisdale appealed for an inquiry into the unresolved and even the unrecognized problems inherent in basic clinical care and the problems inherent in care that are more demanding from an ethical perspective than the usual moral quandaries in medicine. In formal ethical terms, Tisdale saw clinical caring as characterized by the ideals of love and charity and as a form of duty beneficence, a duty to benefit others apart from special relationships and responsibilities. Making certain that expected benefits of a particular procedure outweigh the definite risks is a characteristic of caring for one's patients.

In the highly influential book published in 1970, *Patient as Person,* Paul Ramsey linked care with "covenant fidelity," which he saw as the appropriate norm for the relationship between physician and patient. Covenant fidelity always requires care, which is directed to the person of the patient. But at the end of life, when attempts to cure are no longer appropriate, one must always care even if one only cares—through keeping company and offering comfort—while permissibly withdrawing medical care.

Caring for the sick, the wounded, and the troubled has been characterized through the centuries by altruistic motives and virtues. By the 1920s, an interest had arisen in the virtue of care as the basic moral orientation to healthcare, based in feelings for the other. Practitioners felt that care could provide the grounding for the moral practice of healthcare and for mitigating some of the excesses of medical technique. Still, very little by way of a formal ethic had arisen.

## Caring in Nursing Theory, Philosophy, and Ethics

It required the intellectual and moral energy of feminist perspectives on care in the 1980s to establish a noteworthy movement promoting an ethic of care that reached deep into the field of bioethics.

Nursing theorists, educators, and philosophers explored and applied a more extensive theory and ethic of care prior to 1982 than any other single group had. Their contributions differed considerably from those of physician-writers: The nursing theorists paid much more attention to the meaning and theories of nursing, examined the structures and functions of care, turned occasionally to philosophers who had explained the meaning of care (such as Martin Heidegger and Milton Mayeroff), developed the implications of care for nursing practices and skills, considered the status of caregivers, showed an interest in the historical links between nursing and maternal care, and proposed educational improvements to foster professional care.

The strongest impetus for an examination of the role of caring in nursing came from Madeleine Leininger, who has organized national conferences on caring and published on the topic (1981). Leininger was one of the pioneers who fostered the idea that caring is the essence of nursing and the unique focus of the profession. Leah Curtin went a step further when she claimed that the distinctiveness of nursing cannot be located in functions, but in "the moral art of nursing," in its primary moral conviction, by virtue of which

nurses "are committed to care for, as well as to the care of, other human beings" (p. 26).

Nursing theorists offer a variety of definitions of care: for example, the explanation that caring in nursing is a process in which one shows "compassionate concern for the individual" (Gaut, in Leininger, 1981, p. 18). Leininger suggests this definition of professional nursing care: "those cognitively learned humanistic and scientific modes of helping or enabling an individual, family, or community to receive personalized services through specific culturally defined or ascribed modes of caring processes, techniques, and patterns to improve or maintain a favorably healthy condition for life or death" (1981, p. 9). This definition includes concepts of compassion, concern, nurturance, stress alleviation, comfort, and protection.

The precise historical origins of a concern for caring in nursing are unclear, but a number of authors trace them to the writings of Florence Nightingale. However, nurse theorists have relied not so much on a history of care in nursing as on the writings of social scientists and existentialists such as Buber, Erikson, and Rogers (Gaut, in Leininger, 1981).

Why did nursing theorists turn so strongly to the idea of care in the 1970s? Marilyn Ray explains that as nursing became increasingly technological, bureaucratic, managerial, and supervisory, nurses began experiencing a struggle relative to their central focus as a "direct caring profession" (Ray, in Leininger, 1981, p. 28). Barbara Carper (1979) answers the question by mentioning two factors that have had the effect of eroding care in health generally, not just in the experience of nurses: depersonalization of healthcare due to the fragmentation of specialized treatment, the subdivision of tasks, and highly institutionalized bureaucracy; and technological progress and technical expertise, which she saw as having the potential of overshadowing individuals, "reducing them to objects or abstractions" (p. 13). Within such a system, even when competent, scientifically based care is delivered, it "is often perceived by the client as lacking the 'personally experienced feeling of being cared for'" (p. 13, quoting Menninger, p. 837). This depersonalization of the individual entails the devaluing and loss of identity of the individual. She sees a compelling metaphor for the relationship of technology to care in the novel in which Dr. Frankenstein created a monster. Frankenstein's tragedy was not due to his scientific triumph over nature, but "his *failure to care* for what he had created. He was unable to recognize or experience the humanness of another's self" (Carper, p. 13).

Finally, even prior to the emergence of an ethic of care in other disciplines, nurses were already applying the idea of care both to nursing practice and to nursing ethics. For example, Carper argued that caring is the most essential ingredient in the curative process, because caring acts and decisions "make the crucial difference in effective curing consequences" (Carper, p. 14, quoting Leininger, 1977, p. 2). Anne J. Davis stimulated reflection on the relationship between caring and ethical principles in the context of taking care of the dying. She contrasted the compassionate meaning of care (to undergo with, to share solidarity with) with the technical terms *nursing care* or *medical care*. She argued that situations of serious illness and dying call for putting aside the instrumental meaning of caring and instead manifesting "the most demanding and deeply human aspect of caring: the expressive art of being fully present to another person" (p. 1). A caring attitude would incline the nurse not to turn away from the stranger's world of suffering, but to appreciate the other person's independent existence and enter into and share his or her pain as much as possible. Caring for the sufferer is an ethical obligation inherent in the health professional's role. But caring transcends role obligations: It acknowledges the vulnerable humanness of the other and reinforces the caring of the one who cares. Ethical principles are not at variance with care: They provide specific judgments in the context of caring for another person. A caring disposition inclines caregivers to respect the patient as an autonomous agent and to recognize the patient's considered value judgments, even if they go contrary to what the clinician expects.

The foregoing presents a few indications of the pioneering work in nursing care theory and ethics in the 1970s. As the following entry indicates, the ethics of nursing care expanded considerably after the notion of care came to be more widely acknowledged through the writings of women social scientists.

WARREN THOMAS REICH (1995)
BIBLIOGRAPHY REVISED

SEE ALSO: *Alternative Therapies; Beneficence; Chronic Illness and Chronic Care; Compassionate Love; Emotions; Feminism; Healing; Human Dignity; Long-Term Care; Medicine, Art of; Nursing Ethics; Obligation and Supererogation; Paternalism; Professional-Patient Relationship; Women, Historical and Cross-Cultural Perspectives;* and other *Care* subentries

### BIBLIOGRAPHY

Annas, George J. 1990. *American Health Law.* Boston: Little, Brown.

Benfield, D. Gary. 1979. "Two Philosophies of Caring." *Ohio State Medical Journal* 75(8): 508–511.

Blumgart, Hermann L. 1964. "Caring for the Patient." *New England Journal of Medicine* 270(9): 449–456.

Bonet-Maury, G. n.d. "Hospitality (Christian)." In vol. 6 of *Encyclopaedia of Religion and Ethics,* pp. 804–808, ed. James Hastings. New York: Charles Scribner's Sons.

Cabot, Richard C. 1926. *Adventures on the Borderlands of Ethics.* New York: Harper & Brothers.

Carper, Barbara A. 1979. "The Ethics of Caring." *Advances in Nursing Science* 1(3): 11–19.

Carr, Mark F. 2001. *Passionate Deliberation: Emotion, Temperance, and the Care Ethic in Clinical Moral Deliberation.* New York: Kluwer Academic Publishers.

Clement, Grace. 1999. *Care, Autonomy, and Justice: Feminism and the Ethic of Care (Feminist Theory & Politics).* Boulder, CO: Westveiw Press.

Cluff, Leighton E., and Binstock, Robert H., eds. 2001. *The Lost Art of Caring: A Challenge to Health Professionals, Families, Communities, and Society.* Baltimore, MD: The Johns Hopkins University Press.

Curtin, Leah. 1980. "Ethical Issues in Nursing Practice and Education." In *Ethical Issues in Nursing and Nursing Education,* pp. 25–26. New York: National League for Nursing.

Davis, Anne J. 1981. "Compassion, Suffering, Morality: Ethical Dilemmas in Caring," *Nursing Law & Ethics* 2(5): 1–2, 6, 8.

Grubb, Edward. n.d. "Philanthropy." In vol. 9 of *Encyclopaedia of Religion and Ethics,* pp. 837–840, ed. James Hastings. New York: Charles Scribner's Sons.

Jonsen, Albert R. 1990. *The New Medicine and the Old Ethics.* Cambridge, MA: Harvard University Press.

Laín Entralgo, Pedro. 1969. *Doctor and Patient,* tr. Frances Partridge. New York: McGraw-Hill.

Leininger, Madeleine. 1977. "Caring: The Essence and Central Focus of Nursing," In *The Phenomenon of Caring: Part V.* Washington, D.C.: American Nurses Foundation, Nursing Research Report 12, (1): 2–14.

Leininger, Madeleine. 1981. *Caring: An Essential Human Need: Proceedings of Three National Caring Conferences.* Thorofare, NJ: Charles B. Slack.

Locke, John. 1993 (1690). *An Essay Concerning Human Understanding,* 3rd edition., rev., ed. John W. Yolton. London: Dent.

May, William F. 1983. *The Physician's Covenant: Images of the Healer in Medical Ethics.* Philadelphia: Westminster Press.

May, William F. 1986. "Philanthropy," In *The Westminster Dictionary of Christian Ethics,* pp. 474–475, ed. James F. Childress and John Macquarrie. Philadelphia: Westminster Press.

McGee, Mike, and D'Antonio, Michael. 1999. *The Best Medicine: Doctors, Patients, and the Covenant of Caring.* New York: St. Martins Press.

Menninger, W. Walter. 1975. "'Caring' as Part of Health Care Quality." *Journal of the American Medical Association* 234(8): 836–837.

Miller, Timothy S. 1985. *The Birth of the Hospital in the Byzantine Empire.* Baltimore: Johns Hopkins University Press.

Numbers, Ronald L., and Amundsen, Darrel W. 1986. *Caring and Curing: Health and Medicine in the Western Religious Traditions.* New York: Macmillan.

Peabody, Francis W. 1987 (1927). "The Care of the Patient," In *Encounters Between Patients and Doctors: An Anthology,* pp. 387–401, ed. John Stoeckle. Cambridge, MA: MIT Press.

Ramsey, Paul. 1970. *The Patient as Person: Explorations in Medical Ethics.* New Haven, CT: Yale University Press.

Sigerist, Henry Ernest. 1943. *Civilization and Disease.* Ithaca, NY: Cornell University Press.

Tisdale, William A. 1979. "On Clinical Caring." *Pharos* 42(4): 23–26.

Verkerk, M. 1999. "A Care Perspective on Coercion and Autonomy." *Bioethics* 13(3–4): 358–368

## III. CONTEMPORARY ETHICS OF CARE

A major contemporary impetus to scholarly discussions of caring occurred with the 1982 publication of Carol Gilligan's *In a Different Voice: Psychological Theory and Women's Development.* Nursing theorists—and, to a lesser extent, physicians—were exploring moral dimensions of caring prior to the publication of Gilligan's work; but her book led, for the first time in the history of the idea of care, to widespread efforts to develop a systematic philosophical ethic of care beyond the world of healthcare practitioners.

### Contemporary Elements of an Ethic of Care

*In a Different Voice* begins by contrasting the primary moral orientation of boys and men with the primary orientation of girls and women. Gilligan proposes that females and males tend to employ different reasoning strategies and apply different moral themes and concepts when formulating and resolving moral problems. According to Gilligan's analysis, females are more likely than males to perceive moral dilemmas primarily in terms of personal attachment versus detachment. From this perspective, which she dubs the *care perspective,* central concerns are to avoid deserting, hurting, alienating, isolating, or abandoning persons and to act in a manner that strengthens and protects attachments between persons. In this analysis, the moral universe of girls and women tends to be primarily "a world of relationships and psychological truths where an awareness of the connection between people gives rise to a recognition of responsibility for one another, a perception of the need for response" (p. 30). For example, Amy, an eleven-year-old girl whom Gilligan interviews in her book, describes herself in terms of her connection with other people: "I think that the world has a lot of problems, and I think that everybody should try to help somebody else in some way ..." (Gilligan, p. 34).

By contrast, Gilligan argues that the primary moral orientation of men and boys tends to focus on moral concerns related to inequality versus equality of individuals. Rather than emphasizing the importance of sustaining personal relationships, this approach emphasizes abstract ideals of fairness and rights, and requires abiding by impartial principles of justice, autonomy, reciprocity, and respect for persons. Viewed from this perspective, which Gilligan refers to as the *justice perspective,* moral dilemmas are defined by hierarchical values and impersonal conflicts of claims. The moral agent, like the judge, is called upon to "abstract the moral debate from the interpersonal situation, finding in the logic of fairness an objective way to decide who will win the dispute" (p. 32). To illustrate justice reasoning, Gilligan describes the moral reasoning of Jake, an eleven-year-old boy interviewed for her book. Asked how he would resolve a conflict between responsibility to himself and other people Jake answers, "You go about one-fourth to the others and three-fourths to yourself," and adds that "the most important thing in your decision should be yourself, don't let yourself be guided totally by other people ..." (p. 35–36). Gilligan concludes that Jake understands this moral dilemma as an abstract mathematical equation and perceives his responsibility for others as potentially interfering with his personal autonomy.

Gilligan, a developmental psychologist, argues that an ethic of care has been generally ignored in the past because girls and women have been excluded as subjects in the study of moral development. For example, accounts of moral maturation described by Lawrence Kohlberg (1981, 1984) and Jean Piaget were based entirely on studies and observations of boys and men. These male-based theories of moral psychology, when applied to girls and women, were interpreted as showing girls and women to be deficient in moral development. Gilligan identifies an ethic of care as a distinctive form of moral reasoning.

### Implications for Ethics of Healthcare

The implications of Gilligan's analysis for contemporary bioethics are the subject of ongoing discussion. First, an ethic of care may lead to positive changes in bioethical education, including placing greater emphasis on healthcare providers' communication skills and emotional sensitivity, and on the effects that ethical issues have on relationships (Carse). To the extent that bioethicists with formal training in ethics are inclined to emphasize justice over care, it may be desirable to broaden their training to include an ethic of care (Self et al.).

In addition to producing changes in ethics education, a care orientation within bioethics arguably requires placing greater emphasis on beneficence as the healthcare provider's primary responsibility to the patient (Sharpe). Finally, an ethics emphasizing caring for others may produce substantive changes in the way we resolve moral problems. It may encourage resolutions of moral problems that give greater authority to family members in healthcare decision making (Hardwig, 1990, 1991; Jecker, 1990), or it may lead to paying greater attention to how various relationships are affected by moral decisions (Jecker, 1991).

One area within bioethics where an ethic of care has been studied in some detail is abortion. Gilligan found that women who face abortion decisions tend to frame moral issues in terms of a responsibility to care for and avoid hurting others. These women often base decisions about having an abortion on "a growing comprehension of the dynamics of social interaction … and a central insight, that self and others are interdependent" (p. 74). In other words, rather than conceptualizing abortion in terms of abstract values, such as *life,* or in terms of competing claims or rights, these women tend to see abortion as a problem of how best to care for and avoid harming the particular people and relationships affected by their choices. Considered in this light, the resolution of abortion requires taking stock of how any decision might affect not only the pregnant woman and fetus, but also the relationship between the pregnant woman and biological father, and relationships and persons within the wider family circle (Jecker, 1999). Arguably, an ethic of care illuminates the moral issues abortion raises better than an ethic of justice, because only an ethic of care portrays individuals as uniquely constituted by their connections to others (Gatens-Robinson).

In addition to these proposed changes, introducing a care orientation within bioethics may shed a negative light on more traditional forms of bioethical analysis (Carse). For example, Virginia Sharpe claims that a justice orientation has dominated bioethics in the past, and this has encouraged ethicists to treat provider–patient relationships as free exchanges between equals. She argues that this picture of the provider–patient relationship is seriously distorted. Rather than being equals in relationships with healthcare providers, patients typically experience diminished power and authority as a result of being physically and emotionally vulnerable and in need of the provider's help (Sharpe). Others charge that a justice orientation has traditionally prevailed within bioethics, resulting in too much focus on competition for power, status, and authority and too little focus on the human relationships at stake (Warren). For example, the autonomy–paternalism debate within bioethics concentrates on who has the authority to make treatment decisions. Similarly, when bioethicists emphasize impersonal ethical principles, such as autonomy, nonmaleficence, beneficence,

and justice, the particular persons and relationships involved in ethical dilemmas can become incidental, rather than essential, to the crafting of moral responses.

## Feminist versus Feminine Ethics

Gilligan's ongoing effort (Gilligan et al., 1988; Gilligan et al., 1989; Brown and Gilligan) to characterize the moral reasoning of girls and women in terms of care has occurred in tandem with important developments in feminist ethics. It is useful, however, to distinguish between the care ethic that Gilligan describes, which has been called a *feminine ethic,* and the development of *feminist ethics.* According to Susan Sherwin, the primary concern of feminine ethics is to describe the moral experiences and intuitions of women, pointing out how traditional approaches have neglected to include women's perspectives.

In addition to Carol Gilligan, both Nel Noddings and Sara Ruddick have made important contributions to feminine ethics. Whereas Gilligan emphasizes the unique form of moral reasoning that caring engenders, Noddings focuses on caring as a practical activity, stressing the interaction that occurs between persons giving and receiving care. From this perspective, she identifies two distinctive features of caring: *engrossment* and *motivational shift.* Engrossment refers to a receptive state in which the person caring is "receiving what is there as nearly as possible without assessment or evaluation"; motivational shift occurs when "my motive energy flows towards the other and perhaps … towards his ends" (Noddings, 1984, p. 33, 34). Critics of Noddings's approach raise the concern that her interpretation of caring may lead to exploitation (Houston) or complicity in the pursuit of evil ends (Card, 1990).

Unlike Gilligan and Noddings, Ruddick emphasizes *maternal thinking,* which she says develops out of the activity of assuming regular and substantial responsibility for small children. Although Ruddick acknowledges that the work of mothering falls under the more general category of *caring labor,* she argues that it cannot simply be combined with other forms of caring because each form of caring involves distinctive kinds of thinking arising from different activities (Ruddick). Ruddick delineates maternal thinking as a response to the small child's demands for preservation, growth, and acceptability. These demands elicit in the mothering person the responses of *preservative love, fostering growth, conscientiousness,* and *educative control,* which Ruddick identifies as the hallmarks of maternal thinking.

In contrast to feminine ethics, the primary concern of feminist ethics is to reject and end oppression against women. Susan Sherwin defines *feminist ethics* as "the name given to the various theories that help reveal the multiple, gender-specific patterns of harm that constitute women's oppression," together with the "diverse political movement to eliminate all such forms of oppression" (p. 13). By *oppression,* Sherwin means "a pattern of hardship that is based on dominance of one group by members of another. The dominance involved … is rooted in features that distinguish one group from another" and requires "exaggerating these features to ensure the dominant group's supremacy" (p. 24). Feminism aims, in this interpretation, to show that the suffering of individual women is related because it springs from common sources of injustice. According to Rosemarie Tong, feminist ethics is typically far more concerned than feminine ethics with making political changes and eliminating oppressive imbalances of power (1993).

In many respects, however, feminine and feminist ethics are interrelated. The careful study of women's lives and moral reasoning that feminine ethics undertakes can contribute substantially to dismantling habits of thought and practice that enable women's oppression to continue. Both feminine and feminist ethics share the goal of adding women's voices and perspectives to various fields of scholarly inquiry. Finally, as Ruddick notes, feminist ethics can lend important support to the ideals that feminine ethics upholds. For example, feminist ethics can help to ensure "women's economic and psychological ability to engage in mothering without undue sacrifice of physical health and nonmaternal projects" (p. 236).

## Objections to an Ethic of Care

Since the publication of *In a Different Voice,* the proposal to develop a feminine ethic of care has met with a variety of concerns and objections. One set of concerns is that a feminine ethic of care may unwittingly undermine feminism. These concerns stem, in part, from a belief that the qualities in girls and women that feminine ethics esteems have developed within the context of a sexist culture. Thus, some suspect that women's competency at caring for and serving others is an outgrowth of their subordinate status within modern societies (Sherwin; Moody-Adams), and worry that emphasizing caring as a virtuous feminine quality may simply serve to keep women on the down side of power relationships (Holmes). Susan Moller Okin, for example, cautions that women are often socialized from a very early age into strict gender roles, involving caring for and serving others. This socialization radically limits their future prospects by diminishing women's capacity to choose alternative life plans. We should therefore reject traditional socialization, because it seriously violates the equality of persons basic to liberalism. Others urge women to aspire to assertiveness, rather than caring, in order to challenge conventional

images of women as concerned with serving and pleasing others (Card, 1991). Feminist critics also warn that caring cannot function as an ethic that is complete unto itself. Observing that caring can "be exploited in the service of immoral ends" (Card, 1990, p. 106), Card insists on the need to balance caring with justice and other values. Exclusive attention to caring can also lead to overlooking "the lack of care of women for women" and may preclude "the possibility of our looking at anything but love and friendship in women's emotional responses to one another" (Spellman, p. 216). Finally, excessive focus on caring at the expense of other values can blind us to the critical assessment of the object of caring. As Warren Thomas Reich noted in 2001, care by itself can be easily manipulated, and does not offer tools for analyzing the moral importance of what we care about.

In response, defenders of feminine ethics distinguish between *distorted* and *undistorted* forms of caring (Tong, 1998). Distortions of caring include the exploitation, abuse, or neglect of careers. As Tong notes, just because caring can become distorted does not suffice to show that an ethic of care is inherently distorted. Nor does it establish that "every woman's caring actions should be contemptuously dismissed as yet another instance of women's *pathological masochism* or *passivity*"; instead care should be preserved and celebrated in its undistorted form: "rescued from the patriarchal structures that would misuse or abuse it" (Tong, 1998, p. 171).

A second family of concerns about a feminine ethic of care relates to the belief that caring for others can lead to neglect of self. The phenomenon of *burnout,* for example, refers to the situation of parents, nurses, family caregivers, or other individuals who become utterly exhausted by the physical and emotional demands associated with giving care. Especially when care is conceived to be an ethic that is sufficient unto itself, the tendency may be to continue caring at any cost. Attention to other values, such as respect for the rights of the one caring, may be necessary in order to preserve the integrity of the caregiver: Arguing along these lines, Nancy Jecker notes that "if women are seen as having the same possibility men have to create a plan of life that places central importance [in activities other than caregiving] …, then a duty … [to care] can potentially stand in the way of what a woman wants to do" (2002, p. 128). The idea here is that individuals presumably prefer to protect, as much as possible, their freedom to choose whether or not to devote themselves to caring (2002). Others suggest that in order to care for others—which is an inherently limited ability—one must first be cared for by other individuals, by communities, and by oneself (Reich, 1991).

A third group of objections to developing a feminine ethic of care holds that the concept of care is not helpful at the social and institutional level. This group of objections may acknowledge that an ethic of care serves well within the limited sphere of personal ethics, but finds care unhelpful outside of this sphere. One form this objection takes is to argue that an ethic of care cannot be formulated in terms of the general rights and principles that are necessary for designing public policies. Proponents of a care ethic sometimes acknowledge this limitation. Thus, Noddings states, "to care is to act not by fixed rule but by affection and regard" (1984, p. 24). Similarly, Patricia Benner and Judith Wrubel maintain that caring is always specific and relational; hence, there exist no "context-free lists of advice" on how to care (p. 3). They reject the idea of formulating ethical theories or rules about caring on the grounds that general guides cannot "capture the embodied, relational, configurational, skillful, meaningful, and contextual human issues" that are central to an ethic of care (p. 6). Despite this view, there exist historically important examples of using the vocabulary of general rights and principles to formulate an ethic of care. For example, the UN's *Universal Declaration of Human Rights* identifies "motherhood and childhood" as "entitled to special care and assistance," and that organization's *Declaration of the Rights of the Child* asserts general principles of caring for children, noting that children need "special safeguards and care" on the basis of their "physical and mental immaturity."

Another reason why care may be assumed unworkable at a social or institutional level is that historically, public and private spheres have been distinguished as separate moral domains (Elshtain). During the nineteenth century, for example, the doctrine of separate spheres held that the family constituted a private sphere in which a morality of love and self-sacrifice prevailed; this private domain was distinguished from the public life associated with business and politics, where impersonal norms and self-interested relationships reigned (Nicholson). To the extent that these historical attitudes continue to shape present thinking, they may lead to the mutual exclusivity of care-oriented and justice-oriented approaches. In response to this structural objection, some ethicists have argued that justice and care are compatible forms of moral reasoning (Jecker, 2002).

A final set of objections to a feminine ethic of care does not deny the importance of care, but rather argues that care is not properly interpreted as an ethic that expresses an exclusively feminine form of moral reasoning. Iddo Landau, for example, argues that the significant factors for preferring the use of care or justice ethics are, in fact, not masculinity or femininity, but factors such as education and economic class. Landau concludes that "Justice and care ethics should

be seen as the ethics of certain economic classes and levels of education, not of men and women" (p. 57). Defenders of feminine ethics often meet this objection by claiming that their approach has been misunderstood. Thus advocates of feminine ethics may deny that care is an ethic that only women articulate, or an ethic that is valid only within the moral experience of women. According to Noddings, caring is an important ingredient within all human morality, and moral education should teach all people how and why to care. She concludes that "an ethical orientation that arises in female experience need not be confined to women"; to the contrary, "if only women adopt an ethic of caring the present conditions of women's oppression are indeed likely to be maintained" (1990, p. 171). Gilligan and Jane Attanucci also reject the idea that an ethic of care correlates strictly with gender, and instead report that most men and women can reason in accordance with both care and justice. Gilligan's research supports the more modest claim that care is gender-related. That is, although women and men can reason in terms of both care and justice, women are generally more likely to emphasize care while men generally emphasize justice. Thus she states that the so-called different voice she identifies is characterized "not by gender, but by theme," and cautions that its association with gender "is not absolute" and is not a generalization about either sex (p. 2).

## Caring and Contemporary Nursing

Within healthcare, attention to caring is perhaps most evident within nursing. Emphasizing caring as a central value within nursing often provides a basis for arguing that nursing requires its own description, possesses its own phenomena, and retains its own method for clarification of its own concepts and their meanings, relationships, and context (Jameton; Fry, 1989a, 1989b; Watson; Swanson; Reverby, 1987a, 1987b). For example, Jean Watson holds that nurses should reject the impersonal, objective models that she says currently dominate ethics and choose instead an ethic that emphasizes caring.

Those who invoke caring in developing a theory of nursing ethics often assign caring a privileged or foundational role. For example, Sarah Fry posits caring as "a foundational, rather than a derivative, value among persons" (1989b, p. 20–21). She argues that other ethical values, such as personhood and human dignity, are an outgrowth of nurses's caring activity. Similarly, Benner and Wrubel argue for the primacy of caring on the grounds that skillful technique and scientific knowledge do not suffice to establish ethical nursing in the absence of a basic level of caring and attachment.

Like Fry, Kristen Swanson regards caring as central to nursing ethics. According to her analysis, caring requires acting in a way that preserves human dignity, restores humanity, and avoids reducing persons to the moral status of objects. Specifically, caring requires:

1. knowing, or striving to understand an event as it has meaning in the life of the other;

2. being with, which means being emotionally present to the other;

3. doing for, defined as doing for the other as he or she would do for himself or herself if that were possible;

4. enabling, or facilitating the other's passage through life transitions and unfamiliar events; and

5. maintaining belief, which refers to sustaining faith in the other's capacity to get through an event or transition and to face a future of fulfillment.

Susan Reverby finds caring to be a central ethic throughout nursing's history. Tracing the history of nursing to its domestic roots during the colonial era, when nursing took place within the family, Reverby argues that caring for the sick was originally a duty rather than a freely chosen vocation for women. Reverby suggests that nurses today possess "some deep understandings of the limited promise of equality and autonomy in a healthcare system. In an often implicit way, such nurses recognize that those who claim the autonomy of rights often run the risk of rejecting altruism and caring itself" (1987a, p. 10).

Some have challenged the proposal to consider care as a foundational or unique concept for nursing ethics. Invoking a Nietzchean method of analysis, John Paley rejects the idea that caring is the *core* of nursing on the ground that it bears a striking resemblance to a *slave morality* and thus deteriorates into *a celebration of weakness.* He urges nursing to aspire instead to *noble values,* including competence in the management of recovery and rehabilitation. Other approaches do not reject a care ethic outright, but question the attempt to regard an ethic of care as unique to nursing. Robert M. Veach, for example, suggests that care is essential to human relationships generally. Others hold that care itself is still too broad a concept to demarcate what is unique about ethics in nursing, and instead identify nursing with maternal practice, a specific kind of caring activity (Newton; O'Brien). For example, Patricia O'Brien defends the importance of nursing's maternal function by noting that historically the source of nurses' prestige has been the manner in which nurses blend home and hospital. That is, nursing's strength has come from nurses' skill at the traditionally female tasks of feeding, bathing, cleaning, coaching, and cajoling those in one's care. Just as mothers make a home, it is female nurses who have been able to make a home of the hospital, to personalize an increasingly impersonal environment.

Critics of the maternal paradigm for nursing fault this approach as casting women in traditional and stifling roles. Historically, for example, nurses were socialized into the healthcare field to know their place and were relegated to the bottom of the pyramid and taught not to ask questions (Murphy). Casting nursing practice in terms of mothering potentially reverses progress made in the late 1970s when nurses began to see themselves as shared-decision makers rather than handmaidens to physicians (Stein et al.).

A further objection to identifying ethical ideals of nursing with ethical ideals of mothering holds that nurses's proper function is to serve as patients's advocates, rather than as patients' parents. Gerald Winslow, for example, argues that advocacy of patients' autonomy, rather than paternalistic promotion of patient benefit, should guide nursing ethics.

## Caring and Contemporary Medicine

Whereas nursing is often associated with a caring function, doctoring has traditionally been associated with a curing function. However, the tendency to associate caring exclusively with nursing is misleading for a variety of reasons (Jecker and Self). First, both doctors and nurses are engaged in caring for patients. In addition, assigning caring activities to nurses and curing activities to doctors is misleading because certain meanings of *curing* are actually derived from *caring.* Thus, the Latin definition of *cure* comes from the word *curare,* meaning "care, heed, concern; to do one's busy care, to give one's care or attention to some piece of work; or to apply one's self diligently"(Oxford English Dictionary).

Although there has been less explicit attention to an ethic of care in medicine than in nursing, caring for patients represents a central component of ethics in medicine. Caring is inextricably linked to the physician's obligation to relieve suffering, a goal that stretches back to antiquity (Cassell, 1982).

There are several more specific ways in which an ethic of care becomes manifest in the practice of medicine. First, caring is manifest in the activity of healing the patient. Whereas curing disease typically requires the physician to understand and deal with a physical disease process, healing requires that the physician also respond to the patient's subjective experience of illness (Cassell, 1989). For example, healing a patient who is suffering from a serious infection requires not only administering antibiotics to kill bacteria but also addressing the patient's feelings, questions, and concerns about his or her medical situation. In cases of serious illness where cure is not possible, caring for the patient may become the primary part of healing. For example, when patients are terminally ill and imminently dying, physicians' primary duty may become providing palliative and comfort care. Under these circumstances, healing emphasizes touch and communication, psychological and emotional support, and responding to the patient's specific feelings and concerns, which may include fear, loss of control, dependency, and acceptance or denial of death and final separation from loved ones.

Caring is also evident in what Albert Jonsen calls the "*Samaritan principle*: the duty to care for the needy sick, whether friend or enemy, even at cost to oneself" (p. 39). The tradition of Samaritanism dates to the early Christian era and the parable of the Good Samaritan described in the Gospel according to Luke; it persists during the modern, secular era as a central ethic for medicine. Jonsen argues that although the original Christian parable of the Samaritan refers to giving aid to a particular individual, the ethical tradition of Samaritanism within medicine bears relevance to entire groups of patients. So understood, Samaritanism underlies the physician's broader social duty to care for indigent persons. In contrast to the past, when physicians provided charity care for indigent persons without financial remuneration, universal health insurance is the norm in most developed countries. Therefore, in contemporary times physicians are generally compensated for their services through a private or government health insurance mechanism. In the United States, however, large numbers of patients continue to lack health insurance. A principle of Samaritanism continues to be evident in the legal and ethical requirement that U.S. physicians provide emergency treatment to any patient regardless of the patient's ability to pay for care. A stronger Samaritan ethic, mandating access to all forms of basic healthcare, would require, in the United States, successful implementation of healthcare reform.

A third way in which caring is manifest in the ethics of medicine is through the healing relationship of doctor and patient. Edmund Pellegrino and David Thomasma regard this relationship as one of inherent inequality because the patient is vulnerable, ill, and in need of the physician's skill. In light of the patient's diminished power, Pellegrino and Thomasma argue that the physician incurs a duty of beneficence, a duty requiring the physician to respond to the patient's needs and promote the patient's good. Other ethical values in medicine can presumably be derived from the physician's primary duty of beneficence. For example, according to Pellegrino and Thomasma, a duty to enhance patients' autonomy is based on the duty to benefit patients.

Some, Sharpe for example, have sought to identify the principle of beneficence that Pellegrino and Thomasma delineate with an ethic of care. However, beneficence and care differ in crucial respects. Whereas a principle of beneficence identifies promoting the patient's good as a requirement for right action, an ethic of care is a type of virtue ethic that is basically concerned about the affective orientation and moral commitment—that is, the concern—of the one who cares. For example, a physician may perform actions that promote a patient's good, and thus meet the requirement of beneficence, without caring about or feeling any commitment toward the patient. If this analysis is correct, then actions that fulfill the principle of beneficence do not necessarily fulfill standards associated with an ethic of care. An ethic of care suggests both a feeling response directed to the object of care and a commitment to ensuring that things go well for that person.

Despite the integral role that an ethic of caring plays in medicine, contemporary physicians sometimes neglect to offer adequate palliative and comfort measures to patients. This may stem from a failure to teach and nurture empathy in medical education (Spiro et al.) and from financial incentives that discourage spending time at patients's bedsides and getting to know patients as persons. In addition, physicians may overlook caring for patients when conflicts exist about the use of futile treatments (Schneiderman et al.). For example, members of the healthcare team may become distracted debating the appropriateness of high-technology interventions and neglect to care for patients's spiritual and emotional needs.

## Conclusion

Although the development of theories of an ethic of care for healthcare is new, the idea of care has long presented a moral standard or ideal for healthcare. Although caring has been an abiding concern within nursing practice, within medicine care has sometimes been overshadowed by other ethical values and goals. The emergence of feminine ethics can play an important role in reemphasizing the value and importance of caring within medicine. However, the close association of care with gender and with the feminine voice may hinder efforts to develop a broader human understanding of care, such as the understanding of care that emerged earlier in human history.

NANCY S. JECKER
WARREN THOMAS REICH(1995)
REVISED BY NANCY S. JECKER

SEE ALSO: *Beneficence; Chronic Illness and Chronic Care; Compassionate Love; Emotions; Ethics: Normative Ethical Theories; Feminism; Healing; Human Dignity; Long-Term Care; Medicine, Art of; Narrative; Nursing Ethics; Obligation and Supererogation; Paternalism; Professional-Patient*

*Relationship; Virtue and Character; Women, Historical and Cross-Cultural Perspectives;* and other *Care* subentries

### BIBLIOGRAPHY

Benner, Patricia, and Wrubel, Judith. 1989. *The Primacy of Caring.* Menlo Park, CA: Addison-Wesley.

Brennan, Samantha. 1999. "Recent Work in Feminist Ethics." *Ethics* 109: 858–893.

Brown, Lyn M., and Gilligan, Carol. 1992. *Meeting at the Crossroads: Women's Psychology and Girls' Development.* Cambridge, MA: Harvard University Press.

Card, Claudia. 1990. "Caring and Evil." *Hypatia* 5(1): 101–108.

Card, Claudia. 1991. "The Feistiness of Feminism." In *Feminist Ethics,* ed. Claudia Card. Lawrence: University Press of Kansas.

Carse, Alisa L. 1998. "Impartial Principle and Moral Context: Securing a Place for the Particular in Ethical Theory." *Journal of Medicine and Philosophy* 23(2): 153–169.

Carse, Alisa L., and Hilde Lindemann Nelson. 1996. "Rehabilitating Care." *Kennedy Institute of Ethics Journal* 6(1): 19–35.

Cassell, Eric J. 1982. "The Nature of Suffering and the Goals of Medicine." *New England Journal of Medicine* 306: 639–645.

Cassell, Eric J. 1989. *The Healer's Art.* Cambridge, MA: MIT Press.

Elshtain, Jean Bethke. 1981. *Public Man, Private Woman: Women in Social and Political Thought.* Princeton, NJ: Princeton University Press.

Fry, Sarah T. 1989a. "The Role of Caring in a Theory of Nursing Ethics." *Hypatia* 4(2): 88–103.

Fry, Sarah T. 1989b. "Toward a Theory of Nursing Ethics." *Advances in Nursing Science* 11(4): 9–22.

Gatens-Robinson, Eugenie. 1992. "A Defense of Women's Choice: Abortion and the Ethics of Care." *Southern Journal of Philosophy* 30(3): 39–66.

Gilligan, Carol. 1982. *In a Different Voice: Psychological Theory and Women's Development.* Cambridge, MA: Harvard University Press.

Gilligan, Carol, and Attanucci, Jane. 1988. "Two Moral Orientations." In *Mapping the Moral Domain: A Contribution of Women's Thinking to Psychological Theory and Education,* ed. Carol Gilligan, Janie V. Ward, and Jill M. Taylor. Cambridge, MA: Harvard University Press.

Gilligan, Carol; Lyons, Nona P.; and Hanmer, Trudy J., eds. 1989. *Making Connections: The Relational Worlds of Adolescent Girls at the Emma Willard School.* Cambridge, MA: Harvard University Press.

Gilligan, Carol; Ward, Janie V.; and Taylor, Jill M., eds. 1988. *Mapping the Moral Domain: A Contribution of Women's Thinking to Psychological Theory and Education.* Cambridge, MA: Harvard University Press.

Hardwig, John. 1990. "What About the Family?" *Hastings Center Report* 20(2): 5–10.

Hardwig, John. 1991. "Treating the Brain Dead for the Benefit of the Family." *Journal of Clinical Ethics* 2(1): 53–56.

Holmes, Helen B. 1989. "A Call to Heal Medicine." *Hypatia* 4(2): 1–8.

Houston, Barbara. 1990. "Caring and Exploitation." *Hypatia* 5: 115–119.

Jameton, Andrew. 1984. *Nursing Practice: The Ethical Issues.* Englewood Cliffs, NJ: Prentice-Hall.

Jecker, Nancy S. 1990. "The Role of Intimate Others in Medical Decision Making." *Gerontologist* 30(1): 65–71.

Jecker, Nancy S. 1991. "Giving Death a Hand: When the Doctor and Patient Stand in a Special Relationship." *Journal of the Geriatrics Society* 39(8): 831–835.

Jecker, Nancy S. 1999. "Abortion." In *Ethics Applied,* 2.0 edition, ed. Paul De Vries, Robert Veatch, Lisa Newton, New York: Simon and Schuster.

Jecker, Nancy S. 2002. "Taking Care of One's Own: Justice and Family Caregiving." *Theoretical Medicine* 23: 117–133.

Jecker, Nancy S., and Self, Donnie J. 1991. "Separating Care and Cure: An Analysis of Historical and Contemporary Images of Nursing and Medicine." *Journal of Medicine and Philosophy* 16(3): 285–306.

Jonsen, Albert R., ed. 1990. "The Good Samaritan as Gatekeeper." In *The New Medicine and the Old Ethics.* Cambridge, MA: Harvard University Press.

King, Roger J. H. 1991. "Caring About Nature: Feminist Ethics and the Environment." *Hypatia* 6(1): 75–84.

Kohlberg, Lawrence. 1981. *The Philosophy of Moral Development: Moral Stages and the Idea of Justice.* San Francisco: Harper & Row.

Kohlberg, Lawrence. 1984. *The Psychology of Moral Development: The Nature and Validity of Moral Stages.* San Francisco: Harper & Row.

Landau, Iddo. 1996. "How Androcentric is Western Philosophy?" *The Philosophical Quarterly* 46(182): 48–59.

Moody-Adams, Michele M. 1991. "Gender and the Complexity of Moral Voices." In *Feminist Ethics,* ed. Claudia Card. Lawrence: University Press of Kansas.

Murphy, Catherine P. 1984. "The Changing Role of Nurses in Making Ethical Decisions." *Law, Medicine, and Health Care* 12(4): 173–175, 184.

Newton, Lisa H. 1990. "In Defense of the Traditional Nurse." In *Ethics in Nursing: An Anthology,* ed. Terry Pence and Janice Cantrall. New York: National League for Nursing.

Nicholson, Linda J. 1986. *Gender and History: The Limits of Social Theory in the Age of the Family.* New York: Columbia University Press.

Noddings, Nel. 1984. *Caring: A Feminine Approach to Ethics and Moral Education.* Berkeley: University of California Press.

Noddings, Nel. 1990. "Ethics from the Standpoint of Women." In *Theoretical Perspectives on Sexual Difference,* ed. Deborah L. Rohode. New Haven, CT: Yale University Press.

O'Brien, Patricia. 1987. "All a Woman's Life Can Bring: The Domestic Roots of Nursing in Philadelphia, 1830–1885." *Nursing Research* 36(1): 12–17.

Okin, Susan Moller. 2002. "Mistresses of Their Own Destiny: Group Rights, Gender, and Realistic Rights of Exit." *Ethics* 112: 205–230.

*Oxford English Dictionary,* vol. 1., 1971. Oxford, England: Oxford University Press.

Paley, John. "Caring as a Slave Morality: Nietzschean Themes in Nursing Ethics." *Journal of Advanced Nursing* 40(1): 25–41.

Pellegrino, Edmund D., and Thomasma, David C. 1988. *For the Patient's Good: The Restoration of Beneficence in Health Care.* New York: Oxford University Press.

Piaget, Jean. 1965. *The Moral Judgment of the Child.* New York: Free Press.

Reich, Warren Thomas. 1991. "The Case: Denny's Story," and "Commentary: Caring as Extraordinary Means." *Second Opinion* 17: 43–45.

Reich, Warren Thomas. 2001. "The Care-Based Ethic of Nazi Medicine and the Moral Importance of What We Care About." *American Journal of Bioethics* 1(1): 64–74.

Reverby, Susan. 1987a. "A Caring Dilemma: Womanhood and Nursing in Historical Perspective." *Nursing Research* 36(1): 5–11.

Reverby, Susan. 1987b. *Ordered to Care: The Dilemma of American Nursing, 1850–1945.* New York: Cambridge University Press.

Ruddick, Sara. 1989. *Maternal Thinking: Toward a Politics of Peace.* Boston: Beacon Press.

Schneiderman, Lawrence J.; Faber-Langendoen, Kathy; and Jecker, Nancy S. 1994. "Beyond Futility to an Ethic of Care." *American Journal of Medicine* 96(2): 110–114.

Self, Donnie J. 1993. "The Influence of Philosophical versus Theological Education on the Moral Development of Clinical Medical Ethicists." *Academic Medicine* 68(11): 848–852.

Self, Donnie J.; Skeel, Joy D.; and Jecker, Nancy S. 1993. "A Comparison of the Moral Reasoning of Physicians and Clinical Ethicists." *Academic Medicine* 68(11): 852–855.

Sharpe, Virginia A. 1992. "Justice and Care: The Implications of the Kohlberg-Gilligan Debate for Medical Ethics." *Theoretical Medicine* 13(4): 295–318.

Sherwin, Susan. 1992. *No Longer Patient: Feminist Ethics and Health Care.* Philadelphia: Temple University Press.

Spellman, Elizabeth V. 1991. "The Virtue of Feeling and the Feeling of Virtue." In *Feminist Ethics,* ed. Claudia Card. Lawrence: University Press of Kansas.

Spiro, Howard M.; McCrea, Mary G. M.; Peschel, Enid; et al. 1993. *Empathy and the Practice of Medicine: Beyond Pills and the Scalpel.* New Haven, CT: Yale University Press.

Stein, Leonard I.; Watts, David T.; and Howell, Timothy. 1990. "The Doctor-Nurse Game Revisited." *New England Journal of Medicine* 322(8): 546–549.

Swanson, Kristen M. 1990. "Providing Care in the NICU: Sometimes an Act of Love." *Advances in Nursing Science* 13(1): 60–73.

Thomson, Judith Jarvis. 1990. *The Realm of Rights.* Cambridge, MA: Harvard University Press.

Tong, Rosemarie. 1993. *Feminine and Feminist Ethics.* Belmont, CA: Wadsworth.

Tong, Rosemarie. 1998. *Feminist Thought,* 2nd edition. Boulder, CO: Westview Press.

UN General Assembly. 1948. *Universal Declaration of Human Rights.* New York: Author.

UN General Assembly. 1960. *Declaration of the Rights of the Child.* New York: Author.

Veatch, Robert M. 1998. "The Place of Care in Ethical Theory." *Journal of Medicine and Philosophy* 23(2): 210–224.

Warren, Virginia L. 1989. "Feminist Directions in Medical Ethics." *Hypatia* 4(2): 73–87.

Watson, Jean. 1988. *Nursing: Human Science and Human Care: A Theory of Nursing.* New York: National League for Nursing.

Winslow, Gerald R. 1984. "From Loyalty to Advocacy: A New Metaphor for Nursing." *Hastings Center Report* 14(3): 32–40.

# CASUISTRY

• • •

*Casuistry,* a term derived from the Latin word meaning "event, occasion, occurrence" and in later Latin, "case," was coined in the seventeenth century to refer pejoratively to the practice described by contemporary Christian theologians as "cases of conscience" (*casus conscientiae*). Today the word might be defined as the method of analyzing and resolving instances of moral perplexity by interpreting general moral rules in light of particular circumstances. This entry will relate the origins and development of casuistry in Western culture, its decline, and its revival as a method of ethical analysis, particularly in bioethics.

## Origins of Casuistry

The earliest discussions of morality in Western philosophy reveal the tension between general moral norms and particular decisions. The Sophists of fifth-century Greece maintained that since no universal truths could be affirmed in moral matters, right and wrong depended entirely on the circumstances: ethics consisted in the rhetorical ability to persuade persons about "opportune" action. Plato devoted his *Republic* to a vigorous refutation of this thesis, placing moral certitude only in universal moral truths: ethics consisted in transcending particularities and grasping permanent ideals from which right choice could be deduced. Aristotle proposed that in ethical deliberations, which deal with contingent matters, formal demonstration was not possible. Rather, plausible argument would support probable conclusions. Ethics belongs, he maintained, not in the realm of scientific knowledge but in the domain of practical wisdom (*phronesis*). *Phronesis* is a knowledge of particular facts and is the "object of perception rather than science" (*Nicomachean Ethics,* VI. viii. 1142a). Criticism, interpretation, and amplification of these theses constitutes much of the history of moral philosophy. The Aristotelian viewpoint, which places moral certitude in the domain of practical judgments about what ought to be done in the actual circumstances of a situation, is the remote philosophical ancestor of the casuistry that developed in Western culture.

The Roman philosopher and statesman Marcus Tullius Cicero (106–43 B.C.E.) designed an approach to moral problems that would powerfully influence the casuistic authors of the Middle Ages and Renaissance. Cicero, although a philosophical eclectic, inclined to Stoic thought in ethics. Drawing from the Stoics Panaetius and Posidonius and inspired by the Roman passion for practicality, he held that to be a virtuous person one must become "a good calculator of one's duty in the circumstances, so that by adding and subtracting considerations, we may see where our duty lies" (*On Duties,* I, 59). This adding and subtracting was done by offering and evaluating "probable reasons." The primary moral problem was the continual conflict between duty and utility, a conflict resolved only by examining the circumstances of cases. In his *On Duties,* Cicero proposed a number of cases, some drawn from the Stoic philosophers and others from Roman history. Each case, representing an apparently insoluble conflict between duty and utility, was then analyzed to show how, if circumstances were taken into account, one could discern one's moral duty. Cicero also espoused the Stoic doctrine of natural law and often referred to its overarching precepts in his analyses of cases; but the problem, he affirmed, was how these precepts were to be interpreted in context. *On Duties* remained one of the most studied texts of antiquity through the subsequent centuries. By its organization of material and its methods of reasoning, *On Duties* powerfully influenced the way in which morality was conceived and taught in the Western world, and thus sanctioned subsequent casuistry.

While moral discourse always moves between the broad generalizations of principle and the particular decisions made in specific circumstances, religions that are monotheistic and moral in nature face a particular problem in moving from the general to the particular. The three "religions of the Book"—Judaism, Christianity, and Islam—have in common a Scripture in which the word of God is recorded; that is, in which God speaks to believers in concrete and specific language. Also, the divine message contains imperatives that enjoin moral obligations, sometimes stated in broad terms and sometimes referring to specific forms of behavior. It becomes necessary for believers to understand how the broad general imperatives apply to the great variety of daily life, and to learn how specific commands expressed in the language and cultural setting of the past are to be followed in the circumstances of later times. Thus, each religion of the Book developed a moral teaching that begins with affirmations from the divine text, moves through traditional interpretations of that text by the saintly and the scholarly, and comes, finally, to the task of bringing text and interpretation to bear on particular circumstances of time and place. Each of these religions, then, has developed a casuistry or manner of working at the task of concrete application. The particular forms of Jewish and Islamic casuistry are discussed elsewhere; this entry will relate the development of casuistry in Western Christianity.

Christianity introduced a powerful and original morality into the Greco-Roman world. The thought of its founder, Jesus, both reflected the dedication of Jewish law to the sovereignty of God and refashioned it to include a demanding commitment to himself as Lord as well as self-sacrifice for one's neighbors, spelled out in strenuous, often paradoxical commands. His early disciples, seeking to follow these commands, preached an ascetic repudiation of "the ways of the world." This meant that the moderate virtues prized by the pagans among whom the early Christians lived were often deprecated and the vices of pagan life, which even pagan authors often criticized, were reviled. The morality of the Hebrew Scriptures and the Christian Gospels, which condemned many attitudes and practices common in pagan culture and demanded adherence to self-discipline and altruism, posed profound difficulties to believers. How were they to live in a world that held different values? How were the "hard commandments" of the Gospels to be carried out in daily life? These problems perplexed Paul of Tarsus, the most influential of Jesus' first followers, whose efforts to answer them, especially in his First Letter to the Corinthians, adumbrated the work of later Christian casuists. In addition, early Christian thinkers were suspicious of the philosophical thought of the Greco-Roman world. However, by the third century, many Christian scholars had come to accept that Christian belief and "pagan" philosophy were compatible in important respects. The authors of the patristic era (second to sixth centuries) reflected on Christian moral problems with the help of Plato, Aristotle, and Cicero. The framework of virtues, natural law, and practical reasoning elucidated in these and other pagan authors were modified and incorporated by Christian authors and teachers. They sought, as did their pagan mentors, to understand the nature of the moral life but were concerned, above all, with providing practical advice about how the faithful should live a Christian life in a non-Christian world. Many Christian authors used Cicero's *On Duties* as a model for treatises on morality: St. Ambrose of Milan (339–397), friend and teacher of the great St. Augustine, also titled a book *On Duties* and, closely following Cicero, attempted to refashion the latter's thoughts within the perspective of Christian faith.

Christian teaching does not merely require belief; it strongly stresses the importance of morally correct behavior. While killing, deception, and adultery are condemned as sins, and charity, self-denial, and honesty are commanded, inevitably questions arise about what sorts of behavior belong in these general categories. Early Christians were intensely aware that failure to follow the rigorous commandments of their faith separated them from God and from their fellow believers. The practice of confession of one's sins before the community of believers and the imposition of penance that would once again reconcile the sinner to God and to the community became common in the early centuries. By the eighth century, private confession to a priest, who had the ecclesiastical authority to absolve the repentant sinner from guilt, had been introduced. This practice of sacramental confession and penance enhanced the need for clear descriptions of the moral dimensions of various behaviors and of the ways in which various circumstances excused or aggravated the seriousness of those behaviors. From the eighth to the twelfth centuries, educators of the clergy produced penitential books that presented systematic catalogs of sinful and virtuous actions under various typical circumstances (e.g., the killing of another out of vengeance, in fear, in ignorance, etc.). The motives, the consequences, and the social status of the agent were important considerations in evaluating the responsibility and seriousness of behavior. Appropriate penances were assigned in view of the gravity of the sin.

These penitential volumes, the earliest examples of which came from the Irish and Welsh churches, became widespread throughout Europe. In the course of four centuries, their content became more elaborate and their format more systematic. The first were collections of crudely described cases with simple distinctions, elaborated with biblical or patristic quotations. Later examples incorporated advancing biblical and theological scholarship and, above all, the work of the canon lawyers who, since the rediscovery of Roman law in the eleventh century, had exercised increasing influence over the formulation of church law as it touched the organization and practices of Christian life. The work of Peter the Chanter (d. 1197), Alain of Lille (d. c. 1203), and Thomas Chobham (c.1200) were filled with well-described cases of moral perplexity, analyzed with reference to biblical texts, maxims from the fathers of the church, and the growing body of church law. These books were not only for the education of the parish priest but also to guide the ecclesiastical hierarchy in the formulation of policy and the making of judicial decisions. Some of these books were written for the instruction of the laity in making a proper confession and leading a good life.

During the twelfth through fourteenth centuries, great theological scholars such as Abelard, Peter Lombard, Albert the Great, Thomas Aquinas, Duns Scotus, and William of Ockham elaborated systematic treatises or *summas* in which they attempted to present the full range of Christian belief and to support it with rational argument. In doing so, they placed the questions of morality within larger frameworks of interpretation and justification, drawing heavily on philosophers of antiquity. These treatises did not discuss cases, as did the penitential literature, but created theoretical foundations for the discussion of cases. The relevance of scriptural admonitions, natural law, custom, and civil and canon law to moral decisions was explored in great depth; the relevance of principle, motive, and circumstances was carefully examined. These theologians, while not casuists, greatly influenced the next generations of casuists.

## Casuistic Writings

Through the fourteenth and fifteenth centuries, many books of cases of conscience were published. The *Summa Angelica* (1480) and the *Summa Sylvestrina* (1516) were the most famous. However, these works were staid, unimaginative, and formalistic; many authors simply plagiarized from more celebrated authors. But casuistry properly speaking came into its own in the mid-sixteenth century. In 1556 a Spanish canonist, Martin Azpilcueta, published *A Handbook for Confessors and Penitents,* which revitalized the literature of cases of conscience. This book abandoned the practice of listing moral problems alphabetically and adopted a less frequently used device of organizing various sins under the Decalogue. This allowed for a more flexible and nuanced treatment and for comparison between various categories of moral behavior. Above all, it introduced the analysis of issues from the more clear and obvious to the more complex, a method that later casuists would exploit and that is described below as reasoning by paradigm and analogy.

Azpilcueta's style was widely copied. The Jesuit order, founded in 1534, was dedicated to the work of moral education and guidance of conscience, especially in sacramental confession. The Jesuits introduced Azpilcueta's approach into their own training of priests as ministers of the sacrament of penance. They published many volumes of cases of conscience. John Azor's *Moral Instruction* (1600) was the preeminent work. Jesuit casuistry was, in general, careful, scholarly, sensible, and practical. It was also comprehensive. While the general rubric of the Decalogue was used to organize materials, the duties of various occupations, the obligations of princes and bishops, and the moral dimensions of diplomacy, Jesuit casuistry also dealt with economics, warfare, and exploration. It has been suggested that the origins of modern economics, sociology, and political science lie in the work of the seventeenth-century casuists. Certainly, their advice was often sought by popes and kings in matters that we would today consider political or economic rather than moral. But in the seventeenth century, the moral questions on a king's or pope's conscience often concerned politics and finance.

The seventeenth-century casuists not only analyzed and resolved complex cases. They also elaborated speculative positions, writing treatises on topics such as justice, usually as prolegomena to their analyses of cases of government or trade. Among the central speculative questions was that of the degree of moral certitude required to act in good conscience, that is, how sure a person must be that a casuistic resolution of a moral problem is the correct one before acting upon it. A vigorous intellectual debate on this question took place in the last half of the seventeenth century between the Jesuits and their theological rivals, the Dominicans, and among the Jesuits themselves. From that debate, the position of the leading Jesuit theologians emerged as dominant. That position, *probabilism*, maintained that a person was entitled to act in good conscience if there were probable arguments in favor of the choice; probable arguments are those supported by solidly reasoned opinion and defended by respected authors. Probabilism, while defended with elegant argument and sanctioned by ecclesiastical authority, remained a contentious issue and led to the tarnishing of the casuists' reputation in the seventeenth century, since many critics accused them of being able to find any probable argument to justify their preferences.

The Jesuits were by no means the only authors of casuistry; many other Catholic theologians were so engaged. Anglican divines produced clear and sensible books of casuistry; and since most works of classical casuistry have not been translated from their original Latin, Anglican casuistical books offer the best access to casuistry for English readers (see Perkins). Lutherans were not well disposed toward casuistic analysis: Luther had cast into the flames the *Summa Angelica,* calling it "Summa Diabolica." Still, the Jesuits attained the reputation of being the premier casuists. Since they were deeply involved in the religious and secular politics of the era, they won enemies on every side and their casuistry appeared to many to serve their own interests rather than the good conscience of their penitents. In particular, the genius mathematician Blaise Pascal found distressing the Jesuits' opposition to Jansenism, a particularly rigoristic Catholic theology that he favored; and at the urging of other Jansenists, he set out to destroy the Jesuits' anti-Jansenist arguments.

Pascal's *Provincial Letters* (1656) was a brilliant and wittily written refutation of the Jesuit arguments against Jansenist theology and, in particular, of the casuistry that, he claimed, made a mockery of Christian moral beliefs. He gave numerous examples of Jesuit resolution of cases of conscience and found them tainted by a probabilism that bred moral laxity, intellectual sophistry, and disguised heresy. Despite the fact that Pascal took cases out of context and chose only those that suited his polemical purposes, his diatribe became immensely popular. At best, it can be said that his critique demolished not casuistry itself but the lax casuistry that was counted reprehensible even by the Jesuits whom he accused. It was not only Pascal's popular book that tarnished casuistry's reputation. Certain casuists, few of them Jesuits, did take the skill at case analysis to an extreme: Almost any argument could be presented plausibly and fine distinctions could be drawn to make, as Plato said of the Sophists, "the worse appear the better." Casuistry and sophistry became invidious synonyms, as did casuistry and Jesuitry. And casuistic argument, once quite liberal, became legalistic in tone and content, promoting a morality of observance rather than of conscience. Finally, casuistry was falling out of step with the prevailing intellectual progress. The interest in intellectual systems, seen in Isaac Newton, Gottfried Wilhelm Leibniz, Baruch Spinoza, and Hugo Grotius, made the casuists' interest in particular cases appear disorderly and without solid foundation. By the end of the seventeenth century, casuistry was discredited in the European intellectual world. The word *casuistry* was invented as a term of abuse (earlier the word *casista* was used merely to describe a scholar who presented cases of conscience). Bayle's *Dictionary* (1697) defined *casuistry* as the "art of quibbling with God." At the close of the eighteenth century, Kant, who was familiar with traditional casuistry as a way of teaching ethics, found the only interesting question to be how to transform the limited and probable maxims of moral discourse into categorical certitude.

Casuistic writing continued through the eighteenth and nineteenth centuries within the Roman Catholic tradition, particularly in the education of the clergy, but it was a desiccated casuistry, wary of innovative solutions and bound by ecclesiastical pronouncements on moral matters. The work of the French Jesuit J. Gury (1862) was representative of the fading tradition; a journal titled *The Casuist,* published for American Catholic clergy (1906–1917), shows the tradition at its nadir. Still, casuistry continued to serve the practice of sacramental penance for which it had been created. Outside this tradition, remnants of casuistry lingered in the teaching of ethics. The textbooks of the time included fragments of Aristotle and Cicero and many of the classical cases, loosely grouped around virtues and duties. In 1870, revolted by the untidy and incoherent presentations of these texts, Henry Sidgwick, professor of casuistical divinity at Cambridge University (he had his chair renamed "moral philosophy"), undertook to construct a systematic presentation of an ethical theory, utilitarianism, in which tenets were tightly argued, inconsistencies rectified, and opponents refuted. The progress of moral philosophy from Sidgwick's time until recently has been toward greater articulation of theory and away from analysis of cases of conscience.

## The Practical Need for Casuistry

Casuistry then almost disappeared from the formal academic disciplines that study moral discourse. However, in the 1960s, a number of important moral questions began to trouble the American conscience, and moral philosophers were spurred to attend to the practical application of their discipline. The war in Vietnam required many to examine their consciences concerning support of and participation in what they felt was an immoral war. At the same time, the civil rights movement stimulated consciences concerning discrimination and racial injustice. The analytic moral philosophy current in academic circles had little advice to offer. Even the widely accepted and elaborate utilitarian theory seemed to lead to no firm conclusions.

The emerging interest in the ethics of medical and healthcare also opened vistas for a new casuistry. Medical care is about cases: the illness and the treatment of particular persons with particular diseases. Philosophers and theologians who engaged in this work had initially tried to bring the standard ethical theories to the analysis of medical problems, but they found themselves discussing cases, not theories, and felt the need for an approach that would stay closer to the particulars of the case under discussion than did the standard theories. Above all, they realized that cases were being discussed not merely to elucidate the meaning of concepts but also to arrive at a resolution: physicians, nurses, and patients were interested in what moral philosophy had abandoned: answers to practical moral perplexity. By the late 1970s, talk of "case method" had become common in

bioethics. At the same time, ethical issues in business, government, and journalism seemed to call for study of individual cases rather than flights into ethical theory. Also, influential moral philosophers were beginning to criticize the dominance of moral theory in practical ethics and to call for approaches that were more concrete than speculative.

Albert Jonsen and Stephen Toulmin published *The Abuse of Casuistry* in 1988. Aware that many were interested in inventing a "case method" for ethics, they hoped to show that such a method had been invented long ago and that, although discredited and seemingly outmoded, classical casuistry had much to offer modern ethicists. Case method in ethics might be similar in many respects to the case method in Anglo-American common law, which had developed in parallel with classical casuistry. Both the common law, about which much research has been done, and casuistry, which has been invisible to the scholarly world for several centuries, need to be explored if a case method for ethics, of "morisprudence," is to be re-created. These authors attempted to restore casuistry to intellectual respectability. After a historical survey of the rise and fall of casuistry, they contrast it with current approaches to moral philosophy and define it as follows:

> [T]he analysis of moral issues, using procedures of reasoning based on paradigms and analogies, leading to the formulation of expert opinion about the existence and stringency of particular moral obligations, framed in terms of rules and maxims that are general but not universal or invariable, since they hold good with certainty only in the typical conditions of the agent and circumstances of the case. (p. 257)

## Methodology

The term *methodology* may be too formal a word to describe how casuistry works. The casuists of the past left almost no formal description of their way of working; the casuists of the present, pressed by their critics based in moral philosophy, are still asking themselves questions about methodology. Still, certain characteristics of the casuistic approach can be noted. These characteristics appear to have their origins in the classical discipline of rhetoric rather than in philosophy as such. The historical casuists had, like all educated persons of their time, been educated thoroughly in rhetoric. Aristotle and Cicero, the authors from whom they learned rhetoric, also taught them ethics. Classical rhetoric was defined as having a moral purpose: the persuasion of persons toward right and just action. Indeed, the classical books of rhetoric, because they were so rich in comments about and examples of moral behavior, were often used as texts in ethics. In the centuries during which casuistry flourished, moral philosophy was not a clearly defined discipline. Thus, it is not surprising to find the historical casuists implicitly using the techniques of rhetoric in their analysis of cases of conscience. Both rhetoric and casuistry had morally correct attitudes and action as their ultimate goal.

Two characteristics of rhetorical technique are particularly important for casuistry: topics and the comparison of paradigm and analogy. Rhetoricians taught that discourse in general could be divided into a set of common ideas, such as "causality," "temporal sequence," and so on, which they called "topics." Each of these topics had sets of definitions and forms of argumentation that were invariant. Also, each special realm of discourse, such as discourse about politics, art, or economics, has its own set of "special topics," the features of the field that must be understood and discussed if an adequate argument is to be made about what should be done. A casuistic approach to an ethical problem, then, requires that the field of discourse be analyzed to designate the invariant features. For example, it has been suggested that the topics of clinical ethics are: (1) medical indications, (2) patient preferences, (3) quality of life, and (4) contextual features, such as costs of care and allocation of resources (Jonsen, Siegler, and Winslade). Each of these topics has certain definitions, maxims, and arguments that must be taken into account in discussion of any case. The particular circumstances of time, place, personal characteristics, various behaviors, and so on that are the details of any case are viewed in the light of these topics.

Once the particular case is described by its circumstances and topics, casuistical analysis seeks to place this case into a context of similar cases. The classical casuists were accustomed to line up cases of similar sorts, so that cases describing various sorts of homicide, for example, were aligned in order that the similarities and differences between cases would become clear. This enabled the casuist to see those cases in which the moral principles and maxims appeared to lead to an unambiguous resolution. Thus, the prohibition against killing another human being seemed most obviously to hold if the circumstances described a vicious, unprovoked attack on an unoffending person; the prohibition would allow an exception if the circumstances described a killing that resulted from that unoffending person's self-defense against a lethal attack. This technique of lining up cases, rather than seeing them in isolation, is the essence of casuistical analysis. It is called by some authors the technique of paradigm analogy: The paradigm case is the case in which circumstances allow moral maxims and principles to be seen as unambiguously relevant to the resolution of the case; the analogies are those cases in which particular circumstances justify exceptions and qualifications of the

moral principles. A high degree of assurance, or moral certitude, pertains to the resolution of paradigm cases, while varying degrees of moral probability, or probabilism, attach to the resolution of analogous cases.

Finally, the resolution of each case depends on what Aristotle called *phronesis*, or moral wisdom: the perception of an experienced and prudent person that, in these circumstances and in light of these maxims, this is the best possible moral course. As one commentator on modern casuistry has written, "for casuistry, moral truth resides in the details … the meaning and scope of moral principles is determined contextually through the interpretation of factual situations in relation to paradigm cases" (Arras, p. 37).

Bioethics is the most prominent field in which casuistry is beginning to be reintroduced as a method for ethical analysis. This is not surprising, since a strong interest of bioethics is the clinical care of patients, and many cases that came to the early attention of bioethicists involved life-and-death decisions arising from the use of new medical technologies. Cases about whether life-supporting technologies should or should not be continued for particular patients lend themselves to casuistic analysis. The differing circumstances of individual patients, the topics (the significant categories into which a medical-ethical decision can be factored), and the maxims (such as "do no harm" or "respect the patient's informed choices") are each in their own way crucial to the resolution of any case. The placing of the case in a lineup of paradigm and analogy, from the most obvious—in which the patient is brain dead, or continued care is manifestly futile—to the problematic, in which diminished quality of life or unclear preferences are at issue, allows for discretionary judgment between cases (Jonsen). This sort of casuistry can also be applied to questions of healthcare policy, such as those surrounding the various programs proposed for allocation of resources, although relatively little of such analysis has been done.

Casuistry, then, keeps moral reflection close to cases. Neither classical nor modern casuistry repudiates principles: Casuistry is not merely another name for situationism or contextualism. Rather, principles are seen to be relevant to cases in varying degrees: In some cases, principles will rule unequivocally; in others, exceptions and qualifiers will be appropriate. Modern casuists dislike the description of casuistry as "applied ethics," since they explicitly repudiate the notion that an ethical theory must be elaborated and then "applied to" the circumstances of the case. Still, the relationship between cases and ethical theory is unclear and poses the principal speculative problem that casuists and moral philosophers must ponder, just as the historical casuists pondered the problem of the certitude of practical judgment. On the one hand, casuistry is not simply applied ethical theory; on the other, it is not simply immersion in the factual circumstances of cases, which would reduce it to situationism. Casuistry is not tied to any single theory of ethics but can be comfortable with selected elements of multiple theories. For example, a casuistic argument might draw on utilitarian, deontological, and contractual justifications in a single case. Also, the designation of topics and the selection of paradigms have theoretical presuppositions. Finally, the normative nature of principles and maxims, which must be clarified in order to specify the obligatory nature of casuistic resolutions, requires reference to theory. Casuistry, then, is not "theory free" but is rather, as one commentator has suggested, "theory modest" (Arras, p. 41). Theories, for contemporary casuistry, are not mutually exclusive, a priori foundations for practical ethical discourse but limited and complementary perspectives that illuminate practical judgment. Much work remains to be done on the relationship between theory and practical judgment. Still, as suits the style of casuistry through its history, it can grapple effectively with difficult cases even though all speculative and theoretical questions about its methods and presuppositions have not yet been answered.

ALBERT R. JONSEN (1995)

SEE ALSO: *Bioethics; Conscience; Conscience, Rights of; Ethics: Normative Ethical Theories; Narrative; Natural Law; Principlism; Responsibility*

### BIBLIOGRAPHY

Arras, John D. 1991. "Getting Down to Cases: The Revival of Casuistry in Bioethics." *Journal of Medicine and Philosophy* 16: 29–51.

Carson, Ronald A. 1986. "Case Method." *Journal of Medical Ethics* 12(1): 36–39.

Gury, J. 1862. *Casus conscientiae in Praecipuas Quaestiones, Theologiae Moralis,* 1st edition. Lepuy: Marchesson.

Jonsen, Albert R. 1991. "Casuistry as Methodology in Clinical Ethics." *Theoretical Medicine* 12(4): 295–307.

Jonsen, Albert R.; Siegler, Mark; and Winslade, William. 1992. *Clinical Ethics: A Practical Approach to Ethical Decisions in Clinical Medicine,* 3rd edition. New York: Macmillan.

Jonsen, Albert R., and Toulmin, Stephen E. 1988. *The Abuse of Casuistry: A History of Moral Reasoning.* Berkeley and Los Angeles: University of California Press.

Juengst, Eric. 1989. "Casuistry and the Locus of Certainty in Ethics." *Medical Humanities Review* 3(1): 19–28.

Kirk, Kenneth. 1927. *Conscience and Its Problems: An Introduction to Casuistry.* London: Longman's Green.

Leites, Edmund, ed. 1988. *Conscience and Casuistry in Early Modern Europe.* Cambridge, Eng.: Cambridge University Press.

Mahoney, John. 1987. *The Making of Moral Theology: A Study of the Roman Catholic Tradition.* Oxford: Oxford University Press.

McHugh, John Ambrose, ed. 1906. *The Casuist: A Collection of Cases in Moral and Pastoral Theology.* New York: Joseph E. Wagner.

Pascal, Blaise. 1967. *The Provincial Letters,* ed. and tr. Alban Krailscheimer. Harmondsworth, Eng.: Penguin.

Perkins, William. 1970. *Works.* Abingdon, Eng.: Sutton Courtenay Press.

# CHILDREN

• • •

## I. HISTORY OF CHILDHOOD

Childhood is a culturally determined social construct that might be thought of as a set of expectations for children. The principal dynamic in the history of childhood involves changes in these expectations. The history of childhood can be organized around three fundamental concepts: socialization, maturation, and modernization. Socialization is the process whereby a child incorporates the principal elements of the culture into which she or he is born. Maturation is the biological process of growing up. Modernization is the large-scale transformation of economies and societies—of European countries first, and then others. This process includes industrialization, urbanization, and the expansion of capitalistic systems of economic organization. The most dramatic changes in socialization and maturation of children come from the impact of modernization.

In traditional societies, socialization usually took place within families at a gradual pace and in informal ways. Sons learned the skills and practices of adult males by working alongside their fathers. Similarly, daughters worked and learned in close contact with their mothers. In the modern world, new agencies such as schools appeared and became part of the socialization process; and the process of maturation, formerly a natural process marked, perhaps, by rites of passage from youth to adulthood, now became the focus of serious social thought and practice. Put another way, maturation has been redefined in the modern age as a time of "identity crisis" for youth. In the modern age, youths have a greater range of choices for adult roles than did their ancestors.

The pioneering work in the history of childhood is *L'Enfant et la vie familiale sous l'ancien régime,* published by Philippe Ariès in 1960 (and translated into English as *Centuries of Childhood: A Social History of Family Life* [1962]). Ariès not only wrote one of the first modern scholarly treatments of the history of childhood, he also made the central point that childhood is socially constructed; that is, that ideas about and expectations for children are determined by social leaders and experts (advice-givers). Another early writer on the history of childhood, Lloyd deMause, in a work titled *The History of Childhood,* argued that "The further back in history one goes, the lower the level of child care and the more likely children are to be killed, abandoned, beaten, terrorized, and sexually abused" (p. 1). Professional historians have modified the views of Aries and deMause as they have developed deeper knowledge of the ways earlier societies regarded and treated children. The lasting importance of both scholars is that they founded the field of history of childhood and stimulated others to further investigations and revisions.

## Childhood in the Ancient Western World

We know that childhood, a period of relative freedom from work, existed in the ancient world because children's play was depicted on Greek vases and Roman sarcophagi. There were several ancient treatises on the diseases of children and a recognition that children were to be treated differently from adults. Thus there was a tradition of childhood in the ancient world that saw children as passing through stages of growth, as being malleable, as being fragile, playful, and sometimes headstrong. This tradition saw children as individually different and in need of protection from abuse by adults. Ancient philosophers, particularly Plato and Aristotle, wrote about child-rearing practices and regarded children as a link to the future. Some children's toys have survived—dolls, small versions of weapons, and the like—and they point to adult agendas for future citizens. Epitaphs remind us that ancient parents mourned the death of their children.

The Greeks and Romans devoted special attention to children and child-rearing practices. Women were the child rearers, and a number of other adults worked with children: midwives, teachers, tutors, and physicians. Both Plato and Aristotle recognized five stages of childhood (expressed in modern terms):

1. Babyhood, from birth to about two years—that is, until the child is weaned and can talk;

2. The early preschool age, from two to three years or later—when the child is separating emotionally from the mother, becomes more active physically, and begins to play games alone;

3. Later preschool age, from ages three to seven—a stage when children become more active and more involved in social groups;

4. School-age children (up to puberty)—a time of intense competition, especially among boys; and

5. The stage between puberty and adulthood—which continues into the late teens or early twenties.

The last stage may have been brief or nonexistent for girls, who married at a relatively early age. In their broad outline, however, these stages closely resemble modern child-development theory.

## Threats to Children in the Ancient World

Childhood in the ancient world had a darker side: some people practiced infanticide as a means of birth control or eugenics (French); some children were sold into slavery; and some of the little slaves were maimed so that they could be more pitiable beggars. Additionally, the use of wet nurses for the newborn was common and undoubtedly led to higher infant mortality rates. Wet nursing led to higher infant mortality because there was a greater possibility of disease, the wet nurse had less concern for the child than the mother did, and the amount of nourishment from the wet nurse might have been less. Infanticide was common, and such evidence as there is suggests that it was more common for female children than for male children to be killed by being abandoned and left to starve. A Roman law, for instance, said that all boy children and at least one girl born to a family had to be raised. In Sparta (from 700 to about 350 B.C.E.) infanticide was part of a program of eugenics whereby defective children were exposed. Illegitimate children were also disposed of through infanticide. Most children grew up in small nuclear families with one or two siblings. These small families were of concern to the Romans, who sought to increase the birth rate through incentives.

## Childhood in Medieval and Early Modern Times

Very little is known about child-rearing practices and childhood in the early centuries of the Middle Ages because the historical sources for this period are very scattered and fragmentary. But it is known that children were valued. Among the Visigoths, for example, a male baby had a blood price (*wergild*) of one-tenth that of an adult male. As the child aged, the wergild increased. Female children had a blood price half that of male children, but adult women's wergild was five-sixths that of an adult male. There was some schooling in this period; scattered references attest to schools in palaces and monasteries, although the practice of taking in small boys as oblates by monastic orders was already declining. For much of the population the process of maturation involved a long apprenticeship with children working alongside adults and thereby learning adult roles and responsibilities.

Literary references suggest that adults treated young children in a kindly fashion but that they had little regard for young people in their teens. Laws set the age of criminal responsibility (when a child could be charged with a crime) at seven and the age of majority (when a person could make a binding contract) at eighteen or older. As in the ancient world, medieval parents clearly mourned the deaths of their children. Medieval commentaries on childhood saw three stages in place of the ancient world's five (again expressed in modern terms):

1. Infancy, up to the age of two;
2. The preschool period, from age two to age seven;
3. Puerility, from age seven to age fourteen.

There were texts that stressed the importance of breast-feeding (and by inference pointed to the dangers of wet nurses), but the use of wet nurses was common among the upper classes. An English bishop wrote of the importance of cradles (which would prevent infant deaths resulting from suffocation in the parental bed). Some children's toys—miniature figurines, for example—have survived from the period.

Infanticide was still common for female babies, but illegitimate children were sometimes added to the father's household. To counter the pattern of infant exposure and abandonment, orphanages appeared, the first being established in 787 at Milan. By the early fourteenth century, there were two hospitals in Florence that accepted foundlings, and in 1445 a separate foundling hospital, the Innocenti, was established. Other foundling hospitals appeared in Rome, Bologna, Pavia, and Paris by the end of the fifteenth century.

During the course of the Middle Ages, opportunities for schooling expanded from the limited possibilities offered by palaces, monasteries, or nunneries. Schools began to appear in the major cities of Europe; many of them, such as the grammar school at St. Paul's Cathedral in London, which was revived by John Colet early in the sixteenth century, were founded for the express purpose of training boys in business.

Most medieval children left home fairly early. Girls entered the work force at around age eight as servants, and boys typically were apprenticed to learn a trade. In effect these children traded their labor for their upkeep in their new households.

The death rate for children in the medieval world was extremely high—from 30 to 50 percent of children did not live to maturity. Besides disease, infanticide, and wet nursing, accidents claimed a great many children. There was little supervision of young children. Newborn children were swaddled (tightly wrapped with strips of cloth so that they could not move about or even move their limbs). Older siblings might provide some care, but most children were left alone; many of them suffered accidents, such as falling into an open fire, as a result.

European living patterns in the medieval and early modern period are comparable in some ways with traditional Japanese households. In traditional Japan the household was a residence as well as a legal, economic, affective, and ritual unit. In it children were regarded as treasures, although only one child would remain in the household as heir (the heir could be either male or female). The other children became apprentices or spouses or servants or remained in the household as dependents. The successor inherited all the assets of the household and was responsible for the continuity of the household and its reputation. The household was child-centered and stressed socialization into traditional roles. In recent times, as a result of the modernization of Japanese society, the process of socialization has changed. Japanese children do not remain in the traditional households, and younger families move to cities, where schools and other institutions have replaced the household as the primary agent of socialization because new occupations require different forms of preparation.

A similar transformation occurred in the Muslim Middle East. Ironically, it began with a reemphasis on the traditional household, which had been devalued by Westerners since the modern colonial period began in 1798. The family became a point for resistance to colonialism and strengthened paternal authority at a time when Western families were becoming more democratic. As the nations of the Middle East gained independence in the last half of the twentieth century, these traditional households began to give way before the process of modernization. And, as was the case in Japan and early modern Europe, schools and other institutions supplemented the family as agents of socialization.

## Childhood in the Modern Western World

As modernization transformed western Europe and North America in the eighteenth and nineteenth centuries, a new and distinctive pattern of childhood emerged that was the result of a number of influences—economic changes such as the intensification of a market economy, a decline in family size, the rise of rationalism in public discourse, to name a few. In addition, several important European thinkers were midwives to this new form of childhood. John Locke helped to undermine the dominant Puritan conception of children as innately evil, that is, born in sin, when he published his *Essay Concerning Human Understanding* in 1690. In it he argued that ideas could come from experience and thus were not innate. In 1693 he issued *Some Thoughts Concerning Education,* in which he attacked the doctrine of infant depravity. Locke did not regard children as innately good; rather, he argued that they were morally neutral—blank tablets.

Another central figure was the French philosopher Jean-Jacques Rousseau, whose *Émile* (1762) was the story of a boy and his tutor. Rousseau argued that children should be reared more naturally, making use of their innate curiosity to motivate their learning. For Rousseau both nature and the child were innately good. Evil arose from the corruptions of civilization. One of Rousseau's followers who put his ideas into practice was Johann Heinrich Pestalozzi, who founded a school in Switzerland in 1799.

Yet another important figure in the emergence of the modern concept of childhood was the English novelist Charles Dickens, whose well-known child characters Oliver Twist, Charley Bates, Jack Dawkins, and the Artful Dodger personalized some of the tragic effects of the industrial revolution in England. Dickens vividly described the desperation of the urban working classes and the processes whereby homeless children had to fend for themselves. His writings, supported by the findings of royal commissions and by the work of social reformers, helped transform the social attitudes of the Western world. In 1848 the English established "Ragged Schools" for the children of the urban working classes. Later they created a system of universal public education with the Forster Education Act of 1870.

In the United States in the nineteenth century, Charles Loring Brace, a New York clergyman and reformer, founded the Children's Aid Society in 1853 to ship "surplus" urban children—whether orphaned or not—to rural areas. The Children's Aid Society also founded lodging houses for homeless newsboys and industrial schools for homeless girls of the streets. (It was hoped that by teaching the latter unfortunates a trade such as sewing, they might be rescued from prostitution.) Later in the nineteenth century another New York reformer, Elbridge Thomas Gerry, founded the Society for the Prevention of Cruelty to Children in 1875. Popularly known as "the Cruelty," the organization sought to reduce or eliminate the worst instances of child abuse and neglect.

While these reforms and the expansion of public schools sought to provide opportunities for the child victims of modern society, the problem of child labor proved more difficult to solve. In part this was because few people—and certainly not most parents or employers—regarded child labor as a problem. For one thing, children had always worked before the modern era. Only the sons and daughters of the privileged elite escaped labor during their childhood. In the preindustrial world most families, whether urban or rural, relied on the labor of their children. Children in that world were regarded as a renewable labor supply. They began doing simple chores as early as possible, and they continued to work throughout adulthood and into old age, as long as they were able. Children also functioned as safety nets for parents. As parents became too infirm to work, they relied on their offspring for food and shelter. This family labor system moved with families to industrial cities. Thus, in nineteenth- and twentieth-century factories children joined their parents on the shop floor, first as helpers and later as hands. Industries welcomed child labor because it guaranteed a steady supply of trained workers, and families depended on the income the children produced.

But modern society demanded more skills from its work force than the family labor system was able to deliver. As a result, families had to forgo the income from some of their children so that they could learn the skills necessary to obtain employment. At the same time, reformers began to define child labor as a social problem and to expand the availability of schools. By the 1920s, child labor was on the decline in the Western world as schools, child labor laws, and technological innovation finally reduced the supply of child laborers and the demand for them.

In the process of expanding schools and trying to reduce child abuse and to regulate child labor, Western society was redefining childhood. Childhood now became a special, protected status, a time during which biological maturation could run its course, and children could come to know the complexities of the modern world and find their places in it. Two other social developments were significant in this process of redefinition: the creation of the federal Children's Bureau and a federally funded program to reduce infant mortality in the United States. The Children's Bureau, established in 1912, was an outgrowth of the First White House Conference on Children, convened by President Theodore Roosevelt in 1909. At first it concentrated on the reduction of infant mortality, which led in 1921 to the passage of the Sheppard-Towner Act, a program of matching grants for states. The grants helped states set up programs of education and prenatal clinics. This program of prevention and education had the desired effect, but was killed by lobbying from the American Medical Association in 1929.

Other social advances in the nineteenth and twentieth centuries included the rise of pediatrics as a medical specialty and the rise of child psychologists, psychiatrists, and social workers. By the late twentieth century virtually all advanced industrial countries, including many outside the West, had made significant strides in reducing some of the threats to children's health and well-being.

## Conclusion

The experiences of children in the recent past cannot be reduced to simple generalizations; there are too many variables. But it is obvious that region, economic health, and aspects such as race, class, and gender all have a major impact on children and childhood. Having noted these difficulties, some observations are possible. Abortion is more common in the industrialized world, whereas infant mortality is much lower. Children are less likely to become orphans in industrialized countries, to experience the death of a sibling, or to die before reaching adulthood. Children in industrialized countries will probably know their grandparents, and their parents may well have been divorced; many of them live in single-parent households, a sharp contrast to the extended households of traditional cultures.

Children in industrialized countries will spend more time in schools than children did in the medieval world, or than they do now where traditional cultures prevail. They will spend more time in groups with children of the same age. Their parents will have relied more heavily on experts, and they will probably have only a few siblings and perhaps a room of their own. They will have money of their own, and parts of the media will cater especially to them. They will also have a legal status that is clearly spelled out, although their status will vary from country to country. Of course even in industrialized countries poorer children will enjoy fewer privileges than the children of middle-class or elite parents.

In the twentieth century the improvements in children's lives in industrialized countries have been dramatic. In the United States, for example, in 1900 infant mortality was estimated to be more than 160 per 1,000 live births; by 1990 this rate had dropped to around 10 per 1,000. In Japan the rate was 5 per 1,000. Similar improvements occurred in access to schooling and literacy. In 1900 high school graduates in the United States constituted less than 4 percent of the seventeen-year-old population. By 1990 they represented approximately 75 percent. Similar evidence of significant improvement in children's health and education can be cited for most, if not all, industrialized nations.

In the modern world childhood has been extended, redefined, and supported by an array of experts and social institutions. Maturity, once a biological matter worth little notice, has become a complex process perhaps more social and psychological than physical in nature. Similarly, the process of socialization is now much more complex, reflecting, as always, the society into which children are to be socialized. In complex modern societies, the preparation necessary to become a productive adult is much longer and more intensive than formerly. In recognition of this, students now extend their schooling well into their twenties and even beyond. Maturation, modernization, and socialization as they have interacted have created an entirely new world of childhood.

JOSEPH M. HAWES
N. RAY HINER (1995)

SEE ALSO: *Abuse, Interpersonal: Child Abuse; Adoption; Family and Family Medicine; Feminism; Infanticide; Infants, Public Policy and Legal Issues; Pediatrics, Adolescents; Research Policy: Subjects; Women, Historical and Cross-Cultural Perspectives;* and other *Children* subentries

### BIBLIOGRAPHY

Ariès, Philippe. 1962 (1960). *Centuries of Childhood: A Social History of Family Life,* tr. Robert Baldick. New York: Random House.

deMause, Lloyd, ed. 1974. *The History of Childhood.* New York: Psychohistory Press.

Fingerhut, Lois A., and Kleinman, Joel C. 1989. *Trends and Current Status in Childhood Mortality, United States, 1900–1985.* Washington, D.C.: U.S. Government Printing Office.

French, Valerie. 1991. "Children in Antiquity." In *Children in Historical and Comparative Perspective: An International Handbook and Research Guide,* pp. 3–29, ed. Joseph M. Hawes and N. Ray Hiner. Westport, CT: Greenwood.

Gillis, John R. 1974. *Youth and History: Tradition and Change in European Age Relations, 1770–Present.* New York: Academic Press.

Golden, Mark. 1990. *Children and Childhood in Classical Athens.* Baltimore: Johns Hopkins University Press.

Greenleaf, Barbara Kaye. 1978. *Children Through the Ages: A History of Childhood.* New York: McGraw-Hill.

Hanawalt, Barbara A. 1986. *The Ties That Bound: Peasant Families in Medieval England.* Oxford: Oxford University Press.

Hawes, Joseph M. 1971. *Children in Urban Society: Juvenile Delinquency in Nineteenth-Century America.* New York: Oxford University Press.

Hawes, Joseph M. 1991. *The Children's Rights Movement: A History of Advocacy and Protection.* Boston: Twayne.

Hawes, Joseph M., and Hiner, N. Ray, eds. 1985. *American Childhood: A Research Guide and Historical Handbook.* Westport, CT: Greenwood.

Hawes, Joseph M., and Hiner, N. Ray, eds. 1991. *Children in Historical and Comparative Perspective: An International Handbook and Research Guide.* Westport, CT: Greenwood.

Hiner, N. Ray, and Hawes, Joseph M., eds. 1985. *Growing Up in America: Children in Historical Perspective.* Urbana: University of Illinois Press.

Hunt, David. 1970. *Parents and Children in History: The Psychology of Family Life in Early Modern France.* New York: Basic Books.

Jordan, Thomas E. 1987. *Victorian Childhood: Themes and Variations.* Albany: State University of New York Press.

King, Charles R. 1993. *Children's Health in America: A History.* New York: Twayne.

Korbin, Jill E., ed. 1981. *Child Abuse and Neglect: Cross-Cultural Perspectives.* Berkeley: University of California Press.

Maynes, Mary Jo. 1985. *Schooling in Western Europe: A Social History.* Albany: State University of New York Press.

Pollock, Linda A. 1983. *Forgotten Children: Parent-Child Relations from 1500 to 1900.* Cambridge, Eng.: Cambridge University Press.

Sommerville, C. John. 1990. *The Rise and Fall of Childhood,* revised edition. New York: Vintage.

## II. RIGHTS OF CHILDREN

Since about 1970, philosophical interest in the rights of children has grown substantially. This growth owes much to the social upheavals of the 1960s and 1970s, especially the civil rights and women's movements, both of which employed the rhetoric of rights. When the plights of children, homosexuals, and the disabled began to be highlighted, it was natural that advocates for these groups also used the rhetoric of rights.

The invocation of rights in connection with children, however, predated the 1960s. In 1959 the United Nations General Assembly (1960) adopted a ten-principle *Declaration of the Rights of the Child*, itself a descendant of one adopted by the League of Nations in 1924.

### Why Rights?

Why do activists concerned with the lives of children attempt to protect children's interests by invoking the notion of rights? The key features of the rhetoric of basic rights are (1) that rights are entitlements, and (2) that they impose duties on others. To claim something as a fundamental right is to make the strongest kind of claim one can make; it is to claim that something is an entitlement, not a privilege—something it would be not merely inadvisable or regrettable, but wrong and unjust, to withhold. And, typically, if one person is the bearer of rights, some or all others are the bearers of obligations. In the case of basic rights, the responsibilities fall either on all others as individuals or on the government, which in the case of democracies means on individuals acting as representatives of the citizenry. This is easily seen in the cases of the rights of adults to free speech and to healthcare.

The rights to free speech and healthcare illustrate two broad classes of rights given a variety of names by theorists. These may be designated *option* rights and *welfare* rights respectively (Golding). The idea behind option rights is that there is a sphere of sovereignty within which the individual cannot be intruded upon by government, even for the greater good. This idea is at the heart of classical liberal theory. Option rights are rights to choose. For instance, although persons have the right to speak, they may remain silent if they wish. Welfare rights, on the other hand, are rights to direct provision of services, such as medical care, that meet a basic need.

Do both categories apply to children? The notion of option rights motivated children's rights activists who saw children as oppressed by adults. Psychologist Richard Farson stated, "Children, like adults, should have the right to decide the matters which affect them most directly. The issue of self-determination is at the heart of children's liberation" (p. 27). The authors of the United Nations *Declaration*, on the other hand, focused almost exclusively on welfare rights. For example:

> The child, for the full and harmonious development of his [*sic*] personality, needs love and understanding. He shall, wherever possible, grow up in the care and under the responsibility of his parents, and in any case in an atmosphere of affection and of moral and material security; a child of tender years shall not, save in exceptional circumstances, be separated from his mother. (United Nations, p. 113)

Although some children's advocates urge recognition of both option and welfare rights, the underlying rationales are quite different. While the rationale for according children option rights conceives of minor status itself as a disabling condition that ought to be removed, the rationale for welfare rights urges that various goods and services be provided to minors as minors.

Most sensible people would look askance at putting children, especially young children, on a par with adults, insofar as freedom to live as they wish is concerned. The notion of a protected sphere of autonomous decision making is closely linked to the presence of developed capacities for rational choice, capacities that usually are only potential in young children. It may well be that the development of autonomy is impeded when children are not permitted to exercise choices in their lives, but advocating that children be given some options is a far cry from asserting that children have the same rights as adults to live their lives as they please. Paternalism, the coercion of individuals for their own good, is odious only when those coerced are capable of exercising rational choice.

## Why Not Rights?

Rights discourse does have some limitations in the context of advocacy for children. An initial difficulty lies in identifying universal rights while taking account of the limited resources and diverse values of particular societies. It may not be possible in some countries to fulfill the universal right to grow up in an atmosphere of material security, due to lack of resources. A second difficulty is that alleged welfare rights may be in tension with each other—for example, the right of a child to grow up in material security and the right to love and understanding.

A danger of rights discourse derives from the fact that, taken literally, respect of children's rights may permit substantial intrusion into parents' lives. For example, should government agents monitor parents to make sure they provide their children with the love and understanding they need? A less obvious danger derives from the fact that some of a child's most important needs, such as the need for love, cannot be coerced. If love fails, must the child be taken from the parent and given to another who is known to love the child? It is apparent that the struggle for children's rights may have the potential of making parents and children into adversaries.

## Alternatives to Rights

Given children's vulnerability to abuse and neglect by immediate caregivers and by society at large, what ethical bases other than rights might serve to enhance children's welfare? Philosopher Onora O'Neill (1989) suggests that Immanuel Kant's notion of imperfect duty provides such a basis. An "imperfect" duty—the duty to contribute to charity is an illustration—differs from a "perfect" duty in the latitude allowed for fulfillment; toward whom and how much the duty requires is not specified. Thus, although we all have an obligation to help the next generation not only to survive but also to develop its capacities, we may meet this obligation in different ways—some as parents, some as professional caregivers, some as taxpaying citizens. The idea is attractive philosophically, but it admittedly lacks the

precision, and hence the force, of the language of rights. Since the precise nature of the duty cannot be specified, it will be difficult to determine when people have or have not done enough to help needy children.

Another stream of ethical reasoning centers on character and virtue. So-called virtue ethics takes the focus away from whether particular acts are obligatory, permitted, or forbidden, and explores the notion of a good or virtuous person, a notion it alleges is fundamental. Proponents of virtue ethics would say, for example, that the idea of a virtuous or good mother cannot be reduced to that of a mother who performs or refrains from performing specific actions viewed as duties. A decided advantage of virtue ethics is that it encourages us to ask a key question: What legal and economic structures are conducive to "good parenting"? Virtuous parents, for example, take time to be with their children, especially when they are ill, but such virtuous actions will be more likely if employed parents enjoy legal protection against punitive actions by employers for their taking family leave.

Unlike the children's rights approach, which may pit parents against children, this approach does not put parents on the defensive. But virtue ethics also has theoretical difficulties, chief of which is defining character traits in ways that do justice to the diverse cultural ideals present in a heterogeneous population like that of the United States. Everyone will agree that virtuous parents, for example, need to teach their children to distinguish right from wrong, but may they use corporal punishment in the process? Here, consensus will break down. Another limitation of the approach is that virtue ethics has little to say about what precisely is owed to, or what ought to be done for, children whose primary caregivers have already failed them.

Care ethics, a variant of virtue ethics, is utterly antithetical to the Kantian emphasis on general principles and the development of rational agency. Deriving primarily from the work of feminist psychologists and philosophers, this approach takes close personal relationships, such as that between mother and child, as a model for all moral relations. Emphasis is placed on the need for compassion and empathy in the context of relationships to particular others in concrete settings, rather than on allegiance to abstract principles. Parents, for example, often succeed in meeting the needs of their children because they can empathize with them in particular situations; no abstract duty to care for one's children needs to be evoked. The ethic of care counters a philosophical focus on rationality as the defining essence of humanity.

Is care ethics sufficient to meet the needs of all children? For example, should affluent citizens provide funds for intensive professional care of babies born with drug addictions, babies they never will meet? If the answer to such a question is yes, then the notion of duty may provide a more secure basis for persuading people that such contributions are obligatory, since emotional identification with those one does not know is likely to be weak.

If both justice and care are regarded as virtues, then virtue ethics may have the potential to offer moral grounds for the protection and care of all children. Whether such a reconciliation of alternative approaches is possible remains an open question. If it is not possible, then philosophical ethics offers a number of lenses through which to view the status of children. As in the case of actual lenses, however, there may be no single lens that fits all purposes.

FRANCIS SCHRAG (1995)
BIBLIOGRAPHY REVISED

SEE ALSO: *Abuse, Interpersonal: Child Abuse; Adoption; Feminism; Family and Family Medicine; Human Rights; Infanticide; Infants, Public Policy and Legal Issues; Justice; Natural Law; Pediatrics, Adolescents; Research Policy: Subjects;* and other *Children* subentries

### BIBLIOGRAPHY

Aiken, William, and LaFollette, Hugh, eds. 1980. *Whose Child? Children's Rights, Parental Authority, and State Power.* Totowa, NJ: Littlefield, Adams.

Farson, Richard E. 1974. *Birthrights.* New York: Macmillan.

Freeden, Michael. 1991. *Rights.* Minneapolis: University of Minnesota Press.

Golding, Martin P. 1968. "Towards a Theory of Human Rights." *Monist* 52(4): 521–549.

Houlgate, Laurence D. 1980. *The Child and the State: A Normative Theory of Juvenile Rights.* Baltimore: Johns Hopkins University Press.

Kruschwitz, Robert B., and Roberts, Robert C., eds. 1987. *The Virtues: Contemporary Essays on Moral Character.* Belmont, CA: Wadsworth.

Noddings, Nel. 1984. *Caring: A Feminine Approach to Ethics and Moral Education.* Berkeley: University of California Press.

O'Neill, Onora. 1989. "Children's Rights and Children's Lives." In her *Constructions of Reason: Explorations of Kant's Practical Philosophy,* pp. 187–205. Cambridge, Eng.: Cambridge University Press.

O'Neill, Onora, and Ruddick, William, eds. 1979. *Having Children: Philosophical and Legal Reflections on Parenthood.* New York: Oxford University Press.

United Nations. General Assembly. 1960. *Declaration of the Rights of the Child: Adopted by the General Assembly of the United Nations, New York, November 20, 1959.* London: H.M.S.O.

## III. HEALTHCARE AND RESEARCH ISSUES

Access to good parenting, food, housing, and sanitation is the primary method for enhancing children's well-being and opportunities. The consensus that children also should have basic healthcare and social services grew throughout the twentieth century. Initially, advocates for better health and social care for impoverished, neglected, abused, and exploited children included those active in the women's rights movement, the newly recognized specialty of pediatrics, and the visiting home-health nursing programs. As the century progressed, lawyers and social scientists joined the reform movement, attacking the long-dominant views that children are the property of their parents or guardians and that the state has no authority to intervene even if children are abused or neglected.

Children gained rights to certain medical services and the right to be protected from abuse, poverty, neglect, and exploitation; adolescents gained liberties such as the right to consent to some kinds of treatments or services without parental approval or notification (Holder, 1985, 1989). Scientists helped transform children's programs through studies of children's growth, development, needs, experiences, illnesses, and perspectives, showing the importance of candor and respect for children's views. A distinctive feature of advocacy for improved health and social care for children can be summarized as follows: Others make most decisions for minors in terms of their personal care and the allocation of funds for children's programs.

Moral disputes about healthcare for children will be discussed under four headings: Who should make decisions for children? How should those decisions be made? When should children be enrolled as research subjects? How much of society's healthcare funds should be allocated to children's programs?

### Basic Moral Values

Different solutions to these questions are evaluated herein in terms of basic moral values: Solutions are judged to be superior when they fairly promote children's well-being and opportunities to flourish and help children become empowered, self-fulfilled persons who can develop their potential. The United Nations *Declaration of the Rights of the Child* (United Nations General Assembly) endorsed these basic values, underscoring their wide acceptance.

These values received international support because most adults want to help children and recognize their responsibility to assist them. They also promote stability by helping address inequalities of the "natural lottery" (inequalities caused by nature, such as health status) and the "social lottery" (inequalities caused by social factors, such as wealth, schooling, and family). Children are not responsible for those inequalities, yet they affect whether children will thrive and flourish. Adequate healthcare and social services enhance children's well-being and opportunities by treating diseases, in some cases returning children from the brink of death or permanent disability to full and healthy lives. These services also restore or maintain compromised function, avert or ameliorate suffering, and prevent disease or disabilities through interventions or counseling. Basic prevention, diagnosis, treatment, rehabilitation, and social services not only make children's lives better, they provide society with healthier and more productive citizens.

The focus of this discussion is primarily on preadolescent children, who clearly are not responsible for their quality of life or its inequities and who need help in making prudent decisions.

## Who Has the Authority to Decide for Children?

Adults are presumed competent and minors incompetent to consent to medical treatment or participation in research. Minors generally lack the capacity, maturity, foresight, and experience to make important choices for themselves and cannot determine which choices will promote their well-being or opportunities. In general, the younger and less experienced the child, the greater the presumption that he or she cannot participate competently in healthcare decisions but the trend is to include children as young as five years old. Many older children, especially adolescents, clearly overturn this presumption that they cannot participate.

SHARED DECISION MAKING. Ideally, important healthcare choices should represent a consensus among parents, doctors, nurses, and the child if he or she is mature enough and willing to participate. Together they find the option best suited to the child and the family (U.S. President's Commission, 1982). In the final analysis, however, parents or guardians generally have legal and moral authority to make medical decisions for minor children.

PARENTS' OR GUARDIANS' AUTHORITY. Parents and guardians have the authority to make healthcare decisions for the same general reasons they can select their children's religion and schooling. The philosophers Allen Buchanan and Dan Brock (1989) discuss several reasons for this policy. First, parents and guardians are generally most knowledgeable about and interested in their children and so are most likely to do the best job for them. Second, the family usually bears the consequences of the choices that are made for a child. Some choices and their consequences suit certain families better than others. Third, children learn values and standards within their families, and different values and standards may lead to different healthcare choices. Within limits it is important to honor the standards and values of families because it is primarily in the family structure that people in society learn values. Fourth, families need intimacy with minimal state intrusion. Thus, unless a child is placed at risk, there is reason to tolerate the choices that families make for their children and give families wide discretion in selecting children's healthcare.

Parents or guardians maintain this authority as long as they promote the well-being and opportunities of those under their care and prevent, remove, or minimize harms to their minor children. Their authority can be contested, however (Rodham; Holder, 1985; Kopelman, 1997). Moral disputes over when to challenge parental authority to make healthcare decisions often center on practical and theoretical issues about when harms or dangers to children warrant interfering with parental authority and what restrictions on parental choice are needed to secure a child's well-being.

Parents who abuse, neglect, or exploit their children may lose custody of them temporarily or permanently. Physical, sexual, or emotional abuse inflicted on children constitutes grounds for the loss of parental authority. In addition, parents who make imprudent or neglectful decisions may lose custody temporarily or permanently. For example, parents may lose custody temporarily if they endanger a child by declining standard antibiotic care to treat the child's bacterial meningitis, preferring the use of herbal teas. Parents also may lose custody temporarily if they endanger a child by acting on certain beliefs. For example, Christian Scientists object to surgery and Jehovah's Witnesses object to blood transfusions, yet courts can order either intervention if a child is endangered (Holder, 1985; Rodham; Kopelman, 1997). Because children cannot protect themselves, healthcare professionals, teachers, neighbors, and other members of the community have a duty to report suspected child abuse, neglect, or exploitation to state agencies for investigation. When parental acts or omissions pose an imminent danger to children, doctors, nurses, hospital administrators, and social workers have a moral and legal duty to seek a court order for proper care (Holder, 1985; Kopelman, 1997).

CHILDREN'S ASSENT AND CAPACITY Decisions about when to consult or inform children about their healthcare options usually are important for older children and those with serious illnesses in cases in which distinct choices result in different outcomes. Some, but not all, children want to understand the decisions about their healthcare and often have an opinion about their care (Buchanan and Brock; Holmes; Matthews). Moreover, adolescents do not always need parental consent to obtain services such as treatment for substance abuse, abortion, and contraception (Holder, 1985, 1989).

This trend toward informing or consulting children stems from several sources. First, it results from research about what children of different ages and stages of development can understand. Social-science research has found that many children understand a great deal about their diseases and even their imminent death (Bluebond-Langner). They sense when people are not truthful, and this can cause them to suffer by feeling isolated from discussions, decisions, and support (Bluebond-Langner; Matthews).

When children have capacity and are prepared appropriately, truthfulness usually has good consequences by promoting cooperation and enhancing trust in their caretakers. Truthfulness also can foster decision-making abilities and maturity. When children have life-threatening or chronic illnesses, it may be especially important to them to gain some control over their lives and some respect for their views. For those facing death, opportunities to become self-fulfilled and self-determining persons may be restricted to choices about how they will live their last months.

Second, this trend stems from an understanding that capacity is task-related. In assessing ability the question must be asked: Capacity for what? People are capable of doing some things and not others and thus may have the capacity to make some healthcare decisions but not others (Buchanan and Brock; Faden et al.; Kopelman, 1990; Matthews; U.S. President's Commission, 1982). An eleven-year-old child with cancer may understand a great deal about the illness because he or she has had experiences beyond those of most eleven-year-old children. Consequently, the child may be better able than most children of the same age to understand or participate in healthcare decisions.

Children are increasingly able to participate in healthcare decisions as they become better able to understand and reason about their options and life plans. Although young children cannot do this, some adolescents may be capable as most adults in these respects (Holmes).

In recent literature *competent* and *incompetent* are used as legal categories. The presumption is that unless the courts decide otherwise, adults are legally competent and minors are not. In reality, many legally competent adults lack decision-making capacity and many older minors are as capable as most adults. For the purpose of healthcare, decision-making capacity concerns the individual's ability to understand and appreciate the information needed to make informed decisions, evaluate that information in terms of stable personal values, and be able to use and manipulate the information in a reasonable way (Applebaum and Roth; Buchanan and Brock; Kopelman, 1990). To decide whether minors have the capacity to participate in important healthcare decisions, adults should assess how well children can understand the information, deliberate, appreciate the situation, and make, defend, and communicate choices. In addition, it is important to determine whether a minor has reasonable and stable personal values. The more they have such abilities, the more they should participate.

Many authors favor a sliding scale to determine whether a person is capable of making medical decisions (Applebaum and Roth; Kopelman, 1990). The lower the probability and the magnitude of the risk of harm from the decision, the less the need to scrutinize the decision-making capacity of the person giving consent. However, the greater the probability and the risk of harm from the decision, the higher the level of scrutiny that the decision is rational. The reasoning of parents who refuse chemotherapy for a child with cancer, for example, has to be assessed very carefully.

## How Should Decisions Be Guided?

There are four important standards for healthcare decision making:

1. The first standard—self-determination—applies primarily to the voluntary decisions of legally competent and informed adults who make their own choices about their well-being and opportunities as long as they do not harm or violate the rights of others. As minors become more mature, they should be accorded more self-determination, but their preferences need not be honored as are those of adults (Holder, 1985, 1989). An adolescent with cancer who insists that he or she would rather die than lose a leg needs help to understand that reaction. The degree of irreversibility and the severity of the consequences often determine whether a minor's preferences should be honored. Minors' choices generally become more morally binding on adults when minors show that they understand and appreciate the nature of the situation in relation to their life goals. Adult guidance is needed when minors cannot demonstrate that their choices enhance their well-being and opportunities.

2. Like some adults, older children may prepare advance directives about their healthcare choices if they become incapacitated. Although a minor's choice need not be honored in the same way as an adult's decision, it may be an important consideration or seem morally binding in some circumstances. Dying children may, for example, indicate that they wish to donate organs or plan their funerals. Parents may want to follow such instructions carefully out of respect to the child's wishes.

3. A third standard—substituted judgment—applies to someone who once was able to express preferences. In using this standard, people select the option they believe the person would choose if he or she were able. Families often know their relatives well enough to predict the choices their relatives would have made. Children, especially those with serious or chronic illnesses, also may express general preferences that should guide parental choices. One child who was very sick insisted that he did not want to be maintained in a persistent vegetative state (PVS) "like a zombie."

4. The best-interest standard applies to those who do not have the ability or authority to make decisions for themselves. This standard maintains that decision makers should try to identify a person's immediate and long-term interests and then determine whether the benefits of an intervention or procedure outweigh the burdens. This does not mean that they seek what is absolutely best, because that may be impossible (the best doctor cannot treat everyone), but that they seek the best among the available options. This standard permits complex judgments about what on balance is likely to be best for an individual in light of the available options (Buchanan and Brock; Kopelman, 1993, 1997). For example, the benefit of obtaining a long and healthy life would outweigh the burden of enduring intense pain for a short time. The best-interest standard, however, might be used by parents, doctors, and nurses to withhold or withdraw maximal life-support treatment from children who have intense and chronic pain, with no prospects of improvement or foreseeable pleasures, understanding, or capacities for interaction.

In some cases objectively or intersubjectively confirmable estimates about pain and a well-understood prognosis force parents and doctors to choose between preserving biological life and providing comfort. Some children live in considerable discomfort from the technologies that keep them alive, such as a gastrostomy (a tube through which food goes directly into the stomach), intravenous lines, ventilators (breathing machines), long stays in intensive-care units, and a tracheotomy (a hole in the throat that aids breathing).

One goal of medicine, which should be balanced against others, is to preserve and prolong biological life. Since ancient times this ideal has been understood to mean that one ought to prevent untimely death. However, a question remains regarding the best interests of a person whose life is continued by means of maximal treatment that is a burden to that person (U.S. President's Commission, 1983; Buchanan and Brock; Kopelman, 1993). In cases where doctors and others disagree about what is best, it is hard to apply the best-interest standard. In such situations and for the general reasons discussed above, which give parents wide discretion when doctors disagree about what is best, an established legal and moral consensus using the best-interest standard allows parents to choose from options advanced as best (Buchanan and Brock; Holder, 1985, 1989; U.S. President's Commission, 1982, 1983).

The best-interest standard was challenged by President Ronald Reagan (1986) and Surgeon General C. Everett Koop (1989), who believed that quality-of-life considerations were likely to be abused. Under their influence the federal government in 1984 amended its child-abuse laws and adopted the so-called Baby Doe guidelines ("Child Abuse and Neglect," 1985). These rules forbid withholding or withdrawing lifesaving care from a sick infant unless the child is dying or is in an irreversible coma or when treatment is both virtually futile in terms of survival and inhumane. To forgo lifesaving treatments it is not sufficient that the treatment be inhumane or gravely burdensome, as it would be in the Roman Catholic tradition. Suffering cannot be taken into account except when the child cannot survive even with maximal treatment (Kopelman, 1989a, 1993).

The Baby Doe rules are controversial because they radically restrict parental discretion and standard medical practice. In a 1988 survey U.S. neonatologists indicated that the use of this policy for judging when to withdraw or withhold care for infants would result in overtreatment, poor use of resources, and insufficient attention to suffering (Kopelman et al., 1988).

Defenders maintain that properly understood, the best-interest standard is a useful way to protect children and others who are incompetent (Kopelman, 1997). For example, the U.S. President's Commission states, "This is a very strict standard in that it excludes considerations of the negative effects of an impaired child's life on other persons, including parents, siblings and society" (U.S. President's Commission, 1983, p. 219).

Allen Buchanan and Dan Brock (1989) argue that quality-of-life assessments are not open to abuse if they are limited to judgments about what is best for the individual patient. The courts and others who reject such judgments made on behalf of incompetent people, they argue, do not distinguish two kinds of quality-of-life judgments. Quality of life judgments based on considerations of social worth try to weigh the interests or value of a person's life against the interests or value of other people's lives; they are comparative. In contrast, noncomparative quality of life judgments try to consider the value of the life to the person, comparing the value of living the individual's life to having no life at all. Although this comparison is difficult to make, it can be guided by choices made by competent adults who decide that there are worse things than death, including certain burdensome treatments to keep them alive. Buchanan and Brock (1989) hold that in applying the best-interest standard one should use noncomparative estimates, contemplating only the quality of life for that individual; a person's social value should not be part of the assessment. Noncomparative quality-of-life judgments, then, should be circumscribed very carefully and strictly. It is possible to reflect, for example, on whether most people would want to live such a life.

To some extent the effectiveness of the best-interest standard relies on the degree of social consensus about what is best for children and other persons who lack decision-making capacity. Consequently, it is hard to use in cases in which there is sustained disagreement, as there may be about when and how to use quality-of-life considerations. Arguably, one cannot avoid quality-of-life decisions entirely. For example, the Baby Doe regulations state that one need not provide maximal treatment to those who are permanently comatose, and that is a quality-of-life judgment. The debate also concerns what discretion should be given to parents, physicians, and other clinicians to select the best available option.

Kopelman (1997) has argued that some of the criticisms of the best-interest standard stem from confusing its different meanings. First, it is used as an ideal. For a child to receive a very scarce resource for a marginal benefit may be ideal yet unreasonable once one considers the claims and needs of others and the available resources. Nonetheless, it is important to consider what might be ideal for a child in framing what should be done in light of others' needs and the available resources. Ideals are also important in giving direction to people's efforts. The ideal of no children being abused or neglected gives direction to advocates for children.

Second, the best-interest standard is used in the sense of what is best given the options or what is best all things considered. For example, it may not be possible to give each child ideal healthcare, but it may be realistic to seek basic healthcare for all children. Another example is that some parents are not ideal guardians, but the state does not step in unless their children are endangered. If parents refuse lifesaving healthcare for children, the courts may remove custody from the parents temporarily or permanently; they then may use the best-interest standard to seek what is best for the child given the available options. They are not seeking what is ideal, because that may not be realistic, but what is best, all things considered, for the child given the available options.

## Children as Research Subjects

Children are not responsible for their illnesses. The natural and social lotteries leave some children with diminished opportunities as a result of illness. Good health and social services may be essential to give these children a chance to flourish and develop their potential as self-fulfilled and self-determining persons. In addition, good healthcare helps children by preventing many illnesses and allows for early diagnosis and treatment. Good healthcare, however, is the product of study and research, and the problem is how research should be conducted to help children.

The ethical basis for research policy with children concerns promoting the same primary values that shape treatment decisions: enhancing well-being and opportunities. Because many children, like adults severely impaired with mental illness or retardation, lack the capacity to give informed consent, they are regarded as vulnerable research subjects. Like policy regarding treatment, research policy with children is shaped by different authority principles (who decides) and guidance principles (substantive directions about how decisions should be made). There is, however, an additional problem.

Pediatric research regulations and policy must deal with a dilemma: With too few protections, children selected as subjects may be exploited. If the regulations impose too many protections, however, it may become so difficult to conduct research that the knowledge base for making good decisions for children will erode. Different policy options try to solve this dilemma but do so differently:

1. The *surrogate* or *libertarian* solution allows the same sort of research with children as with other subjects if the parents consent. This solution may not offer adequate protection to children because it permits parents to enroll them in potentially harmful research even if it holds out no direct benefits to them. Parents' legal and moral authority presupposes the promotion of children's opportunities and well-being and the prevention, removal, or minimization of harms to them. Parents have no authority to enroll their children in potentially harmful research that hold out no benefits to them. Volunteering to put another person in harm's way may violate a guardian's protective role.

2. The *no consent–no research* or *Nuremberg* solution excludes children because children are not considered competent to give informed consent to being enrolled as research subjects. This view, expressed in the Nuremberg Code (Germany [Territory under Allied Occupation], 1947), seems too restrictive. It prohibits enrolling a child in a study even if the project could benefit the child directly. Moreover, to test the efficacy of treatments for distinctive groups, some members of those groups must be subjects. Competent, normal adults cannot serve as subjects in projects that test children's growth or maturity, drugs for premature infants, and treatments for children's life-threatening asthma.

3. The "risk-benefit" solution allows research with children if it benefits them directly or does not place them at unwarranted risk of harm, discomfort, or inconvenience. To balance the social utility of research with respect for and protection of children, this option stipulates that the greater the risk, the more rigorous and elaborate the procedural protection and consent requirements. Many countries, such as the United States, Canada, the United Kingdom, South Africa, Australia, and Norway, in addition to international organizations such as the World Health Organization in its *Declaration of Helsinki* and the Council for the International Organizations of Medical Science, favor this solution. Research should be approved by local boards known variously as institutional review boards (IRBs) ethical research committees (ERCS), or research ethics committees (RECs) and in some cases by federal boards as well. Approval is based on findings that subjects have been selected fairly and that the risks to them are minimized and reasonable in relation to the anticipated benefits of the study ("Protection of Human Subjects," 1993). Adequate provisions also must be made for the safety and confidentiality of subjects. Investigators must seek parents' informed consent. When possible, they also must obtain the child's assent, where assent means a positive agreement, not merely failure to refuse. Children's refusals are not binding when their parents and doctors judge that it is in their interests to participate, for example, in studies in which children may obtain a scarce resource to treat a deadly disease. This risk–benefit solution tries to determine whether the risks are proportional to the benefits for each individual and uses risk assessment to try to balance the social utility of encouraging studies that maintain respect for and protection of children's rights and welfare.

Using a likely harms-to-benefit calculation, U.S. regulations ("Protection of Human Subjects," 1993), as outlined below, specify four categories of research with children. As the risks increase, the regulations require increasingly more rigorous documentation of appropriate parental consent, children's assent, direct benefits to the child, or benefits to children with similar conditions. Local IRBs can approve studies only in the first three categories.

The first category of research permits research with no greater than a minimal risk provided that it makes adequate provisions for parental consent and children's assent. Many important studies are safe, such as asking children to perform simple and pleasant tasks. Using this category, investigators might gain approval to study at what ages preschool children can name colors, identify animals, and perform simple tasks such as stacking blocks on request.

The second category of research permits the approval of studies with greater than a minimal risk if (1) the risk is justified by the anticipated benefit to each subject; (2) the risks in relation to these benefits are at least as favorable to each subject as are the available alternatives; and (3) provisions are made for parental consent and the child's assent. This category permits a child to get an investigational drug that is available only in a research study. Moreover, because children have unique diseases and reactions, to study the safety and efficacy of many conventional, innovative, or investigational treatments for children, some children have to serve as subjects in controlled testing.

The third category of research permits research (1) with a minor increase over minimal risk that holds out no prospect of direct benefit to the individual subject; (2) in cases in which the study is like the child's actual or expected medical, dental, psychological, or educational situation; (3) in cases in which the study is likely to result in very important information about the child's disorder or condition; and (4) in cases in which provisions are made for parental consent and the child's assent. In using this category, investigators have been permitted to perform additional lumbar punctures on children with leukemia, who get them anyway, to help study that disease.

Research that cannot be approved under the first three categories may sometimes be approved if (1) it presents a reasonable opportunity to understand, prevent, or alleviate a serious problem affecting the health or welfare of children; and (2) the study is approved by the secretary of the U.S. Department of Health and Human Services (DHHS) after consultation with a panel of experts about the value and ethics of the study and determination that adequate provisions have been made for public comment, parental consent, and the child's assent. In using this category investigators might gain approval to conduct studies to prevent or treat epidemics affecting children, such as the acquired immune deficiency syndrome (AIDS) epidemic, or a new infectious disease like the killers of the past (pneumonia, scarlet fever, diphtheria, and polio).

**DIFFICULTIES.** Unfortunately, the risk–benefit solution leaves key terms undefined or poorly defined, allowing different interpretations concerning when risks of harm are warranted and what constitutes a benefit (Freedman et al.; Kopelman, 2000, 2002; National Bioethics Advisory Commission [NBAC]). For example, consider the pivotal concepts of a "minimal risk" and a "minor increase over minimal risk." The federal rules state: "*Minimal risk* means that the probability and magnitude of harm or discomfort anticipated in the research are not greater in and of themselves than those ordinarily encountered in daily life or during the performance of routine physical and psychological examinations or tests" ("Protection of Human Subjects," 1993, section 102i). The first part of the definition focuses on everyday risks, and the second on routine examinations. (Interestingly, the National Bioethics Advisory Commision [2001] recommended dropping the second part of the definition in favor of the more permissive first part, whereas the Council for International Organizations of Medical Science [CIOMS] omits the first [Council for International Organizations of Medical Science, 2002].)

Kopelman has argued that this definition is morally and conceptually problematic, especially the part using "everyday risk": First, how should people establish thresholds for the probability and magnitude of harm used to identify everyday risks, and even if they solve this problem, why are everyday risks morally relevant for determining acceptable research risk? People's daily risks may include car accidents and terriorist attacks. Is it possible to know the nature, probability, and magnitude of these everyday hazards well enough that they could serve as a baseline to estimate morally acceptable research risks for children? It seems easier to determine that a study asking children to stack blocks is a morally acceptable, minimal-risk study than to estimate the nature, probability, and magnitude of whatever risks of harm people normally encounter.

Second, given the different hazards in different countries and communities, what locale or locales should be used to assess everyday risks in determining morally acceptable research? Some favor a relative standard by which minimal risk is judged against the background of the children's location, environment or condition. Others reject this "relativistic" standard in favor of an absolute standard, saying that all children should have the same standard; otherwise one reaches morally abhorrent conclusions such as that more risks can be taken with children in dangerous neighborhoods than with children in safe and affluent neighborhoods.

Third, why should everyday risks of harm be regarded as morally relevant for determining that research risks are minimal when some everyday risks are great?

Fourth, if this is a useful and clear standard, why has there been sustained disagreement over whether common procedures should be viewed as having a minimal risk, a minor increase over minimal risk, or greater risk? Since the regulations appeared decades ago, there have been sustained and substantive differences among pediatric experts in both treatment and research settings about how to assess the risk of procedures such as venipuncture, arterial puncture, and gastric and intestinal intubation (Janofsky and Starfield). Investigators and others concluded that better standards of risk assessment in children's research had to be formulated (Janofsky and Starfield; Lascari; National Bioethics Advisory Commission; Kopelman, 2002).

In addition, the U.S. regulatory definition of minimal risk offers little guidance about how to assess psychosocial risks such as breach of confidentiality, stigmatization, labeling, and invasion of privacy. Risks are allegedly minimal if they are encountered ordinarily in daily life or during routine examinations. Doctors, nurses, and psychologists, however, "ordinarily encounter" many psychosocially sensitive discussions in routine examinations and testing, including those about family abuse, substance abuse, sexual preference, and diagnoses, any of which could affect how people are viewed or whether they will be able to get jobs or buy insurance. Moreover, psychosocial-risk assessment is an increasingly difficult problem. Some genetic and other testing has low physical risks, such as taking a drop of blood, but high psychosocial risks. For example, Huntington disease is a genetic condition that causes progressive dementia and loss of motor function typically when the person becomes an adult. A person known to have this condition could be denied a job or insurance or be stigmatized in the community. Thinking of risks of harm as merely physical ignores such profound psychosocial risks.

Moreover, there is no definition of "a minor increase over minimal risk," the upper limit of risk that many review boards can approve. The courts have begun to consider what risks of harm are permissible and may help standardize interpretations (Kopelman, 2002).

Even when it is agreed that the ethical basis for research policies with children is to promote their opportunities, well-being, fair treatment, and self-determination, it is difficult to articulate policies that balance the need to protect children and the need to gain knowledge. If research is not conducted with children as subjects, children may be denied the benefits of advances stemming from research and good information about which procedures or interventions promote health and prevent, treat, or diagnose disease. However, if children are enrolled as research subjects, vulnerable individuals who cannot give informed consent are being used.

## Resource Allocation

Many children do not receive basic healthcare or social services. In some cases, countries that can afford to provide those services allocate insufficient funds for them. For example, the main health problems of children in the United States arise from failure to provide such basic care for children's allergies, asthma, dental pathology, hearing loss, vision impairment, and chronic disorders (Starfield; Newachecket et al.). Basic healthcare and social services promote children's well-being, enhancing their opportunities in fundamental ways and correcting some inequities caused by the natural and social lotteries. Children who are sick cannot compete as equals and thus lack equality of opportunity with other children. The more these conditions are easily correctable, as many of them are, the more unjust it is to leave children sick or disabled. Failure to provide children with basic healthcare and social services when a society has sufficient means is unjust on the basis of any of four important theories of justice: utilitarianism, egalitarianism, libertarianism, and contractarianism. This point of agreement among widely divergent positions serves as a powerful indictment and proof that as a matter of justice goods, services, and benefits should be redistributed more fairly to children to provide them with basic healthcare and social services.

Four theories of justice offer different guidance about how to allocate goods, services, and benefits. Proponents have used them to determine children's fair share of healthcare funding in relation to adults (intergenerational allocation) and ways to set priorities for funding within children's healthcare programs (intragenerational allocation). Each theory addresses what kinds of benefits, goods, and services should be provided to people as a matter of justice and how to choose from among programs when not all can be funded. Although there are many variations of these positions, each seeks a defensible standard to help make choices fairly.

UTILITARIANISM. Utilitarianism offers one solution to the problem of allocating healthcare justly between generations and among children's programs. In a well-known version, the philosopher John Stuart Mill (1863) argued that a just allocation provides the greatest good to the greatest number of people; the utility of following principles of justice is so great that these are among the most fundamental moral

principles. People should not consider only the utility of isolated acts, Mill maintained, but also the rules of conduct that, if adopted and adhered to, maximize utility. Actions are right insofar as they fall under such a rule.

In their efforts to maximize utility for the greatest number in accordance with just rules, utilitarians seek to prevent or cure the most common illnesses, adopt programs that help many rather than few persons, and use funds where they will have the greatest impact for the most people. For example, utilitarians would resist funding expensive organ transplantations that help relatively few persons for a short time if those transplantations sidetracked programs that could help many people.

Some of the least expensive and most beneficial interventions are education about the benefits of exercise, a good diet, prevention of teenage pregnancy, and avoidance of alcohol, tobacco, and harmful drugs (U.S. Department of Health and Human Services). Relatively inexpensive interventions can aid in the treatment of many problems common in childhood, including vision impairment, hearing loss, dental pathology, allergies, and asthma, as well as the variety of chronic disorders that cause considerable functional impairment (Starfield; Newachecket et al.). Utilitarians favor providing such healthcare for children because it greatly increases their well-being and opportunities. It is socially useful and cost-effective because it can prevent costly illnesses and benefit the current generation of adults, who, when aged, will need support from a healthy, stable, and productive work force.

Utilitarians might even favor preferential consideration of children. Interventions that benefit both children and adults generally offer children the most years of benefit. Those added years increase the net good and thus could justify some preference toward children. For example, in some countries children receive dental care that is unavailable to adults because it has lifelong benefits and prevents costly future problems. Daniel Callahan (1987, 1990) believes that the young have a stronger claim to healthcare than the old and should be given priority; the healthcare system should see as its first task helping young people become old people and help older people become still older only if money is available. He argues, moreover, that medicine should give its highest priority to the relief of suffering rather than the conquest of death.

In choosing among children's programs for funding, defenders of utilitarianism assess the net benefit for the community of children. A utilitarian would favor funding routine care, mass screening, and prevention programs that help many children rather than the development of costly therapies that help few children. Consequently, utilitarians probably would resist using state funds to give otherwise normal short children growth hormone for many years, at a cost of many thousands of dollars a year, to increase minimally their adult height. Utilitarians, however, might permit private insurance or payment (in a multitiered healthcare system) for these and other services if it increased or did not diminish the net good.

Defenders of utilitarianism presuppose that it is possible to calculate what is best for the greatest number, but critics question that presumption (Brock). Moreover, critics state, whole groups could be excluded from beneficial healthcare for the sake of the common good, such as people with expensive or rare conditions and those with illnesses that are stigmatizing.

Utilitarians might respond that society would suffer from such exclusions, showing that this is not a good option even if one uses utilitarian calculations. This presupposes, however, that enough people would know about the exclusions and be distressed enough to alter the calculation. Sympathy for utilitarianism may depend on beliefs about whether it is possible to make utility calculations and whether a theory is acceptable if it permits people to exclude some groups for the common good regardless of the results of the utility calculation (see Brock). Defenders of rule utilitarianism, a version of utilitarianism that clarifies the role of rules in assessing utility, respond that, properly understood, utility prohibits unfair exclusions of individuals or groups; people adopt rights and justice principles because they are useful, and unjust exclusions undercut the utility of those rights and principles for all (Buchanan; Mill). Even if it is cost-effective or politically expedient to exclude a particular person or group, that exclusion undercuts something more important for all of us, namely, fair rules.

Utilitarians favor basic healthcare and social services for all children because of the utility to the children and to society. For example, suppose society could save a great deal of money by excluding certain children from healthcare services. Although this might save money in the short run, defenders of rule utilitarianism might argue that it is unjust because adapting and adhering to the rule that all should receive basic services are more useful in the long run than is excluding a few to save money. Accordingly, the rule that all children should receive basic care is vindicated because the rule is useful and making exceptions is less useful.

**EGALITARIANISM.** Egalitarianism is a theory of justice whose proponents attempt to solve allocation issues and intergenerational disputes by holding that access to the same benefits, goods, and services should be provided to everyone on the same basis. It is a principle of justice that requires society to try to make all people's objective net well-being or opportunities as equal as possible. Most people do not want dialysis because they do not have kidney disease, but people want access to dialysis if they should need it. Egalitarians, then, do not want exactly the same treatment for everyone as a condition of justice but want everyone to have access to the same goods, services, and benefits on the same footing.

Egalitarians look at outcomes of distribution schemes to determine whether distributions are fair. Accordingly, proponents of egalitarianism judge it to be unfair, for example, that adults over sixty-five can get diabetes and asthma treated free of charge in the United States but children cannot. Age might be a determinant in deciding who gets benefits, goods, and services, but only as one among other prognosticators of success. For example, people over eighty or under two years of age might be excluded from consideration for a certain type of surgery because they are unlikely to survive the procedure.

Defenders of egalitarianism hold that what is provided to one person should be available to all similarly situated persons. The advantages of good healthcare are such that in fairness they should be distributed on as equal a basis as possible. There should not be a multitiered system with one level of goods and services for the rich and another for the poor. If society allows some normal short children to have growth hormone for many years at a cost of thousands of dollars a year, all who are similarly situated should have access to similar services. For expensive or scarce resources, many egalitarians favor lotteries so that all those who are similarly situated have an equal opportunity and are recognized as having equal worth (Childress; Veatch). Consequently, if organs for transplantation can be provided only to some children, there should be a lottery among those who meet whatever standards are set. In this way people acknowledge the value of each person and the importance of fair access of all to scarce or costly benefits, goods, and services. One difficulty for egalitarians is that some people's needs are so great that they could consume most of the resources of a healthcare system. Robert Veatch (1986) tries to defend a commitment to those who are so disadvantaged that they could use unlimited resources while placing limits on their claims on other members of society.

In defending egalitarianism it is difficult to clarify what kind of equality is important. If it is *access* to the same benefits, goods, and services, age bias and discrimination could be introduced through preference for certain benefits, goods, and services. For example, treatment for prostatic hyperplasia and Alzheimer's disease helps only adults; other care helps adults much more than children, such as treatments for heart disease or lung cancer and treatments at the end of life. Some funding choices discriminate by excluding services equally and for all diseases afflicting people with stigmatizing conditions, such as sexually transmitted diseases. This parallels a problem of utilitarianism in which whole groups can be excluded if society decides, to save money, that none will have treatments for certain conditions.

If, however, equality is understood in terms of *outcomes* rather than access, age bias and discrimination also can be introduced through the method of collecting and presenting data (Starfield). In the United States, for example, data collection to determine the health of different populations focuses on life-threatening illnesses and death. Relatively few children have such morbidity or mortality in comparison to adults, giving the impression that children are generally healthy. This impression, however, is a consequence of how the data are collected. Most children's needs stem from problems that are not life-threatening illnesses but have a profound effect on health, such as dental problems, vision impairment, allergies, and asthma. Moreover, although the death rate of children in the United States is low compared with that of adults, it is the highest among equally affluent countries (Starfield). Looking at certain outcomes, then, promotes an unfair view of childhood health and morbidity. Programs based on such data can create unjust age bias against children. Thus, treating everyone as equals is problematic if the measures favor certain groups.

People's willingness to defend egalitarianism depends in part on whether they believe it is fair to restrict choices by insisting that no one can have healthcare that cannot be provided to all on the same basis. If people can squander their assets on entertainment and clothes, it seems unfair to insist that they cannot spend it on marginally beneficial, exotic, or expensive healthcare for their families. Some respond that rich people dread single-tiered systems because it means that they cannot have their usual advantages through money and forces them to live by the same rules as others. They argue that allocation of healthcare (especially in life-and-death situations) is too important to be left to unregulated personal choice and market forces. Some defenders of egalitarianism modify their view to permit people to use their discretionary resources as they wish.

**LIBERTARIANISM.** Libertarians generally agree that competent adults should not be forced to do anything by the state unless it prevents harm to third parties. Coercion is permissible to prevent theft, murder, physical abuse, and fraud; enforce contracts; and punish competent people for harming others (Buchanan). The best-known defender of this view, Robert Nozick (1974), follows the eighteenth-century philosopher John Locke in maintaining that people's right to their fairly obtained property is fundamental and determines the proper functions of the state and the moral interactions among individuals.

People are entitled to their holdings and may dispose of them as they wish, according to this view. They argue that the state should not redistribute people's wealth in accordance with a pattern of distribution that examines outcomes (such as utilitarianism and egalitarianism) or uses coercive measures to take people's holdings, and adults should be free to fashion social arrangements out of their ideas of compassion, justice, and solidarity (Engelhardt). People do not have a responsibility to be charitable, say libertarians, but acts of charity are praiseworthy and should be encouraged.

Libertarians hold that children's healthcare is the responsibility of their guardians, not the state. Market forces of supply and demand and choices about how to use their own money should shape the kind of healthcare people select for themselves and their children. If parents want to pay for special services such as growth hormones or repeated organ transplants, they should be permitted to do so. H. Tristram Engelhardt, Jr., argues that societies can decide morally who is entitled to healthcare of a certain kind within certain limitations. However, a society does not, for example, have "the moral authority to forbid consensual acts among agreeing adults, such as agreement to sell an organ" (Engelhardt, p. 10).

Sympathy for libertarianism depends on whether it is believed to offer enough protection for people, especially children and impoverished or incompetent adults. This view arguably benefits the wealthy and powerful; because most children are neither, it might create an age bias against children. Libertarians argue that competent adults should pay their own way, but when do people really do that? Typically, people's healthcare insurance gives them access to institutions heavily subsidized by public money. People who "pay their own way" may pay just a bit more for many more services. Those who cannot pay more are unfairly excluded. Libertarians might agree that separate institutions should be set up in which people truly pay their full share even if that would mean that few could afford such added care.

Libertarians usually favor special state protection for children, allowing the state to interfere with parents who endanger, neglect, or harm children. This can include providing children with a "safety net" of basic healthcare and social services. A system favoring special benefits based on redistribution of wealth for competent adults, however, is considered unjust. Hence, a system like that in the United States that provides many social and health benefits to competent and even wealthy adults but not to children, for example, in the allocation of healthcare benefits, goods, and services, would be viewed by libertarians as unjust.

**CONTRACTARIANISM.** Contractarians hold that distributions of social goods are fair when impartial people agree on the procedures used for distribution. The best-known defender of this position is John Rawls, who in *A Theory of Justice* (1971) and *Political Liberalism* (1993) contends that people form stable and just societies by building a consensus that merits endorsement by rational and informed people of goodwill.

This entails a commitment to three principles of justice. First, "each person is to have an equal right to the most extensive system of equal basic liberties compatible with a similar system compatible for all." Second, "offices and positions are to be open to all under conditions of equality of fair opportunity—persons with similar abilities and skills are to have equal access to offices and positions." Finally, "social and economic institutions are to be arranged so as to benefit maximally the worst off" (Rawls, 1971, p. 60). These principles are ordered lexically such that the first, the greatest equal-liberty principle, takes precedence over the others when they conflict and the second, the principle of fair equality of opportunity, takes precedence over the third, the difference principle. Nowhere is healthcare as a right mentioned specifically in Rawls's attempt to frame the basic structure of a just society. This is understandable because a society may not have enough healthcare goods, services, or benefits to distribute. In a society that does have such goods, services, and benefits, however, their fair distribution seems central to promoting fair equality of opportunity and benefits to the worst off.

Norman Daniels (1985), building on Rawls's work, argues that society should provide basic care to all but redistribute healthcare goods and services more favorably to children. The moral justification for giving children access to basic healthcare, argues Daniels, rests on a social commitment to what he and Rawls call "fair equality of opportunity" (or affirmative action). Healthcare needs are basic insofar as they promote fair equality of opportunity. Healthcare for children is especially important in relation to other social goods because diseases and disabilities inhibit children's capacity to use and develop their talents, thus curtailing their opportunities. For example, children cannot compete as equals if they are sick or cannot see or hear the teacher. Thus, a society committed to a fair equality of opportunity for children should provide adequate healthcare.

Daniels holds that to assess whose needs are greatest, people have to use objective ways of characterizing medical and social needs; the ranking of needs helps determine what is basic and who profits most from certain services. Using the difference principle, free, additional service might be provided to the poorest children to help level the playing field so that they could compete more effectively with those from more affluent homes. Unlike utilitarians, who would be guided by where money would have the greatest overall impact on the health of the greatest number of children, contractarians try to bring all children of similar talents to the same level of functioning so that they can compete as equals.

Contractarianism has certain difficulties. Some regard it as a method for arriving at ethical principles, not as an alternative to views such as utilitarianism, egalitarianism, and libertarianism (Veatch). Accordingly, those who think it generates a unique theory need to clarify how it has a distinct content. In addition, it is hard to specify what is meant by "people's normal opportunity ranges" or to decide how to apply fair equality of opportunity. This position seems to suggest (arguably similar to egalitarianism) the unsatisfactory consequence that people should fund treatments, however exotic and costly, that offer a chance for the most disadvantaged to improve their normal opportunity range irrespective of the needs of the many; gifted children could be denied opportunities to excel so that others could enhance their normal opportunity range or be brought to the level of well-being and opportunities of average children. Another problem is that contractarianism presupposes, like utilitarianism, that there is a fair and objective system for ranking medical and social needs and deciding who benefits most from services (Brock). It is unclear whether such a comprehensive and objective ranking is possible. Such "objective" choices about appropriate or useful programs might be mixed with social and personal biases. These problems, however, do not undermine the contractarians' commitment to the justice of equal opportunity for children, including the fairness of providing basic health and social care for children.

**A PROPOSED CONSENSUS.** Each of these theories of justice supports the claim that children are entitled to basic healthcare and social services to correct inequalities and promote their flourishing as free and self-determining people who can develop their potential. The fact that defenders of such divergent approaches agree on this entitlement reflects a consensus that children's distress ought to be relieved whether it is related to inadequate healthcare, poverty, abuse, neglect, malnutrition, or exploitation. A primary duty of a just society is to promote fairly its children's well-being and opportunities to become self-fulfilled persons through access to basic healthcare and social services and to address the inequities resulting from life's natural and social lotteries. Children living in low-income homes in the United States are two to three times as likely as children in high-income homes to be of low birth weight, get asthma and bacterial meningitis, have delayed immunizations, and suffer from lead poisoning. Poor children are also three to four times as likely as rich children to become seriously ill and get multiple illnesses when they become sick (Starfield).

The gap between the rich and the poor is increasing, and the rise of poverty is most rapid among children. Healthcare costs, driven higher by an aging population and increased demands for expensive technologies, will make it harder for societies to allocate costs justly. In addition, the AIDS epidemic has left many children sick, orphaned, or both, and many children live in the developing world, where resources that could help them are meager. Consequently, disputes involving intergenerational and intragenerational allocation from national and international funds are likely to continue as programs compete for funding. Because children depend on others to advocate for them, adults should continue to set aside their individual interests and consider children's well-being, needs, and opportunities as a matter of justice.

LORETTA M. KOPELMAN (1995)
REVISED BY AUTHOR

SEE ALSO: *Autonomy; Coercion; Competence; Research, Human: Historical Aspects; Students as Research Subjects; Surrogate Decision-Making;* and other *Children* subentries

### BIBLIOGRAPHY

Appelbaum, Paul S., and Roth, L. H. 1982. "Competency to Consent to Research: A Psychiatric Overview." *Archives of General Psychiatry* 39(8): 951–958.

Bluebond-Langner, Myra. 1978. *The Private Worlds of Dying Children.* Princeton, NJ: Princeton University Press.

Brock, Dan W. 1982. "Utilitarianism." In *And Justice for All: New Introductory Essays in Ethics and Public Policy,* ed. Tom Regan and Donald VanDeVeer. Totowa, NJ: Rowman and Allanheld.

Buchanan, Allen E. 1981. "Justice: A Philosophical Review." In *Justice and Health Care,* ed. Earl E. Shelp. Dordrecht, Netherlands: D. Reidel.

Buchanan, Allen E., and Brock, Dan W. 1989. *Deciding for Others: The Ethics of Surrogate Decisionmaking.* New York: Cambridge University Press.

Callahan, Daniel. 1987. "Terminating Treatment: Age as a Standard." *Hastings Center Report* 17(5): 21–25.

Callahan, Daniel. 1990. *What Kind of Life: The Limits of Medical Progress.* New York: Simon & Schuster.

"Child Abuse and Neglect Prevention and Treatment Program." 1985. *Federal Register* 50(72), April 15, pp. 14878–14892.

Childress, James F. 1970. "Who Shall Live When Not All Can Live?" *Soundings* 53: 339–354.

Daniels, Norman. 1985. *Just Health Care.* Cambridge, Eng., and New York: Cambridge University Press.

Engelhardt, H. Tristram, Jr. 1992. "The Search for a Universal System of Ethics: Post-Modern Disappointments and Contemporary Possibilities." In *Ethical Problems in Dialysis and Transplantation,* ed. Carl M. Kjellstrand and John B. Dossetor. Dordrecht, Netherlands: Kluwer.

Faden, Ruth R.; Beauchamp, Tom L.; and King, Nancy M. P. 1986. *History and Theory of Informed Consent.* New York: Oxford University Press.

Freedman, Benjamin; Fuks, Abraham; and Weijer, Charles. 1993. "In Loco Parentis: Minimal Risk as an Ethical Threshold for Research upon Children." *Hastings Center Report* 23(2): 13–19.

Germany (Territory under Allied Occupation, 1945–1955: U.S. Zone) Military Tribunals. 1947. "Permissible Medical Experiments." In *Trials of War Criminals before the Nuremburg Tribunals under Control Law No. 10,* vol. 2. Washington, D.C.: U.S. Government Printing Office.

Holder, Angela. 1985. *Legal Issues in Pediatrics and Adolescent Medicine,* 2nd edition. New Haven, CT: Yale University Press.

Holder, Angela. 1989. "Children and Adolescents: Their Right to Decide about Their Own Health Care." In *Children and Health Care: Moral and Social Issues,* ed. Loretta M. Kopelman and John C. Moskop. Dordrecht, Netherlands: Kluwer.

Holmes, Robert L. 1989. "Consent and Decisional Authority in Children's Health Care Decisionmaking: A Reply to Dan Brock." In *Children and Health Care: Moral and Social Issues,* ed. Loretta M. Kopelman and John C. Moskop. Dordrecht, Netherlands: Kluwer.

Janofsky, Jeffrey, and Starfield, Barbara. 1981. "Assessment of Risk in Research on Children." *Journal of Pediatrics* 98(5): 842–846.

Koop, C. Everett. 1989. "Mercy, Murder, and Morality: Perspectives on Euthanasia: The Challenge of Definition." *Hastings Center Report* 19(1) (special suppl., January–February): 2–3.

Kopelman, Loretta M. 1989a. "Charlotte the Spider, Socrates, and the Problem of Evil." In *Children and Health Care: Moral and Social Issues,* ed. Loretta M. Kopelman and John C. Moskop. Dordrecht, Netherlands: Kluwer.

Kopelman, Loretta M. 1989b. "When Is the Risk Minimal Enough for Children to Be Research Subjects?" In *Children and Health Care: Moral and Social Issues,* ed. Loretta M. Kopelman and John C. Moskop. Dordrecht, Netherlands: Kluwer.

Kopelman, Loretta M. 1990. "On the Evaluative Nature of Competency and Capacity Judgments." *International Journal of Law and Psychiatry* 13(4): 309–329.

Kopelman, Loretta M. 1993. "Do the 'Baby Doe' Rules Ignore Suffering?" *Second Opinion* 18(4): 101–113.

Kopelman, Loretta M. 1997. "The Best-Interests Standard as Threshold, Ideal, and Standard of Reasonableness." *Journal of Medicine and Philosophy* 22(3): 271–289.

Kopelman, Loretta M. 2000. "Children as Research Subjects: A Dilemma." *Journal of Medicine and Philosophy,* Millennium Issue, 25(6): 745–764.

Kopelman, Loretta M. 2002. "Pediatric Research Regulations under Legal Scrutiny: *Grimes* Narrows Their Interpretation." *Journal of Law, Medicine and Ethics* 30: 38–49.

Kopelman, Loretta M.; Irons, Thomas G.; and Kopelman, Arthur E. 1988. "Neonatologists Judge the 'Baby Doe' Regulations." *New England Journal of Medicine* 318(11): 677–683.

Lascari, Andre D. 1981. "Risks of Research in Children." *Journal of Pediatrics* 98(5): 759–760.

Matthews, Gareth B. 1989. "Children's Conceptions of Illness and Death." In *Children and Health Care: Moral and Social Issues,* ed. Loretta M. Kopelman and John C. Moskop. Dordrecht, Netherlands: Kluwer.

Mill, John Stuart. 1863. *Utilitarianism.* London: Parker, Son and Bourn.

Newachecket, Paul W.; McManus, M.; Foz, H. B.; Hung, Y. Y.; and Halfon, Neal. 2000. "Access to Health Care for Children with Special Health Care Needs." *Pediatrics* 105(4): 989–997.

Nozick, Robert. 1974. *Anarchy, State and Utopia.* New York: Basic Books.

Rawls, John. 1971. *A Theory of Justice.* Cambridge, MA: Harvard University Press.

Rawls, John. 1993. *Political Liberalism.* New York: Columbia University Press.

Reagan, Ronald. 1986. "Abortion and the Conscience of the Nation." In *Abortion, Medicine, and the Law,* 3rd edition, ed. J. Douglas Butler and David F. Walbert. New York: Facts on File.

Rodham, Hillary. 1973. "Children under the Law." *Harvard Educational Review* 43(4): 487–514.

Starfield, Barbara. 1989. "Child Health and Public Policy." In *Children and Health Care: Moral and Social Issues,* ed. Loretta M. Kopelman and John C. Moskop. Dordrecht, Netherlands: Kluwer.

Starfield, Barbara. 1991. "Childhood Morbidity: Comparisons, Clusters, and Trends." *Pediatrics* 88(3): 519–526.

United Nations General Assembly. 1960. *Declaration of the Rights of the Child.* Adopted by the General Assembly of the United Nations, New York, November 20, 1959. New York: United Nations.

U. S. 45 Code of Federal Regulations 46: 401–409. 1983. "Additional Policy for Children Involved as Subjects in Research." (SUBPART D.) *Federal Register* 58: 9816–9820.

U.S. Department of Health and Human Services. 1992. *Healthy People 2000: National Health Promotion and Disease-Prevention Objectives.* Full Report with Commentary. DHHS publication no. (PHS) 91–50212. Washington, D.C.: U.S. Government Printing Office.

U.S. President's Commission for the Study of Ethical Problems in Medicine and Biomedical and Behavioral Research. 1982. *Making Health Care Decisions: A Report on the Ethical and Legal Implications of Informed Consent in the Patient-Practitioner Relationship.* Washington, D.C.: U.S. President's Commission.

U.S. President's Commission for the Study of Ethical Problems in Medicine and Biomedical and Behavioral Research. 1983. *Deciding to Forego Life-Sustaining Treatment: A Report on the Ethical, Medical, and Legal Issues in Treatment Decisions.* Washington, D.C.: U.S. President's Commission.

Veatch, Robert M. 1986. *The Foundation of Justice: Why the Retarded and the Rest of Us Have Claims to Equity.* New York: Oxford University Press.

INTERNET RESOURCES

Council for International Organizations of Medical Science. 1993, 2002. *International Ethical Guidelines for Biomedical Research Involving Human Subjects.* Geneva, Switzerland. 2002 revision. Available from <www.cioms.ch.>.

National Bioethics Advisory Commission. Bethesda, Maryland (August 2001). Recommendation 4.2. See also its "Regulatory Understanding of Minimal Risk, Testimony before the Human Subject Subcommittee of the National Bioethics Advisory Commission Meetings," January 8, 1998, Arlington, VA. Available from <www.bioethics.gov/transcripts/>.

World Medical Association. 2000. *Declaration of Helsinki: Ethical Principles for Medical Research Involving Human Subjects.* Available from <www.faseb.org/>.

## IV. MENTAL HEALTH ISSUES

Conceptualizing a domain of "mental health and children" represents an advance in cultural and societal thinking. The various impediments to this view are well known among students of the history of childhood—at least in Western cultures. These include the concept of children as property, and the broader ignorance and denial of children's affective and cognitive development.

More modern concepts of children and childhood provide a foundation for focusing on the mental health of children as a vital concern. One testament to this development is the passage in 1989 of the United Nations *Convention on the Rights of the Child*. The convention provides a view of children and childhood in which mental-health concerns are central, one that goes beyond the ideas contained in the 1959 *Declaration of the Rights of the Child*.

The convention makes it clear that mental-health issues (e.g., policies that facilitate prevention, and access to services, among others) are primary implications of children's rights. Children, the convention asserts, are entitled to basic psychological resources. These include mandates to ensure family and social identity, empathic and stable care, protection from exploitation, and rehabilitative treatment when experiencing mental-health problems or being exposed to trauma, such as war and abuse.

This rights-focused orientation to the mental health of children reflects a growing appreciation for the scope, depth, range, and subtlety of children's experience. Indeed, in the field of children's mental health there has been a growing recognition and empirical exploration of the existence and characteristics of child variants and precedents of most major adult mental-health problems. Important examples are those of schizophrenia, post-traumatic stress disorder, and depression.

## Schizophrenia

There is evidence that schizophrenia, one of the most devastating mental illnesses with a whole life prevalence rate of about 1 percent, is a developmental disorder, tracing its origin to abnormalities in brain development, which cause subtle and non-specific behavioral changes in childhood and later lead to full blown psychosis, usually in adolescence. Duration of untreated psychosis seems to be a significant predictor of poor outcome (Harrigan et al.), thus making early identification and treatment of first-episode schizophrenia especially important. However, because of the limited specificity and predictive value of the known risk factors for schizophrenia, treatment of asymptomatic subjects with psychotropic drugs is considered unwarranted from a clinical and ethical perspective (Heinssen et al.).

## Childhood Experience of Trauma

Trauma—the overwhelming arousal and cognitive dislocation that results from experiencing horrible events—is an important field of study for those who seek to understand mental health in childhood. As with depression, it was once thought that children were incapable of experiencing genuine psychological trauma (Van der Kolk). But research and clinical experience since 1980 have established that trauma and post-traumatic stress disorder play significant roles in the mental health of children.

Children experience trauma in many settings: televised violence, community violence, domestic violence, war, and homelessness. All point to the need to develop a better understanding of the impact of trauma on childhood as part of a larger commitment to understand the mental health issues facing children.

Children may suffer from post-traumatic stress disorder as a consequence of their experiences at home, in school, or in the community. Symptoms in children include sleep disturbances, daydreaming, re-creating trauma in play, extreme startle responses, diminished expectations for the future, and even biochemical changes in their brains that impair social and academic behavior. Trauma can produce significant psychological problems that interfere with learning and appropriate social behavior in school and the family, the bedrocks for mental health in childhood.

The children least prepared to master trauma outside the home are those who experience psychological, physical, or sexual maltreatment at home. Hundreds of thousands of children face the mental health challenge of living with chronic community violence, whether it derives from war or domestic crime. Some 30 percent of the children living in high-crime neighborhoods of Chicago had witnessed a homicide by the time they were fifteen years old, and more than 70 percent had witnessed a serious assault (Garbarino et al.). In refugee camps around the world, children witness and are subject to violence and exploitation.

The experience of community violence takes place within a larger context of risk for these children. They are often poor; often live in families where the father is absent; often contend with their parents' depression or substance abuse; often are raised by parents with little education or few employment prospects; and often are exposed to domestic violence. This constellation of risk by itself creates enormous mental-health challenges for young children. For them, the trauma of community violence is often literally the straw that breaks the camel's back.

## Depression in Children

Until the 1970s, many clinicians and scholars expressed doubt that children experience *genuine* depression. The common view held that children were incapable of experiencing full-blown depression. It is clear that children do experience depression, but do so and express it differently from adults (e.g., in offering less verbalization concerning mood and symptoms). With proper developmentally appropriate rewording, the same diagnostic criteria for major depression that are used in adults can apply to children. Depression becomes increasing common as the child grows and reaches a prevalence rate among adolescents that is comparable to that in adults. It is estimated that up to 9 percent of adolescents meet current criteria for major depressive disorder (MDD) and up to 25 percent had suffered from it by their late teens (Kessler et al.). While depression seems to equally affect boys and girls before puberty, female teenagers have a substantially higher rate of depression than their male peers. As in adults, in youth depression is a major risk factor for suicide, which in 2003 ranked third among the leading caused of death among adolescents.

Some children mask their depression by denying symptoms to avoid humiliation and embarrassment, to *protect* vulnerable adults who do not appear to be able to tolerate the child's sadness, or to avoid therapeutic intervention that children perceive adversely (e.g., a child may resist the idea of missing recreational activities to attend therapy or may not acknowledge symptoms of depression to avoid causing parental upset or even conflict).

More generally, one of the important breakthroughs in understanding the mental health of children has been the recognition that "what children can tell us depends upon what adults are prepared to hear." That is, children reveal their mental health status in ways that make sense to adults *if* the adults have the technical skill and psychological availability necessary to receive the child's messages. For adults to be responsive to the mental health issues facing children, they need to understand some basic features of child development, particularly the operation of risk and opportunity.

## Risk Factors and Opportunities

Children face a variety of opportunities and risks for mental health and development because of their genetic makeup and because of the social environments they inhabit. Like in other areas of medicine, genetic and environmental factors act in concert in increasing or decreasing the risk for mental disorders. For instance, it has been determined that the risk for antisocial behavior was increased among maltreated boys who also had a genotype resulting in low levels of monoamine oxidase A (MAO), which is an enzyme involved in the metabolism of neurotransmitters (Caspi et al.). The importance of these findings rests on the fact that it was only the coexistence of maltreatment and low MAO expression genotype that conferred an increased risk, whereas either condition in isolation did not. Thus, environment can affect mental health through its impact on the genetically determined makeup of the child. In addition, specific environmental toxins can negatively impact the brain during development. For example, environmental lead poisoning of children may lead to mental retardation and/or behavioral problems. There are also many examples of positive impact of environment during development, such as proper education and non-abusive discipline, which can prevent the emergence of mental disorders even in the presence of an increased genetic risk for these conditions. The complex interaction of risk and protective factors, either environmental or genetic in nature, has profound implications for understanding the mental health of children. The *accumulation of risk factors* is especially important. For instance, the average IQ scores of four-year-old children were found to be related to the number of psychological and social risk factors present in their lives, including socioeconomic conditions as well as intrafamilial, psychosocial factors (Sameroff et al.). But this research reveals that the relationship is not simply additive. Average IQ for children with none, one, or two of the factors is above 115. With the addition of a third and then a fourth risk factor, the average IQ score drops precipitously to nearly eighty-five, with relatively little further decrement as there is further accumulation of five through eight risk factors. This is important because IQ plays an important role in resilience and coping. Thus, low IQ is a risk factor for children's mental health.

*Windows of opportunity* (opportunity that arises at particular points in development) for intervention on behalf of the mental health of children appear repeatedly across the life course. What may be a threat at one point may be harmless or even developmentally good for a child at another. Classic analysis of the impact of the Great Depression of the 1930s in the United States reveals that its mental health effects were felt most negatively by young children (Elder). However, some adolescents, particularly girls, benefited from the fact that paternal unemployment often meant special opportunities for enhanced responsibility and status in the family.

*Opportunities for development* include meaningful relationships in which children find material, emotional, and social encouragement compatible with their needs and capacities at a specific point in their developing lives. For each child, the exact combination of factors depends upon temperament, family resources, potential, skill, and the role of culture in defining the meaning and social significance of specific characteristics or behaviors, within some very broad guidelines of basic human needs that are renegotiated as development proceeds and situations change.

## Participation of Children in Mental Health Research

Like in other areas of health, human research has shown to be the most efficient means of acquiring critical knowledge on how to prevent and treat mental illness among children. Direct participation of children in research is considered necessary as research in adults is neither fully relevant nor sufficient due to developmental differences. Thus, treatments of proven efficacy and safety in adults have been found to lack efficacy or to be toxic in children. Child participation in research is subject to special ethical requirements that are in addition to those common to all human research (Code of Federal Regulations). Based on the type of research activity, the concepts of *favorable risk/benefit ratio, minimal risk,* and *minor increase over minimal risk* are especially important in determining whether a particular study is ethically acceptable (Vitiello et al.).

## Conclusions

The right to mental health is considered an integral part of children's basic rights. Recent years have seen major advances in understanding child development, especially with respect to the interface between neurobiological and psychosocial components and the interaction between genetic endowment and environment. Research on child mental health has emerged as an essential means of developing effective and safe mental health preventive and treatment interventions for children. Participation of children in research raises important ethical issues, thus making child mental health bioethics a particularly lively and rapidly developing area.

JAMES GARBARINO (1995)
REVISED BY BENEDETTO VITIELLO

SEE ALSO: *Abuse, Interpersonal: Child Abuse; Confidentiality; Emotions; Institutionalization and Deinstitutionalization; Mental Health; Mental Illness; Patients' Rights: Mental Patients' Rights;* and other *Children* subentries

### BIBLIOGRAPHY

Caspi, Avshalom; McClay, Joseph; Moffitt, Terrie E.; et al. 2002. "Role of Genotype in the Cycle of Violence in Maltreated Children." *Science* 297: 851–854.

Elder, Glen H. 1974. *Children of the Great Depression: Social Change in Life Experience.* Chicago: University of Chicago Press.

Garbarino, James; Dubrow, Nancy; Kostelny, Kathleen; and Pardo, Carole, eds. 1992. *Children in Danger: Coping with the Consequences of Community Violence.* San Francisco: Jossey-Bass.

Harrigan, Susy M.; McGorry, Patrick D.; and Hrstev, H. 2003. "Does Treatment Delay in First-Episode Psychosis Really Matter?" *Psychological Medicine* 33: 97–110.

Heinssen, Robert K.; Perkins, Diana O.; Appelbaum, Paul S.; and Fenton, Wayne S. 2001. "Informed Consent in Early Psychosis Research: National Institute of Mental Health Workshop, November 15, 2000." *Schizophrenia Bulletin* 27: 571–584.

Kessler, Ronald C.; Avenevoli, Shelli; and Merikangas, Kathleen R. 2001. "Mood Disorders in Children and Adolescents: An Epidemiological Perspective." *Biological Psychiatry* 49: 1002–1014.

Sameroff, Arnold J.; Seifer, Robert; Barocas, Roger; et al. 1987. "Intelligence Quotient Scores of 4-Year-Old Children: Social-Environmental Risk Factors." *Pediatrics* 79(3): 343–350.

U.S. 45 Code of Federal Regulations 46 Subpart A: 101–124 (1991).

U.S. 45 Code of Federal Regulations 46 Subpart D: 46.401–409 (1991).

Van der Kolk, Bessel A., ed. 1987. *Psychological Trauma.* Washington, D.C.: American Psychiatric Press.

Vitiello, Benedetto; Jensen, Peter S.; and Hoagwood, Kimberly. 1999. "Integrating Science and Ethics in Child and Adolescent Psychiatry Research." *Biological Psychiatry* 46: 1044–1049.

# CHRISTIANITY, BIOETHICS IN

• • •

As western culture moves ever deeper into the period characterized in the mid-twentieth century by historian Christopher Dawson as "secularized Christendom," the emerging interdisciplinary field that since 1970 has gone by the name *bioethics* can be understood only as a microcosm of the whole. In certain defining respects the impact of the Enlightenment of the eighteenth century was felt uniquely in the closing decades of the twentieth, in effects good and bad. The effacing of religious discourse from the public square, and the steady fragmentation of the professions under the reductionist pressures of economic and other social forces, show this delayed impact in contexts that have radically shaped the possibility of a bioethics rooted in the Christian vision of the western tradition. If religion is removed from the metaphor of public affairs, it is only in translation that the Christian worldview retains any opportunity to shape the public institutions of the culture. The predicament of Christianity in bioethics at the cusp of this third millennium C.E. lies precisely here. Yet at the same time, the subject matter of bioethics could hardly be of greater moment to those who hold the Christian view of the world.

The core question of which every bioethics issue is ultimately derivative is that of human nature. The vision of human beings defined by their creation in the image of God sets the Christian agenda, to be addressed within public and professional contexts in translation. As has been somewhat ruefully observed (Verhey and Lammers), the exercise of translation has itself led to the *marginalization* of religion. Stephen Lammers notes it at the micro level: The ubiquitous hospital ethics committees, often established under the tutelage of chaplains or other religiously-motivated professionals, immediately take their place in the secular institutional life and language of even religious hospitals. At the macro level, as the ebb tide of the sea of faith runs fast, it has become standard practice to translate Christian moral argument into secular language for public purposes. As a communications strategy in a changing culture, this is perhaps as inevitable as it is estimable. Yet the strangely invidious position in which it places the Christian religion has profound consequences for Christian engagement in bioethics. So it is worth exploring at more length the dynamics of bioethics on "Dover Beach" (Matthew Arnold's elegy on the collapse of the Victorian age of faith).

## History of Bioethics

The half-century history of bioethics is emblematic of the relations of Christianity and the culture of the west. Arising as an interdisciplinary field in the aftermath of World War II, still in its old name of *medical ethics,* it focused the new ethical uncertainties of the generation of Joseph Fletcher. The promulgation of the *Declaration of Helsinki* by the World Medical Association (WMA) was intended to reassert Hippocratic medical values as the foundation for the reconstruction of medicine in light of the Nazi horrors revealed in the so-called "Doctors' Trial" at Nuremberg. Yet its supplanting of the Oath (a pagan document that was nonetheless powerfully theistic in orientation and had long sustained the theological ethics of the Western medical tradition) with a *Declaration* (that could of course be revised by vote, as it would be in response to liberal abortion) set the scene for the reconstruction of medical values on fresh, open-ended, terms. Powered by the continuing cultural weakness of the Christian religion and a succession of new scientific and technical achievements (and corresponding dilemmas) in medicine in the second half of the twentieth century, bioethics has emerged as the quintessentially ambiguous gift of the church to a culture struggling to free itself from the entailments of Christendom. The general failure of a *Christian bioethics* to take hold even within the churches and their educational and medical affiliates has led to a blending of religious and secular in a manner that, for all the good intentions of religious contributors, has tended to extinguish their distinctive character and give primacy to the secular debate and its categories. Thus the most prestigious American graduate program in bioethics is located at an institution of the Society of Jesus (Georgetown); yet its programmatic importance for the development of the discipline is focused in its advocacy of the *principlism* epitomized in Tom Beauchamp and James Childress's influential *Principles of Biomedical Ethics*, the embodiment of secular bioethics.

In Europe, by contrast, where the pattern of religious observance is in general substantially lower than in the United States, Christian participants in the bioethics community tend to be more distinctive in their approach, and in turn the community more accepting of religious perspectives. For example, the Roman Catholic university of Louvain (in the Netherlands) is overtly religious and theological in its approach; and the European Association of Centers of Medical Ethics, the major institutional network, includes a significant minority of explicitly Christian institutions, Catholic and Protestant. The explanation of this contrast lies in

wider European–United States differentia, including assumptions about church–state issues and the public legitimacy of religious speech, and the more tradition-conscious nature of European debate, in which *medical ethics* remained for a generation the default term and bioethics was often noted as an Americanism; though the Council of Europe established in the 1980s an Ad Hoc Committee on Bioethics (CAHBI), its major fruit was the European Convention on Human Rights and *Biomedicine* (a favored European term). In parallel, in Europe the continuance of the idea of bioethics as an interdisciplinary field, in which theology is a legitimate participant, can be observed; this stands in marked contrast to the increasing specialized and reductionist approach to bioethics in the United States as a secularized quasi-discipline of its own.

The *magisterium* has given clear guidance to faithful Catholics on many of the questions of bioethics, but there has not emerged a major *school* of Roman Catholic writers within or even over against the bioethics community. By the same token, the substantial growth of conservative Protestantism in the United States during this period, despite its influential political stance on the question of abortion, has failed to initiate a commensurable intellectual movement in bioethics. The tendency of Protestant and Catholic participants has been to aggregate themselves to the secular bioethics mainstream, as they have played their own ironic part in the marginalization of the dominant tradition of western medical ethics (their own). Harder to explain is their failure to develop in parallel serious centers of intellectual gravity for their distinctive bioethics agendas, especially in the United States. This is more surprising in the case of the Roman Catholic church, possessed as it is of research universities and an extensive system of hospitals that have generally maintained stronger connections with their Catholic roots than their Protestant equivalents. As Albert R. Jonsen comments, even "theologically trained bioethicists … remain, in their bioethical analyses, outside the faith" (p. 58).

## Christian Theology and Bioethics

From its beginnings, Christianity has displayed an interest in questions of health and healing that has verged on preoccupation. The gospels tell the story of one who went about *doing good* often in the form of miraculous interventions in the form of healings (throughout the Gospels) and, in certain cases, resurrections (e.g., Lazarus). In the ensuing story of the church the care and healing of the sick has had a special place, and medical missions have often been at the heart of the church's missionary thrust. In light of what is often taken to be a Christian focus on the life to come and the transitory nature of life in this world, this enduring theme of Christian service to health here and now may seem curious. Though Christian traditions have differed markedly in their approach to *miraculous* healing understood as a spiritual gift—denied absolutely by some, ignored by many, practiced as central to their faith within the Pentecostal and related traditions—the practical focus on medicine and nursing has led to the development of major hospital systems in the United States as well as mission hospitals in many centers of the developing world. Jesus's ministry focus on healing, evidence of miraculous healing in the early church, and the fact that much of the New Testament (Luke, Acts) was written by a physician, lie in a theological context that is not widely understood but sets the place of medicine at the heart of the Christian vision. Within orthodox Christian theology, explicated first and most fully in the Pauline corpus in the New Testament, the origins of human death and the disease that presages mortality are treated as fundamentally unnatural, the consequence of divine judgment on human sin (Romans 5). By the same token, among the benefits of the new order in Jesus Christ, who has stood in as representative and substitute and taken our death penalty as his own, will come not simply the resurrection but, specifically, the *redemption of the body* (Romans 8) as the final undoing of sin and its dire effects. This readily explains the focus on healing, as anticipatory of the final redemption; and the dramatic resurrections even of those who would *die again* like Lazarus. Whatever else these statements mean, they serve as object lessons in the faith that grant a sampling of the kingdom that is to come.

Behind these concerns lies the question that is emerging with increasing candor as the subject matter of contemporary bioethics conversation, the nature of human being. Within the Judeo-Christian tradition the answer has been unambiguous and, in the context of Western culture, profoundly influential. Human beings are constituted by their bearing the divine image (*imago Dei*), and from that fundamental fact flows their unique and inviolable dignity as persons. As the agenda in bioethics shifts from discussion of conditions under which human life may be taken (abortion, euthanasia, embryo experimentation, in the context of what we call here Bioethics 1) to our employment of the fresh manipulative powers that biotechnology is urging into our hands (cloning, inheritable genetic modifications, cybernetics—Bioethics 2), the relevance of this fundamental understanding grows markedly. Whether the churches and their theologian-ethicists will find it within themselves to rise to these immense challenges remains to be seen.

In light of the *imago Dei* question, and a historic commitment to the questions of sickness and healing, it is extraordinary that the distinctively Christian contribution to bioethics has, after an initial firm beginning, rapidly lapsed into a desultory state in which Christian and secular interpreters are generally indistinguishable; only a minority report offers trenchant engagement from within the "distinctive vision" of the Christian worldview. This is all the more surprising since the two most influential figures in the first generation of bioethics were theologians, who actually wrote explicitly theological ethics (from very different perspectives): Joseph Fletcher, whose innovative book *Morals and Medicine* (1954) framed the questions and sought radically fresh approaches in the 1950s, in effect seeking from the inside to subvert the Christian tradition at every key point and prepare the way for the post-Christian bioethics to come; and Paul Ramsay, whose work in the 1960s and 1970s set out a massive defense of Christian ethics even as he engaged the philosophy and emerging jurisprudence of his day.

As commentators have widely noted (Verhey and Lammers; Jonsen), the tendency has been for Christians writing in bioethics to be accommodated to the secular mainstream that since the waning of Ramsay's influence has set the tone for American bioethics. Across Catholic and Protestant thought alike we may note a spectrum of responses. At one end are writers who have essentially been absorbed by the categories and conclusions of the secular bioethics flow. In the center are others who while generally adopting the terminology of secular bioethics have sought to influence or restate it in terms that reflect Christian convictions; or, perhaps, to translate key components in the new bioethics into terms that are related to Christian theology. At the other end are those who take a classical approach from within the Christian tradition. While they sometimes use the public speech of secular bioethics, they are translating distinctively Christian ideas that are developed in explicit theological categories.

Throughout the second half of the twentieth century—from Joseph Fletcher on—much of the bioethics debate focused substantively on the question of the sanctity of human life (abortion, euthanasia, the use of human embryos in research, protocols for organ transplant, definition of death, scare resource allocation, and others), and procedurally on autonomy as the organizing principle of the new bioethics (centered on the role of the patient in decision making, and symbolized by the advanced directive and its culture of individualism in end-of-life choices). Indeed, the movement of bioethics has tended to be from substantive to procedural, and the bioethics literature is little focused on the rights and wrongs of such questions as abortion. The euthanasia debate, potentially of vast significance though on the sidelines of bioethics as a public policy concern, is encapsulated in the focus on *physician-assisted suicide,* which essentially turns substance into protocol. The sanctity of life, long the central feature of our civilization's medical values though seen by many in the bioethics community as perverse, is rarely a locus of bioethics debate; its central place in a Christian bioethics, stemming from the Judeo-Christian doctrine of the creation of human beings in the image of God, has had slight impact on the bioethics mainstream. Peter Singer's *speciesist* challenge—an upending of the *image Dei* that suggests it is as irrational and as unethical as racism—has evoked little Christian response.

## The Future: Emergence of Bioethics 2

A similar spectrum of responses from those writing within the Christian tradition is already evident as the questions of Bioethics 2 begin to focus discussion. The advent of in vitro fertilization in the late 1970s heralded a developing agenda in which the focus would cease to be on the old clinical ethics with its dilemmas grouped around the sanctity of life and move to the new manipulative powers of biotechnology. However, one decisive difference is now evident. As a range of fundamentally new questions is raised for biomedicine and the human good, the Christian mind is one generation removed from the influence of Ramsey and still further from the older tradition of candid theological engagement with the earlier issues of bioethics. The prospect of cloning and germline genetic interventions, coupled with crucial policy issues focused in patent law, reveal the paucity of Christian resources since the fundamental questions of anthropology that are at stake in these debates have been comprehensively neglected by theologians and Christian bioethicists alike. C.S. Lewis's prophetic essay *The Abolition of Man* is widely quoted in the near-absence of more recent and more detailed theological reflection on what is widely agreed to be the most serious set of questions ever to have confronted the human race.

These unfolding questions raise the most profound concerns, both for the Christian understanding of human procreation and of human nature itself. The significance of such basic theological themes as the nexus of marriage/sexuality/family and the nature of human being itself are at stake, as the frontiers of the debate move from whether and when life may be taken to the logic of procreation-reproduction and the manipulative capacities of biotechnology to re-make human nature. It is for Christians an open question whether it is worse for life that is made in God's image to be taken, or for life to be made in an image of our own devising, in a wholly fresh assault on the sanctity and dignity of human being. There is no greater need than for

fresh exploration of the significance of both the *imago Dei* and the incarnation of Jesus Christ for our human nature in light of the new, emerging powers of biotechnology and cybernetics. The challenge to Christian theology is both to articulate the distinctive implications of the Christian understanding of human nature for Christians themselves, and then, with equal vigor, to translate that understanding into public terms, drawing on the common language and values of our cultural tradition and engaging in arguments from natural law. Christian thinkers have so far shown little appetite for either of these tasks.

NIGEL M. DE S. CAMERON

**SEE ALSO:** *Abortion, Religious Traditions: Roman Catholic Perspectives; Abortion, Religious Traditions: Protestant Perspectives; Death: Western Religious Thought; Ethics: Religion and Morality; Eugenics and Religious Law: Christianity; Double Effect, Principle or Doctrine of; Medical Ethics, History of: Europe; Medical Ethics, History of: The Americas; Population Ethics, Religious Traditions: Roman Catholic Perspectives; Population Ethics, Religious Traditions: Protestant Perspectives; Population Ethics, Religious Traditions: Eastern Orthodox Perspectives*

### BIBLIOGRAPHY

Ashley, Benedict M., and O'Rourke, Kevin D. 1986. *Ethics of Health Care.* St Louis, MO: Catholic Health Association of America.

Beauchamp, Tom A., and Childress, James C. 2001. *Principles of Biomedical Ethics,* 5th edition. New York: Oxford University Press.

Bouma, Hessel, III, et al. 1989. *Christian Faith, Health, and Medical Practice.* Grand Rapids, MI: William B. Eerdmans.

de S. Cameron, Nigel M. 1992 (reprint 2001). *The New Medicine: Life and Death after Hippocrates.* London: Hodder and Stoughton.

de S. Cameron, Nigel M., et al., eds. 1995. *Bioethics and the Future of Medicine.* Grand Rapids, MI: Wm. B. Eerdmans.

Cole-Turner, Ronald. 1993. *The New Genesis: Theology and the Genetic Revolution.* Louisville, KY: Westminster/John Knox.

Curran, Charles. 1970. *Medicine and Morals.* Washington, D.C: Corpus.

Englehardt, H. Tristram, Jr. 1991. *Bioethics and Secular Humanism: The Search for a Common Morality.* Philadelphia.: Trinity Press International.

Englehardt, H. Tristram, Jr. 2000. *The Foundations of Christian Bioethics.* Exton, PA: Swets and Zeitlinger.

Fletcher, Joseph F. 1954. *Morals and Medicine.* Princeton, NJ: Princeton University Press.

Gormally, Luke, ed. 1999. *Issues for a Catholic Bioethic.* London: Linacre Centre.

Gustavson, James M. 1996. *Intersections: Science, Theology, and Ethics.* Cleveland, OH: The Pilgrim Press.

Haring, Bernard. 1973. *Medical Ethics.* Notre Dame, IN: Fides.

Hauerwas, Stanley. 1993. *Suffering Presence.* Notre Dame, IN: University of Notre Dame Press.

Jonsen, Albert R. 1998. *The Birth of Bioethics.* New York and Oxford: Oxford University Press.

Kelly, David F. 1979. *The Emergence of Roman Catholic Bioethics in North America.* New York and Toronto: Mellen.

Kilner, John F. 1992. *Life on the Line: Ethics, Aging, Ending Patients' Lives, and Allocating Vital Resources.* Grand Rapids, MI: Wm. B. Eerdmans.

Kuhse, Helga. 1996. *The Sanctity of Life Doctrine: a Critique.* Oxford: Clarendon Press.

Lammers, Stephen E., and Verhey, Allen, eds. *On Moral Medicine: Theological Perspectives in Medical Ethics.* Grand Rapids, MI: Wm. B. Eerdmans.

Lewis, C. S. 1991 (1946). *The Abolition of Man.* London: Collins.

Lustig, B. Andrew. 1991–1997. *Bioethics Yearbook,* vols. 1–5. Dordrecht, Netherlands: Kluwer.

Mahoney, John. 1987. *The Making of Moral Theology.* Oxford: Oxford University Press.

Marty, Martin E., and Vaux, Kenneth, eds. 1982–. *Health/Medicine and Faith Traditions: An Inquiry into Religion and Medicine,* Philadelphia: Fortress.

Meilaender, Gilbert. 1996. *Bioethics: A Primer for Christians.* Grand Rapids, MI: Wm. B. Eerdmans.

McCormick, Richard. 1981. *How Brave a New World?* Washington, D.C.: Georgetown University Press.

Nelson, J. Robert. 1994. *On the New Frontiers of Genetics and Religion.* Grand Rapids, MI: Wm. B. Eerdmans.

O'Donovan, Oliver. 1984. *Begotten or Made?* Oxford: Clarendon Press.

Ramsay, Paul. 1970. *Fabricated Man: The Ethics of Genetic Control.* New Haven, CT: Yale University Press.

Ramsay, Paul. 1970. *The Patient as Person: Explorations in Medical Ethics.* New Haven, CT: Yale University Press.

Ramsay, Paul. 1978. *Ethics at the Edges of Life. Medical and Legal Intersections.* New Haven, CT: Yale University Press.

Shelp, Earl E., ed. 1996. *Secular Bioethics in Theological Perspective.* Boston: Kluwer Academic Publishers.

Shelp, Earl E., ed. 1985. *Theology and Bioethics: Exploring the Foundations and Frontiers.* Boston: D. Riedel.

Verhey, Allen. 1996. *Religion and Medical Ethics: Looking Back, Looking Forward.* Grand Rapids, MI: Wm. B. Eerdmans.

Verhey, Allen, and Cox, John D., ed. 1994. *Christian Scholar's Review* XXIII(3).

Verhey, Allen, and Lammers, Stephen E., eds. 1993. *Theological Voices in Medical Ethics.* Grand Rapids, MI: Wm. B. Eerdmans.

# CHRONIC ILLNESS AND CHRONIC CARE

• • •

This entry traces the ethical topography and presents concepts entailed in chronic illness and chronic care. There is no authoritative definition of chronic illness or chronic care. However, a *consensus definition* for purposes of this entry can be found on the Public Broadcasting System (PBS) web site (Fred Friendly Seminars, 2001b), where chronic illness is defined as "a condition that lasts a year or longer, limits activity, and may require ongoing care." Some persons describe chronic as "illnesses or impairments that cannot be cured" (Institute for the Future, p. 260; Summer, p. 2). An incurable chronic condition can be manifest at birth, as in Down's syndrome.

Chronic illness is contrasted with acute episodes of illness or injury that will either result in death or will be treated and the person restored to *health.* Although chronic diseases differ from acute diseases, they can have acute episodes or flare-ups. Persons with chronic conditions may experience accidents or comorbidity in addition to their ongoing problem(s).

Paradoxically, as various public health measures, pharmacological agents, and other medical interventions become more effective in either preventing or curing diseases and postponing death, the number of persons with chronic conditions increases in both absolute and relative numbers. "Over the past century, the economically more developed countries of the world have gone through considerable change in their population structure and the types of diseases which afflict them—the so-called demographic and epidemiological transitions" (Harwood and Sayer, p. 1).

Care of a person with chronic illness should involve productive interactions between patients and providers; the latter may include medical and social support. Responsive providers and services are key in such care, as are the financial resources to enable the person to utilize them. Three elements seem to differentiate sound chronic *care,* at least in emphasis, from ordinary, good medical practice in general: continuity over time; management of any accompanying frailty and dependency; means to pay for the extraordinary costs of drugs, prosthetic devices, and care both in the home and in alternate living situations.

## Three Related Concepts

**PROGRESSIVE INTERMITTENT FRAILTY.** Frailty can be seen as a condition at a given point in time and as a process over time. It denotes a condition in which a person has difficulty with activities of daily living and is vulnerable to various *assaults* upon his or her person both from within, (e.g., organ failure) or without (e.g., falls). Frailty, especially in the elderly, often continues over time in a progressive fashion with periods of remission and exacerbation until the person becomes substantially dependent and dies.

Persons who are frail may have difficulties with activities of daily living either on a temporary or an ongoing basis. Frailty often accompanies chronic illness, though not all chronically ill persons are frail. Some frailty results from general system(s) failure that is associated with age and the gradual molecular deterioration accompanying it; other frailty can be associated with a transitory illness or trauma.

**DEPENDENCY.** Dependency is a state in which a person requires the assistance of others. It may be temporary or permanent, intermittent or continuous. It may or may not be associated with chronic illness. Chronic illness, depending on severity, may or may not create a dependent state.

**NATURAL DEATH AND DYING.** All will die. Dying occurs in different modes. It may be caused by sudden organ failure or by disease or infection. A relatively new phenomenon is the increasing number of persons with serious chronic illness at the end of life. Certain patients function quite well for a time, with substantial decline in the last few weeks before death, typical of cancer. Others experience a less predictable course, with periods of disease exacerbation interspersed with periods of higher functionality, as in organ system failure of the heart or lung. Some go through a drawn-out course with early loss of function and incremental decrements in function and vigor over many months or years before death, characteristic of frailty and dementia (Lunney, Lynn, and Hogan; and Lynn).

As the trajectory toward death becomes more apparent, even if still somewhat unpredictable as to its exact time, specific medical, psychological, and spiritual interventions become central, emphasizing physical and emotional comfort rather than seeking to cure the underlying cause.

## Seeking to Understand the Challenge

Given the lack of an agreed upon definition of chronic illness, it is difficult to estimate with any precision the aggregate numbers and costs. In addition to the confounding element of what to include as a chronic condition, each possible candidate has its own life course and associated costs. However, all agree there are large numbers of people with chronic illnesses. In fact, virtually all who die in old age will have one or more chronic conditions.

Having noted the imprecision of definitions and insurmountable difficulty of quantifying the extent and costs of chronic illness, some representative statements can contribute to an understanding of the dimensions of the problem:

- Almost one-half of the U.S. population of 276 million people in the year 2000 had a chronic condition in some form (Partnership for Solutions, 2001).

- In 2020, about 157 million people will live with chronic conditions, and about 81 million, more than half of these people, will have multiple chronic conditions (Partnership for Solutions 2002a, pp. 6–7).

- In one listing, thirty-seven conditions are characterized as chronic illnesses (Fred Friendly Seminars, 2001a). There may be more.

- Each chronic condition has its own etiology and course history and is experienced by a person unique in his or her personhood and cultural/social milieu.

- Each person has greater or less access to, or is in command of, a different array of help.

- Chronic conditions may be more or less debilitating at different parts of the course of the illness.

- About *60 million* people experience comorbidity, and more than *3 million* of these have five chronic conditions (Partnership for Solutions, 2001).

- Some chronic conditions can be ameliorated for long periods of time with medications and/or prosthetic devices; others may have a decided trajectory in which increasing, albeit sometimes periodic, disability requires hands-on assistance or a more supportive environment.

- The various treatment regimens for people with multiple chronic conditions can interact to diminish health and increase disability (Partnership for Solutions, 2002b).

- Some chronic conditions can render a person more vulnerable to disease or accidents.

- Not only do poor and disadvantaged people experience greater prevalence of chronic conditions, those who are unemployed, less educated, and uninsured suffer more from these conditions (Bethell, Lansky, and Fiorillo).

- According to a 1998 Medical Expenditure Panel Survey, 78 percent of healthcare dollars was spent on care of chronic conditions for noninstitutionalized persons, and approximately 58 percent of healthcare dollars was spent on the 21 percent of those suffering from more than one chronic condition (Partnership for Solutions 2002a, pp. 17 and 19).

## Commonalities in Chronic Illness

The conceptual embrace of chronic illness has become so broad and varied that the utility in using this concept to inform policy may be compromised. However, all chronic conditions have common threads. Chronic conditions intrude upon the quality of life and life patterns of individuals. They not only alter the life of the persons closest to the afflicted individuals but many with whom these individuals come in contact on a daily basis, for example, employers, fellow employees, neighbors, and even strangers. Chronic illness sufferers need extra, even in some instances extraordinary, resources to ameliorate the effects of their illnesses, and this in turn generates costs to society either in the form of risk-sharing schemes such as insurance (public or private) or through welfare/charitable support.

## Ethical Topography of Chronic Illness

Chronic illness occasions decisions that have an ethical component since it constitutes an interruption for a significant time in the life and life plan of an individual, and by extension, that of those who are closely associated with the individual. Furthermore, it constitutes a societal issue because of the *costs* involved.

**DOMAINS.** A chronic illness evokes responses with ethical implications in various domains. Each choice has implications for the well-being of the person with the chronic condition, those who are part of his or her primary social network, and the broader society.

**THE INDIVIDUAL.** While one must be cautious in blaming the victim, some, but by no means all, chronic illnesses have their origin in lifestyle choices. At the outset of ethical reflection, one must consider individual behavior not only because of a fundamental responsibility to self but also because of its consequences to others, both proximate and remote. For example, 80 percent to 90 percent of chronic obstructive pulmonary disease (COPD) cases are the result of long-term smoking (Ames). A substantial number of cases of human immunodeficiency virus (HIV) disease are caused directly or indirectly by unsafe sexual activity or needle sharing by drug abusers. Refusal to wear seat belts or helmets increases the risk of incurring catastrophic, debilitating injuries.

Regardless of the etiology of the chronic illness, the person suffering with it faces ethical choices that have an impact on his or her well-being, as well as that of other individuals and society in general. For example, one with chronic illness can be compliant with medical regimes or not, behave in a risky manner or not, and make treatment choices that can influence the quality and length of life and entail costs.

**THE PERSON'S SOCIAL NETWORK.** Depending on the severity of the illness and the moral/psychological bonds, the lives of family and psychologically significant others become a party to the disease. Each person impacted confronts ethical choices on how he or she will respond to the person in need.

Friends, neighbors, and even strangers are actors and reactors since physical proximity creates a moral field within which responses are evoked. Persons may or may not come to the assistance of others when that assistance is needed in a particular instance or over time. The need of the person, the relationship to *the other*, the inconvenience or costs (opportunity, monetary and psychological), and the availability of other assistance all enter into the ethical equation facing the potential helpers.

**THE WORK ENVIRONMENT.** Many persons with chronic conditions are employed or employable. While the Americans with Disabilities Act requires reasonable accommodations in the workplace, ethically based attitudes and interactions with co-workers will either enhance or detract from the well-being of persons with chronic conditions. For example, at one end of the spectrum are those co-workers who consistently respond with grace and enthusiasm from day to day. Their personal principles would propel them to risk their lives to help another co-worker in a wheelchair exit the building in an emergency. At the opposite end are those who frequently regard chronically ill co-workers with irritation or agitation; in an emergency situation, compromised co-workers with chronic conditions would not get their attention.

**PRIVATE SECTOR POLICY.** *Insurance.* Insurance in the private sector is driven mainly by marketplace forces and actors. It is also subject to both ethical considerations and to incentives and disincentives provided through public policy for taxation of employee benefits and for the regulation of insurance markets.

Insurance involves the sharing of risk. Paying a certain cost (premium) makes access to care affordable and possible for an expensive event that will occur in a group but not *to all* members of the group. Persons choose certainty over uncertainty and presumably pay premiums that they and their insurers hope will total considerably less than the costs associated with untoward events. However, when these events have already occurred or their imminent onset is highly probable (e.g., when a person over sixty-five pays his or her first premium), then insurance becomes a method of financing burdens that is unlikely to be profitable.

Insurers are economically motivated to exclude very sick and high-risk persons from coverage in order to lessen the cost of premiums and increase their corporate margins. Often they attempt to exclude persons with pre-existing conditions entirely, although this is more difficult to do under 2003 federal law. In lieu of such an option, actuarial considerations dictate a higher premium, which places a burden on all covered persons.

Faced with competitive pressures, major insurers are structuring boutique-type policies for healthcare, and to a lesser extent, long-term care, so that employers can offer lower premiums to presumably low-risk employees. This results in more costly options for those at higher risk. Some employers are moving toward a contribution to the individual for the purchase of insurance in the marketplace rather than offering an employer-sponsored plan. Presumably this will make the purchase of affordable insurance more difficult and costly for higher-risk persons. Such trends disadvantage chronically ill persons because they consign them to high-risk, high-cost pools.

A subset of ethical and public policy issues arises with chronic illnesses and conditions that have been associated with lifestyle choices, for instance, from motor vehicle accidents in which appropriate safety devices were not used (helmets or seat belts) and some AIDS patients. Should such persons be afforded benefits born by others because of their risky behaviors?

While these scenarios are the very stuff of free enterprise, they are not without ethical implications for insurers, group purchasers, and regulators.

*Genetic testing.* The field of genetics is in its infancy and holds promise in the prevention and treatment of all diseases, especially those that tend to be chronic. However, the knowledge gained by testing may identify the person as being at such risk of a particular chronic condition that he or she becomes *uninsurable* and, despite the absence of any indication of the disease, unemployable.

"At present the predictive value of most genetic tests is limited" (Anderlik and Rothstein, p. 425). These authors find scant evidence of discrimination to date on the basis of genetic testing in health insurance markets in the United States. This finding holds for states that do and those that do not regulate the use by insurers of genetic information. However, they note a particular problem for persons seeking long-term care insurance as genetic testing improves to permit discrimination among risks: *Medical underwriting* of long-term care insurance (in contrast to the provision of social insurance) could discriminate against persons with serious chronic disease because coverage is "directly tied to the provision of necessary health care" while the "premium structure … is based on mortality risk" (Anderlik and Rothstein, p. 425).

This potential for future discrimination as genetic testing is perfected is a concern in the insurance field, the popular press, and other countries. Dr. John W. Rowe, Chairman and CEO of Aetna, called for legislation and industry-wide guidelines to promote genetic testing and counseling with provisions for strict confidentiality. Furthermore, he advocated a prohibition of the use of genetic information to establish risk selection or classification (Aetna, Inc.). An editorial in *USA Today* on August 20, 2002, ends with "Medicine is giving people a chance to gaze into their futures—and maybe change them. But until their genetic secrets remain just that, the scientific breakthroughs could cause more problems than they solve" (*USA Today*, p. A.10). In 2001, the Human Genetics Commission of the British House of Commons "concluded that it was important to establish a clear and defensible regulatory system which not only balances the interests of insurers, insured persons, and the broader community but also enjoys the confidence of the public" and thus "decided to recommend to Government an immediate moratorium on the use by insurance companies of the results of genetic tests."

**PUBLIC POLICY.** The costs associated with chronic illness, the possible limitations of earning capacity, and the way others may treat those who have some limitation all make governmental action an important factor. Public policy affects not only access to needed services but continued participation in the life of the community for chronic illness sufferers.

Public policy emanates from the democratic process with its often messy and contentious elements. However, in many instances it finds justification, if not its origins, in widely held ethical perspectives. Among these public values are the convictions that people should not be denied opportunity because of particular characteristics and that the most vulnerable should have at least basic dignity.

*Discrimination.* Government has had a role in protecting the rights of individuals, especially those most at risk as evidenced in affirmation of voting rights, fair housing laws, and nondiscrimination in employment and public accommodations, as well as opportunities for participation for the disabled. While these result immediately from legislation and court decisions, they have foundation in a public ethic.

*Income support.* The costs often involved with chronic illness make governmental support a vital aspect for the well-being of those afflicted.

Based both on pragmatic and ethical considerations, the U.S. has enacted programs of social insurance requiring risk sharing and consequent creation of entitlement to meet basic needs in those areas in which people would be unable or unwilling to make prudent economic decisions about future need.

Social Security was enacted to assure a floor of income for those who cease to work because of age (1934) or disability (1956). It assures continued participation in the economy and offers support for those unable to work and their survivors. Social Security mandates equal contributions by employees and employers to a premium during employment in view of a possibility of unemployment. It offers a greater return to those who have modest employment earnings than to those who have been fortunate enough to have better earnings.

It has been United States policy since the 1930s that income in retirement should be considered to have three sources: Social Security, private pensions, and personal savings. There is growing evidence that income from these sources will be inadequate to meet basic living costs (including the costs of managing chronic illness) for most persons born between 1946 and 1964 who are living alone, and especially the oldest persons (Employee Benefit Research Institute [EBRI] Education and Research Fund and Milbank Memorial Fund; Dugas). The causes of this shortfall, which will be catastrophically expensive for society, include:

- structural problems in the private pension system;
- projected shortfalls in the Social Security Trust Fund that are tempting policy advocates to propose remedies that put individuals at higher risk;
- the difficulty most Americans have in both saving and maintaining their standard of living during their working years; and
- the periodic decline and routine volatility of the financial markets in which pension savings are invested.

Each of these causes raises ethical issues.

*Financing and organizing care during acute episodes of illness.* Most of the health insurance offered by government (Medicare and coverage of public employees most importantly) and the private sector (individual and group coverage) is derived historically from plans to cover infectious disease, injuries, pregnancy and childbirth, and episodes of chronic degenerative diseases requiring hospitalization and medical specialty services. Although this coverage has evolved gradually to include many services for managing chronic illness, payment is still driven mainly by diagnosis and is more generous for invasive procedures than for either counseling or outpatient drugs (Fox). As a result, most persons who experience progressive intermittent frailty (which means, in fact, most persons) are at high risk of receiving care that is discontinuous, fragmented, and inappropriate.

*Financing and organizing long-term care.* The United States has devised a vast system of long-term services based on the organizational concept of the nursing home and the financing assumption that individuals and families will pay for care with government serving as the payer of last resort. This system is a logical counterpart of a health insurance system created to respond to the most serious acute manifestations of disease. Nursing homes, the dominant institutions, are stripped down (or not so stripped down) hospitals in which persons wait, secure against injury but isolated from their community, until the next acute episode of illness returns them to the acute care health sector. Since waiting is deemed a residual activity, it is logical for individuals to pay for it out of income and savings unless (or until) they are too impoverished to do so. Then society (through Medicaid, Supplemental Security Income, and charity) pays the cost. This model for organizing and financing long-term care, like the health insurance model described in the previous paragraph, is deeply flawed: conceptually and financially, and many have argued, ethically. There is growing analysis and advocacy on behalf of alternative models for organizing and financing long-term care that take account of the inevitability of progressive intermittent frailty for most people and recognize the well-documented desire among Americans to spend as much of their later lives as possible in homelike, minimally restrictive settings (U.S. Department of Health and Human Services). One of these models is the Program for All-Inclusive Care of the Elderly (PACE). PACE is a risk-sharing system that provides for all acute, long-term care, and hospitalization needs of frail elderly participants in one program. Participants pay a capitated fee rather than fee for service with their Medicaid and Medicare entitlements. Most of the PACE participants can still live at home or in a community-based setting and are transported to the program's day health center one or more times a week for care of their medical and social needs.

To provide this "all-inclusive" care, the health center is staffed with an interdisciplinary team (Centers for Medicare & Medicaid Services, 2002). Another example allowing for various flexible state-designed alternative models is the Medicaid Home and Community Based Services (HCBS) 1915(c) Waivers Program. The U.S. government allows the states to provide HCBS waiver programs for certain segments of their Medicaid-eligible population. One segment is the elderly. Under an HCBS waiver program for care of the elderly, a state can ask the federal government for waivers of certain Medicaid requirements so that Medicaid benefits can be provided in the home or a community-based setting as well as in an institution (Centers for Medicare & Medicaid Services, 2003).

*Research.* Vast and increasing amounts are spent on research pertinent to chronic disease in the United States, primarily by the federal government, through the National Institutes of Health (NIH) and the Veterans Health Administration (VA), and by the pharmaceutical industry. The two most prominent objects of this research are the mechanisms of chronic disease and the development of drugs and devices to treat, cure, and manage them. Consumer and professional groups are prominent advocates of increased public research budgets for particular diseases, often with overt or covert support from the pharmaceutical industry and manufacturers of medical devices. However, enthusiasm for developing and testing new interventions distracts attention and resources that could be invested in new randomized controlled trials of existing interventions, research on head-to-head comparisons of competing treatments, and replacement of open or arbitrary drug formularies with preferred drug lists based on systematic reviews employing the methods of research synthesis. This hopeful and lucrative focus on new ways to prevent, cure, and manage disease has made it difficult for advocates of the rapidly developing science of research synthesis to make their case. This recently emerged area of research makes it possible to evaluate more confidently than ever before the effectiveness of health and social care interventions, including drugs, devices, diagnostic tools, and methods of organizing services (Chalmers et al.).

## Social Solidarity and Concern for "The Other"

While individual autonomy is inherent in the notion of dignity, humans are social beings who inherit from the past, live in community in the present, and perceive themselves as having responsibility to the future. Humans are free to pursue their own goals as long as they do not interfere with others, a negative right. There is a generally recognized corollary that humans live in community with a positive

obligation to contribute to the common good and share others' burdens. Personal responsibility is indicated not only for the sake of the person but because "no man is an island," and his or her well-being or disorder has social ramifications. Maintenance of health and function is significant not only to the individual but also to all who are part of his or her social network. Aristotle has been credited with teaching that a just society is one in which burdens are shared by equals equally and unequals unequally in accord with capacity and need.

The pluralistic nature of contemporary society makes it easier to identify when and where ethical issues occur than to apply universally accepted approaches to their solution. Yet, at least at the societal level, decisions have and will be made through the democratic process, largely driven by self-interest but often with appeals to a sense of fairness and decency. However, a recent study of policy makers' use of ethicists' advice concluded that persons who emphasize ethics "will always be disappointed by the politics of policy making in any countries that are fit to live in" (Fox and Klein). On the more personal level, however, such decisions are made, for better or worse, on a daily basis, either easing the burden of chronic illness or leaving the chronically ill person ever more isolated in his or her distress. Decisions of fairness and decency and those that ease the burden become ever more vital as the number of people affected by chronic illnesses increases in the first half of the twenty-first century.

CHARLES J. FAHEY
DANIEL M. FOX

**SEE ALSO:** *Aging and the Aged; Care; Dementia; Disability; Healthcare Resources, Allocation of; Health Policy in the United States; Human Dignity; Justice; Life, Quality of; Long-Term Care; Managed Care; Medicaid; Trust*

### BIBLIOGRAPHY

Anderlik, Mary R., and Rothstein, Mark A. 2001. "Privacy and Confidentiality of Genetic Information: What Rules for the New Science?" *Annual Review of Genetics* 35(1): 402–433.

Chalmers, Iain; Hedges, Larry V.; and Cooper, Harris. 2002. "A Brief History of Research Synthesis." *Evaluation and the Health Professions* 25(1): 12–37.

Dugas, Christine. 2002. "Retirement Crisis Looms as Many Come Up Short." *USA Today* July 19, p. A. 01.

Fox, Daniel M. 1995. *Power and Illness: The Failure and Future of American Health Policy.* Berkeley: University of California Press.

Fox, Daniel M., and Klein, Rudolf. 2004. "Ethics and the Politics of Health Policy: Case Studies of Law and Regulation in the United Kingdom and the United States." In *The Cambridge*

*History of Medical Ethics,* ed. R. Baker and L. McCullough. Cambridge, Eng.: Cambridge University Press.

Harwood, Rowan H., and Sayer, Avan Aihie Sayer. 2002. *Current and Future Long-Term Care Needs.* Geneva: World Health Organization.

Institute for the Future. 2003. *Health and Health Care 2010: The Forecast, The Challenge,* 2nd edition, p. 260. San Francisco: Jossey-Bass.

Lunney, June R.; Lynn, Joanne; and Hogan, Christopher. 2002. "Profiles of Older Medicare Decendents." *Journal of the American Geriatric Society.* 50(6): 1108–1112.

Lynn, Joanne. 1997. "An 88-year-old Woman Facing the End of Life." *Journal of American Medical Association* 277(20): 1633–1640.

*USA Today.* 2002. "Genetic Tests Outpace Efforts to Safeguard People's Data" (editorial). August 20, p. A.10.

### INTERNET RESOURCES

Aetna, Inc. 2002. "Aetna Recommends Guidelines for Access to Genetic Testing," press release of June 17. Available from <www.aetna.com/news/2002/pr_20020617.htm>.

Ames, Margaret. Geriatric Services of America. 2002. "Respiratory Disease—The Real Facts." Available from <www.geriatricservices.com/Dr%20Margaret/emailcold.asp?name=test2%20test2>.

Bethell, Christina; Lansky, David; and Fiorillo, John. Foundation for Accountability (FACCT) and Robert Wood Johnson Foundation. 2002. "A Portrait of the Chronically Ill in America, 2001." Available from <www.rwjf.org/publications/publicationsPdfs/report_chronic_illness.pdf>, p. 2.

Centers for Medicare and Medicaid Services. 2002. "Program of All-Inclusive Care for the Elderly (PACE) History." Available from <cms.hhs.gov/pace/pacegen.asp>.

Centers for Medicare and Medicaid Services. 2003. "Home and Community-Based Services 1915(c) Waivers." Available from <cms.hhs.gov/medicaid/1915c/default.asp>.

Employee Benefit Research Institute (EBRI) Education and Research Fund and Milbank Memorial Fund. 2002. "Kansas Future Retirement Income Assessment Project: Third Draft." Available from <www.ebri.org/pdfs/kansas.pdf>.

Fred Friendly Seminars, Inc. 2001a. "Directory of Chronic Illnesses." Available from <www.pbs.org/fredfriendly/whocares/awareness/directory.html>.

Fred Friendly Seminars, Inc. 2001b. "What is Chronic Illness?" Available from <www.pbs.org/fredfriendly/whocares/awareness/what_is.html>.

Human Genetics Commission. 2001. "The Use of Genetic Information in Insurance: Interim Recommendations of the Human Genetics Commission." Available from <www.hgc.gov.uk/business_publications_statement_01may.htm>.

Partnership for Solutions. 2001. "Rapid Growth Expected in Number of Americans Who Have Chronic Conditions." Available from <www.partnershipforsolutions.org/statistics/prevalence.cfm>.

Partnership for Solutions. 2002a. "Chronic Conditions: Making the Case for Ongoing Care." Available from <www.partnershipforsolutions.org/DMS/files/chronicbook2002.pdf>.

Partnership for Solutions. 2002b. "Multiple Chronic Conditions: Complications in Care and Treatment." Available from <www.partnershipforsolutions.org/DMS/files/2002/multiplecoitions.pdf>.

Summer, Laura. 1999. "Chronic Conditions: A Challenge for the 21st Century." National Academy on an Aging Society. Available from <www.agingsociety.org/agingsociety/pdf/chronic.pdf>, p. 2.

U.S. Department of Health and Human Services, Administration on Aging. 2000. "The Future Is Aging." Available from <www.aoa.dhhs.gov/May2000/FactSheets/r3%20-%20life%20course.pdf>.

# CIRCUMCISION, FEMALE

• • •

*Female circumcision* is the term used to identify the practice of removing healthy normal female genitalia by surgical operation. Because of the severity of the operation and its known harmful effects, the term *female genital mutilation* is now generally used. There are three increasingly severe types of this operation, and each makes orgasm impossible. Clitoridectomy, or sunna (Type 1), is the removal of the prepuce of the clitoris and the clitoris itself (Figure 1–1). When excited, the clitoris swells and becomes erect, and it is this excitement that causes female orgasms. Excision, or reduction (Type 2), is the removal of the prepuce, the clitoris, and the labia minora, leaving the majora intact. The labia minora produce secretions that lubricate the inner folds of the lips and prevent soreness when these lips rub against each other (Figure 1–2). Infibulation, or pharaonic circumcision (Type 3), is the removal of the prepuce, the clitoris, the labia minora and majora, and the suturing of the two sides of the vulva, leaving a very small opening for the passage of urine and menstrual blood (Figure 1–3). This type of circumcision is referred to as pharaonic probably because it is identified with circumcision methods of ancient Egypt under the pharaohs.

In a study of the various types of circumcision undergone by women in Sierra Leone (Koso-Thomas), it was found that 39.03 percent of the women had undergone Type 1, 59.85 percent, Type 2, and 1.12 percent, Type 3. In Somalia, 80 percent of the operations are Type 3 (El Dareer). The prevalence of circumcision in Africa ranges from 10 percent in Tanzania to 98 percent in Djibouti (Toubia).

The most common and basic procedure followed during circumcision is the traditional method. In this method, usually employed by circumcisers who have no medical training, the female is firmly held down on dry ground with her legs wide apart to expose the genitalia and the parts to be removed. In some cases, the genital part to be excised is held with a special hemostatic leaf before excision, or the candidates are made to lie near a cold flowing stream so the excised area can be bathed in chilled water to numb the pain. The implements used are often unsterilized razor blades, knives, scissors, broken bottles, or any other sharp implement. Some form of herbal dressing is applied to the raw wound after the operation. The same implement is used for successive operations without sterilization. When the operation is carried out in modern clinics, standard modern surgical practice is followed.

## Origin of the Practice

We do not know with any precision when, why, and how female circumcision began. There is evidence that female circumcision and female genital surgery have been done in many parts of the world, although currently it is mainly done in different communities in parts of Africa, Asia, the Far East, Europe, and South America.

The early Romans, concerned about the consequences of sexual activity among female slaves, adopted the technique of slipping rings through their labia majora (Figure 1–4) to block access to the vagina. In the twelfth century C.E., Crusaders introduced the chastity belt in Europe for the same purpose; the belt prevented girls and women from engaging in unlawful or unsanctioned sex. This method caused little permanent physical damage to the individual. Genital surgery was permitted in North America and Europe in the late nineteenth century with the intention of curing nymphomania, masturbation, hysteria, depression, epilepsy, and insanity. There is no evidence that such surgery was associated with any ritualistic activity. Elsewhere, the surgery has historical links with either religious or ethnic rituals. It is believed that the ancient Egyptians and ancient Arabs practiced this form of surgery. Genital mutilation seems to have been transplanted to Latin America from Africa during the slave trade and may have taken root first in the central part of Brazil, where groups of West Africans were resettled after the abolition of the slave trade in the middle of the nineteenth century, and to eastern Mexico and Peru through migration. In Asia genital mutilation is found among Islamic religious groups in the Philippines, Malaysia, Pakistan, and Indonesia. Where the mutilation exists in the Middle East

and Asia, it is strongly associated with Islam. Female genital mutilation is not practiced in all Islamic countries. Those societies known to practice it, namely, the United Arab Emirates, South Yemen, Oman, and Bahrain in the Middle East, and northern Egypt, Mauritania, Sudan, Somalia, Mali, and Nigeria in Africa, probably inherited it from pre-Islamic cultures.

## Alleged Benefits of Female Circumcision

The modern defense of female circumcision allows us to reconstruct the ancient rules that governed moral action or behavior in polygamous communities. The defense enumerates a wide range of health-related and social benefits alleged to result from the practice:

1. maintenance of cleanliness;
2. maintenance of good health;
3. preservation of virginity;
4. enhancement of fertility;
5. prevention of stillbirths in women pregnant for the first time;
6. prevention of promiscuity;
7. increase of matrimonial opportunities;
8. pursuance of aesthetics;
9. improvement of male sexual performance and pleasure; and
10. promotion of social and political cohesion.

Cleanliness is regarded as a great virtue by women in countries where the practice is common. In some cultures, particularly in Africa, women are required to cleanse their genitalia with soap and water after urinating. Those who justify removing parts of the genitalia that produce secretions cite this preoccupation with the cleanliness of the genital organs. Some traditional circumcision societies claim that circumcised women are generally healthy and that the operation cures women suffering from problems resembling those identified in nontraditional societies as depression, melancholia, nymphomania, hysteria, insanity, epilepsy, and the social disorder of kleptomania. In situations where proof of virginity is essential for concluding a marriage transaction, circumcision is believed to be the guarantee against premarital sex. This guarantee benefits parents who are able to demand a high bridal price for their daughters. Marriage immediately after the transaction ceremony is common, and such marriages, involving pubertal girls, are usually followed by pregnancy within a very short time. Circumcised girls and women are regarded as having an advantage over the uncircumcised in marrying. Where female genital mutilation is an established custom, tradition

**FIGURE 1**

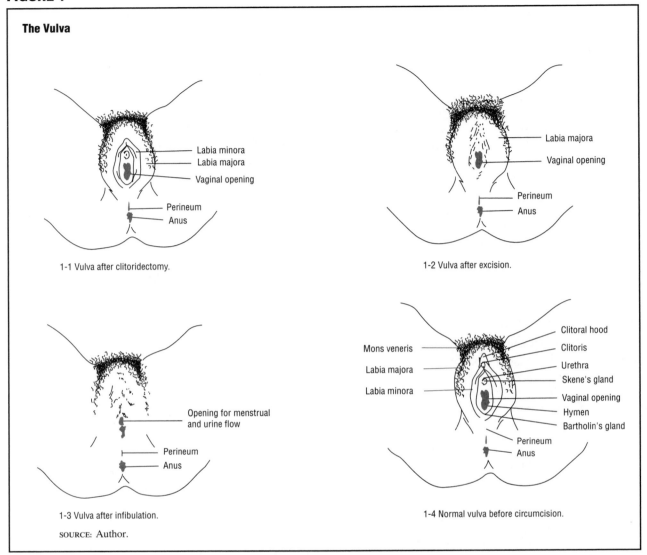

The Vulva

1-1 Vulva after clitoridectomy.

1-2 Vulva after excision.

1-3 Vulva after infibulation.

1-4 Normal vulva before circumcision.

SOURCE: Author.

forbids men to marry uncircumcised girls; hence, circumcision of girls ensures they will be marriageable. Certain traditional communities, such as the Mossi of Burkina Faso and the Ibos of Nigeria, believe that a firstborn child or even subsequent babies will die if their heads touch a mother's clitoris during the birth process. The clitoris is therefore removed at the time of delivery if this has not already been done. Since female genital mutilation reduces or even eliminates sexual pleasure, the practice presumably eliminates the risk of female promiscuity. The justification of the practice to preserve chastity, eliminate promiscuity, foster or improve sexual relations with men, generate greater matrimonial opportunities, protect virginity, and increase fertility reflects the existence in traditional societies of strict controls on social behavior.

The belief that circumcision enhances beauty stems from the claim that the male prepuce or foreskin is removed mainly for aesthetic reasons, and that the clitoris, the female counterpart to the penis, should be removed for the same reason. If left intact, the clitoris is believed likely to grow to an embarrassing and uncomfortable size. In some patriarchal societies, female genital mutilation is also said to benefit the male by prolonging his sexual pleasure, since the clitoris is thought to increase male excitement during sexual intercourse with a female partner and may rush a man's orgasm. Of great importance to women in such cultures is the status circumcision bestows on the circumcised. It entitles them to positions of religious, political, and social leadership and responsibility.

The argument in favor of circumcision serves narrow social interests and does not achieve the goods desired or guaranteed. Failure to achieve these goods, moreover, is often blamed on the woman rather than the ritual. For example, maintaining cleanliness becomes an agonizing task. The hardened scar and stump that result from circumcision are unsightly, and they halt the flow of urine and menstrual blood through the normal channels. This obstruction causes unnecessary fluid retention and results in odors more disagreeable than those from the natural hormonal secretions that tradition teaches are degrading. Associating the death of babies at childbirth with clitoral contact is clearly refuted by the evidence that millions of healthy babies are born to uncircumcised mothers.

While the desire of organized society to maintain control over people's actions may be understandable, not all such control promotes their well-being or self-determination. Such rituals also cause harm to society by increasing morbidity and mortality levels. In addition, although these rites may promote social and political cohesion, they thwart the individual's freedom to determine what is right and in her best interests. Even women who learn that circumcision is an unsafe and harmful practice may feel pressure from society to agree to it for themselves or their children in order to marry or remain members of the group.

## Harmful Effects of Female Circumcision or Female Genital Mutilation

The medical consequences of female genital mutilation are quite grave (El Dareer; Koso-Thomas). In Africa an estimated ninety million females are affected (Hosken). Three levels of health problems are associated with the practice. Immediate problems include pain, shock, hemorrhage, acute urinary retention, urinary infection, septicemia, blood poisoning, fever, tetanus, and death. Occasionally, force is applied to position candidates for the operation, and as a result, fractures of the clavicle, humerus, or femur have occurred. Intermediate complications include pelvic infection, painful menstrual periods, painful and difficult sexual intercourse, formation of cysts and abscesses, excessive growth of scar tissue, and the development of prolapse and fistulae. A fistula is an abnormal passage: a hole (opening) between the posterior urinary bladder wall and the vagina or a hole between the anterior rectal wall and the vagina. Late complications include accumulation of menstrual blood of many months or even years, primary infertility, painful clitoral tumors, recurrent urinary tract infections, and kidney or bladder stone formation. Obstetric complications such as third-degree perineal tear, resulting in anal incontinence and

fissure formation, and prolonged and obstructed labor are also known to occur. Psychological problems of anxiety, frigidity, and depression, as a result of the physical inability to have a clitoral orgasm, may also develop.

Women who undergo circumcision suffer various degrees of emotional and mental distress depending on the nature of complications following their operation. Records show that 83 percent of all females undergoing circumcision are likely to be affected by some condition related to that surgical procedure requiring medical attention at some time during their lives. This level of health risk should be of concern to nations with a large proportion of circumcised women, because such women may never make the progress toward the economic and social development required of them.

## Application of Modern Medical Practice to Female Genital Mutilation

Modern medicine has made impressive strides in investigating, preventing, and treating a wide range of ailments. Through its investigative approaches it has judged that unwarranted surgery is wrong. In the case of female genital mutilation, studies have found that certain of the resulting medical conditions are serious and can lead to complications and permanent health damage requiring both medical treatment and counseling (Koso-Thomas). Awareness of female genital mutilation's harmful effects has encouraged changes in how the operation is performed, changes that may include sterilization of equipment and dressings and administration of local anesthetic, antibiotics, and antitetanus injections prior to circumcision.

## Ethical Aspects

Since some followers of Islam in Africa, the Far East, and the Middle East endorse circumcision, it has been widely identified as an Islamic rite. However, female genital mutilation is not practiced in Saudi Arabia, Algeria, Iran, Iraq, Libya, Morocco, or Tunisia. Many Islamic and Christian religious leaders have categorically denied that female circumcision or female genital mutilation is an injunction in the Qur'an or a "commandment" in the Bible. Since the foundations of the practice lie outside Islamic or Christian religious law, the origins of circumcision and its justification must lie in the moral, social, and religious structure and operation of societies practicing it. Individuals practicing it act within a system of rules that strictly regulate sexual behavior in society. Female genital mutilation generally thrives in communities with strictly enforced conventions and social rules.

With the knowledge of its harmful effects now common, no social system endorsing this kind of mutilation can be said to promote a favorable climate for a fulfilling life.

The attitudes of women toward circumcision depend on their experiences and level of education. Most women affected by the practice are unaware that circumcision is the cause of their health difficulties (Koso-Thomas). Once aware of this relationship, however, many women who have some education and training and who are exposed to a modern environment are better able to assess what is involved in circumcision actions and, on that basis, to make a reasoned judgment of its rightness or wrongness. Many such women have come to believe that the practice is unacceptable and have refused to allow their female children to go through the same traumatic experience. Many feminists and health professionals have openly displayed a higher regard for women's health than for tradition.

It has been shown, however, that some women who admit to suffering under the unexpected effects of the operation still feel obliged to support the practice. A study carried out to obtain opinions on circumcision involving 135 men and 120 women showed that 25 percent were shocked at what happened to them on their circumcision day, as it was not what they had expected (Koso-Thomas). The majority of them, either semi- or nonliterate, believed that they had done the right thing and planned to have their daughters circumcised. Those women who were not shocked by their experiences were also mainly illiterate and did not see why their daughters should not undergo circumcision. The attitude of men in the sample also varied according to their level of education. Illiterate men insisted that all women should be circumcised to keep them in their place, while the literate men argued that women should be given a choice as to whether or not to be circumcised. They felt that to deny women this choice was a violation of their human rights. It has also been found that circumcision is supported in most women's organizations, particularly political and social groups, since these groups reflect the feelings of the majority in the community.

Usually the decision to have a girl circumcised is made by the female elder members of the family/clan who insist on carrying out the procedure. An aura of secrecy, celebration, and pride surrounds the circumcision and encourages voluntarism on the part of recruits by making membership in the group seem more attractive. A few educated women, however, who have had access to modern medical assessment of their health as well as information on the dangers of the practice also support circumcision but advocate changes to reduce its health hazards. A few healthcare personnel have felt that medical intervention at the early stages of the operation might prevent the more serious health consequences of circumcision. Since circumcision cannot take place without health consequences, the position of these women and health practitioners is untenable.

Women who live in a traditional environment tend to judge their actions on the basis of traditional rules and principles of their society. There may be some misogynistic attitudes among such women, but the dominant force directing their actions comes from the society that demands, among other things, that this ritual be performed in order for them to qualify for marriage and social acceptance.

There are also attitudes inherent in African sexuality that not only permit circumcision but foster it. In most African cultures, sexuality is regarded as a gift to be used for the procreation of the human species, and any public or even private display of sex-related feeling or enjoyment is seen as debasing this gift. In some communities, only a token expression of the sexual self is permitted. The issue of sexual fulfillment is unimportant. Thus, controls over the sexual behavior of women are designed to curb female sexual desire and response and to encourage disregard for the sexual aspects of their lives. The removal of the organ or organs responsible for sexual stimulation is therefore taken as necessary for the fixation of certain values within the community and for ensuring the acceptance of rigid standards of sexual conduct. Thus, the underlying concern of those who defend the institution of female circumcision is that women's sexuality will be corrupted if women are allowed the freedom to control it or indeed to pursue the personal satisfaction of their sexual desire. Implicit in this argument is the major premise that it is immoral for a woman to act on her sexual desire. Women who still support the practice continue to promote injury with confirmed medical consequences. In this respect the role of the healthcare practitioner in the society is crucial and may lead to personal dilemmas that have to be resolved. Many feel anger against the executors and supporters of the ritual and sadness at the futility of the exercise and at the intransigence of traditional circumcising communities. Healthcare professionals presented with the choice of treating or not treating women who have chosen to be circumcised are often determined to rescue a life they see as poised on the brink of destruction. On the other hand, traditional circumcisers have no moral dilemmas about the practice. They believe that they have no choice in a matter which concerns the preservation of their cultural heritage. That heritage dictates how women must live, and to them, life should be one of happiness in subservience to the will of the people and in obedience to customary and religious laws.

OLAYINKA A. KOSO-THOMAS (1995)

## BIBLIOGRAPHY

Aune, Bruce. 1979. *Kant's Theory of Morals.* Princeton, NJ: Princeton University Press.

El Dareer, Asma. 1982. *Woman, Why Do You Weep? Circumcision and Its Consequences.* London: Zed.

Francoeur, Robert T. 1983. *Biomedical Ethics: A Guide to Decision Making.* New York: Wiley.

Hosken, Fran P. 1982. *The Hosken Report on Genital and Sexual Mutilation of Females,* 3rd rev. edition. Lexington, MA: Women's International Network News.

Koso-Thomas, Olayinka. 1987. *The Circumcision of Women: A Strategy for Eradication.* London: Zed.

MacIntyre, Alasdair C. 1967. *A Short History of Ethics.* London: Routledge & Kegan Paul.

"Report of the Workshop on African Women Speak." 1984. Khartoum: Scientific Association for Women's Studies.

Schweitzer, Albert. 1947. *Civilization and Ethics,* 3rd rev. edition. London: A. and C. Black.

Thiam, Awa. 1986. *Speak Out, Black Sisters: Feminism and Oppression in Black Africa.* London: Pluto.

Toubia, Nahid. 1993. *Female Genital Mutilation: A Call for Global Action.* New York: New York Women.

Walker, Alice. 1990. *Possessing the Secret of Joy.* New York: Harcourt Brace Jovanovich.

Walker, Alice, and Parmar, Pratibha. 1993. *Warrior Marks: Female Genital Mutilation and the Sexual Blinding of Women.* New York: Harcourt Brace.

## UPDATE

The United Nations International Children's Emergency Fund (UNICEF) estimates that "between 100 million and 130 million women suffered female genital mutilation or cutting as children" and that another 2 million are at risk each year (UNICEF). It calls on all nations to honor their commitments to eliminate those practices by 2010. The World Health Organization (WHO), UNICEF, and United Nations Population Fund (UPFPA) (WHO, 1997) issued a joint statement advocating a zero-tolerance view, but it has not been endorsed universally (WHO, 2000). The worldwide scrutiny of ancient practices in which some or all of women's genitals are removed, usually during infancy or childhood, stems from several movements that began in the 1980s.

### Ongoing Disputes about Zero Tolerance

In the 1980s a growing number of activists in countries where these rites are popular tried to stop these practices or at least substitute less mutilating rites (nicking the labia or the foreskin around the clitoris) for the more mutilating forms, which were and in some cases still are practiced widely, especially in Africa, and some Middle Eastern countries. Those rites include Type 1 (removal of the prepuce with or without removal of all or some of the clitoris), Type 2 (removal of the entire clitoris and all or most of the labia minora), and Type 3, or pharaonic circumcision (removal of all of the clitoris and labia minora and parts of the labia majora) as well as the practice of infibulation (the wound to the vulva from the cutting is stitched closely, leaving a tiny opening so that the woman can pass urine and menstrual flow). Also included among those rites are scraping or cutting tissue at the vaginal opening or the vagina and placing corrosive substances into the vagina to induce bleeding or narrow or tighten it (WHO, 2000).

Prominent African activists, including Olayinka Koso-Thomas (author of the main entry above), Nahid Toubia, and Raquiya Abdalla, have long advocated stopping all forms of genital mutilation and cutting while retaining the cultural and religious rituals that educate and welcome girls into adulthood and the community. They favor "circumcision through words" and family-planning education that includes telling young males about the health hazards to women and asking them to make a vow not to require circumcision as a condition of marriage. Those changes might accommodate important religious, cultural, economic, community, and family considerations without harming girls.

Others argue that a more effective approach to zero tolerance would be to replace the mutilating rituals with removal of the foreskin around the clitoris or tiny nicks in the labia (Davis; El Dareer). This, they argue, might "wean" people away from the more extreme forms of genital mutilation. If there are no complications, the tiny nicks do not preclude sexual orgasm later in life. The chance of success with this tactic is more promising and realistic, they hold, than would be the case with an outright ban; people could maintain many of their traditions and rituals of welcome without causing as much harm, especially if the operations were done by doctors and nurses under sterile conditions. However, Nahid Toubia objects, stating that removal of the clitoral hood invariably causes considerable, even if unintended, harm to the clitoris because tissue from the clitoris is very likely to be taken.

Dena Davis expresses the concern that something other than zero tolerance could send the wrong message to immigrants:

> Because FGA [female genital alteration] in its most common forms around the world is mutilating and life threatening, it is reasonable to adopt a "zero tolerance" policy to make it absolutely clear to immigrants that this practice is never acceptable …

further, an argument could be made that, once a "nick" is allowed, it would be difficult if not impossible for the state to make sure this did not become a loophole through which the worst elements of FGA would slide. As MGA [male genital alteration] is not anywhere close to as mutilating and threatening to life and health as are many forms of FGA, this argument would serve as a constitutionally valid distinction between the two practices. (p. 561)

In the end, however, Davis tries to justify a compromise for the sake of cultural sensitivity, legal consistency, and medical safety, arguing that procedures might be permitted that allow roughly the same harm done to girls as is done to boys in male circumcision: a minor nick in a girl's labia or clitoral hood.

Raquiya Abdalla, however, objects to equating female circumcision with male circumcision because their purposes differ and the degree of harm frequently is drastically different. For some people the best reason for drawing parallels between male and female genital cutting is to help abolish both practices. Even if the timetables do not coincide exactly, they hold, comparisons should not be used to allow some female circumcision in countries that permit male circumcision. Still others maintain that there are health benefits to male circumcision that justify distinguishing the two. Most agree, however, that it is unfortunate that the same word, *circumcision,* is used for the full range of practices, from trivial to mutilating. Removal of the clitoris is comparable to amputation of the penis rather than removal of the foreskin in men.

## Findings about Morbidity and Mortality

In the 1980s some African clinician-activists from countries that practice those rites documented and brought to the world's attention the accompanying morbidity and mortality. Those pioneering medical studies include the ones conducted in the Sudan by Asma El Dareer (1982), in Sierra Leone by Olayinka Koso-Thomas (1987), and in Somalia by Raquiya Haji Dualeh Abdalla (1982). The death, infection, and disabilities associated with the rites are well established, challenging local beliefs that the rites promote health and well-being. For example, as Koso-Thomas (p. 10) pointed out, stable medical evidence discredits the belief that "death could result if, during delivery, the baby's head touches the clitoris," and Abdalla (p.16) pointed to the disutility of regional practices of putting "salt into the vagina after childbirth … [because this] induces the narrowing of the vagina—to restore the vagina to its former shape and size and make intercourse more pleasurable for the husbands."

Some of those studies suggest that many women would prefer not to perform the rites if they were not necessary for the marriage of their daughters and that more younger women are having second thoughts about this cultural practice for their own daughters (Moschovis).

Other epidemiological studies have confirmed the morbidity and mortality associated with those rites and have demonstrated that they are still widespread in some regions. For example, Daphne Williams Ntiri (1993) found that in some African countries most young girls between infancy and ten years of age have received Type 3 circumcision from traditional practitioners who often used sharpened or hot stones, razors, or knives, frequently without anesthesia or antibiotics. The WHO estimates that worldwide about 80 percent of the rites involve excision of the clitoris and labia minora and that infibulation is done in about 15 percent of all cases (WHO, 2000). In some regions, such as Egypt, Guinea, Somalia, Eritrea, and Mali, national surveys indicate that 94 to 99 percent of women are circumcised (WHO, 2000, 2001).

## Oppression of Women

Beginning in the 1980s, despite insistence by people within the culture about their good intentions, voices worldwide condemned the rites as brutal forms of oppression of women comparable to making men eunuchs (removal of the testes or external genitals). International organizations denounced the practices, including UNICEF, the International Federation of Gynecologists and Obstetricians, and WHO, along with the American Medical Association and many women's groups. They deny that this is just a cultural issue, arguing that the rites should be opposed with the same vigor as other violations of human rights (Schroder; Toubia). Pressure from human rights groups, for example, forced some governments to ban all registered health professionals from performing female cutting or infibulation and helped women find political asylum in other countries to avoid genital cutting.

Some countries are more willing to pass laws prohibiting the rites than to enforce those laws. UNICEF (2003) is troubled by governments' lack of will to confront those practices, educate their communities about the risks, and enforce existing laws that prohibit them. UNICEF promotes challenges to the beliefs, attitudes, and customs that support these rites and discrimination against uncircumcised women. Even in the United States, the United Kingdom, France, Canada, and other countries where female circumcision is viewed as child abuse, it is practiced in "back rooms" (Davis). UNICEF praised the European Parliament's launching of an initiative called "Stop FGM" in

December 2002. Whether or not the intent of the rites is to honor women, UNICEF and others regard them as "culturally sanctioned forms of women's oppression, male domination, and control of women's sexuality" (UNICEF, 2003).

## Immigration

After 1980 waves of immigrants from North Africa and southern Arabia made the rites better known and widely condemned. Those immigrants came from regions where most women receive Type 2 and Type 3 forms of circumcision and moved to areas of the world where those rites are viewed as horrific and oppressive practices that put young girls at terrible risk of death and chronic disability. Consequently, families that seek female genital cutting in their adopted countries generally avoid the healthcare system, and the risks of nonmedical circumcision are assumed to be very high (Davis).

## Cultural Sensitivity

The cultural clashes that have resulted from criticisms of female circumcision have centered on whether there is any justification for interfering with the deeply held practices of other cultures. Extreme ethical relativists state that there is no moral or epistemological basis for interfering with popular customs in other countries and that meddling constitutes cultural imperialism (Scheper-Hughes; Ginsberg; Shweder). This view, which once was popular among anthropologists and others, has been challenged on many sides (Kopelman, 1994, 1997).

First, shared goals and methods sometimes can be used to assess other cultures in a way that has moral and epistemological authority. For example, most people share the goal of seeking health for woman and infants and endorse similar methods of logic, science, and medical investigation. Medical research is respected in those communities and their own studies show that the rites cause pain, emotional trauma, infection, chronic disease, disability, and death. These shared goals and methods can be used to help reason with people about destructive cultural practices that involve not just female genital cutting but wars, pollution, and epidemics.

Second, criticism of these practices within those communities is growing (Moschovis), and as a result the depth of the commitment to the rites is changing. As the investigators who originally touched off the contemporary debate over female circumcision illustrate, cultures are not monolithic but contain passionate disagreements and may change rapidly. Moreover, most people do not live in only one culture

but cross easily from one culture to another in their professions, religions, and ethnic groups. People who brought the practice of female genital cutting with them when they moved, for example, live in more than one culture. It no longer is possible to count or separate cultures sharply when world travel and communication are so easily available. Cultural, religious, professional, ethnic, and other groups overlap and have many variations within nation-states. To say that people belong to overlapping cultures or that people cannot distinguish precisely between or count cultures, however, undercuts extreme ethical relativism and its tenet that the only way to determine whether something is right is to see if it has cultural approval (Kopelman, 1994, 1997).

Third, cross-cultural criticism seems to be important and even obligatory when one considers cultures that engage in terrorism, war, torture, mass rape, infanticide, and slavery, and so people should be able to criticize female genital cutting on the same basis. Otherwise, people would be led to the very problematic view that any act is right if it has cultural approval even if it is a culturally endorsed act of war, oppression, enslavement, aggression, rape exploitation, racism, or torture. In this view the disapproval of other cultures is irrelevant in determining whether acts are right or wrong. Even if this version of ethical relativism is defended consistently, its plausibility is eroded by its conclusion that the disapproval of people in other cultures, even victims of war, oppression, enslavement, aggression, exploitation, rape, racism, or torture, is irrelevant in deciding what is wrong in the aggressor culture (Kopelman, 1994, 1997).

## Consistency

Finally, scrutiny has revealed apparent contradictions in the beliefs and attitudes associated with the rites. For example, on the one hand people from those regions say that nothing is given up because women cannot enjoy sex, but on the other hand they say that the rites are needed to control women who mighty be sexually out of control without the surgeries (Kopelman, 1994, 1997). (This fear that girls will be sexually promiscuous is a frequently given reason for doing the surgery in the West, where girls and young women have considerable freedom compared with the situation in their original homelands.) Another apparent inconsistency concerns insistence that respect for cultural mores requires that deeply embedded cultural views about female genital cutting must be respected in the adopted countries even if this means violating the deeply embedded views of the dominant culture of the new land. It is inconsistent to insist that their deeply embedded views must be respected—but not those of other cultures. Finally, some say that there is no way to determine what is right when cultures disagree but also insist on transcultural universal normative principles such as "every culture counts for one," "preserve ancient cultures," and "when in Rome do as the Romans do."

Worldwide attention to female genital mutilation and cutting rituals since the 1980s has made those rites the center of controversy about practical and theoretical issues concerning human rights, ethical relativism, and the limits of tolerance of cultural diversity. Medical studies document the resultant morbidity, mortality, and disabilities and the resulting lack of sexual sensitivity and satisfaction for millions of women. Proposals by activists in those regions include stopping clinicians from participating in the rites and adopting and enforcing meaningful legislation, but many people believe that education about the harms of genital cutting and infibulation may be the most important way to stop the practices (El Dareer; Abdalla; Dirie and Lindmark; Toubia).

LORETTA M. KOPELMAN

SEE ALSO: *Anthropology and Bioethics; Body: Cultural and Religious Perspectives; Children: Rights of; Circumcision, Male; Circumcision, Religious Aspects of; Coercion; Feminism; Harm; Islam, Bioethics in; Judaism, Bioethics in; Medicine, Anthropology of; Sexual Behavior, Social Control of; Women, Historical and Cross-Cultural Perspectives*

### BIBLIOGRAPHY

Abdalla, Raquiya H. D. 1982. *Sisters in Affliction: Circumcision and Infibulation of Women in Africa.* London: Zed.

Davis, Dena. 2001. "Male and Female Genital Alteration." *Health Matrix* 11: 487–569.

Dirie, M. A., and Lindmark, G. 1992. "The Risk of Medical Complications after Female Circumcision." *East African Medical Journal* 69(9): 479–482.

El Dareer, Asma. 1982. *Woman, Why Do You Weep? Circumcision and Its Consequences.* London: Zed.

Ginsberg, Faye. 1991. "What Do Women Want? Feminist Anthropology Confronts Clitoridectomy." *Medical Anthropology Quarterly* 5(1): 17–19.

Kopelman, Loretta M. 1994. "Female Circumcision/Genital Mutilation and Ethical Relativism." *Second Opinion* 20(2): 55–71.

Kopelman, Loretta M. 1997. "Medicine's Challenge to Relativism: The Case of Female Genital Mutilation." In *Philosophy of Medicine and Bioethics in Retrospect and Prospect: A Twenty-Year Retrospective and Critical Appraisal,* ed. Ronald A. Carson and Chester R. Burns. Vol. 50 in the Philosophy of Medicine Series. Dordrecht, Netherlands, and Boston: Kluwer.

Koso-Thomas, Olayinka. 1987. *The Circumcision of Women.* London: Zed.

Moschovis, Peter P. 2002. "When Cultures Are Wrong." *Journal of the American Medical Association* 288(9): 1131–1132.

Ntiri, Daphne Williams. 1993. "Circumcision and Health among Rural Women of Southern Somalia as Part of a Family Life Survey." *Health Care for Women International* 14(3): 215–216.

Scheper-Hughes, Nancy. 1991. "Virgin Territory: The Male Discovery of the Clitoris." *Medical Anthropology Quarterly* 5(1): 25–28.

Schroeder, P. 1994. "Female Genital Mutilation—A Form of Child Abuse." *New England Journal of Medicine* 331: 739–740.

Shweder, Richard. 1990. "Ethical Relativism: Is There a Defensible Version?" *Ethos* 18: 205–218.

Toubia, Nahid. 1994. "Female Circumcision as a Public Health Issue." *New England Journal of Medicine* 331: 712–716.

INTERNET RESOURCES

United Nations International Children's Emergency Fund. 2003. "UNICEF Calls on Governments to Fulfill Pledge to End Female Genital Mutilation: International Day of Zero Tolerance of FGM Is Springboard for Action." UNICEF press release, February 18, regarding meeting in Addis Ababa and Nairobi, February 6, 2003. Available from <www.unicef.org/newsline/2003/03pr08fgm.htm>.

World Health Organization. 1997. "Genital Mutilation: A Joint WHO/UNICEF/UNFPA Statement." Geneva: World Health Organization. Available from <www.who.int/frh-whd/publications/p-fgm1.htm>.

World Health Organization. 2000. "Female Genital Mutilation." Fact Sheet No. 241. Available from <www.who.int./inf-fs/en/fact241.html>.

World Health Organization Estimated Prevalence Rates for FGM. 2001. Available from <www.who.int/frh-whd/FGM/FGM%20prev%20update.html>.

# CIRCUMCISION, MALE

• • •

Male circumcision entails the surgical removal of the foreskin that covers the glans of the penis. The relative simplicity of the surgical procedure itself belies the complexity of the conflicting values surrounding this minor operation. The primary ethical question is whether the pain, risks, and costs of routine neonatal circumcision are justified by the potential medical and social benefits to infants who undergo this procedure. Given the strong opposing opinions surrounding circumcision, there is some question as to whether children should undergo the procedure prior to an age when they can provide informed consent on their own behalf. Circumcision in adults is less common and will not be the focus of discussion here.

## The Prevalence of Male Circumcision

Circumcision is the most common procedure performed on males in the United States—an estimated one million procedures are performed per year. Only about 20 percent of the procedures are performed for religious reasons; the majority are performed in newborns for medical, cultural, or aesthetic reasons. Estimates suggest that circumcision is performed on 60 to 90 percent of boys in the United States. Although observers have noted some variations by region and by cultural group in the use of this procedure, accurate rates for circumcision are not available (Wallerstein). The best documented rates of newborn circumcision in the United States come from a study of infants delivered in U.S. military hospitals (Wiswell, 1992). The rate of circumcision in 1971 was estimated to be 89 percent, falling to 70 percent in 1984, with a subsequent rise to 80 percent in 1990. These differences suggest that parents' decisions about circumcision are influenced by the ebb and flow of social debate over the procedure.

The high rate of nonritual circumcision places the United States in a unique position in the world. In regions where the majority of the world's population lives, including western Europe, the former Soviet Union, China, and Japan, male circumcision is not performed. In 1985, Edward Wallerstein provided the following estimates of circumcision rates: In Great Britain an estimated 1 percent of the male population is circumcised; in New Zealand the figure is about 10 percent; in Australia, 35 to 40 percent; and in Canada, 35 to 40 percent. Circumcision is performed commonly as a religious ritual by Jews, Muslims, many black Africans, and nonwhite Australians.

## The History of Circumcision

The walls of Egyptian tombs depict male circumcision, so the practice is known to be at least 5,000 years old. The Jewish and Muslim traditions of circumcision have their origin in the Old Testament. Jews accept the practice as a sign of the covenant between God and Abraham. In Genesis 17:12, God instructs Abraham: "He that is eight days old shall be circumcised among you, every male throughout your generations." As a Jew, Jesus was circumcised, and the early Christian church debated the need for circumcision as a criterion for joining the Christian fellowship; it was decided that circumcision was not necessary for salvation. According to the apostle Paul, "For in Jesus Christ neither circumcision availeth nor uncircumcision; but faith which worketh by love" (Gal. 5:6). These religious traditions remain strong, although the health debate has led to a questioning of the religious practice by a few members of the Jewish community (Milos and Macris).

The practice of routine neonatal circumcision has been debated within the U.S. medical profession for over a century. Circumcision was initially advocated in the Victorian era as a measure that would reduce masturbation. Medical benefits from the procedure were first widely proposed in 1891 by P. C. Remondino, who claimed that circumcision prevented or cured a host of diseases, including alcoholism, epilepsy, asthma, and renal disease (Wallerstein). More scientific studies of the potential medical benefits of circumcision began to appear in the professional literature in the 1930s. Urologists observed an association between penile cancer and an intact foreskin (Schoen, 1992). During World War II, American troops stationed in the Pacific and in desert climates had problems with irritation and infection of the penis because of sand and the inability to maintain adequate hygiene. The military response was to circumcise many of the affected soldiers. However, the Japanese did not use circumcision despite their war experience in the same environments (Wallerstein).

Circumcision became popular, indeed almost universal, after the war. Rates remained high until the 1970s, when both the medical profession and the general public began to question the widespread use of the procedure for newborns. The American Academy of Pediatrics issued two separate statements, in 1971 and 1975, declaring that there were no valid medical indications for neonatal circumcision (Committee on Fetus and Newborn). Specific concerns were raised over the pain of the procedure and over potential complications in the face of questionable medical benefits. In 1985, the first in a series of papers was published that documented an increased risk of urinary tract infections in uncircumcised neonates (Wiswell et al., 1985). These reports came in association with an apparent increased risk of sexually transmitted disease, specifically the human immunodeficiency virus (HIV), in uncircumcised males (Schoen; Bailey). In 1989 the American Academy of Pediatrics issued a revised statement that concluded that there were both medical advantages and medical disadvantages to the procedure and that full information and informed consent were important for parents who were making this decision.

## Medical and Ethical Issues

The basic ethical question regarding circumcision is whether it is justified to perform a surgical procedure on a healthy, unconsenting child to prevent the possibility of future disease. The primary ethical task is to balance the pain and potential complications with the potential benefits. In addition, there is a strong tradition of respecting parental wishes when their decisions are not clearly contrary to the welfare of the child. Although the full details of the risks and benefits are beyond the scope of this discussion, key issues will be outlined.

Proponents of circumcision claim several advantages for the procedure, including decreased incidence of urinary tract infections in infancy, decreased risk of penile cancer in adults, and decreased risk of sexually transmitted diseases (Wiswell, 1992; Wiswell et al., 1985). In addition, routine circumcision prevents occasional penile problems such as phimosis (a narrowing of the foreskin that prevents its retraction), balanitis (an infection of the head of the penis), and posthitis (an infection of the foreskin). Significant complications of the procedure are quite rare, occurring in less than 1 percent of circumcised neonates (Kaplan). Until the mid-1980s, circumcision was performed commonly without anesthesia. Current techniques permit the pain of circumcision to be reduced with a number of simple techniques. In contrast to female circumcision, the procedure has no significant effect on sexual function or pleasure (Collins et al.).

Social issues are a significant element in the debate. Many parents would like their sons to look like the majority of their peers, and many parents would like their sons to look like their fathers, the majority of whom are circumcised. Finally, parents who have grown up in a society of circumcised men may find a circumcised penis to be more aesthetically agreeable.

Those who question the value of the procedure counter that the case for reductions in urinary tract infections, cancer rates, and sexually transmitted diseases is not convincing, or that many of the same benefits may be achieved through better personal hygiene (Poland; Milos and Macris). While the procedure is generally safe, according to George Kaplan, there are risks of excessive bleeding, infection, removal of too much tissue, tissue damage and scarring, reactions to anesthetic agents, and retention of urine. It is also argued that the penile problems that may arise in uncircumcised males, such as phimosis or balanitis, can be prevented or effectively treated when they occur. Further, it is noted that pain-control measures are not consistently effective, carry their own risks, and are associated with some pain as well. Marilyn Milos and Donna Macris note that some have claimed that the foreskin provides a protective covering for the glans, making the uncircumcised penis more sensitive during sexual activity.

Since the 1960s, a cultural shift has placed a higher value on preserving the natural look. Uncircumcised males are common enough, the argument goes, that the appearance of an uncircumcised penis in a high school locker room will not be cause for embarrassment. Finally, it is claimed that a simple explanation from father to son will prevent a son's confusion about a different look to his penis.

Of all of the potential medical advantages of circumcision, the reduced risk of urinary tract infection in the infant is the best documented, and this is the benefit most likely to be experienced by the child (Wiswell, 1992; Schoen). Urinary tract infections in neonates are potentially serious infections that may be life-threatening and, if recurrent, may lead to the later development of renal insufficiency and hypertension. However, the risk of urinary tract infection in uncircumcised infants is still relatively small, occurring in approximately 1 to 4 percent of infants. Of those infected, only a small minority will suffer long-term kidney damage (Chessare). Further, it is estimated that eighty infants would need to be circumcised to prevent one urinary tract infection (Lerman and Liao).

Parents are thus left with a difficult decision. Circumcision might be delayed until the child is old enough to make his own choice, but this alternative obviates the primary medical advantage of decreasing the risk of urinary tract infection in infancy. In addition, performing the procedure beyond the newborn period may be associated with greater risks (Wiswell et al., 1993). Therefore, reliance on surrogate decision making by the parents for the newborn boy remains an ethically appropriate approach. With all of the current data in hand, many physicians and parents find themselves falling between the polar positions in this debate. The AAP drew the following conclusions in its 1999 policy statement on circumcision:

> Existing scientific evidence demonstrates potential medical benefits of newborn male circumcision; however, these data are not sufficient to recommend routine neonatal circumcision. In the case of circumcision, in which there are potential benefits and risks, yet the procedure is not essential to the child's current well-being, parents should determine what is in the best interest of the child. To make an informed choice, parents of all male infants should be given accurate and unbiased information and be provided the opportunity to

discuss this decision. It is legitimate for parents to take into account cultural, religious, and ethnic traditions, in addition to the medical factors, when making this decision. Analgesia is safe and effective in reducing the procedural pain associated with circumcision; therefore, if a decision for circumcision is made, procedural analgesia should be provided.

For many parents the final decision will be made primarily on cultural and social grounds, with less weight placed on the potential health benefits or risks. Fortunately, there is some evidence that most adult men like the way they are, whether circumcised or not (Lee).

There has also been a vocal debate over the practice of female circumcision (AAP, 1998), which has led some to draws parallels between male and female procedures. While both procedures are performed primarily for cultural reasons, there are dissimilarities worthy of note. There are a few well-documented medical benefits to male circumcision and no long-term morbidities, unlike the female procedure. Further, male circumcision is not associated with sexual control and subjugation, cultural attitudes that are at the foundation of the tradition of female circumcision.

The social debate over the procedure in the United States is likely to continue. In this context, the responsibilities of both the physician and the parents are to make sure that all are fully informed about the benefits and risks of this procedure, and that the procedure, if elected, is performed in a competent and humane manner.

JEFFREY R. BOTKIN (1995)
REVISED BY AUTHOR

SEE ALSO: *Anthropology and Bioethics; Body: Cultural and Religious Perspectives; Children: Rights of; Circumcision, Female; Circumcision, Religious Aspects of; Coercion; Harm; Medicine, Anthropology of; Sexual Behavior, Social Control of*

### BIBLIOGRAPHY

American Academy of Pediatrics Committee on Bioethics. 1998. "Female Genital Mutilation." *Pediatrics* 102(1): 153–156.

American Academy of Pediatrics, Task Force on Circumcision. 1989. "Report of the Task Force on Circumcision." *Pediatrics* 84(2): 388–391.

American Academy of Pediatrics, Task Force on Circumcision. 1999. "Report of the Task Force on Circumcision." *Pediatrics* 103(3): 388–686.

Bailey, Robert C.; Plummer, Francis A.; and Moses, Stephen. 2001. "Male Circumcision and HIV Prevention: Current Knowledge and Future Research Directions." *Lancet Infectious Diseases* 1(4): 223–31.

Chessare, John B. 1992. "Circumcision: Is the Risk of Urinary Tract Infection Really the Pivotal Issue?" *Clinical Pediatrics* 31(2): 100–104.

Collins, Sean; Upshaw, J.; Rutchik, Scott; et al. 2002. "Effects of Circumcision on Male Sexual Function: Debunking a Myth?" *Journal of Urology* 167: 2111–2112.

Committee on Fetus and Newborn. 1975. "Report of the Ad Hoc Task Force on Circumcision." *Pediatrics* 56(4): 610–611.

Elmore, James M.; Baker, Linda A.; and Snodgrass, Warren T. 2002. "Topical Steroid Therapy as an Alternative to Circumcision for Phimosis in Boys Younger Than 3 Years." *Journal of Urology* 168: 1746–1747.

Kaplan, George W. 1983. "Complications of Circumcision." *Urologic Clinics of North America* 10(3): 543–549.

Kirya, Christopher, and Werthmann, Milton W. 1978. "Neonatal Circumcision and Penile Dorsal Nerve Block—A Painless Procedure." *Journal of Pediatrics* 92(6): 998–1000.

Lee, Peter A. 1990. "Neonatal Circumcision." *New England Journal of Medicine* 323(17): 1204–1205.

Lerman, S. E., and Liao, J. C. "Neonatal Circumcision." *Pediatric Clinics of North America* 48: 1539–1557.

Milos, Marilyn F., and Macris, Donna. 1992. "Circumcision: A Medical or a Human Rights Issue?" *Journal of Nurse-Midwifery* 37(2) suppl.: 87s–96s.

Poland, Ronald L. 1990. "The Question of Routine Neonatal Circumcision." *New England Journal of Medicine* 322(18): 1312–1315.

Robson, William Lane, and Leung, Alexander K. 1992. "The Circumcision Question." *Postgraduate Medicine* 96(6): 237–242, 244.

Schoen, Edgar J. 1992. "Urologists and Circumcision of Newborns." *Urology* 40(2): 99–101.

Schoen, Edgar J. 1993. "Circumcision Updated—Indicated?" *Pediatrics* 92(6): 860–861.

Snellman, Leonard W., and Stang, Howard J. 1992. "Prospective Evaluation of Complications of Local Anesthesia for Neonatal Circumcision." *American Journal of Diseases of Children* 146(4): 482.

Stang, Howard J.; Gunnar, Megan R.; Snellman, Leonard; et al. 1988. "Local Anesthesia for Neonatal Circumcision: Effects on Distress and Cortisol Response." *Journal of the American Medical Association* 259(10): 1507–1511.

Taeusch, H. W.; Martinez, A. M.; Partiridge, J. C.; et al. 2002. "Pain during Mogen or Plastibell Circumcision." *Journal of Perinatology* 22: 214–218.

Wallerstein, Edward. 1985. "Circumcision: The Uniquely American Enigma." *Urologic Clinics of North America* 12(1): 123–132.

Wiswell, Thomas E. 1992. "Circumcision: An Update." *Current Problems in Pediatrics* 22(10): 424–431.

Wiswell, Thomas E.; Smith, Franklin R.; and Bass, James W. 1985. "Decreased Incidence of Urinary Tract Infection in Circumcised Male Infants." *Pediatrics* 75(5): 901–903.

Wiswell, Thomas E.; Tencer, Heather I.; Welch, Catherine A.; et al. 1993. "Circumcision in Children beyond the Neonatal Period." *Pediatrics* 92(6): 791–793.

# CIRCUMCISION, RELIGIOUS ASPECTS OF

• • •

Throughout history different cultures have used genital alteration of males and females to express religious identity, inscribe social values, and enforce social norms of marriage, sexuality, and appropriate gender behavior. Societies differ greatly on whether they practice genital alteration on males and females, both, or neither, and on the stage of life at which procedures are done. Male circumcision, for example, is done on the eighth day of life by observant Jews, at around four or five years of age by Muslims in Turkey, and at puberty in some sub-Saharan African cultures.

Genital alteration became the subject of controversy toward the close of the twentieth century for a number of reasons. First, it is primarily performed on children and women, two groups perceived to be especially vulnerable. In the case of children, there is obvious lack of informed consent. Second, as immigrants from cultures that performed female genital alteration settled in Western countries, healthcare providers became aware of the procedures and of their negative effects on women's health. Third, a strong international feminist movement produced critics of the female procedures, both from within and without the indigenous cultures. Fourth, a century-long controversy in the United States over the health benefits of the male procedure began to move the practice away from routine recommendation of male circumcision. Fifth, a nascent *children's rights* movement began to question the ethics of performing surgery to excise healthy, normal tissue, with no proven medical benefit and, some argued, a diminution of sexual function.

The content of the controversy can be categorized into three parts. First, although there is no dispute over the lack of health benefit to females and the terrible impact of these surgeries on women's health, lively controversy exists over the negative and positive impact of male circumcision on males's health and sexual function.

Second, there is serious disagreement over appropriate language, reflecting the competing values in the debate. Male newborn genital alteration is almost always referred to as *circumcision,* a vaguely medical term that signals society's acceptance of this procedure. Conversely, the term *uncircumcised,* as opposed to *intact* or *natural,* signals the normative status of the circumcised male in American culture. When writers use circumcision to refer to the female procedure, there is often an outcry; opponents of the female procedure and defenders of the male procedure alike object to casting them in the same light. The term *female genital mutilation,* preferred by most opponents of the procedure and the term officially adopted by the World Health Organization (WHO), has its own problems. For one, as anthropologists Sandra D. Lane and Robert A. Rubinstein point out, "mutilation implies removal or destruction without medical necessity," which logically ought to refer to routine male circumcision as well (Lane and Rubinstein, p. 35). Further, the term ignores the meanings of female genital alteration in the cultures in which it is practiced, in which not to be circumcised is to look weird and disgusting. Finally, the term polarizes people rather than inviting discussion. *Cosmetic genital surgeries,* as a term for male and female procedures, has the advantage of inviting comparison with more widely accepted surgical interventions, such as breast augmentation, but the disadvantage of misleadingly implying a surgical environment, a far cry from the primitive conditions that attend most female genital surgeries. This entry uses the neutral terms *male and female genital alteration.*

Third, there is debate about whether genital alterations stem from *religion* or *culture,* with the explicit or implicit inference that the former commands more respect.

## Male Genital Alteration

The origins of male genital alteration predate any religion now in existence. It is certain that ancient Egyptians practiced some form of adult male circumcision; there are many theories about how and why the practice made its way from Egyptian culture to the Israelites, who became the first people known to genitally alter infants.

According to the Hebrew Bible, Abraham was the first Israelite to be circumcised; performing the operation on himself at the age of ninety-nine. He then circumcised all the members of his household. The Biblical injunction reads: "Every male among you shall be circumcised. And ye shall be circumcised in the flesh of your foreskin, and it shall be a token of a covenant betwixt Me and you. And he that is eight days old shall be circumcised among you, every male throughout the generations" (Gen. 17: 11–12). Both of Abraham's sons were circumcised: Ishmael, the child of Abraham's servant Hagar, and Isaac, the son of Abraham's wife Sarah.

## Male Genital Alteration in Judaism

While circumcision is the sign of belonging to the covenant, it does not confer Jewishness. Uncircumcised males can still be considered Jewish; Judaism does not practice female circumcision, but females are not thereby excluded from the covenant. In order for the religious obligation of circumcision to be fulfilled, the surgery must be set in the proper context, which includes the blessings, the correct procedure, the appropriate mindset, and the religiously mandated day of performance.

The Jewish ritual of male circumcision is called a *berit milah,* or a *bris.* It has two components: the cutting and the naming of the baby. The cutting is performed by a *mohel,* who may also be a physician. On the eighth day of the baby's life, the *mohel* comes to the home. The *berit milah* is a social occasion; friends and family are invited. Although there are many variations in how the ceremony is performed, the core ritual commonly begins with the lighting of a candle. One or two people have the honor of bringing the baby to the *throne of Elijah,* a special chair set aside for the male (often the baby's grandfather) who will hold the baby during the cutting. Traditionally, the mother remains in another room. After the ritual cutting, the baby is rediapered and allowed to nurse. The baby is given his Jewish name, and the *mohel* or rabbi, if one is present, recites blessings for the rapid healing of the baby and the continued recovery from childbirth of the mother. This is followed by a festive meal. The foreskin may be buried in the earth. In one custom, it is buried beneath a tree whose branches are later harvested to make the boy's wedding canopy.

## Male Genital Alteration in Islam

In Islam male circumcision is performed for reasons of ritual cleanliness or purity; the term used is *fitra,* which implies both physical hygiene and inner purity. Cleanliness is required for prayer to be efficacious; the uncircumcised male faces the possibility that some trace of urine will remain under the foreskin and his prayers will be nullified. Circumcision is not mentioned in the Qur'an, but is part of the second source of Islamic law: *hadith* (the sayings and doings of the Prophet). Further, the obligation of circumcision can be inferred from the fact that Allah (God) told the Prophet Muhammed to follow the religion of Ibrahim (Abraham),

and Ibrahim considered circumcision important enough to rectify his own uncircumcised state even at the advanced age of ninety-nine.

Depending upon the particular Islamic tradition and which scholars are most influential, male circumcision can be considered either obligatory or strongly recommended. The Prophet Muhammed recommended that circumcision be performed at an early age. In many Muslim cultures, the preferred time is on the seventh day after birth, and that is the common practice among North American Muslims.

## Female Genital Alteration

It would be a mistake to assume an identity between Islam and female genital alteration. Saudi Arabia and Iran, two of the most conservative Muslim nations, abjure the practice, while non-Muslim minorities living in predominantly Islamic cultures sometimes embrace it. Further, traditional genital surgeries are performed in some non-Islamic African cultures. Nonetheless, the majority of people who practice some form of this custom identify with Islam, either as a religion or as a culture.

As is the case with male circumcision, the female procedure is not mentioned in the Qur'an, but claims for its legitimacy come from *hadith.* The use of the word *sunna* (meaning to follow the path of the Prophet) as the term signifying one form of the female procedure suggests that the practice is commendatory or virtuous. Similarly, the colloquial Arabic term for female circumcision is *tahara,* referring to a state of ritual purity. The *hadith* include a saying of the Prophet that ritual circumcisers should "not overdo it, because [the clitoris] is lucky for the woman and dear to the husband." This *hadith* (although considered somewhat weak in its authenticity) is used by some Muslims to argue against the more severe forms of female genital alteration (Winkel).

## Religion and Culture Intertwined

The controversies over genital surgeries often include intense debates on the question of whether they are religiously or culturally inspired. In the United States, defining a practice as religious tends to surround it with an aura of heightened respect and protection not granted to those deemed *merely* cultural. However, it is often impossible to distinguish religious motivations from cultural ones.

Among all but the most traditional Jews, it is probably correct to say that the reasons for performing newborn circumcision are made up of religious elements, medical beliefs, and familial and communal motivations. In the United States, where approximately 80 percent of all males are circumcised, the practice of Jews is simply subsumed into the general norms. Although statistics are not available, it is generally believed that the majority of American Jews who have their newborn sons circumcised do not do so in a *berit milah*. Thus the circumcision does not fulfill the religious obligation, and will have to be repeated (in a nominal fashion) should the boy grow up to be a religious Jew. Other American Jews go through the religious ceremony, but do not partake of any other elements of Jewish religious or communal life. A high percentage of Jews genitally alter their sons in response to societal, community, or familial pressures, or simply so that a boy will look like his father. These reasons attest to the way in which male circumcision remains an important element of the communal *glue* that holds Jewish culture together, especially in tolerant America, where assimilation is feared more than anti-Semitism.

Some Jewish feminists have expressed criticism of *berit milah* because it surrounds the birth of a boy with more importance than that of a girl (although naming ceremonies for baby girls are becoming more common), and because it seems to imply a necessary connection between the male body and membership in the Jewish covenant. Miriam Pollack argues that the ritual cutting topples the mother from her rightful role as protector and nurturer of the baby, ignoring her biological instincts and "mother wisdom" (p. 171).

Female genital alteration is also practiced in response to a mix of religious, cultural, nationalist, and quasi-medical beliefs. A good example of this mix occurred in Egypt, where the proportion of genitally altered women is among the highest in the world. In 1994, at the International Conference on Population and Development in Cairo, a horrifying CNN film about female circumcision was shown, depicting the brutal cutting of a little girl. Members of Parliament responded with proposed legislation to criminalize the practice, but conservative religious authorities countered that female circumcision was an Islamic duty, and in integral component of Egyptian national identity. Other religious leaders claimed that female circumcision was a weak duty in Islam, at best, and that the issue should be decided by medical experts.

Anthropologists Lane and Rubinstein comment that, "Although it is not a practice of the majority of Muslims in the world, among those who do practice it female circumcision is nonetheless often considered to be legitimized by religion" (p. 34). Other reasons, often closely interwoven with religious ones, include the belief that without circumcision girls will *run wild*, become sexually active, and besmirch family honor (thus also flouting religious norms). The more extreme forms of genital alteration *guarantee* a daughter's virginity until marriage. In cultures in which some form of alteration is the norm, parents worry that uncircumcised daughters will be unmarriageable.

Group identity and communal cohesiveness are other motivations for female genital alteration. As new national boundaries threaten to disrupt historical tribal dominance in particular geographic areas, a process accelerated by urbanization, genital alteration can be seen as a way of marking and strengthening distinct village and tribal identities. In fact, war and dislocation can stimulate people to defend and display their cultural identity by intensified adherence to the practice. In 1997 women in displaced persons camps in Sierra Leone celebrated the end of war and their imminent return to their homes by holding a series of circumcision rituals. "'I decided to go to the bush and have this done now because I am a mature woman now,' said Bateh Kindoh, a shy 16-year-old who sat with two other recent initiates to speak with a visitor. 'We will go back to our villages soon, and I wanted to become part of the Bondo [women's communal society] first. This is a happy time for us.'" (French, p. A4).

Male and female genital alteration has an abundance of layered meanings: religious, cultural, familial, and political. There are also economic incentives for professional circumcisers to continue to defend their practice. Any discussion of these practices must take these meanings into account.

DENA S. DAVIS

SEE ALSO: *Anthropology and Bioethics; Body: Cultural and Religious Perspectives; Children: Rights of; Circumcision, Female; Circumcision, Male; Coercion; Harm; Feminism; Islam, Bioethics in; Judaism, Bioethics in; Medicine, Anthropology of; Sexual Behavior, Social Control of*

## BIBLIOGRAPHY

Abu-Sahlieh, Sami A. Aldeeb. 1994. "To Mutilate in the Name of Jehovah or Allah: Legitimization of Male and Female Circumcision." *Medicine and Law* 13: 575–622.

Coleman, Doriane Lambelet. 1998. "The Seattle Compromise: Multicultural Sensitivity and Americanization." *Duke Law Journal* 47: 717–783.

Davis, Dena S. 2001. "Male and Female Genital Alteration: A Collision Course with the Law?" *Health Matrix* 11: 487–570.

Eilberg-Schwartz, Howard. 1992. "Why Not the Earlobe?" *Moment* 17(February): 28–33.

French, Howard W. "The Ritual: Disfiguring, Hurtful, Wildly Festive." *New York Times*, January 31, 1997, p. A4.

Goldman, Ronald. 1998. *Questioning Circumcision: A Jewish Perspective.* Boston: Vanguard Publications.

Gollaher, David L. 2000. *Circumcision: A History of the World's Most Controversial Surgery.* New York: Basic Books.

Lane, Sandra D., and Rubinstein, Robert A. 1996. "Judging the Other: Responding to Traditional Female Genital Surgeries." *Hastings Center Report* 26(3): 31–40.

Moss, Lisa Braver. 1992. "Circumcision: A Jewish Inquiry." *Midstream: Monthly Jewish Review* January: 20–23.

Pollack, Miriam. 1995. "Circumcision: A Jewish Feminist Perspective." In *Jewish Women Speak Out: Expanding the Boundaries of Psychology,* ed. Kayla Weiner and Arinna Moon. Seattle: Canopy Press.

Romberg, Henry C. 1982. *Bris Milah: A Book About the Jewish Ritual of Circumcision.* New York: Feldheim Publishers.

Smith, Robin Cerny. 1992. "Female Circumcision: Bringing Women's Perspectives into the International Debate." *Southern California Law Review* 65: 2449–2504.

Winkel, Eric. 1995. "A Muslim Perspective on Female Circumcision." *Women and Health* 23(1): 1–7.

INTERNET RESOURCE

Berit Mila Program of Reform Judaism. Available from <www.rj.org/beritmila/settupbe.html>.

# CLIMATE CHANGE

• • •

In recent years many environmental problems have come to public consciousness. Of all of these problems, global climate change could prove to be the most dramatic and least reversible. It could have profound implications for the health of humans and other beings.

A climate change is quite different from a change in the weather. While weather constantly changes, climate is relatively stable. One can discuss the North American climate during the last ice age, but when one talks about the cold and snow in Boulder, Colorado, yesterday, they are talking about the weather. Weather systems last from a few hours to a few weeks and range from about 10 to 10,000 horizontal kilometers in size. A climate regime may persist for millennia, with variability in temperature and precipitation being part of a stable climate system. The climate system involves complex interactions between the atmosphere, oceans, land surface, snow and ice cover, and the biosphere. Researchers

are learning that human activity is also a part of the dynamic that affects climate.

## The Discovery of Anthropogenic Climate Change

On June 23, 1988, a sweltering day in Washington, D.C., in the middle of a severe drought in the United States, James Hansen of the National Aeronautics and Space Administration (NASA) testified before the U.S. Senate Committee on Energy and Natural Resources. It was 99 percent probable, Hansen contended, that global warming had begun. His testimony, which was covered by media all over the world, appeared to many people to come from nowhere. But like most overnight sensations, speculation about climate change has a history.

In the eighteenth century Benjamin Franklin surmised that the hard winter of 1783 to 1784 was due to excessive dust in the air, either from the destruction of meteorites or from volcanic eruptions. Early in the nineteenth century the French mathematician Jean Baptiste Fourier (1768–1830) speculated that the atmosphere might function like the glass in a greenhouse, warming Earth's surface by preventing heat from escaping. In 1861 British physicist John Tyndall (1820–1893) showed that slight changes in the composition of the atmosphere could significantly raise Earth's temperature. The Swedish Nobel Prize winner Svante Arrhenius (1859–1927) theorized in 1896 that the use of fossil fuels would increase atmospheric carbon dioxide, thereby changing climate and affecting biological processes. He calculated that a doubling of atmospheric carbon dioxide would lead to an increase of four to six degrees centigrade in Earth's mean surface temperature. In the 1930s the British engineer George Callendar revived Arrhenius's ideas and asserted that global warming had already begun. Working in the United States, Gilbert Plass, Roger Revelle, and Hans Suess brought these ideas into the scientific mainstream in the 1950s. A very influential article by Revelle and Suess in 1957 asserted that because of the exponentially increasing use of fossil fuels, an experiment was in progress that could not have happened in the past and that could not be reproduced in the future. Their work led to the establishment of the Mauna Loa Observatory in Hawaii, which has been measuring carbon dioxide concentrations in the atmosphere since 1958.

The climate anomalies of 1972 and the global food shortages of 1972 to 1973 brought the possibility of climate change to the attention of a broader audience. Droughts in the Sahel region of Africa in the late 1960s and early 1970s had reminded people how dependent on climate humans remain. When drought also occurred in the Soviet Union in 1972, world grain prices doubled and global food shortages followed. During the same year, frost destroyed coffee plantations in Brazil, and changes in seawater temperatures (related to a climate anomaly called El Niño) had a severe impact on Peru's anchovy fisheries. U.S. Secretary of State Henry Kissinger raised the possibility of climate change in a 1974 speech to the United Nations.

The climate change scare of the early 1970s was a fear of cooling. From the 1940s through the 1960s, Earth's mean surface temperature had declined; there was concern that another ice age was beginning. The Central Intelligence Agency undertook a study of how such a cooling might affect agricultural production in the Soviet Union; and the same Senate committee that fifteen years later would hold hearings on global warming held hearings on global cooling.

Whether the fear was of a cooling or a warming, climate increasingly came to be viewed as a dynamic system that is vulnerable to human action. By the mid-1970s the possibility of climate change had been discovered.

## The Current Scientific View

Throughout the late 1970s and 1980s, conferences and studies were instituted by a wide range of national and international organizations. The culmination of this activity was the 1990 report of the Intergovernmental Panel on Climate Change (IPCC). The process that led to the development of this report involved 170 scientists from 25 countries; 200 other scientists reviewed the results. The goal of the IPCC process was to determine the international scientific consensus about climate change. The conclusion was that if emissions of *greenhouse gases* (primarily carbon dioxide, methane, chlorofluorocarbons, and nitrous oxide) continue as usual, Earth's mean surface temperature could rise 0.2 to 0.5 degree centigrade per decade, with a likely warming of 1 degree centigrade by 2025, and 3 degrees centigrade by the end of the twenty-first century. This would be the greatest temperature change to have occurred on Earth for at least 10,000 years.

The eight warmest years in the historical record have occurred since the publication of the first IPCC report in 1990. This, combined with scientific advances in the understanding of climate and increasingly sophisticated climate models, has strengthened the case for anthropogenic climate change. This has been reflected in subsequent IPCC reports. The 1995 Second Assessment concluded that "[t]he balance of evidence suggests a discernible human influence on global climate" (p. 5). The Third Assessment, published in 2001, stated categorically that "[a]nthropogenic climate change will persist for many centuries," estimating that the Earth's global mean surface temperature will increase from 1.4 to 5.8°C from 1990 to 2100 (p.17).

Although some remain skeptical, one thing that is certain is that there is a *greenhouse effect.* According to climatologist Stephen Schneider, it is "one of the best, most well-established scientific theories in the atmospheric sciences" (Boyle and Ardill, p. 12). Were it not for the greenhouse effect, all of the planets of the solar system would be cold and lifeless. But as researchers have learned in other areas, such as medicine, too much of a good thing can be a bad thing.

The greenhouse effect occurs when a planetary atmosphere, due to its physical/chemical composition, permits solar radiation to heat the surface of the planet but traps some of the heat that would otherwise radiate back into space. The greenhouse effect explains, at least partially, the differences between conditions on the surfaces of Venus, Mars, and Earth. Venus has an extremely dense, carbon dioxide-rich atmosphere that traps so much heat that life is not possible on the surface of the planet. Mars has a very thin, carbon dioxide–poor atmosphere, and mid-latitude surface temperatures on Mars are about the same as those of Earth's polar winters. Earth is just right for evolving and sustaining life—at least for the moment.

Another fact about which researchers are certain is that human activity is affecting the chemical composition of Earth's atmosphere. From 1860 to 2000 there was an increase of about 34 percent in atmospheric carbon dioxide, more than half of that occurring since the 1960s. Other greenhouse gases have increased by even greater percentages during the same period. Concentrations of these gases have risen as a result of activities that are essential to economic growth and development, at least as they are presently conceived: fossil fuel combustion, deforestation, food-animal production, rice-paddy agriculture, and fertilizer use.

What is certain, then, is that the greenhouse effect exists, and that concentrations of greenhouse gases in the atmosphere are increasing. However, not all scientists agree about the likely effects of these increasing concentrations. There are extremely complicated and ill-understood feedbacks in the climate system. The effects of these feedbacks could be to stabilize climate even in the face of changes in the atmosphere, or to exaggerate the effects of climate change. Since these feedbacks are not well understood, the scientific community's prediction of a significant greenhouse warming is a cautious one.

## The Effects of Climate Change

The image that many people have of a global warming is that all regions of Earth would be warmed equally, as if one turned up the thermostat in the global house. This image is quite misleading. The impacts of global warming would be very diverse. Some regions would warm while others would cool. Precipitation patterns would change, and extreme events (e.g., droughts and hurricanes) would become more frequent. While this much is clear, it is extremely difficult to say how particular regions would be affected. The predictions generally agree about the global effects of climate change but disagree to a great extent about its regional effects.

Impacts of climate change fall into three categories. First-order impacts involve physical changes such as rises in sea level, effects on biological systems and circulation of water and so on. A large number of species will become extinct and many ecosystems will fracture and disintegrate. Some of the most dramatic first-order effects of a global warming would be the inundation of island nations, such as the Maldives, Kiribati (Gilbert Islands), and the Marshall Islands. Egypt could lose 1 percent of its land due to flooding. Second-order impacts involve the direct social, economic, and health effects of first-order impacts. An example would be the economic, social, and cultural consequences of Egypt's loss of 1 percent of its land. The part of Egypt that would be threatened by a sea-level rise is the Nile delta, home to 48 million people and contributor of 15 percent of Egypt's GNP. Third-order impacts of climate change involve the indirect social and political responses to the first- and second-order effects. Third-order impacts might include massive emigration from affected regions such as the Nile delta, and international conflicts resulting from economic dislocations and changing patterns of resource use.

The impact of climate change on human health is an area of research that has been receiving a great deal of attention. In particular, there is concern that infectious diseases such as malaria and dengue fever will become more prevalent, along with water-borne diseases such as cholera. There are already 300 million clinically confirmed cases of malaria in the world, causing more than 1 million annual deaths. Infectious diseases are currently the largest source of mortality in the developing world, and until sometime in the twentieth century they were also the largest killer in most of the developed world. Increases in the prevalence of infectious disease could have devastating effects on the human population.

Until the late 1980s it was commonly said that all people would suffer from climate change. However it has become increasingly clear that climate change will involve winners and losers, and most experts believe that the rich countries will do better than the poor ones. Rich countries can build seawalls and dikes to protect coastal areas against rising sea levels. They can even gain economically by developing and exporting technologies that will help in adapting

to climate change. Rich countries can pay more for food if climate change adversely affects agriculture. In general, their control of capital can be used to shield them from many effects of a changing climate. Poor countries do not have resources to protect themselves in these ways. Moreover, some poor countries (e.g., Bangladesh) already suffer enormously from extreme climatic events.

But even though it may generally be true that the rich would do better than the poor in adapting to climate change, there are still reasons for the rich to be concerned. Rich people are often more averse to risk than poor people, for they have more to lose. Moreover, if climate change occurs, there will be differential effects across both rich and poor countries. For example, according to some scenarios, agriculture in the U.S. Great Plains might dry up and blow away, while in some arid regions of Africa precipitation might increase.

Although the regional effects of global climate change are uncertain, it is clear that there will be winners and losers. When human action has consequences that benefit some and burden others, it becomes a matter for moral evaluation.

## Risk and Insurance

Some commentators have tried to transform the ethical problems implicit in the possibility of climate change into problems of rational choice. One approach has been to think of the possibility of climate change as a risk, and the costs of emission reduction, mitigation, and adaptation as the premium paid for insurance against this risk. However tempting this approach may be, the insurance metaphor is misleading. An insurance company is able to set rational premiums because of actuarial tables that are based on the frequency with which compensable losses occur. But however strong the theoretical reasons are for thinking that climate change will occur, researchers have nothing like actuarial tables that tell them about the frequency of climate change when the atmosphere is loaded with greenhouse gases. Moreover, the idea that society is in a position to reasonably assess the potential damages of climate change is quite absurd. No one knows what all the economic and health effects of a greenhouse warming would be, much less how to attach meaningful economic values to the loss of many wild species and the destruction of societies and cultures. As a result, economists who work on climate change tend to focus on the more easily quantifiable costs of emissions reductions rather than on the damages that such investments might help society to avoid. While it is easy to talk about the importance of taking out insurance against the possibility of a greenhouse warming, at present there is no way to determine what it would be rational to pay for such insurance.

Finally, the insurance metaphor defers rather than evades the ethical questions. Even if one were able to determine a rational premium, the question of how the costs should be distributed would remain. Talk of purchasing insurance against the risk of a greenhouse warming does not free society from the hard ethical discussions.

## Moral and Political Issues

Philosophers often distinguish duties of justice from other sorts of duties. For present purposes, however, one can think of climate change as posing questions of justice with respect to human contemporaries (intragenerational justice), descendants (intergenerational justice), and possibly nonhuman nature. Because climate change is by its very nature global in scope, the questions of justice that it provokes are international.

The rich countries of the world have loaded the atmosphere with the greenhouse gases that may already be changing climate. They have benefited from their actions by developing economically. While rich countries have gained the benefits, the deleterious effects of their emissions will be felt by everyone. If climate change-induced floods occur in Bangladesh, it will not be due to the actions of the Bangladeshis. They will not have caused the floods, nor will they have benefited from the past emissions of greenhouse gases that caused them.

In addition to these historical inequities in emissions, there are important differences in present emissions. A handful of industrial countries emit between one-half and three-quarters of all greenhouse gases. Yet at the United Nations-sponsored Conference on Environment and Development, held in Rio de Janeiro in June 1992, the rich countries were unwilling to agree to timetables and targets even for stabilizing their emissions, much less reducing them, mainly due to the intransigence of the United States. Finally at Kyoto in 1997 the nations of the world did agree to binding timetables and targets for emissions reductions, only to have the United States and Australia jump ship after doing everything they could to weaken the agreement.

Rich countries became rich in part by taking actions that are changing the global climate. This climate change may have devastating impacts on poor countries. What do the rich owe the poor as a consequence of their actions? This question arises against the background of an international system characterized by radical and increasing inequality. According to Sir Crispin Tickell, in 1880 the ratio of real per capita income between Europe, on the one hand, and India and China, on the other, was two to one; in 1965 it was forty to one; and in the 1990s it was seventy to one. Even on the most conservative assumptions, between 1820 and 1970

global inequality doubled (Dollar and Kraay). One way of making this inequality vivid is by considering these examples from the *Human Development Report 1998: Consumption for Human Development* (United Nations Development Programme, p. 29). In 1960, 20 percent of the world's people who lived in the richest countries had thirty times the income of the poorest 20 percent, and by 1995 eighty-two times as much income. The wealth of the fifteen richest people in the world exceeds the total GDP of sub-Saharan Africa. The assets of the eighty-four richest individuals in the world are greater than the GDP of China at the beginning of the twenty-first century. The 225 richest people in the world have combined wealth that is equal to the annual income of the poorest 47 percent of the world's population. In absolute terms, more than 1 billion people live on less than $1 per day, and nearly 3 billion live on less than $2 per day (World Bank).

Underlying these problems of inequality and poverty are an exploding population in some parts of the developing world and increasing overconsumption in the developed world. The United States, with 5 percent of the world's population, annually consumes 25 percent of the world's fossil fuels, 33 percent of its paper, 24 percent of its aluminum, and 13 percent of its fertilizer. A child born in 1994 in the United States will in his or her lifetime drive 700,000 miles, using 28,000 gallons of gasoline; produce 110,250 pounds of trash; eat 8,486 pounds of red meat; and consume enough electricity to burn 16,610 pounds of coal. Earth simply cannot support many Americans. The world population as of 2003 is more than 6.2 billion, and is increasing by 75 million per year. An optimistic scenario calls for world population to stabilize at more than 10 billion in the twenty-third century. Many observers expect population to grow far beyond that.

One way of trying to understand the joint impact of overconsumption and exploding population is to consider the following facts. Sweden is a country that enjoys one of the highest standards of living in the world, yet its per capita carbon dioxide emissions are little more than one-fourth of those of the United States. If Sweden's level of per capita emissions were to be established as an international ceiling, the United States would have to reduce its emissions by vastly more than anyone is willing to even consider. Yet, even given such painful reductions on the part of some countries, on this scenario world emissions would increase by more than one-third, reflecting the large populations of some less developed countries that consume very little energy.

Philosophical theorizing about international justice is underdeveloped, and very little work has been done on international environmental justice. The most influential philosophical theories of justice were formulated with an eye to what constitutes a just national distribution of private goods. Pattern theories such as that of John Rawls, and entitlement theories such as that of Robert Nozick, have received the most attention. Although one can speculate about what these theories might imply with respect to climate change, neither philosopher has had much to say about global justice, much less global environmental justice.

Rawls' principle of distributive justice is the "Difference Principle": Social and economic inequalities are to be attached to positions and offices that are open to all under conditions of fair equality of opportunity, and they are to be distributed to the greatest benefit of the least advantaged members of society. Whether one takes the subjects to be individuals or societies, it seems quite obvious that the global distribution of social and economic benefits is unjust according to this principle. Moreover, if one were to use the Difference Principle as a test for who should benefit from further releases of greenhouse gases and who should bear the costs of reduction, it seems equally clear that current policies would not satisfy this principle.

Nozick argues that the moral acceptability of a distribution depends entirely on how it came about. If the present distribution resulted from a just initial distribution through voluntary exchanges, then it is just, regardless of how unequal it may be. But given the global history of domination, imperialism, and exploitation, it seems clear that the present global distribution is unjust on Nozick's grounds. According to Nozick, any complete theory of justice must include a principle specifying how past injustices are to be rectified, but he has little to say about what such a principle may require.

Although it appears that both Rawls and Nozick are committed to the view that the current international order is unjust, neither deals specifically with this question or with the distribution of environmental benefits and burdens. Moreover, there are reasons for supposing that many environmental goods resist treatment as distributable benefits and burdens. The bad effects of climate change would include spillover effects suffered by some parties who had virtually no role in bringing them about. On reasonable human time scales, a stable climate is irreplaceable and irreversible. Furthermore, modeling aspects of the environment as distributable goods may be misleading and inappropriate. Such an approach neglects the fact that humans are situated in an environment that conditions and affects everything they do, and in part constitutes their identities.

While there is good reason for supposing that both historical and current patterns of greenhouse gas emissions are part of an unjust system of intragenerational relationships, philosophical theories of justice have not yet given the conceptual resources to address these issues in a detailed and meaningful way. More work needs to be done.

In addition to questions about intragenerational justice, global climate change poses moral questions about intergenerational justice. Those who come after us will live in a very different world than the one we inhabit in the early twenty-first century, due in part to actions that we are taking. Some who are influenced by utilitarian philosophers such as Henry Sidgwick may think that we owe just as much to future people as to present ones, since once they come to exist, they will be just as real as present people and will have the same moral status. On this view, the claims of future people should not be treated less seriously than those of present people simply because they are remote from us in time. But barring a complete collapse of Earth's human population, over the course of millennia there will be vastly more people in the future than exist now. If we take each future person as seriously as each present person, it would appear that the interests of the present would be swamped by virtue of the size of our future human population.

Other thinkers, impressed by an argument in Derek Parfit's 1984 book titled *Reasons and Persons*, may conclude that we have no obligations to future people (although this is not Parfit's conclusion). On this view, future people who feel disadvantaged would have no cause for complaint against us because their very existence would be contingent on actions that we have taken. If our present actions were other than they are, then different people would come to exist in the future. Thus, no future person can say that he or she would have been better off had we made different choices; for if we had made different choices, then that person would not have existed at all.

Many economists would grant that we have obligations to those who will follow us, but they would argue that these obligations are easily fulfilled. Suppose that, because in 2003 we act in such a way as to change the climate, our descendants living in 2103 incur damages valued at $N$ dollars. In order for our climate change activities to be justified, we must profit enough from them to provide our descendants with $N$ dollars when they come into existence. Because of the power of compound interest, small present benefits justify large future damages. If $N$ dollars come due in a century and we can obtain a 5 percent return on our investments, our present benefit from climate-changing activities would have to be only $.0068N$ dollars (compounded monthly) in order for them to be justified. In other words, a present benefit of $100,000 would justify inflicting a compensation of $14.68 billion on those living a century hence.

There are many problems with such an approach. Even if we were able to compensate future people adequately in this way, they will have been deprived of the ability to make some significant choices. For example, they will not have been able to choose to preserve a stable climate regime, even if that implies a lower standard of living.

This approach also involves the ludicrous idea that we can attach meaningful economic values to the loss of many wild species, the destruction of societies and cultures, and the unknown health effects of significant climate change. There simply are no credible attempts to carry out a benefit-cost analysis of the warming of Earth's median surface temperature by 3 degrees centigrade. This is hardly surprising, since there is often a great deal of disagreement about such relatively simple questions as the short-term effects of a change in the marginal tax rate of a single country.

Peter Brown and Edith Brown Weiss have argued that we have a fiduciary trust to preserve Earth's natural and human heritage at a level at least as good as that we received. On this basis, Weiss argues that we should reduce greenhouse gas emissions, take steps to minimize the damage that results from climate change, and develop strategies to assist future generations in adapting to climate change. This is a sensible approach that has the virtue of squaring with many people's moral intuitions. It suggests that we have significant obligations to future people, but that they do not entirely swamp the interests of the present.

Unfortunately, the fiduciary view verges on the platitudinous. Among those who believe that the buildup of greenhouse gases poses a threat, not many would deny that we need to reduce emissions, minimize harms, and develop adaptation strategies. What people disagree about is how aggressively we should pursue these policies, what the proper mix of them is, and who should bear the burdens. The fiduciary approach stops short of trying to answer these hard questions.

Furthermore, if we take seriously the idea that each generation has an obligation to preserve Earth's natural and human heritage at a level at least as good as what was received, then we are immediately faced with questions about how to evaluate the goodness of our own heritage and various changes that we might make with respect to it. These are the sorts of questions that economists try to answer, using various techniques of benefit-cost analysis, such as interviewing people about their willingness to pay (or accept compensation) for environmental good, that ethicists typically find unsatisfactory.

In addition to the problems of human health and welfare that are likely to be caused by climate change, nonhuman nature will also be affected. Climate change is likely to be much too rapid for most plants and animals to adapt to or migrate from. Even when migration would in principle be possible, no migration routes will be available for most plants and animals in a densely populated and developed world.

In recent years a powerful literature has developed that argues humans have obligations to nonhuman nature. Some philosophers, such as Peter Singer, argue that our direct obligations end at the border of sentience; others, such as Holmes Rolston III, argue that we have obligations to virtually every element of the natural order. Whatever we may think about this dispute, only someone who believes that our obligations are exhausted by our duties to humanity can remain unmoved in the face of this anticipated destruction of nonhuman nature.

Indeed, even someone who believes that our obligations are only to humans may feel that massive destruction of nonhuman nature is morally appalling. Humans have preferences about what happens to nature, and insofar as nature's destruction is contrary to human preferences, this destruction can be morally condemned. Moreover, anyone can be morally appalled by the character of a culture that would so willingly destroy nature in order to preserve a way of life that is rooted in overconsumption. One might think of nature as being like a work of art. We may not think that works of art are the direct objects of moral concern, yet we may morally condemn those who would vandalize them—say by burning the contents of the Louvre in order to warm their houses by one or two extra degrees for a year or so.

Climate change poses serious threats to human health and welfare and raises questions about our global duties and our duties to nonhuman nature. As the concentration of greenhouse gases in the atmosphere continues to increase, the moral issue of climate change will grow in importance.

DALE JAMIESON (1995)
REVISED BY AUTHOR

SEE ALSO: *Agriculture and Biotechnology; Endangered Species and Biodiversity; Environmental Ethics; Environmental Health; Future Generations, Reproductive Technologies and Obligations to; Hazardous Wastes and Toxic Substances; Justice; Population Ethics; Sustainable Development*

### BIBLIOGRAPHY

Agarwal, Anil, and Nurain, Sunita. 1991. *Global Warming in an Unequal World: A Case of Environmental Colonialism.* New Delhi: Centre for Science and the Environment.

Boyle, Stewart, and Ardill, John. 1989. *The Greenhouse Effect.* London: New English Library.

Brown, Peter G. 1992. "Climate Change and the Planetary Trust." *Energy Policy* 20(3): 208–222.

Dollar, David, and Kraay, Aartt. 2002. "Spreading the Wealth." *Foreign Affairs* 81(1): 120–133.

Glantz, Michael, ed. 1988. *Societal Responses to Regional Climatic Change: Forecasting by Analogy.* Boulder, CO: Westview.

Houghton, J. T., et al., eds. 1996. *Climate Change 1995: The Science of Climate Change* Cambridge, Eng.: Cambridge University Press.

Intergovernmental Panel on Climatic Change (IPCC). 2001. *Climate Change: 2001* 3 vols. Cambridge, Eng.: Cambridge University Press.

Jamieson, Dale. 1992. "Ethics, Public Policy, and Global Warming." *Science, Technology, and Human Values* 17(2): 139–153.

Jamieson, Dale. 1994. "Global Environmental Justice." In *Philosophy and the Natural Environment,* ed. Robin Attfield and Andrew Belsey. Cambridge, Eng.: Cambridge University Press.

Jamieson, Dale. 2001. "Climate Change and Global Environmental Justice." In *Changing the Atmosphere: Expert Knowledge and Environmental Governance,* ed. Clark A. Miller and Paul N. Edwards. Cambridge, MA: MIT Press.

McMichael, Anthony J. 1996. *Climate Change and Human Health.* Geneva: World Health Organization.

Nordhaus, William D. 1994. *Managing the Global Commons: The Economics of Climate Change.* Cambridge, MA: MIT Press.

Nozick, Robert. 1974. *Anarchy, State, and Utopia.* New York: Basic Books.

Parfit, Derek. 1984. *Reasons and Persons.* Oxford: Oxford University Press.

Rawls, John. 1999. *A Theory of Justice,* 2nd edition. Cambridge, MA: Harvard University Press.

Revelle, Roger, and Suess, Hans E. 1957. "Carbon Dioxide Exchange Between Atmosphere and Ocean and the Question of an Increase of Atmospheric CO2 During the Past Decades." *Tellus* 6(1): 18–27.

Rolston, Holmes, III. 1988. *Environmental Ethics: Duties to and Values in the Natural World.* Philadelphia: Temple University Press.

Sidgwick, Henry. 1874. *Methods of Ethics.* London: Macmillan.

Singer, Peter. 2001. *Animal Liberation,* 2nd edition. New York: Ecco Press.

Tickell, Sir Crispin. 1992. "The Quality of Life: What Quality? Whose Life?" *Interdisciplinary Science Reviews* 17(1): 19–25.

United Nations Development Programme. 1998. *Human Development Report 1998: Consumption for Human Development.* Oxford: Oxford University Press.

Weiss, Edith Brown. 1988. *In Fairness to Future Generations: International Law, Common Patrimony, and Intergenerational Equity.* Dobbs Ferry, NY: Transnational Publishers.

World Bank. 2000. *World Development Report 2000/2001: Attacking Poverty.* New York: Oxford University Press.

World Meteorlogical Organization/United Nations Environment Programme, Intergovernmental Panel on Climate Change, The IPCC Response Strategies. 1991. Washington, D.C.: Island Press.

# CLINICAL ETHICS

• • •

I. Development, Role, and Methodologies

II. Clinical Ethics Consultation

III. Institutional Ethics Committees

## I. DEVELOPMENT, ROLE, AND METHODOLOGIES

Formal efforts to address clinical ethics first developed in the United States and Canada, though similar efforts are clearly underway in western and central Europe and Japan. Indeed, interest in clinical ethics has spread to many areas of the world, including parts of Central and South America, eastern Europe, and parts of Africa. Though variously defined, clinical ethics involves the identification, analysis, and resolution of value conflicts or uncertainties that arise in the provision of healthcare in clinical settings (Fletcher and Boyle; Jonsen, Siegler, and Winslade). Clinical ethics activities include examination or formulation of relevant policies, ethics education, and ethics consultation to healthcare professionals, patients, families, surrogates, or organizations. Unlike some solely academic domains of the broader field of bioethics, clinical ethics must take into account the actual context in which clinical ethical issues arise because it aims to make contributions to clinical practice and to policy governing clinical practice. This context includes complex psychosocial, medical, legal, cultural, and political dimensions that have implications both for the types of ethical issues that arise and how those issues may be resolved (Aulisio, Arnold, and Youngner, 2000, 2003; May).

Traditionally, clinical ethics discussions tended to focus on issues related to informed consent, confidentiality and privacy, decision capacity or competence, decision making involving minors, resource allocation, and end-of-life care. Though these issues remain central to clinical ethics, the mid-1990s through early 2000s saw a growing recognition of the important relationship between clinical, organizational, and business ethics (Schyve et al.), along with the development of a number of new areas of concern, including physician-assisted suicide (Battin, Rhodes, and Silvers), palliative care (Barnard et al.), medical mistakes (Rubin and Zoloth; Institute of Medicine), ethics and genetics (Juengst), and even bioterrorism (Gostin).

The typical mechanism for addressing issues in clinical ethics in most healthcare institutions is an ethics committee. Ethics committees are present in most hospital settings in the United States and Canada, and increasingly in other settings, such as long-term care, as well. In some clinical settings, most often academic medical centers, ethics committees are part of a much larger clinical ethics program. Such programs are commonly staffed by full-time ethicists who are responsible for ethics education, service, and research.

## Development

Renée C. Fox and David J. Rothman both argued that bioethics began in the 1960s as a social and intellectual movement. The earliest concerns of bioethics were focused on acute ethical problems in research settings. Influenced by the U.S. civil rights movement, bioethical inquiry also exposed weaknesses in institutional arrangements that no longer adequately protected research subjects or patients (Fletcher). From its origins to the present, the bioethics movement has had two arms: (1) an interdisciplinary dialogue, known as bioethics, that became a new academic subdiscipline in the larger field of ethics; and (2) an agenda for institutional and social change to prevent abuses and enhance the values that guide decision making concerning research subjects and patients. Social changes in research settings to protect human subjects preceded such changes in patient-care settings by almost a decade.

The 1960s saw a number of widely publicized and much debated cases that brought to the fore the value-laden nature of clinical practice and the difficult choices posed, in part, by rapid advances in medical technology (Jonsen, 2000). The invention of a plastic arteriovenous shunt by an American physician, Belding H. Scribner, in 1960 made possible chronic hemodialysis and, simultaneously, created a profound ethical dilemma because there were far more patients in need of chronic hemodialysis than the Seattle Artificial Kidney Center could accommodate. This dilemma led to the establishment of the Admissions and Policy Committee, later infamously referred to as the "Seattle God Committee," which employed "social worth criteria" to select candidates for dialysis. Throughout the decade, successes in organ transplantation created similar ethical dilemmas related to resource allocation. In 1967 South African surgeon Christiaan Barnard's successful transplantation of a

beating heart from a patient with "irreversibly fatal brain damage" raised serious ethical questions about the definition of death. In response, a committee at Harvard Medical School, the following year, formulated a statement that defined "brain death" (Jonsen, 2000).

If the ethical dilemmas raised by chronic hemodialysis and organ transplantation remained a bit removed from the lives of ordinary people, the 1970s were dominated by cases that clearly resonated with the general populace. In the racially charged climate of the early 1970s, the *New York Times'* 1972 expose of the U.S. Public Health Service's forty-year Tuskegee Syphilis Study of the progression of untreated syphilis in African-American men powerfully demonstrated how social values, even disvalues such as racism, can dramatically affect "scientific" practice in clinical settings. The study, which ran from 1932 to 1972, enrolled 600 African-American men from Tuskegee, Alabama. All participants were told that they had "bad blood" and were in need of regular medical exams, including spinal taps. In exchange for these exams, participants were given transportation to and from the hospital, hot lunches, medical care, and free burial (upon the completion of an autopsy). Of the study participants, 200 did not have syphilis, while the other 400 were diagnosed with syphilis but were never told their diagnosis or treated for their disease (even after effective treatment became available) (Jonsen, 2000; Pence). In January 1973, less than a year after the Tuskegee expose, the value-laden nature of clinical practice was again thrust into the public eye when the U.S. Supreme Court handed down its landmark decision in *Roe v. Wade.* In setting off a decades-long struggle over the morality and legality of abortion, the case also introduced extramedical notions such as "personhood," "viability," and "privacy" into the public debate.

Despite the significance of Tuskegee and *Roe,* no single case captured the public imagination or shaped the development of clinical ethics more than the tragedy of Karen Ann Quinlan did (Pence). Quinlan was a twenty-one-year-old patient at St. Clare's Hospital in Denville, New Jersey. Having lapsed into a coma in April 1975 as a result of the combined effects of alcohol, Valium, and, possibly, Librium, she was dependent on a respirator (ventilator) and was eventually deemed to be in a *persistent vegetative state* (sometimes referred to as being *permanently unconscious*). In addition to the respirator, Quinlan was dependent on the technological administration of nutrition and hydration through the use of a nasogastric (NG) tube (one that delivers food and water to the stomach through the nose). After months of anguished deliberation, Quinlan's parents, Julia and Joseph Quinlan, in consultation with their parish priest, decided to remove her from the respirator and let her die. The Quinlan's decision, however, was opposed by hospital officials on the grounds that to remove the patient's respirator support in order to let her die was euthanasia—the moral and legal equivalent of murder (Pence).

Though New Jersey Supreme Court, in a 1976 ruling, ultimately supported the rights of the Quinlans to remove their daughter from the respirator, the tragedy of Karen Ann Quinlan had a dramatic impact on society and, in particular, on the rise of clinical ethics. Quinlan's dependence on a respirator and feeding tube came to symbolize, for many, "an oppressive medical technology, unnaturally prolonging dying" (Pence, p. 31). Once again, technological developments in medical science, this time the respirator and NG tube, had created new and difficult ethical dilemmas. Before the advent of respirators and feeding tubes, patients in Quinlan's situation simply died. There were no questions about "withholding" or "withdrawing" treatment, "active" or "passive" euthanasia, "ordinary" or "extraordinary" means, or who should be allowed to make life-and-death decisions and under what circumstances. If some people could not identify with chronic hemodialysis, organ transplantation, and the like, everyone could identify with the plight of Quinlan. Indeed, the New Jersey Supreme Court seemed to recognize this when it suggested that ethics committees be developed in hospitals so that future cases might be addressed before reaching the courts (*In re Quinlan*, 1976).

Not surprisingly, then, the 1970s saw the first clear growth of formal efforts in clinical ethics. Ethics committees began to be established in major hospitals. Scholars in bioethics increasingly taught new courses as faculty members of medical, nursing, and other professional schools. Bioethics scholars also served developing programs in the "medical humanities." In addition, some academic medical centers began to use bioethics and medical humanities scholars to offer ethics education and even ethics consultation in cases involving patients (Jonsen, 1980).

Throughout the 1980s difficult cases continued to spur the development of clinical ethics. In part because of the *Quinlan* case and a national debate on end-of-life decisions, 1980 saw the establishment of the President's Commission for the Study of Ethical Problems in Medicine and Biomedical and Behavioral Research, which in 1983 issued its groundbreaking report, *Deciding to Forego Life-Sustaining Treatment*. The 1980s also saw the debate about withholding/withdrawing life-sustaining treatment extend to neonatal intensive care medicine with a series of hotly debated "Baby Doe" cases involving impaired newborns. The cases of Nancy Cruzan (*Cruzan v. Director*, 1990) and Elizabeth Bouvia (*Bouvia v. Superior Court,* 1986) raised additional ethical issues concerning end-of-life decisions and adults: Is artificially administered nutrition and hydration medical treatment? What evidentiary standard should be satisfied in making end-of-life decisions for formerly competent, but now incompetent, adults? Who is authorized to set such a standard? Does a competent adult have a right to refuse nutrition and hydration? Finally, the emergence of the HIV/AIDS epidemic raised a host of ethical issues that surfaced throughout the 1980s, including, but not limited to, concerns about: confidentiality and privacy; health professionals' duties to treat HIV-infected patients and duties to disclose their own HIV/AIDS status; duties to warn at-risk third parties; patient duties to disclose HIV/AIDS status to health providers; and mandatory testing for health professionals and others.

During the 1980s, several postgraduate training programs, some textbooks, and one journal declared that they addressed *clinical ethics,* a term that had not been used in the earlier bioethics movement. The practice of ethics consultation began to be defined in the early to mid-1980s (Fletcher, Quist, and Jonsen), and ethics committees multiplied in clinical settings to protect shared decision making with patients and family members.

With the Patient Self-Determination Act of 1991 and the stipulation of the Joint Commission on Accreditation of Healthcare Organizations (1993) that member institutions must have a "mechanism" for "the consideration of ethical issues arising in the care of patients and to provide education to caregivers and patients on ethical issues in health care" (R.1.1.6.1, p. 9), the importance of formal efforts in clinical ethics was given expression through regulatory requirements in the United States. These rules intensified the need for competence and leadership in clinical ethics. Partly in response to this, the 1990s saw efforts by groups in Canada and the United States to address standards for ethics consultants and consultation. From the mid- to late 1990s physician-assisted suicide and palliative care captured much of the clinical ethics debate, and the rise of managed care pushed organizational ethical issues into the clinical domain.

There can be little doubt that clinical ethics is becoming an established subdiscipline of the broader field of bioethics. Highly multidisciplinary, clinical ethics is pursued by clinicians—physicians, nurses, social workers, and other health professionals—as well as by those with backgrounds in the humanities (including philosophy, theology, history, and literature), social sciences (including sociology, anthropology, and public health), and law. By 2001 there were at least forty-seven academic institutions offering graduate training programs (including certificate and fellowship programs) in bioethics or medical humanities; a number had clinical ethics components; and several were specifically devoted to clinical ethics (Aulisio and Rothenberg). Despite the rapid increase in graduate training programs in bioethics and medical humanities, the vast majority of the people offering clinical ethics services at healthcare institutions have little or no formal education and training in clinical ethics (Aulisio, Arnold, and Youngner, 2003). This suggests a continued need for educational and training programs tailored specifically to this group.

## Role and Methodologies

Education and service (e.g., consultation and policy formation) are the foci of clinical ethics efforts in most healthcare institutions. Typically, a clinical ethics program in a healthcare institution, such as a large hospital, will provide staff and community education, policy critique and formulation, retrospective and prospective case review, and case consultation. The most active clinical ethics programs tend to be at academic medical centers that employ clinical ethicists. In the academic medical setting, clinical ethicists may be involved in teaching at all levels of health-professional education (preclinical, clinical, graduate, postgraduate, and continuing education). Some institutions with programs in clinical ethics offer advanced education and training through fellowship or degree programs. They may also have outreach efforts to assist in the formation of clinical ethics programs and the training of leaders for these programs.

Although education and service are central to any clinical ethics program, research can be an important component as well, particularly in an academic setting. Such research may include the type of conceptual and analytic work characteristic of humanities research (e.g., case analysis, conceptual clarification, normative assessment of particular clinical ethics issues) or the type of empirical research more characteristic of the social sciences (e.g., frequency occurrence of various ethical problems; the practical impact of various policies or practices; attitudes and beliefs of specific populations toward particular ethical issues; effectiveness of certain interventions designed to promote informed consent, protect privacy, and so forth) (Singer, Siegler, and Pellegrino). The increasingly vast clinical ethics literature is indicative of the dramatic growth in clinical ethics research since the 1980s.

Like clinical ethics itself, discussions of methodological issues in clinical ethics have evolved and developed over the years. As clinical ethics emerged, the prevailing approach to bioethical inquiry (Beauchamp and Childress) used systematic reflection on moral principles and their relevance for resolving ethical problems in biomedicine by weighing and balancing the claims of competing principles (an approach known as *principlism*). Although this mainstream approach

achieved valuable work, criticisms pointed to three ways in which the approach needed to be strengthened: (1) more attention needed to be given to the nature of diseases and the clinical contexts in which clinicians and patients face ethical problems (Sider and Clements); (2) the criticism that principlism appeared to promote a hierarchical form of reasoning that deduced ethical resolutions for complex clinical problems from fixed moral principles and rules needed to be addressed (Jonsen and Toulmin); and (3) in addition to moral principles, more conceptual and methodological resources for ethical inquiry needed to be developed, because principlism appeared too vague and flexible to yield well-reasoned conclusions (Clouser and Gert).

In response to these perceived inadequacies in the forms of ethical inquiry, Glenn C. Graber and David C. Thomasma attempted to recast the theory and practice of medical ethics in terms of a "unitary ethical theory" founded in clinical medicine itself (Ackerman et al.). Their contribution, with strengths and weaknesses, was expertly reviewed in 1990 by Richard M. Zaner, a philosopher with significant clinical experience, who enriched the literature with narratives of illness and of the ethical conflicts over uses of high technology that are frequent in tertiary-care centers. Other contributors to the clinical ethics literature responded by drawing on the works of feminist (Gilligan; Noddings; Wolf; Tong) and theological (Hauerwas) writers who criticized bioethics for neglecting the ethical significance of specific clinical virtues, such as caring for persons in concrete human relationships.

Additional methodological resources for ethical inquiry appeared in the renewal of interest in casuistry, the art of ethical analysis that compares and contrasts relevantly similar cases (Jonsen and Toulmin; Brody, 1988; Arras). Clinical decision making is case-specific: It is directed at the care of a particular patient faced with a particular illness or injury. Each case has a history: what preceded the problems that needed medical attention, what needed to be done, and what was done to address the problems presented by the patient. Because it focuses on the ethics of clinical practice, clinical ethics strives for the richest possible descriptions of cases and their interpersonal dynamics and power differentials. In this vein, several anthologies of cases have appeared with well-informed clinical discussions (Pence; Crigger), including casebooks with cases drawn from ethics consultations (Kuczewski and Pinkus; Culver). Like the practice of clinical medicine, casuistry builds on the accumulated experience, both of the individual and of the professions, in dealing with a variety of cases. Comparing and contrasting related cases can reveal important ethical considerations that may not be apparent in isolated focus on a particular case.

Yet another response to critiques of earlier bioethics was to deepen and enrich the study of larger issues and themes in clinical practice, both by using cases and by drawing on knowledge available only through the intimacies of the clinician–patient encounter. Authors of such studies tend to be clinician-ethicists or ethicists who have adapted to the clinical setting sufficiently to share in such intimacies. Four examples among many are discussions of informed consent (Katz), life-and-death decision making (Brody, 1988), pain and suffering (Cassell), and the uses of power by clinicians (Brody, 1992). These studies draw on a variety of disciplines and experiential data obtained in clinical settings. As such, they encourage ethical scrutiny and reform of understandings and practices in the clinical encounters between patients and clinicians (Zaner). In this way, clinical ethics strengthens the conceptual underpinnings of bioethics with experiential data and helps motivate clinicians to reform their practices.

The continuing multidisciplinary growth in clinical ethics has, not surprisingly, created a great deal of methodological diversity in approaching clinical ethics issues. Methodological approaches characteristic of various health professions, the humanities, and the social sciences can be found in the literature (McGee; Charon and Montello; Kuczewski; Nelson; Bosk; Moreno). In practice, the approaches of different persons involved in clinical ethics efforts will, naturally, reflect, at least in part, their professional or disciplinary perspective. This is part of the great richness of clinical ethics.

In the face of this rich methodological diversity, clinical ethics, far from being fragmented, is held together by a profoundly practical aim: to make contributions to clinical practice and to policy governing clinical practice. To the extent that it is able to achieve this, clinical ethics must pay careful attention to and take into account certain features of the clinical context. As mentioned at the outset, these features include complex psychosocial, medical, legal, cultural, and political dimensions that have implications both for the types of ethical issues that arise and how these issues may be resolved (Society for Health and Human Values). For example, in the United States, the pluralistic societal context, the rights of individuals to live according to their values, and the value-laden nature of clinical practice make ethical conflict or uncertainty an inevitable feature of the clinical setting. Indeed, these features, in conjunction with advances in medical technology, arguably have created the need for formal efforts in clinical ethics. In the U.S. societal context, therefore, irrespective of the methodological approach employed by any particular person in working to address a given clinical ethics issue, the political rights of individuals must be taken into account if the approach is to make a contribution to actual clinical practice. Thus, in a very real sense, methodological approaches in clinical ethics and the theoretical commitments behind them are subordinated to the practical aim of this discipline.

JOHN C. FLETCHER
HOWARD BRODY (1995)
REVISED BY MARK P. AULISIO

**SEE ALSO:** *Autonomy; Beneficence; Bioethics; Casuistry; Ethics: Normative Ethical Theories; Feminism; Informed Consent; Justice; Narrative; Nursing Ethics; Principlism; Virtue and Character;* and other *Clinical Ethics* subentries

### BIBLIOGRAPHY

Ackerman, Terrence F.; Graber, Glenn C.; Reynolds, Charles H.; and Thomasma, David C., eds. 1987. *Clinical Medical Ethics: Exploration and Assessment.* Lanham, MD: University Press of America.

Arras, John D. 1991. "Getting Down to Cases: The Revival of Casuistry in Bioethics." *Journal of Medicine and Philosophy* 16(11): 29–52.

Aulisio, Mark P.; Arnold, Robert M.; and Youngner, Stuart J. 2000. "Health Care Ethics Consultation: A Position Paper from the Society for Health and Human Values–Society for Bioethics Consultation Task Force on Standards for Bioethics Consultation." *Annals of Internal Medicine* 133(1): 59–69.

Aulisio, Mark P.; Arnold, Robert M.; and Youngner, Stuart J., eds. 2003. *Ethics Consultation: From Theory to Practice.* Baltimore, MD: Johns Hopkins University Press.

Aulisio, Mark P., and Rothenberg, Les S. 2002. "Bioethics, Medical Humanities, and the Future of the 'Field': Reflections on the Results of the ASBH Survey of North American Graduate Bioethics/Medical Humanities Training Programs." *American Journal of Bioethics* 2(4): 3–9.

Barnard, David; Towers, Anna; Boston, Patricia; et al. 2000. *Crossing Over: Narratives of Palliative Care.* Oxford: Oxford University Press.

Battin, Margaret; Rhodes, Rosamond; and Silvers, Anita. 1998. *Physician Assisted Suicide: Expanding the Debate.* New York: Routledge.

Beauchamp, Tom L., and Childress, James F. 2001. *Principles of Biomedical Ethics,* 5th edition. New York: Oxford University Press.

Bosk, Charles. 1995. *All God's Mistakes: Genetic Counseling in a Pediatric Hospital.* Chicago: University of Chicago Press.

Brody, Baruch A. 1988. *Life and Death Decision Making.* New York: Oxford University Press.

Brody, Howard. 1992. *The Healer's Power.* New Haven, CT: Yale University Press.

Cassell, Eric J. 1991. *The Nature of Suffering and the Goals of Medicine.* New York: Oxford University Press.

Charon, Rita, and Montello, Martha, eds. 2002. *Stories Matter: The Role of Narrative in Medical Ethics.* New York: Routledge.

Clouser, K. Daniel, and Gert, Bernard. 1990. "A Critique of Principlism." *Journal of Medicine and Philosophy* 15(2): 219–236.

Crigger, Bette-Jane, ed. 1998. *Cases in Bioethics: Selections from the Hastings Center Report,* 3rd edition. New York: St. Martin's Press.

*Cruzan v. Director, Missouri Department of Health.* 497 U.S. 261; 110 Sup. Ct. 2841 (1990).

Culver, Charles M., ed. 1990. *Ethics at the Bedside.* Hanover, NH: University Press of New England.

*Elizabeth Bouvia v. Superior Court of the State of California of the County of Los Angeles (Glenchur).* 225 Cal. Rptr. 297 (Cal. App. 2 Dist. 1986).

Fletcher, John C. 1991. "The Bioethics Movement and Hospital Ethics Committees." *Maryland Law Review* 50(3): 859–894.

Fletcher, John C., and Boyle, Robert, eds. 1997. *Introduction to Clinical Ethics,* 2nd edition. Frederick, MD: University Publishing Group.

Fletcher, John C.; Quist, Norman A.; and Jonsen, Albert R., eds. 1989. *Ethics Consultation in Health Care.* Ann Arbor, MI: Health Administration Press.

Fox, Renée C. 1976. "Advanced Medical Technology: Social and Ethical Implications." *Annual Review of Sociology* 2: 231–268.

Gilligan, Carol. 1982. *In a Different Voice: Psychological Theory and Women's Development.* Cambridge, MA: Harvard University Press.

Gostin, Lawrence O. 2002. "Law and Ethics in a Public Health Emergency." *Hastings Center Report* 32(2): 9–11.

Graber, Glenn C., and Thomasma, David C. 1989. *Theory and Practice in Medical Ethics.* New York: Continuum.

Hauerwas, Stanley. 1986. *Suffering Presence: Theological Reflections on Medicine, the Mentally Handicapped, and the Church.* South Bend, IN: Notre Dame University Press.

Joint Commission on Accreditation of Healthcare Organizations. 1993. "Patient Rights." In *Accreditation Manual for Hospitals, 1992.* Chicago: Author.

Jonsen, Albert R. 1980. "Can an Ethicist Be a Consultant?" In *Frontiers in Medical Ethics: Applications in a Medical Setting,* ed. Virginia Abernathy and Harry S. Abram. Cambridge, MA: Ballinger.

Jonsen, Albert R. 2000. *A Short History of Medical Ethics.* New York: Oxford University Press.

Jonsen, Albert R.; Siegler, Mark; and Winslade, William J. 2002. *Clinical Ethics: A Practical Approach to Ethical Decisions in Clinical Medicine,* 5th edition. New York: McGraw-Hill.

Jonsen, Albert R., and Toulmin, Stephen E. 1988. *The Abuse of Casuistry: A History of Moral Reasoning.* Berkeley: University of California Press.

Juengst, Eric T. 1995. "Ethics of Prediction: Genetic Risk and the Physician–Patient Relationship." *Genome Science and Technology* 1(1): 21–36.

Katz, Jay. 1984. *The Silent World of Doctor and Patient.* New York: Free Press.

Kuczewski, Mark G. 1999. *Fragmentation and Consensus: Communitarian and Casuist Bioethics.* Washington, D.C.: Georgetown University Press.

Kuczewski, Mark G., and Pinkus, Rosa Lynn B. 1999. *An Ethics Casebook for Hospitals: Practical Approaches to Everyday Cases.* Washington, D.C.: Georgetown University Press.

May, Thomas. 2002. *Bioethics in a Liberal Society: The Political Framework of Bioethics Decision Making.* Baltimore, MD: Johns Hopkins University Press.

McGee, Glenn, ed. 2003. *Pragmatic Bioethics.* Cambridge, MA: MIT Press.

Moreno, Jonathan. 1995. *Deciding Together: Bioethics and Moral Consensus.* New York: Oxford University Press.

Nelson, Hilde Lindemann, ed. 1997. *Stories and Their Limits: Narrative Approaches to Bioethics.* New York: Routledge.

Noddings, Nel. 2003. *Caring: A Feminine Approach to Ethics and Moral Education,* 2nd edition. Berkeley: University of California Press.

Pence, Gregory E. 2000. *Classic Cases in Medical Ethics,* 3rd edition. Boston: McGraw-Hill.

*Quinlan, In re.* 70 N.J. 10; 355 A.2d 647 (1976).

*Roe v. Wade.* 410 U.S. 113; 35 L.Ed.2d 147; 93 Sup. Ct. 705 (1973).

Rothman, David J. 1991. *Strangers at the Bedside: A History of How Law and Bioethics Transformed Medical Decision Making.* New York: Basic.

Rubin, Susan B., and Zoloth, Laurie, eds. 2000. *Margin of Error: The Ethics of Mistakes in the Practice of Medicine.* Hagerstown, MD: University Publishing Group.

Schyve, Paul; Emanuel, Linda L.; Winslade, William; and Youngner, Stuart J. 2003. "Organizational Ethics: Promises and Pitfalls." In *Ethics Consultation: From Theory to Practice,* ed. Mark P. Aulisio, Robert M. Arnold, and Stuart J. Youngner. Baltimore, MD: Johns Hopkins University Press.

Sider, Roger C., and Clements, Colleen D. 1985. "The New Medical Ethics: A Second Opinion." *Archives of Internal Medicine* 145(12): 2169–2173.

Siegler, Mark; Pellegrino, Edmund D.; and Singer, Peter A. 1990. "Clinical Medical Ethics." *Journal of Clinical Ethics* 1(1): 5–9.

Singer, Peter A.; Pellegrino, Edmund D.; and Siegler, Mark. 1990. "Ethics Committees and Consultants." *Journal of Clinical Ethics* 1(4): 263–267.

Singer, Peter A.; Siegler, Mark; and Pellegrino, Edmund D. 1990. "Research in Clinical Ethics." *Journal of Clinical Ethics* 1(2): 95–99.

Society for Health and Human Values–Society for Bioethics Consultation. Task Force on Standards for Bioethics Consultation. 1998. *Core Competencies for Health Care Ethics Consultation: The Report of the American Society for Bioethics and*

*Humanities.* Glenview, IL: American Society for Bioethics and Humanities.

Tong, Rosemarie. 1997. *Feminist Approaches to Bioethics: Theoretical Reflections and Practical Applications.* Boulder, CO: Westview Press.

U.S. President's Commission for the Study of Ethical Problems in Medicine and Biomedical and Behavioral Research. 1983. *Deciding to Forego Life-Sustaining Treatment: A Report on the Ethical, Medical, and Legal Issues in Treatment Decisions.* Washington, D.C.: U. S. Government Printing Office.

Wolf, Susan M., ed. 1996. *Feminism and Bioethics: Beyond Reproduction.* New York: Oxford University Press.

Zaner, Richard M. 1988. *Ethics and the Clinical Encounter.* Englewood Cliffs, NJ: Prentice-Hall.

## II. CLINICAL ETHICS CONSULTATION

The dictionary defines consulting as "providing professional or expert advice." A clinical ethics consultant is defined here as a person who upon request provides expert advice to identify, analyze, and help resolve ethical questions or dilemmas that arise in the care of patients. Although the ethics consultant also may provide ethics education and help formulate policy, the bedside role is central to the definition of an ethics consultant (Jonsen).

In the United States, clinical ethics consultation began in some academic medical centers in the late 1960s and early 1970s (La Puma and Schiedermayer), and was given great impetus by the development of hospital ethics committees in the late 1970s and 1980s. During this period the rapid growth of medical technology confronted critically ill patients, their families, and health professionals with difficult ethical choices. At the same time, the traditional authority of the physician was challenged not only by the patient-rights and consumer-rights movements, but also by changes in the way medical care was delivered in tertiary-care hospitals, where patients were often treated by teams consisting of physicians, nurses, social workers, medical technicians, and others. Decisions about forgoing life-sustaining treatment for incompetent adults or premature infants were being made in a legal vacuum often filled by the fears of civil and even criminal litigation. In this atmosphere there was considerable uncertainty about the optimum process for resolving difficult ethical decisions without resorting to the public arena of the courts.

In its 1976 Quinlan decision, the New Jersey Supreme Court tentatively suggested the use of ethics committees to assist persons who faced difficult end-of-life decisions. In the early 1980s, the federal "Baby Doe" regulations spurred hospitals to develop internal mechanisms for dealing with decision making for severely handicapped infants. In 1983 the U.S. President's Commission for the Study of Ethical Problems in Medicine and Biomedical and Behavioral Research endorsed the notion of shared decision making between patients and physicians. It suggested consultation with an ethics committee as a possible means for resolving disputes that arose in the clinical setting, but noted that the efficacy of such consultation had not been demonstrated (U.S. President's Commission).

In 1985 the National Institutes of Health and the University of California at San Francisco cosponsored a conference in Bethesda, Maryland, for persons designated by their institutions as ethics consultants. The conference was attended by fifty-three invitees, and fifty additional persons expressed interest in attending a future meeting of this group (Fletcher, 1986). By 1987 the Society for Bioethics Consultation was formed for the support and continuing education of clinical ethics consultants. In 1992 the Joint Commission for the Accreditation of Health Care Organizations (JCAHO) published a requirement for healthcare institution accreditation that all healthcare institutions must have in place a mechanism for resolving disputes concerning end-of-life decisions.

### Structures of Clinical Ethics Consultation

Clinical ethics case consultation is provided in several ways: by an ethics consultative group as a whole (such as an ethics committee), by a subgroup of the consultative group, or by individual consultants. Clinical ethics case consultation by a large group has the potential for having diffused accountability and being depersonalized, bureaucratic, insensitive, closed-ended, and removed from the clinical setting. But it has the advantage of providing multiple perspectives and opportunities for queries from persons of diverse backgrounds, and for correcting the potential for narrow or idiosyncratic views of an individual consultant.

In contrast, clinical ethics case consultation by an individual consultant is an open-ended process that can extend over a period of time, and permit ongoing discussion and pursuit of issues that require clarification. The individual consultant can decide what information is necessary and obtain it firsthand. Interviews with patients, families, and health professionals can be scheduled flexibly and conducted in private settings more conducive to diminishing apprehension, establishing trust, sharing information, and allowing the kind of give-and-take that is so important to exploring emotionally powerful and intensely personal issues. Furthermore, an individual ethics consultant is more visible and accountable than a committee (Agich and Youngner). For these reasons, many ethics consultative groups and healthcare professionals have found the individual clinical ethics consultant more effective than the committee. Many ethics consultative groups have created a middle ground that involves small teams who serve as an extension of the ethics consultation group or ethics committee.

Some see an advantage to a relationship between the ethics consultant and an ethics consultative group or committee because the large group regularly can review the individual consultant's activities. This arrangement provides peer review and quality assurance for the consultant as well as education for the larger group or committee. The ethics consultant or consultation team can ask the entire group to become involved in particularly controversial or complex cases.

## The Role of the Clinical Ethics Consultant

Despite the growing interest in and practice of clinical ethics consultation, important questions remain about its purpose, requisite skills, methods, specific responsibilities, evaluation, and effect. Unlike traditional medical consultants, clinical ethics consultants are not subject to widely accepted standards and procedures for training, credentialing, maintaining accountability, charging fees, obtaining informed consent, or providing liability coverage (Purtilo; Agich).

While the role of the ethics consultant generally has been pragmatic, that is, to provide practical assistance with actual patient-care decisions (Cranford; Glover et al.; Siegler and Singer; Fletcher, 1986), there has been little consensus about how this role should be implemented. For example, although some see the ethics consultant, like the traditional medical consultant, as an expert who uses specific skills and knowledge to help "answer" ethical questions, exactly what constitutes the appropriate skills and knowledge base is a matter of debate. Does the expertise come from the wisdom of practical clinical experience (La Puma et al.), or is it derived from a knowledge of moral theory and ethical principles?

Others see the clinical ethics consultant's role not so much as an expert but as someone who facilitates decisions in a "community of reflective persons" (Glover et al., p. 24). This approach stresses the importance of involving all persons connected with the case—the patient, family members, physicians, nurses, medical students and residents, social workers, friends, and clergy. In this view, a shared decision-making process should extend beyond the physician–patient dyad so that a greater range of personal values and interests can be considered. This view is less compatible with the traditional model of medical consultation, which focuses more narrowly on the physician as decision maker.

Some commentators have worried that the individual ethics consultant, the ethics consultative group, or the ethics committee will act as moral "police" or "God Squad" (Siegler and Singer, p. 759), and erode the decision-making authority of the physician. Troyen Brennan has voiced a more subtle concern: that by turning increasingly to ethics consultants and ethics committees, we "run the risk of forcing the ethics of the caring relationship to the periphery of clinical practice as something that is best left to experts" (Brennan, p. 4). Furthermore, the role of the ethics consultant may be confused with other institutional roles, such as risk management, peer review, quality assurance, or resource allocation. Taking on these roles could create a conflict of interest for the ethics consultant.

## Reasons for Ethics Consultation

Ethics consultations are requested for a variety of reasons that include prevention of litigation; mediation of disputes and resolution of conflicts between or among the patient, healthcare professional, and family; confirmation of or challenges to decisions already made; emotional support for difficult decisions; and identification of morally acceptable alternatives. For example, ethics consultation may be requested because physicians and family members disagree about how aggressively to treat a dying, incompetent cancer patient, or because there is difficulty interpreting a patient's living will. Ethics consultants may be called because there is disagreement about the acceptability of a family request to stop tube feeding an Alzheimer patient who refuses to eat. Requests for ethics consultation may come because nurses or house officers are concerned that competent patients are being left out of the decision-making process.

## Goals of Ethics Consultation

There is disagreement about the appropriate goals of ethics consultation. John La Puma and E. Rush Priest have suggested that ethics consultations's primary goal should be "to effect ethical outcomes in particular cases and to teach physicians to construct their own frameworks for ethical decisions making" (La Puma and Priest, p. 17). Patient-rights advocates disagree. They argue that the primary goal of ethics consultation is the promotion of patient autonomy by encouraging shared decision making (Tulsky and Lo). John Fletcher takes a broader view. He identifies four goals of ethics consultation: (1) to protect and enhance shared decision making in the resolution of ethical problems; (2) to prevent poor outcomes; (3) to increase knowledge of clinical ethics; and (4) to increase knowledge of self and others through participation in resolving conflicts (Fletcher, 1992).

## Contributions to the Practice of Ethics Consultation

While the general purpose of clinical ethics consultation is to help resolve ethical questions or dilemmas in patient care, persons who perform ethics consultation come from diverse professional backgrounds and do not share the same problem-solving methods or theoretical assumptions. This diversity has left its stamp on the way clinical ethics consultation is performed, and has profound implications not only for the practice of clinical ethics consultation but also for the training of its practitioners.

Despite this diversity, a common ground can be seen in the shared goal of identifying an ethically supportable solution to a clinical ethical question or dilemma, and in a recognition that the process of arriving at a solution requires knowledge of law, ethics, medicine, psychosocial issues, and at times, religion.

The legal tradition has influenced clinical ethics consultation by placing emphasis on rights and on formal mechanisms of decision making and arbitration, such as due process. The protection and nurturing of individual rights are central to this style (Wolf). Strict adherence to this style, however, may encourage adversarial rather than collaborative or nurturing relationships between patients and healthcare professionals (Agich and Youngner).

The medical tradition has contributed methods, assumptions, and traditions of clinical practice: a combination of technical knowledge and clinical experience (La Puma and Toulmin). Some argue that physicians are best suited to provide clinical ethics consultation because (1) their advice will be easily accepted by their medical colleagues, because they have clinical experience and speak the same language; and (2) only physicians can understand the ethos of physician-patient relationships. Critics caution that because they are "insiders," physicians may promote the values of medicine rather than those of their patients or the larger community. They argue that the ethics consultant should serve as a bridge between medical and other values, and cannot function properly from a position entirely within medicine (Glover et al.; Churchill).

Moral philosophy has offered three major approaches to clinical ethics consultation. The first is principle-based ethics, which argues that the answer to a given ethical question or dilemma may be discovered by applying the correct ethical theory (e.g., utilitarianism) or principle (e.g., autonomy) to the case. The second is virtue ethics, which emphasizes that the possession of certain virtues (e.g., honesty, loyalty, compassion) is essential to sound ethical decision making. The third is a case-based or casuistic ethic, which holds that by examining the particulars of a given case

and comparing them with similar cases, a moral maxim that applies to the case can be discovered. An advantage of casuistry is that it sues a decision-making method already employed by clinicians (Jonsen and Toulmin). Casuistry relies upon teachable medical moral maxims that build upon experience. Because casuistry is not principle-based, it has been criticized as "situational," that is, pragmatically driven to solve individual problems without reference to a broader moral framework.

While principle-based clinical ethics reasoning has the advantage of providing a consistent moral reference point, its principles are necessarily abstract, often conflict with each other, and may create a rigid paradigm that is insensitive to differences in specific cases.

Theology and religion contribute to clinical ethics consultation by recognizing that specific religious positions may either facilitate the resolution of an ethical question or contribute to its intensity. For example, the Jehovah's Witness position on blood transfusions can create serious ethical dilemmas in the case of a Jehovah's Witness patient who is in urgent need of extensive, lifesaving surgery but refuses blood. One of the disadvantages of this perspective is that many physicians are suspicious of or even hostile to religious or theological interpretations of medical problems. However, insight into the religious morality of patients, family members, and healthcare professionals is useful in establishing communication and reaching understanding among physicians, patients, and family members.

Consultation liaison psychiatry and clinical psychology have influenced clinical ethics consultation by addressing dynamic and interpersonal elements of clinical ethics cases. This style involves using insight into the motivations and values of those involved in the ethics case to resolve conflicts among decision makers. The goal is to produce a consensus or compromise solution rather than to evoke rights language, ethical principles, or religious codes. A disadvantage of this approach is that a compromise solution is not always a just one. Its strength is that it skillfully manages confrontation and addresses the emotional needs of the participants.

## Knowledge and Skills Needed for Ethics Consultation

While there is not unanimity about how rigorously schooled in specific academic disciplines or how proficient in specific skills the consultant should be, there is general agreement about the kind of skills, knowledge, and personal qualities ethics consultants require. These include knowledge of ethical language and ethical theory; skills of ethical analysis and reflective moral judgment; knowledge of clinical medicine (e.g., medical terminology, the natural history of disease and its treatment); knowledge of and familiarity with hospital structure, sociology, and politics; knowledge of and familiarity with the professional ethos of physicians and nurses; knowledge of the law and legal reasoning; knowledge of psychological and social theories of behavior; communication and teaching skills; personal qualities such as the ability to establish rapport, empathy, and compassion; and professional attributes such as dedication, ability to maintain confidentiality, and comfort with cultural and ethical diversity.

## Access to Ethics Consultation

Who should be able to request an ethics consultation? The answer to this question has political as well as moral implications. On the one hand, if only physicians have access to ethics consultation, many important ethical issues may never be examined (Tulsky and Lo). On the other hand, permitting patients, families, and other health professionals to request ethics consultation, especially without the physician's concurrence, might discourage more direct communication, disrupt physician-patient relationships, or undermine physician authority. The last possibility would be most threatening to authoritarian-minded physicians and very likely would challenge the traditional power structure of many hospitals. This may explain the gap between the argument in the literature for the ideal—that patients, families, and nurses should be able to request an ethics consultation—and the impression that many institutions do not permit, and almost none actively encourage, patient, family, or other health professional requests for ethics consultation.

The ability to ask for consultation is only one question concerning patient and family access to and control over the consultation process. Other questions include whether the patient or family should have authority to (1) call a consultation when the physician refuses to do so; (2) be informed routinely when consultations are requested by physicians; (3) veto physician-initiated consultation requests; (4) participate in all ethics consultations if they wish; and (5) receive verbal or written information about the consultant's findings and recommendations. Some argue that an insistence on a rights-based approach to these questions would doom ethics consultation services to failure in modern hospitals because of political considerations (Agich and Youngner).

## Standards and Evaluation

The fact that standards and methods for evaluating clinical ethics consultation are not established comes as no surprise.

The infancy of clinical ethics consultation and the disagreement about its goals, as well as the diverse academic and professional backgrounds of its practitioners, account for this lack. Most studies to date have employed physician satisfaction and usage as outcome measures. By this standard, ethics consultations have been judged to be helpful. Critics have pointed out, however, that by not including patient and surrogate satisfaction and reactions of house staff and nurses, an incomplete and perhaps inaccurate picture of ethics consultation is painted (Tulsky and Lo). For example, "it would be hard to argue that it is desirable for an ethics consultant to reject the choices of a competent and informed patient, even if the attending physician expresses satisfaction with such a consultation" (Tulsky and Lo, p. 591). More objective measures like changes in physician behavior, reduction in use of limited resources (Kanoti et al.), and decreased litigation are attractive, but could confuse matters if these goals were achieved at the expense of more traditional values, such as patient autonomy and well-being.

## Credentialing and Accreditation

As ethics consultation becomes more widespread and perceived as part of the standard of medical care, society will hold accountable its practitioners and the institutions that employ them. Individual institutions and national accrediting bodies, such as the Joint Commission for the Accreditation of Health Care Organizations, will undoubtedly become more concerned with setting standards for clinical ethics consultation: consultation through traditional professional methods, such as standardized education and training, accreditation of training programs, and credentialing of ethics consultants. This process will be a major challenge to an interdisciplinary field that has yet to agree on its goals and how to evaluate them.

## Fees

By and large, ethics consultants have not charged patients or third-party payers for their services. This may be explained by at least two factors. First, the efficacy of ethics consultations has not been clearly demonstrated; and second, ethics consultations are called as frequently to assist health professionals as they are to help patients. Generally, ethics consultants have been paid by the institutions where they practice, either directly for their consultations or indirectly, as part of their overall responsibility in directing ethics programs or committees.

As our healthcare system becomes increasingly constrained by economic factors, healthcare institutions may find it more difficult to support clinical ethics consultation.

This will put pressure on ethics consultants to charge patients or third-party payers or to demonstrate that their activities save money by decreasing litigation or reducing resource consumption.

## Conclusion

Clinical ethics consultation arose in the United States in the latter half of the twentieth century amid the moral and legal uncertainty spawned by the rapid expansion of choices produced by medical advances, the emergence of the tertiary-care medical center, and the individual-rights movement that challenged traditional authority structures. Although it holds great promise, clinical ethics consultation remains a nascent profession. Many of the theoretical and practical questions about its goals, training, evaluation, accountability, and support remain unanswered. Nonetheless, clinical ethics consultation is growing and even flourishing. As the U.S. health system evolves over the coming years, the role and place of clinical ethics consultation in the healthcare system certainly will be addressed.

GEORGE A. KANOTI
STUART YOUNGNER (1995)
BIBLIOGRAPHY REVISED

SEE ALSO: *Anthropology and Bioethics; Autonomy; Beneficence; Bioethics, African-American Perspectives; Care; Casuistry; Coercion; Compassionate Love; Competence; Confidentiality; Conscience, Rights of; Death; Ethics; Healthcare Resources, Allocation of; Informed Consent; Life, Quality of;* and other *Clinical Ethics* subentries

### BIBLIOGRAPHY

Agich, George J. 1990. "Clinical Ethics: A Role Theoretic Look." *Social Science Medicine* 30(4): 389–399.

Agich, George J. 1995. "Authority in Ethics Consultation." *Journal of Law and Medical Ethics* 23(3): 273–283.

Agich, George J., and Youngner, Stuart J. 1991. "For Experts Only? Access to Hospital Ethics Committees." *Hastings Center Report* 21(5): 17–31.

Ahronheim, Judith C.; Moreno, Jonathan D.; and Zuckerman, Connie. 2000. *Ethics in Clinical Practice,* 2nd edition. New York: Aspen Publishers.

Andre, J. 1997. "Goals of Ethics Consultation: Toward Clarity, Utility, and Fidelity." *Journal of Clinical Ethics* 8(2): 193–198.

Aulisio, Mark P. 2001. "Doing Ethics Consultation." *American Journal of Bioethics* 1(4): 54–55.

Aulisio, Mark P.; Arnold, Robert M.; and Youngner, Stuart J., eds. 2003. *Doing Ethics Consultation* Baltimore, MD: Johns Hopkins University Press.

Brennan, Troyen A. 1992. "Quality of Clinical Ethics Consultation." *QRB: Quality Review Bulletin.* 18(1): 4–5.

Churchill, Larry R. 1978. "The Role of the Stranger." *Ethicists in Professional Education: Hastings Center Report* 8(6): 13–15.

Cranford, Ronald E. 1989. "The Neurologist as Ethics Consultant and a Member of the Institutional Ethics Committee: The Neuroethicist." *Neurologic Clinics* 7(4): 697–713.

Fletcher, John C. 1986. "Goals and Process of Ethics Consultation in Health Care." *Biolaw* 2(2): 37–47.

Fletcher, John C. 1992. "Needed: A Broader View of Ethics Consultation." *QRB: Quality Review Bulletin* 18(1): 12–14.

Fletcher, John C., and Siegler, M. 1996. "What are the Goals of Ethics Consultation? A Consensus Statement." *Journal of Clinical Ethics* 7(2): 122–126.

Glover, Jacqueline J.; Ozar, David T.; and Thomasma, David C. 1986. "Teaching Ethics on Rounds: The Ethicist as Teacher, Consultant, and Decision–Maker." *Theoretical Medicine* 7(1): 13–32.

Jonsen, Albert R. 1980. "Can an Ethicist Be a Consultant?" In *Frontiers in Medical Ethics: Applications in a Medical Setting,* pp. 157–171, ed. Virginia Abernathy and Harry S. Abram. Cambridge, MA: Ballinger.

Jonsen, Albert R., and Toulmin, Stephen E. 1988. *The Abuse of Casuistry: A History of Moral Reasoning.* Berkeley: University of California Press.

Howe, E. G. "The Three Deadly Sins of Ethics Consultation." *Journal of Clinical Ethics* 7(2): 99–108.

Kanoti, George A.; Gombeski, William; Gulledge, A. Dale; Knorads, Dale; Collins, Robert; and Medendorp, Sharon. 1992. "Impact of Do-Not-Resuscitate Policies on Length of Stay." *Cleveland Clinic Journal of Medicine* 59(6): 591–594.

La Puma, John, and Priest, E. Rush. 1992. "Medical Staff Privileges for Ethics Consultants: An Institutional Model." *QRB: Quality Review Bulletin* 18(1): 17–20.

La Puma, John, and Schiedermayer, David L. 1991. "Ethics Consultation: Skills, Roles and Training." *Annals of Internal Medicine* 114: 155–160.

La Puma, John; Stocking, Carol B.; Silverstein, Marc D.; DiMartini, Andrea; and Siegler, Mark. 1988. "An Ethics Consultation Service in a Teaching Hospital: Utilization and Evaluation." *Journal of the American Medical Association* 260(6): 808–811.

La Puma, John, and Toulmin, Steven E. 1989. "Ethics Consultants and Ethics Committees." *Archives of Internal Medicine* 149(5): 1109–1112.

Perkins, Henry S., and Saathoff, Bonnie S. 1988. "Impact of Medical Ethics Consultation on Physicians: An Exploratory Study." *American Journal of Medicine* 85(6): 761–765.

Phillips, D. F. 1996. "Ethics Consultation Quality: Is Evaluation Feasible?" *Journal of the American Medical Association* 275(24): 1866–1867.

Purtilo, Ruth B. 1984. "Ethics Consultations in the Hospital." *New England Journal of Medicine* 311(15): 983–986.

Siegler, Mark, and Singer, Peter A. 1988. "Clinical Ethics Consultation: Godsend or God Squad." *American Journal of Medicine* 85(6): 759–760.

Society for Health and Human Values, Society for Bioethics Consultation, Task Force on Standards for Bioethics Consultation. 1998. *Core Competencies for Health Care Ethics Consultation: The Report of the American Society for Bioethics and Humanities.* Glenville, IL: American Society of Bioethics and Humanities.

Tulsky, James A., and Fox, Elizabeth. 1996. "Evaluating Ethics Consultation: Framing the Questions." *Journal of Clinical Ethics* 7(2): 109–115.

Tulsky, James A., and Lo, Bernard. 1992. "Ethics Consultation: Time to Focus on Patients." *American Journal of Medicine* 92(4): 343–345.

U.S. President's Commission for the Study of Ethical Problems in Medicine and Biomedical and Behavioral Research. 1983. *Deciding to Forego Life-Sustaining Treatment: A Report on the Ethical, Medical, and Legal Issues in Treatment Decisions.* Washington, D.C.: Superintendent of Documents.

Wolf, Susan M. 1991. "Ethics Committees and Due Process: Nesting Rights in a Community of Caring." *Maryland Law Review* 50: 798–858.

Zaner, Richard M., ed. 1999. *Performance, Talk, Reflection: What Is Going on in Clinical Ethics Consultation.* New York: Kluwer Academic Publishers.

## III. INSTITUTIONAL ETHICS COMMITTEES

Ethics committees have played clinically relevant roles in U.S. healthcare contexts since the 1960s. At that time, some hospitals established committees to approve requests for abortion and sterilization and to allocate scarce dialysis machines. Universities and hospitals created human subjects committees to scrutinize research protocols and consent forms; in the 1970s, these committees became federally mandated institutional review boards (IRBs).

In the 1976 *Quinlan* case, in which parents won the authority to remove a ventilator from an incompetent adult child, the New Jersey Supreme Court recommended that hospitals establish ethics committees to confirm prognoses in cases involving withdrawal of life support. The 1982 "Baby Doe" ruling that allowed parents to withhold a lifesaving operation from an infant with Down syndrome led to the establishment of infant-care review committees in cases of withholding or withdrawing life support from disabled newborns. In 1983, a report from the U.S. President's Commission for the Study of Ethical Problems in Medicine and Biomedical and Behavioral Research encouraged the formation of hospital ethics committees to review cases that raised ethical dilemmas and to resolve ethical conflict.

By the mid-1980s, a movement had begun to establish institutional ethics committees in healthcare facilities, especially in hospitals. In 1982, only 1 percent of all U.S. hospitals had ethics committees; by 1987, over 60 percent did (Fleetwood et al.). Ethics committees were endorsed in this period by leading professional groups, including the American Medical Association, the American Hospital Association, the American Academy of Pediatrics, and the American Academy of Neurologists. Growth in the number of institutional ethics committees continued into the 1990s and spread to nursing homes and hospices (Glaser). It is likely that the number and influence of these committees will grow as the length of stay in hospitals continues to decline and more patient days are spent outside hospitals. Moreover, with the shift of many kinds of care to alternative sites, it is likely that other institutional ethics committees will develop and spread—in home-healthcare agencies and managed-care networks, for example. Hospital ethics committees remain, however, the most common institutional ethics committees and the most closely analyzed in bioethics literature.

There is a paucity of empirical studies of hospital ethics committees. Committees have a "grass-roots" character, reflecting a variety of local circumstances and personalities. These factors make it hard to generalize. Nevertheless, some typical features have emerged. One of these features is interdisciplinary composition. Generally, committees are composed of doctors, nurses, social workers, pastoral-care professionals, and philosophers or theologians trained in ethics. Committee members can also include administrators, hospital attorneys, and consumer or community representatives. Committees are sometimes authorized by the medical staff; sometimes by the hospital governing board; sometimes by the administration.

### Functions of Ethics Committees

Committee functions vary but generally include one, two, or all three of the following. First, institutional ethics committees create a vehicle for education on ethical dimensions of patient care. Committees typically have dual efforts in this respect: education of the committee itself, through discussion of current bioethics literature, for example; and education of the medical staff and hospital employees, by organizing periodic lectures, panel discussions, and "ethics grand rounds."

Second, committees draft institutional policies on ethical questions. This may arise through committee initiative. For example, a hospital panel discussion may reveal the need for a new policy on withholding resuscitation from dying patients, and the ethics committee takes the lead by preparing a first draft. New policies or review of existing policies may also be requested from the ethics committee by the hospital administration, or other hospital committees may route drafts of proposed policies and revisions of existing policies to the committee for review and comment.

Third, many institutional ethics committees offer ethics consultations, prospectively or retrospectively, on difficult clinical cases, often those involving the withholding or withdrawal of life-support measures. This last function—ethics consultation, especially for ongoing cases—has been the main focus of discussion in the bioethics literature. Seven issues have dominated these discussions: questions of competence and authority; impact on the doctor-patient relationship; access to consultation; recordkeeping and charting; problems of evaluation; unsettled legal questions; and questions about the purpose or purposes of consultations.

COMPETENCE AND AUTHORITY. Some committees that offer consultation services, generally smaller committees, consult as a committee of the whole. Larger committees typically have a subcommittee that consults prospectively and reports to the committee as a whole for retrospective review of its work. Some committees offer consultation through a single ethics consultant who may be on the committee or have a formal relationship with it. Some critics have expressed concern that when committees consult, difficult ethical choices will be affected by compromise, hospital politics, professional rivalries, and conformism (Wikler). Concerns about competence have been raised when individuals provide consultations. Clinicians typically have few of the skills of trained ethicists and vice versa.

Continued spread of ethics committee consultation to more hospitals and nonhospital settings is indirect evidence that the challenges to competence and authority are being met successfully. Furthermore, most published concerns about the competence of committees or individuals are from the 1970s "first wave" of writing about institutional ethics committees, at a time when the idea of ethics consultation was new and controversial. The literature of the 1980s and 1990s displays a growing confidence about the concept of ethics consultation and more attention to resolving specific problems. Apparently, committees had learned to negotiate without conformism or loss of principle. Individuals have been acquiring the proper expertise: clinicians gaining the analytic techniques of ethicists, and ethicists learning to apply their analyses in clinically relevant ways.

Gender-related questions have not been raised directly in the bioethics literature on ethics committees. However, they are raised indirectly when the focus is on the role of nurses, given the fact that most nurses are women. Nurses have been excluded from some committees, could not access them for consultation, or have found their special ethical concerns omitted from consideration. In addition to the gender issue, this situation raises questions of professional status in relation to other healthcare providers. In some hospitals, these problems have been addressed by the formation of nursing ethics committees (Edwards and Haddad).

There has also been a suggestion in the literature that ethics committees, especially those that are or function as infant-care review committees, should include persons with disabilities on the committee (Mahowald). This step could help ensure that the quality of life of persons with disabilities is not undervalued in deliberations about treatment decisions.

DOCTOR-PATIENT RELATIONSHIP. Trust in the doctor-patient relationship is grounded in the doctor's professional obligation to the patient. Some have expressed concern that ethics consultations will undermine that obligation and trust by limiting doctors' authority to act for their patients or by encouraging abdication of the responsibility (Siegler). These concerns are addressed or attenuated by the fact that use of a committee's consulting service is generally optional and its findings are advisory (Fost and Cranford). It should be admitted, however, that when an ethics consultation is sought and its findings are received, a de facto "burden of proof" may be imposed on those doctors who choose to reject or ignore the ethics committee's advice. They will probably need to muster strong reasons for doing so.

ACCESS TO CONSULTATION. Who should have the authority to request an ethics consultation? Some committees use a medical model whereby only the attending physician can initiate a consultation; he or she alone joins in the deliberations and receives the advice. But many committees allow other physicians, nurses, other professionals, and the patient and family to initiate consultations.

There are two main reasons why ethics committees reject the medical model. First, ethical dilemmas in patient care, especially those surrounding withholding or withdrawing life support, are felt acutely by all professionals involved. Second, if the consulting process helps to delimit or set priorities for a patient's options, the patient's right of informed consent may require that he or she, or a surrogate, be able to participate in the consultation. There is no clear pattern for such participation in the literature. Some consulting teams interview competent patients; others do not. Some encourage the presence of patients or surrogates at consultations; others do not. While most committees that reject the medical model respond to patient requests for consultation, it is not clear generally whether objection by a patient or surrogate can prevent an ethics consultation or stop one that has been initiated by others.

**RECORDKEEPING AND CHARTING.** Some committees and consultants keep no records in order to ensure patient confidentiality and to prevent the use of committee deliberations in legal proceedings. Plainly, all institutional ethics committees must carefully adhere to the norms of medical confidentiality, but the prevailing wisdom is that ethics committees should keep good records and should enter their advice and reasons for it into the patient's active chart (Cranford et al.). Such procedures build trust in the committee, educate the medical and nursing staffs on ethical issues, and provide accountability for committee advice in what are often literally life-and-death decisions.

**EVALUATION.** The brief history of most ethics committees, the confidential status of what they do, and the ambiguity many of them experience about their roles, especially in consultation, have made it difficult to conduct comprehensive evaluation of their effectiveness. Moreover, there is no independent standard of right and wrong against which the advice of these committees can be measured. However, committees can be evaluated by reference to their own mission statements, by written assessments of those who request consultations, and by the informal measures of success as an interdisciplinary forum: enhanced institutional sensitivity to ethical issues and increased requests for consultation (Van Allen et al.).

Some ethics committees use very explicit regulations or ethical guidelines for consulting. These documents could provide norms for more focused evaluation of consultation. Hospitals in the Veterans Administration system, for example, employ detailed national protocols on withholding and withdrawing life support. Catholic hospitals make explicit use of ethical guidelines contained in the Ethical and Religious Directives for Catholic Health Facilities (Craig et al.).

**UNSETTLED LEGAL QUESTIONS.** A number of legal questions about ethics committees remain unsettled for want of legislation and court decisions. Can an ethics committee and/or its members be sued and held accountable in civil or criminal actions? Are the records of an ethics committee discoverable? If used in court, what weight should they be given (Wolf)? There is also a widely held, but undocumented, view that the availability of an ethics committee can lessen the likelihood of litigation because it provides a forum for resolving conflict and because it allows for thorough examination of ethical issues that frequently have significant legal components.

**THE PURPOSE OR PURPOSES OF CONSULTATIONS.** Several authors have argued that protection of patients' interests should be the single purpose of an institutional ethics committee's consultation (Hoffmann). But it is also clear that consultations often serve other purposes: to assist caregivers, to support patients' families, to negotiate compromise when disputes arise, to protect the hospital, to offer the correct or best moral advice. Sometimes these other purposes can conflict with the purpose of protecting the patients' best interests. Moreover, in some cases a patient's apparent best interest is incompatible with what the patient demands. Clear strategies for dealing with such conflicts have not yet emerged in the bioethics literature, but they are plainly needed.

## Conclusion

Much remains to be done to sharpen the focus of the work of institutional ethics committees and to evaluate the strengths and weaknesses of various committee and consultation models. This area is one of social experimentation and will remain so into the foreseeable future. Nevertheless, in a very short time, ethics committees have contributed greatly to the general bioethics agenda of creating dialogue on ethics issues in healthcare. Most acute-care hospitals in the United States, and many other settings where chronically ill and dying patients receive care, have an established institutional vehicle for explicit, interdisciplinary discussion of difficult ethical issues.

CHARLES J. DOUGHERTY (1995)
BIBLIOGRAPHY REVISED

SEE ALSO: *Anthropology and Bioethics; Autonomy; Beneficence; Bioethics, African-American Perspectives; Care; Casuistry; Coercion; Compassionate Love; Competence; Confidentiality; Conscience, Rights of; Death; Ethics; Healthcare Resources, Allocation of; Informed Consent; Life, Quality of; Nursing Ethics; Patients' Rights; Pastoral Care and Healthcare Chaplaincy;* and other *Clinical Ethics* subentries

### BIBLIOGRAPHY

Aulisio, Mark P.; Arnold, Robert M.; and Youngner, Stuart J., eds. 2003. *Doing Ethics Consultation.* Baltimore: Johns Hopkins University Press.

Craig, Robert P.; Middleton, Carl L.; and O'Connell, Laurence J. 1986. *Ethics Committees: A Practical Approach.* St. Louis, MO: Catholic Health Association.

Cranford, Ronald E.; Hester, F. Allen; and Ashley, Barbara Ziegler. 1985. "Institutional Ethics Committees: Issues of

Confidentiality and Immunity." *Law, Medicine, and Health Care* 15(2): 52–60.

Edwards, Barba J., and Haddad, Amy M. 1988. "Establishing a Nursing Bioethics Committee." *Journal of Nursing Administration* 18(3): 30–33.

Fleetwood, Janet E.; Arnold, Robert M.; and Baron, Richard J. 1989. "Giving Answers or Raising Questions?: The Problematic Role of Institutional Ethics Committees." *Journal of Medical Ethics* 15(3): 137–142.

Fost, Norman, and Cranford, Ronald. 1985. "Hospital Ethics Committees: Administrative Aspects." *Journal of the American Medical Association* 253(18): 2687–2692.

Glaser, John W. 1989. "Hospital Ethics Committees: One of Many Centers of Responsibility." *Theoretical Medicine* 10(4): 275–288.

Hendrick, Judith. 2001. "Legal Aspects of Clinical Ethics Committees." *Journal of Medical Ethics* 27: 50i–53i.

Hoffmann, Diane E. 1993. "Evaluating Ethics Committees: A View from the Outside." *Milbank Quarterly* 71(4): 677–701.

Mahowald, Mary B. 1988. "Baby Doe Committees: A Critical Evaluation." *Clinics in Perinatology* 15(4): 789–800.

McCarrick, P. M. 1992. "Ethics Committees In Hospitals." *Kennedy Institute of Ethics Journal* 2(3): 285–306.

McGee, Glenn; Caplan, Arthur L.; Spanogle, J. P.; and Asch, D.A. 2001. "A National Study of Ethics Committees." *American Journal of Bioethics* 1(4): 60–64.

Milton, C. L. 2001. "Institutional Ethics Committees: A Nursing Perspective." *Nursing Science Quarterly* 14(1): 22–23

*Quinlan, In Re.* 355 A.2d 647 (N.J. 1976).

Schick, I. C., and Guo, L. 2001. "Ethics Committees Identify Success Factors: A National Survey." *HEC Forum* 13(4): 344–360.

Slowther, Anne-Marie; Hill, Donald; and McMillan, John. 2002. "Clinical Ethics Committees: Opportunity or Threat?" *HEC Forum* 14(1): 4–12.

Slowther, Anne Marie, and Hope, Tony. 2000. "Clinical Ethics Committees." *British Medical Journal* 321(7262): 649–650.

Siegler, Mark. 1986. "Ethics Committees: Decisions by Bureaucracy." *Hastings Center Report* 16(3): 22–24.

Society for Health and Human Values, Society for Bioethics Consultation, Task Force on Standards for Bioethics Consultation. 1998. *Core Competencies for Health Care Ethics Consultation: The Report of the American Society for Bioethics and Humanities.* Glenville, IL: American Society of Bioethics and Humanities.

Spicker, Stuart F., ed. 1997. *The Healthcare Ethics Committee Experience: Selected Readings from HEC Forum.* Malabar, FL: Krieger Publishing Company.

U.S. President's Commission for the Study of Ethical Problems in Medicine and Biomedical and Behavioral Research. 1983. *Deciding to Forgo Life-Sustaining Treatment: A Report on the Ethical, Medical, and Legal Issues in Treatment Decisions.* Washington, D.C.: Author.

Van Allen, E.; Moldow, D. G.; and Cranford, Ronald. 1989. "Evaluating Ethics Committees." *Hastings Center Report* 19(5): 23–24.

Wikler, Daniel. 1989. "Institutional Agendas and Ethics Committees." *Hastings Center Report* 19(5): 21–23.

Wolf, Susan M. 1986. "Ethics Committees in the Courts." *Hastings Center Report* 16(3): 12–15.

# CLONING

• • •

I. Scientific Background

II. Reproductive

III. Religious Perspectives

## I. SCIENTIFIC BACKGROUND

The term *cloning* has many meanings. Scientific meanings are reasonably clear, although they have become more complex since technologies for reproducing mammals by cloning from nuclei of somatic cells were demonstrated by Keith H. Campbell and colleagues (1996) and Ian Wilmut and colleagues (1997), the latter resulting in Dolly, the first sheep cloned from an adult somatic cell. Since then, there has been an explosion of research in this area, and the terminology has sometimes been controversial. This entry will cover scientific aspects of both reproductive and therapeutic cloning.

### Definitions

Etymologically, *clone* is derived from the Greek word *klon* (twig). The ancient Greeks already knew that planting a twig from a tree or bush generally resulted in a new organism very similar to the parent tree. Hundreds of species of plants routinely reproduce by cloning, both at the hand of mankind (e.g., potatoes, asparagus) and naturally (e.g., aspen trees). So, what does "reproduction by cloning" mean?

There are two main approaches to biological reproduction: sexual and asexual. In almost all cases, sexual reproduction involves the processes of meiosis and fertilization. Asexual reproduction does not include these processes. For example, seeds are products of meiosis and fertilization by pollen, and planting these embryos results in sexual reproduction. This is fundamentally different from cutting a potato into several pieces and planting them. Thus, cloning can be broadly defined as asexual reproduction.

There is plenty of asexual reproduction in animals, too. If one appropriately bisects a planarian (a flatworm) or various other invertebrates, two normal copies eventually result. The situation becomes less flexible with vertebrates, particularly with mammals. Nevertheless, even in mammals, asexual reproduction occurs when identical twins or triplets (or quadruplets, etc.) are produced. The duplication that occurs when one embryo produces two individuals is asexual reproduction, albeit superimposed on sexual reproduction. The production of identical multiple offspring is the norm in at least two species of armadillos, and probably in several other mammalian species.

Cloning can also be defined as transplantation of a nucleus from a cell (see Figure 1) into an ovum (technically, an oocyte, or egg). To understand this process, a few biological principles will be reviewed. The billions of cells in bodies of animals can be classified into two kinds: somatic cells and germ-line cells. The germ-line cells have an element of immortality; certain early embryonic cells divide to form a lineage of cells that divide to form gametes (sperm or oocytes), which, after fertilization, form embryos of the next generation, and so on *ad infinitum* unless the species becomes extinct. Except for gametes, all cells in the body are diploid, that is they have two similar copies of genetic material, one copy inherited from the sperm, and one copy from the egg. Whenever cells divide, they first duplicate the genetic material so that *each* resulting daughter cell remains diploid. However, the cells that will form sperm divide twice after duplicating their genetic material, resulting in four haploid (one copy of genetic material) sperm, rather than two diploid cells; similar divisions occur to form haploid eggs.

With this background, the basic principle of nuclear transplantation is simple enough. Instead of fertilizing the haploid oocyte with a haploid sperm, one removes the chromosomal genetic information from the oocyte and "fertilizes" it with a diploid cell (see Figure 2).

The first mammals produced via nuclear transplantation were derived from nuclei of cells of early embryos (around the sixteen-cell stage) in the 1980s by Steen M. Willadsen in Cambridge, England. With this approach, one makes a number of genetic copies of an embryo, not an animal. This, of course, changed with Dolly, whose "parent" was a somatic cell derived from differentiated adult mammary tissue. Thus, cloning via nuclear transplantation is fundamentally different when using nuclei from embryonic cells than when using nuclei from adult cells, in that there is considerable uncertainty about the phenotype (visible characteristics) that will result from the embryo, whereas there will be more information about what will result with a nucleus taken from an adult animal, or even a newborn.

Cloning is often defined very broadly as simply making a genetic copy (or copying an organism)—sometimes with the implications of making many copies. Sometimes *clone* is used as a noun to indicate a genetic copy.

## How Identical are Clones with Each Other?

Clonal, or asexual, reproduction, in nature results in nearly genetically identical individuals. This includes two categories of genetic identity: between parent and offspring, and among offspring. However, for numerous traits, genetic identity does not result in phenotypic identity, either due to epigenetic effects or to environmental effects. The environmental effects are well known, particularly from human identical-twin studies. Epigenetic effects are defined as effects due to genes that vary from organism to organism due to random chance, and therefore, cannot ever be predicted exactly. Epigenetic effects are less well known than environmental effects, but can be huge for some traits, such as different coat-color patterns among clones or identical twins. There is no genetic instruction specifying the color of each individual hair in animals with hair of different colors, but only genetic instructions for the general pattern of hair color. These instructions provide general guidelines about how melanoblasts, which differentiate into cells termed melanocytes, migrate and invade hair follicles during fetal development, but not an instruction whether or not to invade an individual hair follicle. Melanocytes reside in hair follicles and add packets of melanin to color each hair as it grows. Numerous other epigenetic phenomena occur during embryonic and fetal development such as random X-chromosome inactivation in female mammals, different methylation (addition of a carbon atom plus 3 hydrogen atoms) patterns of cytosines (see below), and lengths of telomeres, which make up the ends of chromosomes.

There also is considerable variability in embryonic development due to chance effects. Richard C. Lewontin has described how these effects interact with genotype, and with epigenetic and environmental effects, in complex ways so as to generate considerable differences among clonal sets.

One other potential source of differences among animals cloned from genetically identical nuclei is cytoplasmic (see Figure 1) inheritance, illustrated most clearly by mitochondria. Mitochondria are small cytoplasmic bodies located in all cells (with hundreds per cell). They have numerous functions, including generation of energy for such life processes as muscular movement. Mitochondria have their own genetic information in the form of small, circular chromosomes. These almost always are inherited exclusively from mother via the oocyte. Different maternal lines have mitochondria of different genetic makeup, so it is the cytoplasm of the oocyte that determines the makeup of the mitochondrial genome, rather than the chromosomes in the nucleus. Thus, when cloning by nuclear transfer, the mitochondrial genetics will differ from clone to clone unless the oocytes are all derived from the same maternal line of females.

Another source of differences among clones is mutations in the DNA in nuclear chromosomes or mitochondria. DNA is composed of only four kinds of building blocks, known as adenine, thymine, guanine, and cytosine, or A, T, G, and C, respectively. The genetic makeup (DNA) of the nucleus of each mammalian diploid cell has around 12 billion of these building blocks, theoretically hooked together in precisely the same way when DNA is replicated, so that each daughter cell produced has the same genetic makeup, or order of the four building blocks as the "parent" cell that divided. As one might imagine, there is an occasional error when assembling 12 billion items in a specific sequence, and these errors are one source of mutations. Other causes of mutations include background radiation (with which we are constantly bombarded) and chemical reactions, such as peroxidation, which is a chemical process caused by oxygen that can be very detrimental.

The human body is loaded with antioxidants to prevent peroxidation, and its cells contain DNA proofreading and repair enzymes, but these are imperfect at preventing mutations. A common example of mutations is cancer cells, which no longer have true copies of the DNA of normal cells. Most mutations do not cause cancer or have any other noticeable effect, but some cause changes—such as blue rather than brown eyes. Differences among otherwise genetically identical clones due to mutations are usually minor, but nevertheless do occur frequently.

The "gold standard" for genetic identity of mammals is identical twins, triplets, etc. These at least start out with identical chromosomal and mitochondrial genetics and are gestated in the same environment. Even postnatally, identical twins usually grow up in a very similar environment. All man-made clones will be less identical than these, especially in phenotype. Since there are considerable differences between naturally occurring identical twins, such differences will also occur among manufactured clones, in addition to the other differences already discussed.

## Procedures for Cloning Mammals

There are numerous procedures for cloning mammals, but two are the most common. The first concerns making identical copies of embryos from embryonic cells, and the

FIGURE 1

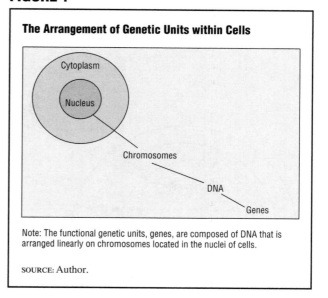

**The Arrangement of Genetic Units within Cells**

Cytoplasm

Nucleus

Chromosomes

DNA

Genes

Note: The functional genetic units, genes, are composed of DNA that is arranged linearly on chromosomes located in the nuclei of cells.

SOURCE: Author.

second creates embryos (with identical nuclear DNA) from cells of embryos, fetuses, young animals, or adult cells.

Conceptually, the simplest approach would be to separate the two cells of a two-cell embryo so that two identical organisms form. This has been done repeatedly in one way or another, even occasionally resulting in identical quadruplets when dividing a four-cell embryo four ways. Success rates are quite high when aiming at identical twins, but become very low when dividing embryos into quadruplets, the practical limit of the technique. For technical reasons, this approach is much more practical at later stages of embryonic development—at the 100-cell stage, for example), when embryos can be bisected. This latter approach has been used to produce thousands of identical twins (and occasionally triplets) commercially, primarily with cattle (as illustrated by Timothy Williams and colleagues [1984]).

Surprisingly, the main reason for splitting embryos to produce demi-embryos is not to produce sets of identical copies, but rather because splitting embryos augments the general technology of embryo transfer, which is designed to increase the reproductive rates of agricultural (and other) females, much like artificial insemination increases the reproduction of males. To illustrate, pregnancy rates for whole bovine embryos are around 65 percent, whereas pregnancy rates for half embryos are around 50 percent. Thus, because there are twice as many demi-embryos after the splitting process, the net pregnancy rate is frequently over 100 percent. Identical twins and triplets produced by these methods make excellent experimental subjects because genetic variation can be controlled, and sometimes they are produced mainly for these purposes.

**FIGURE 2**

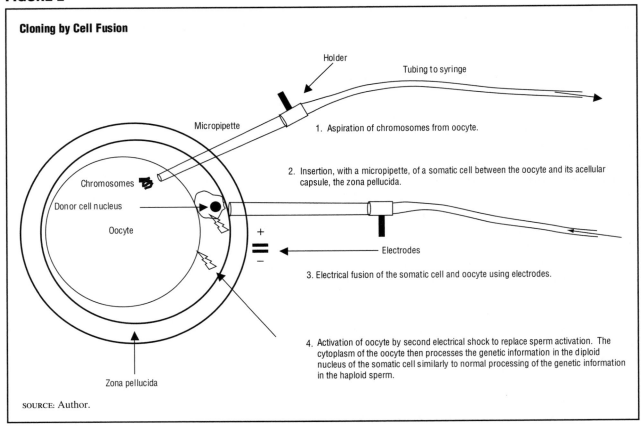

Cloning by Cell Fusion

Holder

Tubing to syringe

Micropipette

1. Aspiration of chromosomes from oocyte.

2. Insertion, with a micropipette, of a somatic cell between the oocyte and its acellular capsule, the zona pellucida.

Chromosomes

Donor cell nucleus

Oocyte

+

=

−

Electrodes

3. Electrical fusion of the somatic cell and oocyte using electrodes.

4. Activation of oocyte by second electrical shock to replace sperm activation. The cytoplasm of the oocyte then processes the genetic information in the diploid nucleus of the somatic cell similarly to normal processing of the genetic information in the haploid sperm.

Zona pellucida

SOURCE: Author.

With nuclear transfer, the main principle is that the ovum, or oocyte is a minifactory designed to produce an embryo, which eventually develops into a term pregnancy. Half of the genetic instructions to make the conceptus normally come from the oocyte, and half from the sperm. With cloning, a complete set of genetic instructions is provided by the nucleus of one embryonic or somatic cell. Of course, those instructions originally were derived from the sperm and oocyte that resulted in the organism that provided the donor cell.

One problem is obtaining oocytes to use as recipients for the diploid nuclei. These cells, the largest in the body (about 1/200 inch in diameter), must be of the same species as the donor nucleus. Usually, they are aspirated from ovarian follicles (large blister-like, fluid-filled structures). In the case of farm animals, oocytes are often obtained from ovaries of slaughtered animals of unknown background. An alternative is to aspirate (remove by suction) oocytes through a large needle inserted into the ovaries in the body cavity of living animals—ultrasound is usually used to visualize the follicles so the needle can be guided into them after piercing the wall of the vagina. This method is used in women to obtain oocytes for routine in vitro fertilization. Oocytes

from laboratory animals such as mice are usually obtained after the oocytes are ovulated (released from the follicles) naturally. The oocytes then are located in the part of the reproductive system called the oviduct, and the body cavity needs to be opened to get them out, either via surgery with anesthesia, or after euthanizing the animal.

After oocytes are obtained, they are cultured under specific conditions with specific chemicals until they have matured appropriately. The length of the maturation period may range from less than an hour to two days, depending on the species, the treatments, and the reproductive status of the animal providing the oocytes.

The next step is to remove or destroy the unwanted chromosomes of the oocyte. This usually is done by aspiration of this material with a micropipette (see Figure 2), although there are other options, such as destroying the chromosomes with a laser. Following this step comes transplantation of the nucleus. This can be done by removing the nucleus from the donor cell and injecting it into the cytoplasm of the oocyte. However, in the vast majority of cases the entire donor cell is simply fused with the oocyte using an electric pulse. This incorporates the nucleus into the oocyte, but it also mixes the cytoplasm of the two cells, which also mixes the mitochondria. This is usually not a problem because the oocyte has more than 100 times the volume of the cytoplasm of the donor cell, so the donor cytoplasm essentially gets diluted out.

When a sperm fertilizes an oocyte, it not only adds its 50 percent contribution of genetic material, it also activates, or turns on, the oocyte. Prior to fertilization the oocyte is a large, slowly dying cell. The sperm adds a specific enzyme that chemically activates the ovum, so it comes to life, starts using more energy, and, among other things, duplicates the genetic material in preparation for division to the two-cell stage. This activation function must be duplicated during the nuclear transplantation process for successful embryonic development. It is accomplished in a variety of ways, depending on the species and other details, such as the degree of maturity of the oocyte. A common approach is to apply a strong electrical shock.

The final step is to allow the cloned embryo to develop *in vitro,* eventually growing from the two-cell stage to a suitable stage for transferring the embryo back to the reproductive tract of a recipient. The length of this culture is usually a few days to a week, depending on the species.

## Potential Applications of Cloning
### Nonhuman Animals

Aside from splitting embryos to produce more offspring, the main application of cloning to date has been to obtain basic biological information that can be applied in other areas. This will continue to be the main value of cloning for some time, and will result in information about causes of birth defects, aging, cancer, and other disease states.

One obvious application of cloning by nuclear transplantation and cell fusion is to make genetic copies of outstanding agricultural animals. As discussed earlier, a genetic copy does not equal a phenotypic copy, so this is not nearly as attractive as most people surmise. For example, the genetic contribution (heritability) to differences between cattle (within breeds) in milk production is on the order of 30 percent, while other factors, mainly environment and random chance, explain the other 70 percent. Thus, if one cloned a cow producing 3,000 gallons of milk annually, selected from a herd averaging 2,000 gallons of milk, on the average only 30 percent of the difference between the production of the individual cow and the herd would show up in the clone. A herd of such clones might average 2,300 gallons of milk, a substantial improvement over the 2,000 gallons average, but not even close to the 3,000 gallons

produced by the animal being cloned. (This example is an oversimplification, for a variety of reasons—including interactions between genotype and environment [see Lewontin]—but the broad idea is correct.)

There is an even more serious problem with using cloning to increase production of milk (or meat, fiber, etc.), which is that it is not economically viable. The value of the extra milk produced by such a cow would be less than $1,000 during her lifetime, and she might eat more feed than other cows because more nutrients are required to make more milk, further decreasing her economic value. Costs of cloning in 2003 are in excess of $10,000 per cow, and while this likely will decrease markedly, it is unlikely that costs will approach economic viability in the foreseeable future. Thus, herds of cloned cows are not likely any time soon. The situation for meat production is even less favorable economically. If one did use this strategy, there would be hundreds of different donor cows cloned due to wanting different optimal genotypes for different environments (e.g. the optimal Vermont cow would be different from the optimal cow for Georgia) not to mention the individual preferences of farmers).

One agricultural application that does make sense is to make copies of genetically (as opposed to phenotypically) outstanding individuals. A good example is a bull whose daughters, on the average, have excellent milk production and are not prone to mammary gland infections. Such a bull might have thousands of daughters demonstrated to be superior to the average population. This bull obviously is essentially worthless phenotypically—copies will not produce any milk—but cloned copies of the bull will produce essentially identical sperm that can be used to produce more daughters by artificial insemination. For this example, one or two clones would likely produce all the semen that could be sold, so large numbers of copies are not needed. In fact, the main application in this context is insurance. Such bulls are extremely valuable, and having one or two copies makes good economic sense. More copies, however, are redundant and expensive to feed and maintain.

Another popular potential application of somatic-cell cloning concerns companion animals, particularly dogs and horses. Again, one will not get a phenotypic copy, so this only makes marginal sense. The resulting cloned animal will often have somewhat similar coat-color patterns and be roughly the same size, but it may have a very different personality, since this is largely influenced by environment. One does not recreate the same animal by cloning, simply a chromosomal genetic copy.

There are myriad experimental uses of cloning, particularly in making transgenic technology more useful. Cloning by nuclear transplantation is thus a powerful experimental tool.

## Potential Applications of Human Cloning

In most cultures there would be huge ethical problems in making genetic copies of human beings—so-called reproductive cloning. Currently, this is ethically unacceptable because of the high incidence of congenital abnormalities in offspring derived from cloning by nuclear transfer. If there were no such problems—if cloned children would be as healthy as those produced naturally—one can concoct scenarios for which reproductive cloning might be ethically acceptable. The classic example is a couple whose baby dies within a day or two of birth due to an accident that also makes the mother incapable of reproducing due to damage to ovaries. One could theoretically take cells from the dead baby and clone them using a donated oocyte, which could then be transferred to the uterus (which is still functional) of the woman. The donor cells from the dead baby could also be frozen for later use, so timing would not be a problem.

Other (very improbable) scenarios could be envisioned that would make reproductive cloning ethically acceptable for most people. In any case, this technology for reproductive cloning of persons would likely work with a similar success rate as occurs in other species (extremely low, as of 2003). It is certainly possible that a century or more in the future this mode of reproduction will be used to some extent, and persons from that era may well consider our current collective thinking quaint. Since chromosomal genetic identity never results in phenotypic identity, one never recreates a person or animal, and even if phenotypic identity were possible, such individuals would still be individuals. Identical twins and triplets provide some guidance on potential problems. Such individuals usually lead fairly normal lives, and they are considerably more identical than manufactured clones will ever be.

## Therapeutic Cloning

A second kind of cloning, therapeutic cloning, is intended to produce tissue and organ replacement parts. There are millions of people worldwide who suffer from debilitating diseases such as diabetes, heart disease, and cirrhosis of the liver. Similarly, millions suffer from accidents that severely damage tissues and organs, including burns, spinal cord damage, and crushed kidneys. In many of these cases, tissue or organ transplants will prolong life and greatly increase quality of life. There are two major problems with this approach: (1) There is a critical shortage of such tissues

and organs, and (2) there is usually immunological incompatibility of donor and recipient, which requires immunosuppressive therapy that is debilitating and greatly increases the incidence of cancer.

A solution to this unfortunate situation is to use nuclei of somatic cells of the subject to make immunologically compatible tissues for replacement parts. This approach is not yet available for practical use, but likely will be developed in one form or another in the near future. What is envisioned is to take cells (e.g., from skin) of the person who needs the replacement tissue, and fuse them with donated oocytes from which original chromosomes are removed to form early embryos. Instead of transferring these to the uterus to form a fetus, they would be induced to develop into various tissues *in vitro*. No fetus would be formed, so there would be no brain, heart, leg, or face, but rather tissues that make up body parts. Quite a bit is known about how to induce the embryonic cells to make muscle, skin, or other tissues, but there is still much to be learned.

This approach likely cannot be used to produce a heart or a kidney, at least in the foreseeable future, but producing heart-muscle cells, nerve cells, pancreatic tissue, liver tissue, or skin does seem feasible. Liver, for example, has a remarkable regenerative capability, so only a small bit of liver may be needed—such as liver stem cells, which might regenerate a whole organ after transplantation. Producing pancreatic tissue to alleviate diabetes would likely be considerably simpler, while producing nerve cells to repair spinal cord damage would likely be more difficult.

It is possible that some tissues can be generated from adult stem cells, circumventing the need for cloning via embryos. However, the embryonic approach has several theoretical advantages—it is the way tissues develop naturally, for example—and it has some practical advantages as well. Furthermore, research into *in vitro* differentiation of tissue, much of which can be done in animal models with or without the cloning steps, will likely produce information that can eventually be used outside of the context of cloning to accomplish the numerous therapeutic objectives.

## Characteristics of Cloned Animals and Related Ethical Consequences

If all goes well, a genetic copy of the animal being cloned is produced, but, again, one clone can vary considerably in phenotype from the donor for numerous traits. Unfortunately, natural reproduction does not go well in every case, and such problems are greatly exacerbated with cloning. In a 2002 summary of all available information on animals cloned from somatic cells (38 studies resulting in 335 subjects in 5 species), Jose B. Cibelli and colleagues found that 77 percent of the resulting animals were normal, while 23 percent were not. The normal subjects, though mostly adults, had not yet lived out their normal life spans, so additional problems (over and above those due to normal aging) could yet develop. Cloning from somatic cells has not resulted in monsters, but, in most cases, reasonably normal individuals.

However, 23 percent abnormalities, mostly neonatal death, is completely unacceptable ethically for producing children, and for most scientists working in this area that ends the ethical debate on human reproductive cloning. In the Cibelli survey it was noted that many of the animals produced represented the initial, or at least early, studies on cloning in respective laboratories, and that the incidence of abnormalities likely would decrease with more experience and improved techniques. This is already being borne out in the scientific literature, but it likely will be many years before the incidence of problems with somatic-cell cloning will decrease to acceptable levels for reproductive cloning of people. However, this ethical crutch will also likely disappear with time.

A complex ethical question is where to set the boundaries on acceptable levels of abnormalities. Interestingly, a 2002 study by Michèle Hansen and colleagues that looked at children produced via *in vitro* fertilization showed that congenital abnormalities were approximately double the 4 percent seen with natural reproduction. Most of these abnormalities were not extremely serious and could be circumvented or repaired. Nevertheless, the abnormalities were doubled, and some were serious. Thus, this ethical problem is already with us.

The question boils down to the right of people to reproduce given an increased risk of an abnormal child. Of course, these questions arise outside of the context of assisted reproductive technology, such as the increased risk of a child with Down's syndrome when older women reproduce. Modern science can minimize such suffering (e.g., by genotyping embryos before transfer back to the uterus, and eliminating those that will result in severely abnormal individuals). Another reality is that, in one sense or another, nearly all persons are abnormal. For example, essentially all humans have lethal or severely debilitating recessive alleles in their genetic makeup, which, if matched with another such allele in a gamete of a mate, will result in death of the conceptus or resulting child.

A frequent abnormality that occurs with cloning by nuclear transfer via embryonic or somatic donor cells is fetal overgrowth. It is not unusual for offspring to be 30 or 40 percent larger than normal at birth. In some studies, up to 30 percent of offspring have this condition, known as *large-offspring syndrome,* and some animals cloned from the same donor are large, some are normal, and some are small—which elegantly illustrates that identical chromosomal identity does not equal identical phenotype. Large-offspring syndrome is not a genetic trait, in that this problem is not transmitted to the next generation when the cloned animals reproduce naturally. Also, Michael Wilson and colleagues showed in 1995 that these excessively large neonates develop into only slightly larger adults. The scientific consensus is that large-offpsring syndrome can be summarized as a genetically normal fetus in an epigenetically abnormal placenta. That is, the placenta from cloned pregnancies is often abnormal, resulting in secondary problems in the fetus that largely correct themselves after birth. Unfortunately, with routine husbandry, the newborns often die because of being debilitated from gestating in an abnormal placenta. Fortunately, with a few days of intensive care starting at birth, such offspring survive reasonably well and develop normally, as shown by Frank B. Garry and colleagues in 1995.

As with human babies, animal offspring derived from *in vitro* fertilization or long-term *in vitro* culture of embryos have a much higher incidence of abnormalities than with normal reproduction, but a lower incidence than with cloning (see Kelley Tamashiro and colleagues). Clearly, some (but not all) *in vitro* manipulations, particularly when the *in vitro* period exceeds several days, lead to increased problems in resulting offspring. Thus, there is a baseline of problems with natural reproduction, which increases with the amount of *in vitro* manipulation (and reaches a higher level with somatic-cell cloning). It is likely that these problems will decrease or be circumvented with improved techniques, and also that the basic information obtained will be useful in decreasing birth defects and neonatal problems that occur with natural reproduction.

There are some special problems with a small percentage of pregnancies from somatic-cell cloning that are not just an increase in incidence of naturally occurring problems. In some cases, the immune system appears to be severely compromised, and there can be major problems with the heart, blood vessels, and kidneys that are extremely rare with normal reproduction. Furthermore, there is an unusual amount of embryonic death and fetal absorption or abortion with cloned pregnancies—over 80 percent embryonic and fetal attrition is not unusual (compared with around 30 percent with normal reproduction). Thus, the incidence of problem conceptuses is very high, and most of these die in early pregnancy. This is still another reason that, as practiced at the beginning of the twenty-first century, reproductive cloning should not be done with human embryos.

A final point is that cloning via nuclei from somatic cells is very inefficient, currently on the order of 2 percent success per oocyte. This is due to the multiplicative attrition (or success) of the various steps. For example, if there is 90 percent successful fusion of donor cell and oocyte, with 50 percent dividing into embryos suitable for transfer to recipients, 30 percent embryonic survival until pregnancy can be diagnosed, 20 percent of diagnosed pregnancies developing to term, and 85 percent surviving the neonatal period, the result is an overall success rate of around 2 percent. These are typical current values, and are one reason why the costs of cloning are so high. While success rates are improving, it will likely be some years until overall success even approaches 10 percent. For human reproductive cloning, dozens of women would need to be involved as donors of oocytes and recipients of embryos to produce even one baby—assuming the procedures worked as well as they do with animal models, which is unlikely. This illustrates another ethical issue, in that undue use of scarce and expensive medical resources would be required for clonal human reproduction.

## Conclusion

The most important conclusions from this scientific overview are that, although cloning procedures for mammals are yielding huge amounts of important scientific information, current procedures are extremely inefficient and result in a high incidence of abnormalities in offspring. These problems severely limit immediate prospects for applications of cloning mammals due to both financial and ethical considerations. Furthermore, cloning does not and will not lead to reincarnation of an animal or person, but rather to a new individual with considerable phenotypic differences from the genetic donor.

GEORGE E. SEIDEL, JR.

SEE ALSO: *Christianity, Bioethics in; Embryo and Fetus; Harm; Reproductive Technologies; Research Policy; Technology;* and other *Cloning* subentries

### BIBLIOGRAPHY

Campbell, Keith H.; McWhir, James; Ritchie, W. A.; et al. 1996. "Sheep Cloned by Nuclear Transfer from a Cultured Cell Line." *Nature* 380(6569): 64–66.

Cibelli, Jose B.; Campbell, Keith H.; Seidel, George E., Jr.; et al. 2002. "The Health Profile of Cloned Animals." *Nature Biotechnology* 20(1): 13–14.

Garry, Frank B.; Adams, Ragin; McCann, Joseph P.; et al. 1996. "Postnatal Characteristics of Calves Produced by Nuclear Transfer Cloning." *Theriogenology* 45(1): 141–152.

Hansen, Michèle; Kurinczuk, Jennifer J.; Bower, Carol; et al. 2002. "The Risk of Major Birth Defects after Intracytoplasmic Sperm Injection and In Vitro Fertilization." *New England Journal of Medicine* 346(10): 725–730.

Lewontin, Richard C. 2000. "Cloning and the Fallacy of Biology Determinism." In *Human Cloning*, ed. Barbara MacKinnon. Urbana: University of Illinois Press.

Seidel, George E., Jr. 2002. "Genetic and Phenotypic Similarity among Members of Mammalian Clonal Sets." In *Principles of Cloning*, ed. Jose Cibelli, Robert P. Lanza, Keith H. S. Campbell, et al. San Diego, CA: Academic Press.

Tamashiro, Kelley L. K.; Wakayama, Toruhiko; Akutsu, Hidenori; et al. 2002. "Cloned Mice Have an Obese Phenotype Not Transmitted to Their Offspring." *Nature Medicine* 8(3): 262–267.

Willadsen, Steen M. 1986. "Nuclear Transplantation in Sheep Embryos." *Nature* 20(6057): 63–65.

Williams, Timothy J.; Elsden, R. Peter; and Seidel, George E., Jr. 1984. "Pregnancy Rates with Bisected Bovine Embryos." *Theriogenology* 22(5): 521–531.

Wilmut, Ian; Schnieke, Angelika E.; McWhir, James; et al. 1997. "Viable Offspring Derived from Fetal and Adult Mammalian Cells." *Nature* 385(6619): 810–813.

Wilson, J. Michael; Williams, J. D.; Bondioli, Kenneth R.; et al. 1995. "Comparison of Birth Weight and Growth Characteristics of Bovine Calves Produced by Nuclear Transfer (Cloning), Embryo Transfer, and Natural Mating." *Animal Reproduction Science* 38(2): 73–83.

## II. REPRODUCTIVE

Reproductive cloning uses the technique of cloning to produce a child. Using technology to assist in "making babies" is nothing new. Artificial insemination has been available since the first part of the twentieth century. The first of many "test-tube babies" produced by *in vitro* fertilization (IVF) was born in England in 1978. Newer technologies include the injection of sperm directly into the egg and the use of frozen and donated eggs and embryos. In 1985 there were thirty fertility clinics in the United States alone, but by 2000 this number had grown to more than 350. More then 1 million couples in the United States seek fertility treatment each year, some of which includes the use of assisted reproductive technologies.

Only recently has producing a child through the technique of cloning become a real possibility. Since the birth of Dolly the sheep at the Roslin Institute near Edinburgh, Scotland in March, 1996, people have wondered whether it would also be possible to produce humans by this method. Dolly was a clone, a genetic copy, of a six-year-old ewe. Rather than coming into being by the joining of sperm and egg, Dolly was created by inserting the nucleus of a cell from the udder of this ewe into a sheep egg from which the nucleus had been removed. After being stimulated to grow, the egg was implanted into the uterus of another sheep from which Dolly was born. Because Dolly was a mammal like humans, people concluded that it might be possible to clone human beings as well. Moreover, Dolly was produced from a body or somatic cell of an adult sheep with already determined characteristics. Because the cells of an adult are already differentiated, have taken on specialized roles, scientists had previously assumed that cloning from such cells would not be possible. After Dolly, it seemed, it might be possible to produce an identical, though younger, twin of an already existing human being.

Reactions to this possibility varied widely. Some hailed it as another marvel of science that could benefit many. Others were horrified at the prospect that this seeming science fiction might become reality. Some thought of it as just another form of assisted reproductive technology, while others viewed it as something radically different. This overview of cloning for the purpose of reproduction will address the following questions:

What is reproductive cloning?

What are the present capabilities in the area of cloning?

What are the proposed uses of this type of cloning?

What are the ethical considerations and objections to it?

What are the public policy implications?

## Cloning: Its Nature and Capabilities

The type of cloning described above is called somatic cell nuclear transfer (SCNT) because it transfers the nucleus of a somatic or body cell into an egg from which the nucleus has been removed. A different type of cloning is achieved through fission or cutting of an early embryo. Through this method it may be possible to make identical human twins or triplets from one embryo. These genetically identical embryos could then be stored for further tries at conception, thus saving a woman from undergoing repeated ovulation during fertility treatment. Here, however, the concentration will be on cloning through SCNT. Also, this entry treats only cloning for reproductive purposes, not what has come to be called research or therapeutic cloning. In the latter, the same process occurs but is not intended to lead to the birth of a child. Rather it is oriented, for example, to the study of the process of development or to the producing of stem cells that might be useful in therapies for Parkinson's, diabetes, and other diseases.

How close are we to being able to produce a human being through cloning? As of the beginning of 2003, to researchers' knowledge there have been no human beings produced through cloning. Clonaid, a company founded by a religious sect called the Raelians, has claimed to have produced five cloned babies. However, no DNA or other evidence has so far been provided to substantiate this. In November 2001, Advanced Cell Technology, a small biotech company in Worcester, Massachusetts, said it had succeeded in producing a human embryo through cloning. Scientists extracted human eggs from seven volunteer women and replaced the nuclei of these eggs with cells from an adult donor, some skin cells and some cumulus cells (the cells surrounding a maturing egg). While none of the eggs that used the skin began the cell division process, three of the eight eggs that were re-nucleated with cumulus cells began dividing. One developed to the two-cell stage, one to the four-cell stage, and the third to the six-cell stage, at which point it too died.

One can also judge something of the potential for human cloning from the progress of animal cloning. In just the past two decades a number of higher animals have been produced through cloning, including cows, sheep, goats, mice, pigs, rabbits, and a cat called CC for carbon copy or copy cat. Cloned animals themselves have produced offspring of their own in the natural way. Dolly had six seemingly normal lambs. Several generations of mice have also been produced through SCNT. Clones have been derived not only from udder cells, but also from cells from embryos and fetuses, and from mice tails and cumulus cells.

However, these experiments have been neither efficient nor safe. In the case of Dolly, 277 eggs were used to produce only one lamb. In March 1996, the Roslin Institute also produced two lambs from mature embryo cells, Megan and Morag. However, they were only two out of five who were born and survived in a project that used over 200 embryos. Alan Coleman, research director of PPL Therapeutics, the company that produced Dolly, reported having cloned five female pigs who were genetically modified to lack a gene that makes pig organs incompatible with the human immune system. However, here the success rate was again quite low. Scientists implanted 300 embryos, producing twenty-eight sows that gave birth to seven live piglets, only four of which survived. In another project involving rabbits, 371 eggs were implanted, using twenty-seven rabbits as foster mothers, but only six rabbits were born and only five of these survived to the state of weaning. CC, the cat mentioned above, was one of eighty-seven embryos implanted in eight surrogate mother cats, and was the only one of two resulting pregnancies that survived.

Cloned animals also have shown various abnormalities. In one study all twelve cloned mice died between one and two years of age. Six of the cloned mice had pneumonia, four had serious liver damage, and one had leukemia and lung cancer. On February 14, 2003, Dolly died. She was euthanized because she suffered from a lung disease that the owners feared would spread. At age five, Dolly had also been diagnosed with arthritis. Some suggest that this may be due to the fact that she was cloned from the cell of an already aged adult sheep. However, in late 2001 Advanced Cell Technology claimed to have cloned thirty cattle from skin cells, twenty-four of which were alive and healthy between one and four years later. Some say that the high failure rate and the prevalence of serious abnormalities in animals means that cloning humans is probably not possible. Others believe that with time the efficiency and safety of animal cloning will improve and then it may be possible to clone human beings as well.

## Uses of Reproductive Cloning

What uses might there be, or what reasons might someone have, for producing a human being through cloning? What follows is a survey of a number of possible uses of this procedure, some of which are obviously more problematic than others. The ethical issues that have been or might be raised regarding the possible uses of reproductive cloning will then be discussed.

One of the probable primary uses, if cloning does become a reality, is for the treatment of fertility problems. For example, if the male or husband is sterile, or does not produce sperm, DNA from one of his cells could be inserted into a de-nucleated egg from the female or wife who would also bear the child. Both would then be contributing to the make up and birth of the child. Many have pointed out that there is a strong desire among people who want a child to have one that is biologically related to them. These parents also may wish to avoid the confusion that can result from the use of donor eggs or sperm. If the woman is infertile, another woman's egg could be used along with the DNA of the infertile woman or her husband or partner. Cloning might also be used to avoid genetic diseases.

Another possible use would be in the fertilization of a woman who wants to have children to whom she is related biologically, but who does not have a partner and does not wish to use donor sperm. The woman might be one who is single and who has not found a suitable partner, or who is divorced and still wants to have children. A cell from her body could be used. In this case the child would be a clone of the woman herself. Or in the case of a lesbian couple, a cell from the body of the other partner could be used. In this case both would have contributed to the make up of the child.

Someone might want to produce a child who is a clone of a much-loved spouse or child who has died. As noted below, while this would not bring back the loved one or duplicate them exactly, there would be some similarities and thus in a way the ability to keep some part of the person alive. One might even want to achieve a certain kind of immortality by cloning oneself. This would be similar in some way to living on through our children and their children.

Cloning could also be used to help ill family members. There have been cases in which parents have conceived a child in the hope that he or she could be a donor match for a sibling who had some serious disorder. A child who was the clone of such a sibling could also be a blood or bone marrow donor for the sibling. Although no one is suggesting that clones would be produced simply as the source of organs, some organ donation might not be objectionable.

Finally, cloned human beings could provide us with further information about the relationship between nature and nurture. A disabled person might want to show or see what he would have been like but for the disability, or someone might simply be curious to see how a clone of himself might grow to adulthood.

## Ethical Objections and Arguments

Ethics judges or evaluates human choices and actions or policies as being, for example, good or bad, right or wrong, and just or unjust. Ethical or moral judgments (the terms being used synonymously here) require reasons that justify them. Many people have raised various ethical objections regarding human cloning. The arguments and the reasons given for them are summarized here as well as the responses of critics of the arguments. However, since what is presented is only a summary, it is not possible to give a full analysis of the kind of reasons that they exemplify and why these might or might not be well-grounded in generally-accepted values or in ethical theory.

It should also be noted at the outset that ethical evaluation is independent of social policy and law. Not everything that is morally bad or wrong ought to be illegal. It takes a separate set of reasons to conclude that because some instances of human cloning might be morally wrong that they should then also be illegal. Nevertheless many of our policies and laws do have ethical bases. First the ethical arguments will be treated and then finally some social policy issues related to them. Some suggestions regarding the relationship between these two domains will also be provided.

## Playing God

One of the objections to human cloning most often raised is that it would be *Playing God*. While it is not always clear just what is meant by this, at least three or four overlapping versions of this objection can be delineated. One is that only God can and should create a human life. This role is specifically reserved to God, such that when humans who try to do it take on a role that is improper for them to play.

Those who hold this view might use religious reasons and sources to support it. However, while this looks like a religious position, it is not necessarily so. For example, it might mean that the coming into being of a new person is a creation, not a making or production. A creation is the bringing into being of something the outcome of which is not known in advance. The coming into being of a human being or person is also a said to be a mysterious thing and something in the face of which humankind should be in awe. When producing a human being, as in cloning, people become instead makers or manipulators of a product that they control and over which they have power. Rather, this argument continues, those who bring a child into the world should do so with an attitude of respect for something wondrous, the coming into existence of a totally unique and new being.

A third version of this objection stresses the significance of nature and the natural. In producing a human being through cloning, scientists act against human nature. In humans, as in all higher animals, reproduction is sexual, not asexual. Cloning, however, is asexual reproduction. Leon Kass is one of the strongest proponents of this view. He alleges that in cloning a human being people wrongly seek to escape the bounds and dictates of their own sexual nature.

A fourth and related version of the "don't play God" argument holds that attempting to clone a human being would demonstrate hubris, thinking we are wise enough to know the effects of one's acts when in fact that is not the case. It is similar to the warning that it is dangerous to "mess with mother nature." When dealing with human beings one should be particularly careful. Above all each person should avoid doing what unknowingly may turn out to be seriously harmful to the individuals produced and to future generations.

Just as there are various possible interpretations of this objection, there are various responses to, or criticisms of, it. On the point that by interfering in nature people take on a role that belongs only to God, the response is to ask how this is any different from other ways that man interferes with or changes nature. One example is medicine. Here science fights off natural threats, disease, and disability, for example, with inoculations, insulin, blood transfusions and prostheses. Others argue that God gave us brains to use and God is honored by that use, especially if it is for the benefit of humans and society. Human intelligence, the argument continues, is in fact a part of nature, so that in using it people do not actually oppose nature but follow it. Critics also point

out that in using technology to assist reproduction, one does not necessarily lose a sense of awe in the face of the coming into being, though with human help, of a unique new being. Objectors may point out, however, that cloning does not create a unique new being, but a copy of one that already exists or has existed. This objection thus overlaps with a second major objection, namely, that cloning is a threat to individuality.

## Threats to Individuality

Some people object to the very idea of cloning a human being because they believe that the person cloned would not be a unique individual. He or she would be the genetic copy of the person from whom the somatic cell was transferred. He or she would be the equivalent of an identical twin of this person, though years younger. Moreover, since dignity and worth is attached to a person's uniqueness as an individual, cloned individuals would lose something that is the basis of the special value each person should have. Some go so far as to claim that each person has in fact a right to a unique identity. Others point out the difficulties that clones would have in maintaining their individuality. People often have difficulty distinguishing identical twins from one another. Sometimes they dress alike and often they are expected to act alike. The implication is that they do not have the freedom or ability to develop their own individual personalities.

This objection is sometimes expressed as the view that a cloned human being would not have a soul, that he or she would be a hollow shell of a person. This version of the objection is probably based on a religious belief that only God should be allowed to create a human being and in doing so directly acts to place a soul in that person. Thus if through cloning man produces a human being, God is prevented from placing a soul in that person.

Again, criticisms of these objections vary with the interpretation. One response is to review the facts about identical twins. Identical twins are more like each other than a clone would be to the person who was cloned. This is because identical twins shared the same nuclear environment as well as the same uterus. This would not be the case with clones. They would have had different mitochondria. This is important because the mitochondrial genes in the cytoplasm surrounding the re-nucleated cell do play a role in development. Clones would have developed in different uteruses and they would be raised in different circumstances and environments. Studies of plants and animals give dramatic evidence of how great a difference the environment makes. For example, plants and some animals vary significantly in structure and characteristics depending on the altitude of the land in which they develop. The genotype does not fully determine the phenotype. CC, the cloned cat mentioned above, does not quite look like its mother, Rainbow, a calico tri-colored female. They have different coat patterns because genes are not the only factor that controls coat color. At one year CC also has a different personality from her mother, being much more playful and curious. Even in the science fiction stories of creation of groups of clones, for instance of Hitler in the movie, *The Boys from Brazil,* the creators try to duplicate the environment. While genes do matter, and thus there would be similarities between the clone and the person who was cloned, the two would not be identical. Furthermore, these critics note, even normally-produced children may look like one or both of their parents and this fact does not prevent them from being individuals.

On the matter of soul, critics wonder why could God not give each person, identical twin or clone, an individual soul. Consider when the soul is supposed to be implanted in an individual. Some medieval writers, for example, held that the soul appeared or was implanted in the fetus when it had developed sufficiently so that it was fit for a human soul. Previous to that point, some held, the developing fetus had a vegetable and then an animal soul. Aristotle held that the soul or psyche was simply the form of the being, that which gave it unity as a particular living being, whether it be a plant or animal or person. Like any living human being, a cloned human being would on this view be a distinct being and so would have a human psyche or soul.

## A Right to an Open Future

Some have argued that cloning a human being is objectionable because the clone is expected to be like the person from whom he or she was cloned and thus would not be free to develop independently. Joel Feinberg has written about what he calls the "right to an open future" and Hans Jonas "the right to ignorance." The idea is that each person should be free to construct his or her own life and develop a unique self. However, a clone would be expected to use the person from whom he or she was cloned as a model. His or her future would already be given and known. Even if such expectations for the clone were not generally accepted, people would be hard pressed not to at least entertain such ideas. The argument also points out that an essential feature of having a child should include accepting whatever the child turns out to be. This would mean accepting the child as a unique being. Children are not objects to be controlled, nor to mold in a particular image. They have their own lives to lead. Parents may try to influence them and teach them while realizing that the children may decide to do or be different, which is their right as individual persons.

Critics of this argument may admit that there might be some inclination to have certain expectations for the clone. However, they argue, this undue influence is a possibility in the case of all parents and children, and not limited to clones. Parents decide on what schools to send their children and what sports or activities they will promote. The temptation or inclination may exist to unduly influence their children, but it is incumbent on parents to control the extent of that influence. The goal is to provide children with opportunities of various sorts from which the children themselves eventually choose. It is not cloning, these critics contend, that would cause a threat to an open future for a child, but the attitudes and character of parents and others.

## Exploitation

Related to the previous objection is one that holds that cloned children or persons would tend to be exploited. If one looks at many of the reasons given for cloning a person, the objection goes, they tend to be cases in which the cloning is for the sake of others. For example, the cloned child could be a donor for someone else. We might make clones that are of a certain sort that could be used for doing menial work or fighting wars. We might want to clone certain valued individuals, stars of the screen or athletic arena. In all these cases the clone would not be valued for his or her own self nor respected as a unique person. He or she would be valued for what they can bring to others. German philosopher Immanuel Kant (1724–1804) is cited as the source of the moral principle that persons ought not simply be used but ought to be treated as ends in themselves.

Critics could agree with Kant, but still disagree that a cloned human being would be any more likely than anyone else to be used by others for their own purposes only. Just because a child was conceived to provide bone marrow for a sick sibling would not prevent her from also being loved for her own sake. Even a case in which a man would clone himself in order to see how such a being might grow could turn out to be a situation in which the clone would be much loved and respected for himself and his own unique characteristics. Furthermore, the idea that we would allow anyone to clone a whole group of individuals and imprison them while training them to be workers or soldiers is not living in the present world in which there are legal protections against such treatment of children or other individuals. So also, critics may contend, the possibility that some group might take over society and create a 'Brave New World' in which children were produced only through cloning is far-fetched and no more than fiction. So also is a world in which there would be widespread cloning of stars and pop idols. While eugenics as a social policy has not been unknown in modern history, it is highly unlikely in open societies. Moreover, cloning is not the only way that eugenics could be practiced, as is demonstrated by the existence of (little-used) sperm banks of Nobel prize winners.

## Effect on Families

Some people believe that if human cloning were a reality, it would only add to the confusion already generated by the use of some other reproductive technologies. When donated eggs and surrogate mothers are used, the genetic parents are different from the gestational parents and the rearing parents, and conflicts have arisen regarding who the *real* parents are. Cloning, objectors contend, would be even more of a problem. It would add to this confusion the blurring of lines between generations. The mother's child could be her twin, or a twin of her own mother or father.

According to Leon Kass in "The Wisdom of Repugnance," this would lead to a confusion of kinship relations. In natural reproduction, two lineages come together to form one new being. "The child is the parents' own commingled being externalized and given a separate and persisting existence" (p. 30). Genetically, the cloned child has only one parent, the provider of the somatic cell. The child is literally the child of only one of a couple. What happens, then, to the traditional relationships with the members of the other side of the family, grandparents, aunts, and uncles? Or to the relationship of the husband to the child who is the twin of the mother or the wife to the child who is the twin of her husband? The answer, according to this objection, is that normal and natural human family relationships would be seriously eroded and harmed.

Critics of these arguments respond that, although there is a traditional type of family that in fact varies from culture to culture, there are also many different kinds of nontraditional families. Among these are single-parent households, adopted families, blended families, and lesbian and gay families. It is not the type of family that makes for a good loving household, the argument goes, but the amount of love and care that exists there. Children can learn new or different ways of relating to others. For example, just as stepparents can find ways of being valued parts of their stepchildren's lives, so also the parent who is not a genetic parent of a cloned child could adapt.

## The *Yuck* Factor

The argument that gives this section its title goes something as follows: Sometimes one has a gut reaction to something regarded as abhorrent. One is offended by the very thought of it and cannot always give reasons for this reaction. Yet instinctively one knows that what is abhorred is wrong. Many people seem to react to human cloning in this way. Such emotional reactions can be described as an expression of a kind of knowledge, as a kind of moral intuition. They could even be viewed as expressions of a kind of deep wisdom. The very idea of someone making a copy of themselves or many copies of a famous star is simply bizarre, revolting, and repulsive, and these emotional reactions tell us that there is something very wrong with it, even if there is no full explanation for what that is.

Any adequate response to this argument would entail an analysis of how ethical reasoning works when it works well. Emotional reactions or moral intuitions may indeed play a role in moral reasoning. However, most philosophers would agree that adequate moral reasoning should not rely on intuition or emotion alone. Reflections about why one might rightly have such gut reactions are in order. People have been known to have negative gut reactions to things that in fact were not wrong—interracial marriage, for example. It is incumbent on those who assert that something is wrong, most philosophers believe, that they provide rational argument and well-supported reasons to justify these beliefs and emotional reactions.

## Rights

Some of the arguments about human reproductive cloning have relied on the use of the language of rights for their conclusions. For example, as noted above, some have objected to cloning on grounds that people have a "right to an open future." In contrast, some argue that human cloning should be allowed because people have a "right to reproduce." And again, because cloning is such a risky process, some argue that it ought to be prohibited because children have a "right to be born healthy." Some attention should be given here, then, to what is meant by a right and why and whether we have certain rights, including these particular rights.

A right is generally understood to be a strong and legitimate claim that people can make to certain things. If the assertion is based on moral grounds, we refer to the right as a moral right, whether or not it is reinforced by law. It is a negative right or claim if it is a claim not to be interfered with. This is sometimes called a liberty right. Thus a right to freedom of speech would be classified primarily as a negative or liberty right, that is, a right not to be prevented from speaking out. But a positive right is a claim to be given certain things. Thus a right to healthcare would be classified as a right to be given certain forms of healthcare. Since rights are legitimate claims, there must be serious reasons or grounds given for their assertion. One view is that only persons have rights (not rocks or plants, while animals are a disputed case) for only persons are moral agents who can be held responsible for their actions. There are certain things that are essential in order for a person to function well as a human being, and these can be legitimately claimed as rights.

Given these clarifications about rights, which of the above mentioned claims might be legitimate claims and of what kind? Being able to produce a child of one's own might well be so important for a full human existence (with certain exceptions perhaps for celibates or others who serve higher or other causes) that one might well be said to have a legitimate claim or right to do so. It would first of all be classified as a negative or liberty right, in other words a right not to be prevented from producing children, and perhaps also producing them through cloning, at least when no one is harmed. Whether it is also so important that it could be considered a positive right such that society ought to provide the means or aids for those who are having trouble reproducing in the natural way due to infertility problems is another matter. While it may not at first seem reasonable to assert a right to reproduce in this or that way, it may make sense if one thinks of it as one thinks of eyeglasses or wheel chairs, namely as necessary aids to seeing and mobility, things that are essential for a satisfying human life and thus legitimate claims that people can make. A right to an open future could most reasonably be claimed as a negative right, namely a right not to be prevented from choosing a life for oneself. Things that would seriously interfere with this would then be morally problematic as threats to that right.

A right to be born healthy would most reasonably be thought of as a negative right. No one should deliberately do what will result in harm to a child, or do what poses an inordinate or undue risk to its life or health. It would be more problematic to claim that a being that does not exist in some requisite sense has a right to be given a life. However, if it is to have a life, then one might well argue that it should if possible have a life with decent chances for development and happiness. One might ground this in notions of equal opportunity and justice, that each person should have a fair chance to develop and to compete for access to life's goods. Given the risks that are associated with animal cloning, grave questions can be raised about human cloning in this regard.

## Safety and Harms

Given the abnormalities so far associated with animal cloning, there is a high likelihood that similar risks would accompany human cloning, at least at present. As described above, animal clones are at a rather high risk for a short life and a life with various diseases and abnormalities. Some have argued that since the alternative for the cloned child is not to

exist at all, one cannot claim that giving birth to a child with abnormalities harms that child. One could only say the child was harmed if it were brought into existence with such difficulties that its life with these conditions would be worse than having no life at all. However, others have questioned this sort of reasoning. They believe that it does make sense to say that doing what one knows will bring into existence a child whose life will be short and encumbered with serious ills is to harm that child. Since the harm is serious and the risk is high, they argue, one would be wrong to take it. However, this is not the same as arguing that the law ought to prevent people from taking such risks for others. This is discussed below.

Other harms to consider relate to the number of oocytes or human eggs that thus far must be used to achieve one cloning success. These eggs would presumably have to be obtained from women volunteers. Care would have to be taken that these donors are not coerced or simply used as egg providers. So also care would have to be taken, as in other cases, that women into whom the enucleated eggs were placed for gestation would not be harmed or unduly influenced into performing that service.

Some people have objected to human cloning on the grounds of possible harm to society. One argument is the possible threat human cloning might pose to genetic diversity. If the human gene pool were seriously restricted, we would be less able than otherwise to adapt or respond to environmental changes and threats. However, this would be a possible problem only if human cloning were widespread. Since the normal method of reproduction is so much more enjoyable and desired, this would be very unlikely.

## Social Policy

Often, when the issue of human cloning is addressed, there is a confusion about whether what is being asserted is that human cloning is morally right or wrong or whether it ought to be legally permitted or prohibited. These two realms are distinct. In particular, not everything that is morally wrong ought to be legally prohibited. Many examples can be provided, such as spiteful thoughts about others. So also, where a particular case of cloning a human being might be morally objectionable, there may or may not be grounds for it to be legally prohibited. This is partially dependent on the relationship between the realms of morality and the law.

Although not all the views on this relationship can be analyzed here, the most generally accepted view is governed by what has been called the harm principle. This is the view that the law ought to restrict people's liberty only to prevent them from harming others. The purpose of law is not to see that people do the morally right thing or that they do not do what causes harm only to themselves (if they are adults), for example. On the basis of the harm principle, the possible harm done to those cloned would be particularly relevant. This is why the safety aspect of human cloning is particularly important with regard to what the law should do. Both the degree and certainty of the harm would be important. If the risk were high and the harm serious, there would be grounds to restrict the cloning of human beings by law, at least until it were safe.

One could also argue that people can be harmed by having their basic liberties restricted (where they are not harming others) or their privacy invaded. Those arguing for procreative liberties may also use this principle in support of their views. However, there would still remain a provision that their liberty or privacy could be restricted to protect others from being seriously harmed.

Some have argued in favor of allowing human cloning to proceed on grounds that science cannot and should not be legally regulated or restricted. However, this view would surely need to be tempered at least by the harm principle. Many laws and policies do restrict science on this ground, including food and drug safety regulations. Moreover, while technology has many benefits, it can also be misused. Concerns regarding the misuse and dangers of technology have probably given rise to objections to human cloning of the "Frankenstein" type. Some fear that the results of human cloning could not be controlled. Why cloning would be less controllable than other technology is an open question. But some argue that it is better to permit certain practices and technologies to develop and even to fund them with public money because of the increased publicity and monitoring that this provides.

At present there are no U.S. federal laws prohibiting human cloning, though a few states have passed such legislation, among them California, Louisiana, Michigan, and Rhode Island. Internationally a number of countries and international groups have banned the cloning of humans, including Great Britain, the European Union, and the General Assembly of the United Nations. In early 2003, the recommendations of the U.S. National Bioethics Advisory Commission in their 1997 Report are still being considered by the U.S. Congress as it addresses the issue of human cloning, both reproductive and research/therapeutic. A key recommendation of this report was that at present human reproductive cloning ought to be prohibited because of the safety issues. Congress may also consider the July 2002 recommendations of a divided Presidential Council on Bioethics for a four-year moratorium on both therapeutic and reproductive cloning. The Council rejected these terms in its report, opting instead for "cloning-for-biomedical-research" and "cloning-to-produce-children." However, there

are also more general existing laws that could govern human cloning such as those protecting human research subjects, especially non-consenting subjects.

This summary of the issues surrounding human reproductive cloning has considered the nature of human cloning, its present capabilities, and some possible uses for it. It has focused on the ethical objections to cloning, responses to them, and has concluded with some discussion of the relation between ethics and public policy.

BARBARA MACKINNON

SEE ALSO: *Christianity, Bioethics in; Embryo and Fetus; Genetic Engineering, Human; Harm; Human Dignity; Natural Law; Reproductive Technologies; Research Policy; Sikhism, Bioethics in; Technology; Transhumanism and Posthumanism; Utilitarianism and Bioethics;* and other *Cloning* subentries

## BIBLIOGRAPHY

Andrews, Lori. 1999. *The Clone Age: Adventures in the New World of Reproductive Technology.* New York: Henry Holt.

Brannigan, Michael C. 2000. *Ethical Issues in Human Cloning.* New York: Seven Bridges Press.

Committee on Science. 2002. *Scientific and Medical Aspects of Human Reproductive Cloning.* Washington, D.C.: National Academy Press.

Dudley, William. 2001. *The Ethics of Human Cloning.* Farmington Hills, MI: Gale Group.

Feinberg, Joel. 1980. "The Child's Right to an Open Future." In *Whose Child? Children's Rights, Parental Authority, and State Power,* ed. William Aiken and Hugh LaFollette. Totowa, NJ: Rowman and Littlefield.

Foley, Elizabeth Price. 2002. "Human Cloning and the Right to Reproduce." *Albany Law Review* 65(3): 625–649.

Foote, Robert H. 1998. *Artificial Insemination to Cloning: Tracing 50 Years of Research.* Ithaca: New York State College of Agriculture & Life Sciences.

Goodnough, David. 2002. *The Debate over Human Cloning: A Pro/Con Issue.* Berkeley Heights, NJ: Enslow Publishers.

Hall, Stephen S. 2002. "President's Bioethics Council Delivers." *Science* 297(5580): 322–324.

Humber, James M., et al. 1998. *Human Cloning.* Totowa, NJ: Humana Press.

Jonas, Hans. 1974. *Philosophical Essays: From Ancient Creed to Technological Man.* Englewood Cliffs, NJ: Prentice-Hall.

Kass, Leon R. 1998. *Ethics of Human Cloning.* Washington, D.C.: American Enterprise Institute for Public Policy Research.

Klotzko, Arlene Judith. 2001. *The Cloning Sourcebook.* New York: Oxford University Press.

Kolata, Gina. 1998. *The Road to Dolly and the Path Ahead.* New York: William Morrow.

Lauritzen, Paul. 2001. *Cloning and the Future of Human Embryo Research.* New York: Oxford University Press.

MacKinnon, Barbara. 2000. *Human Cloning: Science, Ethics and Public Policy.* Urbana and Chicago: University of Illinois Press.

McGee, Glenn. 1998. *Human Cloning Debate.* Berkeley, CA: Berkeley Hills Books.

National Bioethics Advisory Commission. 1997. *Cloning Human Beings.* Rockville, MD: Gem Publishers.

Nussbaum, Martha C., et al. 1998. *Clones and Clones: Facts and Fantasies about Human Cloning.* New York: W. W. Norton & Company, Inc.

Pence, Gregory E. 1998. *Flesh of My Flesh: The Ethics of Cloning Humans.* Lanham, MD: Rowman & Littlefield Publishers.

Pence, Gregory E. 1998. *Who's Afraid of Human Cloning?* Lanham, MD: Rowman & Littlefield Publishers.

Pistoi, Sergio. 2002. "Father of the Impossible Children." *Scientific American* 286(4): 38–39.

President's Council on Bioethics. 2002. *Human Cloning and Human Dignity: An Ethical Inquiry,* July report. Washington, D.C.: Author.

Silver, Lee M. 1997. *Remaking Eden: Cloning and Beyond in a Brave New World.* New York: Morrow/Avon.

Stix, Gary. 2002. "What Clones? Widespread Scientific Doubts Greet Word of the First Human Embryo Clones." *Scientific American* 286(2): 18–19.

U. S. Congress, House Committee on the Judiciary, Subcommittee on Crime. 2001. *Human Cloning: Hearing Before the Subcommittee on Crime of the Committee on the Judiciary, House of Representatives, One Hundred Seventh Congress, First Session on H.R. 1644 and H.R. 2172, June 7 and June 19, 2001.* Washington, D.C.: United States Government Printing Office.

Wilmut, Ian., et al. 1997. "Viable Offspring Derived from Fetal and Adult Mammalian Cells." *Nature* 385: 810–813.

Wilmut, Ian., et al. 2000. *The Human Cloning Debate.* Berkeley, CA: Berkeley Hills Books.

## III. RELIGIOUS PERSPECTIVES

In its 1997 report on human cloning, the National Bioethics Advisory Commission (NBAC) paid significant attention to the views and concerns of the world's religious communities and their traditions. The NBAC recognized that various religions have supported critical and sustained reflection on issues relevant to assessing human cloning, including the relation of humanity to the natural world, the significance of marriage and procreation in human life, the status of the embryo, and others. For that reason, the NBAC commissioned a report, "Cloning Human Beings: Religious Perspectives on Human Cloning," and took testimony from distinguished scholars of various religious traditions. Drawing on the NBAC report, the testimony given before the commission, and other sources, this entry offers a thumbnail sketch of how four world religions understand the issues raised by reproductive human cloning, for the most part ignoring matters of "therapeutic cloning." Of particular interest are the issues of how cloned children are likely to be valued in contrast to children born of "natural" means; the relevance of parental motives; the possibility of cloning for the purposes of securing biological material for therapeutic use, for example, bone marrow for ill siblings; the issue of destroying embryos; and the notions of "playing God" and "cheating death."

### Judaism

Many of Judaism's basic beliefs about humans and God are rooted in the Genesis account of creation. Jewish scholars generally agree that the Biblical account accommodates two views of creation, namely, creation as a completed act, and creation as a transformative process. These disparate views can dramatically influence the way one understands human cloning and the roles of God, humans, and technology in procreation.

Viewing creation as a completed event has led some Jewish ethicists to argue against human cloning on grounds that it violates the structure of nature and impinges on God's sovereignty. According to this line of thought, given that God created the structure of the world, who are humans to tamper with it? Further, the Genesis description of humans created in the image of God begs the question of how that likeness could be improved. From this perspective, human cloning is wrong in that it attempts to improve upon the divine creation that God has called both "good" and "very good." Further, cloning alters and transgresses God's ordained method of human sexual reproduction.

A related argument is that cloning is worrisome in that it fuels a kind of narcissistic fascination with the idea of escaping or cheating death. As such, cloning holds out the promise of rebirth, a second chance for the self to live a better, fuller life. Yet this promise is illusory, and so the quest to clone is a self-deceptive journey and one that distracts humans from pressing moral commitments here and now—for example, the pursuit of justice in healthcare.

The more generally accepted Jewish view suggests that human beings are partners with God in the ongoing act of creation. As such, humans are commissioned with a divine mandate both to steward and to improve the earth through their own creativity and knowledge. Humans thus become responsible, creative agents, cocreators with God, endowed with God-given duties to promote health and healing. Given that cloning may promote human well-being, it is, provisionally, an acceptable method of stewardship and improvement. In this view, humans do not usurp God's sovereignty in pursuing cloning because, if cloning changes the world for the better, this pursuit exercises their God-given freedom properly. Of course, the assumption that human cloning would actually improve the world is key to this view. Recognizing what a large assumption this is, Jewish scholars who endorse this view of creation also urge caution and recognize that cloning seems to possess inherent dangers for individuals, families, and cultures.

Jewish Biblical commentary traditionally recognizes two values with respect to human beings that are especially helpful in thinking about cloning: uniqueness and equality. Attending to these values may lead to important questions about cloning: Will human clones be more or less valuable than humans conceived through sexual reproduction? Are human clones more likely to be treated as commodities than humans conceived naturally?

Such concerns grow organically out of an understanding that humans are created in the image of God rather than as replications or images of an existing human. It is conceivable that human clones may be regarded as mere objects of production or genetically replaceable resources for our own uses and ends. That clones might be considered "made," may in some way devalue their existence. That clones may be replaceable may undermine their uniqueness. That clones may be used to breed genetic wonders may impinge upon the long-held value of human equality under God. That human cloning could jeopardize all of these values simultaneously and, in so doing, lead to a form of human slavery is a concern not taken lightly by Jewish thinkers.

While these cautions and concerns are taken seriously, Jewish thought also recognizes the transcendent character of the human person. Therefore, humans can never be fully controlled by human technology, will, or intervention. Furthermore, some Jewish scholars have argued that because cloning is a biologically natural process, whereby the clone would be born through a natural process of a human mother, cloning is an acceptable form of reproduction. It also follows that any cloned human being should be treated morally and legally as fully human. Indeed, there is rabbinic consensus that human clones would be fully human and have full moral status.

Finally, Jewish commentators have been concerned about public policy restrictions on cloning. Given the commitment of Jewish tradition to pursue scientific research for the betterment of humanity, many Jewish scholars have cautioned against restricting or prohibiting cloning as a matter of public policy. Also, because Jewish law does not grant full moral status to the embryo, Jewish scholars have not been among those advocating restriction on cloning because it will lead to the destruction of embryos.

## Christianity

As with other religious traditions, Christian responses to cloning have been mixed. As early as the mid-1960s, Christian ethicists split sharply over whether cloning was "playing God." Supporting new biotechnologies, Joseph Fletcher famously claimed: "let's play God" (p. 126). Paul Ramsey's equally famous and oft-quoted response cautioned against advancing reproductive technologies: "Men ought not to play God before they learn to be men, and after they have learned to be men they will not play God" (p. 138). The contrast between such different Christian responses to interventions in reproduction continues into the twenty-first century. Some of the diversity in Christian responses to cloning is noted below.

**PROTESTANTISM.** Protestant Christianity shares a number of Judaism's intellectual and textual traditions. For example, some of the principal elements of the Protestant view of humanity are rooted in the biblical accounts of creation, taking seriously the *imago Dei* theme found in Genesis. Within the Protestant tradition, *imago Dei* is often discussed either in terms of "stewardship" or of "created cocreatorship," but unlike the Jewish thinking, the stewardship model understands creation as a completed process in which humans serve as God's appointed stewards overseeing a finished work, while the cocreatorship model sees creation itself as incomplete *creation continua,* a process in which humans are responsible to participate and improve. These two perspectives relate to human cloning when one asks whether cloning exceeds the limits of human createdness, and whether humans attempt to play God through the genetic manipulation of another human. Understood as stewards, humanity is restricted to conserving the created order. In this view, human cloning is problematic because it usurps God's role as creator; humans are not called to be creators but rather stewards of creation. By contrast, emphasizing the theme that humans are created cocreators tends to support the permissibility of cloning by highlighting the idea of creative freedom implied by this view of *imago Dei.*

In their analysis of human reproductive cloning, Protestant scholars also seriously consider the impact that asexual reproduction may have on the societal norms of marriage, childbearing, and how humans are likely to view and value human clones. Protestants often maintain a normative Biblical view of the child as a being conceived within marriage, a gift from God, and the result of a loving relationship between a man and a woman. Human cloning raises Protestant concerns regarding the disjunction of marriage and childbearing, and the fear that such a separation will have a lasting and adverse affect on children and society. As representatives in some Protestant denominations have argued, human cloning allows humans to sever the connection between human reproduction and the marital relationship, a separation considered harmful both to child and culture.

Protestants also fear cloning's potential to change how humans view children, namely from a "gift from God" to a "project." Some scholars distinguish between what is "begotten" and what is "made," arguing that begetting is consistent with human dignity in a way that manufacturing is not. Similarly, some Protestant traditions caution against cloning on grounds that it reduces humanity to raw material to be fashioned in human image rather than the image of God.

It is in this light that some Protestants consider both the parental motives for cloning and some of the possible benefits of reproductive cloning. Sympathetic to suffering and the human condition in a fallen world, Protestants remain skeptical of cloning humans for utilitarian purposes such as cloning to replace a young child killed in an accident or cloning to gain access to biological material. Each of these instances of cloning may violate Protestantism's commitment to the inherent and non-instrumental value of human beings.

Indeed, all of these themes are nicely illustrated in a resolution condemning cloning passed by the Southern Baptist Convention in June 2001. According to the resolution, because cloning involves the "wanton destruction" of human embryos; because it is contrary to the "biblical witness" that children are a gift from God and "not the result of asexual replication"; because cloning "does not meet the biblical standards for procreation in which children are begotten, not made"; and because cloning represents "a decisive step toward substituting human procreation with biological manufacturing of humans," cloning is morally abhorrent.

**CATHOLICISM.** Perhaps the most consistent and vocal opposition to human cloning has come from the Catholic Church. Magisterial (authoritative teaching) documents of the church have regularly and vigorously rejected cloning. For example, in *Donum Vitae,* an "Instruction" issued in 1987, the Vatican examined cloning in the context of other reproductive interventions made possible by the advent of *in vitro* fertilization and concluded that cloning was categorically wrong. *Donum Vitae* is typical of Catholic teaching on topics of bioethics in that it appeals both to beliefs that are shared primarily by the community of the faithful and also

to basic human values and experiences that it takes to be common to all humanity. Thus, according to Catholic tradition, it makes sense to note reasons why cloning is morally wrong both in explicitly religious terms and in more secular terms.

An example of the former is Catholic teaching that life is a gift from God and that humans therefore have a responsibility to appreciate and safeguard the inestimable value of human life. According to the Catholic Church, the embryo should be treated as a person from the moment of conception. It follows that cloning is deeply troubling, for embryos will inevitably be destroyed when human beings are cloned. Cloning thus fails to respect the fact that life is a gift from God that should be treasured. Moreover, Catholic tradition emphasizes the fact that humans are created by God as a union of body and soul, and, for that reason, the human person cannot be treated merely as a complex biological system. Thus, to the degree that cloning defines the human person genetically (that is, largely in bodily terms), it is not consistent with a Catholic vision of the spiritual and bodily union of the person and is problematic. Indeed, according to the Vatican, cloning fails to respect the fact that there are limits on human dominance over nature. According to Catholic teaching, it is one thing for reproductive medicine to study human reproduction to assist society in the good that is procreation, it is another thing to dominate the process of procreation. Cloning crosses that line.

In addition to this religiously-grounded argument, Catholic teaching also appeals to the notion of common human experiences. Thus, for example, in her testimony before the NBAC, Lisa Sowle Cahill noted that although autonomy has become a, if not the, central value in contemporary debates in bioethics, Catholic teaching has always emphasized the importance of the common good in addition to individual liberty. With regard to cloning, therefore, Catholic tradition asks not merely whether this technology might benefit individuals, but whether it will benefit society in the long run. In answering this question, Catholic tradition focuses on the importance of family to social good. According to Catholic teaching, the biological connection between parents and children is a manifestation of the natural connection between sex, marriage, and procreation. In traditional language, natural law requires that sex and procreation go together. Thus cloning is wrong in that it violates natural law by separating sex and procreation. This conclusion, says the Church, should be clear even to those who do not share a commitment to natural law. Careful reflection on the importance of families, historically and cross-culturally, along with an examination of how cloning might fundamentally change the notion of family is enough to show that cloning is deeply worrisome.

## Islam

Just as Jewish and Christian scholars have drawn on accounts of creation in thinking about cloning, so, too, have Muslim scholars. For example, Chapter 23, verses 12–14 in the Qur'an, the Muslim scripture, are frequently cited as relevant to a discussion of cloning. The passage reads: "We created man of an extraction of clay, then We set him, a drop in a safe lodging, then We created of the drop a clot, then We created of the clot a tissue, then We created of the tissue bones, then We covered the bones in flesh; thereafter We produced it as another creature. So blessed be God, the Best of creators!" Supporters of cloning have understood this passage to mean that because humans participate in the act of creation with God, humans may intervene creatively in nature to promote human welfare. Thus, to undertake cloning in an effort to promote human flourishing may be acceptable.

In summarizing the response of Islam to reproductive cloning, it is also important to stress three themes from the *Shari'a* (Islamic law) that regulate individual and social morality for Muslims. First, Islamic law places a high value on the importance of scientific knowledge. Scientific research reveals the complexity of God's creation and for that reason can be understood as a kind of worship of God. Second, Islamic tradition has emphasized the importance of heterosexual marriage and the family to social and communal good. Third, although the tradition has no definitive position on the moral status of the early embryo, there is a well-known hadith (saying of the Prophet) that an angel comes to breathe spirit into a fetus at six weeks.

With these fundamental commitments supporting Islamic reflections on cloning, a number of positions can and have been developed. Consistent with the Qur'anic emphasis on the pursuit of knowledge, scientific research into reproduction that has led to the possibility of cloning is entirely legitimate. Indeed, some verses of the Qur'an have been interpreted to support the claim that God's will is manifest in so-called artificial reproduction because unless God wills the creation of life, there would be no life. Thus, assuming that the knowledge gained by pursuing cloning would be used to benefit humanity and not instead misused, cloning may be supported.

Nevertheless, there are aspects of cloning that give scholars of Islam pause. For example, the fact that cloning allows for reproduction without heterosexual pairing is problematic, for the Qu'ran is understood to be quite explicit about this: "And of everything We have created pairs that you may be mindful" (51:49). Thus, just as Catholicism is concerned about the threat cloning may pose to the traditional family, so, too, is Islam. Given the importance Islam places on the notion of a family that is founded upon heterosexual union, cloning has seemed very problematic to some Muslim jurists.

Finally, Islam also shares the concern raised by other religious traditions that cloning will lead to the reduction of children to commodities. Given the emphasis in Islam on the notion of spiritual equality, cloning may be problematic if it leads us to value some humans more highly than others because they have, or are free of, certain genetic traits. If cloning will lead us to place a market value on human beings, it will be opposed by Islam. Moreover, given the tradition that the moral status of the fetus changes approximately six weeks after conception, cloning will be problematic to the degree that it results in a substantial loss of fetal life after this point in gestation.

## Buddhism

In order to understand Buddhist responses to cloning, it is important to note that Buddhist teaching generally emphasizes the centrality of individual judgment and discretion informed by reflection on Buddhist texts and the opinion of respected teachers. Thus, on cloning as on other issues, it is difficult to speak of a Buddhist position.

Nevertheless, the tradition clearly emphasizes a number of values that are helpful in framing a Buddhist response to cloning. First, in Buddhism, human existence is particularly valuable because only human beings can achieve enlightenment and thereby escape perpetual rebirth. The birth of a human being is therefore important because it affords a sentient being the possibility of release from suffering. Reproductive cloning may be viewed positively from a Buddhist perspective because it appears to facilitate the process of rebirth and liberation. The fact that such cloning would involve asexual reproduction does not appear to be significant in Buddhist tradition, which clearly contains stories of other kinds of asexual generation.

In contrast to several Protestant, Catholic, and Islamic objections to human cloning, Buddhists do not argue that asexual reproduction and cloning are human attempts to play God, or that they in any way infringe upon God's sovereignty as creator. Nor do Buddhists fear that human cloning, through genetic manipulation, might deprive cloned individuals of their right to an open future. Buddhism rejects the kind of physical reductionism that such genetic determinism implies, and scholars have been careful to note that human cloning does not determine or control the life of another being. The Buddhist conception of human life maintains that while cloning does determine the genotype of an individual, one's genetic construction does not and cannot determine the complete life of the human being, usually thought to comprise the body, sensation, thought, dispositions, and consciousness.

Buddhism does look upon cloning with skepticism and caution for other reasons. The universal value shared by all Buddhist traditions remains ego-transcending thought and behavior. Egocentric conduct and its motives are considered great moral wrongs. Buddhism is likely to analyze the morality of human cloning in terms of the motives, intentions, and desires of those engaged in genetic engineering and cloning. Should the motives behind cloning in general, or cloning in a specific instance, be found to be purely self-centered or self-gratifying, then the practice would be immoral and contrary to Buddhist values. This point is nicely illustrated by the classic Buddhist narrative, the "Parable of the Mustard Seed." According to the parable, a mother who is grieving over the death of her child approaches the Buddha to ask that he bring her dead child back to life. The Buddha instructs the woman that she will be able to accomplish her goal if she prepares tea from mustard seeds that have come from a house not touched by death. Of course, the woman is unable to find such seeds, and that is indeed the point; all life is impermanent. In the face of this fact, the woman needs to reflect on her desires and attachments to things that are necessarily impermanent.

Given this parable, Buddhist tradition raises serious questions about the wisdom of one form of reproductive cloning, namely, cloning to replace a lost loved one. Such cloning might be acceptable if one can find a physician whose family has not been touched by death, but seeking to replace a loved one appears to interfere with a Buddhist commitment to seek enlightenment through freedom from bondage to the self and its attachments. The parable thus points to the significance of attending to the motives or desires for cloning in rendering a Buddhist assessment of the practice. Many of the reasons that have been advanced for reproductive cloning, for example, to resolve infertility, to replace a lost child, to replicate oneself, appear to be profoundly egocentric. As such, they would be morally problematic according to Buddhist teaching.

Nevertheless, scholars remain divided on this line of thinking. Some have argued that should cloning benefit the couple wishing for a child, and provided it does not cause pain or suffering, then such cloning should be supported. Others have noted, however, that even the least objectionable motivations for cloning, such as the desire to avoid passing down hereditary disease, remain egocentric and self-serving. In this view, the decision to clone instead of using donor cells or adopting a child in need of a family, for example, seems rooted in a desire to have a genetically related child and does not truly look to ease the suffering of another, but has a self-gratifying aim. Accordingly, the argument goes, virtually all rationales for reproductive cloning stem from this desire.

While the motivation behind cloning is of primary significance in assessing its moral value, there is some concern among Buddhists that the inevitable destruction of early human embryos in cloning's experimental phases and in the successful process itself runs contrary to Buddhism's objection to the taking of human life. Although as a non-sentient being the early embryo would not suffer, Buddhism does view the early embryo as a human being and, as previously noted, the human is highly valued for its role in one's attainment of nirvana and the release from suffering. Thus, destroying human life, however early or insentient, may violate one of Buddhism's highest values.

## Conclusion

This survey of religious responses to cloning suggests that there is significant misunderstanding of how major religious traditions have reacted to the possibility of reproductive cloning, at least in the popular media. For example, when the story broke that the British House of Lords had legalized therapeutic cloning for the purpose of deriving stem cells in 2001, the Reuters news service described Parliament as "turning a deaf ear to religious leaders from across the spectrum who had urged them to oppose the measures." Reuters's characterization of religious leaders as uniformly opposed to cloning is fairly typical. The reality is quite different. As this survey attests, Judaism, Christianity, Islam, and Buddhism take subtly different positions on the status of the embryo, on the appropriate motives for even considering cloning, on the notion of "playing God" and manipulating nature, and other matters.

Add to this the fact that, within each tradition, there are disagreements about these matters and the picture becomes very complex. What can safely be said is that none of these traditions appears to embrace cloning as an unqualified good, and, with the exception of official Catholic teaching and that of some evangelical Protestant groups, none appears to condemn cloning as intrinsically and unqualifiedly wrong.

PAUL LAURITZEN
NATHANIEL STEWART

SEE ALSO: *African Religions; Buddhism, Bioethics in; Christianity, Bioethics in; Daoism, Bioethics in; Islam, Bioethics in; Jainism, Bioethics in; Judaism, Bioethics in; Mormonism, Bioethics in; Native American Religions, Bioethics in; Reproductive Technologies; Transhumanism and Posthumanism;* and other *Cloning* subentries

## BIBLIOGRAPHY

Barnhart, Michael. 2000. "Nature, Nurture, and No-Self: Bioengineering and Buddhist Values." *Journal of Buddhist Ethics* 7: 126–144.

Cohen, Jonathan. 1999. "In God's Garden: Creation and Cloning in Jewish Thought." *Hastings Center Report* 29(4): 7–13.

Cole-Turner, Ronald, ed. 1997. *Human Cloning: Religious Responses.* Louisville, KY: Westminster John Knox Press.

Cole-Turner, Ronald, ed. 2001. *Beyond Cloning: Religion and the Remaking of Humanity.* Harrisburg, PA: Trinity Press International.

Fletcher, Joseph F. 1974. *The Ethics of Genetic Control: Ending Reproductive Roulette.* Garden City, NY: Anchor Press.

Hughes, James, and Keown, Damien. 1995. "Buddhism and Medical Ethics: A Bibliographic Introduction." *Journal of Buddhist Ethics* 2: 107–124.

Lauritzen, Paul, ed. 2001. *Cloning and the Future of Human Embryo Research.* New York: Oxford University Press.

Lipschutz, Joshua. 1999. "To Clone or Not to Clone—a Jewish Perspective." *Journal of Medical Ethics* 25(2): 105–108.

Meilaender, Gilbert. 1997. "Begetting and Cloning." *First Things* 74: 41–43.

Post, Stephen. 1997. "The Judeo-Christian Case against Human Cloning." *America* 176(21): 19–22.

Ramsey, Paul. 1970. *Fabricated Man: The Ethics of Genetic Control.* New Haven, CT: Yale University Press.

Walter, James. 1999. "Theological Issues in Genetics." *Theological Studies* 60(1): 124–135.

## INTERNET RESOURCES

Cahill, Lisa. 1997. "Testimony before the National Bioethics Advisory Commission." Available from <www.georgetown.edu/research/nrcbl/nbac/>.

Campbell, Courtney. "Cloning Human Beings: Religious Perspectives on Human Cloning." Available from <www.georgetown.edu/research/nrcbl/nbac/>.

Dorff, Rabbi Elliot. 1997. "Testimony before the National Bioethics Advisory Commission." Available from <www.georgetown.edu/research/nrcbl/nbac/>.

Meilaender, Jr., Gilbert. 1997. "Testimony before the National Bioethics Advisory Commission." Available from <www.georgetown.edu/research/nrcbl/nbac/>.

"National Bioethics Advisory Commission: The Charter of the National Bioethics Advisory Commission expired on October 3, 2001." Available from <www.georgetown.edu/research/nrcbl/nbac/>.

Reuters. 2001. "Green Light for Embryo Cloning." Available from <www.cnn.com/2001/world/europe/uk/01/22/cloning.reut/>.

Sachedina, Abdulaziz. "Islamic Perspectives on Cloning." Available from <www.people.virginia.edu/~aas/issues/cloning.htm>.

Sachedina, Abdulaziz. "Islamic View on Cloning: Recommendations of the 9th Fiqh-Medical Seminar." Available from <www.islamset.com/healnews/cloning/view.html>.

Sachedina, Abdulaziz. 1997. "Testimony before the National Bioethics Advisory Commission." Available from <www.georgetown.edu/research/nrcbl/nbac/>.

Southern Baptist Convention. "Resolution on Human Cloning." Available from <www.sbc.net/resolutions/amResolution.asp?ID=572>.

Tendler, Rabbi Moshe. 1997. "Testimony before the National Bioethics Advisory Commission." Available from <www.georgetown.edu/research/nrcbl/nbac/>.

# COERCION

• • •

Is it ever acceptable for the government to coerce someone into receiving healthcare? Is it acceptable for healthcare professionals to do so? Equally important, if an individual is coerced to do something including, for example, consenting to treatment, does the coercion invalidate responsibility for the act? Are prisoners and other institutionalized persons able to freely decide whether to enroll as subjects in experiments, or should they be seen as coerced, and, if so, does that invalidate their consent? Is paying research subjects to participate in research acceptable, or is that practice coercive?

These questions are basic to many of the ethical dilemmas faced in healthcare and healthcare research. To answer them, it is necessary to answer a number of more general questions. What is coercion? Are coercive acts ever morally legitimate? If so, how can they be distinguished from illegitimate coercion? Are there types of coercive acts that are always illegitimate, or do their moral natures vary with the context in which they occur? This entry aims to answer these and other related questions. A clear definition of coercion is a mandatory first step.

## What Is Coercion?

In their 4th edition of *Principles of Biomedical Ethics,* published in 1994, Tom L. Beauchamp and James F. Childress provided a definition of coercion that is consistent with common usage: "Coercion … occurs if and only if one person intentionally uses a credible and severe threat of harm or force to control another" (Beauchamp and Childress, p. 164). This definition has three critical elements: a person acting intentionally, a threat of harm, and an effort to control another. Perhaps the prototype of this image of coercion is the robber who approaches a victim and says, "Your money or your life." Note that the robber is not forcing the victim to hand over the money. The victim still has options, but the robber has manipulated the options in such a manner that most people would agree to hand over the money.

If Beauchamp and Childress's definition is correct, most constraints on freedom should not be thought of as coercion. In their definition only other people can coerce. Someone who lacks resources should not be thought of as being coerced by the lack of resources. The poor are not coerced into homelessness no matter how much their situation may be out of their control. A nation that lacks oil is not coerced into trading with a country that has oil simply because of its need. Similarly, an environment, such as a prison, cannot be thought to be coercive. Thus the regulatory restrictions on research with prisoners cannot be justified by limitations on coercion.

Similarly, threats are a fundamental feature of this definition; other pressures do not produce coercion. This position is controversial. In his 1986 volume, *Harm to Self,* Joel Feinberg, like Beauchamp and Childress, used the term *compulsion* rather than *coercion* to refer to the actual use of force, because compulsion reduces options and coercion only changes the attractiveness of the options. Michael D. Bayles, like others, however, did not consider this distinction important (Bayles).

Force is not the only type of pressure that is sometimes included in coercion. Positive pressures such as inducements and persuasion may be seen as "excessive." Many commentators on research ethics have suggested that excessive inducements may well constitute a form of coercion (Macklin; Levine; Ackerman; Dickert and Grady). For example, in his 1986 book, *Ethics and the Regulation of Clinical Research,* Robert J. Levine suggested that almost all bioethics support this view. The U.S. Food and Drug Administration's (FDA) information sheets require institutional review boards to ensure that payments not be "unduly influential" (FDA). Indeed, Neal Dickert and Christine Grady suggested in a 1999 article that whether or not a payment is unduly influential is largely determined by the strategy used to establish the amounts to be paid. Several others, including Beauchamp and Childress and Robert Nozick (1969), exclude positive incentives from the concept of coercion.

It should also follow from Beauchamp and Childress's definition that if the threatener has no intention of controlling the behavior of the other party, there is no coercion.

Thus a physician who tells an individual seeking help for what might be a gunshot wound that he must report any gunshot wounds to the authorities is not coercing the potential patient, because there is no attempt to alter that person's behavior.

The question of coercion can be stated as follows: If *A* proposes to do something to *B*, what are the conditions that make the act coercive or not? Several commentators have suggested that the relevant question is whether the proposed act leaves *B* better off or worse off. If better off, it is a legitimate offer; if worse off, it is coercive (Zimmerman). Nevertheless, this does not entirely solve the problem. Consider a physician who tells a sick patient that she will provide treatment but only with the payment of $100 (or some other reasonable fee). This is an entirely reasonable offer and not coercive at all. If, however, the patient belongs to an HMO to which the physician belongs and which forbids this sort of co-pay, this "offer" might be coercive. Put more generally, whether an act is a legitimate offer or coercion depends on the right of the offerer to make the offer.

Such problems can be handled better by what Alan Wertheimer, in his 1987 book, *Coercion* called a "moralized theory" of coercion. Wertheimer objected to views suggesting that what is coercive can be determined simply by looking at the pressure applied to the individual. In his view, coercion is an inherently moralized judgment. One cannot determine whether or not an act is coercive except on the basis of understanding the normative context of the actions. Wertheimer argued that coercion judgments come down to whether the possible coercer has the right to make the proposal and whether the possible coercee has the obligation to resist it.

## Coercion and Autonomy

The view in Western culture that coercion is a bad thing reflects a deep commitment to the principle of autonomy. Starting with the German philosopher Immanuel Kant (1724–1804) and his 1785 work, *Groundwork of the Metaphysics of Morals,* secular ethics has taken the respect for the autonomous actions of others as a primary point of orientation. In this context, coercion is wrong because it interferes with autonomy. Thus the nineteenth-century English philosopher and economist John Stuart Mill argued in *On Liberty* (1859) that there were inherent limitations on the power that the state or other authorities should exercise over individuals:

[T]he sole end for which mankind are warranted, individually or collectively, in interfering with the liberty of action of any of their number, is self-protection.... the only purpose for which power can be rightfully exercised over any member of a civilized community, against his will, is to prevent harm to others. His own good, either physical or moral, is not a sufficient warrant. (Mill, p. 494)

Although this often quoted passage seems to prohibit many coercive actions that Western society accepts routinely today, it is worth noting that Mill made exceptions for children and for adults not of sound mind. His vision of autonomy is so rationalistic that there appears to be no basis for respecting the autonomy of those who are lacking in reasoning ability.

## Is Coercion Always Wrong?

At least in the context of Western values, it is hard to defend coercive behaviors per se. Nonetheless, there are many examples of coercive behaviors that are generally accepted. Indeed, political scientists general acknowledge that the governmental monopoly on the use of force is a fundamental feature of civil order. The ability of the authorities to threaten the use of force seems essential. There are innumerable examples, both in and out of medicine, in which coercion is accepted. The courts routinely tell people who are thought to have a mental illness that they can either take their prescribed medicine or be involuntarily committed to a hospital. In this case, the courts are still consistent with Mill's viewpoint. But when parents are told that if they want their children to attend public schools, the children must have certain vaccinations, this appears to go beyond Mill's limits on coercion.

The viewpoint that coercion is sometimes justified is referred to as *paternalism*. Here the authority, be it the state or the medical professional, justifies the use of threats and force based on the best interests of the individual. Although few ethicists have expressly focused on justifying paternalism per se, there has been considerable discussion of the circumstances under which paternalism might be acceptable.

Feinberg (1971) distinguished between weak paternalism and strong paternalism. The former depends for its legitimacy on an individual's compromised ability to decide, based on, for example, the influence of psychotropic drugs, some forms of mental illness, severe acute pain, or acute neurological injuries. Strong paternalism, by contrast, justifies actions that are simply intended to benefit a competent rational individual who is, in the view of the paternalist, making the wrong decision. Strong paternalism may take the form of either restricting what is disclosed to an individual or simply overriding the person's autonomous choices.

## Empirical Findings: The Example of Psychiatric Admission

Empirical data cannot resolve ethical issues, but experience in bioethics has shown that ethical issues often look quite different when they are embedded in complex situations. Likewise, empirical data can render problematic assumptions about the nature of the ethical decisions that occur in healthcare contexts.

There have not been very many efforts to study coercion in healthcare. The exception is psychiatric care. There has been considerable research into coercion in psychiatric admissions and in other aspects of psychiatric care that are mandated by courts or other legally constituted authorities. Precisely because such situations use the coercive power of the state and yet occur within the context of medical care, they have been of special interest to ethicists and policymakers. For this reason, research on coercion in psychiatry can also be helpful in understanding some of the general issues concerning coercion in healthcare.

Research on coercion in psychiatry was relatively unorganized until the MacArthur Foundation funded a series of studies in the 1990s. These studies contributed a number of important empirical findings, but their most important contribution was to create a measure of perceived coercion that has been widely adopted and that has allowed comparisons across international boundaries and among different types of psychiatric care. It is important to recognize, however, that this scale measures *perceived* coercion and that it is based on an understanding of coercion as a restriction on the ability to make decisions for oneself (Gardner et al., 1993).

Among its findings, the MacArthur group reported several that have important implications for understanding coercion in healthcare. First, there is surprising agreement among the participants in hospitalization decisions (patients, family, and clinicians) about what happened (Hoge et al., 1998; Lidz et al., 1998). The differences are in how the events are evaluated. Thus the different participants often disagreed about the level of coercion even when they agreed about the acts involved.

Perhaps the most surprising MacArthur finding was that being legally involuntarily committed is not necessarily perceived by patients as coercive. Indeed, almost a third of the people who were legally committed reported that they did not feel coerced. Conversely, more than 10 percent of those who were admitted "voluntarily" felt coerced (Hoge et al., 1997). These finding have been confirmed by other investigators (Nicholson, Ekenstam, and Norwood; Hiday et al.). Similar findings have been found in different countries (McKenna, Simpson, and Laidlaw), in involuntary outpatient treatment (Swartz et al.), and in drug treatment (Wild, Newton-Taylor, and Alletto).

Perhaps the most interesting of the MacArthur group's findings involved the issue of moralized versus nonmoralized concepts of coercion. In a 1993 study, Nancy S. Bennett and her colleagues examined the transcripts of interviews with admitted patients and noted that the patients' descriptions of their experiences with admission and their perceptions of coercion appeared to be substantially related to their perception of what came to be called procedural justice. This concept included the sense that patients had a chance to express their own thoughts on the hospitalization, that they were listened to, and that the motives of others involved in the hospitalization decision were benign (Bennett et al.). Subsequent follow-up studies, both from the MacArthur group (Lidz et al., 1995) and others (Hiday et al.), showed that both procedural justice and what the researchers called negative pressures (force and threats) were strongly related to perceived coercion but that "positive pressures" such as inducements were not.

## Conclusion

Coercion may be defined in a purely behavioral manner as the use of a threat to control the behavior of another. Other thinkers have argued that coercion is inherently a moralized judgment that can be understood only in the normative context in which it is made. From this perspective, there can be no such thing as approved coercion. Indeed, coercion is almost universally condemned in the abstract, but there are many instances in which actions that fit behavioral definitions of coercion are approved. The empirical studies of coercion appear to support a view of coercion that involves both behavioral and moral components. There appears to be little empirical support, however, for the idea that offers or other inducements are experienced as coercive.

CHARLES W. LIDZ

SEE ALSO: *Authority in Religious Traditions; Autonomy; Behaviorism; Behavior Modification Therapies; Conscience; Conscience, Rights of; Ethics; Informed Consent; Paternalism; Psychosurgery, Medical and Historical Aspects of; Public Health*

### BIBLIOGRAPHY

Ackerman, Terrance F. 1989. "An Ethical Framework for the Practice of Paying Subjects." *IRB: A Review of Human Subjects Research* 11(4): 1–4.

Bayles, Michael D. 1972. In *Coercion,* ed. J. Roland Pennock and John W. Chapman. Chicago: Aldine Atherton.

Beauchamp, Tom L., and Childress, James F. 1994. *Principles of Biomedical Ethics,* 4th edition. New York: Oxford University Press.

Bennett, Nancy S.; Lidz, Charles W.; Monahan, John; et al. 1993. "Inclusion, Motivation, and Good Faith: The Morality of Coercion in Mental Hospital Admission." *Behavioral Sciences and the Law* 11(3): 295–306.

Dickert, Neal, and Grady, Christine. 1999. "What's the Price of a Research Subject? Approaches to Payment for Research Participation." *New England Journal of Medicine* 341(3): 198–203.

Feinberg, Joel. 1971. "Legal Paternalism." *Canadian Journal of Philosophy* 1: 105–124.

Feinberg, Joel. 1986. *The Moral Limits of the Criminal Law,* vol. 3: *Harm to Self.* New York: Oxford University Press.

Gardner, William; Hoge, Steven K.; Bennett, Nancy S.; et al. 1993. "Two Scales for Measuring Patients' Perceptions of Coercion during Hospital Admission." *Behavioral Sciences and the Law* 11(3): 307–322.

Hiday, Virginia Aldigé; Swartz, Marvin S.; Swanson, Jeffrey; and Wagner, H. Ryan. 1997. "Patient Perceptions of Coercion in Mental Hospital Admission." *International Journal of Law and Psychiatry* 20(2): 227–241.

Hoge, Steven K.; Lidz, Charles W.; Eisenberg, Marlene; et al. 1997. "Perceptions of Coercion in the Admission of Voluntary and Involuntary Psychiatric Patients." *International Journal of Law and Psychiatry* 20(2): 167–182.

Hoge, Steven K.; Lidz, Charles W.; Eisenberg, Marlene; et al. 1998. "Family, Clinician, and Patient Perceptions of Coercion in the Mental Hospital Admission: A Comparative Study." *International Journal of Law and Psychiatry* 21(2): 131–146.

Kant, Immanuel. 1956. *Groundwork of the Metaphysics of Morals,* tr. H. J. Paton. New York: Harper and Row.

Levine, Robert J. 1986. *Ethics and the Regulation of Clinical Research.* New Haven, CT: Yale University Press.

Lidz, Charles W.; Hoge, Steven K.; Gardner, William; et al. 1995. "Perceived Coercion in Mental Hospital Admission: Pressures and Process." *Archives of General Psychiatry* 52(12): 1034–1039.

Lidz, Charles W.; Mulvey, Edward P.; Hoge, Steven K.; et al. 1998. "Factual Sources of Psychiatric Patients' Perceptions of Coercion in the Hospital Admission Process." *American Journal of Psychiatry* 155(9): 1254–1260.

Macklin, Ruth. 1981. "'Due' and 'Undue' Inducements: On Paying Money to Research Subjects." *IRB: A Review of Human Subjects Research* 3(1): 1–6.

McKenna, B. G.; Simpson, A. I. F.; and Laidlaw, T. M. 1999. "Patient Perception of Coercion on Admission to Acute Psychiatric Services: The New Zealand Experience." *International Journal of Law and Psychiatry* 22(2): 143–153.

Mill, John Stuart. 1961 (1859). "On Liberty." In *The Utilitarians.* Garden City, NY: Dolphin Books.

Nicholson, R. A.; Ekenstam, C.; and Norwood, S. 1996. "Coercion and the Outcome of Psychiatric Hospitalization." *International Journal of Law and Psychiatry* 19(2): 201–217.

Nozick, Robert. 1969. "Coercion." In *Philosophy, Science, and Method: Essays in Honor of Ernest Nagel,* ed. Sidney Morgenbesser, Patrick Suppes, and Morton White. New York: St. Martin's Press.

Swartz, Marvin S.; Wagner, H. Ryan; Hiday, Virginia Aldigé; et al. 2002. "The Perceived Coerciveness of Involuntary Outpatient Commitment: Findings from an Experimental Study." *Journal of the American Academy of Psychiatry and the Law* 30(2): 207–217.

U.S. Food and Drug Administration (FDA). 1998. *Information Sheets: Guidelines for Institutional Review Boards and Clinical Investigators.* Rockville, MD: Author.

Wertheimer, Alan. 1987. *Coercion.* Princeton, NJ: Princeton University Press.

Wild, T. Cameron; Newton-Taylor, Brenda; and Alletto, Rosalia. 1998. "Perceived Coercion among Clients Entering Substance Abuse Treatment: Structural and Psychological Determinants." *Addictive Behaviors* 23(1): 81–95.

Zimmerman, David. 1981. "Coercive Wage Offers." *Philosophy and Public Affairs* 10(2): 121–145.

# COMMERCIALISM IN SCIENTIFIC RESEARCH

• • •

Scientific research has never been entirely insulated from the incentives provided by the profit motive and the need to secure financial support. Scientists have always required funding, whether it be from personal funds, patrons, universities, or industry. Similarly, opportunities for scientific entrepreneurship have always existed. Since the early 1800s, however, scientific research has both required increasing amounts of capital investment and promised progressively greater financial returns. Consequently, scientists have been forced to rely on a broader range of funding sources and have become more willing to involve themselves in the financial implications of their work. This incremental "commercialization" of science has increased markedly since the early 1980s and poses challenges for both society and the research community.

Well into the early nineteenth century most scientists were indifferent to the commercial potential of their work and typically did not pursue large-scale or external financial support. Research then did not require huge expenditures, and many researchers believed that scientific research was the work of disinterested amateurs devoted to the pursuit of truth. In the mid- to late nineteenth century the development of the large-scale laboratory in Europe and ultimately in the United States increased the costs of research and foreshadowed the decline of the solitary, amateur researcher. At the same time, a variety of connections between industry and science developed. Many businesses employed their own scientists, but an increasing number established relationships with universities and employed academic scientists as consultants and researchers. While this trend continued in the early twentieth century, industry-sponsored research typically focused on applied-science projects. Basic research areas had yet to be viewed as fruitful areas of investment (Etzkowitz).

In the last half of the twentieth century, several developments enhanced the commercial aspects of science. The cost of basic science research continued to soar, requiring sophisticated equipment and resources, larger laboratories, and more staff. Basic research therefore has become increasingly dependent on financial support from either the government or the private sector. Scientific research, especially in the biomedical fields, promises to generate tremendous profits for those who control new discoveries. Moreover, the gap between basic and applied science has narrowed, so that discoveries can be translated into usable and profitable products with less energy and over a shorter span of time (Etzkowitz).

## Commercialization, the Ideals of Science, and the Public Good

Despite the need for broad-based and generous funding and the right of scientists to reap rewards for their efforts and ingenuity, financial incentives may create conflicts of interest that can undermine and corrupt the ideal of disinterested scientific inquiry. A conflict of interest exists when any professional judgment or activity relating to a primary interest (e.g., intellectual honesty, validity, openness, or objectivity), equivalent to the scientific norms articulated by Robert K. Merton and others, may be influenced by secondary interests (e.g., financial gain, profit, position, or fame). The mere existence of a conflict of interest does not mean that unethical behavior has occurred; the scientist may honor the primary interests and refuse to be influenced by the secondary interests. Conflicts of interest instead signal cases in which the danger of unethical behavior is increased. In some cases the conflicts can be managed by restricting the secondary interests; in more extreme cases ethical outcomes can be assured only if the secondary interests are entirely removed (Thompson; Merton; Cournand).

Conflict of interest may exist at an individual or at an institutional level. For example, one primary interest of a university is to serve the public good. Financial incentives may induce researchers and institutions to behave in ways detrimental to society (Angell). For example, a scientist may forgo research on an important project in favor of another that is more profitable. Comprehensive ethical policies would ideally address both possible levels of conflict, though they require different forms of remedies.

## Industry Investment in Academic Research

Private investment in university research may take a number of forms. Companies may offer universities large grants in exchange for patent rights to anticipated discoveries or establish lucrative consulting arrangements with faculty members who provide sponsoring corporations with priority access to valuable research. Faculty members sometimes own equity interests in biotechnology firms related to their work, or they may found their own corporations. And in what is so far a rare agreement, a corporation may provide an academic research institute generous payments in exchange for the right to market all the institution's discoveries. These secondary—financial—interests threaten to undermine the university's primary interests of advancing basic knowledge, promoting the open exchange of ideas, providing a source of expertise for society, and training future scientists (Etzkowitz; Ashford).

In 2003 Justin E. Bekelman, Yan Li, and Cary P. Gross provided a systematic review of the extent and nature of commercial influence on biomedical research. The researchers found that about one-fourth of biomedical scientists at academic institutions receive research funding from industry, while two-thirds of academic institutions hold equity interests in biotechnology firms. According to the survey findings, it is likely that such relationships bias scientific outcomes because published studies sponsored by industry are substantially more likely than nonindustry studies to reach conclusions favorable to the sale of the sponsors' products. Faculty sponsored by industry are more likely than other faculty to report that publication of their research results was delayed, and more than half of the firms surveyed reported that their contracts typically demand delays in publication of more than six months. Between 12 percent and 34 percent of investigators reported that they had tried to obtain and had been denied access to research results by industry sponsors.

If free exchange through traditional scholarly mediums of conferences and publications is blunted, scientists will be unable to examine and replicate experiments, and scientific progress may be endangered. Some contractual agreements with industries specifically require scientists to withhold submission of their findings to professional journals until the corporation has determined if the information warrants patent protection. After patent protection is secured, the findings can be released to the general scientific community. The propriety of these arrangements depends in part on the length and impact of the delay of release of scientifically important information and varies from contract to contract. It is possible that much of the research that is withheld from the scientific community as trade secrets has little intrinsic scientific value or applicability and is limited to information such as scientifically unimportant formulas for products, scientific instrument calibrations, or engineering tolerances (Snapper).

Commercial considerations can distort academic life in other respects. Researchers may be tempted to devote time earmarked for the university to their commercial projects and to use university resources, including graduate assistants and laboratory staff, for their own financial benefit. Graduate students are particularly vulnerable to the availability of funds; the entire course of their careers may be guided by the source of their mentors' grants (Porter 1992a; Blumenthal). The prospect of large infusions of money into a cash-starved university might make an institution less scrupulous when evaluating potential research projects. For example, an institutional review board (IRB) might be less likely to point out problematic aspects of an experimental study if they believe that the corporate sponsor will withdraw its funds and go elsewhere with the proposal. An existing or potential grant might influence a university's decision on the composition of its faculty, the structure of a department, and the granting of tenure (Nelkin and Nelson). Financial incentives have encouraged some university researchers to redirect their work toward projects that are more likely to yield financial rewards. Such a redirection of research might encourage researchers to value applied projects with clear commercial ends and patentable uses over basic science projects whose practical applications are uncertain. While society benefits from applied research, fundamental breakthroughs and scientific progress are predicated on a strong commitment to basic research.

Despite these caveats, private funding of university research serves as an effective and essential supplement to government funding. Some reports demonstrate that, in general, industry-funded scientists publish more, produce more patentable discoveries, and still manage to teach as much and to serve as many administrative roles as colleagues without corporate financial support (Blumenthal). Industrial subsidies allow universities to support a more talented and larger faculty and to improve their facilities. Therefore, some authors argue that the danger of increased commercial presence in universities must be weighed against the positive contributions made by industry funding (Blake).

## Conflicts and Scientists' Social Duties

Professional researchers are the public's and policymakers' most important source of scientific expertise. Government agencies that evaluate biomedical proposals and projects must rely on scientists to analyze the safety and efficacy of research and products. Scientists also serve as reviewers for governmental grant applications and as authors, editors, and referees for professional publications. Conflicts of interest arise when industry, regulatory agencies, government committees, and editors all seek out the same individuals—a likely prospect when many of the most talented researchers have already-established commercial interests (Culliton).

Few scientists will purposely present biased conclusions, but researchers' commercial interests may influence their professional life in other respects. Scientists might be hesitant to participate in the evaluation of an industry with which they maintain a financial connection. Following a large oil spill on the California coast in the late 1960s, for example, government investigators found it difficult to recruit scientists willing to testify against the oil companies. Most qualified scientists had commercial ties to the industry (Kenney). When a medical journal sought independent reviewers to judge the quality of a research study showing the lack of benefits of a popular drug—a study whose publication the company manufacturing the drug was attempting to suppress on the grounds that the study was badly designed— the editors discovered that virtually all scientific experts in that field had existing financial ties to the company (Rennie). Corporations frequently employ researchers as consultants to determine if their facilities meet governmental health standards or if their new product induces disease. A researcher's desire to please the employer and to preserve the potential of future affiliations may influence the study design and methodology selected for the investigation. A study that monitors employee health for only a short time, for example, would be less likely to uncover an occupation-related disease with a long latency period. A corporation facing liability for a suspect drug would prefer its researchers to find that the product presented no danger and was not responsible for the maladies suffered by current users (Ashford; Porter, 1992a, 1992b).

Similarly, reviewers of grant applications may have commercial interests that unconsciously lead them to undervalue a potential competitor's proposal. Journal referees may denigrate articles or reports that threaten their commercial interests or their industry employer. A researcher with a consulting arrangement or an equity interest in a new development might tend toward findings that would laud the benefits of the innovation. In one egregious case, a researcher who owned over 500,000 shares of biomedical stock altered a study design to delay the release of negative findings until he could sell his holdings for a tremendous profit (American Medical Association). Physician-researchers with commercial interests in innovative treatments or research protocols bear additional responsibilities. A central tenet of medical professionalism holds that the welfare of the patient be placed before any benefit to the physician. If a physician-researcher is testing an experimental therapy, the patient must be protected from risks of undue harm from either the experimental drug itself or from withholding standard therapy. Physician-researchers with financial interests in their protocol might tend to recruit subjects aggressively, playing down the risks and exaggerating the benefits associated with the research. In a highly publicized case in which a young man died during experimental gene therapy, both the investigator and the university had financial interests in the biotechnology firm that planned to market the drug if it proved successful, and it was charged that substantial, known risks were not disclosed to the subject (2001).

During the 1990s a considerable change in pharmaceutical research funding occurred in the United States. Companies began to shift research grants away from universities and toward for-profit contract-research organizations (CROs). The CROs promised quicker research results and hence faster licensing of new drugs, compared to the more cumbersome, bureaucratic university system. Between 1991 and 1998, the portion of pharmaceutical industry research funds going to academic medical centers fell from 80 percent to 40 percent (2000). For-profit commercial IRBs sprang up to service the CROs, creating questions as to the adequacy of ethical review when both the IRB and the investigating organization had such strong financial incentives to speed the progress of research and to produce positive results (Lemmens and Freedman). As research funds were shifted to the private sector, university investigators had to compete more vigorously for the remaining funds, increasing the likelihood that both institutions and individuals would ignore serious conflicts of interest in their eagerness to secure funding.

## Remedies and Safeguards

The integrity of individual researchers is clearly the most important guard against the malevolent potential of conflicts of interest. But honesty alone may sometimes be insufficient, as damage can occur from unconscious bias and error as well as from conscious falsification. While all conflicts of interest have the potential to undermine a scientist's or an institution's primary goals of truth, objectivity, and openness, all conflicts do not pose the same degree of danger or require the same response. The danger of a particular conflict of interest depends both on how likely the arrangement is to corrupt the scientist's professional duty and on how much damage that corruption is likely to cause. Larger financial payments, and longer and closer relationships between researchers and business, will typically pose greater dangers than small financial incentives and one-time contacts with corporations (Thompson). While supervisory and regulatory measures can usually be tailored to the degree of the risk, there may be some situations in which the danger of harm to scientific integrity and society is so high that no protective measure can remedy it.

Universities might limit the amount of support they accept from industry, limit the amount of time that faculty may devote to outside endeavors, or prohibit particularly suspicious arrangements. In addition, research institutes can require the disclosure of all commercial links and interests and establish prospective administrative review of all proposals for outside funding (Varrin and Kukich; AAMC, 1990). Disclosure rules not only assist university officials and peers in policing conflicts of interest but may also make researchers more scrupulous in evaluating the potential bias in their own work. Researchers sometimes end or eschew questionable relationships rather than disclose them to the academic community. Some have argued, however, that today's institutional policies tend to advocate, inappropriately, disclosure alone, treating it as if it were a panacea. A number of prestigious universities and organizations in the United States proposed stringent conflict of interest policies in the early 2000s (Kelch; Kassirer). Many focus on individual conflicts of interest to the exclusion of institutional-level conflicts. By contrast, a group of Canadian authors, stimulated by widely publicized cases in their country of egregious institutional violations of academic freedom, have proposed elements of a conflict of interest policy that offers remedies for both levels of conflict (Lewis et al.). A policy on institutional conflicts of interest proposed in 2002 by the Association of American Medical Colleges (AAMC) locates responsibility for policing potential conflicts of interest within each university, whereas the Canadian group suggested that an appellate process involving a national group independent of any one university would be desirable (Lewis et al.; AAMC 2002). After developing a policy considered one of the most stringent in the nation, Harvard Medical School came under pressure to loosen its requirements, lest some of its most prestigious researchers move elsewhere (Angell). Bioethics programs in universities are part of the research enterprise and, according to some, should have policies to prevent conflicts of interest. Concerns have been expressed about paid consulting relationships between bioethics faculty and industry (Brody et al.).

Government agencies and professional publications also institute policies to guard against conflicts of interest.

The U.S. Food and Drug Administration and the National Institutes of Health require extensive disclosure of all advisers' commercial interests. Some professional journals demand that authors and reviewers disclose any commercial relationships that might be construed as creating conflicts of interest. According to this view, conflicts of interest should not automatically disqualify a reviewer or author, but the revelation will allow readers, editors, and administrators to scrutinize conclusions more carefully (Koshland). Other publications have adopted somewhat more stringent guidelines. The *New England Journal of Medicine,* for example, has required that authors disclose their financial conflicts, that its editors have no financial interest in any business related to clinical medicine, and that authors of review articles and editorials have no financial connection to their topics (Relman). The *Journal* was later forced to admit, however, that many of its authors of review articles had evaded these requirements (Angell, Utiger, and Wood). A few observers warn that excessive concern over conflicts of interest and safeguards may hinder scientific progress and undermine the scientific objectivity that they are designed to preserve. These writers claim that focusing reviewers' and readers' attention on potential outside influences instead of the content of the data, findings, and ideas generates a subjective skepticism unrelated to the objective merit of the work (Rothman). In 2001, however, the editors of thirteen major medical journals decided that the problem was serious enough to demand a unified and even more stringent disclosure policy (Davidoff et al.).

Some observers argue that the physician-researcher's commercial ties should be revealed to the patient-subject through the mechanism of informed consent and to the investigator's institution through a formal reporting mechanism (Finkel). Finally, IRBs can scrutinize protocols that promise great financial rewards for physician-investigators.

## Patents and the Public Interest

Patenting is another commercially motivated practice that may create conflicts between the primary interests of good science and the secondary interests created by the profit motive. Patenting is based on the theory that innovators will be more likely to share their knowledge because they know that they will receive remuneration and credit and that entrepreneurs will be more willing to invest in the development of discoveries because they know that they have exclusive or protected access and will recoup their expenditures in profits. Patenting's skeptics, however, argue that the very nature of patenting undermines the traditional scientific norm of openness. Researchers may be tempted to withhold socially valuable information until they are certain that their pecuniary interests are protected by a patent (Kass; Wiener). Especially in the biomedical fields, a delay in the release of information can lead to postponed development and dissemination and the loss of lives. Others speculate that potentially patentable, lucrative discoveries will lead researchers away from less profitable yet socially important projects. Finally, some critics claim that entrepreneurs who purchase rights to a basic discovery often do not use or develop it in a socially responsible way. Furthermore, their monopoly advantage makes it impossible for the market to force them to distribute the breakthrough in an equitable and useful manner (Goldman).

The federal Bayh-Dole Act of 1980 provided the legal basis for universities to patent genetic and other biotechnology products and discoveries. When passed by Congress, the act seemed uncontroversial, because the public would benefit both from the quicker marketing of the fruits of new research and also from a lower tax burden as universities made more money from patents and licenses. In retrospect, some provisions of the act appear to have had undesirable consequences. Besides the dangers of turning so big a percentage of research funding over to corporate interests, some fear that the ease with which one can patent each separate step of a complex sequence needed to create genetic tests or therapies will actually pose a barrier to future advances, because the manufacture of any gene product may require negotiating license fees with the owners of dozens of patents (Nelkin and Andrews; Merz et al.).

The government can also provide patentlike incentives to encourage the development of products with marginal profitability that are intended to treat a small patient population or that are ineligible for normal patent protection— so-called orphan drugs. Orphan-drug programs might include research grants, investment tax credits, expedited approval processes, and exclusive licenses to produce and distribute the drug. Critics of orphan-drug programs argue that the policy excessively favors drug manufacturers, inflates the costs of lifesaving medications, and delays the development of lower-cost alternatives. Private corporations sometimes reap profits far in excess of their expectations and effort while effectively denying life-sustaining remedies to patients through monopoly pricing practices (Ackiron). Incentives are sometimes overgenerous, and corporations are able to enrich themselves on drugs that serve only a small number of patients and occasionally produce limited benefits (Wagner). It is important to scrutinize the incentive structure of the orphan-drug policy in an attempt to eliminate unnecessary windfall profits for drug manufacturers. Policymakers must balance the cost of the incentives, including monopoly pricing practices and tax abatements,

against the benefits provided by the new drug (i.e., the number of people served and the efficacy of the remedy).

## Marketable Products from Human Sources

Another challenging problem arises when an individual's body parts or cells are transformed into valuable commodities. In one such case, a patient's removed spleen contained unique cells that a physician-researcher cultured into a patented cell line. Should the patient have been apprised, as part of the informed-consent procedure, that the cells had potential commercial value? Fully informed consent would have allowed the patient to evaluate the physician's potential conflict of interests and choice of treatments more effectively. Because society and the law have typically been hesitant to "commodify" the body and do not allow the sale of organs, it might seem inappropriate to grant the patient a share of the profits based on the theory that the tissue is his or her "property." In contrast, the system appears to allow the biomedical entrepreneur to benefit from the sale of body parts. Developers of such innovative products might argue that the resulting cell line is not a body part but rather the result of their labor and ingenuity and that these efforts deserve to be rewarded and encouraged by traditional patents. Even granting this argument, it may be unjust to allow others to benefit from an innovation while the person upon whose existence the development rests receives nothing. Consequently, it seems fair and equitable that individuals receive some benefit from their unique physical characteristics that have been used to create great profits. The amount of remuneration could depend upon the nature of the informed-consent agreement, the degree to which the body tissue contribution was changed by the researcher before it was offered as a product, and the uniqueness of the physical material used (Murray).

## Conclusion

It would be unrealistic to expect modern capital-intensive scientific research to thrive entirely without the support and influence of commercial interests and incentives. Similarly, it would be unwise and impractical to suggest that scientists who maintain commercial connections, and therefore have potential conflicts of interest, should disqualify themselves from all advisory duties. The trend toward adoption of explicit and stringent conflict of interest policies suggests a growing consensus that individuals, institutions, and professional groups have all been too tolerant in the past of ethically questionable but lucrative practices. It remains to be seen how effective these new policies will prove in policing the problem. The U.S. public, moreover, may be forced to reexamine the wisdom of allowing so great a percentage of the total research endeavor to be governed by private commercial interests.

KENNETH ALLEN DE VILLE (1995)
REVISED BY HOWARD BRODY

SEE ALSO: *Conflict of Interest; Corporate Compliance; Pharmaceutical Industry; Private Ownership of Inventions; Profit and Commercialism*

### BIBLIOGRAPHY

Ackiron, Evan. 1991. "Patents for Critical Pharmaceuticals: The AZT Case." *American Journal of Law and Medicine* 17(1–2): 145–180.

American Medical Association (AMA). Council on Scientific Affairs and Council on Ethical and Judicial Affairs. 1990. "Conflicts of Interest in Medical Center/Industry Research Relationships." *Journal of the American Medical Association* 263(20): 2790–2793.

Angell, Marcia. 2000. "Is Academic Medicine for Sale?" *New England Journal of Medicine* 342(20): 1516–1518.

Angell, Marcia; Utiger, Robert D.; and Wood, Alastair J. J. 2000. "Disclosure of Authors' Conflicts of Interest: A Follow-Up." *New England Journal of Medicine* 342(8): 586–587.

Ashford, Nicholas A. 1983. "A Framework for Examining the Effects of Industrial Funding on Academic Freedom and the Integrity of the University." *Science, Technology, and Human Values* 8(2): 16–23.

Association of American Medical Colleges (AAMC). Ad Hoc Committee on Misconduct and Conflict of Interest in Research. 1990. *Guidelines for Dealing with Faculty Conflicts of Commitment and Conflicts of Interest in Research.* Washington, D.C.: Author.

Association of American Medical Colleges (AAMC). Task Force on Financial Conflicts of Interest in Clinical Research. 2002. *Protecting Subjects, Preserving Trust, Promoting Progress II: Principles and Recommendations for Oversight of an Institution's Financial Interests in Human Subjects Research.* Washington, D.C.: Author.

Bekelman, Justin E.; Li, Yan, and Gross, Cary P. 2003. "Scope and Impact of Financial Conflicts of Interest in Biomedical Research: A Systematic Review." *Journal of the American Medical Association* 289(4): 454–465.

Blake, David A. 1992. "The Opportunities and Problems of Commercial Ventures: The University View." In *Biomedical Research: Collaboration and Conflict of Interest,* ed. Roger J. Porter, Thomas E. Malone, and Christopher C. Vaughn. Baltimore, MD: Johns Hopkins University Press.

Blumenthal, David. 1992. "Academic–Industry Relationships in the Life Sciences: Extent, Consequences, and Management." *Journal of the American Medical Association* 268(23): 3344–3349.

Bodenheimer, Thomas. 2000. "Uneasy Alliance: Clinical Investigators and the Pharmaceutical Industry." *New England Journal of Medicine* 342(20): 1539–1544.

Brody, Baruch; Dubler, Nancy; Blustein, Jeff; et al. 2002. "Bioethics Consultation in the Private Sector." *Hastings Center Report* 32(3): 14–20.

Cournand, André. 1977. "The Code of the Scientist and Its Relationship to Ethics." *Science* 198(4318): 699–705.

Culliton, Barbara J. 1982. "The Academic–Industrial Complex." *Science* 216(4549): 960–962.

Davidoff, Frank; DeAngelis, Catherine D.; Drazen, Jeffrey M.; et al. 2001. "Sponsorship, Authorship, and Accountability." *Journal of the American Medical Association* 286(10): 1232–1234.

Dettweiler, Ulrich, and Simon, Perikles. 2001. "Points to Consider for Ethics Committees in Human Gene Therapy Trials." *Bioethics* 15(5–6): 491–500.

Etzkowitz, Henry. 1983. "Entrepreneurial Scientists and Entrepreneurial Universities in American Academic Science." *Minerva* 21(2–3): 198–233.

Finkel, Marion J. 1991. "Should Informed Consent Include Information on How Research Is Funded?" *IRB: A Review of Human Subjects Research* 13(5): 1–3.

Goldman, Alan H. 1987. "Ethical Issues in Proprietary Restrictions on Research Results." *Science, Technology, and Human Values* 12(1): 22–30.

Kass, Leon R. 1981. "Patenting Life." *Commentary* 72(6): 45–57.

Kassirer, Jerome P. 2001. "Financial Conflict of Interest: An Unresolved Ethical Frontier." *American Journal of Law and Medicine* 27(2–3): 149–162.

Kelch, Robert P. 2002. "Maintaining the Public Trust in Clinical Research." *New England Journal of Medicine* 346(4): 285–287.

Kenney, Martin. 1986. *Biotechnology: The University–Industrial Complex.* New Haven, CT: Yale University Press.

Koshland, Daniel E., Jr. 1992. "Conflict of Interest Policy." *Science* 257(5070): 595.

Lemmens, Trudo, and Freedman, Benjamin. 2000. "Ethics Review for Sale? Conflict of Interest and Commercial Research Review Boards." *Milbank Quarterly* 78(4): 547–584.

Lewis, Steven; Baird, Patricia; Evans, Robert G.; et al. 2001. "Dancing with the Porcupine: Rules for Governing the University–Industry Relationship." *Canadian Medical Association Journal* 165(6): 783–785.

Lind, Stuart E. 1986. "Fee-for-Service Research." *New England Journal of Medicine* 314(5): 312–315.

Merton, Robert K. 1942. "Science and Technology in a Democratic Order." *Journal of Legal and Political Sociology* 1: 115–126.

Merz, Jon F.; Kriss, Antigone G.; Leonard, Debra G. B.; and Cho, Mildred K. 2002. "Diagnostic Testing Fails the Test." *Nature* 415(6872): 577–579.

Murray, Thomas H. 1985. "Ethical Issues in Genetic Engineering." *Social Research* 52(3): 471–489.

Nelkin, Dorothy, and Andrews, Lori. 1998. "Homo Economicus: Commercialization of Body Tissue in the Age of Biotechnology." *Hastings Center Report* 28(5): 30–39.

Nelkin, Dorothy, and Nelson, Richard. 1987. "Commentary: University–Industry Alliances." *Science, Technology, and Human Values* 12(1): 65–74.

Porter, Roger J. 1992a. "Conflicts of Interest in Research: Investigator Bias—The Instrument of Conflict." In *Biomedical Research: Collaboration and Conflict of Interest,* ed. Roger J. Porter, Thomas E. Malone, and Christopher C. Vaughn. Baltimore, MD: Johns Hopkins University Press.

Porter, Roger J. 1992b. "Conflicts of Interest in Research: Personal Gain—The Seeds of Conflict." In *Biomedical Research: Collaboration and Conflict of Interest,* ed. Roger J. Porter, Thomas E. Malone, and Christopher C. Vaughn. Baltimore, MD: Johns Hopkins University Press.

Relman, Arnold S. 1990. "New 'Information for Authors'—and Readers." *New England Journal of Medicine* 323(1): 56.

Rennie, Drummond. 1997. "Thyroid Storm." *Journal of the American Medical Association* 277(15): 1238–1243.

Rothman, Kenneth J. 1993. "Conflict of Interest: The New McCarthyism in Science." *Journal of the American Medical Association* 269(21): 2782–2784.

Snapper, John W. 1992. "Doing Science while Keeping Trade Secrets." *Phi Kappa Phi Journal* (winter): 22–25.

Thompson, Dennis F. 1993. "Understanding Financial Conflicts of Interest." *New England Journal of Medicine* 329(8): 573–576.

Varrin, Robert D., and Kukich, Diane S. 1985. "Guidelines for Industry-Sponsored Research at Universities." *Science* 227(4685): 385–388.

Wagner, Judith L. 1992. "Orphan Technologies: Defining the Issues." *International Journal of Technology Assessment in Health Care* 8(4): 561–565.

Wiener, Charles. 1987. "Patenting and Academic Research: Historical Case Studies." *Science, Technology, and Human Values* 12(1): 50–62.

# COMMUNITARIANISM AND BIOETHICS

• • •

In the 1990s, communitarian approaches to bioethics became increasingly common and explicit in the literature. This evolution was the result of the prominence of the communitarian philosophical critiques of liberalism that occurred in the 1980s, particularly works by Alasdair MacIntyre, Michael Sandel, Charles Taylor, and Michael Walzer.

Communitarianism is a neo-Aristotelian philosophy that focuses on the common good and is concerned with the relationship between the good person or good citizen and the good of the community or society. As would be expected, it has much in common with other neo-Aristotelian approaches, such as casuistry and virtue ethics. Communitarianism is both a critique of the dominant Western ideology of liberal individualism and an orientation to ethical problem solving.

Communitarians often argue that the notion of human nature and the concept of the self behind liberalism are insufficient to make possible a shared common understanding of values among members of society. Similarly, communitarians sometimes argue that liberal society is committed to neutrality toward all notions of the good life, and thereby cannot adequately address ethical issues. As a result, communitarians often stress an orientation toward ethical questions that relies on the establishment, or re-establishment, of a shared common understanding, a shared notion of the good life, or a shared notion of the self.

Only a few bioethicists have openly embraced the communitarian label in their writings (Emanuel; Brennan; Loewy; Nelson; Callahan, 1996; Kuczewski, 1997). However, much work in bioethics shares community-oriented assumptions—that healthcare is special and different from market commodities, for example (Daniels), and may be seen as a good that is part of the common good (even by those who do not embrace communitarianism in other spheres of distributive justice) (Jecker and Jonsen). Similarly, many writers take relationships as the starting point of their ethic, rather than the individual (Murray).

Furthermore, even if society tries to remain neutral toward visions of the good life, ethical issues arise within the context of healthcare and require that the public institutions that provide medical treatment and conduct biomedical research somehow address such ethical dilemmas. As a result, pragmatists such as Jonathan Moreno embrace communitarian strands of thought in an effort to resolve such questions through the production of consensus (e.g., the creation of shared common understandings) (Moreno).

## Communitarian Critiques of Liberalism

Communitarian critiques of liberalism have an intuitive appeal, and the nature of the critiques determine the kind of solutions that communitarians seek. It is again important to note that these critiques were developed mainly in the philosophical and political-theory literature and then imported to bioethics, often in a compressed fashion. Two different, but related, starting points form the basis of the communitarian criticisms.

### LOSS OF SHARED COMMON UNDERSTANDING. Some communitarians, most notably the philosopher Alasdair MacIntyre, claim that liberalism will always fail to settle

ethical disagreements because of the loss of a shared common understanding, or of a shared view of the good life (MacIntyre, 1981). According to this view, ethical and moral concepts are only understandable within the framework of the traditions within which the concepts developed. Such traditions are marked by a shared vision of the good life. This vision is thought to contain a shared hierarchy of goods, and ethical disagreements are supposed to be resolved by reference to this hierarchy.

Such communitarians see the contemporary moral situation as dire. Because there is no shared vision of the good life within a liberal democratic society, they claim, there is no such thing as moral discourse. Although there may be the appearance of moral debate, such arguments tend to have a back-and-forth nature, mostly between rival conceptions that share few common assumptions. MacIntyre characterizes such discussions within our society as "shrill" and "interminable" (MacIntyre, 1981, pp. 8–12) The debates are shrill because, lacking the rational basis of a shared hierarchy of goods, rival conceptions can only advance their conclusions by the force of emotion. The debates are interminable because the force of emotion can produce no enduring consensus.

Societal discussion regarding bioethical issues is characterized as essentially being in bad faith. That is, bioethics must put forth public policy and some point to the developing of widespread consensus on several issues, but such consenses are said to be forced and sociological in nature (MacIntyre, 1984; 1990, pp. 226–227). For MacIntyre, the solution to the contemporary moral fragmentation is to build up from particular communities that share a vision of the good life, perhaps through sectarian universities, to the restoration of a shared common understanding of the good life (MacIntyre, pp. 220–223).

Similarly, a number of communitarians echo MacIntyre's criticism by highlighting the fact that liberal political theory embraces the *neutrality thesis* toward views of the good life. It is not that visions of the good life have mysteriously been lost from moral discourse. Rather they are, in principle, not allowed to form the basis of ethical quandaries or social policies (Larmore, 1987, pp. 42–55). The neutrality thesis can be illustrated by the suspicion with which religion is treated in the public sphere. Policy positions that are seen to emanate mainly from religious sentiments, sentiments that are expressions of a particular vision of the good life, are generally not considered viable options within public policy debates. Similarly, such positions, should they become the law of the land, can and are sometimes struck down by courts if they infringe on the liberty interests of the non-religious.

Communitarians note that the state cannot remain neutral toward all elements of the good life. It is the role of the state to protect the life and liberty of its citizens and to foster opportunity among them (i.e., to foster the "pursuit of happiness"). Although safeguarding life, liberty, and the pursuit of happiness does not logically entail a vision of the good life, questions of what kind of life a society wishes to foster can be unavoidable in practice. Simply providing and mandating a specific minimum amount of such a value neutral commodity as education can be more conducive to some visions of the good life than to others. Given the inevitability of impacting on visions of the good life, communitarians often seek ways to produce consensus regarding the values to be fostered, or to create policy solutions that balance widely shared values.

## LIBERALISM'S IMPOVERISHED VIEW OF THE PERSON.
Communitarians can also begin by showing that liberal democracy is based on a certain view of human nature, and that this view is inadequate even for the purpose of establishing the moral aspirations that liberal democratic theorists hold dear.

Liberal theorists do not wish to set forth a vision of the good life. Nevertheless, thinkers such as John Rawls posit a view of what is essential to human nature. Rawls puts forward such a vision in order to provide support for the rationality of the choice of certain principles of justice to govern the basic institutions of society (Rawls, 1971, pp. 54–60). In other words, although no vision of the good life is essential to humans, *choosing* a vision of the good is what is essential to human beings. This self that is defined by choice and will, i.e., this *volitional self* is the justification for a view of society as fostering opportunity to pursue one's vision of the good life.

The communitarian critique of the volitional self points to the fact that this concept fails on its own terms. The political theorist Michael Sandel argues that this vision of human beings is too thin to actually justify the kind of contractarian liberalism that rests upon it. Liberalism typically includes a distributive or redistributive role for government to assist the least advantaged, an aspiration that is viewed as not justifiable when based on such a thin concept of the self. Justifying such an aspiration requires a view of human beings as deliberative and interrelational, not merely volitional and contractual. People are not static and fixed entities who mysteriously have a set vision of the good life that they pursue; they develop and refine values and preferences in social processes. As a result, political processes should be arranged to foster the deliberative capacities of citizens, not to count the preferences in a voting procedure (Emanuel, p. 232).

Liberalism includes a principle of sharing. John Rawls expresses this as the "difference principle" (Rawls, 1971, pp. 75–83). According to this principle, inequalities are allowed as long as they work to benefit the least advantaged. Because liberal theorists wish for a sharing principle to follow from the description of the volitional self, Rawls argues that citizens would choose this principle if they did not know which arbitrary advantages or disadvantages they would have by accident of birth or luck. This derivation of the difference principle follows deductively only if we assume that persons are highly risk-averse creatures and will go to great lengths to avoid being in the worst position, even if such an outcome would be unlikely. This is the position Rawls took in his early development of the "maximin principle" (Rawls, 1971, pp. 152–157).

One could also say that that the choice of the difference principle reflects the kind of choice that persons in a certain kind of historical community would make in virtue of their self-understanding. This is the position toward which Rawls moved in his later work. But, if reflection on the ideals of a community's self-understanding can be the basis for ethics, ethics can be based on more contentful concepts of the self, such as the communitarian's ideal of the self as deliberative and rational.

## The Communitarian Concept of the Self

For the communitarian self, the pursuit and choice of the good life is a process that is interpretive and deliberative. Persons are born into, or thrown into, situations that contain fragments of traditions, values, customs, norms, and habits. However, these raw materials are continuously reinterpreted and reappropriated as circumstances evolve and change. Similarly, persons make choices, accumulate experience, and receive a variety of kinds of feedback. They modify, refine, or change their ends, or the means to those ends, based upon these life processes. In so doing, they come to know who they are. Being a "self" is therefore a process of self-discovery.

Being a person is also a process of mutual self-discovery (Kuczewski, 1997, pp. 51–56, 108–112). That is, a person not only makes his or her own plans and gathers feedback, but is also shaped by his or her response to, and participation in, the process of self-discovery of others. A person's identity is thereby inseparable from the life of the communities and societies in which the person participates. Of course, this is not the mere alignment of the projects and values of the person with the community. The person's identity is partially constituted by his or her community, even in the person's rejection of the community's values.

The essence of a person comes from the person's participation in the process of mutual self-discovery. Thus, for the communitarian, the ultimate question is always how to foster the development of a person's deliberative powers and create appropriate opportunities for exercising meaningful participation in communal deliberation. This heuristic applies to deliberation on levels of interpersonal encounters such as clinical decision making as well as societal decisions regarding the use of common resources.

Communitarian thought is obviously closely related to another neo-Aristotelian ethic, virtue theory. Communitarians hold that the concept of the person includes the notion of capacities that need to be developed to be a good citizen and good person. Virtue ethics takes the development of excellence of character as its end-point, its *telos*. That is, the virtuous person is what the community and social practices should aim to produce. There are few obvious points of tension between communitarianism and virtue ethics, and disputes would seem to be a matter of emphasis and tone. Communitarians are generally oriented to process, virtue theorists to outcome (i.e., character). But both emphasize the relationship and interdependence of the community and the deliberative capacities of its members.

## The Methods of Communitarianism: Consensus from Fragmentation

Communitarianism is probably best characterized as a philosophy of public deliberation that tries to produce consensus on public matters—matters that include the topics typically considered in the field of bioethics. Of course, the important question is how to actually produce that consensus. Three general approaches predominate: the whole-tradition method, liberal communitarianism, and consensus in public judgment.

### THE "WHOLE-TRADITION" METHOD: REVIVAL AND REVITALIZATION OF PARTICULAR TRADITIONS. The "whole tradition" method of communitarianism sees the fragmentation of values and traditions as an almost insurmountable problem. Communitarians such as the philosopher Alasdair MacIntyre and the Christian theologian Stanley Hauerwas view moral concepts as only intelligible within the traditions in which they originated. Moral traditions, therefore, contain concepts that are incommensurable with those of other traditions, and that are untranslatable because they only make sense within their respective traditions. As a result, moral method must take the form of reviving particular traditions.

MacIntyre proposes that moral discourse take the form of a competition among revitalized traditions. Each tradition would express itself through a university in which the tradition would express and develop its worldview across the disciplines. The ultimate test of a tradition is the degree to which it can create a comprehensive worldview that accounts for the facts of the contemporary world and can respond to new challenges and crises that arise. MacIntyre also holds open the possibility that one worldview may simply be developed that is comprehensive enough to encompass the truths and strengths of other traditions. He clearly believes that the Aristotelian-Thomistic tradition is the most promising in this regard (MacIntyre, 1990, p. 81).

The whole-tradition movement in communitarianism is the most radical and pessimistic form of communitarianism. It holds that there is (and can be) no genuine moral discourse in a pluralistic liberal society—and that the revival of whole traditions in toto is the only possible solution. Once such traditions are developed, people can choose among the views of the good life that are contained therein. The work required to bring this about is described by MacIntyre as being akin to the service that Saint Benedict and the monastic orders provided in keeping civilization alive during the medieval period.

**LIBERAL COMMUNITARIANISM.** Communal deliberation is intrinsic to communitarianism. So it is natural that some communitarians should propose that community members gather and deliberate to develop consensus. In bioethics, this approach is notably associated with the early work of Ezekiel J. Emanuel.

In his highly regarded book, *The Ends of Human Life: Medical Ethics in a Liberal Polity* (1991), Emanuel suggests that ethical decisions regarding medical care are best handled by the members of small cooperatives called Community Health Plans (CHPs). Members would have a choice of a variety of CHPs in their geographic area. In the early stages of the founding of the plan, members would articulate the fundamental value assumptions behind the plan. For instance, some CHPs could have a philosophy that is strongly geared toward preservation of biological life, while others might maximize palliative care options. Similarly, some might strongly favor choice in reproductive and contraceptive options, while others would promote religious approaches to family life. By organizing the CHPs according to nonnegotiable value choices, the CHP progresses easily beyond the shrill and interminable debates to the more subtle choices involved in developing a health plan.

In Emanuel's plan, each person would have a voucher that would be brought to the plan. As a result, the deliberation about values and coverage of treatments is also a resource-allocation process. Each member must think not only about his or her values in the abstract, but must consider how to balance the fiscal implications of those commitments against other values and potential needs. This discussion takes place within a communal dialogue among the approximately 10,000 members of the plan. In such a dialogue, a person comes to develop his or her deliberative capacities and refine and clarify his or her values.

The strength of such a proposal is that it embodies the virtues of a genuine deliberative democracy. Such a plan brings together the rights and responsibilities of each person, granting each the right to be true to his or her most fundamental value commitments, and to be self-determining in devising a health plan to meet those commitments. But, more importantly, it demands personal responsibility in accepting the allocation consequences of one's choices. One may choose to be part of a plan that explicitly provides a maximum amount of some services and minimizes other services, and one must live with the minimal services provided should he or she develop an illness that might benefit from a higher level of services. Because the plan respects the rights of each within a communal framework, it is sometimes called *liberal communitarianism*.

Of course, the proposal for CHPs suffers from the practical difficulties of any community-based initiative. Although our best selves may develop in a context of dialogue and deliberation, many persons will simply not wish to devote the time and energy needed to participate meaningfully. Emanuel acknowledges that the model of the New England town meeting (the model on which the CHP is based) usually becomes dominated by a small, highly participatory group in whom the silent majority comes to have confidence (Emanuel, pp. 231–232). However, if stable communal consensus can be developed in ways that do not require the direct participation of most citizens, such approaches may recommend themselves to communitarians.

**CONSENSUS IN PUBLIC JUDGMENT.** *Proxy dialogue and balancing values.* One of the striking facts concerning bioethics is that public debate has produced areas of stable consensus, most notably in the United States, concerning informed consent to treatment and the principles concerning end-of-life decision making. Similarly, some studies have suggested that the American people may, in general, be less fragmented in reference to their values than is usually thought to be the case. Contrary to the radical communitarians such as MacIntyre, there may be empirical reason to be optimistic that a society can achieve stable consensus on moral problems that occur within public and quasi-public institutions.

The public debate concerning informed consent and end-of-life decisions has not been one with a clearly identifiable locus, but has taken a variety of forms, including court decisions, state referenda, and the policy deliberations of institutions such as professional societies and accreditation agencies. The public has been informed in a variety of ways, including media coverage of court decisions, public education efforts when referenda are introduced, and portrayal of these issues in entertainment programming such as television medical dramas. Somehow, over time, a consensus has taken shape.

Consensus, in this context, has tended to mean a set of principles that are widely accepted. It does not mean unanimity, for a large pluralistic society will always include those who disagree. Similarly, the interpretation and application of the principles will constantly require refinement because of the wide variety of possible circumstances in which they may be needed. As a result, debate may seem to be ceaseless, but the object of the debates actually becomes more refined. For instance, the consensus on forgoing life-sustaining treatment includes a distinction between forgoing treatment and assisted suicide (though the state of Oregon does not adhere to this distinction in a substantive way). The consensus also holds that patients who have lost their decision-making capacity (i.e., they have been deemed "incompetent") have the same rights as other patients. While all U.S. states adhere to this general principle, the evidentiary standards regarding the incapacitated patient's prior wishes can differ substantially among states (Meisel, Snyder, and Quill). Although these are important disputes, they do not undermine the widely shared areas of agreement.

Of course, identifying that a society has achieved a stable consensus is not always a simple task. Public opinion polls can measure the public's views, but it is not always obvious when the data reflect a stable consensus. It is often the case that responses to poll questions reflect mere fleeting preferences. Although communitarianism is premised on the idea that people must come to discover their wishes, or how their values translate into preferences, how this happens on a grand scale is somewhat mysterious. However, some suggestions have been made.

First, a consensus is probably more stable if it is able to balance several competing values that are important to a society. For instance, the consensus on forgoing life-sustaining treatment has been relatively stable for more than a decade because it reflects the balancing of important values and considerations (Kuczewski, 2002). A patient's ability to participate in the decisions regarding his or her medical care, especially as one nears death, is fostered and balanced against the duty of society and the medical profession to protect patients, especially those who are vulnerable due to lack of decisional capacity. Policy proposals that tip the balance heavily in favor of patient self-determination, such as those for legalizing assisted suicide, have met with limited success. Similarly, proposals that eschew patient autonomy in favor of the physician's duty to do no harm, such as futility policies, continue to remain outside the consensus (Helft, Siegler, and Lantos).

Second, in situations in which the content of consensus gains widely shared acceptance without direct participation by the citizenry, some sort of "proxy dialogue" might have served as a substitute for direct participation (Yankelovich, 1999, p. 167). That is, representatives of various positions and interests might achieve recognition, and their interaction might forge a position that accommodates the major values at stake. By having the process play out publicly, the solution is internalized by much of the citizenry. Furthermore, consensus is semiperformative (Moreno, p. 52).

A consensus is furthered when an announcement is made that there is a consensus on certain points. People generally do not wish to overturn consensus for its own sake. Thus, when one announces consensus and proceeds to state the specific points, people will probably prefer to assent. This assent would seem more likely to be freely given if the citizens are able to recognize their values as being respected in the points of consensus. Dissent would seem more likely to follow if the consensus is ideological in the sense that it traces all its points to only one value or principle, rather than representing the array of values that are relevant to the issues under consideration. These values may be identified *a priori* by surveying the goods generally considered characteristic of a particular sphere of human activity (Walzer, pp. 6–10), or by empirical approaches that assess the values of the community involved.

***Relationships, casuistry, and pragmatism.*** On the most pragmatic level, communitarians often approach ethical issues by beginning with the norms of the relationships involved, rather than the rights of the individual. In this way, communitarianism provides the foundational philosophical assumptions for the customary workings of popular methods in bioethics, such as casuistry, pragmatism, and the four-principles method. Bioethics, especially clinical bioethics, has often proceeded as if a number of persons have a stake in the outcome of the case, and that dialogue and negotiation leading to consensus are better than a simple assertion of one person's rights. These practices are more easily justified within a communitarian conception of the person as being essentially related to those around him or her than on the liberal conception of the individual. However, this does not necessarily result in a tyranny of the interests of the majority, as there may be spheres of being in which individual rights are more authoritative, and irreconcilable conflicts may have to be resolved in favor of certain individuals no matter in which sphere of endeavor it takes place.

Casuists such as Albert Jonsen and Stephen Toulmin assert that that the kinds of norms that predominate in various types of cases result from the nature of the relationships involved in the particular case under examination. Cases in which the relationships are intimate are more generally decided in favor of values such as beneficence and caring. In these kinds of cases the boundaries between persons are fluid, and looking out for the good of the other is often called for by the situation. In impersonal situations, in which persons are more likely to be strangers, solutions are more often found in the direction of autonomy and individual rights. Nevertheless, specific circumstances can render these generalizations inapplicable, and some spheres of interaction (e.g., healthcare) can embody elements of both an ethics of strangers and an ethics of intimacy. As a result, paradigm cases for each kind of bioethical issue must be sought and taxonomies of paradigms and variations established (Jonsen and Toulmin, pp. 291–292).

Similarly, the famed *four principles* approach, also known as principlism, takes the physician-patient relationship as the starting point of medical ethics (Beauchamp and Childress, pp. 12–13). Principlists argue that ethical problems arise when any of the four main obligations of physicians to patients (respect for autonomy, nonmaleficence, beneficence, and justice) come into conflict with another of the principles. The goal then becomes to resolve this conflict of principles. This method assumes that members of society share a common morality, and that it is interpretable within the confines of the healthcare system (Beauchamp and Childress, pp. 401–405). These same assumptions are shared by many communitarian bioethicists. However, communitarian philosophers have made advances on the static understanding of the moral principles of the principlists. For instance, Emanuel's communitarianism includes a theory of the physician-patient relationship. This relationship, in its highest expression, focuses on helping the patient to interpret and discover his or her health-related values and how they apply to the choices before the patient (Emanuel and Emanuel). In this framework, patient autonomy is an essential element, but in many situations it is seen as the outcome of an interpersonal process rather than as the starting point of the interaction. Others with communitarian leanings focus on familial relationships as the starting point of an ethic.

Thomas Murray, a sociologist by training, argues that bioethics will make more progress toward consensus on controversial issues by starting with a tapestry of relationships that are prized by persons in a society. He notes that familial relationships are often among those that give distinctiveness to life. By creating such a tapestry, and describing the goods fostered therein, he believes that some of the so-called unending debates in bioethics can be defused. For instance, Murray asserts that conclusions in the abortion debate often exceed the premises and are inconsistent with other practices of adherents of the conclusions. Murray believes that the strength of the conclusions is probably a derivative from perceived threats to valued relationships (Murray, pp.173–174).

James and Hilde Nelson have begun the work of developing an ethics of intimate relationships that takes familial relationships as the starting point. This kind of work exemplifies the nuances of contemporary communitarian bioethics in that it results in generalizations about specific spheres of relationships. Furthermore, the kinds of generalizations that are developed give moral weight to those whose interests are most affected by situations, rather than invoking individual rights.

## Applications

Radical whole-tradition communitarianism results in the most radical prescriptions, since it nullifies all rights claims and counsels a return to separate communities to work out a shared ethic. As we have seen, most communitarians have far more subtle prescriptions for facilitating the kind of public deliberation that they seek.

There are few attempts in the literature by communitarians to directly deduce conclusions from communitarian premises. One might expect that communitarians will be more sympathetic to the common good in weighing solutions to ethical problems. It is true that some communitarians have favored aggressive approaches to organ procurement for transplantation (Nelson), mandatory rationing to resolve resource-allocation problems (Callahan, 1990), and public health concerns over individual privacy and choice (Etzioni). However, none of these positions are necessarily entailed by communitarian sympathies as one can easily argue that these same policies foster values the community should reject. As a result, communitarianism continues to be an approach to bioethics that is more about process than particular outcomes.

MARK G. KUCZEWSKI

**SEE ALSO:** *Consensus, Role and Authority of; Contractarianism and Bioethics; Feminism; Healthcare Resources, Allocation* *of; Human Nature; Justice; Law and Morality; Managed Care; Natural Law; Patients' Responsibilities; Public Health: Philosophy; Sustainable Development; Virtue and Character*

## BIBLIOGRAPHY

Beauchamp, Tom L., and Childress, James F. 2001. *Principles of Biomedical Ethics.* New York: Oxford University Press.

Brennan, Troyen A. 1991. *Just Doctoring: Medical Ethics in the Liberal State.* Berkeley, CA: University of California Press.

Callahan, Daniel. 1990. *What Kind of Life: The Limits of Medical Progress.* New York: Simon & Schuster.

Callahan, Daniel. 1996. "Bioethics: A Pious Hope?" *Responsive Community: Rights and Responsibilities* 6(4): 26–33.

Daniels, Norman. 1985. *Just Health Care.* New York: Cambridge University Press.

Emanuel, Ezekiel J. 1991. *The Ends of Human Life: Medical Ethics in a Liberal Polity.* Cambridge, MA: Harvard University Press.

Emanuel, Ezekiel J., and Linda L. Emanuel. 1992. "Four Models of the Physician-Patient Relationship." *Journal of the American Medical Association* 267(16): 2221–2226.

Etzioni, Amitai. 1999. *The Limits of Privacy.* New York: Basic Books.

Hauerwas, Stanley. 1983. *The Peaceable Kingdom: A Primer in Christian Ethics.* Notre Dame, IN: University of Notre Dame Press.

Helft Paul R.; Siegler, Mark; and Lantos, John. 2000. "The Rise and Fall of the Futility Movement." *New England Journal of Medicine* 343(4): 293–296.

Jecker, Nancy S., and Jonsen, Albert R. 1995. "Healthcare As a Commons." *Cambridge Quarterly of Healthcare Ethics* 4(2): 207–216.

Jonsen, Albert R., and Toulmin, Stephen. 1988. *The Abuse of Casuistry: A History of Moral Reasoning.* Berkeley, CA: University of California Press.

Kuczewski, Mark G. 1997. *Fragmentation and Consensus: Communitarian and Casuist Bioethics.* Washington, D.C.: Georgetown University Press.

Kuczewski, Mark G. 2002. "Two Models of Ethical Consensus or What Good is a Bunch of Bioethicists?" *Cambridge Quarterly of Healthcare Ethics* 11(1): 27–36.

Larmore, Charles E. 1987. *Patterns of Moral Complexity.* New York: Cambridge University Press.

Loewy, Erich H. 1993. *Freedom and Community: The Ethics of Interdependence.* Albany: State University of New York Press.

MacIntyre, Alasdair. 1981. *After Virtue: A Study in Moral Theory.* Notre Dame, IN: University of Notre Dame Press.

MacIntyre, Alasdair. 1984. "Does Applied Ethics Rest on a Mistake?" *Monist* 67(4): 498–513.

MacIntyre, Alasdair. 1988. *Whose Justice? Which Rationality?* Notre Dame, IN: University of Notre Dame Press.

MacIntyre, Alasdair. 1990. *Three Rival Versions of Moral Enquiry: Encyclopedia, Genealogy, and Tradition.* Notre Dame, IN: University of Notre Dame Press.

Meisel A.; Snyder, L.; and Quill, T. American College of Physicians and American Society of Internal Medicine End-of-Life Care Consensus Panel. 2000. "Seven Legal Barriers to End-of-Life Care: Myths, Realities, and Grains of Truth." *Journal of the American Medical Association* 284(19): 2495–2501.

Moreno, Jonathan D. 1995. *Deciding Together: Bioethics and Moral Consensus.* New York: Oxford University Press.

Murray, Thomas H. 1996. *The Worth of a Child.* Berkeley: University of California Press.

Nelson, Hilde L., and Nelson, James L. 1995. *The Patient in the Family: An Ethics of Medicine and Families.* New York: Routledge.

Nelson, James L. 1994. "Routine Organ Donation: A Communitarian Organ Procurement Policy." *Responsive Community: Rights and Responsibilities* 4(3): 63–68.

Pellegrino, Edmund D., and Thomasma, David C. 1993. *The Virtues in Medical Practice.* New York: Oxford University Press.

Rawls, John. 1971. *A Theory of Justice.* Cambridge, MA: Belknap Press.

Rawls, John. 1993. *Political Liberalism.* New York: Columbia University Press.

Sandel, Michael. 1982. *Liberalism and the Limits of Justice.* New York: Cambridge University Press.

Taylor, Charles. 1989. *Sources of the Self: The Making of Modern Identity.* Cambridge, MA: Harvard University Press.

Walzer, Michael. 1983. *Spheres of Justice: A Defense of Pluralism and Equality.* New York: Basic Books.

Wolfe, Alan. 1998. *One Nation, After All: What Middle-Class Americans Really Think About God, Country, Family, Racism, Welfare, Immigration, Homosexuality, Work, the Right, the Left, and Each Other.* New York: Viking.

Yankelovich, Daniel. 1991. *Coming to Public Judgment: Making Democracy Work in a Complex World.* Syracuse, NY: Syracuse University Press.

Yankelovich, Daniel. 1999. *The Magic of Dialogue: Transforming Conflict into Cooperation.* New York: Simon & Schuster.

# COMPASSIONATE LOVE

• • •

Compassionate love describes attitudes toward and service for others, motivated by a desire for the good of the other. It includes caring for, valuing, and respecting the person so loved. The combination of the two words "compassionate" and "love" highlights features in both words: this combination describes sympathy towards the other, in a way that is caring, respectful, and appropriately emotionally engaged, which leads to appropriate action in service of the other person. Compassionate love can operate through the relief of suffering, but also through acknowledging life's full possibilities and making space for each human being to reach his or her potential. Compassionate love encourages fullness of life in the other. By the early twenty-first century, compassionate love was also bolstered by scientific research and incorporated into a social science model. It provides a sound concept to guide action benefiting those who are in need, in various situations. Compassionate love is a valuable quality to bring to the care of those who are sick, and would be beneficial to include in treatment, care, and decision making.

## Definitional Issues

Some of the most noble human actions are those that express compassionate love. A person acting with compassionate love perceives the suffering, needs, or potential of another, and chooses to act in ways that can better the condition of the other, placing the other's needs in higher priority. There are other moments when one sets aside selfish needs for those of others, when one expresses to others, by words or actions, that they are of value. This occurs in both professional and personal relationships. To contribute to a better understanding of the concept, some definitional points are helpful. Important features of compassionate love include:

(1) free choice;
(2) some degree of cognitive understanding of the situation;
(3) some understanding of self;
(4) fundamentally valuing the other;
(5) openness and receptivity; and
(6) a response of the heart (heart is here defined as "core," where emotions and cognition integrate).

The particular nature of individual personalities, social setting, cultural setting, genetic predisposition, and other factors limit the freedom of individuals. This makes up the substrate, the basic starting situation, in which individuals begin to act with compassionate love. This starting point is different for each person, and situations in which action takes place differ as well.

The full expression of compassionate love towards those who are ill relies on appropriate motive. Although helpful behaviors are good and useful, and can contribute to the well-being of another, motives focused more on the self than on the other can decrease the positive effect on the person being served, as well as on the moral growth of the individual giving the love. There are many attitudes that can diminish motives, such that they are less likely to result in

compassionate love being fully expressed. These include a variety of possible needs or wants for the self: guilt, fear, needs for love and success, fears of failure, desire to claim the upper hand, reputation. Motives are usually mixed, but when self-centered needs predominate, compassionate love cannot be fully expressed.

## Research Model

Research specifically on compassionate love is needed in order to determine how best to foster this quality in people's lives, and to assess the particular impact of this quality in the care of the sick. Results from research can help to give appropriate priority to this quality in the training of healthcare providers, and in the settings and circumstances provided for those who are sick. In order to do adequate research on compassionate love, it is important to clearly articulate the various essential components, the conditions that might foster and those that might impede its expression, and to develop methodologies for assessment. There are over fifty large research projects specifically gathering data on this topic, some in healthcare settings.

Figure 1 illustrates a research model that has shown promise in this area. It starts with the substrates discussed previously. Given those starting points, as one encounters a specific person in a specific situation, one must make a decision to act (shown centrally in the figure), and a motive drives that decision. Motive is particularly hard to research, but there are some ways to begin to investigate it, such as experimental models (especially those from economics and social psychology), implicit-explicit models, observational studies with multiple actions, insightful self-report, and neural imaging. When motives for self outweigh those for others, or there is an inappropriate action given the various factors to be considered, the result is frequently negative for the person being served. Good actions can also emerge from motives not full of compassionate love, such as the motive to look good in the eyes of others or to feel needed, but ultimately the feedback of repeating these kinds of behaviors on the moral development of the healthcare provider can be detrimental. It is also possible that the more self-centered, condescending, or less respectful motive is noticed by the sick person, and care is not as effective. These kinds of motives can also adversely affect discernment of appropriate care for the sick person.

In the center of the model is both motive and discernment. Compassionate love fully expressed is not just good intentions, but doing what is really good for the other. This kind of discernment occurs continually in healthcare settings. Short-term distress may be necessary to serve the longer-term interests of a sick person. Weighing the relative

**FIGURE 1**

**Research Model for Expression of Compassionate Love**

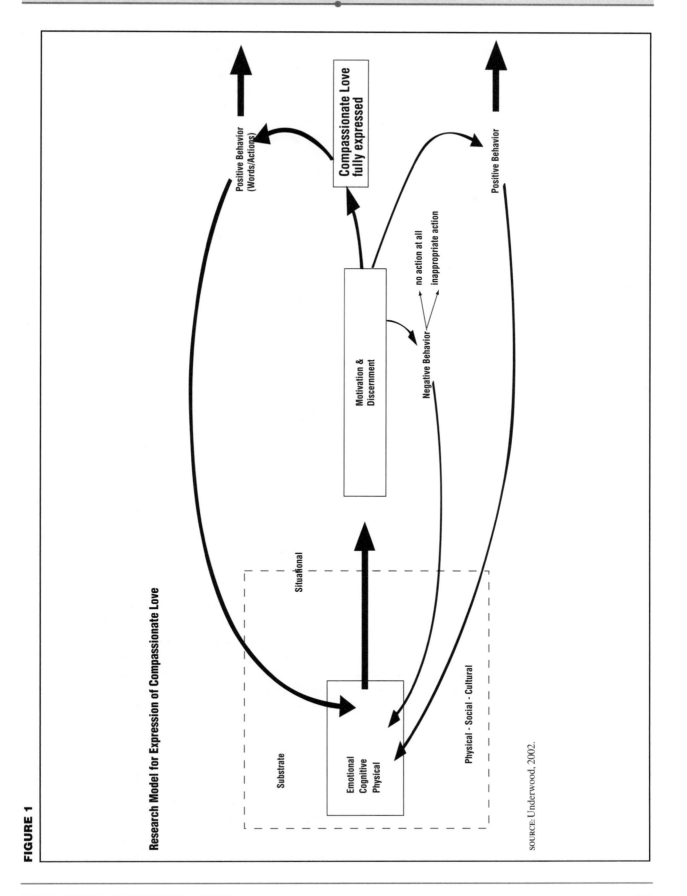

SOURCE: Underwood, 2002.

needs of others, including appropriate care for self, is also critical to good discernment leading to effective actions.

## Revised "Professional Distance"

Compassionate love is not the same as romantic love, familial love, or affection, although it can accompany these other forms of love and blend with them. The professional in a healthcare setting needs to avoid becoming too attached to the patient, and compassionate love allows for this. In fact, one critical aspect of compassionate love is that it is not a "need love," the kind of love that focuses on the needs of the person giving love. In its focus on the needs of the other, compassionate love's non-attachment is very harmonious with the concept of "professional distance," but actually can be more satisfying to both the patient and healthcare provider: it enables an emotional component to be appropriately engaged, if that is called for in the specific setting.

## Improving Well-Being and Health

In the United States and many other medical healthcare systems, a fee for service operating basis, or fee for time, results primarily in action from duty and obligation. However, there is leeway even within this operating system that provides opportunity to "go the extra mile for the patient," or engage in compassionate caring for the sick person.

Initial research has shown that empathy, valuing the patient, and giving the patient a sense that he or she is understood can be powerful factors in contributing to improvements in health outcomes, both through increases in adherence to regimens and more direct effects. Ongoing research is exploring whether increasing compassionate love on the part of the healthcare provider can improve patient outcomes.

It is generally acknowledged that there exists a placebo effect in medical treatments, such that placebos, usually inert substances, are included in most major clinical trials; the various constituents of this effect are currently unknown. Conditioning, optimism, improved self-efficacy, and natural regression to the mean are some of the most frequently cited mechanisms, but the role of the patient-provider relationship on outcomes is just beginning to be explored fully as a part of the placebo effect. Compassionate love is one of the components patients report as being important to them: being valued, feeling understood, feeling cared for, having a provider that goes beyond mere duty. This attitude of the healthcare provider can encourage the sick person to better adhere to medication regimes, and with a more positive attitude toward themselves, exert better efforts

towards self-care and preventive measures. There may also be additional effects on health.

The therapeutic relationship is important for the person who is ill, as has long been asserted in psychotherapy. From the ill person's point of view, feeling valued, cared about, and understood is important, and this works synergistically with the actual treatment—even in treatment for physical illness. This kind of care also can contribute significantly to the well-being of the ill person in areas where health cannot be significantly improved, such as chronic progressive illness and end of life care. This is not a minor issue for healthcare in the twenty-first century context of a continually aging population, and extensive chronic diseases.

## Effects on the Healthcare Provider or Administrator

As described in the model (Figure 1), various substrate factors affect the ability to give compassionate love. Supportive factors can be provided by the healthcare organizational structure, cultural setting, family, religious background, relationships, and others in the healthcare organization. Support from these sources helps to avoid the burnout problem that can occur when one's work focuses continually on those in need. Supportive elements can provide the strength needed to sustain those who care for others.

Outside of the work setting, social relationships, community involvement, family, and religious institutions encourage the healthcare provider's ability and desire to act with compassionate love. Many religions and particular social micro-cultures value this quality, and the nesting of the impetus to act within a religious or social context is useful, as it can provide an infrastructure and additional reinforcement for attitudes and actions.

One who gives compassionate love is also significantly affected by feedback from the one helped. When a good balance (see Figure 2) exists as decisions are made, and the motivation is well grounded, giving compassionate love fully can be satisfying and strengthening to the one who gives it. Feedback from patients can provide a real, positive input for this kind of work, and the ability to express this quality and engage the self more fully in care can be satisfying and add to one's own well-being. This can enable the healthcare provider or administrator to gain more joy from their job.

## Compassionate Love within the Social Network

Social support can contribute positively to a person's health. Compassionate love is nested within social relationships, and it is not only the healthcare provider who improves health and quality of life, but also people within the sick person's social support network. This idea is central to providing healthcare systems and healthcare that value and nurture supportive relationships. Although material support in and of itself is important, scientific literature continually illustrates the value of emotional support. The concept of compassionate love as a contribution to quality of life and well-being can be particularly powerful, and in 2003 is being studied in a variety of social contexts, including a World Health Organization study of contributors to quality of life.

Both the giving and receiving of support can improve well-being and quality of life. Those who are sick generally do not want pity; they want others to help them and understand them and care about them, but also, unless totally incapacitated, they want to give to others, and want to feel of use. One study of pain patients conducted by Frank Keefe, Ph.D at Duke University, is examining the use of a "loving kindness meditation," a Buddhist-inspired practice that has patients dwell on compassionate love for themselves, close friends, those they have trouble with, and the whole world, to help those with pain experience less suffering. When sick people are enabled and encouraged to have good relationships with those around them, they can give to others within the constraints of their situation and this can be an additional positive outcome.

## Making Healthcare Decisions

During a National Institutes of Health conference with the goal of setting a research agenda for end of life care in November of 2001, the physicians and nurses involved in care for patients and their families, the qualitative researchers, the economists, and those representing hospice and nursing homes identified a central theme: the importance of what the patient values, and what society values, as decisions needed to be made. Compassionate love, which includes valuing the other fully, action and attitude driven by other-centered motivations, and clear discernment as to the most caring action, can effectively guide healthcare decisions and policies. In a study of over four thousand people from various cultures and religions worldwide, conducted by the World Health Organization, and presented by Kate O'Connell at the International Quality of Life meeting in Amsterdam in November of 2001, it was found that issues of being loved, cared for, and accepted contribute significantly to overall quatiy of life, over and above basic health indicators.

Compassionate love requires that decisions be considered through a lens that views the other as having significant value. Decision-making based in compassionate love also can include various more consciously-articulated ways of

**FIGURE 2**

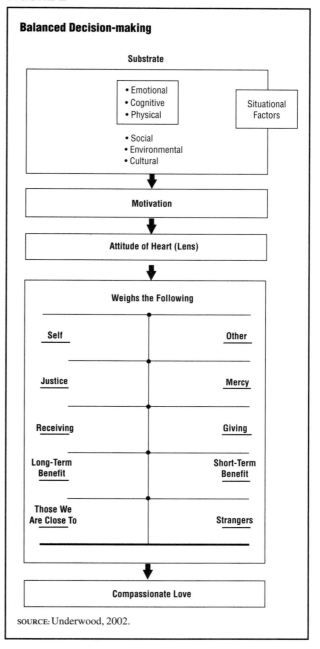

SOURCE: Underwood, 2002.

weighing competing factors (Figure 2). For example, the immediate desires of the patient may not be in the patient's long term interest, and therefore immediate relief of suffering is not always the most compassionately loving act. Decision-making that incorporates these qualities and complexities into the process can result in better decisions for both the cared-for and the caregiver. By including compassionate love in decision-making, the caregiver can better address the needs of the patient and enable a fuller expression of the humanity of the healthcare provider.

## Conclusion

As a guide for action in healthcare settings, compassionate love can lift the care of the sick from a duty to be carried out to satisfying caring with joy. Attitudes toward and care for those who are ill are enriched by taking a respectful, caring, understanding approach that values each individual. The sick person can benefit substantially from this, and various social and behavioral sciences are contributing to a body of literature demonstrating how compassionate love positively affects health. Structural changes in healthcare environments and payment models need to adopt the value of compassionate love in order to improve care.

LYNN G. UNDERWOOD

SEE ALSO: *Buddhism, Bioethics in; Care; Emotions; Feminism; Hinduism, Bioethics in; Human Dignity; Human Nature; Medical Codes and Oaths; Narrative; Responsibility; Transhumanism and Posthumanism; Virtue and Character*

### BIBLIOGRAPHY

Buckwalter, Kathleen C., ed. 2002. "End-of-life Research: Focus on Older Populations: Papers from a National Institutes of Health Workshop." *The Gerontologist* special issue 42(3): 4–134.

Carmel, Sara, and Glick, Shimon. 1996. "Compassionate-Empathic Physicians." *Social Science and Medicine* 43(8): 1253–1261.

Cohen, Sheldon; Underwood, Lynn; and Gottlieb, Benjamin, eds. 2000. *Measuring Social Support and Intervention Development: A Guide for Health and Social Scientists.* New York: Oxford University Press.

de Wit, Han F. 1991. *Contemplative Psychology.* Pittsburgh: Duquesne University Press.

Di Blasi, Zelda; Harkness, Elaine; Ernst, Edzard; Georgiou, Amanda; and Kleijnen, Jos. 2001. "Influence of Context Effects on Health Outcomes: A Systematic Review." *Lancet* 357: 757–762.

Dixon, Michael, and Sweeney, Kieran. 2000. *The Human Effect in Medicine: Theory, Research and Practice.* Abingdon, UK: Radcliffe Medical Press.

Lewis, Clive Stapleton. 1991 (1960). *The Four Loves.* New York: Harcourt Brace Jovanovich.

Mermann, Alan C. 1993. "Love in the Clinical Setting." *Humane Medicine* 9(4): 268–273.

Mitteness, Linda S. 2001. "Compassion in Health Care: An Anthropological Lens." *Park Ridge Center Bulletin* (March-April): 5–6.

O'Connell, Kate. 2001. "World Health Organization Measure of Subjective Quality of Life: Inclusion of Values, Meaning and Spiritual Aspects of Life: Instrument Development and Testing," presentation November 7, 2001. Amsterdam, Netherlands: International Society of Quality of Life Research.

Redelmaier, Donald; Molin, Jean-Pierre; and Tibshirani, Robert. 1995. "A Randomized Trial of Compassionate Care for the Homeless in an Emergency Department." *Lancet* 345: 1131–1134.

Saxena, Shekar; Underwood, Lynn G.; and O'Connell, Kate. 2001. "Spiritual, Religious and Personal Belief Aspects of Quality of Life: A Cross-Cultural Study," presentation. Amsterdam: International Society of Quality of Life Research.

Sen, Amartya. 1987. *On Ethics and Economics.* Oxford: Blackwell.

Squier, Roger. 1990. "A Model of Empathic Understanding and Adherence to Treatment Regimens in Practitioner-Patient Relationships." *Social Science Medicine* 30: 325–333.

Sulmasy, Daniel. 1997. *The Healer's Calling.* Mahwah, NJ: Paulist Press.

Underwood, Lynn G. 1995. "A Working Model of Health: Spirituality and Religiousness as Resources: Applications for Persons with Disability." *Journal of Religion, Disability and Health.* 3(3): 51–71.

Underwood, Lynn G. 2002. "The Human Experience of Compassionate Love: Conceptual Mapping and Data from Selected Studies." In *Altruism and Altruistic Love: Science, Philosophy, and Religion in Dialogue.* Oxford, UK: Oxford University Press.

Vacek, Edward Collins. 1994. *Love, Human and Divine: The Heart of Christian Ethics.* Washington, D.C.: Georgetown University Press.

Vanier, Jean. 1998. *Becoming Human.* Mahwah, NJ: Paulist Press.

# COMPETENCE

• • •

Competence is a necessary condition before a physician can accept a patient's treatment consent or refusal. Competence confers decision-making authority on those who are competent, while disenfranchising those who are not (Beauchamp). A determination of patient competence promotes respect for self-determination as well as patient participation in healthcare and other decision making. In most nonemergency situations, those who are legally competent may consent to or refuse healthcare. A patient maintained for years on outpatient hemodialysis, for example, may be allowed to terminate hemodialysis, resulting in death, if the patient decides that he or she can no longer tolerate the stress of the procedure (Neu and Kjellstrand). And based upon religious reasons, a Jehovah's Witness may even refuse a blood transfusion that would otherwise save his or her life. In contrast, the consent or refusal of those who are legally incompetent or clinically incapacitated need not be respected. A psychotic woman who refuses to have a cardiac pacemaker inserted because she believes that others could then monitor and control her activities would not be permitted to refuse this lifesustaining surgical procedure. Competence is usually not a relevant issue in healthcare emergencies, when treatment delay would be substantially harmful to the patient.

Competence and autonomy are often conflated, although their meanings are quite distinguishable (Beauchamp). Competence allows a person to exercise his or her autonomy. One must be autonomous to be competent, yet competent persons may act nonautonomously when, for example, compelled to do so by another person. Further, an autonomous person may act incompetently (e.g., a professional negligent at work).

This entry considers some of the issues in defining, determining, and assessing competence, as well as some of the applications of competence to the field of mental healthcare.

## Definitions

Generically, "competence" means simply the ability to perform a particular task (Beauchamp), although it has often been used loosely in several senses. In healthcare contexts, competence is the capacity to make autonomous healthcare decisions (Morreim). In most accounts of competence, competence is specific to the task or issue, since a person may be able to perform one task but not another. Few people are globally competent or incompetent. Since one's abilities change over time, in either direction, competence is also specific to time. Abilities may also be a function of the conditions or the situation in which they are tested or the person who tests them.

Competencies, of course, relate to all areas of function (Grisso). While competence to consent to healthcare or research is of primary concern in the present context, issues are often raised about a person's ability to work, manage personal finances, make a contract, write a will, live independently, drive a car, marry and divorce, parent a child, or testify in court. In legal contexts, competence questions arise in civil actions as well as in criminal litigation (competence to stand trial, commit a crime, enter a plea, or be sentenced) (Bonnie). Legal competencies implicate past decision making (e.g., competence to write a will), present decision

making (e.g., competence to stand trial), or future decision making (e.g., competence to manage one's financial affairs).

A person's competence may be questioned in more than one area. In the case of a mother with cancer and a psychotic depressive disorder who is separated from her husband, for example, questions may arise about her capacity to parent her children, manage her finances, and consent to medical or psychiatric care. If she were employed, questions may arise about her ability to function at work if she failed to meet deadlines or otherwise fulfill her job duties due to a medical or psychiatric disorder. Her or her husband's attorney may question her ability to consult with her attorney and participate in the divorce litigation.

This contextualized, decision-specific notion of competence may be contrasted with a more generalized conception that reflects the general legal and moral autonomy enjoyed by most adults in contemporary Western cultures (Wear). Many more adults are considered competent under the general conception than the task-specific one; therefore, establishing that a person is incompetent is more difficult under the former than the latter.

"Incompetence" has come to mean the loss in court of a person's legal right to function in some particular area. Such a narrow legal definition of competence or incompetence contrasts with the more common clinical use of incompetence according to which a person has a legal right to function but is unable to do so. Clinical and legal competence may not correspond. An elderly, demented person, for example, may have the legal right to drive a car or make his or her own healthcare decisions but may no longer be substantially able to do so. Similarly, an adolescent may not be legally competent to consent to healthcare but may be clinically or functionally able to do so.

The increasingly prevalent view is that individuals have various specific abilities or capacities as well as incapacities, each along a continuum. A person is considered incapacitated when the person is no longer able to perform that specific function and incompetent when a court has so ruled. Legally, there is a presumption of competence, which may be overcome when the court is presented with adequate evidence of incapacitation. In the clinical literature, however, competence refers either to an individual's capacities (a descriptive definition) or to whether that individual's particular capacities are sufficient to render legal decision-making authority to him or her (a threshold definition).

Finally, although competence usually refers to a person's abilities, it may also refer to his or her actions or behavior (Beauchamp). For example, a person of general competence may autonomously choose to act incompetently in a given situation (e.g., intentionally fail an examination).

## Managing Incompetence

Because functional or decision-making capacities occur on a continuum and because a person's capacities can be expected to fluctuate over time, in most cases a clinician need not be resigned to accept a patient as permanently incapacitated. The clinician frequently has opportunities to enhance the person's functional or decision-making capacity. Hearing aids, eyeglasses, psychotropic medication, counseling and psychotherapy, and specific behavioral training in the area of incapacity are examples of remedial efforts that can be made to improve a person's capacity. When such efforts fail, disposition of those who are incapacitated is a complex matter and varies with the context in question. In a case where life-saving treatment may be needed, the clinician may have to obtain an adjudication of legal incompetence in order to treat an incompetent refusing patient.

Although competence is a necessary precondition to respecting patient choice, incompetence is not a sufficient condition to overriding it, contrary to much clinical and lay understanding. The clinician may wish to, and often should, respect a person's preferences even if the person is legally incompetent or functionally incapacitated. The clinician may ask a young boy with which parent he prefers to live following his parents' divorce; the clinician probably will ask an elderly, demented woman whom she prefers to manage her estate should the appointment of a legal guardian be authorized.

Before intervening over the person's objection, the clinician needs to specifically assess the risks, benefits, and alternatives; this includes an evaluation of the potential harms of a proposed intervention to the person. Overriding treatment refusals, whether by a healthcare professional, family member, or court, ethically and legally requires evidence that (1) such treatment would benefit the patient (the "best interests" test); (2) such treatment would have been the decision of the patient had he or she been able to make the decision (the "substituted judgment" test); or (3) the patient had provided some previous direction or instruction about the treatment in question ("expressed interest" test). The test of substitute decision making varies with the decision, the decision maker, and the legal jurisdiction. Use of the substituted-judgment or the expressed interest test, in contrast to the best-interests test, better respects the person's autonomy and self-determination.

## Competence Criteria

There is no international clinical, legal, philosophical, or ethical consensus about competence criteria or standards,

and many are in use. In other words, there is no agreement about the threshold of decision-making or functional capacity necessary to consider a person legally or morally competent. In a given case, there may be wide consensus among clinicians, legal professionals, and ethicists that a particular person is, or is not, competent in some respect; however, disagreement is likely in many cases. In part, this derives from the fact that competence determinations are not essentially factual, objective, or empirical matters but rather are value-laden judgments about the relative importance of autonomy and beneficence to the person, as assessed by the clinician or others. Competence is typically inferred from the person's behavior and thinking rather than observed directly, and evaluators may differ in their judgment of the person's competence. Such differences about the person's competence occur in part due to evaluators' varying perceptions of the person's values or of the person's rationality. Under the most common view, competence is not a fixed property of an individual applicable to all decisions and all potential risks; rather, competence is a context-dependent, decision-specific, interpersonal process (Buchanan and Brock; Drane).

Criteria for competence involve whether the person can make a choice, communicate that choice, understand relevant information about the choice and its alternatives, and rationally manipulate information about the choice and its alternatives (Appelbaum and Grisso). The person must be able to apply the relevant information about a prospective decision to his or her own case rather than in the abstract or as applied to someone else.

The influential U.S. President's Commission for the Study of Ethical Problems in Medicine and Biomedical and Behavioral Research adopted a standard of capacity that requires (1) possession of a set of values and goals; (2) the ability to communicate and to understand information; and (3) the ability to reason and to deliberate about one's choices (U.S. President's Commission). This standard emphasizes the process of reasoning or decision making rather than the particular outcome of the decision. A competence standard that focuses upon the outcome of the decision can be faulted for granting greater priority to the values of the person assessing the patient's competence than to the values of the patient.

A similar definition of competence is offered by the Canadian province of Ontario: "Mentally competent means having the ability to understand the subject-matter in respect of which consent is requested and able to appreciate the consequences of giving or withholding consent" (Ontario Ministry of Health). This "appreciation" component, however, involves emotional rather than strictly cognitive considerations, and broadens the competence standard.

As noted by the U.S. President's Commission, assessment of the individual's current and previous personal values is an essential component of evaluating competence. Obtaining a values history for the individual provides critical information about the person's past major life decisions relevant to the present decision making. Judgments about a person's competence must be individualized according to his or her attitudes and values history rather than reflect only the person's knowledge, skills, and cognitive capacities.

It is unrealistic to expect that competence criteria are, or will remain, fixed over time. Competence criteria are likely to evolve as society seeks to resolve the conflict between the competing principles of respect for autonomy and concern for the person's well-being.

SLIDING SCALE OF COMPETENCE CRITERIA. The predominant approach to selecting competence criteria, at least with regard to competence to consent to healthcare, depends on the actual decision at issue. In this scheme, named the "sliding scale," the criteria for competence vary with the particular decision and its risks and benefits. As the risks of the proposed healthcare increase or as the benefits to the proposed healthcare decrease, more capacity is required for the patient to be considered competent to consent to the healthcare (Drane; Roth et al.). For example, it is less difficult to decide to consent to a course of conventional antibiotic medication for a urinary tract infection than a course of experimental chemotherapy for stomach cancer, and less capacity should be required to do so. Likewise, more capacity is required for the patient to be considered competent to refuse healthcare when its risks decrease or its benefits increase.

Although the sliding-scale approach to competence criteria is commonly used in healthcare decision making, some problems accompany its use. Given the strong bias of healthcare professionals—and society—in favor of treatment, one concern is that professionals will manipulate or selectively use those competence criteria that result in labeling competent someone who consents to healthcare, while labeling incompetent someone who refuses care. Another concern of the variable standard approach is that, counterintuitively, a patient could be considered competent to consent to a particular intervention but incompetent to refuse that same intervention (Buchanan and Brock). This may occur because refusing healthcare is more complicated than consenting to it, but here too a protreatment bias is evident.

## Competence Assessments

Clinicians frequently make informal judgments about a patient's competence in their daily work; but some cases, such as treatment refusals or consents by questionably competent patients, necessitate formal, detailed assessments. Competence assessments should focus on the specific area of function in question. Assessments of global or general competence are unlikely to adequately respond to the presenting question. Among the procedural considerations in conducting competence assessments, the time and place of examination and the need for reexamination are especially important (Weiner and Wettstein). These assessments sometimes use written structured or formal assessment inventories of functioning, observational functional assessments (e.g., observing a patient grocery shopping and preparing a meal), psychological testing, or formal psychiatric interviews. History taking and collateral reports from third-party informants such as family, friends, and other healthcare personnel can be valuable additions to individual contact with the person being assessed. The examiner pays particular attention to eliciting information about the patient's decision-making history and the values he or she has placed on personal autonomy, healthcare, disability, and death. Consultations with colleagues or second opinions may also be helpful to the examiner in difficult cases. In general medical hospitals, competence assessments are conducted initially by nonpsychiatric physicians; if necessary, psychiatric consultants are called to assist in the evaluation.

Competence assessments raise many problematic clinical issues including denial of illness; subtle forms of incapacity; impact of elevated or depressed mood on decision-making capacity; fluctuating mental status (due to intermittent treatment compliance, the natural course of the disorder, or side effects of treatment); treatment refusals based on religious reasons; lack of information about the patient, including personal values and goals or history of treatment refusals; lack of formal staff training to do competence assessments; and disagreements among staff about the appropriate competence criteria or threshold. Typically, competence is not challenged, investigated, or formally assessed in clinical practice until a patient refuses treatment or is noncompliant with it.

## Competence and Mental Healthcare

The presence of a mental disorder does not automatically negate the presumption of a person's competence. Although some severely mental ill persons are indeed incapacitated in many areas of their functioning, most mentally ill persons have only some discrete areas of decision-making incapacity, often confined to episodes of their illness. A paranoid delusional patient who denies that he is mentally ill, for example, may be unable to rationally decide whether or not to consent to antipsychotic medication while he is mentally ill but may have adequate decision-making ability to consent to treatment for diabetes and heart disease. In such a case, the content of the patient's paranoid delusions would be irrelevant to the patient's diabetes and heart disease, and the patient would not deny the fact of his medical illnesses. A patient in a manic episode may be unable to manage his finances because he will rapidly dissipate them, but his decision-making capacity will return as the episode ends. Subtle forms of decision-making incapacity can also arise from mildly altered mood states (depression, hopelessness, anxiety, euphoria), from cognitive dysfunction (impairment in memory or attention from head injury), or from personality traits (guilt, self-punishment, feelings of worthlessness).

COMPETENCE TO REFUSE PSYCHOTROPIC MEDICATION. In contrast to admission to a medical-surgical hospital, admission to a psychiatric hospital may be accomplished by voluntary or involuntary means. In either facility, however, there may be uncertainty about the patient's ability to consent to voluntary hospitalization. Patients who are demented or seriously depressed or psychotic often have difficulty understanding that they are ill, need treatment, or should be hospitalized. They may have difficulty comprehending the risks and benefits of treatment and hospitalization. Nevertheless, decisions about the person's ability to consent to voluntary hospitalization precede, and differ from, decisions about the person's ability, once hospitalized, to consent to treatment with medication.

Managing a person's refusal of psychotropic medication (e.g., antipsychotic or antidepressant medication), once he or she has been hospitalized, has been one of the most controversial issues in mental healthcare in recent years. Before the 1980s, many rejected the notion of a psychiatric patient's right to refuse medication, suggesting that the purpose of psychiatric hospitalization would be defeated if patients were permitted to refuse treatment with medication (Appelbaum, 1988). In part, the controversy about involuntary treatment of psychiatric inpatients with medication arose from the nature and effects of psychotropic medication. Psychotropic medications have been viewed somewhat inaccurately as powerful and dangerous substances whose use is akin to "mind control." Their risks, whether short-term dry mouth and constipation or long-term involuntary movement disorders, relative to their benefits, the treatment of the mental disorder, have been greatly exaggerated, at least by many attorneys and courts (Gutheil and Appelbaum).

Once patients enter psychiatric hospitals, especially on an involuntary basis by court order, they sometimes refuse recommended treatment with psychotropic medication, particularly antipsychotic medication. Patients refuse treatment based on problems in the physician-patient relationship, such as rebelliousness towards authority figures and reality-based side effects of medication (e.g., dry mouth, constipation, weight gain, restlessness), or most relevant in the present context, symptoms of the patient's illness, such as a delusional belief that the medication is poison. Decisions about hospitalizing a person involuntarily differ from those about medicating that person involuntarily once hospitalized; the former are largely a function of the person's future risk of violence to self or others due to a mental disorder, while the latter usually depend upon the person's ability to make decisions about accepting medication or his or her best interests. An involuntarily hospitalized patient, even one committed by a court, is not necessarily deemed unable to consent to medication. In most cases, a person who has been involuntarily hospitalized does not lose the legal right to object to or to refuse medication.

Voluntarily hospitalized patients who refuse medication for whatever reason may not be medicated involuntarily, except briefly in emergency situations. It is argued that patient autonomy regarding treatment refusal should be respected despite the consequences of continued illness, hospitalization, and incapacity. This legal right to refuse medication is based on the patient's right to free speech and thought, to freedom from bodily intrusion, the right to bodily integrity, a ban on cruel punishment, and the right to autonomy and self-determination.

Nevertheless, involuntarily hospitalized patients who refuse medication may sometimes be medicated involuntarily in nonemergency situations, as well as briefly in emergencies. Many states in the United States use a judicial model for these cases in which forced medication of involuntarily hospitalized patients may be accomplished only after a judicial hearing and court determination that the patient is incompetent to refuse the mediation because of the mental illness (Weiner and Wettstein). A substitute decision maker is sometimes appointed by the court to determine whether the patient should be compelled to take medication. This is the same procedure that would be followed if the physician sought involuntary surgery (e.g., amputation of a gangrenous extremity) on the patient. In contrast, in some U.S. states and in some Canadian provinces, the attending physician or a medical or administrative review panel decides whether or not to override the patient's refusal; the patient may then appeal the physician or panel's decision to involuntarily medicate to a court (Weiner and Wettstein; Ontario

Ministry of Health). In England, the Mental Health Act of 1983 permits the treating physician to authorize medication for up to three months to an incompetently refusing, involuntarily hospitalized patient (section 56); after that, a second physician opinion is needed to continue the involuntary treatment (section 58) (Appelbaum, 1985). In this nonjudicial model, the patient's decision-making capacity about medication as assessed by the attending physician may still be the most important factor in the disposition of the case. However, the U.S. Supreme Court has held that decision-making capacity is not relevant to determining whether prisoners should be medicated involuntarily with psychotropic drugs (*Washington v. Harper*).

According to empirical data about the right to refuse psychotropic medication, the judicial-review model, using a formal incompetence declaration, carries substantial fiscal costs, given the delays inherent in obtaining the required court hearing. It also involves prolonged periods of nontreatment pending the hearing, which often results in injuries to the patient, other patients, and staff (Ciccone et al.; Hoge et al.). Few courts ultimately grant the patient a right to refuse medication.

COMPETENCE FOR EXECUTION. According to U.S. law civil or criminal litigants must be legally competent before they can bring suit or have suit brought against them. In criminal law, defendants must be competent to stand trial, plead guilty, be sentenced, or be executed before those proceedings can occur.

Executing a person who is considered incompetent (i.e., "insane") at the time of execution, as opposed to at the time of the crime, has been ruled unconstitutional by the U.S. Supreme Court (*Ford* v. *Wainwright*). Execution in such cases offends humanity, has no deterrent value to others, and offers no retribution to the condemned person. The courts, however, have yet to articulate a competence standard by which to adjudicate a death-row inmate as incompetent (Winick).

The courts have not yet decided whether, once death-row inmates have been found incompetent, the state may involuntarily medicate them to restore competence and then execute them (*Louisiana* v. *Perry*). Such an eventuality places the treating psychiatrist, who ethically must not participate in an execution, in a difficult dilemma: Medicate the inmate to relieve suffering, which leads to the inmate's death, or do not medicate the inmate, which spares the inmate's life but fails to reduce suffering (Heilbrun et al.). Only automatic commutation of an incompetent death-row inmate to life in prison would definitively resolve the matter.

## Conclusion

Whether in healthcare, financial, legal, or any other area of decision making, the stakes for both persons and professionals in competence definitions are substantial. Identifying and labeling someone as incompetent can be stigmatizing and deprives the person of self-determination. Legal and healthcare delivery systems are then confronted with, and disrupted by, the need for surrogate decision making for the incapacitated or incompetent person. On the other hand, failure to protect the incapacitated person from making erroneous and harmful decisions (e.g., refusing necessary medical care) may not honor the person's best interests. The question then is when and how to respect people's choices and maximize their decision-making autonomy while protecting them from their own harmful choices (Drane). In most cases in the healthcare system, clinicians agree that the person should, or should not, be considered competent, even if there is no universal consensus on how much rationality and understanding are sufficient for the person to be considered legally competent and granted authority to decide for him- or herself. Still, there are other cases in which judgments about the person's decision-making capacity are problematic, and clinicians, administrators, patients, families, and the courts become involved in emotionally charged disputes about how to manage the person's medical care. Such cases are unlikely to abate in the future as long as our society continues to value, and attempts to balance, autonomy and beneficence.

ROBERT M. WETTSTEIN (1995)
BIBLIOGRAPHY REVISED

SEE ALSO: *Advance Directives and Advance Care Planning; Aging and the Aged: Healthcare and Research Issues; Autonomy; Informed Consent; Law and Bioethics; Mental Illness; Patients' Rights; Pediatrics, Adolescents; Professional-Patient Relationship; Research Policy: Subjects; Responsibility; Sexism; Surrogate Decision-Making*

### BIBLIOGRAPHY

Appelbaum, Paul S. 1985. "England's New Commitment Law." *Hospital and Community Psychiatry* 36(7): 705–706, 713.

Appelbaum, Paul S. 1988. "The Right to Refuse Treatment with Antipsychotic Medications: Retrospect and Prospect." *American Journal of Psychiatry* 145(4): 413–419.

Appelbaum, Paul S. 1998. "Ought We to Require Emotional Capacity as Part of Decisional Competence?" *Kennedy Institute of Ethics Journal* 8(4): 377–387.

Applebaum, Paul S. 1999. "Competence and Consent to Research: A Critique of the Recommendations of the National Bioethics Advisory Commission." *Account Resolution* 7(2–4): 265–276

Appelbaum, Paul S., and Grisso, Thomas. 1988. "Assessing Patients' Capacities to Consent to Treatment." *New England Journal of Medicine* 319(25): 1635–1638.

Beauchamp, Tom L. 1991. "Competence." In *Competency: A Study of Informal Competency Determinations in Primary Care,* pp. 49–78, ed. Mary Ann Gardell Cutter and Earl E. Shelp. Dordrecht, Netherlands: Kluwer.

Berg, Jessica W.; Appelbaum, Paul S.; Parker, Lisa S.; and Lidz, Charles W., eds. 2001. *Informed Consent: Legal Theory and Clinical Practice,* 2nd edition. New York: Oxford University Press.

Bonnie, Richard J. 1992. "The Competence of Criminal Defendants: A Theoretical Reformulation." *Behavioral Sciences and the Law* 10(3): 291–316.

Buchanan, Allen E., and Brock, Dan W. 1989. *Deciding for Others: The Ethics of Surrogate Decision Making.* Cambridge, Eng.: Cambridge University Press.

Buller, T. 2001. "Competence and Risk-Relativity." *Bioethics* 15(2): 93–109

Ciccone, J. Richard; Tokoli, John F.; Gift, Thomas E.; and Clements, Colleen D. 1993. "Medication Refusal and Judicial Activism: A Reexamination of the Effects of the Rivers Decision." *Hospital and Community Psychiatry* 44(4): 555–560.

Drane, James F. 1985. "The Many Faces of Competency." *Hastings Center Report* 15(2): 17–21.

*Ford* v. *Wainwright.* 477 U.S. 399 (1986).

Grisso, Thomas. 1986. *Evaluating Competencies: Forensic Assessments and Instruments.* New York: Plenum.

Grisso, Thomas, and Appelbaum, Paul S. 2000. *Assessing Competence to Consent to Treatment: A Guide for Physicians and Other Health Professionals.* New York: Oxford University Press.

Gutheil, Thomas G., and Appelbaum, Paul S. 1983. "'Mind Control,' 'Synthetic Sanity,' 'Artificial Competence,' and Genuine Confusion: Legally Relevant Effects of Antipsychotic Medication." *Hofstra Law Review* 12: 77–120.

Gutheil, Thomas G., and Bursztajn, Harold. 1986. "Clinicians' Guidelines for Assessing and Presenting Subtle Forms of Patient Incompetence in Legal Settings." *American Journal of Psychiatry* 143(8): 1020–1023.

Heilbrun, Kirk; Radelet, Michael L.; and Dvoskin, Joel. 1992. "The Debate on Treating Individuals Incompetent for Execution." *American Journal of Psychiatry* 149(5): 596–605.

Hoge, Steven K.; Appelbaum, Paul S.; Lawlor, Ted; Beck, James C.; Litman, Robert; Greer, Alexander; Gutheil, Thomas G.; and Kaplan, Eric. 1990. "A Prospective, Multicenter Study of Patients' Refusal of Antipsychotic Medication." *Archives of General Psychiatry* 47(10): 949–956.

*Louisiana* v. *Perry.* 498 U.S. 38 (1990).

Morreim, E. Haavi. 1991. "Competence: At the Intersection of Law, Medicine, and Philosophy." In *Competency: A Study of Informal Competency Determinations in Primary Care,* pp. 93–125, ed. Mary Ann Gardell Cutter and Earl E. Shelp. Dordrecht, Netherlands: Kluwer.

National Bioethics Advisory Commission. 1998. *Research Involving Persons with Mental Disorders That May Affect Decision-Making Capacity Vol I: Report and Recommendations of the National Bioethics Advisory Committee.* Rockville, MD: National Bioethics Advisory Commission.

Neu, Steven, and Kjellstrand, Carl M. 1986. "Stopping Long-Term Dialysis: An Empirical Study of Withdrawal of Life-Supporting Treatment." *New England Journal of Medicine* 314(1): 14–20.

Ontario Ministry of Health. 1987. *Mental Health Act: Revised Statutes of Ontario.* Toronto: Queen's Printer for Ontario.

Roth, Loren H.; Meisel, Alan; and Lidz, Charles W. 1977. "Tests of Competency to Consent to Treatment." *American Journal of Psychiatry* 134(3): 279–284.

U.S. President's Commission for the Study of Ethical Problems in Medicine and Biomedical and Behavioral Research. 1982. *Making Health Care Decisions: A Report on the Ethical and Legal Implications of Informed Consent in the Patient-Practitioner Relationship.* Washington, D.C.: Author.

*Washington* v. *Harper.* 110 S. Ct. 1028 (1990).

Wear, Stephen. 1991. "Patient Freedom and Competence in Health Care." In *Competency: A Study of Informal Competency Determinations in Primary Care,* pp. 227–236, ed. Mary Ann Gardell Cutter and Earl E. Shelp. Dordrecht, Netherlands: Kluwer.

Weiner, Barbara A., and Wettstein, Robert M. 1993. *Legal Issues in Mental Health Care.* New York: Plenum.

Winick, Bruce J. 1992. "Competency to Be Executed: A Therapeutic Jurisprudence Perspective." *Behavioral Sciences and the Law* 10(3): 317–337.

# CONFIDENTIALITY

• • •

Confidentiality has its roots in the human practice of sharing and keeping secrets (Bok). For children, the desire to keep a secret is a manifestation of an emerging sense of self; the desire to share a secret stems from a need to retain or establish intimate relationships with others (Ekstein and Caruth). The willingness to share secrets presupposes an implicit trust or an explicit promise that they will be dept. Keeping and sharing secrets is a more complex social practice among adults. Some adults keep secrets simply to preserve their personal privacy; others may have something illegal or immoral to hide. Some persons do not reveal private thoughts, feelings, or behavior for fear of embarrassment, exploitation, stigmatization, or discrimination. Still others feel a need to disclose secrets to others to help resolve emotional conflicts or seek solutions to problems arising out of interpersonal relationships. The sharing and keeping of secrets among friends, for instance, creates a context in which ethical issues concerning promises, trust, loyalty, and interests of others may come into conflict. For example, I may promise a friend to keep a secret that she feels an urgent need to tell me. She trusts me not to tell anyone else about her revelation. Out of loyalty to my friend, I promise in advance to keep her secret. But I am thrown into a moral conflict when she unexpectedly discloses her impulse and plan to kill a family member who she believes is plotting against her. I realize that my obligations to keep my promise and preserve loyalty and trust conflict with a desire, if not a responsibility, to prevent my friend's harm to herself as well as serious harm to another. Do I preserve confidentiality or protect others? Similar ethical conflicts arise for health professionals and their clients or patients.

The following discussion clarifies the concept of confidentiality and the related ideas of privacy and privileged communication in healthcare settings. The rights of clients/patients and the responsibilities of health professionals to their clients, their professions, and society bring out key ethical issues. Legal regulations both protect and limit confidentiality, sometimes in ways that create ethical conflicts for clients as well as professionals. In healthcare contexts neither absolute protection nor total abandonment of confidentiality is plausible. Yet sometimes it is uncertain where boundaries should be drawn because legitimate interests come into conflict. Personal privacy, professional integrity, effective care, economic considerations, and public health and safety influence both general policies and specific practices concerning confidentiality.

## Conceptual Analysis

Confidentiality is closely related to the broad concept of privacy and the narrower concept of privileged communications. All three concepts share the idea of limiting access of others in certain respects (Gavison; Allen). Privacy refers to limiting access of others to one's body or mind, such as through physical contact or disclosure of thoughts or feelings. The idea of limited access describes privacy in a neutral way. But privacy is closely linked to normative values. Privacy is usually thought to be good; it is something that individuals typically desire to preserve, protect, and control. Thus privacy and a right to privacy are sometimes not clearly distinguished. In law and ethics "privacy" usually refers to privacy rights as well as limited access. Thus, privacy in law is linked to freedom from intrusion by the state or third persons. It may designate a domain of personal decision, usually about important matters such as personal associations, abortion, or bodily integrity.

Confidentiality concerns the communication of private and personal information from one person to another where it is expected that the recipient of the information, such as a health professional, will not ordinarily disclose the confidential information to third persons. In other words, other persons, unless properly authorized, have limited access to confidential information. Confidentiality, like privacy, is valued because it protects individual preferences and rights.

Privileged communications are those confidential communications that the law protects against disclosure in legal settings. Once again, others have limited access to confidential information. A person who has disclosed private information to a spouse or certain professionals (doctor, lawyer, priest, psychotherapist) may restrict his or her testimony in a legal context, subject to certain exceptions (Smith-Bell and Winslade; Weiner and Wettstein).

Privacy and confidentiality are alike in that each stands as a polar opposite to the idea of "public": what is private and confidential is not public. Yet privacy and confidentiality are not the same. Privacy can refer to singular features of persons, such as privacy of thoughts, feelings, or fantasies. Confidentiality always refers to relational contexts involving two or more persons. Privacy can also refer to relational contexts, such as privacy of personal associations or private records. Thus, in this respect the concepts overlap. In many relational contexts the terms "privacy" and "confidentiality" are used interchangeably and sometimes loosely. Professional codes of ethics, for example, often use these terms in this way (Winslade and Ross).

It should be noted, however, that privacy and confidentiality are significantly different in one important respect. Relinquishing personal privacy is a precondition for establishing confidentiality. Confidentiality requires a relationship of at least two persons, one of whom exposes or discloses private data to the other. An expectation of confidentiality arises out of a special relationship between the parties created by their respective roles (doctor-patient, lawyer-client) or by an explicit promise. Confidentiality, as with its linguistic origins (*con* and *fides:* with fidelity), assumes a relationship based on trust or fidelity< Between strangers there is no expectation of trust. Privacy is given up because confidentiality is assured; unauthorized persons are excluded.

Yet confidentiality does not flow simply from the fact that personal or private information is divulged to another. If persons choose to announce their sexual preferences in street-corner speeches, in books, or on billboards, this information, though private in its origin, is not confidential. Confidentiality depends not only on the information, but also on the context of the disclosure as well as on the relationship between the discloser and the recipient of the information. Confidentiality applies to personal, sensitive, sometimes potentially harmful or embarrassing private information disclosed within the confines of a special relationship. It should be noted, however, that the disclosure of private information from client to professional is one-way, unlike other interpersonal confidentiality contexts (Winslade and Ross).

## Rights of Patients/Clients

When clients enter into a healthcare relationship, they relinquish some personal privacy in permitting physical examinations, taking tests, or giving social and medical histories. Usually this information is documented in a medical record, often stored electronically and held by the health professional or an institution. In exchange for the loss of privacy, clients expect and are promised some degree of confidentiality. In general, all personal medical information is confidential unless the client requests disclosure to third parties or a specific exception permits or requires disclosure. For example, clients may request disclosure to obtain insurance coverage or permit disclosure to a scientific researcher. The law requires health professionals to report certain infectious diseases to public-health departments or to report suspected child abuse to appropriate agencies. Unilateral disclosure of otherwise confidential information to third parties by health professionals or institutions is unethical unless it is authorized by the client or by law.

In the United States and other Western societies, the values of privacy, confidentiality, and privileged communications are closely tied to the values of personal rights and self-determination. These rights include freedom from the intrusion of others into one's private life, thoughts, conduct, or relationships. Interest in protection of personal rights has grown in response to public and private surveillance of individuals through the use of data bases to collect, store, and transmit information about individuals (Flaherty). In the United States the ideas of privacy and confidentiality have generated much legal and philosophical scholarship, influenced important judicial decisions, and prompted federal and state legislation (Winslade and Ross). The legal doctrine and ethical ideal of informed consent in healthcare reinforces the importance of personal autonomy (Beauchamp and Childress). The right to informed consent, applied specifically to confidentiality, gives patients/clients the right to control disclosure of confidential information. Other countries with less individualistic traditions do not place such high ethical value on privacy or personal rights. Even persons in cultures where privacy is not a prominent value

can be harmed, however, by revelations of personal information (Macklin).

Traditional ethical theories can be interpreted to provide additional support for the values of privacy and confidentiality. Deontology stresses the rights of persons and the duties of others to respect persons as ends in themselves, to respect especially their personal rights. To the extent that the social practices tied to privacy and confidentiality enhance the welfare of all, utilitarianism may also be invoked on behalf of individuals. Virtue theory advocates personal moral aspiration and achievement. Privacy and confidentiality provide a context and an opportunity for cultivation of virtues without outside interference.

Despite the value of privacy and confidentiality to individuals, however, other values—such as collective need for information or public health and safety—limit individual rights. Confidentiality conflicts often arise about information contained in medical records. Clients usually want information to remain confidential. Others—such as employers, insurers, family members, researchers, and litigants—exert pressure to limit confidentiality and to gain access to personal information. Health professionals are often pulled in both directions by their professional loyalty to patients/clients and their broader social responsibilities.

## Responsibilities of Health Professionals

The responsibilities of health professionals, as articulated in codes of professional ethics, reinforce the value of confidentiality. For example, the Hippocratic oath states:

> What I may see or hear in the course of the treatment or even outside of the treatment in regard to the life of men, which on no account one must spread abroad, I will keep to myself, holding such things shameful to be spoken about. (see Appendix)

Modern codes of professional ethics, like the Principles of Ethics of the American Medical Association, instruct physicians to "safeguard patient confidences within the constraints of the law" (see Appendix). Similarly, ethics codes for psychotherapists, nurses, and other allied health professionals make general, though not always coherent, reference to protection of professional-client confidentiality (Winslade and Ross). The American Psychiatric Association, however, has also issued detailed official Guidelines on Confidentiality pertaining to special situations, records, special settings, and the legal process (Committee on Confidentiality). The American Bar Association has offered a handbook, *AIDS/HIV and Confidentiality Model Policy and*

*Procedures,* that addresses the value of confidentiality, consent to disclosures, third-party access to information, and penalties for unauthorized disclosures (Rennert). The Council on Ethical and Judicial Affairs of the American Medical Association (1992) outlines the scope and value of confidentiality and addresses in detail confidentiality in the context of computerized medical records. These documents stress individual rights and specify professional responsibilities concerning confidentiality.

Despite the explicit attention given to confidentiality in oaths and codes, practical ethical problems arise, occasionally causing heated controversy. For instance, in 1991 an authorized biography of the deceased poet Anne Sexton relied in part upon audiotapes of psychotherapy sessions. One of Sexton's psychiatrists permitted the biographer to listen to some 300 hours of psychotherapy tapes. Prior to the publication of the biography, a front-page story in the *New York Times* about the disclosure of the tapes to the biographer generated a furious ethical debate. On the one hand, some critics believed that release of the tapes violated the deceased patient's privacy. Others pointed out the harm to surviving family members. Still others stressed the duty of the psychiatrist not to reveal anything about the content of therapy. Unless the therapist was required by law to release the information on the tapes, these critics argued, confidentiality should have been preserved. On the other hand, the psychiatrist claimed that his duty was primarily to protect his patient's interests—including her interest in self-revelation, in being understood, and in helping others. The psychiatrist believed that the patient, when competent, had specifically authorized him to use his own best judgment about what to do with the tapes. He also believed that he should cooperate with the request of the patient's literary executor—her daughter—to help make the biography accurate and complete. None of the relevant ethics codes sufficiently clarified or specifically addressed a case of this kind. Although charges were brought that the psychiatrist violated the code of ethics of the American Psychiatric Association, eventually a decision was reached that no ethics violation occurred. But a still-unsettled controversy swirls around these issues.

Professionals are often more aware of confidentiality issues than patients or clients. Professionals realize that privacy and confidentiality may give way to the institutional, governmental, and other third-party pressures for specific information about patients or clients. Health professionals desire to protect the integrity and special value of the professional-client relationship itself. Confidentiality is one basis of professionals' reciprocity with clients who reveal private information. (Other aspects of reciprocity include the clients' payment for the professionals' services in response to the professionals' expertise to meet the clients' needs.)

It should be emphasized that the primary justification for confidentiality is derived from the individual rights of clients and is supplemented by the responsibilities of professionals and the benefits of the healthcare relationship. This is why the client, rather than the health professional, determines what information is to remain confidential. Except where laws or other rules limit clients' rights to confidentiality, the client may not only request but require professionals to disclose otherwise confidential information. It is, after all, the client's private information that has been revealed to the professional.

Some recent critics, including feminist theorists, have questioned the adequacy of rights-based approaches. They argue that an ethics of care or caring must take account of a web of relationships, emotions, and values that include but go beyond individual rights. A care-based ethics stresses the interactive relationships, not only of patients and clinicians, but also families and society. Within the context of caring, humans—especially those who experience special suffering or discrimination—need more than just protection of their legal rights. In the specific context of privacy and confidentiality in medical genetics, for example, an ethics of care rather than rights may better explain the moral reasoning of geneticists (Wertz and Fletcher). This is discussed further in the later section on genetic and other medical screening.

Other critics think that the preservation of confidentiality should take priority over clients' and professionals' autonomy. This idea is based on the idea that total confidentiality is essential to protect both the integrity and the effectiveness of the professional-client relationship. No third parties should ever be permitted to penetrate the boundaries of a protected professional relationship. Neither the client nor the professional, according to this view, should be required or even permitted to disclose confidential information. Something close to this extreme position was considered but rejected by the California Supreme Court in *Lifshutz* (1970). Neither professional organizations nor their ethics codes endorse this idea, but it does highlight the importance that can be ascribed to confidentiality.

Even if the ideal of complete confidentiality cannot be justified in theory, it can sometimes be achieved in practice. A dyadic, exclusive relationship between client and health professional can sometimes fully preserve confidentiality. For example, a client establishes a relationship with a psychotherapist to explore the meaning of a significant personal loss. The client may not want others to know about the consultation. It is nobody else's business.

The therapist's office may have a separate entrance and exit to decrease the likelihood that clients will encounter each other. The therapist may answer personally all phone calls. The therapist may keep no client-specific records and take no notes. The client may pay cash, not file a claim for insurance coverage, explicitly request that all discussions be kept confidential, and take other precautions to prevent others from learning even that the relationship with the therapist exists at all. The client reveals his or her feelings, fantasies, thoughts, or dreams only to the therapist, who seeks to understand and help interpret their meaning only to the client.

If client confidentiality and professional secrecy were always as unambiguous as the foregoing scenario, there would be little more to say. However, professionals as well as clients have widely divergent attitudes, beliefs, expectations, and values concerning confidentiality (Wettstein). A few professionals espouse the absolute value of confidentiality in dyadic therapeutic relationships while many others acknowledge only its limited and relative value. Others lament the declining value of confidentiality while accepting the encroachment of legal, economic, public-health and safety, or research interests. A few others view confidentiality as an inflated value that some professionals or clients use as a shield to conceal fraud, malpractice, or even criminal activity.

Rather than a simple dyadic relationship, a more complex, polycentric model is necessary to capture the nuances of confidentiality in healthcare. Clients, health professionals, and third parties may have varying claims on ethical grounds to protection of or access to confidential information. Clients may waive their rights to confidentiality to obtain other benefits such as insurance coverage or employment. Professionals may discern a conflict between ethical obligations to their clients and legally required reports. Third parties may have a legitimate need to know otherwise confidential information to assess quality of healthcare services, uncover fraud, or determine appropriate allocations of healthcare resources. Loss of confidentiality may result not only from ethical, legal, or economic factors, but also because of client ignorance or misunderstanding, professional or institutional carelessness, or third-party overreaching. The interplay of those various factors can best be understood by examining in more detail selected problem areas where confidentiality comes into conflict with competing ethical and social interests.

## AIDS

The acquired immunodeficiency syndrome (AIDS) epidemic brings with it a full range of confidentiality issues. Patients who think that they might be HIV-positive are reluctant to be tested for fear that disclosure of such sensitive information may cause them to lose employment or insurance coverage or may make them subject to other types of discrimination. Yet if they are not tested, the benefits of clinical care to diminish the damage of the disease are not available. Patients who know that they are HIV-positive may not want others to know of their status to prevent discrimination. But third parties, such as sexual partners, who are at risk of being infected with a lethal virus, have a legitimate interest in access to otherwise confidential information. If the infected person is unwilling to inform others who may be at risk of getting AIDS, health professionals may be permitted or even required to warn persons who have been or may be put at risk of being infected. Family members may want to know why their relative is sick; they may need to know if they become caretakers. But patients may not be willing to disclose their diagnosis. Healthcare workers want to know their patients' HIV status just as patients want to know if their caretakers are infected. Both desire to avoid becoming infected themselves. Those who are at risk of infection may have a justifiable need to know; others may not.

Confidentiality is not the only value at stake, but it does impose substantial burdens on others. For example, in institutional settings, confidentiality of personal information, such as a patient's diagnosis, must be protected by written policies and actual practices. In a recent court case in Maryland, a hospital failed to protect adequately a patient's medical record that included a diagnosis of AIDS. It is not sufficient to state a policy that access to medical records is limited. It is also necessary to have and implement policies that actually restrict physical access to the records (Brannigan). The hospital was negligent because it did not go far enough to limit physical access of unauthorized persons to the records.

## Required Reporting

Legal rules that require health professionals to report child or elder abuse, infectious diseases, or gunshot wounds preempt many of the specific ethical conflicts between confidentiality and public health or safety. However, not all ethical issues are resolved by legal rules. For example, some child-abuse-reporting laws are overly broad; health professionals may fail to make mandated reports in part because of the value ascribed to client confidentiality. Other reporting laws are so narrow that protection of threatened victims is undermined by confidentiality rules and practices (Miller and Weinstock). Some commentators have pointed out, for example, the conflicts created by statutes that require the reporting of not only actual but also suspected child abusers. Some parents alleged to have abused their children have been required to undergo therapy; but to require them to admit abuse before conducting therapy conflicts with the constitutional privilege against self-incrimination.

Professionals, caught between the need for confidentiality in therapy and the legal demand for reporting abuse, sometimes underreport abuse; they protect therapeutic relationships at the risk of legal liability. Other professionals may overreport child abuse because of their concerns about legal liability, strained therapeutic relationships, vulnerability of potential victims, or uncertainty about the value of confidentiality. Some commentators have suggested that child-abuse statutes should be revised to be more specific and limited, requiring professionals to report only when their patients are victims of child abuse, but to give professionals greater discretion about whether to report abusers who are in treatment (Smith-Bell and Winslade).

Another ethical problem for health professionals that arises in connection with legally required disclosures of otherwise confidential information is what to tell clients prior to or near the outset of therapy. If clients are inadequately apprised about the limits of confidentiality, their trust in health professionals is damaged and their relationship may be ruptured. If clients are fully advised of the legal limits placed on confidentiality, they may withhold essential information, terminate therapy, or not even start it. A further problem is that professionals may not know precisely where legal lines have been drawn. For example, a therapist may know that notification must be made to authorities but may not know how much, if any, of the content of therapy must he disclosed.

## Genetic and Other Medical Screening

Genetic and other types of medical screening by epidemiologists, physicians, employers, schools, and other public and private agencies give rise to situations in which confidentiality is threatened by a demand for personal medical information. Individuals who are screened want to control information about themselves to prevent stigma, loss of insurance or employment, or other forms of discrimination. Screeners desire access to such information to promote their interests in knowledge, scientific discovery, publication, or economic considerations as well as therapeutic purposes. Control over the information raises moral issues as well as practical problems. These values must be balanced against individuals' rights to preserve their informational privacy. Blood tests, family medical histories, personal medical histories, DNA assays, and data banking, for instance, all raise questions about confidentiality, access, and control of personal

information (De Gorgey). Lack of consensus about ethical priorities, gaps in legal policies and remedies to individuals, and political uncertainty about jurisdiction and control over medical screening combine to create controversy. Protection of individual rights of privacy and confidentiality requires careful monitoring of the use of data banks to store information obtained by the Human Genome Project (Macklin).

Health professionals in genetics differ in their beliefs about the value of privacy and confidentiality. Considerable disagreement has been documented, for example, in an international study in nineteen countries of the attitudes of geneticists toward privacy and disclosure. These health professionals were asked to respond to vignettes concerning disclosure of false paternity; of a patient's genetic makeup to a spouse; to relatives at genetic risk; of ambiguous test results; and to institutional third parties, such as employers and insurers (Wertz and Fletcher). Some consensus as well as numerous differences were discovered among the geneticists' opinions about what disclosures are appropriate. Dorothy Wertz and John Fletcher also found that geneticists' reasoning was more likely to be based on the complex needs and relationships of the various parties rather than the rights of individuals. A care-based ethics approach poses a theoretical and practical alternative to a rights-based approach.

## Legal Protections and Limitations

Legal protection of confidentiality in the United States has been sporadic and uneven. The 1974 Federal Privacy Act (P.L. 93–579) included some medical information and records; its passage signaled heightened congressional awareness of threats to privacy and confidentiality. The National Privacy Commission's report (U.S. Domestic Council, 1976) seemed to set the stage for further protective federal legislation. Several subsequent attempts to pass comprehensive federal laws to protect medical information failed; a patchwork of state statutes provides only limited protection of patients' confidentiality. The reason is that patients' interests in confidentiality are balanced against powerful interests of third parties, such as healthcare payers, governmental agencies, researchers, and law-enforcement agencies, who wish to have access to otherwise confidential medical information (Hendricks et al.).

Courts have been as hesitant as federal and state legislatures to provide stringent protection of patient confidentiality. The U. S. Supreme Court considered but rejected the idea that patients enjoy a constitutional right to "informational privacy" with regard to treatment records (*Whalen* v. *Roe*). This decision was rendered when the rhetoric of privacy was prominent in Supreme Court opinions; in the

1980s the right to privacy was restricted, and the rhetoric of privacy diminished. State courts, such as those in Florida and California, whose constitutions make explicit reference to a right to privacy, have been more inclined to protect confidentiality of medical information. But state laws provide infrequently enforced bureaucratic protections or opportunities for recovery of damages only after confidentiality has been violated. Even then, litigation is rare because patients are reluctant to further expose confidential matters, damages are difficult to prove, and awards are often limited by statute (Winslade).

In some settings, such as substance-abuse treatment programs, the federal government has established special rules to protect confidentiality. To encourage persons in need of treatment to enter substance-abuse programs, records are not disclosed to law-enforcement agencies that might otherwise seek to prosecute substance abusers. In sensitive human subject research, special "privacy certificates" can be obtained by researchers from the federal government to give added protection to confidential information. Similarly, coded and locked files, limited access even to authorized personnel, and other precautionary measures against leakage further enhance confidentiality (McCarthy and Porter).

Public concern about confidentiality surfaces periodically, especially concerning the potential evils of misuses of patient-identifiable information. For example, implications of the Human Genome Project and healthcare reform have most recently evoked anxiety about discrimination, violation of personal rights, and commerce in patient information. The potential for a new healthcare information infrastructure that relies heavily on computer technology to facilitate the flow of medical information dramatically increases the threat to confidentiality of medical records (Brannigan). Recent commentaries remind us that current legal policies are inadequate to protect individuals against unwarranted disclosure, to provide security for complex medical-information systems, and to preserve individuals' rights to consent and control the uses of personal medical information (Alpert; Gostin et al.).

A specific area of law that directly affects confidentiality concerns the obligations of psychotherapists whose potentially violent patients place other individuals at risk of harm. The California Supreme Court, in the case of *Tarasoff* v. *Regents of the University of California* (1974), ruled that psychotherapists of dangerous patients have a duty to use reasonable care to protect threatened victims from harm. To do so may require the disclosure of otherwise confidential patient information. In balancing public safety and confidentiality, the Court observed that "the protective privilege ends where the public peril begins."

In the *Tarasoff* case, a psychotherapist believed that his patient was potentially dangerous to a young woman who had rejected his interest in her. The patient was obsessed with her at the expense of his studies, his work, and his friends. When the patient talked of revenge and was thought to have a gun, the therapist sought to have his patient evaluated for involuntary hospitalization. But the police declined to bring the patient in for an assessment of his mental status. The patient, angry with his therapist, abruptly terminated treatment. A couple of months later the former patient killed the young woman. Her parents sued the therapists and their employer for failing to warn the victim or her family about the dangerous patient. Although this case was settled out of court without a trial, the reasonable-protection rule was articulated by the court for future cases.

Subsequently, a series of judicial decisions have elaborated the duty of psychotherapists to third parties. Some courts have restricted the duty to situations in which there is an imminent threat of serious violence toward an identifiable victim. Others have focused on the broader duty of health professionals to control the conduct of the dangerous patient. Still others have applied the *Tarasoff* standard even when the risk to others is neither serious nor specific. And a few courts have protected confidentiality rather than endorse the *Tarasoff* standard (Felthous).

The complexity of particular cases and the variability of judicial interpretations of facts and laws inevitably cause some uncertainty. In this context, as in many others, confidentiality is limited by other important values. For example, suppose a voluntary psychotic in-patient with no history of violence leaves the hospital against medical advice. He leaves behind some written notes that include violent fantasies about a family member. His therapist discovers the notes (which were left unsealed). Assume the therapist consults the patient, who demands confidentiality; but the therapist is concerned that the patient may be dangerous. The therapist must assess the probability of harm to the patient or the potential victim, consider alternatives to revealing confidential information, and decide what, if anything, to tell the patient, the threatened victim, or others. This delicate balancing inevitably occurs in contexts where information is incomplete, contextual nuances are elusive, and human behavior is notoriously difficult to predict. Nevertheless, decisions must be made and actions taken that will affect the scope of confidentiality as well as bring about other consequences.

## Information about Limits of Confidentiality

When entering into a professional-client relationship, clients have a right to receive explicit information about the scope and limits of confidentiality. Most nonprofessionals assume that disclosures made in the context of healthcare are confidential (Weiss). Most clients are uninformed about the limits of confidentiality and pressures to reveal presumably confidential information to third parties. Some clients realize that there are legal and ethical restrictions on confidentiality in healthcare, but others learn of them only after an undesired disclosure (Siegler).

Clients for whom confidentiality is especially important may take steps to preserve it. For example, a medical patient who chooses to file an insurance claim may request the right to review all documents released to the insurance carrier. Or the patient may pay privately rather than file an insurance claim. Other clients may be less concerned with confidentiality. Clients have a responsibility to inform themselves about what expectations about confidentiality are reasonable; then they will not be surprised or dismayed because of false assumptions about confidentiality.

Professionals have a responsibility to inform themselves as well as their clients about legal, ethical, and practical aspects of confidentiality. For example, neither patients nor health professionals usually are familiar with the practices of insurance companies concerning redisclosure of confidential information. Patients often sign a blanket waiver of confidentiality in order to obtain insurance benefits. This information may then be sold by the insurer to the Medical Information Bureau, a clearinghouse to protect against insurance fraud. This goal is laudable, but the data-banking process may include erroneous information that is difficult to detect or correct. In addition, many other interests outside healthcare—such as employers, government agencies, educational institutions, and the media—may gain access to information contained in these data bases (Linowes; Alpert).

At the very least, professionals should ask their clients what they want to know about confidentiality. Some professionals prepare a disclosure statement to give each new client, that is, a document that outlines confidentiality practices the particular professional follows. Policies and procedures concerning written medical records might be given to each new client. Further conversation, including clients' questions and professionals' answers, can clarify details that written statements may not address. Because professionals, like their clients, may differ in their attitudes toward confidentiality, it is important that disclosures about confidentiality be particularized. For example, the values of a psychoanalyst in private practice who never publishes patient case reports significantly differs from those of a research-oriented psychoanalyst who tapes and transcribes every session and publishes detailed case reports. Each

should fully inform clients about the nature of his or her practice (Stoller).

Professionals have an obligation to take precautionary measures to protect confidentiality even if their clients have not requested it. Professionals should assume that all client information (including the very existence of the professional-client relationship as well as personal and private information revealed is strictly personal and private information revealed) is strictly confidential unless the client has requested or waived disclosure or unless the law requires it. Professionals should advise their clients of required disclosures, inform them of waivers, explore with them the consequences of disclosing or not disclosing information, and examine the reasons for and against disclosure. But clients retain the authority to decide what voluntary disclosures are to be made to third parties (Winslade and Ross).

Professionals also have a special responsibility to protect confidential client information from leakage through lax office procedures, professional or personal gossip, or the inappropriate inquiries of unauthorized persons. This is particularly problematic in institutional settings, where many individuals may have routine access to patient information contained in medical records (Siegler). As computerization of medical records expands further and information storage, retrieval, and distribution technologies become more sophisticated, the need for professionals' vigilance increases.

Many third parties—government officials and agencies, insurance interests, employers, family members, researchers, and others—seek specific information about particular patients. Third parties should not assume, however, that mere interest gives them legitimate authority to have access to confidential information. Third parties have a responsibility to justify to patients and professionals their need for access to confidential information. In some instances, this may require only a routine inquiry and documentation, but in other situations, professionals may find it necessary to confirm that their patients have requested, waived, or forfeited their rights to confidentiality. Too often, professionals, especially in an institutional setting, capitulate to pressure to disclose more information than necessary to third parties. At the very least, third parties as well as professionals should notify patients when access is sought, how it will be used, and whether the information will be redisclosed to anyone else. If appropriate disclosures are made to patients before access to confidential information is granted to third parties, not only will confidentiality be better preserved, but patients will also be better served.

WILLIAM J. WINSLADE (1995)
BIBLIOGRAPHY REVISED

SEE ALSO: *Autonomy; Beneficence; Genetic Testing and Screening: Predictive Genetic Testing; Healing; Healthcare Systems; Human Dignity; Human Rights; Paternalism; Pediatrics: Adolescents; Profession and Professional Ethics; Public Health Law*

## BIBLIOGRAPHY

Allen, Anita L. 1988. *Uneasy Access: Privacy for Women in a Free Society.* Totowa, NJ: Rowman & Littlefield.

Alpert, Sheri. 1993. "Smart Cards, Smarter Policy: Medical Records, Privacy and Health Care Reform." *Hastings Center Report* 23(6): 13–23.

Beauchamp, Tom L., and Childress, James F. 1989. *Principles of Biomedical Ethics,* 3rd edition. New York: Oxford University Press.

Bennet, Rebecca, and Erin, Charles A., eds. 2001. *HIV and AIDS: Testing, Screening, and Confidentiality (Issues in Biomedical Ethics).* New York: Oxford University Press.

Bloch, Sidney; Chodoff, Paul; and Green, Stephen., eds. 1999. *Psychiatric Ethics.* New York: Oxford University Press.

Bloche, M. G. 1997. "Managed Care, Medical Privacy, and the Paradigm of Consent." *Kennedy Institute of Ethics Journal* 7(4): 381–386.

Bok, Sissela. 1984. *Secrets: On the Ethics of Concealment and Revelation.* New York: Oxford University Press.

Brannigan, Vincent M. 1992. "Protecting the Privacy of Patient Information in Clinical Networks: Regulatory Effectiveness Analysis." *Annals of the New York Academy of Sciences* 670: 190–201.

Committee on Confidentiality. American Psychiatric Association. 1987. "Guidelines on Confidentiality." *American Journal of Psychiatry* 144(11): 1522–1527.

De Gorgey, Andrea. 1990. "The Advent of UNA Databanks: Implications for Information Privacy." *American Journal of Law and Medicine* 16(3): 381–398.

Dennis, Jill Callahan. 2001. *Privacy and Confidentiality of Health Information* (An AHA Press/Jossey-Bass Publication.) San Francisco: Jossey-Bass.

Ekstein, Rudolf, and Caruth, Elaine. 1972. "Keeping Secrets." In *Tactics and Techniques in Psychoanalytic Therapy,* pp. 200–215, ed. Peter L. Giovacchini. New York: Science House.

Felthous, Alan R. 1989. *The Psychotherapist's Duty to Warn or Protect.* Springfield, IL: Charles C. Thomas.

Flaherty, David H. 1989. *Protecting Privacy in Surveillance Societies: The Federal Republic of Germany, Sweden, France, Canada, and the United States.* Chapel Hill: University of North Carolina Press.

Gavison, Ruth. 1980. "Privacy and the Limits of Law." *Yale Law Journal* 89(3): 421–472.

Gostin, Lawrence O.; Turek-Brezina, Joan; Powers, Madison; Kozloff, Rene; Faden, Ruth; and Steinauer, Dennis. 1993. "Privacy and Security of Personal Information in a New Health Care System." *Journal of the American Medical Association* 270(20): 2487–2493.

Hendricks, Evan; Hayden, Trudy; and Novik, Jack. 1990. *Your Right to Privacy: A Basic Guide to Legal Rights in an Information Society,* 2nd edition. Carbondale: Southern Illinois University Press.

*Lifshutz, In re.* 467 P.2d 557 (Cal. 1970).

Linowes, David F. 1989. *Privacy in America: Is Your Private Life in the Public Eye?* Urbana: University of Illinois Press.

Macklin, Ruth. 1992. "Privacy and Control of Genetic Information." In *Gene Mapping: Using Law and Ethics as Guides,* pp. 157–172, ed. George J. Annas and Sherman Elias. New York: Oxford University Press.

McCarthy, Charles R., and Porter, Joan P. 1991. "Confidentiality: The Protection of Personal Data in Epidemiological and Clinical Research Trials." *Law, Medicine and Health Care* 19(3–4): 238–241.

Miller, Robert D., and Weinstock, Robert. 1987. "Conflict of Interest Between Therapist-Patient Confidentiality and the Duty to Report Sexual Abuse of Children." *Behavioral Sciences and the Law* 5(2): 161–174.

Rennert, Sharon. 1991. *AIDS/HIV and Confidentiality: Model Policy and Procedures.* Washington, D.C.: American Bar Association.

Rothstien, Mark A., ed. 1999. *Genetic Secrets: Protecting Privacy and Confidentiality in the Genetic Era.* New Haven, CT: Yale University Press.

Siegler, Mark. 1982. "Confidentiality in Medicine—A Decrepit Concept." *New England Journal of Medicine* 307(24): 1518–1521.

Smith-Bell, Michele, and Winslade, William J. 1994. "Privacy, Confidentiality, and Privilege in Psychotherapeutic Relationships." *American Journal of Orthopsychiatry* 64(2): 180–193.

Stoller, Robert J. 1988. "Patients' Responses to Their Own Case Reports." *Journal of the American Psychoanalytic Association* 36(2): 371–391.

Sweeney, L. 1998. "Privacy and Medical-Records Research." *New England Journal of Medicine* 338(15): 1077–1078.

*Tarasoff* v. *Regents of the University of California.* 529 P.2d 553 (Cal. 1974); 551 P.2d 334 (Cal. 1976).

U.S. Domestic Council. Committee on the Right of Privacy. 1976. *National Information Policy: Report to the President of the United States.* Washington, D.C.: Author.

Weiner, Barbara A., and Wettstein, Robert M. 1993. "Confidentiality." In *Legal Issues in Mental Health Care.* New York: Plenum.

Weiss, Barry D. 1982. "Confidentiality Expectations of Patients, Physicians, and Medical Students." *Journal of the American Medical Association* 247(19): 2695–2697.

Wertz, Dorothy C., and Fletcher, John C. 1991. "Privacy and Disclosure in Medical Genetics Examined in an Ethics of Care." *Bioethics* 5(13): 212–232.

Wettstein, Robert M. 1994. "Confidentiality." *Review of Psychiatry* 13: 343–364.

*Whalen v. Roe.* 97 S. Ct. 869 (1977).

Winslade, William J. 1982. "Confidentiality of Medical Records: An Overview of Concepts and Legal Policies." *Journal of Legal Medicine* 3(4): 497–533.

Winslade, William J., and Ross, Judith Wilson. 1985. "Privacy, Confidentiality, and Autonomy in Psychotherapy." *Nebraska Law Review* 64: 578–636.

# CONFLICT OF INTEREST

• • •

In a conflict of interest, one's obligations to a particular person or group conflict with one's self-interest. A physician, for example, is ordinarily obligated to provide his or her patients with only the care that is reasonable and medically necessary, even if the physician may earn more money through unnecessary interventions. Conflicts of interest should be distinguished from conflicts of obligation, in which one's obligations to one person or group conflict with one's obligations to some other person or group. The latter need not necessarily involve any threat to the agent's own interests. For example, a physician is normally obligated to keep patients' medical problems confidential; however, when a patient poses a danger to others (by transmitting AIDS to a spouse, for example) the physician may have an obligation to protect that third party by violating the confidentiality that would otherwise be owed to the patient. In a healthcare context, conflicts of interest can arise for individual providers, such as physicians, dentists, nurses, or physical therapists, or for institutions, such as hospitals, health maintenance organizations (HMOs), insurers, or pharmaceutical companies.

Conflicts of interest can be found in any human endeavor; indeed, the clash between self-interest and altruism lies at the heart of morality. However, conflicts of interest in healthcare are especially serious because of the patient's vulnerability. Illness can impair a patient physically, emotionally, and rationally. To secure treatment, patients must expose physical and emotional intimacies normally reserved for loved ones, and they frequently face further risks from invasive diagnostic and therapeutic technologies. Patients usually have no choice but to submit to such exposure and risk, because typically they lack the knowledge and skill to identify and treat the illness or to ascertain whether care is being rendered appropriately. This vulnerability creates ample opportunities for providers to exploit patients for personal gain. Physicians or dentists might recommend costly, unnecessary care, or an insurer or

an HMO might attempt to lure subscribers by promising more than it can deliver.

Accordingly, providers such as physicians and dentists are often regarded as fiduciaries, in both a moral and a legal sense. Fiduciaries hold beneficiaries' (the patients') interests in trust and are obligated to promote the latter's interests, even above their own hospitals, insurance companies and HMOs. Nursing and allied health professions are not ordinarily considered fiduciaries in the legal sense, but they do share a strong ethic of dedication to patients' interests.

For many years, a serious commitment to professionalism and an effacement of self-interest seemed sufficient to manage conflicts of interest. The traditional fee-for-service system admittedly encouraged unnecessary services, but prior to the mid-twentieth century providers had relatively few interventions to offer, beyond their own care and concern. As technologies emerged, a relative shortage of providers meant that each had more than enough to do. Furthermore, in the long-term relationships that characterized most healthcare, providers had to live with the consequences of their decisions, right alongside their patients. Exploitive or abusive practices thus carried strong disincentives.

Since about the mid-1960s, however, healthcare has become high cost and big business. Providers now face a plethora of conflicts of interest, ranging from the traditional but much-exacerbated conflicts implicit in fee-for-service to powerful pressures to cut the cost of care by doing less for patients.

## Conflicts of Interest for Physicians

For physicians, conflicts of interest can arise in two distinct realms: the clinical setting, where medical care is primarily designed to help the patient, and the research setting, where physicians seek scientific knowledge that will only sometimes benefit the patient or research subject.

THE CLINICAL SETTING. In the clinical setting, a number of factors could encourage a physician to alter a patient's optimal care, whether it be to secure a personal gain or to avoid a loss. Conflicts can be posed by third-party payers, institutional healthcare providers, private industry, the legal system, and physician investment.

*Third-party payers.* Traditional fee-for-service reimbursement encourages physicians to deliver as many services as possible and, in a maneuver called "unbundling," to break down each service into as many separately billable small interventions as possible. Maximizing income may thus mean excessive care, which in turn threatens needless inconvenience, expense, and iatrogenic injury for patients.

Partly because fee-for-service is an inflationary reimbursement system, healthcare costs grew at an alarming rate from the mid-1960s through the early 1990s. In response, those who pay directly for healthcare—government, businesses, and insurers—placed powerful pressures on physicians to do less for their patients. Payers sometimes offered bonuses to physicians to discharge patients earlier than normal, and they often refused to pay for various tests and treatments unless they were performed in an outpatient setting. Through extensive *utilization review* (UR), many payers reimbursed only hospitalizations or medical interventions that met their criteria of medical necessity. Physicians therefore spent large amounts of time (usually uncompensated) justifying their plans of care to payers in order to secure reimbursement.

As a supplement, or sometimes an alternative, to such controls, many health plans instituted financial incentives. Capitation systems, for instance, attempt to save money by paying a single fee for a large unit of care, thereby creating an incentive to avoid rendering care beyond the budgeted fee. Medicare inaugurated its *diagnosis related group* (DRG) system in the early 1980s, paying hospitals a set amount for a specific episode of illness, based on such factors as the patient's diagnosis, age, and coexisting illnesses.

HMOs, in a broader capitation concept, began to provide all necessary healthcare for each subscriber in exchange for a single annual premium. In order to ensure that their physicians delivered services within the year's budget, most HMOs, in turn, applied downstream financial incentives to their physicians, often withholding 20 percent or more of the physician's salary or fees until the end of the year, when they would be paid (or not) depending on the HMO's financial health. HMOs also have commonly set aside a special fund for diagnostic tests, consultants, and hospitalization. Primary-care physicians, acting as gatekeepers whose permission is required for the patient to gain access to these services, would share any surplus funds (or debts) remaining at the end of the year. Other HMOs placed physicians under subcapitation systems in which the physician provided a range of services for a set fee per patient. These arrangements could make a substantial difference in a physician's year-end income, thereby providing a powerful incentive for physicians to economize on the level of care they provide or authorize for patients.

The mid-1990s saw a brief reprieve from healthcare cost inflation, which, combined with a booming economy and widespread horror stories about the abuses of managed care, prompted most health plans to scale back these cost controls and incentive arrangements. However, as healthcare costs began rising rapidly again in the early twenty-first century, health plans and providers again struggled to keep them in check through a variety of mechanisms.

Although these mechanisms have evolved, certain features have remained constant. Ultimately, all payment systems create conflicts of interest by creating an incentive to provide more of the services that are most profitably reimbursed, and less of those that generate less income. However, the challenge is markedly exacerbated in the healthcare setting. Every medical decision is a spending decision, yet payers ordinarily cannot control their costs by directly dictating what care the physician will and will not provide. To do so would be to practice medicine in the physician's stead. Rather, payers attempt to influence physicians, who control up to 80 percent of healthcare costs through their power of prescription and their professional influence over patients. That influence is almost always gained by placing physicians' personal interests in peril as they are rewarded or penalized for fiscally (im)prudent healthcare decisions.

*Institutional providers.* Institutional healthcare providers, such as hospitals and clinics, can establish incentives to encourage physicians to do more (or less), depending on the institution's economic status (proprietary or charitable) and the patient's financial status (well-insured or not). A for-profit walk-in clinic, for instance, makes its money through the tests and treatments its physician-employees order. Hence, high-profit physicians may be praised and invited to share profits, or even to own a share of the business, while low-profit physicians may receive administrative warnings or lose their jobs if they do not improve . In other cases, physicians and proprietary hospitals may enter into joint ventures to share both the profits and risks of running the facility.

Whether proprietary or charitable, all institutional providers need to contain costs. Monthly printouts comparing the costs of each physician's care may be shared with medical staff in an attempt to shame the high spenders into delivering more conservative care. And those whose patients consistently leave too many unpaid bills may lose their staff privileges in a strategy called *economic credentialing.*

Such incentives systematically place physicians in conflicts of interest. The potential loss of income, peer esteem, staff privileges, or even one's job creates powerful pressures to align one's judgment with the institution's interests, even at some cost to patients' interests.

*Private industry.* Many medical drugs and devices are sold only with the prescription of a licensed physician and, notwithstanding some notable exceptions, are often not readily advertised to the general public. Therefore, manufacturers' marketing typically targets physicians. Because physicians tend to be busy people with substantial incomes, pharmaceutical companies can go to great lengths to get their attention. Promotions over the years have included all-expense-paid trips to exotic locations, ostensibly to hear a lecture on a new product; cash payments to physicians who agree to read literature describing nonapproved uses of a drug; "frequent prescriber" programs that award frequent-flyer points with the physician's preferred airline for every prescription of the company's drug; lavish parties and tickets to entertainment events; costly gifts such as luggage and decorative arts; inexpensive gifts such as pens and notepads; and subsidies for local educational colloquiums and travel to professional meetings.

The conflicts of interest are obvious. Such gifts reward physicians for prescribing drugs and devices whether or not they are necessary, and whether or not that particular product choice is most appropriate and least costly for the patient. Acceptance of gifts can engender a sense of personal gratitude and indebtedness that can put corporate loyalty above patients' interests. Furthermore, patients ultimately bear the costs of such promotions and gifts, whether through higher costs of the drugs and devices, higher costs for health insurance, or by forgoing higher salaries or fringe benefits because their employers are paying higher insurance premiums.

*Legal system.* Parallel to the escalation of healthcare costs, both the frequency and cost of medical malpractice litigation have increased. Physicians fearful of lawsuits may order extra diagnostic tests and more potent therapies to ensure that no one can accuse them of missing a diagnosis or doing too little for their patients. The cost of such "defensive medicine" has been estimated at up to 15 percent of the total cost of physicians' services. When physicians order procedures that are not medically necessary in order to protect their actual or imagined legal interests, they expose patients to extra inconvenience and iatrogenesis—at the patient's expense and usually without the patient's knowledge. It is a clear conflict of interest.

*Physician investment.* In some cases physicians create their own conflicts of interest by investing in facilities to which they refer their patients. Examples include freestanding diagnostic imaging centers, home health services, clinical laboratories, and physical therapy services. Although such investments can enhance the availability and quality of healthcare facilities in a particular locale, the physician owners of such facilities nevertheless have an incentive to refer patients there, even when the care is unnecessary, costly, or of poor quality. In the 1990s a series of federal laws and administrative regulations forbade many, but not all, of these arrangements.

The conflicts embedded in investments are not limited to freestanding facilities. One study found that physicians who owned radiographic equipment in their own offices tended to use it four times more often (generating costs seven times higher) than physicians who referred patients to independent radiologists for those services.

**THE RESEARCH SETTING.** The research context sometimes involves testing new treatments on ill patients, but it can also involve healthy volunteers when researchers look for toxicities of the very newest drugs. In many instances there is no expectation that participation in research will benefit the patient at all, whether because the subject is a normal control subject, because many people in the study will receive a placebo instead of active medication, or because the patient is too hopelessly ill to benefit from any treatment. Whatever the research protocol, however, the physician must respect the research subject's rights and interests.

Physicians can enjoy many personal rewards for successful research. Private companies such as drug manufacturers commonly sponsor research, in some cases paying the physician-investigator a fixed fee of several thousand dollars per person enrolled. The sum is intended to cover the costs of each subject's participation in the study, but in fact can result in a considerable surplus of money pocketed by the investigator. The more patients one enters in a study, the higher one's rewards, and an overzealous recruiter may be tempted to understate the inconvenience, discomfort, or risk that research participation may present for the patient, or to compromise the integrity of the study by signing up patients who are not truly eligible for the protocol.

Research that is funded by the government or other nonprofit sources can mitigate some, but not all, of the conflicts of privately sponsored research. Physician researchers still have strong incentives to gain the prestige, larger laboratory, increased technical support, academic promotion, science awards, and institutional power that come with securing grants and producing publishable research. In addition, some research projects have paid finders' fees to those who recruit patients for studies. As a result, investigators have powerful incentives to recruit patients into studies without necessarily taking full account of the patients' best interests.

Physicians can also create their own conflicts of interest. Sometimes physicians invest in corporations that are sponsoring their research, or they may serve as the corporations' paid spokespersons when research is completed. They may earn money from producing a valuable commodity, such as a cell line, by using tissues that patients either knowingly or unwittingly donate (see *Moore v. Regents of the University of California*). In a few cases physicians performing for-profit scientific research have charged subjects a fee to participate. Although such entrepreneurial research is controversial, the conflicts embedded in for-profit research are not necessarily worse than those found throughout the high-pressure world of medical research.

## Other Health Professionals

Whereas physicians and dentists often are private practitioners or independent contractors, nurses, physical therapists, dietitians, and allied health professionals usually are employees of hospitals, HMOs, clinics, home health services, or public health agencies. These professionals' conflicts of interest most often arise where their contractual duty to administer the therapies ordered by a physician or to follow established institutional rules clash with their own beliefs about what is best for a patient. Such health professionals may suffer personal retaliation if they violate institutional mandates in order to do what they deem best for the patient.

In these cases the problem begins with a conflict of obligation in which one's obligations to the institution do not match one's obligations to the patient. The conflict of interest arises as one faces a personal price, perhaps in the form of retaliation, for favoring the patient over the institution. Thus, though conflicts of obligation are not the same thing as conflicts of interest, in these cases they are connected. For example, in one instance a nurse was fired for informing a patient about alternative cancer treatments (the dismissal was later vacated on procedural grounds (see *Tuma v. Board of Nursing*). In another case a nurse was discharged for refusing to dialyse a patient for whom she believed the treatment was pointless and inhumane (see *Warthen v. Toms River Community Memorial Hospital*). Such clashes between administrative requirements and one's professional judgment are probably the greatest, though not the sole, source of conflicts for allied health professions.

## Institutions

The interests of institutions and their administrators, like those of individual professionals, often mesh with patients' best interests. Ideally, in a competitive market where consumers seek quality and value for their dollars, a healthcare institution will prosper by serving patients well. However, such a happy match does not always occur, partly because ill patients are often not equipped to appraise and challenge the quality of their care, and because generous insurance policies insulate many patients from caring about the costs of care. Accordingly, the financial best interests of a hospital might prompt excessive charges, inadequate staffing and equipment, bloated advertising, or the premature "dumping" of uninsured patients into public institutions. Similarly, a pharmaceutical company may be financially rewarded for producing and marketing new drugs as early and as vigorously as possible, even if the drugs and their production methods are not as refined as they could be. As a result, some drugs may have more side effects, or cost more, than is necessary.

## Managing Conflicts of Interest

The existence of a conflict of interest does not mean that a provider has done anything wrong, or has mistreated or will mistreat any patient. It means only that while there is a mandate to promote the patient's (or someone else's) best interest, there are self-interested reasons to do otherwise. To be tempted is not necessarily to succumb.

Providers cannot escape conflicts of interest. If they are paid according to how many services they provide, their interest is to provide more services, with the concomitant dangers of excessive interventions, costs, and risks of iatrogenesis. If they are paid according to how many patients they care for, their financial advantage lies in taking on too many patients. Physicians who are strictly on a salary have an adverse incentive to minimize their own labor, even if they cannot increase their income, by seeing fewer and less-needy patients.

Formal protections can help. Regulatory agencies, such as state boards of medicine, nursing, and dentistry and the Joint Commission on Accreditation of Healthcare Organizations, can establish standards of performance for individuals and institutions, and the legal system can redress individual cases where providers' self-interest injures patients. Fiduciary law, for example, requires a fiduciary in a conflict of interest to disclose that conflict fully to the beneficiary (here, the patient) and also empowers the latter to determine how the conflict should be resolved (see *Fulton National Bank v. Tate*). Patients thus can have common-law remedies for breach of fiduciary duty, lack of informed consent, and other causes.

Although regulation and litigation can thus provide important protections, they cannot supplant personal integrity. The prospective employee of an HMO, a hospital, or other institutional provider should check carefully into its incentive structure and refuse to join any organization that links financial consequences too closely to individual patient-care decisions. The physician in private practice can refuse to accept costly gifts from drug company representatives. Those who would invest in ancillary facilities within or outside of their offices can ensure that there is a genuine need for the facility, and they can empower their patients with information and freedom to make their own choices regarding their ancillary healthcare providers. Researchers can refrain from investing in corporations sponsoring their research, and they can work with other research-sponsoring institutions to minimize conflicts. Where private industry pays university-based physicians a large per-patient fee, for example, that fee can be put into a general fund to benefit the institution after research costs are paid. Nurses and allied health professionals can work individually or collectively for contract terms that protect their right to exercise professional integrity.

Institutions must ensure that they do not create inordinate conflicts of interest for the professionals they employ. HMOs, for instance, should refrain from instituting incentive systems that unduly influence individual patient-care decisions. They and other payers should likewise disclose to current and potential subscribers any such incentives or limits on care. Informed subscribers are better empowered to guard their own interests. Institutions can also ameliorate their conflicts by pursuing ongoing quality improvement as a way of promoting quality care while economizing on costs. A focus on the success that comes from long-term quality should replace any preoccupation with short-term profitability.

Conflicts of interest affect providers pervasively, powerfully, and personally. Where fiduciary duty once consisted mainly of refraining from vulgar exploitation, the obligation to place the patient's interests before one's own can no longer be an unlimited obligation. Providers must exercise great care to avoid conflicts where possible, and to uphold a strong fiduciary presumption to favor patients' interests over their own. However, they cannot be expected to commit professional self-sacrifice in what may be a futile unilateral attempt to battle economic forces beyond their control. Therefore, one of the most important and difficult moral challenges of medicine's new economics is to consider not just what providers owe their patients but also the limits of those obligations. As healthcare systems continue to evolve, one important remedy will be to provide patients with greater choice and control over the content of their healthcare benefits, and thereby with more power to make their own trade-offs between the cost and quality of care. This will alleviate at least some of the conflicts of interest that arise as providers attempt to make these trade-offs on their patients' behalf.

E. HAAVI MORREIM (1995)
REVISED BY AUTHOR

SEE ALSO: *Commercialism in Scientific Research; Divided Loyalties in Mental Healthcare; Healthcare Resources, Allocation of; Just Wages and Salaries; Managed Care; Maternal-Fetal Relationship; Nursing Ethics; Pharmaceutical Industry; Pharmaceutics, Issues in Prescribing; Profession and Professional Ethics; Surrogate Decision-Making; Whistleblowing in Healthcare*

## BIBLIOGRAPHY

Ansell, David A., and Schiff, Robert L. 1987. "Patient Dumping, Implications and Policy Recommendations." *Journal of the American Medical Association* 257(11): 1500–1502.

*Batty v. Arizona State Dental Board.* 112 P.2d 870 (1941).

Berenson, Robert A. 1987. "In a Doctor's Wallet." *New Republic* May 18, 11–13.

*Berkey v. Anderson.* 82 Cal. Rptr. 67 (Cal. App. 2 Dist. 1969).

Berwick, David M. 1989. "Continuous Improvement as an Ideal in Health Care." *New England Journal of Medicine* 320(1): 53–56.

Blum, John D. 1991. "Economic Credentialing: A New Twist In Hospital Appraisal Processes." *Journal of Legal Medicine* 12: 427–475.

Bock, Randall S. 1988. "The Pressure to Keep Prices High at a Walk-In Clinic: A Personal Experience." *New England Journal of Medicine* 319(12): 785–787.

*Brown v. Blue Cross and Blue Shield of Alabama.* 898 F. 2d 1556 (11th Cir. 1990).

Butler, Stuart M., and Haislmaier, Edmund F., eds. 1989. *A National Health System for America: Critical Issues.* Washington, D.C.: Heritage Foundation.

Chittenden, William A. 1991. "Malpractice Liability and Managed Health Care: History and Prognosis." *Tort and Insurance Law Journal* 26: 451–496.

Chren, Mary-Margaret; Landefeld, C. Seth; and Murray, Thomas H. 1989. "Doctors, Drug Companies, and Gifts." *Journal of the American Medical Association* 262(24): 3448–3451.

*Darling v. Charleston Community Memorial Hospital.* 211 N.E. 2d 253 (Ill. 1965).

Eddy, David M. 1990. "What Do We Do About Costs?" *Journal of the American Medical Association* 264 (9): 1161–1170.

Figa, S. Fred, and Tag, Howard M. 1990. "Redefining Full and Fair Disclosure of HMO Benefits and Limitations." *Seton Hall Legislative Journal* 14: 151–157.

*Fulton National Bank v. Tate.* 363 F.2d 562 (4th Cir. 1966).

Garber, Alan M. 1992. "No Price Too High?" *New England Journal of Medicine* 327(3): 1676–1678.

Hillman, Alan L. 1987. "Financial Incentives for Physicians in HMOs: Is There a Conflict of Interest?" *New England Journal of Medicine* 317(27): 1743–1748.

Hillman, Bruce J.; Joseph, Catherine A.; Mabry, Michael R.; et al. 1990. "Frequency and Costs of Diagnostic Imaging in Office Practice—A Comparison of Self-Referring and Radiologist-Referring Physicians." *New England Journal of Medicine* 323(23): 1604–1608.

Institute of Medicine. 1986. "Committee Report." In *For-Profit Enterprise in Health Care,* ed. Bradford H. Gray. Washington, D.C.: National Academy Press.

Institute of Medicine. 2001. *Crossing the Quality Chasm: A New Health System for the 21st Century.* Washington, D.C.: National Academy Press.

Jonsen, Albert R. 1983. "Watching the Doctor." *New England Journal of Medicine* 308(25): 1531–1535.

Kessler, David A. 1991. "Drug Promotion and Scientific Exchange. The Role of the Clinical Investigator." *New England Journal of Medicine* 325(3): 201–203.

Lind, Stuart E. 1990. "Finder's Fees for Research Subjects." *New England Journal of Medicine* 323(24): 192–195.

*Lockett v. Goodill.* 430 P.2d 589 (Wash. 1967).

*Moore v. Regents of the University of California.* 793 P.2d 479 (1990).

Morreim, E. Haavi. 1989. "Conflicts of Interest: Profits and Problems in Physician Referrals." *Journal of the American Medical Association* 262(3): 390–394.

Morreim, E. Haavi. 1991. *Balancing Act: The New Medical Ethics of Medicine's New Economics.* Dordrecht, Netherlands: Kluwer.

Morreim, E. Haavi. 1991. "Economic Disclosure and Economic Advocacy: New Duties in the Medical Standard of Care." *Journal of Legal Medicine* 12: 275–329.

Morreim, E. Haavi. 1991. "Patient-Funded Research: Paying the Piper or Protecting the Patient?" *IRB* 13(3): 1–6.

Morreim, E. Haavi. 1993. "Am I My Brother's Warden? Responding to the Unethical or Incompetent Colleague." *Hastings Center Report* 23(3): 19–27.

Morreim, E. Haavi. 1993. "Unholy Alliances: Physician Investment for Self-Referral." *Radiology* 186(1): 67–72.

Oldham, Robert K. 1987. "Patient-Funded Cancer Research." *New England Journal of Medicine* 316(1): 46–47.

Randall, Teri. 1991. "Kennedy Hearings Say No More Free Lunch—or Much Else—from Drug Firms." *Journal of the American Medical Association* 265(4): 440–441.

Relman, Arnold S. 1983. "The Future of Medical Practice." *Health Affairs* 2(2): 5–19.

Reynolds, Roger A.; Rizzo, John A.; and Gonzalez, Martin L. 1987. "The Cost of Medical Professional Liability." *Journal of the American Medical Association* 257(20): 2776–2781.

Robinson, James. 2001. "The End of Managed Care." *Journal of the American Medical Association* 285: 2622–2628.

Rodwin, Mark A. 1993. *Medicine, Money, and Morals: Physicians' Conflicts of Interest.* New York: Oxford University Press.

Shimm, David S., and Spece, Roy G. 1991. "Conflict of Interest and Informed Consent in Industry-Sponsored Clinical Trials." *Journal of Legal Medicine* 12: 477–513.

*Tuma v. Board of Nursing,* 593 P.2d 711 (1979).

*Warthen v. Toms River Community Memorial Hospital.* 488 A.2d 229 (N.J.Super.A.D. 1985).

*Wohlgemuth v. Meyer.* 293 P.2d 316 (Cal. 1956).

# CONFUCIANISM, BIOETHICS IN

• • •

Confucianism draws its name from the latinized honorific title of its founder, Kong Chiu or *Kong fuzi* (562–479 B.C.E.), an independent scholar and unsuccessful political advisor who believed moral self-cultivation and the practice of ritual were the cornerstones of an ideal society. Initially espoused by no more than a few dozen students, Confucius's teachings—expanded and significantly elaborated over time—ultimately became the dominant sociopolitical ideology of much of East, Northeast, and Southeast Asia.

Other traditions, notably Mahayana Buddhism and Taoism, successfully rivaled Confucianism for state support over the centuries, but none—not even Maoist atheism in China—ever seriously threatened the Confucian tradition's pervasive cultural dominance. Carried beyond its historical Asian boundaries by merchants, laborers, and refugees, Confucianism also maintains a strong hold on diasporic Chinese, Korean, Japanese, and South-Vietnamese populations the world over.

In considering the complexities of the Confucian tradition, the following must be borne in mind:

1. the tradition is not monolithic, that is, historical era, regional variation, and differential class appropriation inform Confucian practice;

2. the tradition does not exist in conceptual isolation, that is, within any given local culture at any particular historical moment, Confucianism has always been practiced by individuals as part of a constellation of personal practice, including Mahayana Buddhism and local folk religions;

3. although there is a sense of authority residing in the canonical texts and commentaries of the Confucian classics, there is no central governing body, no clergy, and no history of religious jurisprudence within the tradition to dictate orthodoxy or legislate orthopraxy;

4. there is neither a concept of evil nor an absolute dichotomy between right and wrong as understood in Western monotheisms; rather, it is ignorance, self-delusion, and a tendency to gratify selfish desires that pose the greatest obstacles to moral improvement;

5. Comparative discussion of certain contemporary topics, for example, human rights and abortion, is

complicated by the absence of notions of individual "rights"; in the Confucian view, humans are defined by their capacity to fulfill duties and responsibilities rather than by any sense of inherent possession of rights.

## Origins of the Classical Tradition

Core concepts are found in brief statements attributed to the Master himself, recorded by others in the verses of the *Analects,* the *Great Learning,* and the *Doctrine of the Mean.* Modern scholars, notably E. Bruce Brooks and A. Taeko Brooks in their *The Original Analects,* have shown these texts to contain significant interpolations and emendations. As received tradition, however, the aphorisms ascribed to Confucius and his early followers continue to exert considerable authority. At the heart of Confucius's vision was the sense that an individual can become truly human only through a deliberate process of moral education. The cultivation of virtues and their expression in ritual forms yields a *gentleman* (or, in current terminology, a *perfected person*) who stands ready to fulfill the responsibilities of living in concert with others and of establishing a peaceful, just, and aesthetically pleasing society. Ritual without virtue is ornament without substance; virtue without ritual can lead to unbounded good intentions that may ultimately do harm.

Confucian society is built upon a set of five reciprocal relationships, each of which is characterized by particular virtues and specific responsibilities:

1. ruler-subject;
2. parent-child;
3. husband-wife;
4. older-younger (brothers); and
5. friends.

Confucius's primary concern was with the creation of a stable and prosperous state, but he understood that it was the family that would ultimately produce the individuals dedicated to establishing his ideal society. Of the five relationships, therefore, three are located within the family; of these, by far the most important is that between parent and child. For having given life, one's parents are owed an enduring debt of gratitude—an obligation that extends even beyond the temporal boundaries of this lifetime. The practice of filiality, or filial piety, is therefore the starting point for Confucian moral cultivation, and the family is the foremost focus of religious practice.

An individual's relationship with people outside the family is determined by interlocking considerations of age, social and educational position, gender, and degree of professional and personal connection—all of which determine relative seniority and significance, and thus the degree of deference and potential obligation owed. However, how one acts within the resulting relationship is far more flexible and less hierarchical than might be assumed. Much has been made in Western philosophical literature about the Golden Rule found in *Analects* 5:12 and 12:2, but Confucius himself indicated another *single thread* that bound his ethical teachings (*Analects* 4:15). Two strands comprise the single thread, namely, *chung* and *shu,* usually translated as *loyalty* and *reciprocity.* These terms refer to a dialectical process that requires that one first center oneself in the relationship at hand, clearly understanding its attendant responsibilities and privileges. One then imaginatively takes the other's position in the relationship. Then—and only then, from this enlarged and empathetic perspective—one acts, in full awareness of the consequences for the other of one's actions.

In the centuries after Confucius's death, new questions arose to challenge the tradition. A particularly vexatious problem was how to account for people's varying capacities to learn (or even to want to learn) to become truly human. The ensuing debate was ultimately settled in favor of the view espoused by Mengzi (also latinized as Mencius, 372–289 B.C.E.). According to Mengzi, all people possess the four seeds of humaneness, righteousness or duty, propriety, and wisdom. If nourished properly through environment and education, these seeds mature into the moral attitudes and ritual behavior of true humanity. It is worth noting, however, that extrapolation from this claim yields the conclusion that those who do not exhibit these seeds or their outgrowth are not entirely human—a conclusion with potentially troubling ramifications in discussions of capital punishment, euthanasia, and human rights.

## The Han Synthesis

After China was united under the relatively stable administration of the Han dynasty in 206 B.C.E., training in Confucian principles was established as the basis for participation in the state's meritocracy. Over the course of the Han rule (through 221 C.E.), Confucianism's purview expanded beyond philosophical-political discussions of virtue and ritual to encompass cosmological theories derived from ancient divination forms, and from *yin-yang* and the so-called Five Elements systems. The goals were to discern macrocosmic and microcosmic correspondences and then to regulate human actions to ensure harmony with heaven and earth. Although many of the theories incorporated into this syncretic Confucian cosmology are frequently associated with Taoism, they are more accurately described as belonging to a pre-sectarian worldview that underlies all Chinese religio-philosophical traditions.

The hexagrams of the *I Ching* (*Book of Changes*) provided glimpses of the flow of natural processes, especially *qi*, the animating *breath* of the cosmos. The alternation of *yin* (darkness, passivity, decay, emotionality, and femininity) and *yang* (light, activity, growth, rationality, and masculinity) underscored notions of complementarity. The Five Elements (fire, water, wood, metal, and earth) explained a thing's inherent characteristics as well as its patterns of growth and decline. Elaborate correspondences were constructed among these classificatory systems, such that hours of the day, seasons of the year, foods and tastes, colors, sounds, organs of the body, stages of life, heavenly constellations, and virtually all human activities could be mapped and harmonized. A dislocation or inappropriate item in any one part of the schema would lead to disharmony and inauspiciousness elsewhere. In the political realm, disharmony breeds revolution; in the personal realm, disharmony breeds illness. The goal of Chinese medicine is to restore the natural balance of one's internal environment and to harmonize it with external environmental circumstances. This requires that a patient's food, medicines, and therapies be dictated not only by symptoms, but also by individual psychophysiology and local environmental factors such as season of the year. In the Confucian view, maintaining one's good health is dictated by filial responsibility, as one's parents should have no cause for worry.

## Neo-Confucianism

After the collapse of the Han, China fragmented into several smaller kingdoms and parts of north China fell under non-Chinese rule. During the following centuries of disunion, the Confucian tradition was somewhat eclipsed by Taoist sectarian traditions and by the rise of Buddhism. Beginning in the Song dynasty (960–1279), a Confucian revitalization movement gathered momentum. Meditation, visualization, and other interior spiritual techniques were borrowed from Buddhism and Taoism, and traditional Confucian ethical concerns were now linked formally to a notion of the cosmos as inherently inclined toward moral good. Mengzi's view that human nature is essentially good was reaffirmed by the great Neo-Confucian, Zhu Xi (1130–1200). Together with the *Analects*, the *Great Learning*, and the *Doctrine of the Mean*, Zhu Xi promoted the *Mengzi* as comprising the Four Books, the basic course of education in Confucian ideology. Indeed it was Zhu Xi's editions of these and other classical Confucian texts that formed the basis for the imperial Chinese civil service examinations.

Zhu Xi further contributed to the development of Confucian practice through his preparation of detailed *jiaxun,* or family regulations. In addition to providing minute descriptions of ritual preparations, he admonished would-be filial sons and daughters-in-law to acquire medical knowledge adequate to the care of their parents (-in-law). Not only should they know how to prepare certain medicines, but they should also be able to select reputable physicians—practitioners who, in Zhu Xi's day, were viewed as little different from barbers and masseurs. Filial duty also entailed assumption of the primary burden of care. Down to the present, the sense that eldercare is the responsibility of the family remains deeply ingrained in Confucian societies, but with the decline of the extended family, reports of abandoned seniors are increasingly common.

## New Confucianism

After the fall of the Qing dynasty in 1911, Confucianism was widely derided by Chinese intellectuals as a remnant of a feudal past that hindered China's rightful advancement into the modern world. Much of the blame for women's oppression, for example, was allocated to *Confucius and Sons,* and study of the canon was replaced by scientific and technical training. Nonetheless there were some scholars who believed that Confucianism, freed from its feudal origins and centuries of accreted (and erroneous) practice, could be rehabilitated. An international revitalization movement, known as *New Confucianism,* arose in the 1920s at Peking University under the intellectual leadership of Xiong Shili and continued to develop through the 1940s at New Asia College in Hong Kong under Tang Junyi. During the 1960s, the movement gained added momentum by the efforts of Mou Zongsan and Xu Fuguan at Tunghai University in Taiwan. These New Confucians asserted that the tradition holds spiritual resources sufficient to meet the challenges of industrialization, urbanization, and bureaucratization, and to combat the depersonalization of the modern world.

Contemporary New Confucians draw inspiration from Lee Sang-eun (South Korea), Okada Takehiko (Japan), and, especially, Tu Weiming at Harvard University. Following his teacher Mou Zongsan, Tu Weiming has championed Confucianism as a world religious tradition—its ideals and practices open not only to those of East- and Southeast-Asian ethnic background, but to anyone who shares its anthropocosmic vision. And there are many who do. Robert C. Neville, author of *Boston Confucianism,* is a prominent example of those who claim a dual religious orientation and who write persuasively on the significance of Confucian tradition for the West.

## Women

There is nothing in the Confucian tradition inimical to women. Confucius had little to say about women other than, like uneducated men, they "were difficult to deal with" (*Analects* 17: 25). It was only later, with the Han dynasty grafting of cosmological speculation onto the tradition, that women became ineluctably identified with yin and its associated qualities in a negative way. Mengzi, for example, accepted the social mores of his day but did not see women as disposable or unworthy of regard:

> Chunyu Kuan asked, "In giving and receiving things, is it not the rule that men and women should not touch?"
>
> Mengzi repled, "That is the rule."
>
> "If my sister-in-law is drowning, then should I use my hand to save her?"
>
> "Anyone who wouldn't is a wolf. That men and women shouldn't touch in giving and receiving things is the rule; to use your hand to save your sister-in-law transcends rules." (4A17)

Yet it was Mengzi who underscored the filial necessity of producing an heir in order to ensure the care of elderly parents and the maintenance of ancestral veneration. He said, "There are three ways to be unfilial, and the greatest of these is to be without posterity" (4A26). In the premodern world, posterity meant a son or, preferably, sons. The resultant pressures on a woman were great. She was to bear children early and often; to continue bearing children until at least one son was born; and, in cases where she failed in this requirement or seemed likely to do so, to accept divorce or the introduction of concubines into the household.

The imperative to produce a son remains strong and has had a profound impact on the growth of certain reproductive technologies. The desire for male offspring, coupled with restrictive population control measures in China, and with trends toward smaller nuclear families in the industrialized nations of Japan, Taiwan, Korea, and Singapore, has led to increased use of sonograms for fetal sex determination, often followed by elective abortion if the fetus is female. Of course, to describe abortion as *elective* in this context is to gloss over the many pressures—economic, spousal and familial, societal—that may accompany the decision; use of the term here indicates only that the procedure is not medically necessary.

Abortion itself is condemned within the Confucian tradition as a mutilation of familial flesh. Buddhist notions of karma and the Buddhist prohibition against the taking of life compound the sense that a fetus should be protected. However, there is widespread ambiguity in the popular imagination about the ontological status of the fetus, as noted in studies of fetus-ghost appeasement rituals in Japan and Taiwan, conducted by William LaFleur, Helen Hardacre, and Marc Moskowitz. Most people believe the fetus to have a soul at conception, yet there is also the belief that this soul is not solidly anchored, meaning that it is extremely susceptible to fright—and flight—during the first 100 days of infancy. A soul that escapes its body in this way will likely make its way to another, but the specter of a free-floating vengeful spirit has fueled a lucrative fetal-ghost appeasement industry.

It must also be noted that nominally Confucian cultures have long embraced a pragmatic ethical relativism, sometimes attributed to Taoism, which seeks to maximize personal and familial benefit while avoiding inauspicious residual effects. In late-twentieth-century China, an alternative to abortion and female infanticide has emerged: After birth unwanted infant females are anonymously left at local orphanages or social welfare offices, or else they are quickly sold to baby brokers who then deliver them to state facilities. In this way, the state has found itself with a seemingly inexhaustible supply of a highly desirable commodity: infant girls for the international adoption market.

In some areas the male-female sex ratio of recorded live births is severely and increasingly skewed in favor of males. In Korea use of ultrasound screening to determine fetal sex is illegal but widely practiced. In China the overall male-female ratio of recorded births is between 117:100 and 120:100, whereas the average should be 105:100. In certain rural areas, the ratio rises to 144:100, the highest imbalance in the world. It is impossible to know with certainty the exact percentages of the *missing girls* who were aborted or were victims of infanticide, or the number of girls who were born and kept by their families but whose births were not recorded on official rosters. What is known is that decades of increasingly unbalanced male-female ratios have given rise to kidnappings, mail order marriages of children, and wholesale trafficking in women (Rosenthal, Eckholm).

## Ownership of the Body

Of particular relevance to bioethics is the Confucian understanding of ownership of the body. Confucian tradition holds that one's body is not truly one's own; rather, it is held in custody for one's parents and ancestors. In a particularly gendered illustration of this notion, the historical records contain many examples of filial daughters and daughters-in-law who, charged with the care and feeding of parents and parents-in-law, cut flesh from their arms or legs in order to make nourishing broth in times of war or famine. In other circumstances, however, to harm or mutilate one's body might render it insufficient to its purpose of care for preceding generations. To a Confucian, therefore, preserving the integrity of the body is of great importance. This holds true even after death, for although the deceased becomes an ancestor him- or herself, he or she remains at the service of still earlier generations.

Here too, the complexity of Confucian interaction with other traditions becomes apparent: Internal organs are only valued for their functions, and thus the donation of a sample of bone marrow or of a single kidney would seem permissible. However, the general Confucian sense of the body remaining intact in order to serve one's family is compounded by the popular Buddhist notion that a body must be complete in order to move through its karmic destiny. For many people in Confucian cultures, therefore, the combination of these beliefs has precluded acceptance of organ donation and transplantation up until quite recently.

One organization that has been working to change this view is the Tzu Chi Buddhist Compassion Foundation, a lay organization that claims 4 million members worldwide. Founded in rural Taiwan in 1966 by Dharma Master Cheng Yen, a self-ordained nun, the Tzu Chi Foundation exhorts women to fulfill their traditional Confucian role of dutiful wife and mother—even as it promotes women's volunteer efforts outside the home, particularly in medical care and disaster relief. In 1994 Tzu Chi established a bone marrow registry, the third largest in the world in 2003. Tzu Chi encourages organ and tissue donation (and even body donation for the training of medical students) as examples of Buddhist compassion. Although these teachings are at odds with traditional Confucian-Buddhist attitudes toward the body, Master Cheng Yen emphasizes the interconnectedness of all beings and the importance of practicing compassion to save lives. At Tzu Chi hospitals, hospices, free clinics, and medical and nursing schools, healthcare workers are trained to view patients holistically and humanely, seeing them as teachers and as providers of opportunities to serve.

## Current Directions of Contemporary Scholarship

For scholars *of* Confucianism, the implications of studying Confucianism as a world religion are that its texts and interpretive traditions are open to literary critical study; its history is scrutinized for gender, class, and other biases; its ideal figures are analyzed with historical, sociological, and psychological tools; and its entire ethos is set in a comparative framework. The profoundly transformative aspects of its humanistic project can be appreciated as overtly religious, and discussions of Confucian spirituality are increasingly common.

For scholars *in* the tradition, new questions abound. What is the Confucian response to environmental degradation? Can traditional relationships be recast to address new configurations of the nuclear family, for example, same-sex unions, one (female)-child households, or blended families? What is the nature of lateral relationships, that is, what is one's relationship to other members of a civil society? What is the Confucian perspective on various reproductive technologies, or on genetic screening? Such issues are fraught with ambiguity.

For people in cultural China, Korea, Japan, and Vietnam, Confucianism is perhaps best understood as providing a substratum of belief, complementing or complicating other beliefs and values, whether sectarian or secular. Although scholars can debate Confucian responses to any issue, a single Confucian judgment is probably impossible to construct. In the syncretic and diasporic world of Confucian cultures, a Korean Christian Confucian may hold one opinion, a Japanese Buddhist Confucian another, and a *Boston Confucian* may hold yet another view altogether.

VIVIAN-LEE NYITRAY

SEE ALSO: *Aging and the Aged: Old Age; Beneficence; Buddhism, Bioethics in; Daoism, Bioethics in; Death: Eastern Thought; Feminism; Medical Ethics, History of South and East Asia: China; Paternalism; Trust; Women, Historical and Cross-Cultural Perspectives*

### BIBLIOGRAPHY

Brooks, E. Bruce, and Brooks, A. Taeko. 1998. *The Original Analects: Sayings of Confucius and His Successors.* New York: Columbia University Press.

Eckholm, Erik. 2002. "Desire for Sons Drives Use of Prenatal Scans in China." *The New York Times,* June 21, Late Edition—Final, A: 3.

Furth, Charlotte. 1998. *A Flourishing Yin: Gender in China's Medical History: 960–1665.* Berkeley: University of California Press.

Hardacre, Helen. 1997. *Marketing the Menacing Fetus in Japan.* Berkeley: University of California Press.

Hay, John. 1993. "The Body as Microcosmic Source." In *Self as Body in Asian Theory and Practice,* ed. Thomas P. Kasulis. Albany: State University of New York Press.

Koh, Byong-ik. 1996. "Confucianism in Contemporary Korea." In *Confucian Traditions in East Asian Modernity: Moral Education and Economic Culture in Japan and the Four Mini-Dragons,* ed. Wei-ming Tu. Cambridge, MA: Harvard University Press.

LaFleur, William R. 1993. *Liquid Life: Abortion and Buddhism in Japan.* Princeton, NJ: Princeton University Press.

Moskowitz, Marc L. 2001. *The Haunting Fetus: Abortion, Sexuality, and the Spirit World in Taiwan.* Honolulu: University of Hawaii Press.

Neville, Robert C. 2000. *Boston Confucianism: Portable Tradition in the Late-Modern World.* Albany: State University of New York Press.

Nyitray, Vivian-Lee. 2001. "The Single Thread of a New Confucianism: Public Virtue and Private Responsibility." In *Taking Responsibility: Comparative Perspectives,* ed. Winston B. Davis. Charlottesville: University Press of Virginia.

Rosenthal, Elisabeth. 2001. "Harsh Chinese Realities Feed Market in Women." *The New York Times,* June 25, Late Edition—Final, A: 8.

Sivin, Nathan. 1995. *Medicine, Philosophy, and Religion in Ancient China.* Brookfield, VT: Variorum.

Taylor, Rodney L. 1990. *The Religious Dimensions of Confucianism.* Albany: State University of New York Press.

Yao, Xinzhong. 2000. *An Introduction to Confucianism.* Cambridge, England: Cambridge University Press.

# CONSCIENCE

• • •

Matters of conscience arise with some frequency in bioethics. A health professional may cite considerations of conscience in declining to perform or participate in a certain procedure. A patient may refuse a particular treatment on grounds of conscience. And new or unanticipated circumstances may create conflicts of conscience for patients and health professionals alike. What do we mean by "conscience" in these and related contexts? Is conscience an internal moral sense sufficient for distinguishing right from wrong? Is the "voice" of conscience simply the echo of parental and social prohibitions? Or does conscience differ in important ways from either of these? How much weight should be given in ethical reflection to claims of conscience? To what extent and for what reasons should health professionals compromise personal convenience, institutional efficiency, or medical effectiveness in order to respect individual conscience, their own or their patients'?

## Three Conceptions of Conscience

The idea of conscience has a long and complex history (D'Arcy, 1961; Mount). The word "conscience" derives from the Latin *conscientia,* introduced by Christian Scholastics. Most generally, it refers to conscious awareness of the moral quality of some past or contemplated action and the disposition to be so aware (conscientiousness). In what follows we consider three main conceptions: (1) conscience as an inner sense that distinguishes right acts from wrong; (2) conscience as the internalization of parental and social norms; and (3) conscience as the exercise and expression of a reflective sense of integrity.

MORAL SENSE. Conscience is sometimes conceived as an internal moral sense sufficient for distinguishing right from wrong. The reliability of this inner sense is usually attributed to its divine origin, its reflection of our true nature, or some combination of the two. There are, however, difficulties with this conception.

Consider, first, a variation of an argument developed by Plato in his *Euthyphro.* Is what makes an act right the fact that it is endorsed by one's conscience? Or does conscience recommend a certain course of conduct because it is right? If the former, the promptings of conscience appear to be arbitrary. Whatever is urged by a person's conscience would, in this view, be right. There would be no way to assess the deliverances of conscience or to compare the consciences of, say, Hitler and Mother Teresa. If, on the other hand, conscience directs us to perform certain acts because they are right, it cannot be the principal source of moral knowledge. We must, in this event, have prior, independent criteria of rightness and wrongness that allow us to distinguish those acts that should be recommended by conscience from those that should not—in which case conscience is not sufficient to guide conduct.

A related difficulty is the prevalence of conflicts of conscience, both within persons and between them. Such conflicts are especially pronounced in bioethics, where advances in knowledge and technology confront us with unprecedented, consequential choices ranging well beyond our ethical traditions. The limitations of conscience, if it is conceived as a sufficient guide to moral decision making, may not be so noticeable in static, homogenous, insular cultures and subcultures. But where new circumstances require members of pluralistic societies to come to some agreement on bioethical questions, appeals to an internal, self-validating sense of right and wrong are apt to generate more heat than light.

INTERNALIZED SOCIAL NORMS. The most plausible explanation for the limitations of conscience in resolving ethical conflicts is that the "voice" of conscience is simply the echo of social and parental admonitions impressed upon the developing psyches of young children (i.e., the Freudian superego). Whatever its psychological and developmental significance, conscience so conceived has little normative import. That we have certain moral compunctions as a result of our socialization does little to establish their validity. We are bound by the voice of conscience only if we can provide independent justification of its dictates. It is the adequacy of the justification, not the persistence of the voice, that carries moral authority. Conceived as internalized social norms, then, conscience plays no direct role in ethical deliberation.

SENSE OF INTEGRITY. "I couldn't live with myself if I were [or were not] to perform the abortion in these circumstances." "I can no longer participate in this treatment plan in good conscience." "How could I continue to think of myself as a Jehovah's Witness if I were to consent to the blood transfusion?" Each of these sentences expresses an appeal to conscience that is neither a deliverance of an internal moral sense nor an internalization of an external social norm. What is expressed in each case is the culmination of conscientious reflection about the relationship between a certain course of action and a particular conception of the self. So understood, appeals to conscience are closely connected to reflective concern with one's integrity. The focus is not so much on the objective or universal rightness or wrongness of a particular act as on the consequences for the self of one's performing it.

There is something absurd, Gilbert Ryle has observed, in saying "My conscience says that *you* ought to do this or ought not to have done that" (Ryle, p. 31). I may be troubled by your wrongdoing, but unless I have advised or assisted you, or culpably failed to prevent you from performing the act in question, my conscience will be clear. The same is not true, however, about those of my acts that I have determined, for one reason or another, were or would be morally wrong. Having judged a certain act to be wrong, an appeal to conscience stresses the added wrongness of my performing it. Appeals to conscience therefore presuppose a prior determination of the rightness or wrongness of an act (Childress, 1979). Moreover, one may or may not extend the standards one employs in making this assessment to others in similar situations. If, for example, the standards are universalizable principles of respect for persons, justice, or beneficence, one will maintain that anyone would do wrong in performing the act in question. But if one's standards are grounded in religious convictions, personal ideals, or a particular worldview and way of life, one may not hold everyone else to them. What is at stake in all such appeals is one's wholeness or integrity as a person.

## Integrity

"It would be better for me," Socrates says in the *Gorgias,* "that my lyre or a chorus I directed should be out of tune and loud with discord, and that multitudes of men should

disagree with me rather than that I, *being one,* should be out of harmony with myself and contradict me" (Arendt, 1971, p. 439). One cannot lead a good and meaningful life, Socrates suggests, unless the self is reasonably unified or integrated—unless, that is, one's words and deeds cohere with one's basic, identity-conferring, moral, religious, and philosophical convictions. Hence the importance of critical reflection on one's life as a whole. The words, deeds, and convictions of an unexamined life are unlikely to be sufficiently integrated to constitute a singular life—let alone one worth living.

Conscience should not, therefore, be conceived as a faculty or component of the self. It is, rather, the voice of one's self as a whole, understood temporally—as having a beginning, a middle, and an end—as well as at a particular moment. Operating retrospectively, what Christian tradition calls "judicial" conscience makes judgments about past conduct. Operating prospectively, what the same tradition calls "legislative" conscience anticipates whether a prospective utterance or course of action is likely to be at odds with one's most basic ethical convictions (D'Arcy, 1961). In each case, the signal that something is wrong—that one's integrity has been, is currently, or would be compromised—is an actual or anticipatory feeling of guilt, shame, or remorse.

Consider, in this connection, the words of Aleksandr N. Chikunov, a veteran of the 1968 Soviet invasion of Czechoslovakia, as he explains sharing his experience with young soldiers called to Moscow to suppress democratic reforms during the abortive coup of August 1991: "I entered Prague in 1968 and I still have an ill conscience about it. I was a soldier then, like these guys. We were also sent like they are now, to defend the achievements of socialism. Twenty-three years have passed, and I still have an ill conscience" (*New York Times,* August 20, 1991, p. A13). Here Chikunov draws upon the lessons of his "ill" judicial conscience to inform and alert the legislative consciences of the young soldiers. His motivation, it seems, is not only to spare them the pangs of an ill conscience but also to help heal his own (and thus to heal himself).

The authority and sanctions of conscience are, Mr. Chikunov suggests, self-imposed. No external source can create or directly relieve a troubled conscience. Nor may we easily rationalize or evade its judgments. "Other judges," as D'Arcy points out, "may be venal or partial or fallible; not so the verdict of conscience" (D'Arcy, 1961, p. 8). The oppressiveness of a guilty conscience is due in part to its identity with the self.

## Conscience in Bioethics

Three factors contribute to the prevalence of appeals to conscience in bioethics: (1) bioethical decision making often involves our deepest identity-conferring convictions about the nature and meaning of creating, sustaining, and ending life; (2) healthcare professionals and patients and their families will occasionally have radically differing beliefs about such matters; and (3) the complexity of modern healthcare often requires agreement and cooperation on a single course of action.

**CONFLICTS OF CONSCIENCE.** Conflicts of conscience arise not only between individuals but also within them. Consider a physician whose patient, suffering greatly from the ravages of the last stages of a terminal illness, is also a longtime friend. The patient requests the physician to provide both the substance and the instruction for taking his own life. The physician finds herself torn. On the one hand, her conception of medicine and professional identity is incompatible with what appears to be physician-assisted suicide. On the other hand, the bonds of friendship and her natural sympathies strongly incline her to accede to her patient's request. The situation has, as a result, precipitated a crisis of conscience, and the physician must engage in what Charles Taylor has called "strong evaluation"—reflection about the self by the self in ways that engage and attempt to restructure one's deepest and most fundamental convictions (Taylor). Such reflection manifests an admirable concern for wholeness or integrity.

**CONSCIENTIOUS REFUSAL.** From Socrates to Sir Thomas More to Henry David Thoreau, individuals have appealed to conscience in refusing to comply with a wide range of legal or socially mandated directives. In some cases such noncompliance may be covert and evasive—for example, a physician's providing contraceptive information to married couples in Connecticut before that state's anticontraceptive law was declared unconstitutional (Childress, 1985). In most cases, however, health professionals and patients give reasons of conscience in openly seeking personal exemption from certain standard practices.

Physicians may appeal to conscience in refusing to do procedures that are both legal and performed by their colleagues. Consider an obstetrician's refusal to perform a legal abortion or a pediatrician's refusal to prescribe human growth hormone for short, but normal, children at the behest of their anxious parents. In each case the physician's decision may be based on moral convictions or personal ideals. The obstetrician need not believe that abortion ought to be illegal or that women who request, or physicians who perform, abortions are deeply immoral. The pediatrician may neither urge the legal prohibition of administering human growth hormone to short, but normal, children nor

regard parents who request this treatment, or other pediatricians who administer it, as unethical. Both agree, however, that it would be a violation of conscience—a betrayal of their deepest personal convictions about life or the nature of medicine—if they were to perform the act in question.

Similarly, nurses appeal to conscience in seeking exemption from procedures or care plans that threaten their sense of integrity. For example, a nurse may conscientiously refuse to follow a physician's directive to remove medically administered hydration and nutrition from a patient in a persistent vegetative state. Regardless of the act's legality, the family's concurrence, and the physician's directive, given her deepest identity-conferring convictions about the nature and value of life, the nurse may be unable to carry out the action. Her reasoning, she might add, is not strong enough to condemn others who believe differently; but as for herself, she must refrain.

Patients, too, may appeal to conscience in refusing forms of medical treatment. When informed, mentally competent Jehovah's Witnesses refuse blood transfusions on religious grounds, they do not at the same time urge that blood transfusions be legally prohibited, nor do they condemn those who gratefully accept blood transfusions. What they want is not so much respect for the content of their particular convictions as much as respect for their consciences. The same is true of other patients who refuse or request certain forms of treatment on the basis of fundamental moral and religious convictions.

## Respect for Conscience

Respect for conscience is a corollary of the principle of respect for persons. To respect another as a person is, insofar as possible, to respect the expression and exercise, if not the content, of a person's most fundamental convictions. A society's respect for individual conscience may extend not only to religious toleration but also, for example, to exempting conscripted pacifists from direct participation in war.

In the biomedical context, respect for conscience may be inconvenient, inefficient, or detrimental to medical outcomes. Still, it must always be taken seriously and often should prevail. In some cases, respect for conscience may be balanced with biomedical goals. At a certain level of abstraction, the purpose of healthcare is strikingly similar to that of protecting individual conscience. Although healthcare is usually focused on the body, emphasis on informed consent implies that the principal function of medicine is the health or wholeness of the patient as a person. Yet a person's sense of health or wholeness may also be threatened by what the former Soviet soldier, Aleksandr Chikunov, revealingly called an "ill" conscience. The values underlying appeals to conscience within the healthcare system are not, therefore, radically at odds with the values underlying medical and nursing care. In each case the aim is to preserve or restore personal wholeness. Insofar, then, as appeals to conscience and the healthcare system share a fundamental commitment to preserving and restoring personal wholeness or integrity, we ought in cases of conflict to seek some sort of balance or accommodation between them.

Health professionals who refuse, withdraw, or dissociate themselves from certain practices or procedures on grounds of conscience may well be among the more thoughtful and effective members of a healthcare team. Thus a healthcare institution intent on retaining such nurses and physicians has prudential as well as ethical grounds for accommodating their claims of conscience even at the cost of some inconvenience or expense. Respect for conscience requires going to greater lengths for patients, however, than it does for healthcare professionals. This is in part because an individual's role as a healthcare professional is voluntary in a way that being a patient is not. It is one thing, for example, to respect a Jehovah's Witness patient's conscientious refusal of a blood transfusion; it is quite another to respect the conscientious refusal of a physician who is a Jehovah's Witness to administer blood transfusions. An individual whose moral or religious convictions are incompatible with a common, essential type of healthcare has no business seeking a position in which such care is a routine expectation.

## Problems and Limits

At least two important questions remain. First, how do we distinguish genuine claims of conscience from claims serving as smoke screens for laziness, cowardice, distaste for certain procedures, or dislike or prejudice toward certain patients? Second, given that a genuine act of conscience may be morally wrong, should individuals always (or always be permitted to) follow their conscience?

GENUINENESS. Understanding the nature and justification of conscientious refusal allows us to distinguish genuine from spurious or self-deceived appeals to conscience. In assessing the authenticity of such appeals we may, for example, inquire into (1) the underlying values and the extent to which they constitute a core component of the individual's identity; (2) the depth of the individual's reflective consideration of the issue; and (3) the likelihood that he or she will experience guilt, shame, or a loss of self-respect by performing the act in question. Such criteria have been employed with reasonable success by the U.S. Selective

Service System in identifying those whose deep and long-standing moral convictions forbid direct participation in war. They can be used with similar success in identifying genuine appeals to conscience in the healthcare setting (Benjamin and Curtis).

CONSCIENTIOUS BUT WRONG. Conscience is not an infallible guide to conduct. Even those who attend carefully to matters of integrity and who critically examine their basic convictions may, at a later date, judge some of their conscientious acts as wrong. Should one, then, always follow one's conscience? If by "conscience" we mean the exercise and expression of good-faith efforts to integrate conduct with reflective ethical conviction, the answer is "yes." Following conscience is obligatory, even if one's act turns out to be wrong, because one is doing what one reflectively believes to be right. Conversely, deliberately acting contrary to conscience is blameworthy, even if one's act turns out to be right, because one is doing what one reflectively believes to be wrong.

We must therefore distinguish the character of an agent from the rightness of a particular act. That an act is required by conscience entails neither that it is right nor that others must endorse the agent's convictions or permit the act to occur. It is difficult, for example, to question the character of Jehovah's Witness parents when they conscientiously refuse to consent to a life-saving blood transfusion for a young child. Yet if we have good reasons for believing that withholding the transfusion would be seriously wrong, we may try to persuade the parents to consent and, if necessary, seek a court order mandating treatment. Distinguishing the conscientiousness of the parents from our judgment of the act, though not eliminating the difficult question of whether, and if so, how, to intervene, enables us to attend more adequately to its complexity.

MARTIN BENJAMIN (1995)

SEE ALSO: *Autonomy; Conscience, Rights of; Emotions; Ethics, Religion and Morality; Freedom and Free Will; Human Dignity; Human Nature; Principlism; Profession and Professional Ethics*

### BIBLIOGRAPHY

Arendt, Hannah. 1971. "Thinking and Moral Considerations: A Lecture." *Social Research* 38: 417–446. Reprinted in *Social Research* 51: 7–37 (1984).

Arendt, Hannah. 1972. "Civil Disobedience." In her *Crises of the Republic: Lying in Politics, Civil Disobedience, On Violence, Thoughts on Politics and Revolution*, pp. 51–102. New York: Harcourt Brace Jovanovich.

Beauchamp, Tom L., and Childress, James F. 1984. *Principles of Biomedical Ethics,* 3rd edition. New York: Oxford University Press.

Benjamin, Martin. 1990. *Splitting the Difference: Compromise and Integrity in Ethics and Politics.* Lawrence: University Press of Kansas.

Benjamin, Martin, and Curtis, Joy. 1992. *Ethics in Nursing.* 3rd edition. New York: Oxford University Press.

Broad, Charlie Dunbar. 1940. "Conscience and Conscientious Action." *Philosophy* 15: 115–130.

Butler, Joseph. 1900 (1726). *Fifteen Sermons. In The Works of Bishop Butler,* vol. 1; ed. John Henry Bernard. New York: Macmillan.

Childress, James F. 1979. "Appeals to Conscience." *Ethics* 89(4): 315–335.

Childress, James F. 1985. "Civil Disobedience, Conscientious Objection, and Evasive Noncompliance: A Framework for the Analysis and Assessment of Illegal Actions in Health Care." *Journal of Medicine and Philosophy* 10(1): 63–83.

D'Arcy, Eric. 1961. *Conscience and Its Right to Freedom.* New York: Sheed and Ward.

D'Arcy, Eric. 1977. "Conscience." *Journal of Medical Ethics* 3(2): 98–99.

Fuss, Peter. 1964. "Conscience." *Ethics* 74(2): 111–120.

Garnett, A. Campbell. 1966. "Conscience and Conscientiousness." In *Insight and Vision: Essays in Philosophy in Honor of Radoslav Andrea Tsanoff,* pp. 71–83, ed. Konstantin Kolenda. San Antonio: Trinity University Press.

Gillon, Raanan. 1984. "Conscience, Virtue, Integrity, and Medical Ethics." *Journal of Medical Ethics* 10(4): 171–172.

May, Larry. 1983. "On Conscience." *American Philosophical Quarterly* 20(1): 57–67.

McGuire, Martin. 1963. "On Conscience." *Journal of Philosophy* 60(10): 253–263.

Mount, Eric, Jr. 1969. *Conscience and Responsibility.* Richmond, VA: John Knox Press.

Ryle, Gilbert. 1940. "Conscience and Moral Convictions." *Analysis* 7: 31–39.

Taylor, Charles. 1976. "Responsibility for Self." In *The Identities of Persons,* pp. 281–299, ed. Amelie Oksenberg Rorty. Berkeley: University of California Press.

Wand, Bernard. 1961. "The Content and Function of Conscience." *Journal of Philosophy* 58(24): 765–772.

# CONSCIENCE, RIGHTS OF

• • •

The phenomenon of a *right of conscience* arises only in a society that takes seriously the autonomy of individual persons. Philosopher James Childress has described appeals to conscience as "a person's consciousness of and reflection on his own acts in relation to his standards of judgment." (Childress, 1979) Rights of conscience are political rights that protect people's ability to do what they believe is morally best: they are political *autonomy rights.* Common scenarios for the exercise of a right of conscience in healthcare include seeking an exemption from mandatory vaccination and, for physicians, refusing to participate in morally controversial procedures like abortion.

## Political Significance

To understand the political role of rights of conscience, it helps to think of the activities a person might engage in as falling into one of three political categories: (1) prohibited, (2) permitted, or (3) required. In Western societies, the vast majority of possible activities are permitted, meaning people may engage in that activity if they wish (it is not prohibited), but they do not have to engage in that activity (it is not required). A person may exercise autonomy, then, in deciding whether to engage in the activity. Likewise, some activities (e.g., murder, robbery) may be prohibited, and some activities (e.g., military service in times of war) may be required.

An autonomy right ensures that protected activities are not unduly prohibited or required. For example, one prominent autonomy right protects the practice of religion: the autonomy right of freedom of religion means that a person's religious practice cannot be unduly prohibited or required. This allows a person to practice religion, but also allows a person to decide not to practice a religion. Thus, the practice of religion is neither prohibited nor required, allowing a person to exercise autonomy in the practice of religion. Other examples of autonomy rights include freedom of speech (which protects against state prohibition of the expression of opinions, but does not require a person to express their opinion), freedom of assembly (which protects against state prohibition of people's ability to assemble), and, in the United States, the right to own firearms (which protects a person's ability to own a gun).

## The Focus of Autonomy Rights

In Western societies, most political autonomy rights focus on ensuring that certain activities are not unduly prohibited (thus protecting a people's ability to engage in that activity if they should choose). This can be seen in the way such rights are normally phrased:

Congress shall make no law respecting an establishment of religion, or prohibiting the free exercise thereof; or abridging the freedom of speech, or of the press; or the right of the people peaceably to assemble, and to petition the Government for a redress of grievances. (Bill of Rights, U.S. Constitution, Amendment I)

Rights of conscience, however, protect a person from mandatory participation in an activity if the activity in question threatens the fundamental values of an individual person. This focus can be seen in the way conscience clauses are typically phrased: "No person shall be required to …" In a clinical context, rights of conscience are exercised against a backdrop of a professional duty to treat a patient once a provider-patient relationship is established. Thus, rights of conscience claim an exemption to participation in activities that one would otherwise be expected to undertake. The most common example is a claim to be exempt from participation in abortion procedures.

## Conditions of a Right of Conscience

The primary conditions necessary for the legitimate exercise of a right of conscience consist of: (1) the lack of harm posed to others by the exercise of a right of conscience; and (2) strength and sincerity of beliefs that are the basis for a claim of conscience. The exercise of a right of conscience does *not* require a demonstration of the truth of beliefs that are the basis of a right-of-conscience claim, as requiring the truth of a belief to be demonstrated would trivialize the right itself. The first of these conditions represents a straightforward balancing of the rights of individuals through recognition that autonomy rights must be restricted when significant harm is posed to others. Thus, for example, a right to freedom of speech does not include a right to shout "Fire!" in a crowded theater. Similarly, seeking an exemption from mandatory vaccination is restricted in circumstances of epidemic disease, where failure to be vaccinated could pose a threat of harm to others.

Such a balancing of autonomy rights and social harm was clearly recognized in the U.S. Supreme Court case of *Jacobson v. Massachusetts*. Henning Jacobson argued that he should not be forced to receive a vaccination during a smallpox epidemic because "compulsory vaccination is … hostile to the inherent right of every free man to care for his own body and health in such a way as to him seems best." The Supreme Court rejected this argument in the context of an epidemic, however, stating, "The liberty secured by the Constitution of the United States does not import an absolute right.... There are manifold restraints to which

every person is necessarily subject for the common good" (*Jacobson v. Massachusetts*).

The second condition listed above is less commonly required for the exercise of an autonomy right. It requires that rights of conscience only be exercised on the basis of values that are central to one's life. As Childress describes it, "In appealing to conscience I indicate that I am trying to preserve a sense of myself, my wholeness or integrity … and that I cannot preserve these qualities if I submit to certain requirements of the state or society" (Childress, p. 327). To legitimately exercise a right of conscience, one must show that participation in the required activity would threaten values that play a central role in the way one has chosen to live.

Because the majority of people in Western societies are religious, and their religious convictions normally represent their most fundamental values, claims to rights of conscience most commonly arise in the context of religious convictions, though rights-of-conscience claims need not be based upon religion. The most prominent example is conscientious objection to participation in war. During the Vietnam War era, the U.S. Supreme Court ruled that a person may qualify for an exemption to participation in war if the person's opposition stems from "moral, ethical, or religious beliefs about what is right and wrong, and that these beliefs be held with strength of traditional religious convictions" (*Welsh v. U.S.*).

The type and significance of harm to others that might negate the ability to exercise a right of conscience, as well as the abstract notion of *strength of conviction* necessary to qualify for a right of conscience, represent the key points of contention in how to distinguish legitimate from illegitimate claims to a right of conscience. The most prominent debate in the literature concerns the consequences of recognizing rights of conscience relevant to access to abortion services. In some areas, conscientious refusal by physicians to participate in abortion services has limited access to abortion services, or made them unavailable. Use of this type of harm to negate rights of conscience, however, is met with substantial skepticism. The argument requires that the conscience of a woman seeking access to abortion takes precedence over that of a physician, and also assumes that a right to not be prohibited from having an abortion is tantamount to a right of access to abortion services. These issues remain at the center of this ongoing debate.

A second type of harm that is discussed in the literature consists of psychological and moral harms associated with the necessity of transfer of care from a provider a patient has chosen, due to that provider's refusal to participate in a particular treatment plan. The significance of this should not be overlooked: while transfer of care leaves a patient with continued access to care in the abstract, the patient may not feel as comfortable with the caregivers to whom he or she is transferred. Thus, one should only necessitate such a transfer if the values threatened are significant.

## The Exercise of Rights

Recognition of the types of harms described above is closely tied to attempts to outline the scenarios in which a right of conscience should (and should not) be exercised. While it is desirable to recognize rights of conscience in matters of central moral importance to a person, rights of conscience should not be used, for example, to discriminate against a racial or ethnic group by refusing services to that group, or to undermine informed consent by pressuring a patient to agree to a treatment plan through threat of transfer of care. Conscience clauses that offer blanket protection and simply require transfer of care fail to address these concerns, so criteria to distinguish when a right of conscience is appropriately exercised become important.

Most of the literature recognizes that entering into a profession imposes some level of moral duty that may at times conflict with a person's own judgment. While it is important to recognize moral diversity within a profession, and thus allow for some cases of conscientious objection, it is also important to recognize the weight of professional obligations, such as respect for patient autonomy and informed consent. Because professional obligations to respect informed consent do carry moral weight, rights of conscience are, in general, more appropriately exercised over patient requests for services than over patient refusals, since objection to a patient's refusal fails to respect that patient's evaluation that the treatment does not offer desired benefits (this is a general guideline, however, and may admit of exceptions). So, for example, a physician's right of conscience (for refusal of services) is appropriately exercised over a patient's request for an abortion or for assistance in committing suicide (physician-assisted suicide). A right of conscience is not appropriately exercised, however, over a patient's refusal of a ventilator. Similarly, it is widely recognized that rights of conscience should not be exercised over simple disagreement with a patient's treatment choice. These general guidelines still leave a lot of gray area, however. For example, does a request by a Jehovah's Witness for surgery without blood products constitute a refusal of blood products or a request for a specific surgical procedure (one that does not involve the use of blood products)?

Professional obligations of nondiscrimination are also important in formulating criteria for the legitimate exercise of a right of conscience. The conscientious objection in question should not be based on *who* is to receive the treatment or procedure. Instead, conscientious refusal should be based on the *type* of treatment or procedure in question, rather than, for example, provision of this treatment or procedure to members of a particular racial or ethnic group. Here, too, the general guidelines leave room for debate; such as when an objection is based on the fact that a procedure is particularly dangerous for a certain segment of the population (e.g., organ transplant recipients, elderly patients).

## Summary

While several points of debate continue to remain contentious, some general observations can be made concerning the appropriate exercise of a right of conscience. First, such rights should only be exercised if doing so does not pose a threat of significant harm to others. Second, the exercise of a right of conscience should be based upon values that play a central role in the life of the person claiming a right of conscience. Related to this, rights of conscience should not be exercised on the basis of simple disagreement about a treatment plan. Third, conscientious objection to patient requests will be, in general, more appropriate than objection to patient refusals. Finally, professional obligations to respect patient autonomy and to avoid discriminatory practices should be weighed against the exercise of a right of conscience. In this context, conscientious objection should be exercised only when based upon an objection to the *type* of activity in question.

THOMAS MAY

**SEE ALSO:** *Autonomy, Beneficence; Clinical Ethics; Conscience; Informed Consent; Surrogate Decision-Making; Warfare: Medicine and War; Whistleblowing in Healthcare*

### BIBLIOGRAPHY

Blustein, J. 1993. "Doing What the Patient Orders: Maintaining Integrity in the Doctor-Patient Relationship." *Bioethics* 7(4): 289–314.

Cannold, Leslie. 1994. "Consequences for Patients of Health Professionals' Conscientious Actions." *Journal of Medical Ethics* 20: 80–86.

Childress, James. 1974. "Appeals to Conscience." *Ethics* 89: 315–335.

Daniels, Norman. 1991. "Duty to Treat or Right to Refuse?" *Hastings Center Report* 21: 36–46.

Dresser, Rebecca. 1994. "Freedom of Conscience, Professional Responsibility, and Access to Abortion." *Journal of Law, Medicine, and Ethics* 22: 280–285.

Feinberg, Joel. 1984. *Harm to Others.* New York: Oxford University Press.

Greenawalt, Kent. 1989. *Conflicts of Law and Morality.* Oxford: Clarendon Press.

*Jacobson v. Massachusetts.* 197 U.S. 11 (1905).

May, Thomas. 2002. *Bioethics in a Liberal Society: The Political Framework for Bioethics Decision Making.* Baltimore: Johns Hopkins University Press.

Meyers, Christopher, and Woods, Robert. 1996. "An Obligation to Provide Abortion Services: What Happens When Physicians Refuse?" *Journal of Medical Ethics* 22: 115–120.

Raz, Joseph. 1979. *The Authority of Law.* Oxford: Clarendon Press.

Richards, David A. J. 1989. *Toleration and the Constitution.* New York: Oxford University Press.

Silverman, Ross, and May, Thomas. 2001. "Private Choice Versus Public Health: Religion, Morality, and Childhood Vaccination Law." *Margins* 1: 505–521.

Wardle, Lynn D. 1993. "Protecting the Rights of Conscience of Health Care Providers." *The Journal of Legal Medicine* 14: 177–230.

Wear, Stephen; LaGaipa, Susan; and Logue, Gerald. 1994. "Toleration of Moral Diversity and the Conscientious Refusal by Physicians to Withdraw Life-Sustaining Treatment." *Journal of Medicine and Philosophy* 19: 147–159.

*Welsh v. U.S.* 398 U.S. 333 (1970).

Wicclair, Mark. 2000. "Conscientious Objection in Medicine." *Bioethics* 14: 205–227.

# CONSENSUS, ROLE AND AUTHORITY OF

• • •

Consensus plays a paradoxical role in bioethics: Although the weight of opinion is traditionally thought to have little or no merit in the resolution of moral problems, practical moral problems beg for a modus operandi that enables activity to proceed. Upon analysis, consensus also reveals a complex conceptual structure as well as a murky etiology in the history of ideas. Yet it seems difficult, if not impossible, to avoid the pursuit of consensus in the face of a morally troubling situation, however obscure the object of that pursuit might be. The impetus for a consensus is acute in a field like bioethics, which often expresses itself in such settings as clinical or research ethics committees (Moreno, 1988) and governmental policy commissions (Walters).

## The History of Consensus

It is not easy to get clear on the idea of consensus, and particularly the idea of moral consensus. One reason is that relevant discussions in the history of philosophy do not always use those terms. For example, Plato's political philosophy can be taken as a treatise on consensus, but he would understand a consensus (a Latin term, of course), as a common or shared opinion. Thus the findings of the jury in Socrates's trial represent a shared opinion, and to Plato a deeply flawed one, that led to the death of his beloved teacher and seems to have inspired his elaboration and extension of Socratic philosophy in the *Republic.*

Literary and philosophical references to consensus seem first to have appeared with some frequency only since the nineteenth century. By then the political conception of consent of the governed had of course been subjected to close examination prior to the American and French revolutions and played a key role in those epochal events. Consensus might be regarded as the sociological cousin of political consent, not always as explicit in its manifestation nor as definitive, but nevertheless a key element in a well-functioning society. In contrast to the philosophical notion of consensus exemplified in social contract theories, sociological understandings of consensus emphasize acquiescence to extant norms.

For social scientists consensus emerged as an important category of analysis in the era of industrialization, as it helped account for the social harmony required of complex bureaucracies in the private and public sectors. Increasingly, societies in the process of pluralizing also had reason to be more aware of consensus as they encountered an unaccustomed diversity of basic values. By the late twentieth century consensus had become very nearly an end in itself among policy makers intent on finding common ground in postmodern societies rent by divisive issues, such as abortion.

Bioethics is certainly a result of this emerging process. In the early 1960s, when dialysis machines were developed to the point that they could extend life indefinitely but remained in short supply, the need to formulate an acceptable allocation arrangement was acute. Other matters of concern followed rapidly, including organ transplants, genetic engineering, human experimentation, and discontinuing life-sustaining treatment. In each case bioethics gained social standing through its participation in the formulation of a consensus. Conspicuous in its absence from this list is abortion, and it may be significant that this is the only one of these topics that was resolved almost solely in the legal system. Although the law is often an excellent instrument for consolidating a moral consensus, this is evidently not always the case.

## The Paradox of Consensus in Bioethics

The emergence of consensus as a category of moral discourse flies in the face of some deeply held cultural assumptions, at least in the West. Plato's version of consensus as shared opinion was intimately related to his devastating critique of democracy as mob rule, a view that arguably required more than a millennium to overcome. His philosopher-kings knew the Good, they did not have a mere opinion about it. The great moral heroes of Western culture, from Moses to Jesus to St. Joan to Gandhi and Martin Luther King, Jr., embodied the Platonic ideal of the individual who knows the Good, confronting the mob, possessed only of an opinion.

Although one can hardly gainsay the salutary societal effects of moral heroism, the confidence it implies has its pitfalls. What American philosopher and educator John Dewey (1859–1952) so penetratingly labeled a quest for certainty characterizes much of subsequent thought, philosophical and scientific, as well as theological, all under the sway of Platonism. With the emergence of modernity, moral certainty in particular has been in tension with what another American philosopher, Charles Sander Peirce (1839–1914), called fallibilism: the doctrine that assertions must be revisable in light of further evidence, and that in the final analysis belief statements are certified as true by a community, not an individual. Fallibilism is the underlying philosophy of experimental science. Dewey especially argued that there is an experimental quality to the moral life, and that longstanding moral values have proven themselves over long experience and cross-culturally. On this view, the adaptation of values to new circumstances requires literal re-evaluation, much as scientific communities revise hypotheses in light of new evidence. In direct contrast to Platonism, this position valorizes community opinion, or consensus.

As bioethics both draws from traditional moral values and concerns itself with emerging and often quite novel problems, this tension between Platonic and Deweyan views of moral consensus underlies all bioethical discourse. It is perhaps especially well illustrated in the contrasting outcomes of two early bioethics debates. In the recombinant DNA controversy of the 1970s, the first generation of bioethicists allied with scientists to undermine theological critiques of science unleashed on unique human qualities (Evans). By contrast, at the same time bioethicists added their voices to those protesting the high degree of discretion permitted medical scientists in human experiments (Moreno, 2001).

## Modes of Consensus

The moral paradox of consensus in bioethics may therefore work itself out in surprising ways, but on the whole, and especially when it engages in developing public policy, bioethics is largely a consensus-oriented field (Moreno, 1995). These consensus processes may occur in various contexts and may be more or less self-conscious. Patient management conferences often involve ethical issues that may not be acknowledged as such, in contrast to the more formal setting of an ethics committee. The most formalized and public context for moral consensus is the governmental ethics commission. Lying somewhere in between are ethics advisory boards for private entities.

Whatever the context, insofar as consensus is the preferred outcome it can be distinguished from compromise, in which the parties seek to defend and retain certain underlying principles though they may be willing to modify elements of their viewpoints that are less central (Benjamin). In a truly consensus-oriented situation the members of the group do not arrive with fixed positions but each appreciates a genuine puzzlement at the problem and the optimal solution. They then work together to find what seems to be the most ethically justifiable way to manage the problem. Although the common language refers to *seeking* and *achieving* consensus, these terms imply a static series of events while in fact consensus is more accurately described as a process through which a certain shared sense emerges.

Considering that the problems addressed in bioethics tend to be novel in at least some important ways and are often controversial, it may be surprising that consensus is ever realized. In this respect a focus on particular cases or rather highly specified issues can be critical. Frequently consensus characterizes a group discussion of a specific moral problem though the members of the same group may harbor substantial differences concerning general moral views. One may therefore contrast deep with superficial consensus, where the latter is not dependent on the former. Various moral systems may lead to the same conclusion in particular cases. Efforts to reach a deep consensus may even backfire if they fail and the group's solidarity is thereby undermined. The somewhat counter-intuitive conclusion is that, when consensus is the concern, superficial agreement is often quite adequate and efforts to resolve deeper differences should be approached with caution.

Because bioethics is a social institution that often expresses itself in appointed or self-appointed committees, panels, task forces, commissions or some other small group, an important question arises about the relation between that group and its stakeholders. Many ethics panels include members of the community, apparently in contrast to the experts who generally make up the majority of the group. The presence of community members is presumably intended to help ensure that the views of the wider society are represented. But the precise sense of representation at work here raises further questions. One way of modeling this activity is that of democratic deliberation, in which those actually engaged in the discourse are taken to be stand-ins for all those who do not have the resources or opportunity to immerse themselves in the issues at hand.

## Consensus and Its Critics

The rapid growth of the bioethics profession and its close association with consensus processes expose it to the Platonic critique of shared opinion, particularly as these opinions are often received as a kind of moral expertise (Tong). The notion of expertise suggests that there is a certain body of information available to those who have certain training and experience, but not to others. If this information is taken to be at least partly factual in nature, then the consensus of moral experts must be limited to description rather than prescription. That is, on pain of violating the fact-value distinction, moral expertise can do no more than identify what is and has in fact been valued, not what ought to be valued.

Descriptive moral consensus is a form of social science, perhaps of survey research, that leaves little room for the dynamic public and professional discourse that characterizes bioethics. Without running afoul of the fact-value distinction, it appears that bioethicists must reconstruct their activity as a kind of social reform movement (Moreno, 1995). Their expertise lies not in the privileged status of their recommendations but in the arguments they put forward in support of these recommendations. Within these arguments is evidence drawn from many sources and principles derived from various sources, secular and theological, that are viewed as more or less authoritative.

Defenders of the role of consensus in bioethics, such as D. Micah Hester and Bruce Jennings, develop the notion of the individual as inherently a member of a community, so that values are embedded in social life. Rarely does any group speak with a single voice, however, and bioethicists themselves have diverse moral understandings regarding central moral issues. Even among these ethics experts there is often no common moral vision. In fact, it may be argued that this diversity is often ideological in nature, and therefore as suspect as any assertions about morality delivered by anyone with a partisan purpose (Engelhardt, 2002).

Similarly, no professional group can hope to speak for all moral viewpoints. Bioethicists have both adopted and helped articulate a certain ethical framework that valorizes individual self-determination. But many cultural subgroups, both in the developing world and within the developed world, do not accept the standard bioethical doctrines of truth telling and informed consent. Thus even if bioethicists as a professional class share some very broad consensus, they can hardly claim to speak for those groups that do not share their liberal sentiments with respect to individualism. Even a weak consensus seems hard to achieve across the board in a pluralistic society, and it is an impoverished morality that imposes self-determination on those who reject it (Trotter).

Yet a consensus among bioethical experts, however the latter term is defined, is not guaranteed to influence social policy. As Mark Kuczewski has pointed out, in the areas of foregoing life-sustaining treatment and the conduct of biomedical research, bioethicists have had extraordinary success in helping to develop a social consensus. But, as he notes, the same cannot be said for the questions concerning universal health insurance, even though many bioethicists are on record as supportive of such a program. This fact suggests that a bioethical consensus is perhaps not as weighty in public life as the critics of consensus may fear, nor as bioethicists may wish were the case.

## Constraining Consensus

Considering both the moral hazards inherent in consensus and its practical inevitability in a field of ethics oriented toward practice and group decision making, careful attention must be given to the conditions under which consensus processes take place. As Kuczewski notes, in itself agreement among bioethicists means nothing. Acquiescence to expertise for its own sake would be an instance of the naturalistic fallacy, the derivation of a normative statement from a descriptive one. At the extreme, the widespread adoption of a collective bioethical soundbite that moves the public owing to its rhetoric would be emotivism in the guise of reflection.

What does count is the quality of arguments provided. These can and should be formulated, evaluated and revised by a community of bioethical inquirers. The environment must be one that fosters the exchange of reasoned views, further presupposing the peaceful resolution of moral controversy (Engelhardt, 1995). What emerges is a set of side constraints on moral consensus processes. Besides peaceable and reasoned argument there are also elements of democratic deliberation, such as a willingness to entertain unpopular points of view, mutual respect among the protagonists, and the assurance that the voices of all stakeholders have an opportunity to be heard. Strict attention must therefore be paid to the quality of the process. A self-critical consensus process should worry not about whether the outcome approximates an objectively right solution but whether the proceedings have satisfied the requirements of fairness and accuracy.

## The Future of Consensus in Bioethics

If consensus is an intrinsic part of bioethics as a social institution, especially in its capacity as a forum for the development of institutional and public policy, then there will be a continuing need to examine the way consensus processes operate both within bioethics and in the larger society that incorporates the views offered by bioethicists. A field concerned with the construction of moral standards should not be ignorant of the ways its procedures and products may be distorted, whether intentionally or not. This conclusion argues not only for a degree of self-consciousness about bioethical discourse. It also commends the need to develop a sophisticated understanding about those social psychological and political processes that set bioethics apart from other forms of moral inquiry.

JONATHAN D. MORENO

SEE ALSO: *Authority in Religious Traditions; Autonomy; Clinical Ethics: Institutional Ethics Committees; Coercion; Communitarianism and Bioethics; Conscience, Rights of; Ethics: Social and Political Theories; Managed Care; Natural Law; Public Health Law; Trust*

### BIBLIOGRAPHY

Benjamin, Martin. 1990. *Splitting the Difference: Compromise and Integrity in Ethics and Politics.* Lawrence: University Press of Kansas.

Dewey, John. 1929. *The Quest for Certainty: A Study of the Relation Between Knowledge and Action.* New York: Minton, Balch and Co.

Engelhardt, H. Tristram, Jr. 1995. *The Foundations of Bioethics,* 2nd edition. New York: Oxford University Press.

Engelhardt., H. Tristram, Jr. 2002. "Consensus Formation: The Creation of an Ideology." *Cambridge Quarterly of Healthcare Ethics* 11: 7–16.

Evans, John. 2002. *Playing God? Human Genetic Engineering and the Rationalization of Public Bioethical Debate.* Chicago: University of Chicago Press.

Hester, D. Micah. 2002. "Narrative as Bioethics: The 'Fact' of Social Selves and the Function of Consensus." *Cambridge Quarterly of Healthcare Ethics* 11: 17–26.

Jennings, Bruce. 1995. "Possibilities of Consensus: Toward Democratic Moral Discourse." *The Journal of Medicine and Philosophy* 16: 447–463.

Kuczewski, Mark. 2002. "Two Models of Ethical Consensus, or What Good Is a Bunch of Bioethicists?" *Cambridge Quarterly of Healthcare Ethics* 11: 27–36.

Moreno, Jonathan. 1988. "Ethics by Committee: The Moral Authority of Consensus." *Journal of Medicine and Philosophy* 13: 411–432.

Moreno, Jonathan. 1995. *Deciding Together: Bioethics and Moral Consensus.* New York: Oxford University Press.

Moreno, Jonathan. 2001. "Goodbye to All That: The End of Moderate Protectionism in Human Subjects Research." *The Hastings Center Report* 31: 9–17.

Peirce, Charles Sanders. 1934. *Collected Papers of Charles Sanders Peirce,* Vol. 5: *Pragmatism and Pragmaticism,* ed. Charles Hartshorne and Paul Weiss. Cambridge, MA: Harvard University Press.

Tong, Rosemarie. 1991. "The Epistemology and Ethics of Consensus: Uses and Misuses of 'Ethical' Expertise." *The Journal of Medicine and Philosophy* 16: 409–426.

Trotter, H. Griffin. 2002. "Bioethics and Healthcare Reform: A Whig Response to Weak Consensus." *Cambridge Quarterly of Healthcare Ethics* 11: 37–51.

Walters, LeRoy. 1999. "Commissions and Bioethics." *The Journal of Medicine and Philosophy* 14: 363–368.

# CONTRACTARIANISM AND BIOETHICS

• • •

The idea of the social contract has been a central feature of Western moral and political thought since the seventeenth century. Theories that follow that tradition claim that the legitimate source of moral or political authority is mutual agreement. Contractarianism had widespread influence through the writings of Thomas Hobbes, Jean-Jacques Rousseau (1973 [1762]), Immanuel Kant (1965 [1797]), and John Locke (1960 [1706]) and has had a recent revival in the work of John Rawls (1971, 1993), David Gauthier (1986), and Thomas Scanlon (1998). Contemporary contractarians continue to drive discussions about topics such as the nature of democratic principles, the distribution of scarce resources in healthcare, the provision of public goods and services, the current generation's duties to future generations, and the current generation's obligation to preserve and protect the environment.

## The Tenets of Contractarianism

Contractarianism includes a diverse family of theories that share a basic understanding about the nature of normative justification: When faced with questions such as the following—What is just? What is right? What should I do?—contractarianism seeks an answer rooted in agreement. The motivating force behind the contract approach is the idea that consent confers legitimacy on particular moral decisions, the policies and laws of a particular society, and the basic principles of a just society.

The metaphor of the social contract represents people's willingness to enter into a society or a system of moral rules for mutual benefit, agreeing to bind themselves to the rules that make cooperative life possible. The social contract sometimes is characterized as a general agreement to keep more specific agreements. This idea is rooted in a form of skepticism about competing sources of normative authority, such as theories about human nature, theories of natural law, perfectionist theories, virtue theory, and other theories that attempt to offer more objective or foundational support for the content of moral principles and theories of justice.

Within the family of theories contractarians tend to be divided over questions about how to characterize agreement and the mechanisms of choice. For example, does moral justification stem from actual historical agreement, or is it more appropriate to reason hypothetically about what people would have reason to agree to in certain ideal conditions? The former approach to moral questions traces moral justification to actual agreements. The latter approach reflects on the hypothetical agreements of imagined agents in idealized circumstances. Both variants posit a starting point or initial position from which people have historically or hypothetically emerged to contract with one another for the sake of mutual benefit. Both mechanisms make it possible to evaluate current conditions in society or current moral practices by reference to a more ideal historical or hypothetical situation. For the contractarian, social and political institutions are human conventions that are open to criticism, rejection, revision, and ultimately acceptance.

Both the actual and the hypothetical contractarian approaches to moral and political theory have played a central role in bioethics. People who are interested in carrying on the contractarian tradition within bioethics must contend with some of the problems inherited by the more general theory as it has been developed in moral and political philosophy. What follows is an overview of contractarian approaches to the special problems of bioethics, including consideration of the strengths and weaknesses of those approaches.

## Contractarian Approaches to Bioethics

If morality and politics are understood as joint enterprises that are entered into for mutual advantage, as contractarians

understand them, one can begin to see a natural affinity between bioethics and contract theory. The patient-physician relationship, the practice of informed consent, the use of advance directives, the conducting of medical and scientific research, the obligation to take care of the elderly, systems of medical insurance and national healthcare, and many other aspects of health policy are central issues in bioethical debates. In an important way contractarianism attempts to make health policy, scientific institutions, and individual practitioners answerable to the individuals they serve.

Howard Brody (1989) has drawn a parallel between the rise of contractarianism in political philosophy and the rise of contractarianism in medical ethics. Just as Enlightenment philosophers challenged the idea of the divine right of kings to rule over subjects without consent, bioethicists from the early 1960s through the 1970s challenged the idea of paternalism in medicine. If patients are viewed in the way Enlightenment philosophers viewed the citizens of a state—as being autonomous and worthy of respect—treating patients paternalistically—considering them as being ignorant and inherently dependent on physicians—violates patients' autonomy.

**THE PATIENT-PHYSICIAN RELATIONSHIP.** Robert Veatch (1991), one of the earliest proponents of contract theory in bioethics, posed the following question: What type of patient-physician relationship would the parties to that relationship rationally consent to, assuming they were placed in a starting position of equal power? The resulting contractual model allows for important differences in knowledge and decision-making capacities between a patient and a physician but requires that equal respect be given to the interests and goals of both parties. The model grants physicians control over technical decisions and grants patients control over the aspects of a decision that involve personal values. If a patient in renal failure is faced with the options of ongoing renal dialysis and kidney transplant surgery, it is the physician's responsibility to present the risks and benefits of those options and explain the relevant medical information. It is up to the patient to decide what degree of risk she or he is willing to accept with either option and weigh the options in light of his or her own values.

The contractual model of medical ethics views the patient-physician relationship as one of respectful communication and negotiation. The specific list of rights and duties is arrived at through the hypothetical contract mechanism. If physicians and patients were negotiating the terms of the patient-physician contract, what terms would all the interested parties include in the contract? Certain rights, such as the patient's right of self-determination, and certain corresponding duties, such as the physician's duty to disclose all the information needed by the patient to make a fully informed choice, would make up the content of the contractual model. Consistent with this model is the idea that a patient may willingly delegate his or her choices to a physician.

Norman Daniels (1981), following the political philosopher John Rawls (1971), relies on a Rawlsian model of the hypothetical social contract to construct a specific theory of healthcare needs. In the classic Rawlsian model it is imagined that a number of impartial observers are charged with the task of choosing basic principles of justice that will shape the constitution and laws of the society into which the observers will be born. These hypothetical agents do not know what place they will occupy within the society or even the generation to which they will belong. The thought is that the resulting principles of justice will be fairly chosen, unlike principles chosen by actual, biased, and self-interested parties in a real society. Rawls (1971) argues that rational agents in the original position will want to increase the amount of primary social goods available to them, consistent with an equal share of liberty. He assumes that such agents would be risk-aversive in a certain sense: They would not be willing to risk losing a certain basic amount of primary social goods in exchange for the possibility of seeking greater amounts of those primary goods.

**HEALTHCARE NEEDS.** Expanding on Rawls's general theory of justice, Daniels (1988) places healthcare goods under the principle of fair equality of opportunity, including healthcare needs among the primary needs of a society's members. One of the most interesting results of the theory as it is applied to health policy is the way in which Daniels attempts to solve the problem of age-group bias. In attempting to determine a just allocation of scarce health resources most real agents are deeply biased in favor of the scheme that will maximize the resources of their age group, heavily discounting the present over the future. If, however, people place themselves behind a Rawlsian veil of ignorance and imagine that they are blind to their particular generation, they will arrive at fair principles of healthcare distribution. The hope is that the resulting principles of resource allocation will ensure the well-being of all persons as they pass through various health institutions through the course of their lives. A healthcare system designed in accordance with the principle of equal opportunity will attempt to balance, for example, the need for services in critical care, preventive care, and long-term care. If the institutions at each stage are designed prudently, the hope is that all generations will benefit from the overall health system.

**THE REQUIREMENT FOR PERMISSION.** Against the Rawlsian contractrarian approach to bioethics, Tristram Engelhardt (1996) has offered a theory of bioethics rooted in the Kantian philosophical tradition, which relies centrally on the requirement of permission between persons. Engelhardt's approach to the specific problems of bioethics stems from deep skepticism about the possibility of achieving consensus about the substantive questions in morality and politics. He argues that all competing approaches to bioethics rely in some way on prior substantive assumptions about what is good or right. Such assumptions, he claims, cannot reasonably be made in a pluralistic world filled with competing ideas of justice and fairness, understandings of rationality, and visions of the good life.

Engelhardt offers an alternative model of bioethics that rests on a very minimal assumption salvaged from the Enlightenment project and the contractarian tradition. The basic assumption is that the only justifiable ground for dealing with moral controversies in a world of moral diversity is to appeal to actual agreement as the source of moral authority; any other appeal is illegitimate because it involves acceptance through force or coercion. To avoid imposing substantive moral views on those who are strangers to a group of people's views, Engelhardt urges people to appeal to consent as the mark of legitimate moral authority.

Rather than design a healthcare system that is based on the hypothetical agreement of hypothetical agents who must be assumed to have certain substantive views about what is just or good, Enghelhardt proposes that decisions about the allocation of health-resources be made directly by real parties to real agreements. In this model market mechanisms generally will guide decisions about the allocation of health resources on the national level, with the assumption that those who participate in the market implicitly if not explicitly consent to the practice and its outcomes.

Engelhardt leaves open the possibility that smaller groups and communities will agree to set up health institutions, such as private hospitals and long-term-care facilities, that are governed by more substantive goals of justice or visions of the good life. A Catholic hospital, for example, might have an internal policy against performing abortions and also might have a policy of offering a certain amount of charity care to indigent patients. In this model the relationship between the patient and the physician is characterized fundamentally in terms of permission and consent. Agreements between patients and their caregivers, such as those struck through the process of filling out advance directives, play a central role in ensuring that the minimal moral requirement of permission is secured. Similar to Veatch's account, the relationship between patient and physician is, in Engelhardt's model, understood as one of respectful negotiation between the different parties to the decision-making process.

## Critiques of Contractarian Approaches to Bioethics

Several important criticisms have been lodged against contractarian approaches to bioethics. Those criticisms have a common theme: The moral relationships and contexts that characterize the healthcare and research settings are too complex and subtle to be understood solely in terms of a contract. The general concern is that contract theory is too minimal in its approach to the rich and complicated moral terrain of bioethics.

Critics have objected that the physician-patient relationship rarely begins with an agreement or involves explicit negotiating. More often the beginning of the relationship is characterized by surprise, stress, a lack of time, fear, hope, an imbalance of knowledge, and a great need for trust. It is not typically a calm encounter between equal partners in a negotiation. This objection speaks primarily against the actual-contract model offered by Engelhardt because the hypothetical model is attempting to ask what principles should guide this stressful, complex encounter, and these principles are chosen in a calmer hour by philosophers, bioethicists, and health-policy makers.

This objection can be extended to the hypothetical model, however, by pointing out the disparity between the ideal situation in which principles of bioethics are hypothetically chosen and the real world. If the disparity is significant, it is not clear what binding force hypothetically chosen principles should have in actual practice. A great deal depends on the content of the hypothetical situation of choice and the substantive principles of rationality that will guide choice. If too much is packed into the descriptions of the initial position, the resulting choice will be biased and arbitrary, exactly the pitfall the contract tradition was designed to avoid. If one provides no structure and content to the nature of rationality guiding choosers in the initial position, the resulting principles will be empty and meaningless. This is a serious problem for contract theory in general that has been inherited by those hoping to apply that model to bioethics.

The unique relationship between patient and physician, others have argued, is not best characterized by the economic-political metaphor of the contract because the contract model relies too narrowly on rights and permission and overlooks other important goals and duties, such as compassion and trust. From the perspective of virtue theory, for example, the contractarian model of bioethics fails to address important issues about the character of physicians and other healthcare workers. What does it mean to be a good physician or a good nurse? Certainly there is more to being a good health professional or a good researcher than making sure that one negotiates the permission of one's patients and research subjects thoroughly. William May (1996), for example, suggests that the religious idea of a covenant compared with the secular metaphor of the contract is better able to capture the rich sense of duty and obligation inherent in the physician-patient relationship.

What drives this objection is a deeper concern that the minimal moral requirements of the contract model will not encourage a lasting and dedicated relationship with patients but instead will encourage physicians to ask, "Has the consent form been signed?" Although beneficence and compassion are clearly compatible with contractarian requirements in bioethics, there is a sense in which such moral goals remain "optional" because they are not the central focus of the theory.

Along a similar line communitarians have argued that the contract model is too individualistic in its focus. Moral issues in bioethics, even in the narrower domain of medical ethics, involve complicated social systems, shared and unspoken understandings, deep-seated cultural beliefs, and common expectations. Explicit contracts account for only a small part of the moral dealings in this context. Especially in areas such as public health, many decisions are best made in terms of what is best for the community or what maximizes the overall health of the community over and above the desires and preferences of individuals. Sometimes the only way to stem the immediate threat of an infectious disease such as tuberculosis may require practices, such as reporting and quarantine, that infringe on principles of individual consent and permission.

A final objection to the contractarian model, especially as it is applied to bioethics, is that it is centrally a theory about persons, whereas bioethics involves important ethical issues about nonpersons or semipersons, including animals, embryos, fetuses, children, adults with serious mental deficits, brain-dead patients, and the dead. Some of the most interesting and challenging issues in bioethics involve subjects one does not easily imagine sitting at the negotiating table. Because the contract model focuses on what rational, conscious agents would choose, there is concern that the focus on rational agreement excludes the moral concerns of more vulnerable members of society.

A morality based on mutuality and rational consent certainly can deliver principles for addressing the needs of children, the mentally ill, and animals, but only insofar as the agents to the agreement deem those more vulnerable subjects worthy of consideration. Because moral duties and obligations emerge from mutual agreement, any duties that people have toward research animals, for example, could result only from the agreement of the human parties involved. The obligation is indirect: If animals and other vulnerable subjects are thought by human parties to an agreement to be worthy of care and respectful treatment, people will have indirect duties toward those animals. For some critics indirect consideration is too unstable a moral requirement, especially for subjects that cannot be parties to the agreement and are particularly susceptible to being overlooked in the moral calculus of rational consent.

## Conclusion

Despite these objections the metaphor of the contract remains a powerful heuristic tool for reflecting on the existing conventions and practices of medicine and science. The lasting insight of contract theory is that the willingness of individuals, rather than force or rigid appeals to human nature, is a powerful legitimating force in morality and politics in a world where individuals disagree deeply about foundational moral issues. Thus, contract theory remains a particularly useful insight and starting point in the diverse field of contemporary bioethics.

MAUREEN KELLEY

SEE ALSO: *Casuistry; Communitarianism and Bioethics; Consensus, Role of; Ethics; Freedom and Coercion; Obligation and Supererogation; Pragmatism; Principalism; Rights; Utilitarianism*

### BIBLIOGRAPHY

Ackerman, Bruce. 1980. *Social Justice in the Liberal State.* New Haven, CT: Yale University Press.

Brody, Howard. 1989. "The Physician-Patient Relationship." In *Medical Ethics,* ed. Robert Veatch. Boston: Jones and Bartlett.

Buchanan, James, and Tullock, Gordon. 1965. *The Calculus of Consent.* Ann Arbor: University of Michigan Press.

Daniels, Norman. 1981. "Health-Care Needs and Distributive Justice." In *Medicine and Moral Philosophy,* ed. Marshall Cohen, Thomas Nagel, and Thomas Scanlon. Princeton, NJ: Princeton University Press.

Daniels, Norman. 1985. *Just Health Care.* New York: Cambridge University Press.

Daniels, Norman. 1988. *Am I My Parents' Keeper? An Essay on Justice between the Young and the Old.* New York: Oxford University Press.

Engelhardt, Tristram. 1996. *The Foundations of Bioethics,* 2nd edition. New York: Oxford University Press.

Gauthier, David. 1986. *Morals by Agreement.* Oxford: Oxford University Press.

Green, Ronald. 1976. "Health Care and Justice in Contract Theory Perspective." In *Ethics and Health Policy,* ed. Robert Veatch and Roy Branson. Cambridge, Eng.: Ballinger.

Habermas, Jürgen. 1990. *Moral Consciousness and Communicative Action,* tr. Christian Lenhardt and Shierry Weber Nicholsen. Cambridge, MA: MIT Press.

Hampton, Jean. 1986. *Hobbes and the Social Contract Tradition.* Cambridge, MA: Cambridge University Press.

Hobbes, Thomas. 1948 (1651). *Leviathan,* ed. Michael Oakeshott. Oxford: BasilBlackwell.

Hume, David. 1985 (1748). "Of the Original Contract." In *Essays: Moral, Political and Literary,* ed. Eugene Miller. Indianapolis: Liberty Classics.

Kant, Immanuel. 1965 (1797). *The Metaphysical Elements of Justice,* tr. John Ladd. Indianapolis: Bobbs-Merrill.

Locke, John. 1960 (1706). *The Second Treatise on Government,* ed. Peter Laslett. Cambridge, Eng.: Cambridge University Press.

Masters, R. D. 1975. "Is Contract an Adequate Basis for Medical Ethics?" *Hastings Center Report* 5(6): 24–28.

May, William F. 1996. *Active Euthanasia and Health Care Reform: Testing the Medical Covenant.* Grand Rapids, MI: William B. Eerdmans.

Nozick, Robert. 1974. *Anarchy, State and Utopia.* New York: Basic Books.

Rawls, John. 1971. *A Theory of Justice.* Cambridge, MA: Harvard University Press.

Rawls, John. 1993. *Political Liberalism.* New York: Columbia University Press.

Rousseau, Jean-Jacques. 1973 (1762). *The Social Contract,* tr. G. H. Cole. New York: Dutton.

Scanlon, Thomas M. 1998. *What We Owe to Each Other.* Cambridge, MA: Harvard University Press.

Silvers, Anita. 1998. "Formal Justice," In *Disability, Difference, Discrimination,* ed. Anita Silvers, David Wasserman, and Mary Mahowald. New York: Rowman & Littlefield.

Vallentyne, Peter, ed. 1991. *Contractarianism and Rational Choice.* New York: Cambridge University Press.

Vandeveer, Donald. 1981. "The Contractual Argument for Withholding Medical Information." In *Medicine and Moral Philosophy,* ed. Marshall Cohen, Thomas Nagel, and Thomas Scanlon. Princeton, NJ: Princeton University Press.

Veatch, Robert. 1981. *A Theory of Medical Ethics.* New York: Basic Books.

Veatch, Robert. 1991. *The Patient-Physician Relationship: The Patient as Partner, Part 2.* Bloomington and Indianapolis: Indiana University Press.

# CORPORATE COMPLIANCE

• • •

The word compliance can be defined as the act of adhering to or conforming with a law, rule, demand, or request. In a business environment, conforming to the laws, regulations, rules and policies is the part of business operations often referred to as "corporate compliance." Corporate compliance involves keeping a watchful eye on an ever-changing legal and regulatory climate, and making the changes necessary for the business to continue operating in good standing within its industry, community, and customer base. In a broader sense, corporate compliance extends beyond mere legal and regulatory conformity into the realm of promoting organizational ethics and corporate integrity.

The roots of corporate compliance efforts are found in the government contracting scandals of the 1980s. During those years, the Department of Defense received extraordinary charges for commonplace equipment. Investigations led to criminal convictions and monetary settlements for a number of companies providing equipment and supplies under contract to the U.S. government. In response to these events, defense industry companies wishing to contract with the government were required to develop corporate compliance programs to prevent such abuses in the future. Shortly thereafter, the U.S. Sentencing Commission established Organizational Sentencing Guidelines that offered more lenient fines and penalties for corporate violators that created voluntary programs to prevent and remedy violations of law and regulation.

Leniency under the Sentencing Guidelines is calculated. Upon a finding of guilt, the court considers the company's compliance efforts. This is done through the use of a culpability scoring formula set forth in the Sentencing Guidelines and applied to corporate conduct. Documented evidence of compliance efforts such as monitoring, auditing, corrective actions, and system modifications or redesign to prevent future problem behavior reduces the culpability score or degree of "guiltiness." Fines and penalties are then assessed based upon this score.

Beyond the Sentencing Guidelines, indirect incentives exist for businesses to create compliance programs. A company's intolerance for wrongdoing, evidenced by corporate action taken consistent with its corporate compliance effort, can speak volumes to federal prosecutors conducting an investigation of alleged wrongdoing. Where prosecutors determine that a company has high standards of conduct demanding employee compliance with law and regulation, it may be inferred there was minimal or no criminal intent by the organization to commit a wrongful act. The absence or reduction of evidence of intent then translates into a lesser charge or citation, particularly in a case where intent is a critical element of the crime or offense. Corresponding to the reduced charge, the fines and level of penalty are less than would be associated if a more serious (in degree) offense were claimed.

Compliance programs may also impact civil enforcement fines or penalties. If a company is found liable for wrongdoing (rather than guilty as in a criminal action), the existence of a compliance program may reduce the risk of a full-scale government investigation of the company. Short of a civil trial seeking monetary recovery, the existence of an effective compliance program often prompts government agency auditors to find human error rather than conscious misconduct led to a failure to comply with a set of rules. In these instances, leniency can be granted in the form of more favorable repayment terms and interest rates, and reduced civil fines and penalties.

A well-developed, established compliance program also helps a company avoid the imposition of probation or a corporate integrity agreement (CIA). The CIA is a mandated type of compliance program where timeframes for achieving targeted performance are aggressively short. Components of a CIA include staff education on general and specific compliance issues, establishing specific policy and procedures to minimize recurrence of the misconduct, auditing, and monitoring activities. Quite often these mandatory compliance programs call for the use of outside consultants to support business operations and/or provide objective documentation of progress toward fulfillment of the terms set forth in the agreement. CIA implementation is often expensive. Aggressive deadlines for achieving compliance milestones, multiple compliance targets, complexity of compliance issues, and the use of government-approved outside agencies are factors influencing cost.

## Healthcare Compliance

With the decade of the 1990s came a warning from the Office of the Inspector General (OIG) for the U.S. Department of Health and Human Services (HHS). The healthcare industry was not immune from prosecution and liability for fraudulent and abusive practices. OIG audits demonstrated that as much as 10 percent of U.S. government-funded healthcare expenditures were related to care that was not billed correctly, was not medically necessary, or was never delivered to the patient. There were additional concerns about the adequacy of care being delivered in the United States and concern about the reporting of health organization costs. Fraud and abuse are the terms often used in reference to these types of practices.

HHS and the OIG projected savings to be billions of dollars per year if concerted efforts were made to minimize such practices. Several initiatives were considered. One was a curative approach, whereby fraudulent or abusive practices would be investigated and prosecuted. Another was enlisting the voluntary aid of the healthcare industry to implement prevention programs. Given the magnitude of the problem, and the high cost of investigating and prosecuting fraud, the OIG determined that a cost-effective solution to minimize fraud and abuse was to emphasize prevention over law enforcement investigation and prosecution. With this thought, HHS and the OIG embraced the defense industry's compliance concept along with the Sentencing Guidelines and established the first government healthcare compliance guidance in 1997.

The initial guidance was written for laboratories. OIG compliance guidance is available for other care delivery settings such as hospitals, long-term care, home healthcare, hospice, physician offices, and support services such as medical coding and billing companies. On April 23, 2003, the OIG issued compliance program guidance for pharmaceutical manufacturers.

## Early Healthcare Compliance Efforts

Initial OIG-written commentary for healthcare compliance programs focused on internal controls. Healthcare organizations were encouraged, for example, to develop protocols for insurance claim processing and billing, to properly use codes (e.g., diagnosis related group assignments for inpatient hospital service classification and payment), and to ensure patient freedom of choice. Hospital contracts with physicians that encouraged over-utilization of services prohibited by anti-kickback law were also high on the regulatory list of concerns. Yet other compliance efforts focused on provider or entity compliance with governmental and private insurer documentation guidelines, medical need for service, timely refunding of overpayments for services (e.g., refunding credit balanceS), and document retention and destruction policy.

By 2003, it was not unusual to find defined compliance departments within healthcare organizations. The actual name of the department may vary from simply the "corporate compliance department" to the "business practices office." In some organizations, corporate compliance, internal audit, and corporate ethics are combined or maintain close working relations. Independence of review and periodic reporting to senior company officials are two key aspects of any compliance function. Some compliance offices also have advisory committees to assist in various compliance endeavors. At least one organization is known to have a combined compliance and corporate ethics advisory committee. Consistent with the OIG guidance, compliance officers are instrumental in developing or assisting to develop comprehensive policy on OIG target areas, staff training, monitoring, and auditing.

## Effective Healthcare Compliance Programs

Little has been published as to what constitutes an "effective" healthcare compliance program. The OIG initiative broadly encourages healthcare providers and entities to conduct business in a manner that conforms to federal and state law and regulations. Similarly, regulatory agency expectations of compliance initiatives vary with the size and complexity of the entity and monies available to fund compliance efforts. For example, a small family practice physician operating an office in a rural location is not expected to have the same size, scope, and sophistication in terms of a compliance program as a healthcare organization with 1,000 or more beds spread over multiple care delivery sites in a highly populated urban setting. Recent enforcement activities, however, demonstrate that staff compliance education and an entity's ongoing commitment to "following the rules" are key components to proving effectiveness, regardless of the entity's size and complexity. Ineffective programs may not provide the same leniency and opportunities as have been discussed above.

Development of an effective program includes ongoing review and revision of the program based on the emphasis found in the annual OIG work plan. A review of current and prior work plans reveals a continuing focus on payment, billing, and claims processing issues. The OIG also releases a number of publications and opinions throughout the year that advise healthcare providers and entities such as hospitals, home health agencies, extended care facilities, etc., on prevention, detection, and resolution methods for suspect practices. Other OIG publications and opinions clarify subject areas to better enable compliant conduct by health organizations.

Consistent with the expansion of regulatory agency focus, areas of compliance concern have expanded to include issues such as quality of care, maintaining patient privacy, eliminating healthcare errors, maintaining occupational safety, enhancing staff understanding of clinical and business ethics, and eliminating or minimizing conflicts of interest. Specialty areas of the law that were topics for compliance discussion in the early twenty-first century encompass employment law, environmental law, tax law, and intellectual property law. This broadened scope has prompted many organizations to revise and reprioritize compliance programs to incorporate standards of behavior that address organization expectations on existing as well as new focal areas.

## Essential Elements of a Healthcare Compliance Program

Common elements of any healthcare compliance program incorporate the following:

1. designation of a high-level entity officer to lead the compliance program;
2. documented standards of behavior that are described in more detail in the entity's policies and procedures;
3. compliance training for staff with regular updates to maintain awareness;
4. establishment and maintenance of a readily available anonymous communication process for receiving complaints and concerns (i.e. telephone hotline, suggestion boxes);
5. procedures for protecting healthcare whistleblowers;
6. maintenance of a system for responding to complaints in a timely manner;
7. documented disciplinary action procedures for violations of law, regulation, or compliance policies of the entity;
8. planned auditing and monitoring activities to reveal areas where compliance issues exist, and to monitor correction actions for effectiveness;
9. defined investigation processes;
10. a procedure for initiating the entity's process improvement procedure to correct system process problems;
11. a process to address employment decisions for persons who are temporarily or permanently barred from participating in the care of patients who are beneficiaries of a federally-funded healthcare program.

## Operating a Healthcare Compliance Program

Using OIG guidance materials, the compliance officer and compliance committee members develop and direct activities based on governmental and organizational identified areas of concern. The compliance officer should have direct access to both the chief executive officer and the governing board of the organization whenever necessary to ensure timely communication of pertinent issues.

It is important for the organization leadership to grant oversight authority to the compliance officer and committee members for monitoring, auditing, and corrective action activities of the corporate compliance program. Additionally, leadership should support the compliance officer's establishment of alternate methods of communicating with employees to encourage anonymous reporting of compliance issues. It is essential for employees to view the compliance officer as a non-threatening source of education and empowerment, a person they may seek out to resolve concerns without fear of discipline, retaliation, or retribution for reporting a concern.

## Establishing a Corporate Culture of Compliance

An organization must be committed to compliance efforts in order for the program to be effective. Establishing written standards, policies, and procedures demonstrates acceptance by senior leadership and delineates behavioral expectations for all employees, governing body members, officers, management, physicians, contractors, and business associates of the organization. Beginning with a statement describing the organization's mission and vision (goals for the future), the organization guides conduct by defining a potential compliance issue along with the conduct standard and examples of appropriate behavior. An illustration of this concept:

- Mission statement: To provide excellent healthcare for our patients and the communities we serve.
- Vision statement: We are committed to the highest level of organizational and professional excellence and will serve others with respect for individual dignity.
- Performance Standards: Greet everyone with direct eye contact and a smile; At the end of an interaction, "ask is there anything else I can do for you?"; Provide information and give updates at specific intervals as promised.

It is important to write components of a compliance program at a reading level that the majority of staff can understand. It is also important to make the conduct requirements accessible to employees so they can be easily referenced. Since laws and regulations change and the OIG, HHS, professional review agencies, fiscal intermediaries, and carriers identify different areas of concern over time, compliance requirements must be updated to reflect behaviors required for the organization to remain in compliance.

A significant portion of the compliance officer and committee members' roles involve establishing and maintaining positive relationships with others in the organization. In maintaining a level of visibility and collegiality, the compliance officer is more likely to be in a position where opportunities for improvement can be identified and ethical behaviors can be positively reinforced. Likewise, visible, approachable committee members are likely to find less resistance to monitoring and auditing activities. Without these positive relationships, compliance activities may be impeded by efforts to thwart data access and collection for fear of poor audit results and the demand for time-consuming responsive action plans by management. While the compliance officer and committee members are often the most visible leaders of corporate compliance efforts, it remains important for organization leadership and management to mentor employees, encouraging responsible and ethical behavior in the workplace.

## Strategies for Maintaining a Compliance Program with Limited Resources

The number of personnel assigned to the compliance department or to assist with compliance functions varies from organization to organization. The size of the compliance department and level of sophistication of the compliance program is not directly proportionate to organizational size and complexity. Given the limited size of many departments, a compliance officer must often utilize a variety of strategies to maintain the continuity of compliance program activities.

One strategy involves enlisting managers and supervisors of other departments to join in conducting and evaluating daily monitoring activities, and participate in development and implementation of solutions to issues raised. Compliance department staff or internal audit personnel may check on these efforts through quarterly or annual audits. If needed, in-depth analysis may be conducted by outside consultants.

Another strategy involves using work groups or task forces to assist with monitoring and auditing functions. The groups are formed from members of departments with specific but related functions (i.e. patient registration, patient accounts, collections, and coding). By doing this, members are exposed to the compliance program in action. Work group members engaged in program activities often become ambassadors and assist in enhancing the compliance culture within the organization.

Improved organizational performance can be a practical result from compliance work group efforts. Compliance initiatives may reduce payment collection times and rejections rates. Compliance initiatives may also resolve long-festering issues that impede work completion and flow. With the compliance officer acting as a mentor, information resource, and support person, multiple work groups may simultaneously be engaged in compliance activities, thus improving organizational compliance effectiveness in an efficient, thoughtful manner.

## Providers Excluded from Federal Health Programs

Compliance initiatives must also implement steps to ensure practitioners and entities excluded from federal health program participation are not employed or used by the company. By partnering with numerous departments in an organization, a small compliance program can coordinate the monitoring of governmental databases to ensure excluded persons or entities rules are followed. If a monitoring process is ineffective, the organization is likely to realize a significant financial impact because federal programs such as Medicare, Medicaid, or Tri-Care will not reimburse services ordered or performed by these excluded providers.

The monitoring requires that the compliance officer or designee review the Health and Human Services Office of the OIG Excluded Provider database and the General Services Administration database at periodic intervals. The review process and subsequent response activities incorporate human resource, medical staff credentialing, materials management vendor selection, and contractor selection functions within the organization. Legal counsel must be included in these compliance activities to ensure that organization contracts incorporate provisions that impose an affirmative duty on contracting parties to communicate anticipated or actual government action that may result in the party becoming an excluded provider. Action in response to a finding of exclusion may involve, for example, contract termination, termination of employment, or loss of medical staff membership and privileges at the organization.

## Corporate Compliance Programs and Organizational Ethics

Partnering within and among organization departments and functions appears consistent with OIG commentary on effective compliance plans. OIG writings suggest that organizations create and foster compliance efforts that conform to legal and regulatory directives as well as enhance the commitment to ethical clinical and business practices within the corporate culture. Though some similarities exist, ethicists caution that corporate compliance must be viewed as distinct from organizational ethics; each has a unique focus.

Corporate compliance programs focus on establishing a floor or minimum level of appropriate behavior for the organization in order for the organization to conform to legal and regulatory requirements for a given industry. The appropriate behaviors are communicated through the compliance program's conduct standards, policies, and procedures. In behaving appropriately, the organization avoids sanctions and maintains its reputation within the community.

Alternatively, organizational ethics focuses on the realm of behavior where no legal or regulatory requirements exist; where equal priorities compete and where individual values, interests, and beliefs differ to the extent that no "right" answer is readily available. In healthcare entities, organizational ethics faces the additional challenges of reconciling priorities often at the level of life and death seriousness. Individual, professional, and societal values and beliefs; competing interests among parties involved in a controversy; the rights of the patient, other individuals, and the organization must be considered in organizational ethics activities.

Unlike corporate compliance programs, organizational ethics is not a new concept in the business world. The curriculum in secondary education and beyond has included courses in business ethics and corporate responsibility, and coursework in these areas has existed for decades. There are, however, few healthcare industry examples of formal organizational ethics functions. Organizational ethics programs should not to be confused with clinical ethics functions.

## Healthcare Clinical Ethics and Institutional Review Boards

In contrast with organizational ethics efforts, a number of healthcare organizations established clinical ethics programs within their organizations in the 1970s and 1980s. These efforts were often driven by the need to address ethical and legal dilemmas associated with patients or families seeking to terminate care or refuse care associated with the end of life, often in the absence of state law. In other cases, there was a need to address differing family and patient perspectives on what care should be given outside terminal illness settings. Even with greater clarity on the patient's right to refuse treatment, organizations still needed a defined, deliberate

process to address the bioethical and legal issues associated with such decisions.

Another catalyst for establishing a clinical ethics program was the Federal Drug Administration requirement that called for creating an institutional review board (IRB) to protect the patient's rights in clinical research activities. For example, IRB members review research proposals to ensure the patient receives pertinent information about a study prior to agreeing to participate in it, and that adequate safeguards are in place to protect the patient.

## Unscrupulous Activities Toll

In 2002, a number of U.S. corporations were fraught with business practice scandals. The "ripple effect" caused people across the country to watch helplessly as their retirement plans and stock portfolios withered after an international accounting firm and several major corporations ceased operations. Senior executive interest in the business practices of their industries and their organizations was heightened. A nationwide focus developed whereby corporations looked to ensure that their staff understood that compliance with industry-specific accepted business practices was an expectation. Likewise, staff were to conduct themselves in an ethically responsible manner in workplace activities.

It is clear that the federal and state governments were alarmed by these business scandals and the subsequent effects felt by the citizenry. Consequently, government began scrutinizing corporate business practices in an unprecedented manner. Thus, it may be prudent for all organizations, for-profit and nonprofit alike, to expand compliance programs to include an organizational ethics function as well.

## Single Purpose

For one healthcare organization, the foregoing concerns coupled with a discussion of other real-life scenarios and case studies prompted senior leadership and the governing board to encourage the development of a coordinated approach to these issues. By expanding the scope of corporate compliance activities to incorporate organizational ethics and responsible business practices, the organization hopes to operate compliant with law, regulation, and ethical principles (Oakwood Healthcare Inc.). By 2003, a committee had been formed including compliance, ethics, finance, legal, religious, human resource, operations, and internal audit representatives. By appointing members with different perspectives, the committee provides a balanced approach to complex legal, regulatory, and ethical issues. Uniting ethics and compliance supports the effort to do the "right thing," and that, as many say, is the essence of ethics and compliance.

JONATHAN P. HORENSTEIN

SEE ALSO: *Conflict of Interest; Environmental Policy and Law; Genetic Engineering, Human; Healthcare Institutions; Healthcare Management Ethics; Hospital; Law and Bioethics; Managed Care; Medicaid; Whistleblowing in Healthcare*

## BIBLIOGRAPHY

Davis, Joe and Vann, Rita. 2001. "Quality of Care Receives Increased Emphasis by Enforcement Authorities." *Journal of Health Care Compliance.* 3(6): 28, 62.

Josephs, Al. 2001. "A Conversation with Kristin Jenkins, Compliance and Quality Officer." *Compliance Today* 3(5): 13–19.

Kohn, Linda T., et al., eds. 2000. *To Err Is Human: Building a Safer Health System.* Institute of Medicine.

Randall, Deborah. 2001. "Compliance Concerns in the Home Health Prospective Payment System." *Compliance Today* 3(5): 6–9.

St. John Health System. 1998. *Corporate Compliance Training Manual: Facilitator's Guide.* Detroit: SMS Inc.

Weber, Leonard J. 2001. *Business Ethics in Healthcare: Beyond Compliance.* Bloomington: Indiana University Press.

### INTERNET RESOURCES

United States Department of Health and Human Services — Office of Inspector General. *Fraud Prevention & Detection Compliance Guidance.* Available from <www.oig.hhs.gov/fraud/complianceguidance.html>.

United States Department of Health and Human Services — Office of Inspector General. *Work Plan Fiscal Year 2003.* Available from <www.oig.hhs.gov/publications/workplan>.

United States Sentencing Commission. *Federal Sentencing Guidelines Manual and Appendices.* 2002. Available from <www.ussc.gov.guidelin.htm>.

# CYBERNETICS

• • •

Cybernetics, in its purest definition, is the science of control and communication in the animal and the machine. The word was devised by Norbert Wiener in the 1940s and is derived from the Greek word *kybernetes*, meaning "steersman." In his book *The Human Use of Human Beings* (1950), Wiener wrote that "society can only be understood through a study of the messages and the communication facilities which belong to it; and that in the future development of these messages and communication facilities, messages between man and machines, between machines and man, and between machine and machine, are destined to play an ever-increasing part" (Wiener, p. 16). In 1957, W. Ross Ashby described the focus of this theory of machines as focusing not on what a thing is, but on what it does: "Cybernetics deals with all forms of behavior in so far as they are regular, or determinate, or reproducible. The materiality is irrelevant" (Ashby, p.1). Recognizing that there are significant similarities in biological and mechanical systems, subsequent researchers have pursued the ideal of merging biological and mechanical/electrical systems into what Manfred Clynes and Nathan Kline termed *cyborgs* or *cybernetic organisms.* In this sense, cybernetics has taken on the meaning of adding prostheses to the human or animal body to either replace lost function or augment biological activity.

Humans have long used tools to augment various functions, and for centuries have attached some of these tools to their bodies. Filled or artificial teeth, glasses and contact lenses, hearing aids, pacemakers, and artificial limbs are all examples of this phenomenon. By the late twentieth century, significant advances in the fields of neuroscience and computer technologies allowed the direct interface of animal or human nervous systems with electromechanical devices. Examples of this evolving field include the creation of neural-silicon junctions involving transistors and neurons to prepare neuronal circuits, the re-creation of visual images from signals transmitted in the optical pathways of a cat, the remote control of mechanical manipulator arms by implants inserted into the motor cortex of owl monkeys, and a remote control that can move rats over a directed path via implanted electrodes.

While the above are examples of direct internal interfaces between a nervous system and a cybernetic prosthesis, another approach to cybernetic augmentation is through the use of external or wearable computing devices. In this approach, prosthetic enhancement is achieved via miniaturization of traditional computing devices, interface mechanisms, and optical projection devices, and then seamlessly incorporating these devices into clothing, glasses, and jewelry. This form of cybernetic enhancement has moved from the academic to the commercial stage. Aside from allowing the user/wearer of such devices wireless access to the Internet and other databases on a continuous basis, they may also be used for *augmented reality,* which is the concept of supplementing traditional sensory input with augmented senses or new types of sensory data. Examples include retrograde vision (seeing to one's rear), distant or projected hearing, and infrared vision. Further visual input may be analyzed and correlated with other information such as Global Positioning System (GPS) location identification. Buildings and streets could be labeled, hours of business accessed, and people visually identified (with demographic information provided), with all of this information directly projected on the user's retina.

While these developments may sound like something out of a Star Trek episode, cybernetic technology has developed at a rapid pace, and will no doubt continue to be a growing field of investigation, therapeutic intervention, and commercial development. In June 2002, the National Science Foundation and the U.S. Department of Commerce issued a report recommending substantial U.S. government investment in the development of cybernetic technologies, with the specific goal of augmenting human performance. These technologies will be produced by the synergistic convergence of biotechnology, nanotechnology, information technology, cognitive science, and neurotechnology through a proposed Human Cognome Project.

## Healing versus Augmentation

As has already been indicated, the mechanical or prosthetic manipulation of human beings is not a new idea or practice. In the past, however, such interventions have almost always been in the context of repair or replacement of absent, diseased, or disordered function. The goal of visual lenses is to restore vision to biological norms, not to augment or improve function beyond normal. Similarly, prosthetic limbs replace those congenitally absent, malformed, or traumatically severed or injured. Pacemakers replace the electrical pacing of heart contractions lost through injury, aging, or disease. In this context, new tools to restore sight to the blind, hearing to the deaf, and movement and normal function to the lame or paralyzed are tremendous advances fully in keeping with the traditional goals of medicine (healing, restoring, palliation, and prevention of injury). Yet humans also use telescopes, microscopes, night vision, and other means of augmenting visual function for specific purposes. The difference is that these tools are not permanent fixtures of the body. Wearable computing devices and implantable brain chips, however, are being produced and marketed to enhance the normal, not necessarily heal the afflicted. This raises a number of challenging ethical questions, including whether or not human augmentation should even be permitted, let alone pursued?

Before the question of whether augmentation should be permitted, promoted, or prohibited can be addressed, a more basic issue must be considered: Can a distinction between healing and augmentation be delineated? This question poses equal challenges to a variety of areas in addition to cybernetics, particularly the more immediate possibilities of genetic therapy or enhancement and pharmacotherapy for behavior control, mood enhancement, and cognitive enhancement.

The difficulty lies in trying to define a clear line of demarcation between a disease state and normal structure and function. It is sometimes easy to pick out extremes of phenotype, particularly if an underlying pathophysiological mechanism for the deviation can be demonstrated. Examples include hemophilia, congenital dwarfism, and impaired vision. Other situations raise difficulties, illustrating that many times the definition of disease or abnormality can be socially, rather than objectively or scientifically determined. How much deviation from ideal body weight is within the bounds of normal variation, and when does the deviation become pathologic? While anorexia nervosa and morbid obesity are clearly pathologic in that they can influence survival and other health issues, a significant number of individuals are on the edges of the norms, where the threshold of pathology is unclear.

A striking example of the cultural variation in the definition of disease is the response of many congenitally deaf individuals to the suggestion that they are afflicted and in need of therapy. Many deaf parents of deaf children have refused to allow their children to receive cochlear implants to correct the deafness because this would remove the children from the deaf community. At a 1997 conference of deaf individuals, 16 percent of the delegates were interested in prenatal diagnosis for deafness, but, of that group, 29 percent indicated that they would use these techniques to select for deafness in the child (see Middleton, et al.).

Cognitive and neurological function, the areas most impacted by cybernetics, are particularly fraught with difficulty, in part because certain deviations from the norm may impart certain functional advantages in addition to social or behavioral liabilities. For instance, while attention-deficit/hyperactivity disorder (ADHD) and autism are diseases, many of the individuals who have these conditions also manifest significant brilliance and creativity in mathematics, music, art, science and engineering. Both the positive and negative manifestations are part of the same disease entity, and what degree of negative manifestation requires treatment becomes subjective. The treatments employed may suppress the undesired manifestation, but they may also impair the desirable expressions. The situation becomes even more complex when these challenges are extended to a measure of cognitive function such as memory, mathematical calculation, musical ability or language processing. Who doesn't think of himself or herself as being deficient in cognitive abilities or able to benefit from enhancement of cognitive function?

In addition, necessary cognitive function may be very task or profession specific. Should individuals who would be considered cognitively normal be allowed to receive enhancing technologies to permit them to pursue a career otherwise beyond their intrinsic ability? And, as these technologies become available, should professions that demand high levels of cognitive excellence be allowed to require the use of enhancing technologies? Given that books and computers are forms of information exchange enhancement that are currently required for education in the professions, one could argue that the only thing that has changed is the intimacy of the enhancing method. Because, these technologies may intrinsically carry certain risks that are absent from current information technologies, however, many believe that such means should never be mandated, but only available by free choice. The reality, however, is that competition with peers will serve as a strong coercive force to pursue enhancement.

## Safety Questions

The answers to these questions require the consideration of additional issues. At the most basic, cybernetic technologies, both implantable and wearable, must demonstrate physical, emotional, and cognitive safety. While physical safety will, in general, be the most easily addressed, there are still new challenges beyond those typically encountered by medical devices. Traditional medical-device safety issues include the risk of infection, local reaction, tissue injury, and involuntary or undesired neural or muscular stimulation. Current devices, however, tend to function in isolation in the specific local environment of the recipient body. Cybernetic devices, on the other hand, will often be connected to a shifting network environment, dependent upon software and the exchange of external information as well as hardware. As such, viral code could potentially disrupt function of the device, and possibly injure the user. Even wearable devices could potentially be turned into weapons, and so need to be strongly regulated, with proof of software and hardware safeguards against injury by rogue software agents.

The issues of emotional and cognitive safety will be more challenging to understand and regulate. In the era of the Internet there is a growing literature addressing problems with personality fragmentation, breakdown of direct personal interaction in favor of cyber relationships, increasing dissatisfaction with reality, addiction to cybersex and pornography, and other psychosocial concerns. These concerns can only increase when individuals are cybernetically connected most, if not all, of the time. The long-term consequences of virtual environments are unknown. The variability of involvement and susceptibility to dysfunctional utilization will vary tremendously between individuals, making generalized regulation difficult. However, some form of registered informed consent as to potential negative consequences, with mandatory, periodic, and long-term follow-up, may be helpful.

## The Nature of Medicine

The issue of safety introduces yet another question: What sorts of individuals should be involved in implanting devices for internal cybernetic enhancements or for fitting wearable devices with optical interfaces? Because of the invasive nature of the implants, it would seem a logical requirement that physicians, particularly neurosurgeons, place these devices in humans. This certainly would be necessary for cybernetic devices of a therapeutic nature, but what about devices that are solely for enhancement purposes? Placing devices for nonmedical indications leads the physician into participating in interventions that are potentially harmful, have no therapeutic necessity, and thus are outside the traditional goals of medicine. A strong argument could be made that physicians should not participate in applying these technologies for other than therapeutic purposes. Yet few would want someone with less training than a neurosurgeon to invade their nervous system.

An analogy can be made to cosmetic surgery. Some ethicists, such as Franklin Miller and Howard Brody, contend that such interventions are outside the bounds of appropriate goals of medicine and should not be performed. Others counter that an individual should have the freedom to manipulate his or her own body, and, if a physician is willing to provide the service, restriction would be wrong and counter to the cherished goals of autonomy. Anders Sandberg takes the argument further, stating that each person has the fundamental right to pursue whatever means are available that might enhance or prolong life. The implications of this approach for medicine, however, are to change the profession from a group committed to healing (with a dominant ethos of beneficence in trust and nonmaleficence) to individuals skilled in surgical technique who are merely technicians providing whatever service may be requested.

## Justice and Social Values

In the end, safety considerations may mandate that physicians and healthcare resources be used to implant cybernetic devices for nontherapeutic purposes, but justice may require that third-party healthcare dollars not be used to cover the costs of the devices or resources utilized. This raises concerns that access to enhancement technologies will be accessible only to those who already possess economic, educational, and technical advantages, further widening the gap between the haves and have-nots. As some members of society become incrementally enhanced and plugged in to cybernetic communities, these individuals will share less and less in common with the unenhanced, fragmenting society; potentially generating decreasingly compatible, or even competing, separate societies.

This is not necessarily a new phenomenon, for technologies have created boundaries between social groups in the past, the Amish and some Native Americans being notable examples. The difference is that the Amish have always wished to remain a distinct society, while some individuals who wish to reject personal enhancement may still desire participation in and access to the goods of the larger social structure. Deliberate efforts to maintain tolerance of individuals and groups who choose to forgo the use of certain technologies must be pursued if democratic-republican ideals are to be preserved, and inclusive means of communication must remain available to all members of society.

Cognitive cybernetic devices must also be equipped with reliable means of filtering incoming information, especially against information that might be designed for repetitive or subliminal influence. Privacy is a similar critical issue, and must be deliberately and prospectively defended in the cybernetic age. Technologies such as functional magnetic-resonance imaging are being proposed to sense, process, and interpret thought patterns. Not only is the accuracy of such technology a critical requirement, but the concept of invading the mind is at issue.

## To Prohibit, Permit, or Pursue?

Cybernetics offers wonderful devises of healing for significant, age-old disabilities, and it can be welcomed when utilized in that context. It is likely that using such tools to enhance normal function will be possible, but great caution is needed, as well as a commitment to the preservation of privacy and justice. Rigorous safeguards for demonstrating the safety of cybernetics devices, and requirements for government approval and licensing, need to be set in place.

The government, the academy, and industry should commit significant resources to the exploration of the ethical and social implications of these technologies, and to the development of appropriate analysis and preparation of guidelines for implementation.

C. CHRISTOPHER HOOK

**SEE ALSO:** *Enhancement Uses of Medical Technology; Human Dignity; Human Nature; Nanotechnology; Technology; Transhumanism and Posthumanism*

### BIBLIOGRAPHY

Ashby, W. Ross. 1957. *An Introduction to Cybernetics.* London: Chapman & Hall.

Bell, David, and Kennedy, Barbara, eds. 2000. *The Cybercultures Reader.* New York: Routledge.

Clynes, Manfred, and Kline, Nathan S. 1960. "Cyborgs and Space." *Astronautics* September, 1960: 26–27, 74–75.

Fink, Jeri. 1999. *Cyberseduction: Reality in the Age of Psychotechnology.* Amherst, NY: Prometheus.

Geary, James. 2002. *The Body Electric: An Anatomy of the New Bionic Senses.* New Brunswick, NJ: Rutgers University Press.

Gray, Chris Hables. 2001. *Cyborg Citizen: Politics in the Posthuman Age.* New York: Routledge.

Hillis, Ken. 1999. *Digital Sensations.* Minneapolis: University of Minnesota Press.

Hook, C. Christopher. 2002. "Cybernetics and Nanotechnology." In *Cutting-Edge Bioethics,* ed. John Kilner, C. Christopher Hook, and Diann Uustal. Grand Rapids, MI: Eerdmans.

Jenker, Martin; Muller, Bernt; and Fromherz, Peter. 2001. "Interfacing a Silicon Chip to Pairs of Snail Neurons Connected by Electrical Synapses." *Biological Cybernetics* 84: 239–249.

Kurzweil, Ray. 1999. *The Age of Spiritual Machines.* New York: Viking.

Mann, Steve. 2001. "Wearable Computing: Toward Humanistic Intelligence." *IEEE Intelligent Systems.* May/June 2001: 10–15.

Middleton, Anna; Hewison, J.; and Mueller, R. F. 1998. "Attitudes of Deaf Adults Toward Genetic Testing for Hereditary Deafness." *American Journal of Human Genetics.* 63: 1175–1180.

Miller, Franklin; Brody, Howard; and Chung, Kevin. 2000. "Cosmetic Surgery and the Internal Morality of Medicine." *Cambridge Quarterly of Healthcare Ethics* 9: 353–364.

Parens, Erik, ed. 1998. *Enhancing Human Traits: Ethical and Social Implications.* Washington, D.C.: Georgetown University Press.

Stanley, Garrett; Fei, F. Li; and Yang, Dan. 1999. "Reconstruction of Natural Senses from Ensemble Responses in the Lateral Geniculate Nucleus." *Journal of Neuroscience* 19: 8036–8042.

Talwar, Sanjiv; Xu, Shaohua; Hawley, Emerson; et al. 2002. "Rat Navigation Guided by Remote Control." *Nature* 417: 37–38.

Vassanelli, S., and Fromherz, Peter. 1997. "Neurons from Rat Brain Coupled to Transistors" *Applied Physics A.* 65: 85–88.

Wessberg, Johan; Stambaugh, Christopher; Kralik, Jerald; et al. 2000. "Real-Time Prediction of Hand Trajectory by Ensembles of Cortical Neurons in Primates." *Nature* 408: 361–365.

Wiener, Norbert. 1950. *The Human Use of Human Beings: Cybernetics and Society.* Boston: Houghton Mifflin; reprint, 1988. New York: Da Capo.

Wiener, Norbert. 1961. *Cybernetics: or, Control and Communication in the Animal and the Machine,* 2nd edition. Cambridge, MA: The MIT Press.

INTERNET RESOURCES

"Accelerating Intelligence News." Available from <www.kurzweilAI.net>.

"Principia Cybernetica Electronic Library." Available from <paspmcl.vub.ac.be/LIBRARY.html>.

MIT Media Lab. "Wearable Computing." Available from <www.media.mit.edu/wearables>.

Roco, Mikail, and Baindridge, William Sims, eds. 2002. "Converging Technologies for Enhancing Human Performance." Available from <wtec.org/ConvergingTechnologies/>.

Sandberg, Anders. "Morphological Freedom—Why We Not Just Want It, but Need It." Available from <www.nada.kth.se/~asa.Texts/MorphologicalFreedom.htm>.